# Heart Failure
# Pathogenesis and Treatment

# Heart Failure
# Pathogenesis and Treatment


Edited by

**Jagat Narula, MD, DM, PhD, FACC**
*Thomas J. Vischer Professor of Medicine, Vice-Chairman for Research,*
*Department of Medicine, Hahnemann University School of Medicine*
*Philadelphia, Pennsylvania, USA*

**Renu Virmani, MD**
*Chairperson, Division of Cardiovascular Pathology*
*Armed Forces Institute of Pathology*
*Washington, DC, USA*

**Manel Ballester, MD, PhD**
*Cardiomyopathy and Transplantation Unit*
*Hospital de la Santa Creu i Sant Pau*
*Sant Antoni, Barcelona, Spain*

**Ignasi Carrió, MD, PhD**
*Chief of the Service of Nuclear Medicine*
*Hopital Sant Pau, Barcelona, Spain*

**Stephen Westaby, BSc, FRCS, MS**
*Consultant Cardiothoracic Surgeon, Oxford Heart Centre*
*John Radcliffe Hospital, Oxford, UK*

**O. H. Frazier, MD, FACS, FACC**
*Chief, Cardiopulmonary Transplantation*
*Texas Heart Institute, Houston, Texas, USA*

**James T. Willerson, MD, FACC**
*Chief, Adult Cardiology, St Luke's Episcopal Hospital,*
*Texas Heart Institute Houston, Texas, USA*



MARTIN DUNITZ

First published in the United Kingdom in 2002
by Martin Dunitz Ltd, The Livery House, 7–9 Pratt Street, London NW1 0AE

Tel.: +44 (0) 20 74822202
Fax.: +44 (0) 20 72670159
E-mail: info.dunitz@tandf.co.uk
Website: http://www.dunitz.co.uk



A CIP record for this book is available from the British Library.

ISBN 1 901865 84 3

Distributed in the USA by
Fulfilment Center
Taylor & Francis
7625 Empire Drive
Florence, KY 41042, USA
Toll Free Tel.: +1 800 634 7064
E-mail: cserve@routledge_ny.com

Distributed in Canada by
Taylor & Francis
74 Rolark Drive
Scarborough, Ontario M1R 4G2, Canada
Toll Free Tel.: +1 877 226 2237
E-mail: tal_fran@istar.ca

Distributed in the rest of the world by
ITPS Limited
Cheriton House
North Way
Andover, Hampshire SP10 5BE, UK
Tel.: +44 (0)1264 332424
E-mail: reception@itps.co.uk

Cover: Miquel Barcel (1957), Sistole Diastole, 1987. Collection capcMusée, Bordeaux

Produced and typeset by Gray Publishing, Tunbridge Wells, Kent
Printed and bound in Spain

# Contents

# List of contributors

**Maha Abdellatif, MB, ChB, PhD**
*Center for Cardiac Development*
*Section of Cardiology*
*Department of Medicine*
*Houston, Texas, USA*

**Eloisa Arbustini, MD**
*Department of Pathology,*
*IRCCS-Policlinico San Matteo,*
*Pavia, Italy*

**Leonard C. Archard, PhD, DSc(Med), FIBiol, FRCPath**
*Division of Biomedical Sciences*
*Faculty of Medicine*
*Imperial College of Science,*
*Technology and Medicine, London, UK*

**Michael Argenziano, MD**
*Assistant Professor of Surgery,*
*Columbia University College of Physicians and Surgeons*
*Director, Robotic Cardiac Surgery*
*Director, Arrhythmia Service, New York-Presbyterian Hospital, Columbia, New York, USA*

**Ragavendra R. Baliga, MD, MRCP**
*University of Texas Southwestern Medical Center,*
*Dallas, Texas, USA*

**Manel Ballester, MD, PhD**
*Cardiology Department*
*Hospital Universitari Arnau de Vilanova*
*Chairman of Cardiology*
*Faculty of Medicine*
*Universitat de Lleida*
*Lleida, Spain*

**William H. Barry, MD**
*Nora Eccles Harrison Professor*
*Cardiology Division*
*University of Utah Medical Center*
*Salt Lake City, Utah, USA*

**Michael Böhm**
*Medizinische Klinik und Poliklinik*
*der Universität des Saarlandes*
*Innere Medizin III*
*Homburg/Saar, Germany*

**Christian Brilla, MD, PhD**
*Professor of Medicine*
*Division of Cardiology*
*Philipps University of Marburg*
*Marburg, Germany*

**Vincens Brossa, MD**
*Cardiomyopathy and Heart Transplantation Program,*
*Department of Cardiology,*
*Hospital de la Santa Creu i Saut Pau,*
*Barcelona, Spain*

**Allan P. Burke, MD**
*Department of Cardiovascular Pathology,*
*Armed Forces Institute of Pathology,*
*Washington, DC, USA*

**Marta Campreciós, MD**
*Cardiomyopathy and Heart Transplantation Program,*
*Department of Cardiology,*
*Hospital de la Santa Creu i Saut Pau, Barcelona, Spain*

**Josep M. Caralps-Riera**
*Hospital de la Santa Crei i Sant Pau, Barcelona, Spain*

**Ignasi Carrió, MD, PhD**
*Professor of Nuclear Medicine,*
*Autonomous University of Barcelona,*
*Director, Nuclear Medicine Department,*
*Sant Pau Hospital, Barcelona, Spain*

**Y. Chandrashekhar, MD, DM**
*Associate Professor, University of Minnesota*
*Minnesota, Minneapolis, USA*

**Derek Chin, MBBS, MRCP**
*Consultant Cardiologist*
*The Glenfield Hospital,*
*Groby Road, Leicester, UK*

**Wilson S. Colucci, MD**
*Boston University Medical Center*
*Boston, Massachusetts, USA*

**Edecio Cunha-Neto, MD, PhD**
*Laboratory of Immunology*
*Heart Institute (InCor)*
*and*
*Division of Clinical Immunology and Allergy*
*Department of Internal Medicine*
*University of São Paulo School of Medicine*
*São Paulo, Brazil*

**Barbara Dal Bello, MD**
*Department of Pathology,*
*IRCCS-Policlinico San Matteo, Pavia, Italy*

**Federica del Monte, MD, PhD**
*Sceintist and Instructor of Medicine*
*Harvard Medical School*
*Boston, Massachusetts, USA*

**Reynolds Delgado, MD**
*Cardiology Research*
*Texas Heart Institute/St. Luke's Episcopal Hospital*
*University of Texal Medical School at Houston*
*Houston, Texas, USA*

**Eric Eichhorn, MD**
*The Cardiac Catheterization Laboratory (IIIA2)*
*Dallas VA Medical Center, Dallas, USA*

**Diane Fatkin, MD**
*Department of Genetics*
*Harvard Medical School*
*Boston, Massachusetts, USA*

**Thomas L. Force**
*Cardiovascular Tesearch Center and Cardiac Unit,*
*Massachusetts General Hospital,*
*Harvard Medical School, Boston,*
*Massachusetts, USA*

**O. H. Frazier, MD, FACS, FACC,**
*Chief, Cardiopulmonary Transplantation,*
*Texas Heart Institute, Houston,*
*Texas, USA*

**Michael Fu**
*Wallenberg Laboratory*
*Sahlgenska University Hospital,*
*Göteborg, Sweden*

**Anne Carla Goldberg, PhD**
*Laboratory of Immunology,*
*Heart Institute (InCor)*
*University of São Paulo*
*School of Medicine*
*Andar, São Paulo, Brazil*

**Luíza Guilherme, PhD**
*Laboratory of Immunology,*
*Heart Institute (InCor)*
*University of São Paulo*
*School of Medicine*
*Andar, São Paulo, Brazil*

**Judith K. Gwathmey, VMD, PhD, FACC**
*Gwathmey Inc., Cambridge*
*Massachusetts, USA*

**Roger J. Hajjar, MD**
*Cardiovascular Research*
*Center and Cardiac Unit*
*Massachusetts General Hospital*
*Harvard Medical School*
*Boston, Massachusetts, USA*

**Ahvie Herskowitz, MD**
*Clincal Professor of Medicine,*
*University of California, Staff Cardiologist,*
*San Francisco VA Medical Center*
*Chief Operating Officer,*
*Institute for OneWorld Health*
*San Francisco, California, USA*

**Joanne Ingwall, PhD**
*Professor of Medicine (Physiology)*
*NMR Laboratory for Physiological Chemistry*
*Cardiovascular Division,*
*Department of Medicine*
*Brigham & Women's Hospital and*
*Harvard Medical School,*
*Boston, Massachusetts, USA*

**Ami E. Iskandrian, MD**
*William Penn Snyder III*
*Professor of Medicine*
*Director, Section of Nuclear Cardiology*
*Director, Cardivascular Research Institute*
*Hahnemann School of Medicine*
*Philadelphia, Pennsylvania, USA*

**Stefan Kääb, MD, PhD**
*Department of Cardiology*
*University of Munich*
*Munich, Germany*

**Jorge Kalil, MD, PhD**
*International Scholar,*
*Howard Hughes Medical Institute*
*Director, Laboratory of Immunology,*
*Heart Institute (InCor)*
*and Professor and Head*
*Division of Clinical Immunology and Allergy*
*Department of Internal Medicine*
*Faculty of Medicine,*
*University of São Paulo, Brazil*

**Arnold M.D. Katz, MD, DMed(Hon), FACP, FACC**
*Professor of Medicine Emeritus*
*University of Connecticut School of Medicine*
*and Visiting Professor of Medicine*
*Dartmouth Medical School*
*Hanover, New Hampshire, USA*

**Roger Kaprielian, PhD**
*Postdoctoral Fellow*
*Massachusetts General Hospital*
*Boston, Massachusetts, USA*

**Takahiro Katsumata, MD, PhD**
*Oxford Heart Centre*
*Department of Cardiac Surgery*
*John Radcliffe Hospital, Oxford, UK*

**Issei Komuro, MD, PhD**
*Department or Cardiovascular Science*
*and Medicine*
*Chiba University Graduate School of Medicine*
*Chiba, Japan*

**Bernhard Maisch, MD**
*Director of the Department of Internal Medicine and*
*Cardiology*
*Heart Center of Philipps-University Marburg*
*Marburg, Germany*

**Douglas Mann, MD**
*Veterans Administration Hospital and*
*Baylor College of Medicine, Houston*
*Texas, USA*

**Eduardo Marban, MD, PhD**
*Section of Molecular and Cellular Cardiology*
*The Johns Hopkins University*
*Division of Cardiology*
*Department of Medicine*
*Baltimore, Maryland, USA*

**Vincens Martí**
*Cardiomyopathy and Transplantating Program*
*Department of Cardiology*
*Hospital de la Santa Creu i Saut Pau*
*Barcelona, Spain*

**Patrizia Morbini, MD**
*Department of Pathology,*
*IRCCS-Policlinico San Matteo*
*Pavia, Italy*

**Michael Näbauer, MD, PhD**
*Department of Cardiology*
*University of Munich*
*Munich, Germany*

**Jagat Narula, MD, DM, PhD, FACC**
*Thomas J. Vischer Professor of Medicine*
*Vice Chairman, Department of Medicine*
*Director, Heart Failure/Transplant Center*
*Director, Center of Molecular Cardiology*
*Hahnemann University Hospital*
*Philadelphia, Pennsylvania, USA*

**Georg Nickenig**
*Medizinische Klinik und Poliklinik*
*der Universität des Saarlandes*
*Innere Medizin III*
*Homburg/Saar, Germany*

**Guillem Pons-Lladó**
*Director, Noninvasive Imaging Laboratories*
*Division of Cardiology*
*Sant Pau Hospital, Barcelona, Spain*

**Mireia Puig**
*Cardiomyopathy and Heart Transplantation*
*Department of Cardiology*
*Hospital de la Santa Creu i Saut Pau*
*Barcelona, Spain*

**Shahbudin H. Rahimtoola, MD**
*Distinguished Professor*
*George C. Griffith Professor of Cardiology*
*Professor of Medicine*
*Keck School of Medicine of the*
*University of Southern California*
*Los Angeles,*
*California, USA*

**Peter Richardson, MD, FRCP**
*Consultant Cardiologist and Honorary Senior Lecturer*
*King's College Hospital,*
*Denmark Hill*
*London, UK*

**Michael Ritter, MD**
*Division of Cardiology*
*University of Marburg*
*Baldingerstrasse*
*35033 Marburg*
*Germany*

**Eric A. Rose, MD**
*Milstein Hospital Building, New York, USA*

**Anthony Rozensweig, MD**
*Cardiovascular Research Center*
*Massachusetts General Hospital*
*Charlestown, Massachusetts, USA*

**Heinz Rupp, PhD**
*Professor of Physiology, Division of Cardiology*
*Philipps University of Marburg*
*Marburg, Germany*

**Kjella Saatvedt, MD, PhD**
*Oxford Heart Centre*
*Department of Cardiac Surgery*
*John Radcliffe Hospital, Oxford, UK*

**Junichi Sadoshima, MD, PhD**
*Cardiovascular and Pulmonary Research Institute*
*Alleghony University of Health Sciences*
*Pittsburgh,*
*Pennsylvania, USA*

**Satoshi Saito, MD, PhD**
*Oxford Heart Centre*
*Department of Cardiac Surgery*
*John Radcliffe Hospital, Oxford, UK*

**Louis E. Samuels, MD**
*Assistant Professor of Cardiothoracic Surgery*
*MCP-Hahnemann University School of Medicine*
*Surgical Director, Heart Transplant Center*
*Director, Center for Artificial Heart and Assist Devices*
*Director of Clinical Research, Department of Cardiothoracic Surgery*
*Hahnemann University Hospital*
*Philadelphia, Pennsylvania, USA*

**Petra Schnabel**
*Klinik III für Innere Medizin der*
*Universität zu Köln, Köln, Germany*

**Michael D. Schneider, MD**
*Center for Cardiac Development*
*Section of Cardiology*
*Department of Medicine,*
*Houston, Texas, USA*

**Christine E. Seidman, MD**
*Department of Genetics*
*Harvard Medical School*
*Boston, Massachusetts, USA*

**J. G. Seidman, PhD**
*Department of Genetics*
*Harvard Medical School*
*Boston, Massachusetts, USA*

**Mark R. Starling, MD**
*Professor of Internal Medicine,*
*Director, Cardiology Training Program Association.*
*Chief, Division of Cardiology*
*University of Michigan*
*Chief, Cardiology Section*
*VA Ann Arbor Healthcare System*
*Ann Arbor, Michigan, USA*

**Francisco Torrent-Guasp, MD**
*Dènia, Alicante, Spain*

**Renu Virmani, MD**
*Chairperson,*
*Division of Cardiovascular Pathology*
*Armed Forces Institute of Pathology*
*Washington, DC, USA*

**Finn Waagstein**
*Wallenberg Laboratory*
*Sahlgenska University Hospital*
*Göteborg, Sweden*

**Stephen Westaby, BSc, FRCS, MS**
*Consultant Cardiothoracic Surgeon*
*Oxford Heart Centre*
*Department of Cardiac Surgery*
*John Radcliffe Hospital, Oxford, UK*

**James T. Willerson, MD, FACC**
Chief, Adult Cardiology
St Luke's Episcopal Hospital
Texas Heart Institute
Houston, Texas, USA

**Yoshio Yazaki**
*Department of Cardiovascular Medicine*
*University of Tokyo Graduate School of Medicine*
*Tokyo, Japan*

**Hongyi Zhang, MBBS, MM, PhD**
*Clinical Lecturer/Honorary Senior Registrar*
*Division of Biomedical Sciences*
*Faculty of Medicine*
*Imperial College of Science,*
*Technology and Medicine, London, UK*

**Oliver Zolk**
*Department of Pharmacology*
*University of Erlangen,*
*Erlangen, Germany*

# Preface

Congestive heart failure threatens to evolve into an epidemic as we step into this new century. Advances in the prevention and management of the most aggressive cardiovascular diseases of the last century (such as coronary artery disease and hypertension) have predominantly contributed to the rising population of heart failure. However, advancing age expectancy has added to the magnitude of the problem. Cardiovascular diseases associated with infection and poverty in the developing nations (such as rheumatic fever, rheumatic heart disease and Chagas' disease) also contribute to widen the pool of heart failure patients.

The prognosis of the disease continues to be grim and quality of life is rendered limited. Approximately 5 million people in the United States suffer from heart failure. Every year 700 000 new cases are seen and there are a million hospitalizations and 250 000 deaths associated with heart failure necessitating at least $22.5 billion expenditure annually. While these demographic statistics appear somewhat depressing, heart failure has witnessed the most well-organized and carefully designed clinical trials targeted at arresting and reversing ventricular remodelling. These trials have most critically assessed the efficacy and outcome of therapeutic interventions and have offered a promise of substantial reduction in morbidity and mortality. At the same time, technological advances in the development of mechanical devices have helped to manage end-stage heart failure and have raised hopes that an artificial heart is within the realm of possibility.

The unparalled advances in the field have been supported by exquisite basic research. Copious literature emerging from laboratory experiments, trials of novel pharmaceutical agents, and application for mechanical devices warrant the preparation of a well-organized, multi-authored text that offers a comprehensive and balanced view. Various books have admirably responded to this demand in the recent past, and the need for a new book on this subject may be justifiably questioned.

Readers will note that this new volume has tried to move away from the orthodox texts. We have attempted to provide a comprehensive anatomic, pathophysiologic and molecular basis of primary and secondary cardiomyopathic disorders, and used the pathogenetic basis to explain the evolution of medical and surgical intervention strategies. We have purposely avoided inclusion of details of clinical trials, and experimental studies which are available to readers at the click of the mouse. We are fortunate to obtain contributions from the stalwarts in the field and were able to fill the chapters with vivid illustrations in colour. We sincerely hope that this volume will attract those involved in cardiovascular healthcare in adult and geriatric populations. We have especially tried to simplify the text so that it could be used by medicine residents and cardiology fellows and entice them to the field, which so richly deserves urgent attention.

Jagat Narula, Renu Virmani, Manel Ballester,
Ignasi Carrió, O. H. Frazier, Steven Westaby
and James T. Willerson

# SECTION I

# Basic concepts of myocardial architecture and physiology

# Cellular and molecular basis of myocardial contraction 1

A. M. KATZ

## Introduction

Cardiac contraction and relaxation depend on interactions between the heart's contractile proteins and a number of membrane proteins that regulate their activity. The contractile proteins transform chemical energy released by the hydrolysis of adenosine triphosphate (ATP) into the mechanical work that moves blood under pressure from the systemic veins into the pulmonary artery, and from the pulmonary veins into the aorta. Excitation–contraction coupling, the process that activates contraction, begins when an action potential depolarizes the plasma membrane and ends when ionized calcium enters the cytosol to become bound by regulatory proteins in the contractile apparatus. Relaxation, which involves membrane transport processes that remove calcium from the cytosol, is effected by energy-dependent mechanisms that are entirely different from those responsible for excitation–contraction coupling.

Calcium entry into the cytosol during excitation–contraction coupling results from passive (downhill) fluxes in which this ion crosses phospholipid membranes through ion-specific channels. Activator calcium enters the cytosol by passage through two different families of ion channels: one is found in the plasma membrane, the other in the internal membranes of the sarcoplasmic reticulum. The active (uphill) flux of calcium out of the cytosol, which relaxes the heart, is effected by ion pumps and ion exchangers in both the plasma membrane and sarcoplasmic reticulum. Ion pumps are membrane proteins that utilize energy provided by ATP hydrolysis to transport calcium out of the cytosol against an electrochemical gradient, while ion exchangers use the energy of the sodium gradient for the uphill movement of calcium (and other substances) into the extracellular space. This sodium gradient is maintained by the ATP-dependent sodium pump ($Na^+K^+$-ATPase). Energy is therefore used in both contraction and relaxation, although it is used by different systems and in different ways.

This chapter focuses on the mechanisms responsible for excitation–contraction coupling, contraction, and relaxation by the working cells of the atria and ventricles. These processes control the interactions between the contractile proteins that determine myocardial contractility, and thus the emptying of the heart's cavities during systole, as well as the rate and extent of relaxation, which determine the ability of the heart to fill during diastole. General reviews of these topics can be found in references [1–6].

## Excitation and plasma membrane channels

The heart is a complex organ made up of several different cell types. In addition to the working myocardial cells of the atria and ventricles, which are specialized for contraction, other cell types participate in the initiation and transmission of the electrical signals that initiate systole. The latter include the Purkinje fibres, which provide for rapid conduction of the wave of depolarization throughout the ventricles, and smaller nodal cells in the sinoatrial (SA) and atrioventricular (AV) nodes, which are responsible for pacemaker activity and atrioventricular conduction, respectively.

Depolarization of all of these cell types occurs when ions cross the hydrophobic barrier in the centre of the plasma membrane. The resulting ionic currents depend on the opening of voltage-gated ion channels, a family of membrane proteins that provide for the highly regulated control of membrane potential [for review see refs. 7–13]. In the working myocytes of the atria and ventricles, and the rapidly conducting cells of the His–Purkinje system, the flux of sodium ions into the cell interior carries the major inward (depolarizing) currents. In nodal cells, where action potentials are smaller and rise more slowly, depolarization depends mainly on the inward movement of calcium ions. Resting potential in all of these cell types is restored by outward (repolarizing) currents that are generated when potassium moves out of the cell through a diverse group of potassium channels. The structures of these channels are discussed below, after a brief review of the gating mechanisms that open and close their pores.

## Ion channel gating

The ion channels responsible for impulse generation and propagation in the heart are proteins with pores that open and close in response to changes in membrane potential, i.e. channel opening is voltage-dependent. Because various ion channels cycle at different rates, in addition to their voltage dependence these channels also exhibit time-dependent properties. The sodium and calcium channels that depolarize the heart, once opened, do not remain in the open state, but instead cycle through at least two closed states (Fig. 1.1). In the first, which immediately follows the open state, the channel becomes refractory (the closed, inactive state), while in the other, which is seen in the resting heart, the channel can be reopened by physiological stimuli (the closed, resting state). In the case of the sodium and calcium channels that carry depolarizing currents, the transition from the closed (resting) to the open state, called *activation*, is initiated when an approaching wave of depolarization reduces resting potential. The resulting depolarization modifies the conformation of the channel proteins so as to increase the probability of channel opening. At the same time, but more slowly, depolarization increases the probability that these channels will assume their closed (inactive) state. The latter process, called *inactivation*, causes the channels to become unresponsive to additional depolarizing stimuli, i.e. to become refractory. Because activation is much faster than inactivation, depolarization gives rise to a brief opening event. The ability of the same depolarizing signal that opens the channel (activation) to cause the channel to become refractory (inactivation) is made possible by the movements of different charged molecular structures that are initiated by the change in membrane potential (see below). Channel recovery, the transition from the closed (inactive) to the closed (resting) state, requires an additional stimulus. In the case of cardiac sodium and calcium channels, this return to the resting state (reactivation) is brought about by membrane

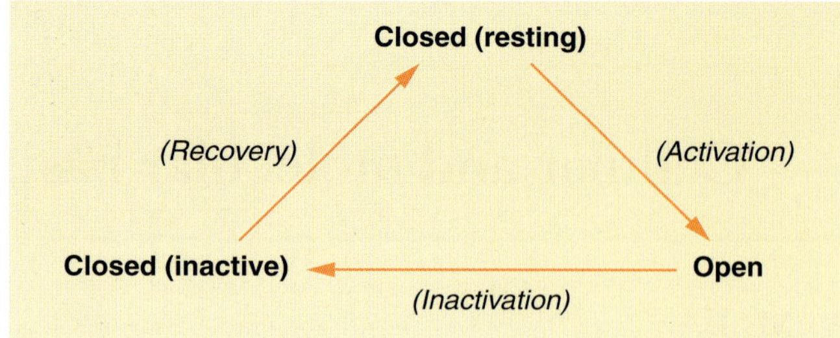


**Figure 1.1** *Three states of a voltage-gated ion channel. Two closed and one open state are indicated, along with the transitions between these states* (arrows). *(Adapted from Katz, Physiology of the Heart (Ref. 1, with permission).)*

**Table 1.1** Sodium channel gating

| State of the channel | State of the m-gate | State of the h-gate |
|---|---|---|
| Closed (resting) | Closed | Open |
| Open | Open | Open |
| Closed (inactive) | Open | Closed |

repolarization, which occurs when the opening of potassium channels generates outward (repolarizing) currents.

In the 1950s, Hodgkin and Huxley [14] carried out a classic study of the ionic basis for the action potential in squid giant axons, and postulated that two different regulatory systems, which they referred to as 'gating mechanisms', open and close the ion channel pores (Table 1.1). In the sodium channel, the transitions between different states were attributed to two distinct molecular structures, called m- and h-gates. According to the Hodgkin–Huxley model, the initial response to depolarization occurs when movement of the m-gates opens the pore to generate an inward sodium current. Because the h-gates are open in the resting sodium channel, opening of the m-gates in response to an approaching wave of depolarization changes the channel from the closed (resting) state to the open state. At the same time, but more slowly, depolarization closes the h-gates. Because sodium ions can cross the membrane only when both m- and h-gates are open, the channels are able to carry depolarizing currents only during the brief period between the rapid opening of the m-gate and the slower closing of the h-gate. The Hodgkin–Huxley model therefore defines the three channel states mentioned above: an open state in which both gates are open, and two closed states, one where the m-gate

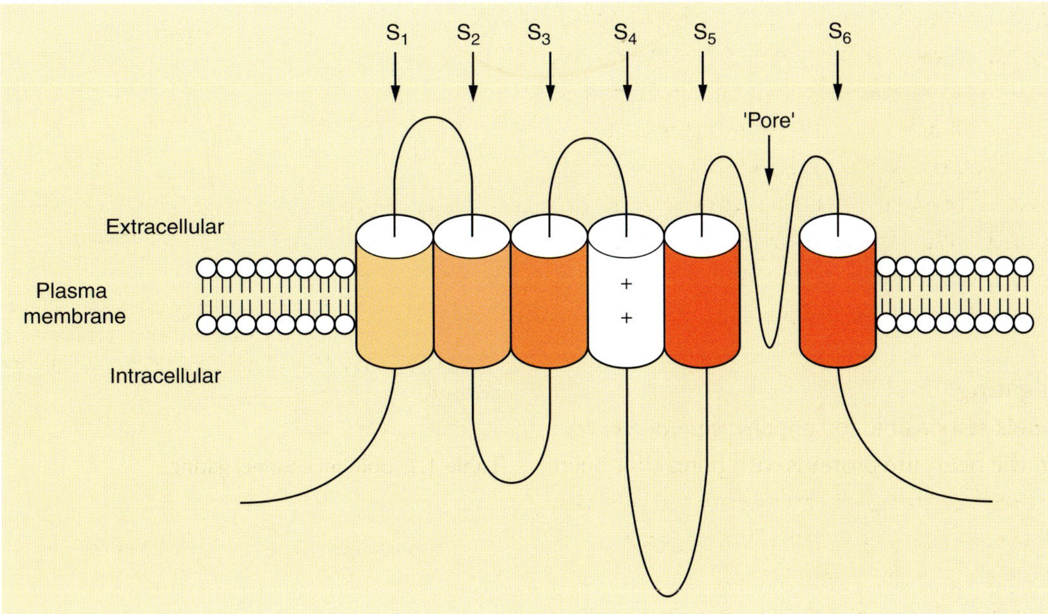


**Figure 1.2** *An ion channel domain. The ion channels depicted in Fig. 1.3 are tetramers made up of four domains, each of which contains six α-helical membrane-spanning segments ($S_1$–$S_6$). The $S_4$ segment, which is rich in positively charged amino acids, opens the channel in response to membrane depolarization. The membrane-spanning segments $S_5$ and $S_6$, along with the intervening peptide chain that dips into the hydrophobic core of the membrane bilayer, line the pore through which ions cross the lipid barrier in the core of the membrane bilayer. (Adapted from Katz,* Physiology of the Heart *(Ref. 1, with permission).)*

is closed and the h-gate open (closed, resting), the other where the m-gate is open and the h-gate is closed (closed, inactive) (Table 1.1). The most important functional difference between the two closed states reflects the fact that the m-gate is opened by membrane depolarization while the h-gate opens only when membrane potential returns to its resting level in the repolarized cell. The remarkable insights contained in the Hodgkin–Huxley model led to several predictions that have been confirmed by recent studies of channel structure. These studies, as discussed below, have identified the molecular basis for ion channel gating.

## Ion channel structure

Ion channels are proteins, embedded in the plasma membrane, which surround a pore that, when open, allows ions to cross the hydrophobic barrier in the phospholipid bilayer. Elucidation of the structures of these ion channel proteins has revealed hitherto unimagined molecular complexities that explain how ion channels open, close, and become refractory, and how disease can affect the way in which these transitions are controlled [for reviews see refs. 7–13].

Plasma membrane ion channels can contain as many as five subunits, called $\alpha_1$, $\alpha_2$, β, γ, and δ. Most important are the large tetrameric α- and $\alpha_1$-protein subunits that, in most voltage-gated ion channels, surround the ion-selective pore. The other channel subunits are smaller proteins that serve mainly to regulate ion channel function; for example, some mediate the effects of cyclic adenosine monophosphate (AMP)-dependent protein kinases, which generally promote channel opening [15, 16].

The large α-subunits of sodium and calcium channels contain four domains (Fig. 1.2) that are connected covalently in a tetrameric structure by relatively short linking segments (Fig. 1.3). Each domain in most ion channels contains six α-helical transmembrane segments, designated $S_1$–$S_6$. The $S_5$ and $S_6$ segments, along with the connecting peptide chain, constitute the pore region of the channel (see below). Most potassium channels are also tetrameric structures made up of domains such as shown in Figure 1.2; however, unlike the sodium and calcium channels, the four domains are not linked covalently. Some classes of potassium channels are assembled from smaller proteins that contain only two transmembrane segments (Fig. 1.4).

The domains of the α-subunits of most plasma membrane ion channels are organized in the phospholipid bilayer so that in the open state of the channel, the four $S_5$ and $S_6$ segments, along with the intervening peptide chains, line

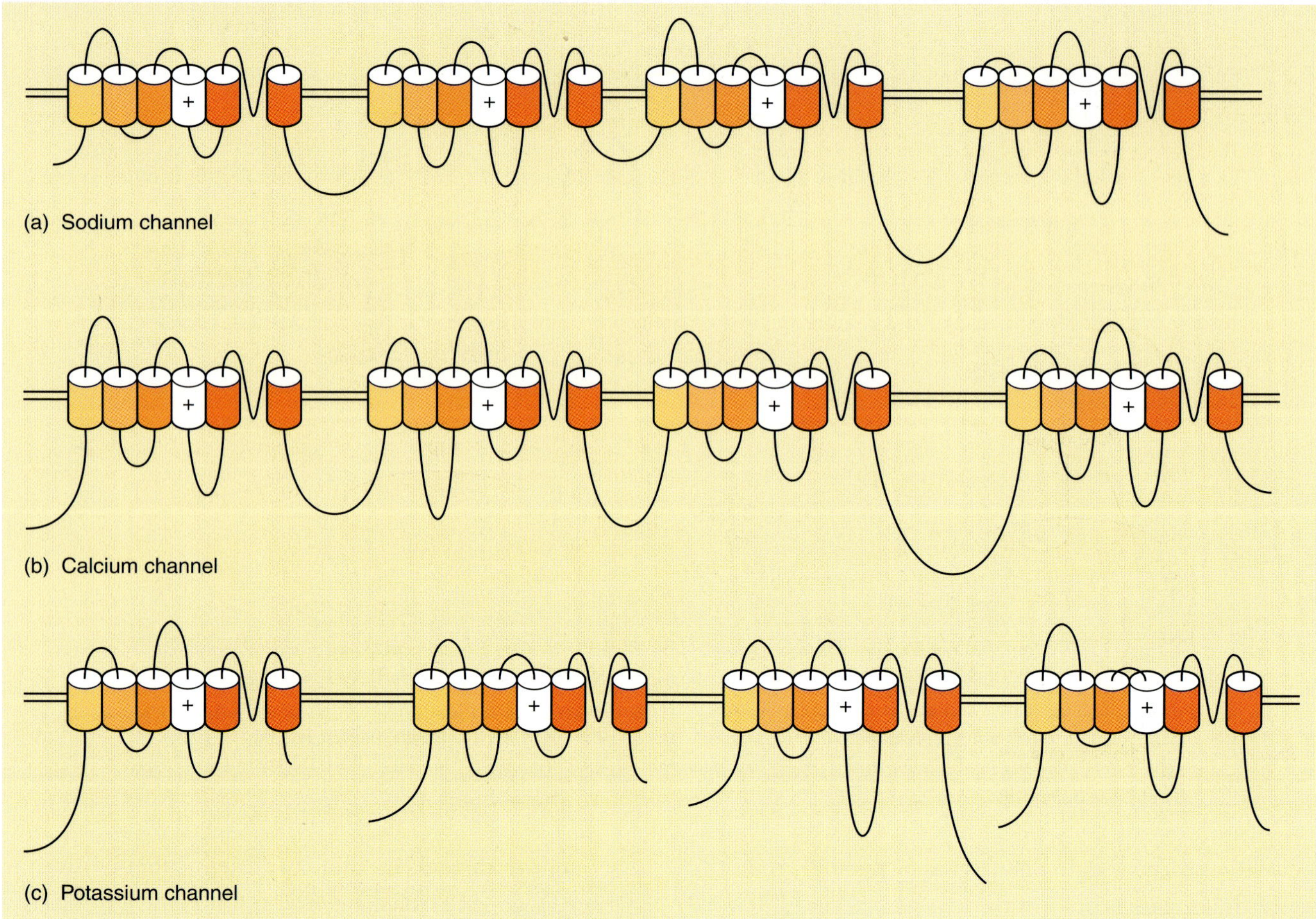


**Figure 1.3** *Three types of voltage-gated ion channel. Sodium and calcium channels are tetramers made up of four covalently linked domains (see Fig. 1.2). Potassium channels are also tetrameric structures, but unlike calcium and sodium channels, the four domains are not covalently linked. (Adapted from Katz,* Physiology of the Heart *(Ref. 1, with permission).)*

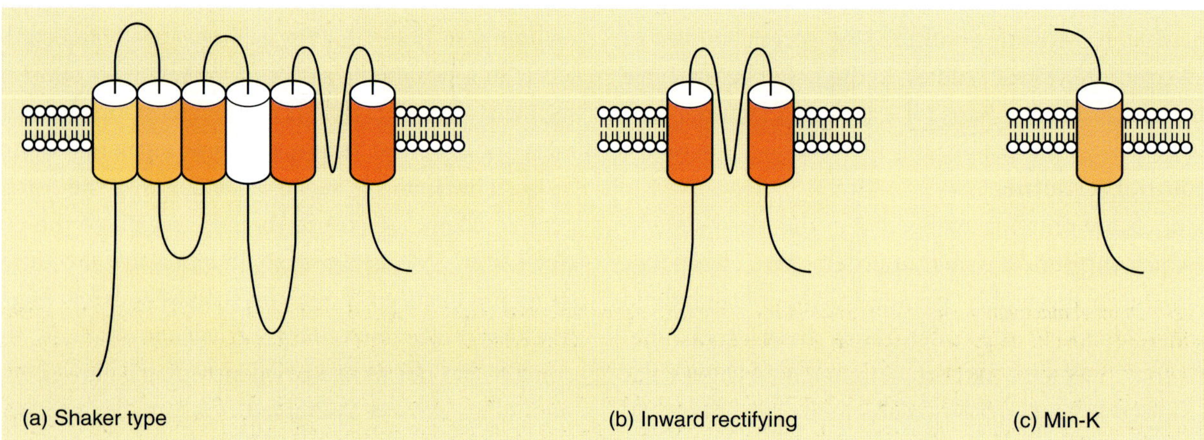


**Figure 1.4** *Three potassium channel structures. (a) The Shaker type channel (named after a* Drosophila *mutant that shakes when this class of channel is abnormal) contains four domains, each of which is made up of the six membrane-spanning segments shown in Fig. 1.2. (b) Inward rectifying potassium channels are made up of four smaller domains that include only the pore regions of the domains shown in Fig. 1.2. (c) An even smaller protein, called Min-K (minimal potassium), includes only a single membrane-spanning segment; this is a regulator of potassium channel function. (Adapted from Katz,* Physiology of the Heart *(Ref. 1, with permission).)*

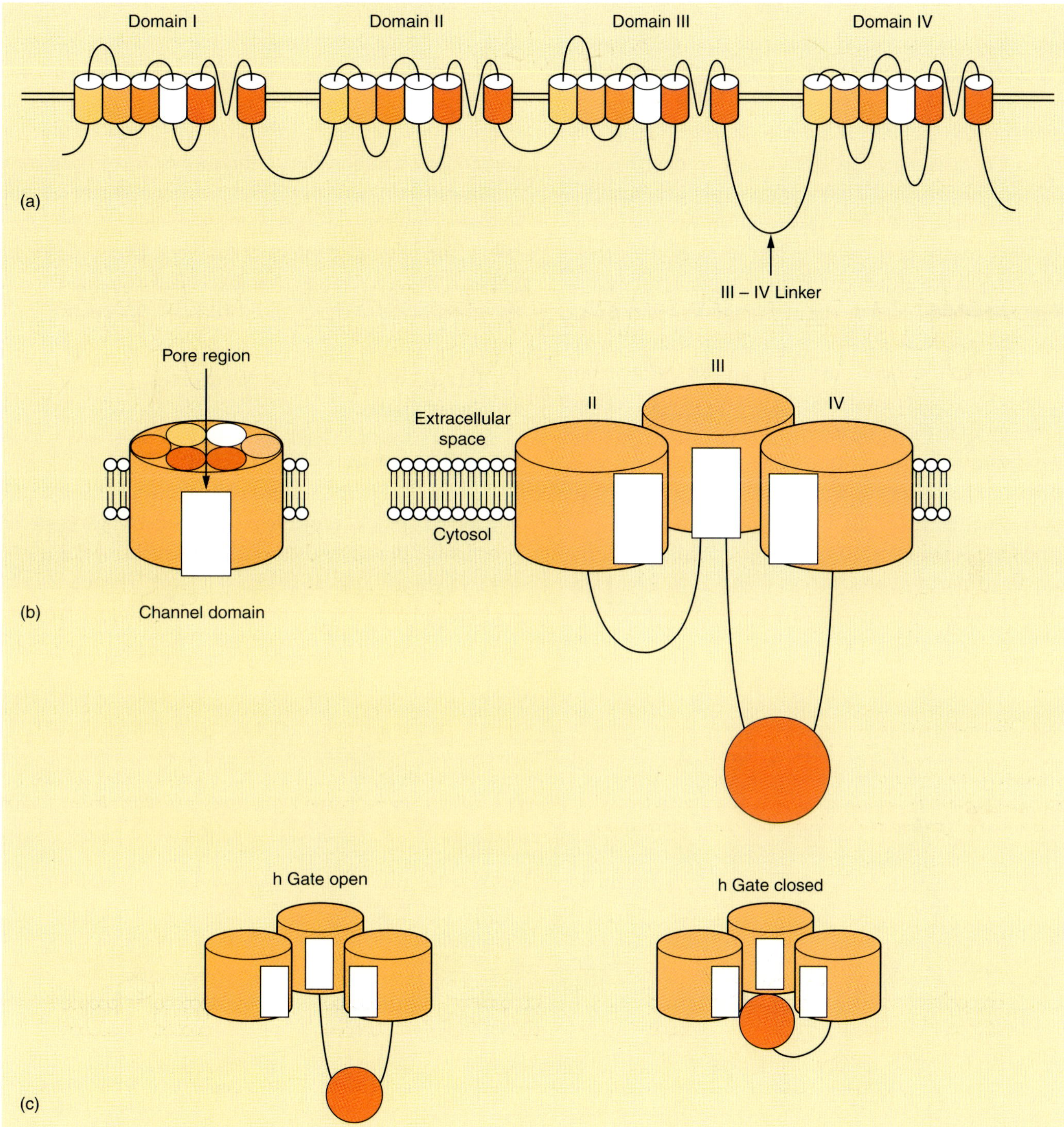


**Figure 1.5** *Channel inactivation. (a) The four domains of the tetrameric channels depicted in Fig. 1.3 are numbered I–IV. The peptide chain linking domains III and IV (the III–IV linker), which can be viewed as a ball at the end of a chain, is the h-gate in the Hodgkin–Huxley model of channel function. (b)* Left: *A single domain made up of six membrane-spanning segments. The pore region is depicted as a light rectangle.* Right: *The pore regions of domains II, III, and IV surround the channel opening (domain I, not shown, would lie in front of these three domains). The ball floats in the cytosol, its position depending on membrane potential. (c)* Left: *In the open state of the h-gate, the ball lies in the cytosol.* Right: *Membrane depolarization causes the ball to move into the pore so as to occlude the channel. (Adapted from Katz,* Physiology of the Heart *(Ref. 1, with permission).)*

a water-filled pore. A selectivity filter, determined by the amino acid sequence of this pore region, restricts passage to a given ion species. The $S_4$ transmembrane segments contain positively charged arginine and lysine residues that represent the voltage sensor, a charged region that responds to membrane depolarization by opening the channel. In sodium channels, this voltage sensor corresponds to the m-gate described by Hodgkin and Huxley (see below). Channel inactivation occurs when intracellular peptide chains that link the domains of the α-subunit, called inactivation particles, occlude the inner mouth of the channel pore. The inactivation particles in sodium channels, which correspond to the h-gate, are made up of the cytoplasmic peptide chain that connects the $S_6$ transmembrane segment of domain III to the $S_1$ segment of domain IV [17–20]. The mechanism responsible for channel inactivation can be viewed as a ball swinging at the end of a chain, in which the inactivation particle (the ball) responds to a change in membrane potential by swinging into the inner mouth of the pore to inactivate the channel (Fig. 1.5). In some potassium channels, a similar mechanism uses portions of other intracellular peptide chains to plug, and so inactivate, the channel [21–23].

The co-ordinated opening and closing of the heart's ion channels generate changes in membrane potential that control the calcium entry responsible for excitation–contraction coupling. Key to this process is the opening of L-type calcium channels that trigger a much larger calcium release from the sarcoplasmic reticulum. As described below, the subsequent steps in this activation process are initiated when activator calcium released from these internal stores binds to the cardiac contractile proteins.

## Contraction and the working myocardium

### Overall structure

More than half of the volume of working myocardial cells is made up of the contractile proteins, which are organized in a manner that gives rise to a characteristic repeating pattern of light and dark striations (Fig. 1.6). The more darkly staining A-bands contain the thick filaments, whereas

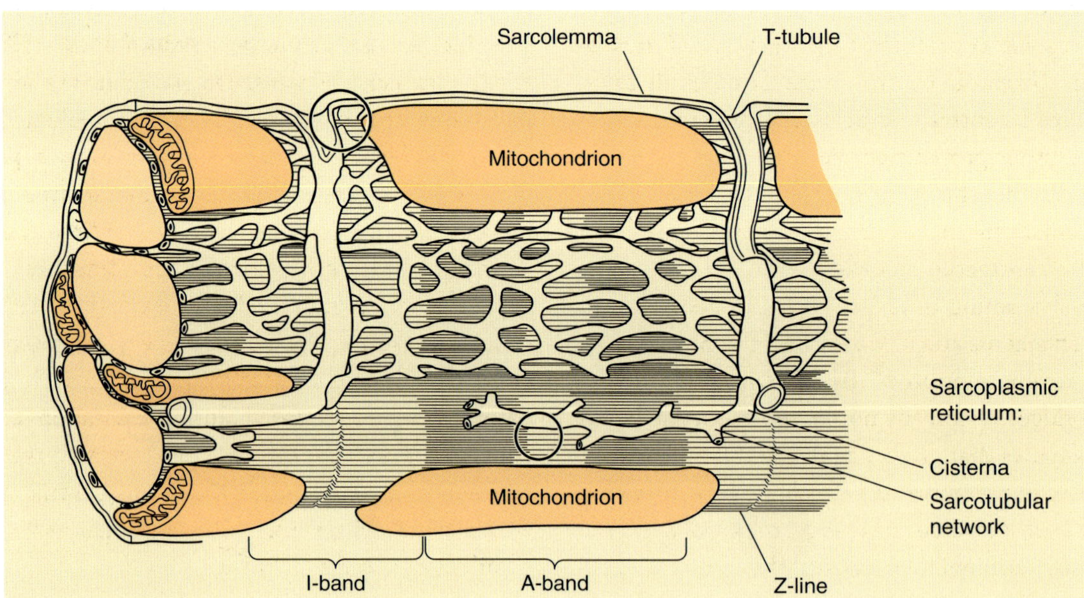


**Figure 1.6** *Ultrastructure of the working myocardial cell. Contractile proteins are arranged in a regular array of thick and thin filaments (seen in cross-section on the left). The A-band represents the region of the sarcomere occupied by the thick filaments into which thin filaments extend from either side. The I-band is the region of the sarcomere occupied only by thin filaments; these extend toward the centre of the sarcomere from the Z-lines, which bisect each I-band. The sarcomere, the functional unit of the contractile apparatus which is defined as the region between adjacent Z-lines, contains two half I-bands and one A-band. The sarcoplasmic reticulum, a membrane network that surrounds the contractile proteins, consists of the sarcotubular network at the centre of the sarcomere and the cisternae, which abut on the t-tubules and the sarcolemma. The transverse tubular system (t-tubule) is lined by a membrane that is continuous with the sarcolemma, so that the lumen of the t-tubules carries the extracellular space toward the centre of the myocardial cell. Mitochondria are shown in the central sarcomere and in cross-section on the left. (Adapted from Katz,* Physiology of the Heart *(Ref. 1, with permission).)*

the lightly staining half I-bands at either side of each A-band contain only thin filaments. Each I-band is bisected by a narrow, darkly staining Z-line that delimits the sarcomeres, the fundamental morphological units of striated muscle. Each of the latter, which is defined as the region between two Z-lines, consists of a central A-band plus the two adjacent half I-bands. The A-bands of the contracted heart contain not only thick filaments but also the ends of thin filaments that penetrate from the Z-lines at either end of the sarcomere. At physiological sarcomere lengths, the thin filaments of the resting heart extend almost to the centre of the A-band, so that when the sarcomere shortens, the extent of overlap between the thick and thin filaments increases.

The A bands are composed largely of myosin, which is arranged so that the active sites of these molecules project from the thick filament as the cross-bridges (see below). The thick filaments contain several additional supporting proteins, including titin, nebulette, and myosin-binding protein C. Titin and nebulette are orientated along the long axis of the filament, while myosin-binding protein C links adjacent thick filaments to each other. The thin filaments are strands made up of actin polymers to which are attached the regulatory proteins: tropomyosin and the troponin complex. Troponin C, one of the latter, binds calcium and so plays a central role in excitation–contraction coupling. The other proteins of the thin filament, along with myosin in the thick filament, participate in cooperative interactions that regulate both the onset and intensity of the contractile process.

Sarcomere shortening in the contracting heart occurs when the thin filaments are pulled towards the centre of the A-band by a rowing motion of the myosin cross-bridges. These cross-bridges, as already noted, represent the heads of myosin molecules that project from the thick filaments. The interactions between the cross-bridges and actin in the thin filaments are powered by energy released from the hydrolysis of the terminal high-energy phosphate of ATP; this occurs when actin activates catalytic sites in the myosin cross-bridges [24, 25].

## Excitation-contraction coupling and relaxation: the plasma membrane and sarcoplasmic reticulum

Two key membrane structures, the plasma membrane and the sarcoplasmic reticulum, regulate excitation–contraction coupling and relaxation. The heart's plasma membrane, which separates the cytosol from the extracellular space, is divided structurally into the sarcolemma, which surrounds the body of the cell, and the transverse tubular (t-tubular) system, which penetrates the cell interior (Fig. 1.6). The lumens of the t-tubules open freely to the extracellular space, which allows these plasma membrane extensions to activate the centre of the myocardial cell by transmitting the action potential into the cell interior.

The sarcoplasmic reticulum is an intracellular membrane system that contains the large supply of calcium needed for rapid activation of cardiac contraction. Proteins associated with these membranes take up, store, and release this activator calcium. The sarcoplasmic reticulum in the adult mammalian heart is divided into two regions. The first is the network of subsarcolemmal cisternae, which are dilated extensions of the sarcoplasmic reticulum that abut the t-tubules and sarcolemma. The cisternae contain both the calcium-binding proteins that store this activator and the calcium release channels through which calcium is delivered into the cytosol at the onset of systole. The second region is the more extensive sarcotubular network which surrounds the contractile proteins in the centre of the sarcomere. This network contains a dense array of calcium-pump ATPase proteins that use the energy obtained from ATP hydrolysis to relax the heart by transporting calcium out of the cytosol into the interior of the sarcoplasmic reticulum.

A critical link in excitation–contraction coupling is provided by the dyads, which are composite structures made up of membranes of the sarcolemma (and its extensions, the t-tubules) and the subsarcolemmal cisternae of the sarcoplasmic reticulum (Fig. 1.7). These structures bring portions of these two membranes into close proximity, and contain the calcium release channels through which activator calcium is released during excitation–contraction coupling. The mechanisms that control the interplay between the sarcolemma and sarcoplasmic reticulum, which is critical for excitation–contraction coupling, are detailed later in this chapter.

## The contractile proteins

Six proteins found in the myofilaments are responsible for the contractile process and its control (Table 1.2): myosin, actin, tropomyosin, and the three components of troponin. Additional proteins provide structural support to the myofilament lattice; these include the actinins, titin, nebulette, and myosin-binding protein C. Myosin and actin suffice to convert the chemical energy of ATP into the

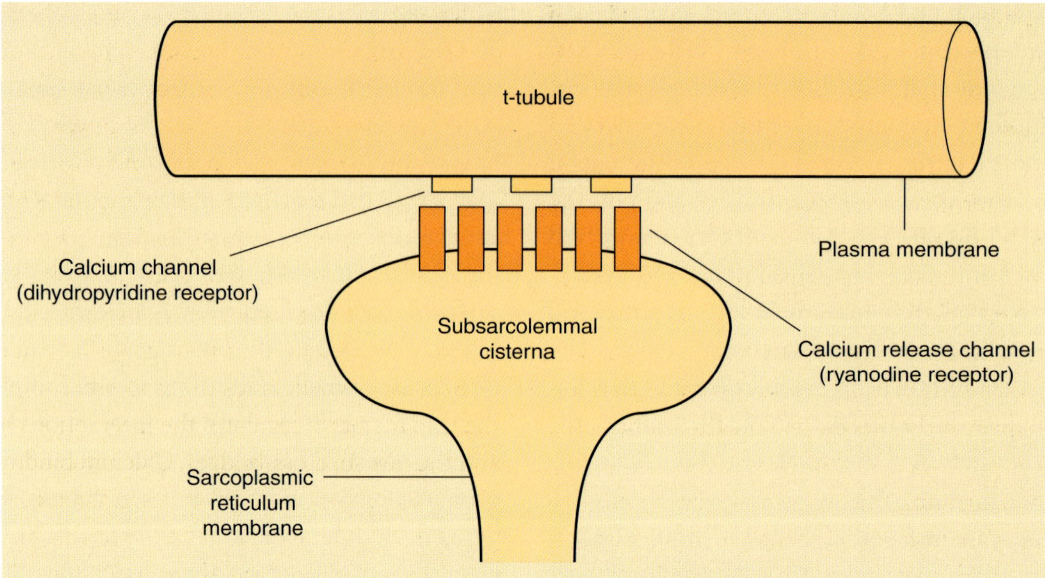


**Figure 1.7** *Schematic diagram of a dyad, a composite structure made up of the membranes of the t-tubule* (above) *and the subsarcolemmal cisternae of the sarcoplasmic reticulum* (below)*. The t-tubules, which are invaginations of the sarcolemma, are lined by extensions of the plasma membrane. Excitation–contraction coupling in the heart occurs when a small amount of calcium enters the space between these membranes through calcium channels in the plasma membrane. When this calcium is 'sprayed' on the calcium-release channels (also called foot proteins or ryanodine receptors) of the sarcoplasmic reticulum, the latter open. As shown in this sketch, there are about half as many plasma membrane calcium channels as calcium release channels in the dyad. (Adapted from Katz,* Physiology of the Heart *(Ref. 1, with permission).)*

**Table 1.2** Contractile proteins of the heart

| Protein | Location | Salient properties |
|---|---|---|
| Myosin | Thick filament | Hydrolyses ATP; interacts with actin |
| Actin | Thin filament | Activates myosin ATPase; interacts with myosin |
| Tropomyosin | Thin filament | Modulates actin–myosin interaction |
| Troponin C | Thin filament | Binds calcium |
| Troponin I | Thin filament | Inhibits actin–myosin interactions |
| Troponin T | Thin filament | Binds troponin complex to tropomyosin and thin filament |

mechanical work that pumps blood out of the heart's cavities. Physiological control of these interactions is provided by co-operative rearrangements within the thin filament that involve tropomyosin and troponins C, I, and T.

### *Myosin*

Myosin is an elongated molecule with a filamentous 'tail' and a globular 'head'. In living muscle, myosin is aggregated in the thick filament so that the myosin heads, which contain both the ATPase and actin-binding sites, project as the cross-bridges. Shortening and tension development occur when the cross-bridges, which in resting muscle are perpendicular to the long axis of the thick filament, bind to the thin filaments and, using energy derived from ATP hydrolysis, shift towards the centre of the sarcomere. In the ventricles, the energy released in this rowing motion can be used to develop pressure or to eject blood. The extent of either is determined by the manner in which the muscle is loaded. If afterload is very high, as occurs in a skeletal muscle preparation when the ends of the muscle are fixed, the sarcomeres cannot shorten, but developed tension is high. In the ventricle, this represents an isovolumic contraction such as occurs in aortic stenosis, a condition in which developed pressure is high, but ejection is impaired. At low afterload, as in an unloaded skeletal muscle fibre, the energy released by the contractile proteins is used for sarcomere shortening; in the left ventricle after massive vasodilation, systole leads to ejection but little pressure development. Afterload, therefore, is a major determinant of the haemodynamic manifestations of the contractile process.

The intrinsic rate at which myosin hydrolyses ATP is of considerable functional importance as it determines both muscle shortening velocity and myocardial contractility [26–28]. This property is determined largely by the cardiac myosin heavy chains. The higher ATPase myosin heavy chain, called α, determines a rapid shortening velocity and high myocardial contractility, whereas the lower ATPase myosin heavy chain, called β, is associated with a weaker, slower contraction. The latter, however, yields a more efficient contraction when the heart ejects against a heavy afterload. The role of the cardiac myosin light chains is less clear; most regulate the intensity of the contractile process.

In the human atrium, the myosin heavy chains are mostly a high ATPase isoform, whereas the human ventricle contains about 90% slow myosin heavy chain [29]. In chronically overloaded human atria, an isoform shift replaces the fast atrial myosin heavy chains with the low ATPase isoform [30, 31]. A similar, but less extensive isoform shift occurs in the failing human ventricle [29].

### *Actin*

Actin is a much smaller globular protein that forms a double-stranded macromolecular helix which represents the backbone of the thin filament. As already noted, the interaction of actin with the myosin cross-bridges allows the chemical energy released by ATP hydrolysis to power the physicochemical changes responsible for the contractile process. Like myosin, actin is found in several isoforms.

### *Tropomyosin*

Tropomyosin, an elongated molecule made up of two helical peptide chains, lies in each of the two longitudinal grooves between the two strands of actin in the thin filament. The major function of tropomyosin, along with the troponin complex, is to regulate the interactions between actin and myosin.

### *The troponin complex*

Troponin includes three discrete proteins. Troponin I, in concert with tropomyosin, reversibly inhibits the interactions between actin and myosin, troponin T binds the troponin complex to tropomyosin, while troponin C contains the high-affinity calcium binding sites that recognize the appearance of calcium in the cytosol as a signal to initiate excitation–contraction coupling. All of these proteins work together to regulate contraction in the living heart.

*Troponin C* is a member of a family of calcium-binding proteins called E–F hand proteins because their calcium-binding sites resemble a hand. In these proteins, the cation is bound by negatively charged oxygen atoms located between two α-helices (E and F) that resemble the extended thumb and forefinger of a right hand [32]. Other E–F hand proteins include calmodulin and the myosin light chains [for review, see 6]. Cardiac troponin C contains the key calcium binding site that recognizes the appearance of calcium in the cytosol as the signal that initiates systole.

*Troponin I*, which binds the troponin complex to actin in the thin filament, regulates the interactions between actin and the myosin cross-bridges. Calcium binding to troponin C causes conformational changes in the proteins of the thin filament that loosen the bond linking troponin I to actin, resulting in a shift in the position of the elongated tropomyosin molecules in the grooves between actin chains. This conformational change plays a central role in excitation–contraction coupling by exposing binding sites on actin that interact with the myosin cross-bridges. Cardiac troponin I also participates in regulatory responses. For example, this protein can be phosphorylated by cyclic AMP-dependent protein kinase in a reaction that, by reducing the calcium sensitivity of troponin C, participates in the lusitropic response to β-adrenergic stimulation.

*Troponin T*, which binds the troponin complex to tropomyosin, does not bind calcium. However, this protein, like the other proteins of the myofibrils, participates in important allosteric reactions. Switches involving the more than 30 isoforms of this protein can modify the calcium sensitivity of tension development. One such change depresses contractility in the chronically overloaded, failing heart by desensitizing the contractile apparatus to calcium [33].

## Interactions between the contractile proteins

The contractile proteins interact in a highly co-operative manner that allows subtle changes in one protein to have marked consequences in terms of the intensity of the contractile process. The response to the major physiological regulator of these interactions, which is the calcium released by excitation–contraction coupling, has already been discussed. Other variables that regulate these interactions include allosteric effects of ATP, which are described later in this chapter, and changing muscle length (see below). Another example is the response to a change in pH. Protons compete with calcium for protein-binding

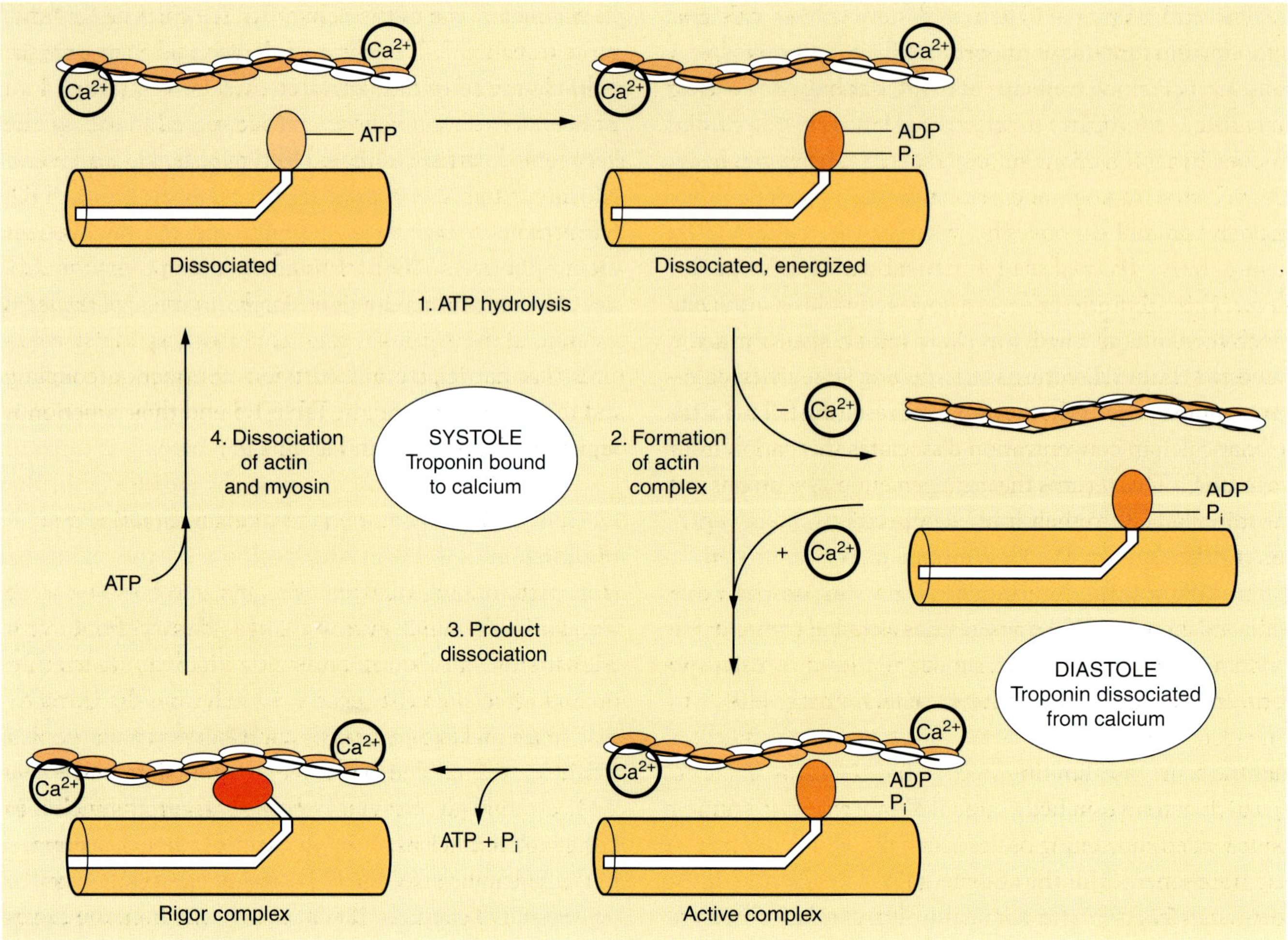


**Figure 1.8** *Reaction mechanism for actomyosin ATPase. During systole* (left)*, the interactions between actin and myosin can be simplified as four steps. These occur repetitively when actin in the thin filament is free to interact with the myosin cross-bridges, which occurs when troponin is bound to calcium. During diastole* (right)*, calcium removal from troponin initiates a conformational change in the thin filament that prevents actin from interacting with myosin. The steps that occur during systole begin at the upper left, where ATP bound to the myosin cross-bridge has dissociated the thick and thin filaments. Hydrolysis of myosin-bound ATP (step 1) transfers the energy of the nucleotide to the cross-bridge, which assumes a dissociated, energized state* (upper right)*. Interaction of the cross-bridge with actin in the thin filament (step 2) leads to the formation of the active complex* (lower right)*; although actin is bound to the myosin cross-bridge in this state, the energy derived from ATP is still associated with the cross-bridge. Dissociation of ADP and $P_i$, the products of ATP hydrolysis (step 3), leads to the formation of a rigour bond. In this step, chemical energy is expended to perform mechanical work and this is depicted as a change in the position of the cross-bridge that shifts the thin filament to the left. The cycle ends when ATP binds to the rigour complex (step 4), which dissociates the cross-bridge from the thin filament. These four reactions cannot take place when calcium is dissociated from troponin because actin is no longer able to interact with the myosin cross-bridges. (Adapted from Katz,* Physiology of the Heart *(Ref. 1, with permission).)*

sites, so that the acidosis which occurs in the energy-starved heart impairs the response to a given rise in cytosolic calcium, thereby reducing myocardial contractility [34].

Control of cardiac performance by changing end-diastolic volume (the Frank–Starling relationship) is due mainly to sarcomere length-dependent changes in the calcium sensitivity of the contractile proteins [35] and, to a lesser extent, to length-dependent changes in calcium release from the sarcoplasmic reticulum [36]. The effects of sarcomere length on the calcium sensitivity of the E–F hand region of troponin C is another example of an allosteric effect involving the contractile proteins. Myocardial contractility, the other physiologically important determinant of the interactions among the heart's contractile proteins, is regulated largely by changes in the level of cytosolic calcium achieved during excitation–contraction coupling.

The physiological control of the contractile process by calcium is due to the ability of this activator cation to modify co-operative interactions among the proteins of the thin filament. In resting muscle, where cytosolic calcium levels are low and troponin C is not bound to this calcium, actin–myosin interactions are inhibited largely by a blocking action of tropomyosin and troponin I. Binding of calcium to cardiac troponin C initiates a series of co-operative interactions among troponin C, troponin I, troponin T, tropomyosin, and actin that shift the position of tropomyosin in the grooves between the two strands of the actin polymer that makes up the backbone of the thin filament. This allosteric effect exposes active sites on actin, which then interacts with myosin to initiate the contractile process. The muscle returns to its resting state when calcium is pumped out of the cytosol. The resulting fall in intracellular calcium concentration dissociates this cation from troponin C. This returns the arrangement of the proteins of the thin filament to their inhibitory positions, thereby preventing further interactions between actin and myosin.

The reaction mechanism of the interactions between actin and myosin ATPase activity has assumed considerable functional significance because of the direct relationship between myosin ATPase activity and shortening velocity in unloaded muscle (see above). This correlation indicates that the same rate-limiting steps in the chemical reactions by which actomyosin hydrolyses ATP are also rate limiting for unloaded shortening of the intact muscle. A number of elaborate schemes for the actomyosin ATPase reaction has been described, but for simplicity this chapter considers only four steps in the reaction mechanisms that allow the contractile proteins to use ATP to generate mechanical work (Fig. 1.8). These steps are the binding of ATP to myosin, hydrolysis of myosin-bound ATP during which the hydrolytic products [adenosine diphosphate (ADP) and inorganic phosphate ($P_i$)] remain bound to myosin, formation of an active actomyosin complex, which begins mechanochemical transduction, and release of hydrolytic products, the step in which the myosin cross-bridge changes position. In the active muscle, this sequence is repeated when ATP again binds to myosin. The physiological control of the contractile process by calcium, which as already discussed reflects conformational changes in the thin filament that result from the binding of this activator to troponin C, reflects shifts in the orientation of tropomyosin that can prevent actin from interacting with the myosin cross-bridges (Fig. 1.8).

## Excitation–contraction coupling and relaxation

Excitation–contraction coupling, as already noted, is the name given to the processes that link depolarization of the plasma membrane to the delivery of the calcium for binding by troponin C. In working adult mammalian myocardial cells, almost all of this activator calcium is released from intracellular stores; in more primitive cells, such as the embryonic heart and most smooth muscle, most activator calcium enters the cytosol from the extracellular fluid. Relaxation, an energy-dependent process that is brought about by entirely different structures than those that activate the heart, is therefore not simply a reversal of the steps involved in excitation–contraction coupling. Major structures that participate in excitation–contraction coupling and relaxation are listed in Table 1.3 and their function is depicted schematically in Figure 1.9.

### *Calcium cycles in excitation–contraction coupling and relaxation*

Most of the activator calcium that binds to the contractile proteins of the adult human heart is derived from intracellular stores in the sarcoplasmic reticulum; the smaller amount of calcium that enters the cell from the extracellular space makes only a small contribution to this pool of activator calcium. The major role of the calcium that enters the heart through plasma membrane calcium channels is to trigger calcium release from the sarcoplasmic reticulum.

The calcium fluxes into and out of the cytosol can be viewed as two distinct calcium cycles, one from the extracellular fluid, the other from within the sarcoplasmic reticulum (Fig. 1.9). In the extracellular cycle, calcium enters the cytosol across the plasma membrane from what is, in effect, an unlimited supply of extracellular calcium, whereas the calcium that enters the cytosol via the intracellular calcium cycle is derived from much more limited stores within the sarcoplasmic reticulum. The latter is a specialization of the endoplasmic reticulum, so that the generic term for these internal membranes is sarco(endo)plasmic reticulum; this is why the sarcoplasmic reticulum calcium pump is generally abbreviated as SERCA.

Calcium crosses the plasma membrane by downhill fluxes through the voltage-gated calcium channels discussed above, while the calcium fluxes out of the sarcoplasmic reticulum are mediated by an entirely different family of proteins called calcium release channels (Table 1.3). The uphill transport of this cation into the extracellular space and lumen of the sarcoplasmic reticulum is effected by calcium pumps and calcium exchangers that are embedded in these membranes. The ATP-dependent calcium pumps in

**Table 1.3** Structure–function relationships in working cardiac myocytes

| Structure | Role in excitation–contraction coupling | Role in relaxation |
|---|---|---|
| Plasma membrane | | |
| Sarcolemma | | |
| Sodium channel | Depolarization<br>Opens calcium channels | |
| Calcium channel | Action potential plateau<br>Calcium-triggered calcium release | |
| Calcium pump (PMCA) | | Calcium removal |
| Sodium/calcium exchanger | Calcium entry | Calcium removal |
| Sodium pump | | Establishes sodium gradient |
| Transverse tubule | | |
| Sodium channel | Action potential propagation | |
| Calcium channel | Calcium-triggered calcium release | |
| Sarcoplasmic reticulum | | |
| Subsarcolemmal cisternae | | |
| Calcium release channel | Calcium release | |
| Sarcotubular network | | |
| Calcium pump (SERCA) | | Calcium removal |
| Myofilaments | | |
| Actin and myosin | Contraction | |
| Troponin C | Calcium receptor | |
| Tropomyosin, troponins I and T | Allosteric regulation | |

the plasma membrane (PMCA) and sarco(endo)plasmic reticulum (SERCA) are members of a family of ATPases that also includes the sodium pump ($Na^+/K^+$-ATPase). The sodium/calcium exchanger, which uses the large sodium gradient across the plasma membrane to transport intracellular calcium uphill out of the cytosol in exchange for extracellular sodium, belongs to yet another family of membrane proteins.

### *Coupling of membrane depolarization to calcium release from intracellular stores*

The functional link between plasma membrane depolarization (the action potential) and the opening of intracellular calcium-release channels is provided by plasma membrane calcium channels. In skeletal muscle, these channels operate through a mechanical coupling, in which plasma membrane depolarization removes a plug that in the resting muscle blocks the intracellular calcium-release channel. This plug is part of an L-type plasma membrane calcium channel that, while it cannot form a calcium-permeable pore, regulates the opening of the intracellular calcium-release channel in skeletal muscle. In the heart, a different L-type plasma membrane calcium channel opens to cause a localized increase in cytosolic calcium concentration that couples membrane depolarization to calcium release from the cardiac sarcoplasmic reticulum. This localized area of high calcium concentration, called a 'calcium spark' [37], then opens adjacent intracellular calcium-release channels in the sarcoplasmic reticulum to cause a much greater release of calcium, a process that is often referred to as $Ca^{2+}$-induced calcium release [38, 39].

### *Structures involved in excitation–contraction coupling and relaxation*

*Plasma membrane calcium channels.* The plasma membrane calcium channels are members of the family of ion-selective channels discussed above. The most important members of this family in the heart are the L-type calcium channels, which bind the familiar classes of calcium channel blockers (dihydropyridines such as nifedipine, phenylalkylamines such as verapamil, and benzothiazepines such as diltiazem). These are sometimes called dihydropyridine receptors because of their high affinity to bind to this class of calcium channel blockers. Other types of plasma membrane calcium channels have recently been described; these are referred to as T, N, P, Q, and R [6, 40, 41].

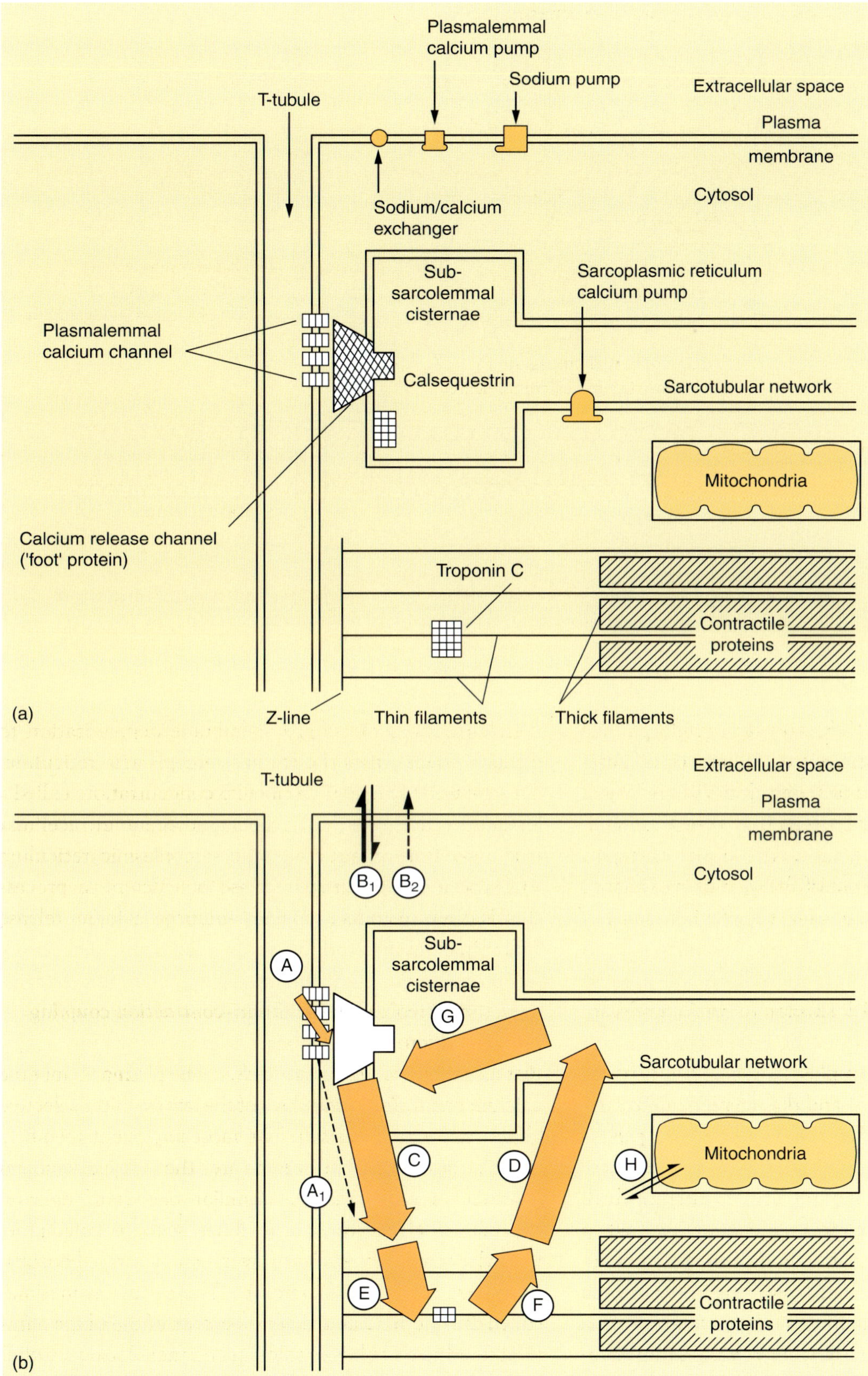


**Figure 1.9** *Schematic diagram showing: (a) key structures and (b) major calcium fluxes involved in cardiac excitation–contraction coupling. The thickness of the arrows indicates the magnitude of the calcium fluxes, while their directions describe the energetics of the calcium fluxes: downward arrows describe passive calcium fluxes and upward arrows describe energy-dependent calcium transport. Calcium enters the cell from the extracellular fluid via plasma membrane calcium channels. (Arrow A). While most of this calcium triggers calcium release from the sarcoplasmic reticulum, a small portion directly activates the contractile proteins (arrow $A_1$). Calcium transport back into the extracellular fluid involves two plasma membrane systems: sodium/calcium exchange (arrow $B_1$), and the plasma membrane calcium pump (arrow $B_2$). The sarcoplasmic reticulum membrane regulates two calcium fluxes: calcium release from the subsarcolemmal cisternae (arrow C) and active calcium uptake by the calcium pump (arrow D). Calcium diffuses within the sarcoplasmic reticulum in a third calcium flux (arrow G), returning to the subsarcolemmal cisternae where it is stored in complex with calsequestrin and other calcium-binding proteins. The contractile proteins are regulated by calcium binding to (arrow E) and dissociation from (arrow F) the high-affinity calcium-binding sites of troponin C. Movements of calcium into and out of mitochondria (arrow H) buffer cytosolic calcium concentration during calcium overload. (Adapted from Katz, Physiology of the Heart (Ref. 1, with permission).)*

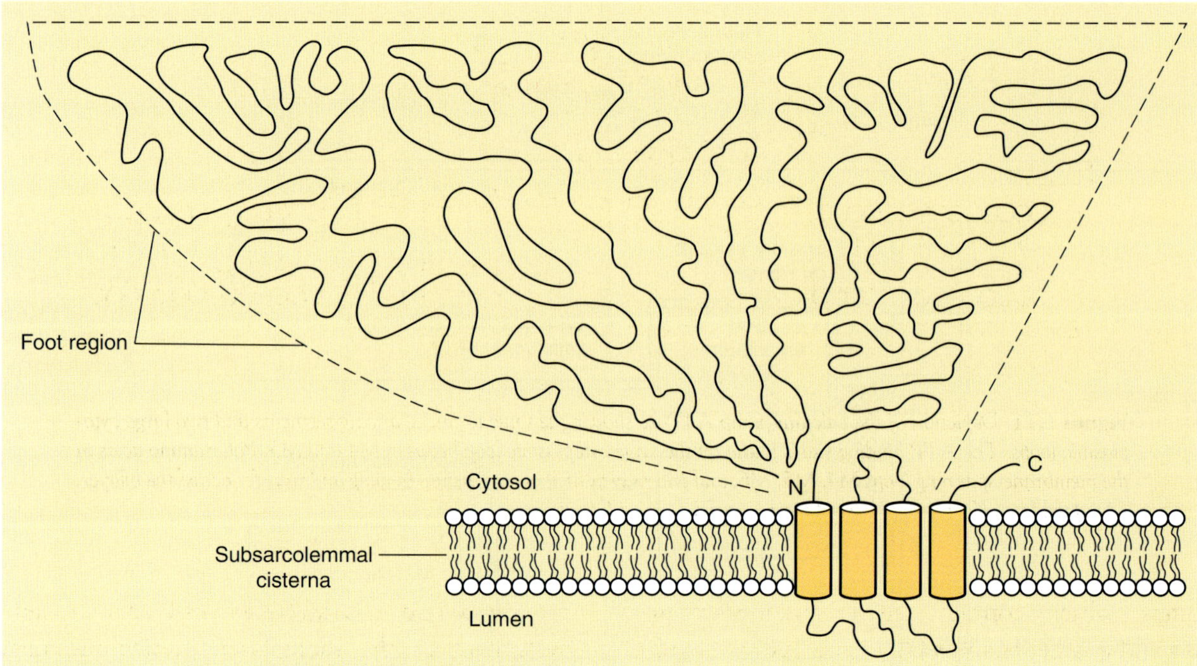


**Figure 1.10** *Structure of one subunit of the tetrameric calcium release channels (foot protein) in the membrane of the subsarcolemmal cisterna* (below), *showing four membrane-spanning regions and the large asymmetrical cytoplasmic domain. The latter make up the foot proteins of the dyad, which are located adjacent to L-type calcium channels in the t-tubular membrane (see Fig. 1.7). The complete calcium release channel is made up of four of the subunits depicted in this figure. (Adapted from Katz, Physiology of the Heart (Ref. 1, with permission).)*

*Intracellular calcium-release channels.* The structure of the intracellular calcium-release channels in the sarcoplasmic reticulum differs considerably from that of the calcium channels in the plasma membrane. The former are members of a family that includes at least two classes of related proteins [for review see refs. 42–44]: the ryanodine receptors, so named because they bind to this plant alkaloid, and the $InsP_3$ receptors, which bind to and are activated by inositol trisphosphate ($InsP_3$). The ryanodine receptors are located in the dyads across from the L-type plasma membrane calcium channels discussed earlier (Fig. 1.7). By releasing calcium from the sarcoplasmic reticulum, the ryanodine receptors mediate the final step in excitation–contraction coupling.

The ryanodine receptors and $InsP_3$ receptors are tetrameric structures, in which each subunit includes a large cytosolic domain and four α-helical transmembrane segments (Fig. 1.10). Although $InsP_3$ receptors are only about half the size of the ryanodine receptors, there is considerable homology between these two classes of intracellular calcium-release channel. Their three-dimensional structures are similar in that the four subunits in both ryanodine receptors and $InsP_3$ receptors surround a central pore through which activator calcium is released when the channel is opened. The single channel conductance of the $InsP_3$ receptors is less than that of the larger ryanodine receptors [45], which means that the former carry less current.

It is clear that the opening of the ryanodine receptor calcium-release channels provides the major source of activator calcium in working myocardial cells. The $InsP_3$ receptors are the predominant calcium channels that initiate the slower contractile responses in smooth muscle [46], but their role in the heart is less clear. As $InsP_3$-activated calcium-release channels release slowly only a small amount of calcium, they cannot participate in the calcium cycles that trigger excitation–contraction coupling in the heart. Cardiac $InsP_3$-regulated calcium channels have recently been found to participate in signal transduction systems that are activated by such neurohumoral mediators as α-adrenergic agonists and angiotensin II, and so may play a role in regulating cellular growth. $InsP_3$ receptors may also contribute to the slow calcium release that regulates diastolic tension.

*Calcium pump ATPases* The calcium pump ATPases are members of a family of closely related proteins, called P-type

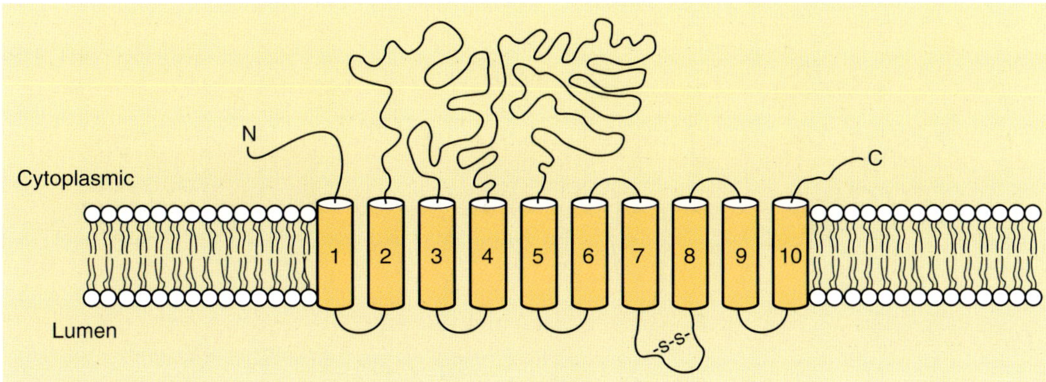


**Figure 1.11** *Depiction of the calcium pump ATPase showing ten membrane-spanning segments and two large cytoplasmic loops. The ATP binding site is found on the large cytoplasmic loop between M4 and M5. Polar amino acids in the membrane-spanning loops M4, M5, M6, and M8 may participate in calcium binding and transfer across the bilayer. (Adapted from Katz, Physiology of the Heart (Ref. 1, with permission).)*

ion pumps, which contain ten membrane-spanning α-helices and a large 'head' that projects into the cytosol (Fig. 1.11). All use a similar reaction mechanism to couple the hydrolysis of the high-energy phosphate bond of ATP to the uphill transport of calcium out of the cytosol [for review, see refs. 47, 48]. In the heart, the plasma membrane calcium pump is larger than that of the sarcoplasmic reticulum; although both share a similar reaction mechanism that allows the energy released by ATP hydrolysis to pump calcium out of the cytosol, they are regulated differently.

The rate of calcium pumping by sarcoplaemic reticulum is stimulated when cyclic AMP activates a protein kinase that transfers a phosphate group to phospholamban. The latter is an inhibitory membrane protein that is distinct from the calcium pump ATPase. As the dephospho form of phospholamban inhibits the calcium pump of the cardiac sarcoplasmic reticulum, phosphorylation of phospholamban accelerates calcium uptake from the cytosol and so accelerates relaxation [for review, see refs. 49–51]. The plasma membrane calcium pump is stimulated when the calcium–calmodulin complex binds to an inhibitory site located on the C-terminal domain of the molecule [47]. This binding peptide, which is not found in the homologous protein SERCA, exerts effects similar to those of phospholamban in that both regulate the transport of calcium out of the cytosol. However, the roles of these regulatory systems differ. Cyclic AMP-activated phosphorylation of phospholamban accelerates cardiac relaxation during β-adrenergic stimulation, whereas the calcium–calmodulin-activated phosphorylation of the plasma membrane calcium pump promotes calcium efflux from the cell under conditions of calcium overload. Phospholamban in the sarcoplasmic reticulum membrane can also be phosphorylated by a calcium-calmodulin-dependent protein kinase, thereby providing the cardiac myocyte with an additional mechanism by which to rid the cytosol of excess calcium.

*The sodium/calcium exchanger* Sodium/calcium exchange plays a major role in the active transport of calcium out of the cytosol and into the extracellular space. The sodium/calcium exchanger, which is a large membrane protein that contains 12 α-helical transmembrane segments [52, 53], differs markedly from that of the calcium pump ATPases (Fig. 1.12). The mechanisms of action of the exchangers and the ATPases also differ markedly. In contrast to the pumping action of the sarcoplasmic reticulum and plasma membrane, which directly couples ATP hydrolysis to osmotic work, the sodium/calcium exchanger uses the osmotic energy of the sodium gradient across the plasma membrane for this active transport. The ultimate energy source for the active calcium transport out of the cell by the sodium/calcium exchanger is ATP hydrolysed by the $Na^+/K^+$-ATPase (sodium pump), which establishes this sodium gradient.

The sodium/calcium exchanger generates a small ionic current because each calcium ion is exchanged for three sodium ions. As a result, calcium efflux via the exchanger generates an inward current in which a positive charge enters the cell. The currents generated by the sodium/calcium exchanger are relatively small and probably contribute less a few millivolts to membrane potential.

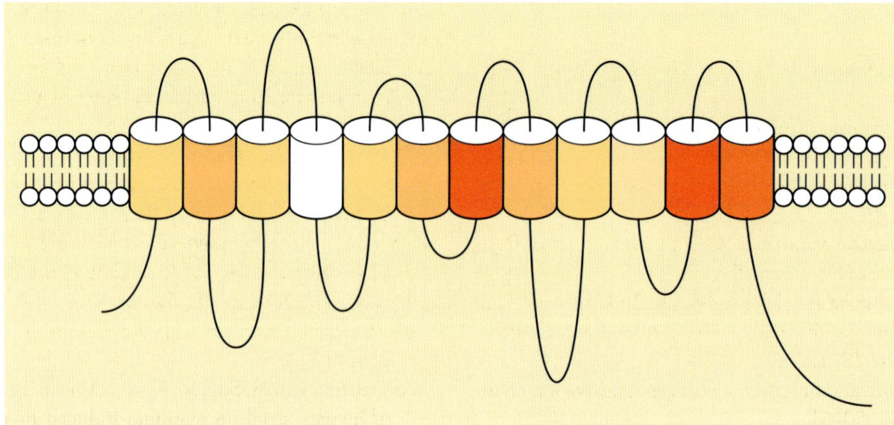

**Figure 1.12** *Structure of the sodium/calcium exchanger. This membrane protein contains 12 membrane-spanning peptides, and so differs from the ion pumps and channels discussed above. (Adapted from Katz, Physiology of the Heart (Ref. 1, with permission).)*

*The sodium pump* The sodium pump, like the calcium pump ATPases described above, uses energy derived from ATP hydrolysis to exchange the small amount of sodium that enters the cell during each action potential for the small amount of potassium lost from the cytosol during repolarization [54]. Because three sodium ions are exchanged for only two potassium ions moved in opposite directions during each turnover, the sodium pump, like the sodium/calcium exchanger, is electrogenic, generating a small, repolarizing current that is normally less than 10 mV. In addition to restoring the intracellular concentrations of sodium and potassium after each action potential, the sodium gradient across the plasma membrane generated by the sodium pump provides a source of osmotic energy that can be coupled to the transport of a number of molecules, including calcium by the exchanger described above.

*Calcium storage within the sarcoplasmic reticulum* While some of the calcium stored in the sarcoplasmic reticulum is in a free, ionized form, much of it is associated with calcium-binding proteins within this intracellular membrane system [48]. The most important of these proteins is calsequestrin, a 45 000 mol. wt protein that traps calcium within this membrane system. Other calcium-binding proteins found in smaller amounts include the 44 000 mol. wt protein calreticulin and a 170 000 mol. wt histidine-rich calcium-binding protein. These calcium-binding proteins are concentrated in the subsarcolemmal cisternae, where they maintain a calcium store that is readily released through the calcium-release channels during excitation–contraction coupling.

## Role of ATP

In addition to its role as an energy donor for the tension-generating interactions between myosin cross-bridges and actin, and the ion pumps that relax the heart, ATP has important allosteric effects on many of these systems [for review, see ref. 55]. The substrate and allosteric effects are seen at quite different ATP concentrations. In the range of 0.1–10 μM, ATP provides the substrate for the energy-consuming reactions involved in muscle contraction and relaxation, whereas the allosteric effects of ATP, which do not require ATP hydrolysis, are seen in the range above 100 μM. Because the ATP concentration in the living heart is well above 1 mM, which is several orders of magnitude higher than needed to saturate the hydrolytic sites that mediate the energy-consuming effects of ATP, the major effects of energy starvation are to attenuate these allosteric effects, as well as to cause a rise in ADP levels that decreases the free energy of ATP hydrolysis.

Most of the allosteric effects of ATP maintain the heart in a relaxed state. These include dissociation of actin and myosin, and acceleration of the sarcoplasmic reticulum calcium pump and the sodium/calcium exchanger. As all of these exert lusitropic effects, a major consequence of energy starvation is to impair relaxation. Other allosteric effects promote contraction: these include acceleration of calcium fluxes through the plasma membrane calcium channels and the calcium-release channels of the sarcoplasmic reticulum. Another consequence of a fall in ATP levels is a reduction in the free energy of ATP hydrolysis, due mainly to a rise in ADP and inorganic phosphate levels [56].

## References


1. Katz AM. *Physiology of the heart*. 2nd edition. New York: Raven Press, 1992.
2. Opie LH. *The heart, physiology from cell to circulation*. 3rd edition. Philadelphia, PA: Lippincott/Raven, 1998
3. Bers DM. *Excitation–contraction coupling and cardiac contractile force*. Dordrecht: Kluwer, 1991.
4. Rüegg C. *Calcium in muscle contraction. Cellular and molecular physiology*. 2nd edition. Berlin: Springer, 1992.
5. Clapham DE. Calcium signalling. *Cell* 1995; 80: 259–68.
6. Katz AM. Calcium channel diversity in the cardiovascular system. *J Am Coll Cardiol* 1996; 28: 522–8.
7. Catterall WA. Structure and function of voltage-sensitive ion channels. *Science* 1988; 242: 50–61.
8. Hille B. *Ionic channels of excitable membranes*. Sunderland, MA: Sinauer, 1992.
9. Catterall WA. Cellular and molecular biology of voltage-gated sodium channels. *Physiol Rev* 1992; 72 (Suppl): S15–48.
10. Jan LY, Jan YN. Tracing the roots of ion channels. *Cell* 1992; 69: 715–18.
11. Katz AM. Cardiac ion channels. *N Engl J Med* 1993; 328: 1244–51.
12. Clapham DE, Ackerman MJ. Ion channels — basic science and clinical disease. *N Engl J Med* 1997; 336: 1575–86.
13. Katz AM. Selectivity and toxicity of antiarrhythmic drugs: molecular interactions with ion channels. *Am J Med* 1998; 104: 179–95.
14. Hodgkin AL, Huxley AF. A quantitative description of membrane current and its application to conduction and excitation in nerve. *J Physiol (Lond)* 1952; 117: 500–44.
15. Nunoki K, Florio V, Catterall WA. Activation of purified calcium channels by stoichiometric protein phosphorylation. *Proc Natl Acad Sci USA* 1989; 86: 6816–20.
16. Ruth P, Röhrkasten A, Biel M *et al.* Primary structure of the β subunit of the DHP-sensitive calcium channel from skeletal muscle. *Science* 1988; 245: 1115–18.
17. Stühmer W, Conti F, Suzuki H *et al.* Structural parts involved in activation and inactivation of the sodium channel. *Nature* 1989; 339: 597–603.
18. Hartmann HA, Tiedeman AA, Chen S-F *et al.* Effects of III–IV linker mutations on human $Na^+$ channel inactivation gating. *Circ Res* 1994; 75: 114–22.
19. Bennett PB, Valenzuela C, Chen L-Q, Kallen RG. On the molecular structure of the lidocaine receptor of cardiac $Na^+$ channels. Modification of block by alterations in the α-subunit II–IV interdomain. *Circ Res* 1995; 77: 584–92.
20. Kellenberger S, Scheur T, Catterall WA. Movement of the $Na^+$ channel inactivation gate during inactivation. *J Biol Chem* 1996; 271: 30971–9.
21. Isacoff EY, Jan YN, Jan LY. Putative receptor for the cytoplasmic inactivation gate in the *Shaker* $K^+$ channel. *Nature* 1991; 353: 86–90.
22. Antz C, Geyer M, Fakler B *et al.* NMR structure of inactivation gates from mammalian voltage-dependent potassium channels. *Nature* 1997; 385: 272–4.
23. Jan LY, Jan YN. Potassium channels and their evolving gates. *Nature* 1994; 371: 119–22.
24. Spudich JA. How molecular motors work. *Nature* 1994; 515–18.
25. Huxley AF. Crossbridge tilting confirmed. *Nature* 1995; 375: 631–2.
26. Swynghedauw B. Developmental and functional adaptation of contractile proteins in cardiac and skeletal muscles. *Physiol Rev* 1986; 66: 710–71.
27. Schwartz K, de la Bastie K, Mercadier J-J *et al.* The biochemistry and molecular biology of the sarcomere. In: B Swynghedauw (ed.) *Cardiac hypertrophy and failure*. London: John Libby, 1990, 105–35.
28. Schwartz K, Chassagne C, Boehler KR. The molecular biology of heart failure. *J Am Coll Cardiol* 1993; 22 (Suppl A): 30–3A.
29. Nakao K, Minobe W, Roden R *et al.* Myosin heavy chain gene expression in human heart failure. *J Clin Invest* 1997; 100: 2362–70.
30. Tsuchimochi H, Sugi M, Kuro-o M *et al.* Isozymic changes in myosin of human atrial myocardium induced by overload. Immunohistochemical study using monoclonal antibodies. *J Clin Invest* 1984; 74: 662–5.
31. Mercadier JJ, de la Bastie D, Menasche P *et al.* Alpha-myosin heavy chain isoform and atrial size in patients with various types of mitral valve dysfunction: a quantitative study. *J Am Coll Cardiol* 1987; 9: 1024–30.
32. Kretsinger RH. Evolution of the informational role of calcium in eukaryotes. In: RH Wassermann, RA Corradino, E Carafoli *et al.* (eds) *Calcium binding proteins and calcium function*. New York: North Holland, 1977, 63–72.
33. Anderson PAW, Malouf NN, Oakeley AE *et al.* Troponin T isoform expression in humans. A comparison among normal and failing adult heart, fetal heart, and fetal skeletal muscle. *Circ Res* 1991; 69: 1226–33.
34. Jacobus WE, Pores IH, Lucas SK *et al.* Intracellular acidosis and contractility in the normal and ischemic heart as examined by $^{31}P$ NMR. *J Mol Cell Cardiol* 1982; 14 (Suppl 3): 13–20.
35. Hibberd MG, Jewell BR. Calcium- and length-dependent force production in rat ventricular muscle. *J Physiol (London)* 1982; 329: 527–40.
36. Fabiato A, Fabiato F. Dependence of the contractile activation of skinned cardiac cells on the sarcomere length. *Nature* 1975; 256: 54–6.
37. Cheng H, Lederer WJ, Cannell MB. Calcium sparks: elementary events underlying excitation–contraction coupling in heart muscle. *Science* 1993; 262: 740–3.
38. Fabiato A. Calcium-induced release of calcium from the cardiac sarcoplasmic reticulum. *Am J Physiol* 1983; 245: C1–14.
39. Wier WG, Egan TM, López-López JR, Balke CW. Local control of excitation–contraction coupling in rat heart cells. *J Physiol (London)* 1994; 474: 463–71.
40. Tsien RW, Tsien RY. Calcium channels, stores, and oscillations. *Annu Rev Cell Biol* 1990; 6: 715–60.
41. Zhang J-F, Randall AD, Ellinor PT *et al.* Distinctive pharmacology and kinetics of cloned neuronal $Ca^{2+}$ channels and their possible counterparts in mammalian CNS neurons. *Neuropharmacology* 1993; 32: 1075–88.
42. Fleischer S, Inui M. Biochemistry and biophysics of excitation-contraction coupling. *Annu Rev Biophys Biophys Chem* 1989; 18: 333–64.
43. Henzi V, MacDermott AB. Characteristics and function of $Ca^{2+}$- and inositol 1,4,5-trisphosphate-releasable stores of calcium in neurons. *Neuroscience* 1992; 46: 251–73.
44. Berridge M. Inositol trisphosphate and calcium signalling. *Nature* 1993; 361: 315–25.

45. Ehrlich BE, Watras J. Inositol 1,4,5-trisphosphate activates a channel from smooth muscle sarcoplasmic reticulum. *Nature* 1988; 336: 583–6.
46. Somlyo AP, Somlyo AV. Smooth muscle structure and function. In: H Fozzard, E Haber, AM Katz (eds). *The heart and cardiovascular system*. 2nd edition. New York: Raven Press, 1991, 1295–324.
47. Carafoli E. Calcium pump of the plasma membrane. *Physiol Rev* 1991; 71: 129–53.
48. Lytton J, MacLennan DH. Sarcoplasmic reticulum. In: H Fozzard, E Haber, A Katz *et al.* (eds). *The heart and circulation*. 2nd edition. New York: Raven Press, 1991; 1203–22.
49. Katz AM. Role of the contractile proteins and sarcoplasmic reticulum in the response of the heart to catecholamines: an historical review. *Adv Cyclic Nucl Res* 1979; 11: 303–343.
50. Tada M, Katz AM. Phosphorylation of the sarcoplasmic reticulum and sarcolemma. *Annu Rev Physiol* 1982; 44: 401–23.
51. Kim HW, Steenaart NAE, Ferguson DG, Kranias EG. Functional reconstitution of the cardiac sarcoplasmic reticulum $Ca^{2+}$-ATPase with phospholamban in phospholipid vesicles. *J Biol Chem* 1990; 265: 1702–9.
52. Nicoll DA, Longoni S, Philipson KD. Molecular cloning and functional expression of the cardiac sarcolemmal $Na^{+}$-$Ca^{++}$ exchanger. *Science* 1990; 250: 469–71.
53. Levitsky DO, Nicoll DA, Philipson KD. Identification of the high affinity $Ca^{2+}$-binding domain of the cardiac $Na^{+}$-$Ca^{++}$ exchanger. *J Biol Chem* 1994; 269: 22 847–52.
54. Horisberger JD, Lemas V, Krähenbuhl JP, Rossier BC. Structure–function relationship of Na, K-ATPase. *Annu Rev Physiol* 1991; 53: 565–84.
55. Katz AM. Is the failing heart an energy-starved organ? (Editorial). *J Cardiac Failure* 1996; 2: 267–272.
56. Tian R, Ingwall JS. Energetic basis for reduced contractile reserve in isolated rat hearts. *Am J Physiol* 1996; 270 (*Heart Circ Physiol* 39): H1207–16.

# Mechanics, determinants and regulation of cardiac contraction 2

M. R. STARLING

## Introduction

The regulation of cardiac contraction is highly complex; however, an understanding of the mechanics and determinants of this process in the normal environment provides the basis for understanding the complexities during maladaptation that develop with myocardial dysfunction. The overriding principle that guides cardiac performance is the adequate provision of oxygenated blood and nutrients to peripheral tissues to meet their metabolic demands. This is accomplished through an interaction with the systemic arterial and venous systems, which serve as the conduits for providing oxygenated blood to the peripheral tissues and returning deoxygenated blood to the pulmonary system for replenishment. This chapter, explores the physiological framework for normal cardiac contraction and relaxation, and the interaction of the heart with the systemic arterial and venous systems. The concepts described include the mechanics and determinants of cardiac contraction, diastolic relaxation properties, contractility, the contribution of arterial properties to afterload, myocardial energetics, and neural control of contractility. These complex concepts are developed into an integrated whole, to provide the infrastructure for understanding alterations in cardiac contraction, relaxation, and interactions with the vascular system in pathophysiological conditions as perturbations from the normal physiological framework.

## Mechanisms of cardiac contraction

### Muscle models

Several muscle models have been proposed in an attempt to obtain a better understanding of cardiac contraction [1]. Each of these models is composed of at least three elements. First, there is a contractile element, which is assumed to be capable of generating force and shortening with activation; at the same time, it is freely distensible at rest and provides no resistance when the muscle is distended. There are two elastic elements: one or two series elastic elements and a parallel elastic element. Both of these are characterized by their respective length–tension curves. In contrast to the length–tension curves of the series and parallel elastic elements, the contractile elements are described by a force–velocity relationship. During isometric or isovolumic contraction, stimulation of the model theoretically leads to shortening of the contractile element, thereby stretching the series elastic element and developing force in accordance with the length–tension relationship of this element. The rate at which force develops is, therefore, determined by the contractile element velocity and the stiffness of the series elastic element. In the classic model of Hill, the properties of the parallel elastic element are defined by the passive length–tension curve. In other muscle models proposed by Voight and Maxwell, both the parallel elastic and series elastic elements contribute to the passive length–tension curve. Recent studies have suggested that a more complex muscle model may be needed to characterize the true complexities of cardiac muscle [2].

### Isometric contraction

Examination of the length–tension relationship in an isolated papillary muscle during isometric contraction provides insight into the relationship between the developed force and total force generated at different muscle lengths as a reflection of the series elastic element [3]. Previous studies have examined this relationship during two contractile conditions, one produced by altering calcium concentrations and the other by changing noradrenaline concentrations [3]. Alteration in the concentration of either produced no effect on the passive length–tension relationship, despite changing contractile conditions. An increase in calcium concentration produced an increase in both developed and total tension at each muscle length, and the time to peak tension development was shortened, reflecting an increase in tension development in a shorter time-frame, consistent with enhanced contractile element velocity. Similarly, noradrenaline enhanced both peak and developed force, and the time to peak tension was achieved even more rapidly than during an increase in calcium concentration. Thus, both calcium and noradrenaline enhanced contractility, which was reflected by an increase in developed force or total force of the series elastic element and an increase in the velocity of the contractile element.

## Force–velocity–length relationship

A more direct assessment of contractile element velocity can be obtained from the force–velocity or force–shortening relationship during alterations in preload or contractility with calcium and noradrenaline [3]. With an increase in preload, there is an increase in isometric tension development. This is further illustrated for isotonic shortening by examining the effects of an increase in preload on shortening and shortening velocity at a fixed afterload. As preload is increased, there is an increase in both the extent and velocity of shortening at any fixed afterload. Extrapolation of the force–velocity relationship back to maximum velocity, reveals that at all levels of preload there is no effect on the maximum velocity of the contractile element. Furthermore, during any preload for which shortening is allowed to occur, the performance of work and power is increased as a function of preload. Work in this context is defined as the product of load and the change in muscle length, and power as the product of load and the rate of change of length. Thus, within this construct, at zero load both work and power are zero and, with an isometric contraction, both work and power similarly are zero. Therefore, maximum work and power occur at some value of preload at which shortening is allowed to occur at an intermediate load.

In comparison to the effects of initial muscle length on the force–velocity and force–shortening relationships, the effects of calcium and noradrenaline on these relationships in the isolated papillary muscle differ [3, 4]. With an increase in either calcium or noradrenaline concentration, there is an increase in the velocity of shortening and the extent of shortening at each afterload. However, in contrast to the effects of changes in the initial muscle length or preload alone, the effect of calcium or noradrenaline is to increase contractile element velocity, which is evident by extrapolation of the force–velocity relationship to zero load and observing a marked increase in the maximum velocity. Thus, it is important to recognize that, consistent with enhancement in contractile element velocity, there is an increase in shortening and shortening velocity at each afterload, which is then associated with increases in work and power.

The interdependence of force, velocity and length in an isolated papillary muscle can be used to illustrate basal, enhanced, and depressed contractile conditions in a three-dimensional representation of the force–velocity–length relationship [3, 5]. This relationship is shown in Figure 2.1 for the basal contractile condition: the length of the isolated papillary muscle is shown on the *x*-axis, velocity is shown on the *y*-axis, and force is shown on the *z*-axis. As load increases, there is an offset to correct for reduced extension of the series elastic element. A hypothetical afterloaded isotonic contraction is demonstrated by the solid line beginning at point A, where the length–tension relationship of the passive elastic element has been maximized at the initial muscle length. When developed force equals load at point $B_{CE}$, external shortening can proceed with a velocity that is inversely related to the load from $B_{CE}$ to $C_{CE}$. If this is accomplished over several loading conditions, the force–velocity relationship can be extrapolated to a zero load to obtain $V_{max}$. Thus, a projection on to the *y*–*z* plane produces the force–velocity relationship, and a projection on to the *x*–*z* plane produces the length–tension relationship. Therefore, if there is an increase in contractile element performance, there would be an increase in the projections on to the force–velocity and length–tension planes, such that the force–velocity relationship is displaced upwards on the *y*–*z* plane to a larger extrapolated $V_{max}$ and the extrapolation of the length–tension relationship on to the *x*–*z* plane is displaced to the right. Consequently, the hypothetical isotonic contraction would reach total load at $B_{CE}$ and proceed at a greater velocity to a shorter muscle length. In contrast, a depressed muscle would do the opposite, such that, at a comparable muscle length, a hypothetical isotonic contraction would proceed at a much slower velocity and maintain a much longer muscle length. Consequently, the force–velocity projection on to the *y*–*z* plane would be displaced downwards to a reduced $V_{max}$, while extrapolation on to the *x*–*z* plane would be displaced to the left. Therefore, both muscle length and contractili-

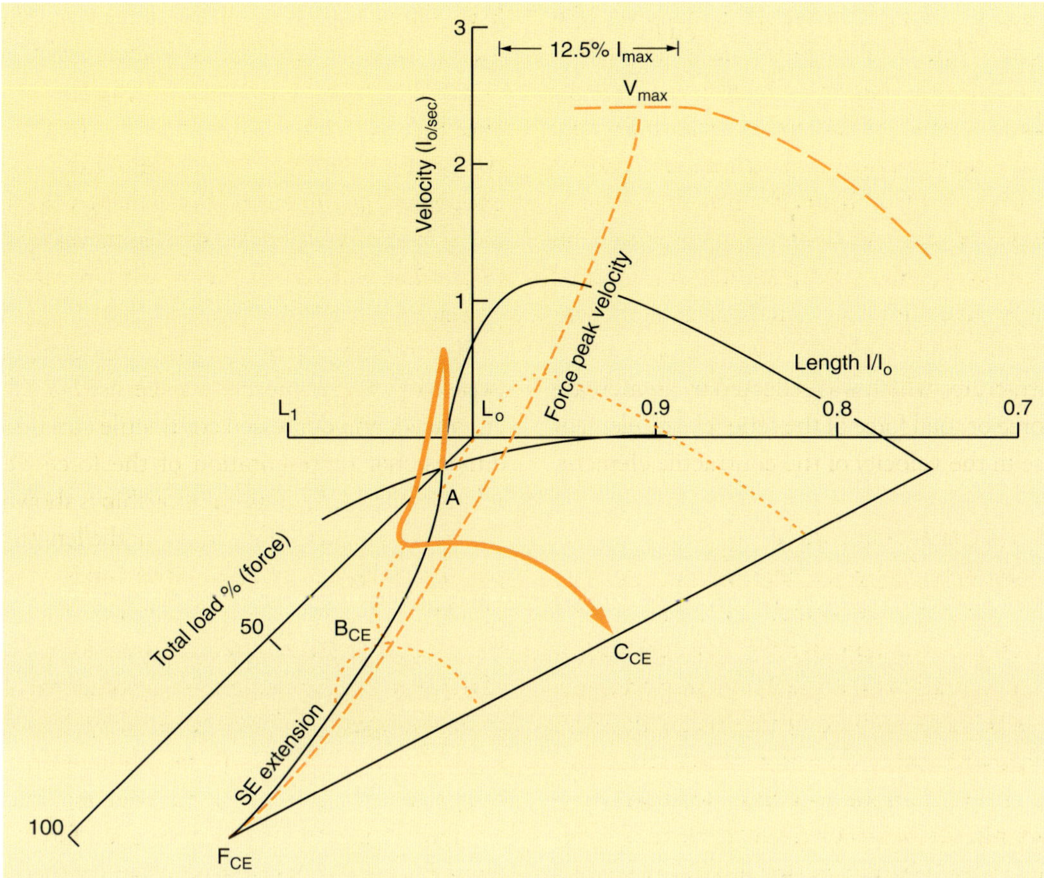


**Figure 2.1** *Three-dimensional representation of the force–velocity–length relationships from an isolated papillary muscle. x-Axis = muscle length or preload; y-axis = velocity of shortening; z-axis = total load or force. The solid line represents a hypothetical isotonic contraction under basal contractile conditions beginning at point A, developing internal load by shortening of the contractile element and extension of the series elastic element to $B_{CE}$, then shortening to point $C_{CE}$. (From ref. 5 with permission.)*

ty contribute to muscle performance [3–7]. Muscle length may do so by allowing calcium to be more actively bound, by increasing triggered calcium release from the sarcoplasmic reticulum, or by enhancing the sensitivity of the myofilaments to calcium [7]. Accordingly, whereas changes in contractility are related to the quantity and rate of calcium availability, changes in muscle length are related to the sensitivity of the cross-bridge units to calcium.

## Structural basis of contraction

The capacity of the intact heart to vary the force of contraction on a beat-to-beat basis as a function of preload as reflected in sarcomere length constitutes one of the major principles of cardiac performance, and is referred to as the Frank–Starling phenomenon [8–12]. This fundamental property of the heart is based on the myocardial length–tension relationship, in which the development of force with each contraction or the extent of shortening is dependent on the initial muscle length which, in turn, is dependent on the ultrastructural relationship between the myofilaments of the sarcomeres. The relationship between myofilament disposition and tension development in skeletal muscle is illustrated in Figure 2.2 [8]. The thin filaments are approximately 1.0 μm and the thick filaments are approximately 1.6 μm in length. The relationship between the tensions that develop at specific sarcomere lengths represents the extent to which there is optimal overlap of the myofilaments. It is apparent that no overlap exists at 3.56 μm and, therefore, there is no tension development. Optimal overlap of the myofilaments for the development for tension occurs at sarcomere lengths between 2.0 and 2.25 μm. As sarcomere lengths fall below 2.0 μm, the

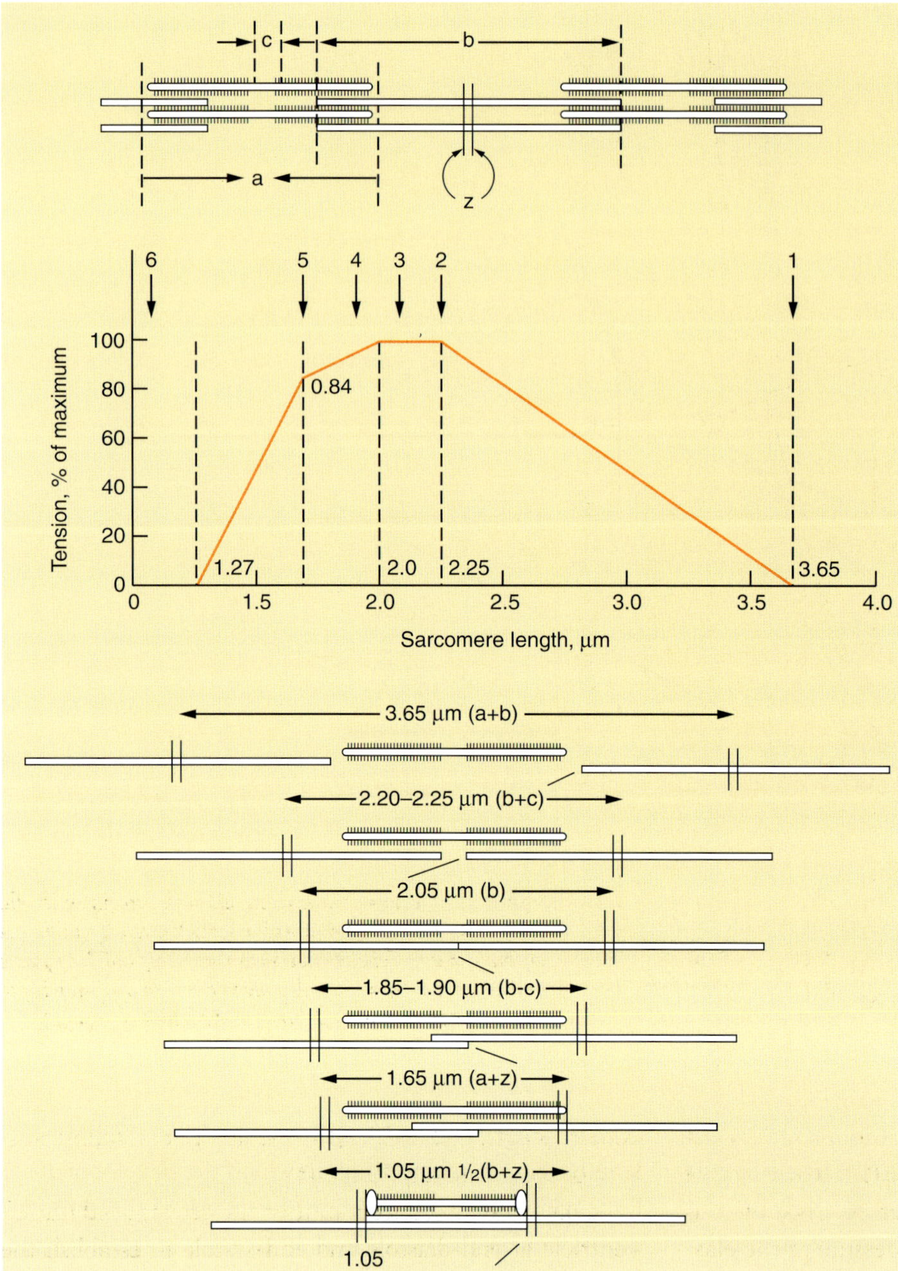


**Figure 2.2** *The capacity of the left ventricle to vary the force of contraction on a beat-to-beat basis is a fundamental property of cardiac muscle known as the Frank–Starling phenomenon. This is a reflection of sarcomere length and interaction of the thin filaments (b) and thick filaments (a). Note that optimal tension development occurs at a sarcomere length ranging from 2.0 to 2.25 μm. (From ref. 8 with permission.)*

thick and thin filaments begin to overlap. At approximately 1.25 μm, no tension has developed because the thick and thin filaments are completely overlapped and compressed below the length of the thick filaments. Thus, as the thick and thin filaments begin to overlap below 2.0 μm, there is interference with cross-bridge cycling and, therefore, with the ability of the thick and thin filaments to bind calcium. This reduces the sensitivity of the thick and thin filaments to calcium and may generate significant internal loads that impede shortening of the sarcomere and, therefore, impede the development of tension.

This relationship between mid-wall sarcomere length and developed pressure from the left ventricle in both the dog and cat, and its effect on tension development, are illustrated in Figure 2.3 [10]. When the left ventricle is empty, the sarcomere length is approximately 1.8–1.9 μm. As the left ventricle fills and distends to a more optimal size, sarcomere lengths increase. As the distending pressure on the left ventricle increases to approximately 12 mmHg, the sarcomere length approaches 2.2 μm. This length of 2.0–2.2 μm is the optimal sarcomere length for the generation of force. In contrast to skeletal muscle, the stiffness

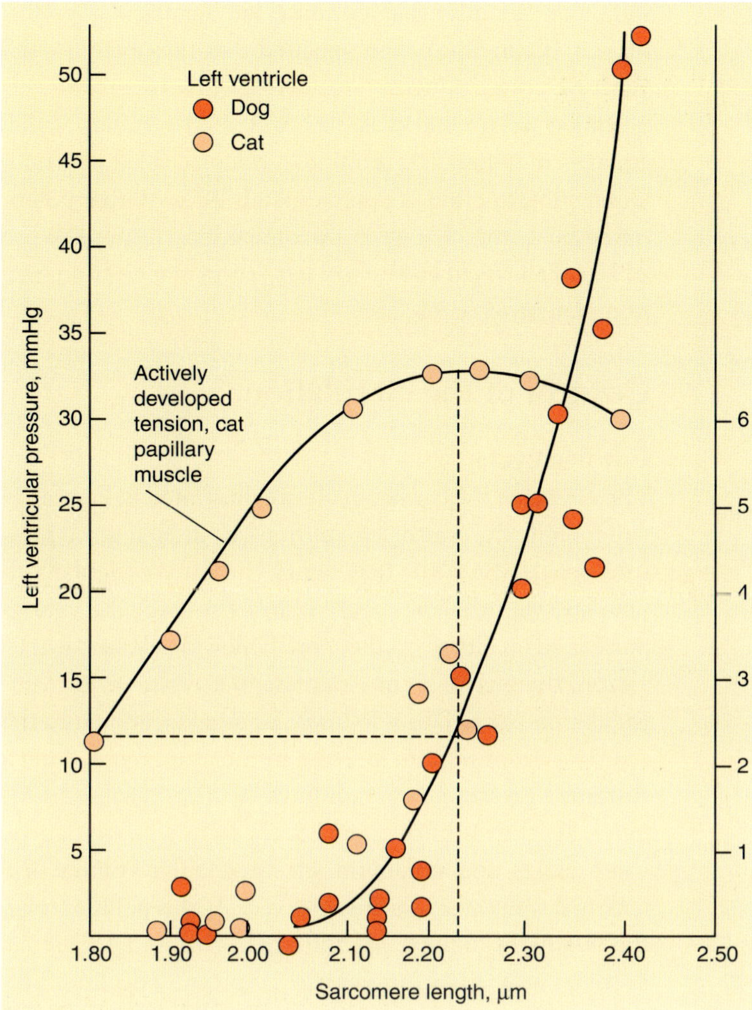


**Figure 2.3** *Relationship between mid-wall sarcomere length, filling pressure, and left ventricular developed tension in the cat papillary muscle. The optimal sarcomere length of 2.25 µm is established at a left ventricular filling pressure of 12 mmHg to develop maximal tension. (From ref. 10 with permission.)*

of the passive elastic element, with or without a series elastic element in combination, impedes further distension of the left ventricle. This limit in increased distension is reflected in a sharp increase in filling pressure as the elastic elements attempt to resist overdistension of the sarcomeres and prevent disengagement of the myofilaments. While the passive elastic element may predominate in resisting overdistension at normal distending pressures of the left ventricle, the series elastic element may become an important contributor to this resistance at higher distending pressures. The relationship between development of the tension in this papillary muscle over the same range of sarcomere lengths is illustrated by superimposition of the active length–tension relationship. This confirms the information that the optimal sarcomere length for maximal tension development is approximately 2.2 µm. Thus, the apex of the active length–tension relationship occurs at a sarcomere length of 2.2–2.25 µm and an optimal filling pressure of approximately 12 mmHg.

To illustrate this concept further, two groups fixed the left ventricle at end-diastole and end-systole to establish the relationship between sarcomere length and ventricular performance in an intact ejecting left ventricle [11, 12]. They confirmed that in the ejecting left ventricle at end-diastole the disposition of the thick and thin filaments averaged approximately 2.1 µm and at end-systole they averaged approximately 1.8 µm. Thus, the left ventricle at end-diastole optimized mid-wall sarcomere length to maximize tension development and shortening. On a potentiated beat, the end-diastolic sarcomere length increased to 2.25 µm and the end-systolic sarcomere length decreased to 1.6 µm. This defined a new active length–tension curve that had shifted to the left and had a steeper slope. Thus, the intact left ventricle operates under basal contractile conditions at

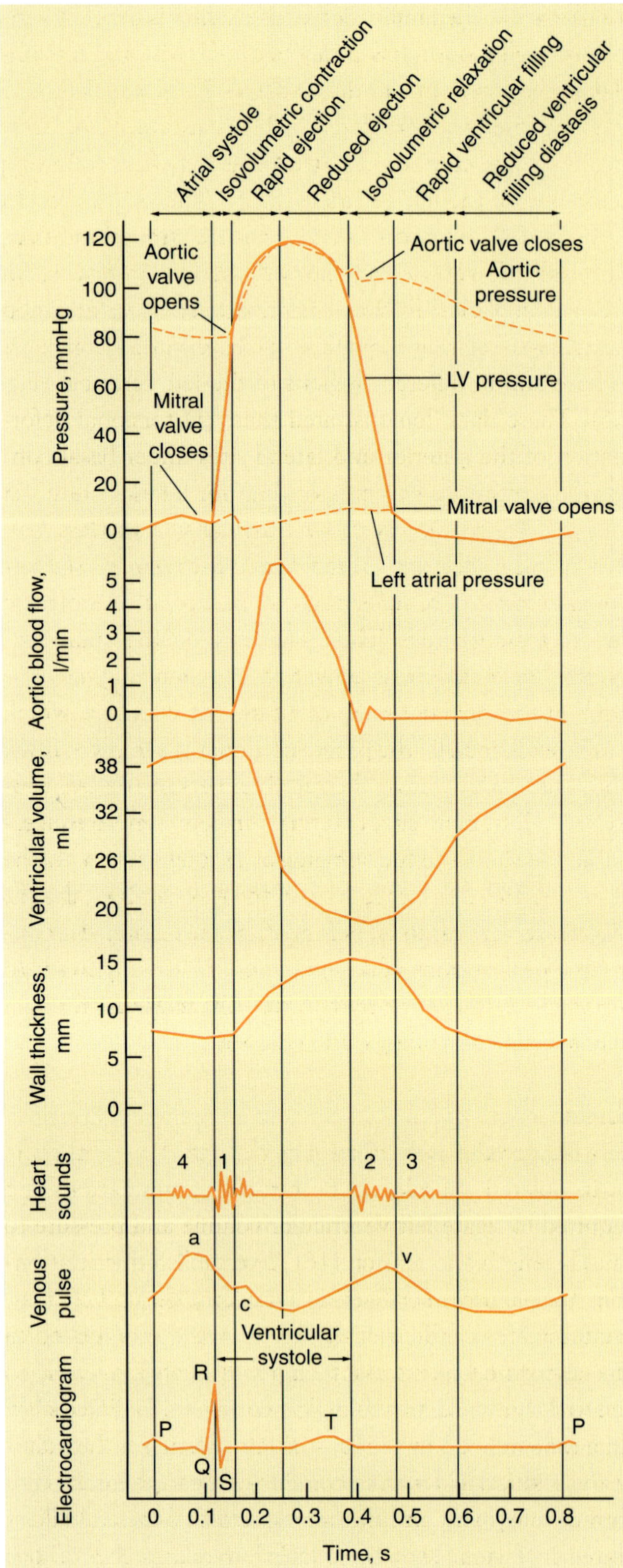


**Figure 2.4** *Events of the cardiac cycle. (From ref. 13 with permission.)*

sarcomere lengths that optimize left ventricular performance. It can also be extrapolated that the operating left ventricle has a change in sarcomere length of approximately 13% between end-diastole and end-systole, which equates, in volumetric terms, to a calculated left ventricular ejection fraction of approximately 50%. With a potentiated beat, the change in sarcomere length increased to 21%, which would equate to a left ventricular ejection fraction of approximately 75%.

## Control of the circulation

### Cardiac cycle

The events of the cardiac cycle are illustrated in Figure 2.4 and include the aortic, left ventricular, and left atrial pressure signals, the aortic flow signal, the left ventricular volume and wall thickness curves, heart sounds, the venous pulse, and an electrocardiogram. Following electrical activation, there is an abrupt increase in isovolumic left ventricular pressure. This is followed by rapid ejection into the arterial system with an increase in the arterial pulse and a sustained pressure elevation until ejection reaches maximum. As flow into the aorta declines to zero, the aortic valve closes and minimum left ventricular volume and maximal wall thickness are achieved. At this point in time, the events of diastole are initiated. The initial diastolic event is early, active left ventricular pressure decline. This is followed once the left ventricular pressure crosses the left atrial pressure by rapid left ventricular filling and left atrial emptying, manifested by a rapid increase in left ventricular volume and thinning of the left ventricular wall. Diastasis is then achieved and passive distension of the left ventricle occurs. Diastole is completed with atrial contraction to distend the sarcomeres of the left ventricle to the desired length to achieve optimal tension development.

### Torsion development

In the intact left ventricle, the orientation of myocardial fibres across the left ventricle varies [14], changing progressively from the epicardium to the endocardium. Only at the mid-wall are the myocardial fibres orientated perpendicular to the long axis. This implies that contraction may not be uniform or directionally similar in myocytes across the full thickness of the left ventricular wall. Moreover, the stresses that the myocytes must overcome before shortening is initiated may also vary across the left ven-

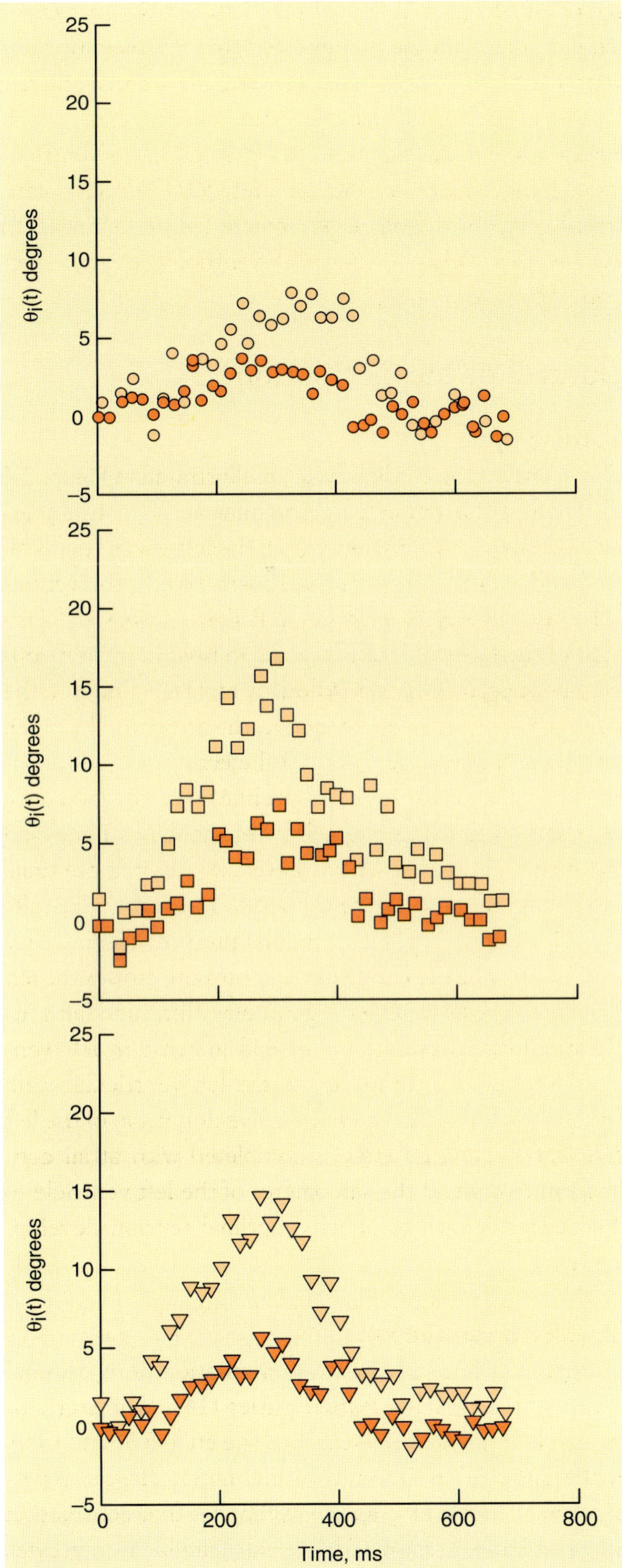


**Figure 2.5** *Torsional deformation angle (θ) for the inferior* (top), *anterior* (middle), *and lateral* (bottom) *segments during basal contractile conditions and with increases in heart rate. (From ref. 15 with permission.)*

tricular wall. The implication of these data is that left ventricular wall motion has components of twist and torsional deformation from end-diastole to end-systole. This issue was examined in more detail by Hansen *et al.* [15]. They examined the counter-clockwise twisting effect following activation of the left ventricle due to fibre orientation in patients following orthotopic cardiac transplantation, who had left ventricular mid-wall markers implanted in orthogonal planes. Torsional deformation angles, measured relative to a referenced point at the base, varied from apex to base and in different regions of the left ventricle (Fig. 2.5). These data demonstrated that: (1) torsional deformation of the anterior and lateral sites under basal contractile conditions was greater than for inferior sites; (2) torsional deformation at mid-ventricular sites was less than that at apical sites; and (3) rapid atrial pacing increased torsional deformation, reflecting the mild positive inotropic effect of tachycardia. Thus, not only do the short axis length shorten following activation, but there is also a non-uniform torsional deformation of the left ventricle, which can be explained by the progressive changes in myocardial fibre orientation across the full thickness of the left ventricle [14]. In more simple terms, this represents a squeezing action similar to the wringing of a sponge. It can also be related to the contractile state of the myocardium, that is, the greater the tortional deformation the greater the contractile performance of the myocytes. This is important to recognize because it may have implications for the dynamics of early filling during diastole.

## Stress

To compare the performance of the intact left ventricle with isolated muscle, more complex formulations are required to relate left ventricular volume and pressure to muscle length and tension [16]. To establish this relationship, the concept of wall stress or the force per unit of cross-sectional area of the wall should be used and is related to the intraventricular pressure and radius, and inversely to the wall thickness. In its simplest construct, La Place's law for a thin-walled sphere is $T = PR/2h$, where $r$ is the radius at the endocardial surface of a thin-walled sphere, $P$ is the intracavitary pressure, and $h$ is the wall thickness. As illustrated in Figure 2.6a, La Place's law relates the various stresses to the internal pressure, $P$, by the equation: $\sigma_1/R_1 + \sigma_2/R_2 = P/h$, where $\sigma_1$ and $\sigma_2$ represent stresses acting on the surface perpendicular to each other in this thin-walled sphere, $R_1$ and $R_2$ represent the radii of curvature of the surface, which would be similar in a thin-walled sphere, and $h$ represents the wall thickness, which would be negligible [17].

Although this has been widely applied in general conceptual terms to the heart, the left ventricle is not a thin-walled sphere; rather, it is more appropriately related to an ellipsoid of revolution, which has a thick wall and where the stresses are not equal [19, 20]. Therefore, two different stress concepts have been developed: meridional stress, which acts perpendicular to the short axis, and circumferential stress, which acts perpendicular to the long axis in line with the direction of the mid-wall circumferential fibres [16]. These two stresses can be expressed by the equations $Pb/2h(1-h/2b)^2$ and $Pb/h(1-h/2b-b^2/2a^2)$, respectively. In the calculation of meridional and circumferential stress ($\sigma_m$ and $\sigma_c$), $a$ and $b$ represent the mid-wall semi-major and semi-minor axes of a thick-walled ellipsoid of revolution. Thus, not only do the calculations of meridional and circumferential stress vary, but they may vary in a non-linear fashion, which changes with left ventricular geometry.

Although left ventricular pressure during ejection may be closely related to afterload, geometric factors and wall thickness must also be considered throughout the ejecting period in the calculation of wall forces in the intact left ventricle. To illustrate this phenomenon, on left ventricular pressure–volume and stress–volume loops generated over a wide range of loading conditions in an intact dog heart are presented in Fig. 2.6b [18]. It is apparent that the left ventricular pressure–volume loops and the stress–volume loops have different configurations when left ventricular wall thickness and geometry are included in the calculation (Fig. 2.7). Nevertheless, at end-systole, the points from each pressure–volume series or stress–volume series are linear over the operating range of pressures, stresses, and volumes. Similarly, the diastolic pressure–volume and stress–volume relations are both curvilinear over the same range of loading conditions and also appear to be little affected by loading conditions. Consequently, both left ventricular pressure–volume and stress–volume relationships provide a basis for assessing contractility in the intact left ventricle at end-systole and diastolic function during late, passive diastolic relaxation.

## The intact circulation

The determination of cardiac output and the various influences upon it, both positive and negative, are complex [17, 22–24]. Optimization of preload, maintenance of contractility, and prevention of afterload excess determine a normal stroke volume which, in combination with heart rate, produce an adequate cardiac output to meet the needs for oxygen and nutrient flow to the tissues. Cardiac output in combination with arterial resistance determines arterial pressure. There are several feedback mechanisms which affect an inherent modulation in this system. Arterial pressure can affect carotid and aortic arch baroreceptors. This input to the medullary vasomotor and cardiac centres can be influenced by higher nervous system centres and yield

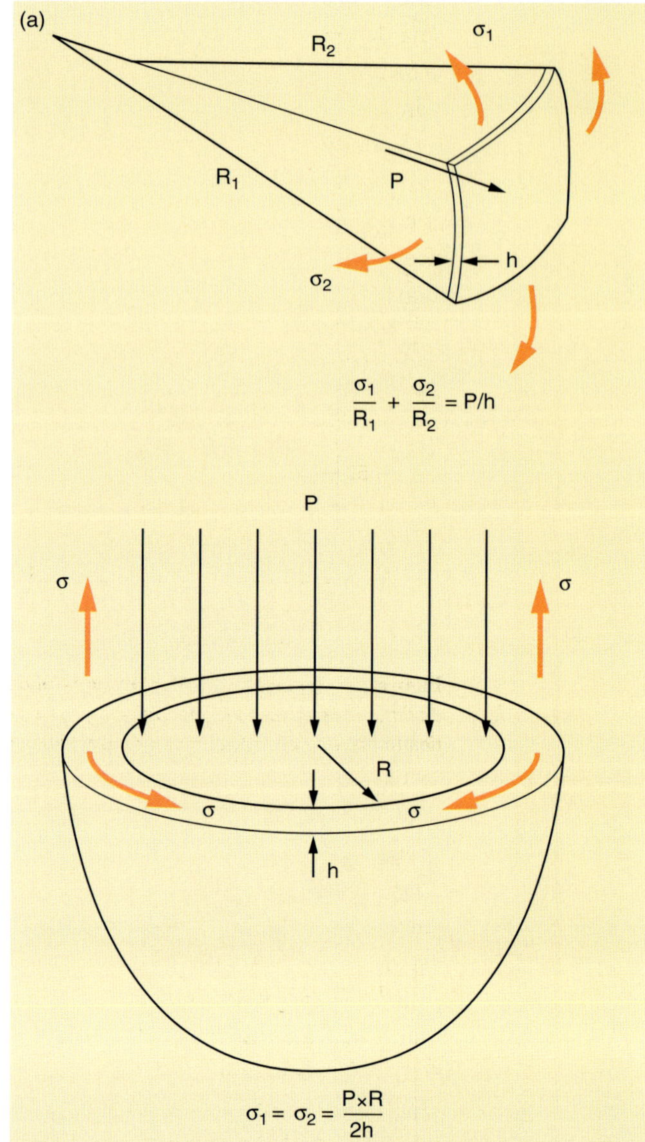


**Figure 2.6** *(a) La Place's law for a thin-walled surface relating stress to internal pressure and wall thickness. (From ref. 17 with permission.). (b) Shown opposite.*

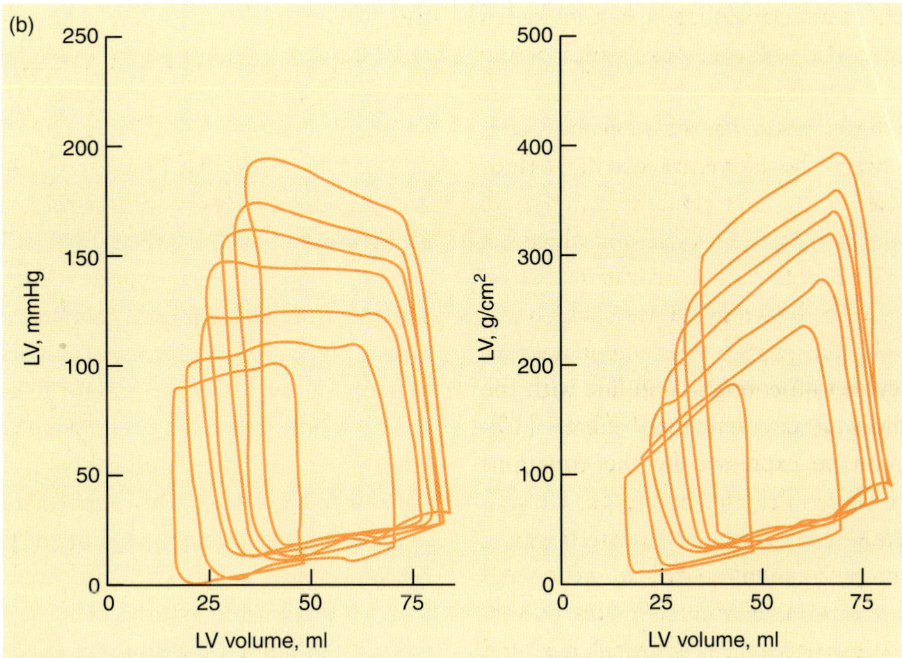


**Figure 2.6** *(b) Left ventricular pressure–volume and stress–volume loops over a range of loading conditions, demonstrating the implications of considering left ventricular wall thickness and geometry in addition to pressure on left ventricular shortening. (From ref. 18 with permission.)*

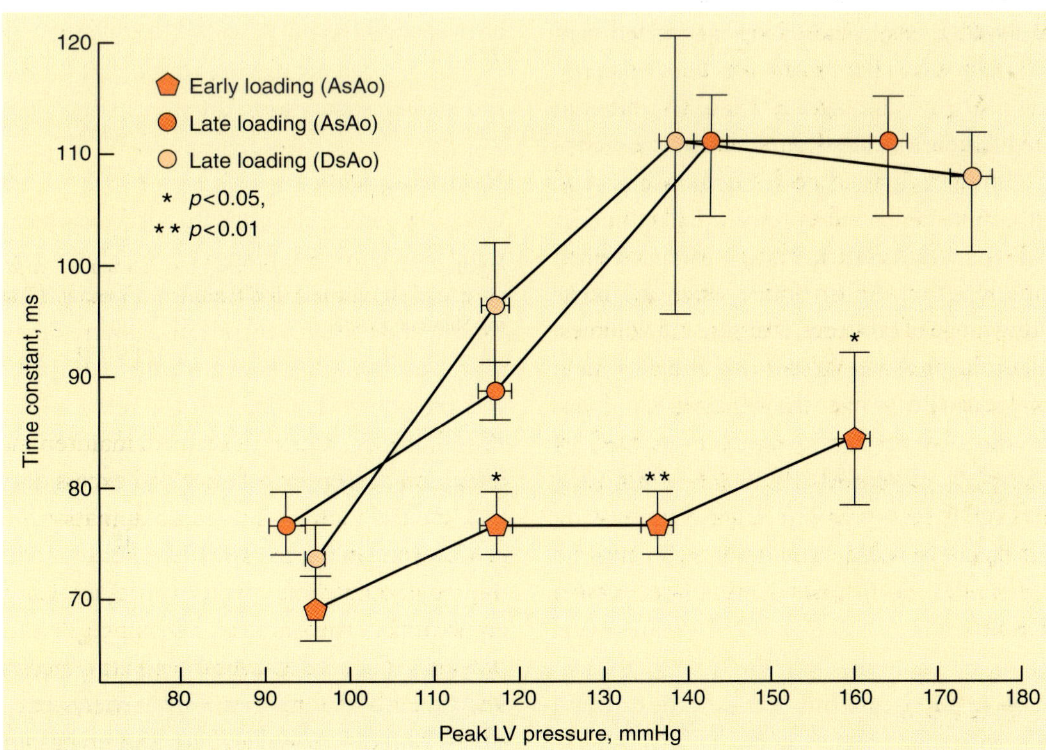


**Figure 2.7** *Effects of early pressure alterations on early, active left ventricular relaxation, contrasted with those of late systolic pressure loading of the left ventricle. (From ref. 21 with permission.)*

variable accommodations in heart rate, peripheral vascular resistance and thus afterload, venous return and thus preload, and contractility. Thus, these complex interactions are intrinsically fine-tuned to regulate beat-to-beat changes in the cardiovascular system to adapt to varying energy demands.

## Diastole

Diastole is composed of four phases: early, active isovolumic relaxation; early, rapid left ventricular filling; late, passive relaxation; and the atrial contribution to sarcomere distention. Throughout these four phases, various factors may influence one or more of them: the rate of left ventricular relaxation, the extent of left ventricular relaxation, early restoring forces, the geometry and elastic properties of the left ventricle, the viscoelastic properties of the left ventricle, ventricular interaction, pericardial restraint, venous return, and, finally, coronary vascular engorgement [25, 26].

### Early, active isovolumic relaxation

Isovolumic relaxation (tau, $\tau$) has been defined as the rate of pressure decline from $(-)dP/dt_{min}$ to 5 mmHg above left ventricular end-diastolic pressure of the subsequent beat. This time is estimated to avoid the effects of rapid left ventricular filling at the point of left ventricular–left atrial pressure cross-over in this calculation. Several different constructs have been used to assess early, active isovolumic relaxation [27–29]. The method described by Weiss *et al.* [27] assumes that left ventricular pressure falls monoexponentially to a zero pressure ($P_0$). Thus, it can be defined using the equation: $\ln P = -1/T(t) + \ln P_0$, where $\ln P$ is the natural logarithm of pressure and $T$ is time. Additional investigators have, however, suggested that the decline in left ventricular pressure may not always proceed to a zero pressure asymptote. An alternative method proposed by Raff and Glantz [28], described the linear relationship between $dP/dt$ and $P$ incorporating a variable pressure asymptote ($P_b$). This relationship was established using the equation: $dP/dt = -1/T(P-P_b)$, where $dP/dt$ is the rate of decline in left ventricular pressure. Tau ($\tau$) is represented by the negative reciprocal of the slope ($-1/T$) in both constructs. Although, in the normal human heart, the rate and duration of left ventricular pressure decline is little affected by modest alterations in left ventricular pressure, irrespective of the approach used [30], several studies suggest that isovolumic relaxation may be pressure dependent. In animals, where the alteration in loading sequences can be controlled [21], it does not appear that the absolute left ventricular systolic pressure is important in determining the rate of left ventricular pressure decline during this early, active phase of relaxation; it is the loading sequence that is important in affecting the rate of left ventricular pressure decline (Fig. 2.7). Early systolic loading, similar to steady-state pressure alterations in humans, produces little if any change in the time-constant of isovolumic left ventricular pressure decay. However, when the aorta is clamped late during systole, there is a progressive and pronounced prolongation in the time-constant that is directly related to the increase in late systolic left ventricular pressure. These data suggest that the afterload-dependent slowing of isovolumic relaxation rates in the dog heart cannot be attributed solely to an increase in systolic pressure, but may be related more to an altered loading sequence associated with the increase in afterload. It is probably reasonable to assume that modest, steady-state alterations in arterial pressure have little effect on the rate of isovolumic left ventricular pressure decline; however, because the loading sequence of the left ventricle may be altered by changes in the peripheral vasculature through wave reflections in the system, indices of early, active isovolumic relaxation may need to be normalized to the pressure that occurs at end-systole, i.e. $(-)dP/dt_{min}$, in an attempt to account for the variations in the loading sequence in different pathological conditions.

### Restoring forces

Once left ventricular pressure falls below left atrial pressure, rapid left ventricular filling occurs. This is dependent on the rate of left ventricular relaxation, the impact of venous return, and the left ventricular–left atrial pressure gradient, as well as restoring forces intrinsic to the myocardium. This was previously described by the relationship between the myofilaments during contraction, where sarcomere lengths may decrease below approximately 1.8 μm [8, 9, 23, 24]. At these short sarcomere lengths, the potential for compression of the thick filaments exists. This compression and the interaction of the thin filaments may generate forces within the sarcomere that accelerate restoration of normal sarcomere lengths. In addition, as a result of twist and torsional deformation within the myocardium, release of this stored potential leads to an untwisting or restoration of the left ventricle to its normal shape, thereby accelerating filling during this early phase of diastole [15]. Thus, restoring forces may be very important in the normal left ventricle, both at rest and, particularly, during states of enhanced contractility, where acceleration of left ventricular filling may be important of maintaining optimal filling.

### Late, passive left ventricular relaxation

Materials that conform to Hooke's law are characterized by a linear relationship between pressure and volume or stress and strain [25–27, 31–33]. However, for biological materials such as the left ventricle and myocardium, these relationships usually assume an exponential form. Thus, the relationship between left ventricular pressure and volume during the passive filling phase of diastole is non-linear and determined by the length–tension relationship of the passive elastic element. Similarly, the relationship between left ventricular stress and strain during the late, passive filling phase of diastole is non-linear. It is important to differentiate the effects of disease processes on left ventricular chamber stiffness and myocardial stiffness, since several factors can affect left ventricular chamber stiffness independently of alterations in myocardial stiffness. Left ventricular chamber stiffness can be assessed using the relationship $dP/dV$ versus $P$, which is linear and can be used to compare late, passive diastolic properties of the left ventricle during this passive filling phase between normal hearts and hearts of patients with pathological disease states. Unfortunately, left ventricular chamber stiffness can be difficult to compare between hearts of widely varying sizes and, therefore, normalization for volume should be used to estimate the left ventricular volume elastance, which is provided by the relationship $dP/dV/V$ versus $P$. This can be used to compare left ventricular chamber stiffness at a common diastolic pressure without the confounding influences of volume. Similarly, plotting the differential of stress and strain versus stress provides a linear function relating the incremental modulus, $E$, to stress. Thus, myocardial stiffness is given by the relationship $d\sigma/d\varepsilon$ versus $\sigma$. The use of left ventricular chamber stiffness and myocardial stiffness has the potential to demonstrate the impact of pathological processes on diastolic performance of the left ventricle.

### Viscoelastic properties

Although simple muscle models would predict that late, passive left ventricular diastolic filling is determined by the passive elastic element, the contribution of dynamic viscoelastic properties of the left ventricular wall to this phase of filling may be substantial [2, 34, 35]. Using a variable rate stretch during dynamic diastolic filling, Rankin *et al.* [2] demonstrated that the simple elastic model differed significantly from the data, whereas a more complex, integrated viscoelastic model incorporating a parallel viscous element in the equation fitted the observed data more closely. Thus, the contribution of dynamic viscoelastic properties to late, passive diastolic filling may be of substantial importance and require a modification of the muscle models by incorporating a parallel viscous element, at a minimum, to characterize fully the passive filling characteristics of the ventricle. Using a viscous element makes it is easier to account for the resistance to distension determined by the rate of an applied stretch. Specifically, as it relates to the left ventricle, viscous properties within the left ventricular myocardium would be expected to result in a greater wall force and rise in chamber pressure when a volume increment is transferred rapidly than when the same incremental volume is transferred slowly. In this conceptualization, viscous elements provide drag forces to resist distention in proportion to the rate of the applied stress or force.

This more complex formulation of late, passive diastolic properties of the left ventricle provides an explanation for two important concepts: stress relaxation and creep. Stress relaxation is the decrease in stress that occurs over time after a sudden applied increase in stretch. LeWinter *et al.* [36] explored this concept in an animal model where the effects on stress of a sudden increase in muscle length produced by saline and phenylephrine infusions were examined. They observed that for any given left ventricular end-diastolic segment length, there was a greater increase in left ventricular end-diastolic pressure, resulting in a greater increase in end-diastolic stress for any given strain during the rapid saline- and phenylephrine-induced stretch compared with recovery (Fig. 2.8, top). During the recovery period at matched left ventricular end-diastolic segment lengths, the left ventricular end-diastolic pressure and stress were lower. When a sudden increase in end-diastolic segment length is maintained, the viscous element was permitted to rearrange internally and decrease pressure and stress for any given segment length or strain. The phenomenon of stress relaxation is consistent with the behaviour of the left ventricle predicted by a more complex viscoelastic model.

Creep describes the increase in deformation of the left ventricle that may occur following a protracted application of a constant stress. During a rapid increase in left ventricular end-diastolic pressure, there is resistance to deformation of the left ventricle that is presumably related to the stress–strain relationships of the passive elastic element (Fig. 2.8, bottom). This leads to a steep relationship between left ventricular end-diastolic pressure and segment length. When the increase in left ventricular end-diastolic pressure is slower, there is a greater increase in left ventricular segment length for any given left ventricular end-diastolic pressure. With a slower change in pressure, the greater increase in left ventricular segment length is, therefore, a reflection of the slow extension of the vis-

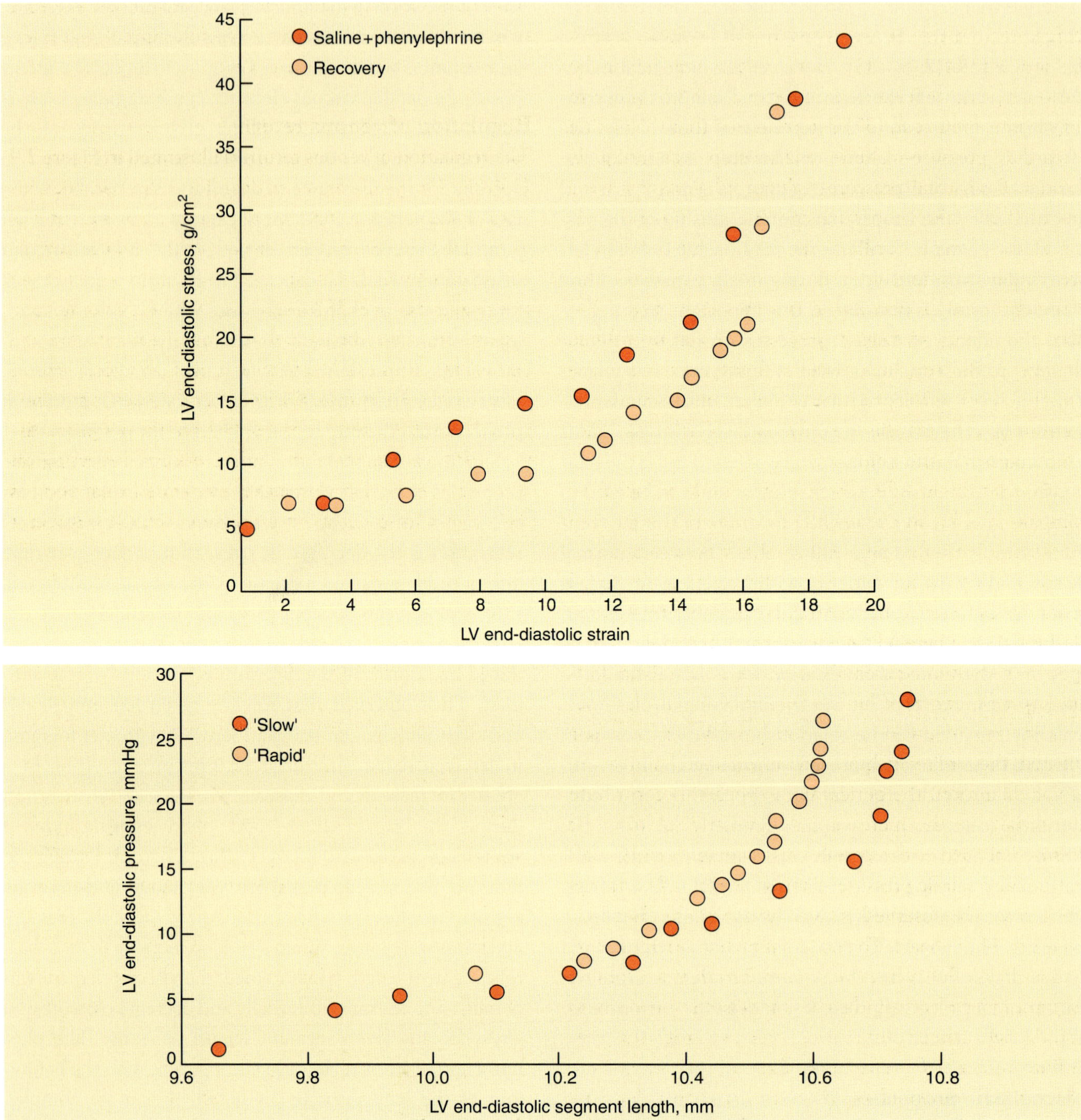


**Figure 2.8** (Top) *Relationship between left ventricular end-diastolic stress and strain during a rapid infusion of saline and phenylephrine demonstrating the concept of stress relaxation.* (Bottom) *Impact of a rapid increase in segment length or increase in left ventricular end-diastolic pressure on segment length illustrating the concept of creep. (From ref. 36 with permission.)*

coelastic element in the muscle model. Thus, the concepts of both stress relaxation and creep that were demonstrated by LeWinter *et al.* [36] in an animal preparation provide strong support for the requirement of a viscoelastic element in addition to a parallel elastic element within the muscle models to explain these unique late, passive diastolic filling characteristics of the left ventricle.

## Pericardial restraint and ventricular interaction

The pericardium plays a substantial role in establishing the relationship between left ventricular end-diastolic pressure and volume. Hess *et al.* [37] demonstrated that the canine pericardial pressure–volume relationship was uniquely bimodal. Pericardial pressure–volume relationships were generated as right ventricular volume was progressively increased: at low pericardial volumes, the pericardial pressure–volume relationship was quite flat, but it became extremely steep at pericardial volumes exceeding 225–250 ml. This suggests that the pericardial pressure–volume relationship has very little effect on late, passive left ventricular diastolic filling properties at low or normal pressures and volumes, but may have a substantial restraining effect at high pressures and volumes.

This restraining effect was amply demonstrated by Shirato *et al.* [38] in chronically instrumented dogs with and without an intact pericardium analysed during acute volume loading. Acute volume loading superiorly displaced the late, passive left ventricular diastolic pressure–volume relationship in a parallel fashion, so that there was a much higher left ventricular diastolic pressure at any given diastolic segment length. When in the same animal, the pericardium was removed and acute volume loading was repeated, these relationships were not affected. With acute cardiac dilatation, the pericardium appears to contribute substantially to the increase in left ventricular diastolic pressure because of the parallel displacements in the left ventricular diastolic pressure–segment length relationship. This can also be observed with dilatation of the chambers of one side of the heart. The effects of increasing right heart volume on the left ventricular diastolic pressure–volume relationship have been studied in postmortem canine hearts [37]. As right heart volumes were increased with the pericardium intact, left ventricular diastolic pressures were incrementally increased for any given left ventricular diastolic volume. This led to an upward displacement of the late, passive left ventricular diastolic pressure–volume relationship. Consequently, at a comparable left ventricular diastolic volume, the left ventricular pressure was disproportionately elevated and would, therefore, have provided an inadequate determination of left ventricular filling pressure. In contrast, when transmural left ventricular pressure, which takes into account both the left ventricular pressure and pericardial pressure, was used there were no differences in transmural pressure across the full range of right and left ventricular volumes, suggesting that transmural pressure may represent a better measure of left ventricular distending pressures in some disease states.

## Regulation of venous return

The regulation of venous return is illustrated in Figure 2.9 [39, 40]. The *y*-axis represents cardiac output and venous return, and the *x*-axis right atrial pressure. It is evident that as right atrial pressure falls, the gradient from the peripheral tissues to the heart increases and, therefore, venous return also increases. With superimposition of a normal cardiac output curve, the cross-over of the cardiac output and venous return is the 'equilibrium point' at which venous return to the heart from the peripheral tissues is matched with the cardiac output from the heart to the peripheral tissues. With an increase in cardiac output, reflecting an increase in cardiac performance, this equilibrium point is shifted to a lower right atrial pressure, since it requires a

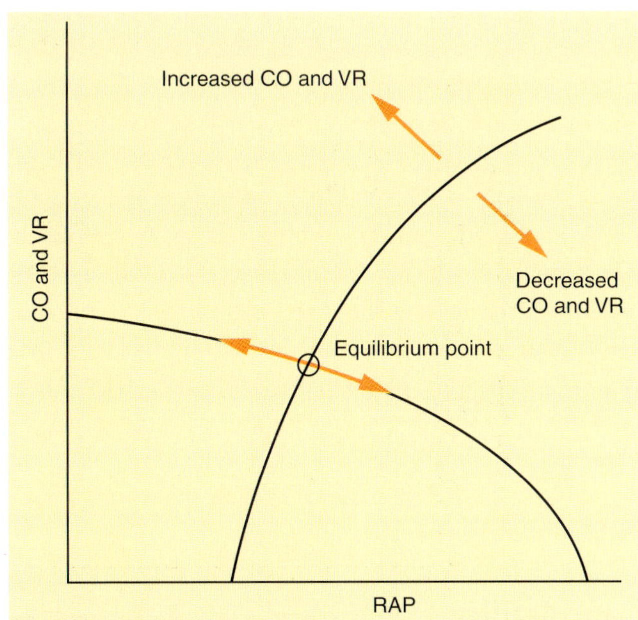


**Figure 2.9** *Relationship between right atrial pressure, cardiac output, and venous return. The intersection of the venous return curve and normal cardiac output curve represents the equilibrium point.*

higher venous return to maintain this output. In contrast, with a reduction in cardiac output reflecting a decrease in cardiac performance, this point is shifted to a higher right atrial pressure, which reflects a decrease in venous return. Depending on the cardiac performance, venous return is then adjusted to match output. The dynamic equilibrium between cardiac output and venous return is finely regulated on a beat-to-beat basis to maintain cardiac output and tissue perfusion.

### Preload reserve and afterload mismatch

Lee *et al.* [41] provided data from conscious dogs to explain the descending limb of the Starling curve. The concept of exhausting preload reserve and afterload mismatch, conceived by Ross [42], suggests that preload may increase to adapt to an increase in afterload with the objective of maintaining stroke volume, but only to a point. Once preload has been called upon to the extent that a steep portion of the diastolic pressure–volume relationship has been achieved, the increment in end-diastolic segment length may be insufficient to maintain stroke volume to accommodate for a further increase in afterload. Thus, an afterload mismatch will occur, such that stroke volume falls because preload reserve has been exhausted.

### Atrial contribution to filling

Linderer *et al.* [43], in an open-chest dog preparation, studied the contribution of atrial contraction to the increase in left ventricular segment length as measured by left ventricular diameter with and without the pericardium intact. For any given volume condition, atrial contraction contributed significantly to an increase in left ventricular diameter or segment length. With the pericardium intact, atrial systole significantly shifted the left ventricular stroke volume/end-diastolic pressure relationship upwards, indicating a significant contribution of left atrial systole to left ventricular systolic performance through its effect on increasing preload, consistent with studies in isolated muscle strips. Thus, there may be a substantial contribution of atrial systole to optimizing left ventricular sarcomere lengths and affecting an adjustment in left ventricular stroke volume and, therefore, cardiac output on a beat-by-beat basis.

## Contractility

### β-Adrenergic receptor modulation of contractility

Modulation of left ventricular contractility through β-adrenergic receptor mechanisms is an important control mechanism for altering myocardial contractility [44–47]. As illustrated in Figure 2.10 [44], the effects of β-adrenergic receptor agonists and antagonists on left ventricular contractility are evident using both left ventricular pressure–volume and stress–strain relationships. β-Agonist administration significantly increased the slope of the left ventricular pressure–volume and stress–strain relationships, indicating enhanced left ventricular contractile performance, while β-antagonists decreased the slope of the left ventricular pressure–volume and stress–strain relationships, indicating a decrease in left ventricular contractility. The slopes of the left ventricular end-systolic pressure–volume and stress–strain relationships are unique to the inotropic state and reflect, in this particular experiment, the intense modulation of contractility that occurs through β-adrenergic receptor mechanisms.

### Heart rate dependence of contractility and the force–frequency relationship

Variations in heart rate over the physiological range can have a substantial effect on left ventricular contractility [48–54]. Maughan *et al.* [48] examined this effect by measuring the left ventricular end-systolic pressure–volume relationship in isolated, ejecting, canine left ventricular preparations over a wide range of heart rates. Contractility increased as the heart rate increased from 60 to 120 beats/min; however, above 120 beats/min, there was no significant effect on left ventricular contractility. Thus, variation in heart rate within the physiological range experienced with normal activities or with limited exercise has a significant impact on left ventricular contractility.

This is further illustrated by the force–frequency relationship which was demonstrated in isolated cardiac muscle preparations by Mulieri *et al.* [51, 52]. An increase in the frequency of contraction in isolated muscle strips from normal donor hearts led to an increase in force generation over a wide range of rates, which was maximal at 160–200 beats/min (Fig. 2.11). However, in a cardiomyopathic or mitral regurgitant heart, there was flattening or actual inversion of the force–frequency relationship, indicative of no effect of heart rate on contractility. In fact, there may be a detrimental effect on contractility at higher heart rates. Because of these data, Ross *et al.* [55] proposed a three-part method of controlling contractility in the intact circulation composed of the length dependence of force development, the force–frequency relationship, and control of contrac-

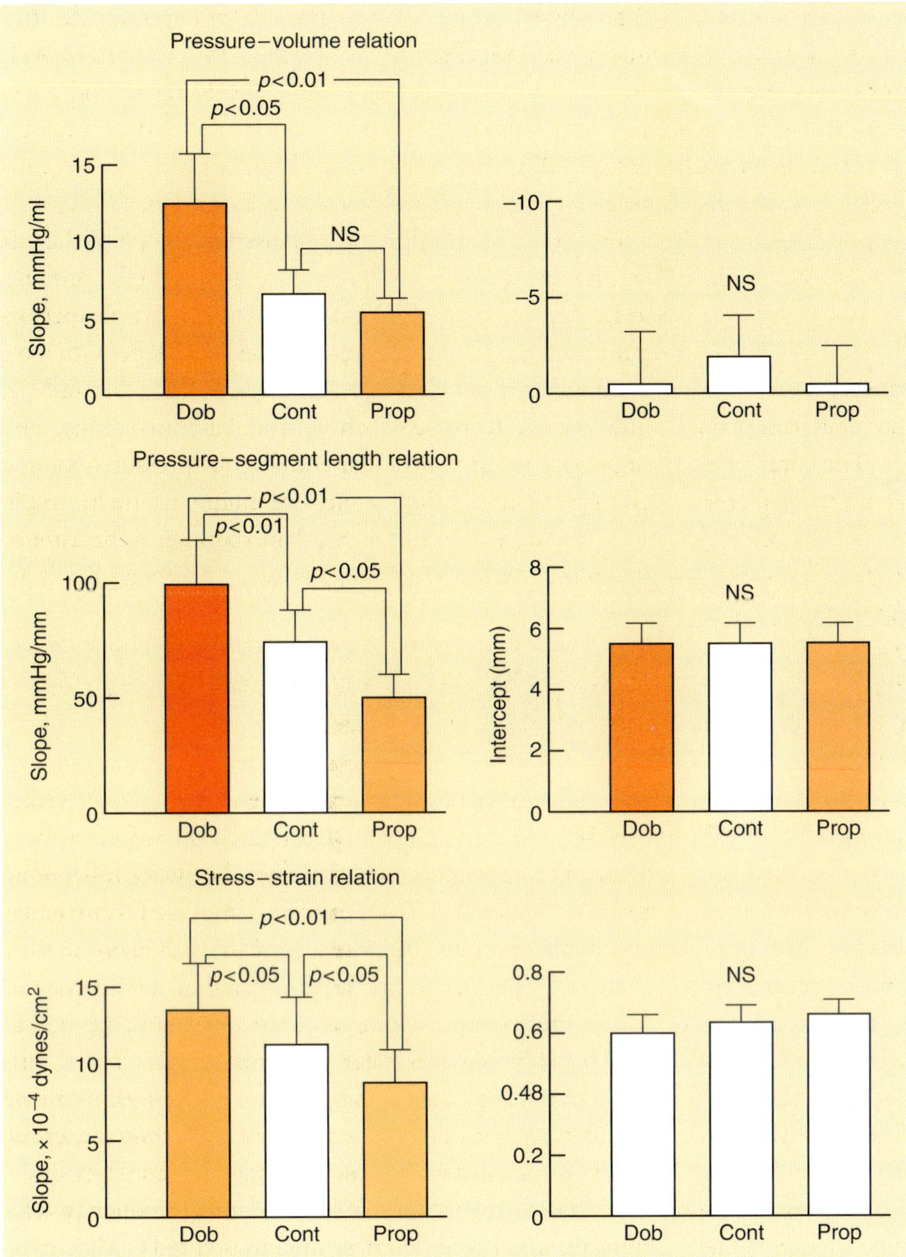


**Figure 2.10** *Left ventricular pressure–volume relation, pressure–segment length, and stress–strain relations under basal contractile conditions and during β-adrenergic receptor agonist stimulation and antagonist administration. Note that both the pressure–volume and stress–strain relations at end-systole increase with the β-agonist dobutamine, and decrease with the β-antagonist propanolol, indicating that both approaches are adequate for assessing left ventricular contractility. (From ref. 44 with permission.)*

tility through β-adrenergic receptor mechanisms. Data have also suggested that β-adrenergic mechanisms may modulate the force–frequency relationship and, therefore, represent a fully integrated series of mechanisms for control of contractility.

### Effects of myocardial perfusion on contractility

Alterations in myocardial perfusion may have a general negative effect on left ventricular contractility. This was demonstrated by Sunagawa *et al.* [56], who showed that a decrease in coronary artery perfusion pressure below 60 mmHg caused a substantial reduction in the end-systolic pressure–volume relationship, suggesting a detrimental effect on myocardial contractility. This effect may also be consistent with the detrimental effects of general anaesthetics, anoxia, acidosis, and other myocardial depressant agents on the performance of the left ventricle.

## Afterload

In classic terms, afterload can be defined as the tension or load that the myocytes must generate before shortening

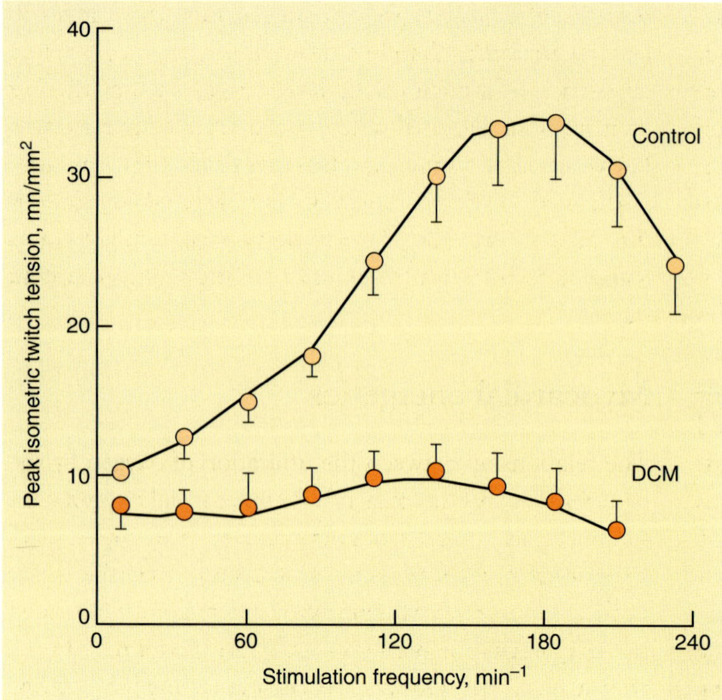


**Figure 2.11** *Force of contraction and frequency of contraction in control hearts and in hearts with contractile depression. (From ref. 51 with permission.)*

occurs. Afterload is, therefore, composed of internal stresses, i.e. stress, viscous resistance, and inertial components that the myocytes must carry, and external vascular load, which is composed of compliance, impedance, and resistance characteristics of the arterial vasculature. The components of stress, left ventricular pressure, mass, and geometry have been described. However, the characteristics of vascular load, their contribution to stress and, therefore, their effects on left ventricular ejection and contractility cannot be ignored because they contribute to the internal forces that the myocytes must carry during each contraction.

## Arterial characteristics

Systemic arterial impedance moduli and phase spectra have been used to characterize the vascular tree. The impedance concept is an effort to present a quantitative description of the opposition to blood flow presented by the arterial vasculature [57–60]. Once again, impedance should not be equated to afterload, the term that has been defined and developed to describe the load that the myocytes must carry during shortening. Nevertheless, impedance can contribute to afterload through its influence on pressure, loading sequence, and geometry. In addition, both resistance and compliance are properties of the arterial vasculature that contribute to, but are not equivalent to, total vascular impedance or opposition to blood flow. Two specific terms have been used to differentiate the total opposition to blood flow: input impedance, when there are no wave reflections in the system, and characteristic impedance, or the average of impedance moduli over the second to tenth harmonic frequencies, when there are wave reflections in the system. Thus, under control conditions, the input impedance, i.e. total opposition to blood flow, falls from a high value at zero frequency (mean aortic pressure divided by mean flow or vascular resistance) to a minimum and then oscillates around a mean characteristic impedance ($Z_0$). The impedance phase over this range of time is negative, indicating that flow is leading pressure. When a pressor agent is administered, the moduli for characteristic impedance increase, indicating an increase in wave reflections in the system and in the complexity of oscillations in phase. When a vasodilator is administered, these phase oscillations and characteristic impedance moduli decrease. These kinds of observation have been made in the non-human primate, as well as the normal human systemic vasculature [59, 60]; they appear not to be affected by heart rate or respiratory variation [59].

## Arterial effects on ejection and contractility

Nishioka *et al.* [61] examined the effects of alterations in arterial resistance and compliance on left ventricular end-systole and end-ejection. When arterial resistance was altered over a four-fold range, the left ventricular end-systolic pressure–volume relationship was not affected; however, there was a substantial effect on the end-ejection pressure–volume relationship. At a high resistance level, the end-systolic and end-ejection relationships were similar, but as arterial resistance was reduced, there was a substantial disassociation of end-ejection from end-systole. This indicates that arterial resistance has little effect on end-systolic indices, but has a substantial effect on ejection characteristics of the left ventricle. Similarly, when compliance was altered over a six-fold range, similar variations remained, although in an opposite direction. At reduced compliance or enhanced stiffness of the arterial tree, end-systolic and end-ejection pressure–volume relationships were similar; when compliance was increased, improving arterial properties, a substantial disassociation of end-ejection from end-systole occurred. Thus, alteration in arterial characteristics, in this case, compliance, affected the ejection characteristics of the left ventricle but not the time of end-systole [62].

### Left ventricular–arterial coupling

The left ventricular–arterial coupling relationship was proposed by Sunagawa *et al.* [63, 64] to understand regulation of left ventricular performance by analysing the contracting left ventricle as it interacts with the arterial system. They evaluated a ventricular model and an arterial model over multiple afterloaded and preloaded conditions, and were able to develop a system that integrated the left ventricular end-systolic pressure–volume relationship with the arterial pressure–volume relationship to predict a measured stroke volume (Fig. 2.12).

This model was used by Burkhoff and Sugawa [65] to analyse the interaction of left ventricle and arterial system to derive analytical expressions for left ventricular stroke work and mechanical efficiency in terms of left ventricular contractility and arterial properties (Fig. 2.13). When left ventricular contractile properties were quantitated in terms of the elastance concept and arterial properties in terms of effective arterial elastance, the model predicted that maximal left ventricular stroke work would occur when the left ventricular and arterial elastances were equal, irrespective of the contractile state. In contrast, the effective arterial elastance that resulted in the greatest myocardial efficiency was less than that which provided maximal left ventricular stroke work. Moreover, as left ventricular contractile properties decreased, left ventricular stroke work and myocardial efficiency were more sensitive to changes in arterial properties than in a heart with normal contractile properties. Although others have suggested that the left ventricular and arterial systems are controlled to maximize left ventricular output, i.e. stroke work [66, 67], this analytical model indicates that under normal physiological conditions, the left ventricle may operate more in a balance somewhere between maximum efficiency and maximum output.

## Myocardial energetics

The relationship between the utilization of oxygen by the myocardium and the demands for myocardial oxygen consumption have ranged from the simple to the complex. Irrespective of these formulations, it is clear that the major determinants of myocardial oxygen demand have remained the frequency of contraction, the work performed during contraction, and inotropy. Brittian and Levine [68] studied the relationship between myocardial oxygen consumption and demand by measuring cardiac output, left ventricular and aortic pressures, heart rate, left ventricular volumes, coronary sinus blood flow, and coronary sinus oxygen extraction in a number of experiments during altered left ventricular loading conditions and contractile states in 23 animals. They demonstrated that over a wide range of loading conditions and contractile states, contractile element work was the major determinant of myocardial oxygen utilization. They concluded that the ultimate formulation of myocardial energetics must include consideration of the energy costs of resting cardiac muscle, excitation–contraction coupling, and isovolumic and ejection work.

Suga *et al.* [69] took this concept into the pressure–volume plane. They regressed myocardial oxygen consumption against the pressure–volume area, which was defined by isovolumic and ejecting beats in the excised, contracting left ventricular preparation. The pressure–volume area was enclosed by the end-systolic pressure–volume relationship during systole, the diastolic curve, and the systolic portion of each pressure–volume trajectory. Although this differed somewhat from the initial formulation of Monroe and French [70], the pressure–volume area had two components in the ejecting heart, the external work performed by the left ventricle and the potential energy stored within the contractile element to perform external work [71, 72]. If this relationship was generated only by isovolumic beats, then only potential energy stored within the

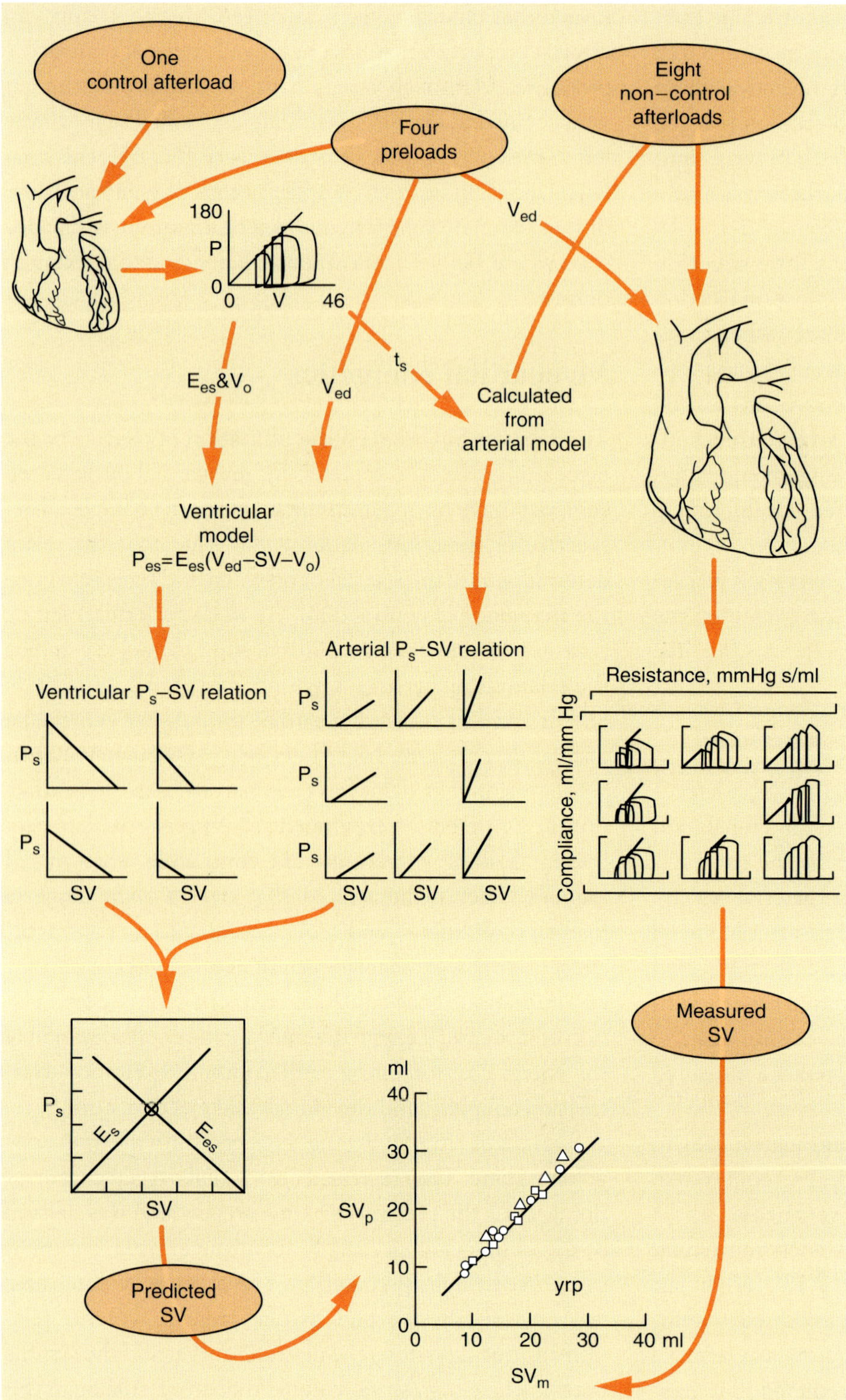


**Figure 2.12** *Relationship between the left ventricular end-systolic pressure–volume relations, a measure of contractility, and total arterial elastance, a measure of arterial load, and their ability to predict measured left ventricular stroke volume under varying compliance and resistances of the arterial tree and contractile states. (From ref. 63 with permission.)*

contractile element was available. When myocardial oxygen consumption was regressed against either the pressure–volume area or its component parts, a highly linear relationship was established between the pressure–volume area and myocardial oxygen consumption. Thus, the pressure–volume area which incorporates external work and the potential energy stored in the contractile element could reliably predict myocardial oxygen consumption. They also demonstrated that over a wide range of heart rates this relationship was maintained [73], that is, the relationship

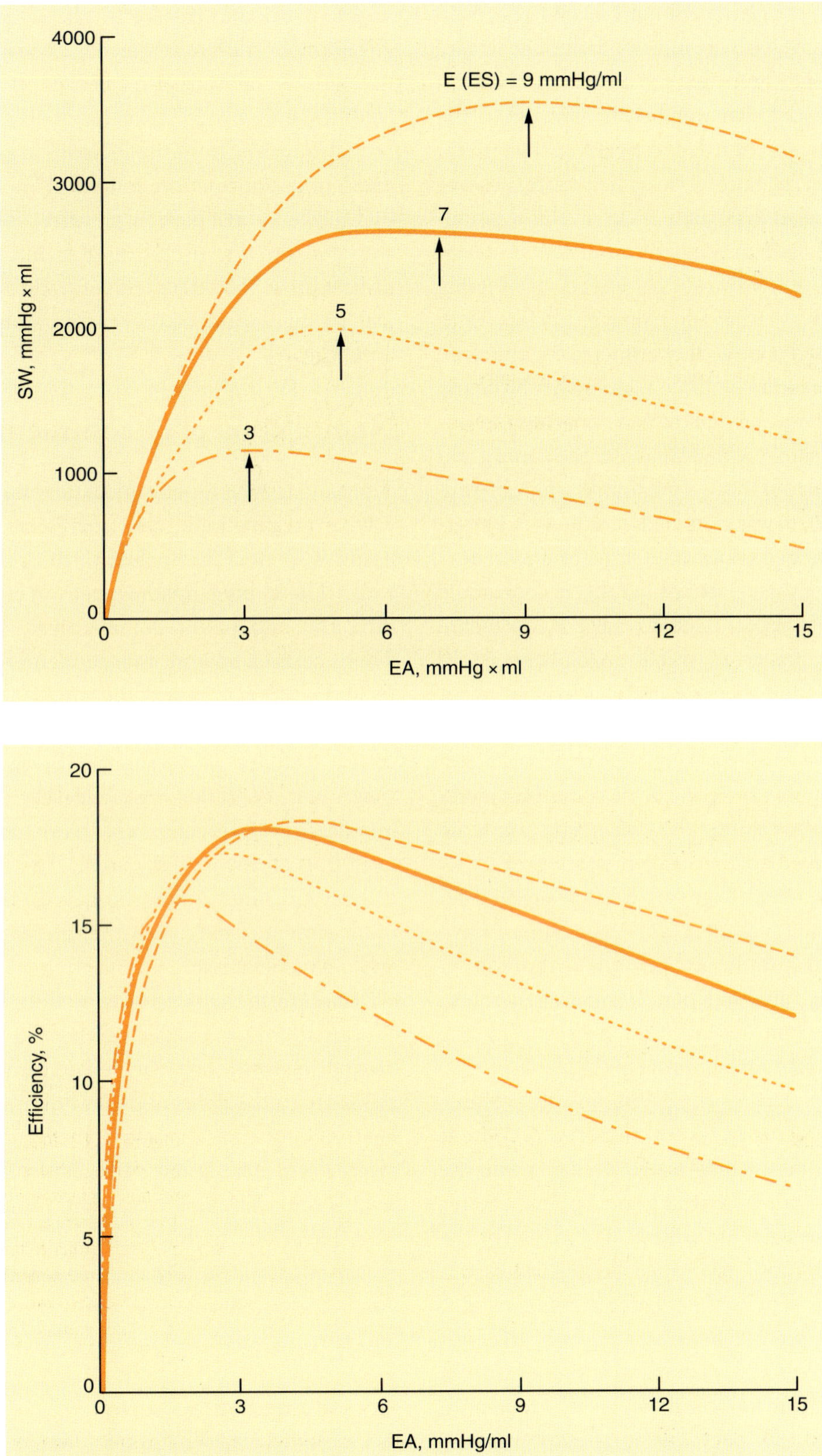


**Figure 2.13** *Relationship between the production of left ventricular stroke work at a matched left ventricular end-systolic elastance* ($E_{es}$) *and total arterial elastance* ($E_a$), *and relationship between myocardial efficiency and* $E_a$. *Note that maximal stroke work occurs when these two elastances are matched* (top), *while maximal efficiency occurs at a somewhat lower ratio* (bottom). *(From ref. 65 with permission.)*

between myocardial oxygen consumption and the pressure–volume area was essentially independent of heart rate when these parameters were expressed on the basis of beat per 100 g of myocardial weight. In contrast to the independence of the myocardial oxygen consumption/pressure–volume area relationship from heart rate, positive inotropic agents have an important effect on this relationship. Suga *et al.* [74] used an isolated canine left ventricular preparation to demonstrate the effects of altering contractile conditions by either adrenaline or calcium. Both agents clearly increased contractility by increasing the slope of the end-systolic pressure–volume relationship by nearly 70%. However, when myocardial oxygen consumption was regressed on the pressure–volume area from the control and enhanced contractile states, comparable slopes were achieved; however, there was an increase in the *y*-axis intercept during the enhanced contractile state. Since the reciprocal of the slope of this relationship reflects contractile efficiency, there would appear to be no effect of contractile state on myocardial efficiency, which ranged between 30 and 35%. In contrast, an increase in the *y*-axis intercept reflects the increment in myocardial oxygen consumption needed for excitation–contraction coupling and basal metabolic rate during the enhanced contractile state. This incremental energy utilization during the enhanced contractile state has been ascribed to the oxygen-wasting effect of inotropic agents, an effect that has been related to an increase in shortening velocity [75, 76]. Others have ascribed the same effect to the augmented energy requirements wasted during force-independent heat generation associated with calcium release and retrieval in the excitation–contraction coupling process [77].

The myocardial oxygen consumption/pressure–volume area relationship is unique in several respects. Because it can examine independently myocardial efficiency and the energy costs of excitation–contraction coupling, better understanding is achieved of the utilization of oxygen by the contractile element and the subcellular contractile machinery. Since the slope of the relationship is constant, the myocardial efficiency of converting energy by the contractile machinery is reasonably constant across contractile states. Nevertheless, this independence of the slope and, therefore, myocardial efficiency during alteration in the contractile state, has not been observed in all animal preparations [78, 79]. Further, since excitation–contraction coupling requires large amounts of energy utilization by the sarcoplasmic reticulum and both adrenaline and calcium augment calcium uptake by the sarcoplasmic reticulum, although by different mechanisms, it is clear that the increase in myocardial oxygen consumption that results from the enhanced contractile state in these experiments probably results from the increase in energy utilization for excitation–contraction coupling. Therefore, the myocardial oxygen consumption/pressure–volume area relationship can provide useful insights into myocardial energy utilization in the intact left ventricle during pharmacological manipulation of contractile state and pathological conditions.

## Neural control of contractility

The cardiac sympathetic and parasympathetic neural pathway of preganglionic cells represents the final common pathway of neural impulses to the cardiovascular system [80]. These preganglionic cells receive excitatory and inhibitory impulses predominantly from medullary centres. These centres operate independently and are capable of regulating cardiac contractility and heart rate, arterial pressure, and regional blood flow. Tonic excitatory medullary centre activity is constantly being modulated under steady-state conditions by cortical centres and by inhibitory impulses from mechanoreceptors and chemoreceptors from the cardiovascular system. An increase in activity in the carotid sinus and aortic nerves, for example, reflexly reduces neural activity in the efferent sympathetic fibres and augments efferent vagal activity. Similarly, vagal afferent fibres from the heart may produce similar modulations of sympathetic and vagal activity. The sympathetic nerves originating from the right stellate ganglion are distributed primarily to the sinus node and right atrium, and control heart rate, whereas those from the left stellate ganglion supply the left atrium and ventricle for the control of contractile state. Terminal sympathetic innervation of the heart is a plexiform architecture surrounding muscle cells. Parasympathetic outflow via the vagal nerve influences predominantly sinoatrial and atrioventricular nodal activity and only sparsely innervates the myocardium.

### Accentuated antagonism

Accentuated antagonism is a concept whereby an interaction of postganglionic sympathetic and parasympathetic neural fibres may affect the balance of the myocardial contractility state, depending on the balance of activity in the two systems [81–83]. Under basal contractile conditions when sympathetic activity is low and parasympathetic restraint is dominant, further activation of the parasympathetic nervous system does not significantly affect contractility function. When the sympathetic postganglionic neural activity is heightened, particularly through the left stellate ganglion, left atrial transfer function is increased, left ventricular preload is, therefore, increased, and stroke volume increases. Myocardial contractility is also increased, thereby enhancing the generation of pressure and improving shortening. During this heightened sympathetic neural activity, an increase in parasympathetic neural activity becomes more apparent and may decrease left ventricular contractility in a measurable way, consistent with the concept of accentuated antagonism.

Several studies have examined the augmentation in left ventricular contractility produced by peripherally administered sympathomimetic amines after muscarinic blockade [84–86]. After muscarinic blockade, there was a greater increase in contractility, the development of left ventricular tension, and shortening than during the basal state, suggesting that the parasympathetic nervous system can exert a tonic inhibitory influence on inotropic responses to peripherally administered sympathomimetic amines (Fig. 2.14). The striking augmentation of inotropic potential may be mediated through the vagal release of acetylcholine which may inhibit the action of sympathomimetic amines at a postsynaptic β-adrenergic receptor site.

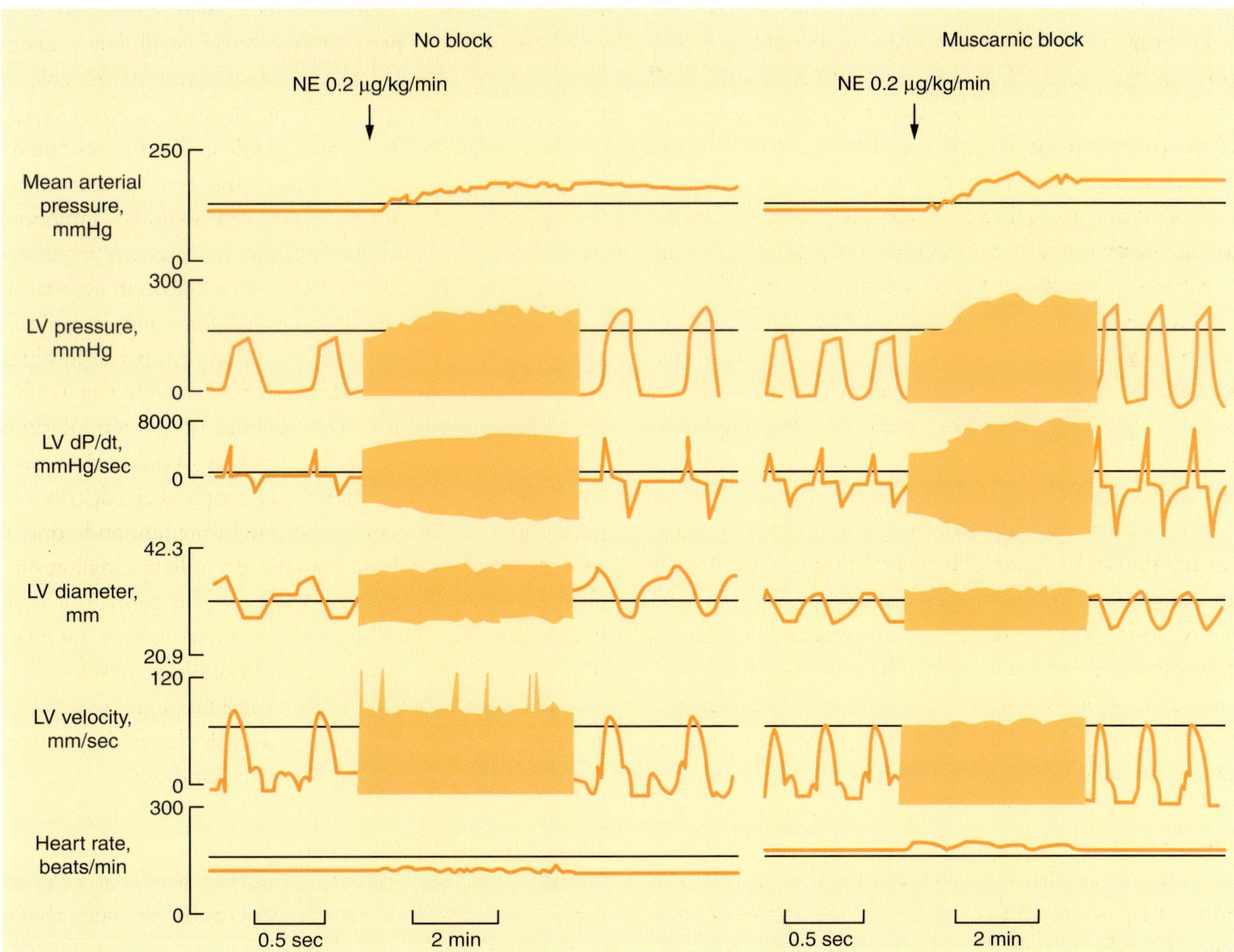


**Figure 2.14** *Augmentation of contractility produced by peripherally administered sympathomimetic amines after muscarinic blockade.* (*From ref.* 84 *with permission.*)

## Conclusions

A clear comprehension of the complexities of myocardial contraction, the interplays among preload, contractility, and afterload, and the modulation of this system by neural mechanisms is important before attempting to understand the pathophysiological processes that affect these functions. The cardiovascular system is clearly a highly integrated and finely tuned system, which can be affected by any one of a number of processes, leading to significant perturbations and abnormalities in the system. The importance of understanding normal cardiovascular physiology is fundamental to interpreting these perturbations in the system, identifying their cause, and establishing the appropriate intervention.

## References


1. Parmley WW, Sonnenblick EH. Series elasticity in heart muscle: Its relation to contractile element velocity and proposed muscle models. *Circ Res* 1967; 20: 112–23.
2. Rankin JS, Arentzen CE, McHale A *et al.* Viscoelastic properties of the diastolic left ventricle in the conscious dog. *Circ Res* 1977; 41: 37–45.
3. Sonnenblick EH. Force–velocity relations in mammalian heart muscle. *Am J Physiol* 1962; 202: 931–9.
4. Burns JW, Covell JW, Ross J. Mechanics of isotonic left ventricular contractions. *Am J Physiol* 1973; 224: 725–32.
5. Brutsaert DL, Sonnenblick EH. Force–velocity–length–time relations of the contractile elements in heart muscle of the cat. *Circ Res* 1969; 24: 137–49.
6. Ter Keurs HE, Rijnsburger WH, Heuningen RV, Nagelsmit MJ. Tension development and sarcomere length in rat cardiac trabeculae. *Circ Res* 1980; 46: 703–14.
7. Kentish JC, Wrzosek A. Changes in force and cytosolic $Ca^{2+}$ concentration after length changes in isolated rate ventricular trabeculae. *Am J Physiol* 1998; 506: 431–44.
8. Gordon AM, Huxley AF, Julian FJ. The variation in isometric tension with sarcomere length in vertebrate muscle fibres. *J Physiol* 1966; 184: 170–92.
9. Sonnenblick EH, Skelton CL. Reconsideration of the ultrastructural basis of cardiac length–tension relations. *Circ Res* 1974; 35: 517–26.
10. Spotnitz HM, Sonnenblick EH, Spiro D. Relation of ultrastructure to function in the intact heart. Sarcomere structure relative to pressure-volume curves of intact left ventricles of dog and cat. *Circ Res* 1966; 18: 49–66.
11. Sonnenblick EH, Ross J, Covell JW *et al.* The ultrastructure of the heart in systole and diastole. *Circ Res* 1967; 21: 423–31.
12. Ross J Jr, Sonnenblick EH, Covell JW *et al.* Changes in Sarcomere length: Architecture of the heart in systole and diastole technique of rapid fixation and analysis of left ventricular geometry. *Circ Res* 1967; 21: 409–21.
13. Starling MR. Myocardial mechanisms and neurohumoral regulation of the circulation. In: E Braunwald, WS Colucci: (eds). *Atlas of heart failure: cardiac function and dysfunction.* 2nd edition. Philadelphia: Current Medicine, Inc., 1999, 2.1–2.19.
14. Streeter DD, Spotnitz HM, Patel DP *et al.* Fiber orientation in the canine left ventricle during diastole and systole. *Circ Res* 1969; 24: 339–47.
15. Hansen DE, Daughters GYT, Alderman EL *et al.* Torsional deformation of the left ventricular midwall in human hearts with intramyocardial markers: Regional heterogeneity and sensitivity to the inotropic effects of abrupt rate changes. *Circ Res* 1988; 62: 941–52.
16. Mirsky I. Left ventricular stresses in the intact human heart. *Biophys J* 1969; 9: 189–208.
17. Badke FR, O'Rourke RA. Congestive heart failure. In: JH Stein (ed.) *Cardiovascular physiology in internal medicine.* 1st edition. Boston, MA: Little, Brown and Co., 1983; 407–23.
18. Ross J. Applications and limitations of end-systolic measures of ventricular performance. *Fedn Proc* 1984; 43: 2418–22.
19. Dodge HT, Sandler H, Ballew DW, Lord JD. The use of biplane angiography for the measurement left ventricular volume in man. *Am Heart J* 1960; 60: 762–76.
20. Hutchins GM, Bulkley, Moore GW *et al.* Shape of the human cardiac ventricles. *Am J Cardiol* 1978; 41: 646–54.
21. Hori M, Inoue M, Kitakaze M *et al.* Loading sequence is a major determinant of afterload-dependent relaxation in intact canine heart. *Am J Physiol* 1985; 249: H747–54.
22. Braunwald E, Sonnenblick EH, Ross J. Mechanisms of cardiac contraction and relaxation. In: E Braunwald (ed.) *Heart disease: a textbook of cardiovascular medicine.* 3rd edition. Philadelphia, PA: WB Saunders, 1988, 383–425.
23. Berne RM, Levy MH. *Cardiovascular physiology.* 3rd edition. St Louis, MO: CV Mosby, 1977.
24. Potts JT, McKeown KP, Shoukas AA. Reduction in arterial compliance alters carotid baroreflex control of cardiac output in a model of hypertension. *Am J Physiol* 1998; 274: H1121–31.
25. Glantz SA, Parmley WW. Factors which affect the diastolic pressure–volume curve. *Circ Res* 1978; 42: 171–80.
26. Gilbert JC, Glantz SA. Determinants of left ventricular filling and of the diastolic pressure–volume relation. *Circ Res* 1989; 64: 827–52.
27. Weiss JL, Frederiksen JW, Weisfeldt ML. Hemodynamic determinants of the time-course of fall in canine left ventricular pressure. *J Clin Invest* 1976; 58: 751–8.
28. Raff GL, Glantz SA. Volume loading slows left ventricular isovolumic relaxation rate. Evidence of load-dependent relaxation in the intact dog heart. *Circ Res* 1981; 48: 813–21.
29. Mirsky I. Assessment of diastolic function: Suggested methods and future considerations. *Circulation* 1984; 69: 836–41.
30. Starling MR, Montgomery DG, Mancini GB, Walsh RA. Load independence of the rate of isovolumic relaxation in man. *Circulation* 1987; 6: 1274–81.
31. Mirsky I, Parmley WW. Assessment of passive elastic stiffness for isolated heart muscle and the intact heart. *Circ Res* 1973; 33: 233–43.
32. Mirsky I, Cohn PF, Levine JA *et al.* Assessment of left ventricular stiffness in primary myocardial disease and coronary artery disease. *Circulation* 1974; 50: 128–36.
33. Gaasch WH, Levine HJ, Quinones MA, Alexander JK. Left ventricular compliance: Mechanisms and clinical implications. *Am J Cardiol* 1976; 38: 645–53.

34. Pouleur H, Karliner JS, LeWinter M, Covell JW. Diastolic viscous properties of the intact canine left ventricle. *Circ Res* 1979; 45: 410–19.
35. Grossman W, McLaurin LP. Diastolic properties of the left ventricle. *Ann Intern Med* 1976; 84: 316–26.
36. LeWinter MM, Engler R, Pavelec RS. Time-dependent shifts of the left ventricular diastolic filling relationship in conscious dogs. *Circ Res* 1979; 45: 641–53.
37. Hess OM, Bhargava V, Ross J, Shabetai R. The role of the pericardium in interactions between the cardiac chambers. *Am Heart J* 1983; 106: 1377–83.
38. Shirato K, Shabetai R, Bhargava V *et al.* Alteration of the left ventricular diastolic pressure–segment length relation produced by the pericardium. *Circulation* 1978; 57: 1191–7.
39. Guyton AC, Jones CE, Coleman TG. Graphical analysis of cardiac output regulation. In: AC Guyton, CE Jones, TG Lobman (eds) *Circulatory physiology: cardiac output and its regulation*. 2nd edition. WB Saunders: Philadelphia, PA, 1973; 237–52.
40. Rothe CF. Physiology of venous return. An unappreciated boost to the heart. *Arch Intern Med* 1986; 146: 977–82.
41. Lee JD, Tajimi T, Ptritti J, Ross J. Preload reserve and mechanisms of afterload mismatch in normal conscious dog. *Am J Physiol* 1986; 250: H464–73.
42. Ross J. Afterload mismatch and preload reserve: A conceptual framework for the analysis of ventricular function. *Prog Cardiovasc Dis* 1976; 18: 255–64.
43. Linderer T, Chatterjee K, Parmley WW *et al.* Influence of atrial systole on the Frank–Starling relation and the end-diastole pressure–diameter relation of the left ventricle. *Circulation* 1983; 67: 1045–53.
44. Kaseda S, Tomoike H, Ogata I, Nakamura M. End-systolic pressure–volume length and stress–strain relations in canine hearts. *Am J Physiol* 1985; 249: H648–54.
45. Suga H, Sagawa K. Instantaneous pressure–volume relationships and their ratio in the excised supported canine left ventricle. *Circ Res* 1974; 35: 117–26.
46. Suga H, Sagawa K, Shoukas A. Load independence of the instantaneous pressure–volume ratio of the canine left ventricle and effects of epinephrine and heart rate on the ratio. *Circ Res* 1973; 32: 314–22.
47. Sagawa K, Suga H, Shoukas A, Bakalar KM. End-systolic pressure/volume ratio: A new index of ventricular contractility. *Am J Cardiol* 1977; 40: 748–53.
48. Maughan WL, Sunagawa K, Burkhoff D *et al.* Effect of heart rate on the canine end-systolic pressure–volume relationship. *Circulation* 1985; 72: 654–9.
49. Mitchell JH, Wallace AG, Skinner NS. Intrinsic effects of heart rate on left ventricular performance. *Am J Physiol* 1963; 205: 41–8.
50. Covell JW, Ross J, Taylor R *et al.* Effects of increasing frequency of contraction on the force–velocity relation of left ventricle. *Cardiovasc Res* 1967; 1: 2–8.
51. Mulieri LA, Leavitt BJ, Hasenfuss G *et al.* Contraction frequency dependence of twitch and diastolic tension in human dilated cardiomyopathy (tension–frequency relation in cardiomyopathy). *Basic Res Cardiol* 1992; 87: 199–212.
52. Mulieri LA, Leavitt BJ, Martin BJ *et al.* Myocardial force–frequency defect in mitral regurgitation heart failure is reversed by forskolin. *Circulation* 1993; 88: 2700–4.
53. Higgins CB, Vatner SF, Franklin D, Braunwald E. Extent of regulation of the heart's contractile state in the conscious dog by alteration in the frequency of contraction. *J Clin Invest* 1973; 52: 1187–94.
54. Klautz RJ, Baan J, Teitel DF. The effect of sarcoplasmic reticulum blockade on the force/frequency relationship and systolic contraction patterns in the newborn pig heart. *Pflugers Arch* 1997; 435: 130–6.
55. Ross J Jr, Miura T, Kambayashi M *et al.* Adrenergic control of the force–frequency relation. *Circulation* 1995; 92: 2327–32.
56. Sunagawa K, Maughan WL, Friesinger G *et al.* Effects of coronary arterial pressure on left ventricular end-systolic pressure–volume relation of isolated canine heart. *Circ Res* 1982; 50: 727–34.
57. Latham RD, Rubal BJ, Sipkema P *et al.* Ventricular/vascular coupling and regional arterial dynamics in the chronically hypertensive baboon: Correlation with cardiovascular structural adaptation. *Circ Res* 1988; 63: 798–811.
58. Finkelstein SM, Collins VR. Vascular hemodynamic impedance measurement. *Cardiovasc Dis* 1982; 24: 401–18.
59. Nichols WW, Conti CR, Walker WE, Milnor WR. Input impedance measurement. *Prog Cardiovasc Dis* 1982; 24: 451–8.
60. Murgo JP, Westerhof N, Giolma JP, Altobelli SA. Aortic input impedance in normal man: Relationship to pressure wave forms. *Circulation* 1980; 62: 105–16.
61. Nishioka O, Maruyama Y, Ashikawa K *et al.* Effects of changes in afterload impedance on left ventricular ejection in isolated canine hearts: Dissociation of end-ejection from end-systole. *Cardiovasc Res* 1987; 21: 107–18.
62. Maughan WL, Sunagawa MK, Burkhoff K, Sagawa K. Effect of arterial impedance changes on the end-systolic pressure–volume relation. *Circ Res* 1984; 54: 592–602.
63. Sunagawa K, Maughan WL, Burkhoff D, Sagawa K. Left ventricular interaction with arterial load studied in isolated canine ventricle. *Am J Physiol* 1983; 245: H773–80.
64. Sunagawa K, Maughan WL, Sagawa K. Optimal arterial resistance for the maximal stroke work studied in isolated canine left ventricle. *Circ Res* 1985; 56: 586–95.
65. Burkhoff D, Sagawa K. Ventricular efficiency predicted by an analytical model. *Am J Physiol* 1986; 250: R1021–7.
66. van den Horn GH, Westerhof N, Elzinga G. Optimal power generation by the left ventricle. A study in the anesthetized open thorax cat. *Circ Res* 1985; 56: 252–61.
67. Elzinga G, Westerhof N. Matching between ventricle and arterial load. An evolutionary process. *Circ Res* 1991; 68: 1495–500.
68. Britman NA, Levine HJ. Contractile element work: A major determinant of myocardial oxygen consumption. *J Clin Invest* 1964; 43: 1397–408.
69. Suga H, Hayashi T, Shirahata M *et al.* Regression of cardiac oxygen consumption on ventricular pressure–volume area in dog. *Am J Physiol* 1981; 240: H320–5.
70. Monroe G, French GN. Left ventricular pressure–volume relationships and myocardial oxygen consumption in the isolated heart. *Circ Res* 1961; 9: 362–74.
71. Suga H, Yasumura Y, Nozawa T *et al.* Prospective prediction of $O_2$ consumption from pressure–volume area in dogs' hearts. *Am J Physiol* 1987; 252: H1258–64.
72. Suga H. External mechanical work from relaxing ventricle. *Am J Physiol* 1979; 236: H494–7.

73. Suga H, Hisano R, Hirata S *et al.* Heart rate-independent energetics and systolic pressure–volume area in dog hearts. *Am J Physiol* 1983; 244: H206–14.
74. Suga H, Hisano R, Goto Y *et al.* Effect of positive inotropic agents on the relation between oxygen consumption and systolic pressure–volume area in canine left ventricle. *Circ Res* 1983; 53: 306–18.
75. Graham TP, Covell JW, Sonnenblick EH *et al.* Control of myocardial oxygen consumption: Relative influence of contractile state and tension development. *J Clin Invest* 1968; 47: 375–85.
76. Sonnenblick EH, Ross J, Covell JW *et al.* Velocity of contraction as a determinant of myocardial oxygen consumption. *Am J Physiol* 1965; 209: 919–27.
77. Gibbs CL, Gibson WR. Isoprenaline, propranolol and the energy output of rabbit cardiac muscle. *Cardiovasc Res* 1972; 6: 508–15.
78. Nozawa T, Yasumura Y, Futaki S *et al.* Relation between oxygen consumption and pressure–volume area of *in situ* dog heart. *Am J Physiol* 1987; 253: H31–40.
79. Starling MR, Mancini GBJ, Montgomery DG, Gross MD. Relation between maximum time-varying elastance pressure–volume areas and myocardial oxygen consumption in dogs. *Circulation* 1991; 83: 304–14.
80. Corr PB, Yamada KA, Witkowski FX. Mechanisms controlling cardiac autonomic function and their relation to arrythmogenesis. In: HA Fozzard, E Haber, RB Jennings *et al.* (eds) *The heart and cardiovascular system.* 1st edition. New York: Raven Press, 1986, 1357–71.
81. Levy MN, Martin PJ. Neural control of the heart. *Physiology and Pathophysiology of the Heart*, ed 1. Edited by Speilakis N. Boston: Martinus Mijhoff Publishing; 1984: pp. 337–54.
82. Levy MN. Sympathetic–parasympathetic interactions in the heart. *Circ Res* 1971; 29: 437–45.
83. DeGeest H, Levy MN, Zieske H, Lipman RI. Depression of ventricular contractility by stimulation of the vagus nerves. *Circ Res* 1963; 17: 222–35.
84. Vatner SF, Rutherford JD, Ochs HR. Baroreflex and vagal mechanisms modulating left ventricular contractile responses to sympathomimetic amines in conscious dogs. *Circ Res* 1979; 44: 195–207.
85. Vatner SF, Rutherford JD. Control of the myocardial contractile state by carotid chemo- and baroreceptor and pulmonary inflation reflexes in conscious dogs. *J Clin Invest* 1977; 61: 1593–601.
86. Fujii AM, Vatner SF. Sympathetic mechanisms regulating myocardial contractility in conscious animals. In: HA Fozzard, E Haber, RB Jennings *et al.* (eds) *The heart and cardiovascular system.* 1st edition. New York: Raven Press, 1986, 1119–32.

# Myocardial energetics and cardiac contractility 3

J. S. INGWALL

## Introduction

The absolute requirement of mechanical performance, synthesis of biological molecules and transport of ions in cardiac myocytes for adenosine triphosphate (ATP; structure shown in Fig. 3.1) is well established. All processes in the heart depend either directly or indirectly on chemical energy in the form of ATP. When the ATP concentration ([ATP]) falls and the products of ATP hydrolysis, namely adenosine diphosphate (ADP) and inorganic phosphate ($P_i$), accumulate, the heart is unable to maintain normal pump function. The subject of this chapter is the chemistry of ATP and the relationship between energetics and contractile function. First, the importance of preserving the ATP pool and the capacity for ATP resynthesis is described, followed by the relationship between ATP and its metabolites for driving the contractile apparatus. Some aspects of the energetics of two clinically important conditions, ischaemia and heart failure, as well as that of the normal heart, are used to illustrate some of the basic principles. Many of these examples come from the author's laboratory; exciting aspects of energetics being pursued in other laboratories are not presented here, including some of the emerging evidence suggesting that

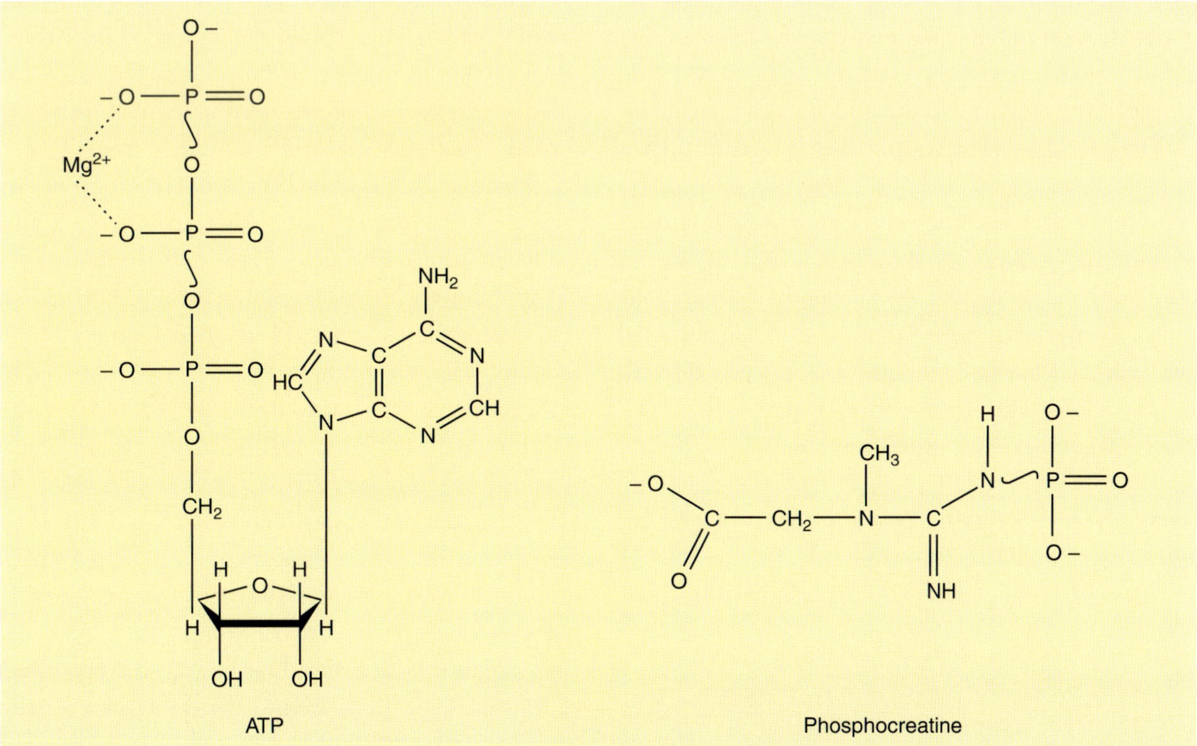


**Figure 3.1** *Structure of ATP and phosphocreatine. The bonds in ATP linking the $\gamma$-, $\alpha$-, and $\beta$-phosphates are curved to denote that chemical energy is released when they are broken. These bonds are referred to as phosphoryl bonds in the text.*

nitric oxide (NO) regulates energetics and the use of [$^{13}$C]nuclear magnetic resonance (NMR) spectroscopy to study intermediary metabolism. The fundamentals of intermediary metabolism for the heart have been described elsewhere [1] and are not presented here.

## ATP and the capacity for ATP synthesis

### Relationship between ATP content and ATP turnover rates: changing workloads

Mammalian ventricular tissue contains about 5 μmoles/g wet weight, which corresponds to a concentration of 8–10 mmoles/l of intracellular water (mM) or 30–35 μmoles/g cardiac protein. In the normal myocardium, the concentration of ATP is maintained essentially constant. The amount of ATP in the heart, about 0.6 g for a 250 g human heart, is sufficient to maintain pump function for less than 50 beats. Using a value for the rate of ATP synthesis (and utilization) of about 1.0 mM/s, a person uses about 7 kg of ATP in a day. Because the amount of ATP in the heart is small, the myocardial cell must continually resynthesize it to maintain normal pump function and cellular viability. Based on these estimates, the heart replenishes the ATP pool 10 000 times a day. The metabolic machinery needed to accomplish this formidable task without allowing the ATP concentration to fall is impressive.

The distinction between the concentration of ATP and ATP turnover rate is central to the understanding of bioenergetics. The energetics of increasing cardiac work illustrates this principle. As the workload of the heart increases, oxygen consumption (a good index of the rate of ATP synthesis via oxidative phosphorylation in the mitochondria) proportionately increases, yet ATP content is essentially unchanged. Thus, the rate at which ATP is made and used (turnover rate) but not its concentration increases as work increases. This illustrates the important principle that ATP synthesis rate matches ATP utilization rate.

### Preservation of the purine pool: a central issue in managing myocardial ischaemia

The primary pathway for ATP degradation in heart (Fig. 3.2) is:

$$\text{ATP} \rightarrow \text{ADP} \rightarrow \text{AMP} \rightarrow \text{adenosine} \rightarrow \text{inosine} \rightarrow \text{hypoxanthine} \rightarrow \text{xanthine.}$$

The purine nucleotides ATP, ADP, and adenosine monophosphate (AMP) are highly charged molecules and do not easily cross the cell wall. The purine nucleosides and nucleobases adenosine, inosine, and hypoxanthine, in contrast, are not charged and readily diffuse across the cell wall. In the normal heart, flux down this pathway occurs constantly, but there is no measurable change in the ATP concentration because the pathways for ATP resynthesis (supply) balance the rate of ATP degradation (demand). The balance is severely disrupted during acute ischaemia or hypoxia, however, and, as a consequence, the ATP concentration decreases. Under these conditions, the metabolites adenosine, inosine, and hypoxanthine are lost from the cell, depleting the total purine pool. This occurs during hypoxia and low-flow ischaemia and upon restoration of flow in areas of no-flow ischaemia. Because *de novo* synthesis of the purine ring in mammalian myocardium is very slow, in the order of nM/s [3], resynthesis of ATP under these conditions occurs only by rephosphorylation of the remaining pool of cytosolic adenine nucleotides, mainly AMP. Therefore, preservation of the adenine nucleotide pool, especially the AMP pool, during hypoxic and ischaemic episodes is essential to maintain cell function and viability.

The size of the AMP pool in ischaemic heart cells is determined primarily by the activity of the cytosolic AMP-specific 5′-nucleotidase (5′-NT). By dephosphorylating AMP to adenosine, this enzyme plays a major role in ATP degradation in mammalian myocytes (Fig. 3.2). Indeed, it is the gatekeeper of the purine pool. Surprisingly, this enzyme has received little attention, especially in contrast to the ecto-5′-NTs. Thus, a brief description of its properties is given. The cytosolic AMP-specific 5′-NT has been well characterized *in vitro*. In the late 1980s, two groups [4, 5] studying the enzyme isolated from pigeon, rat, and rabbit hearts showed that the enzyme requires $Mg^{2+}$ for its activity, has a pH optimum near 7, and is inhibited by $P_i$ and $H^+$. More recent studies of highly purified enzyme isolated from hearts of large mammals, dog [6] and human [7], have shown that the enzyme is activated by AMP, ADP, and $Mg^{2+}$, and is active between pH 6.8 and 7.8. If the same regulation occurs *in vivo*, then intracellular pH has an important role in the determination of the size of the AMP pool in the ischaemic myocardium.

Using isolated perfused rat hearts and a combination of [$^{31}$P] NMR spectroscopy and chemical assay, the regulation of this enzyme was studied in the intact heart [2, 8]. The results show that 5′-NT is activated early during hypoxia and ischaemic stress but is inhibited during prolonged

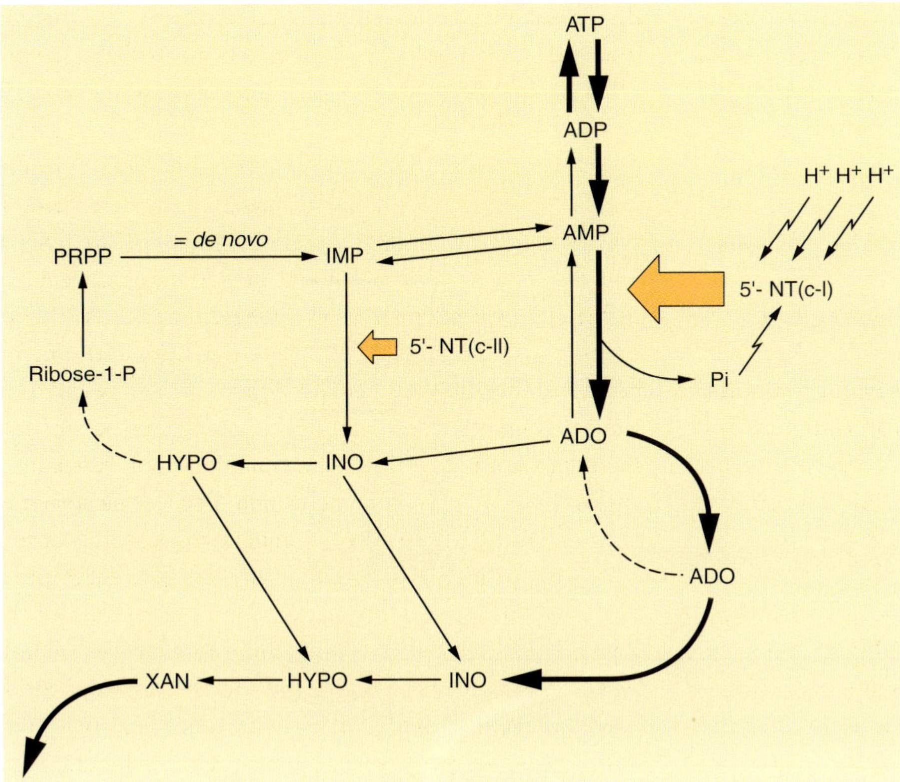


**Figure 3.2** *Principal pathway of purine metabolism in the mammalian heart.* De novo *refers to the synthetic pathway for inosine monophosphate (IMP) synthesis from non-purine precursors. Thick lines represent dominant pathways; thin lines and dashed lines represent quantitatively minor pathways. All phosphorylated compounds remain in the myocyte, whereas inosine (INO), hypoxanthine, (HYPO), and adenosine (ADO) diffuse from the myocyte to the extracellular space and vessels. The multistep reactions important for* de novo *purine synthesis using HYPO, ribose-1-phosphate (ribose-1-P) and 5-phosphoribosyl-1-pyrophosphate (PRPP) are indicated by dashed lines. The broken arrows show the inhibitory effects of* $H^+$ *and* $P_i$*. (Reprinted from ref. 2 with permission.)*

ischaemia. Intracellular pH is likely to be the primary inhibitor of 5′-NT and the difference in pH between high-flow hypoxia (where pH remains near 7) and zero-flow ischaemia (where pH falls to near 6) is sufficient to explain the differences in the capacity for net ATP resynthesis in ischaemic and hypoxic tissues [8]. By taking advantage of the ability to manipulate the intracellular pH in the hyperthyroid rat heart during ischaemia, and analysing all the known regulators of 5′-NT, the hypothesis that intracellular acidosis is the primary regulator of this important enzyme has been strengthened [2]. This salutary effect of intracellular acidosis on preserving the adenine nucleotide pool is a novel role of $H^+$ in protecting ischaemic tissue which merits consideration in planning new strategies for myocardial preservation in the settings of acute ischaemia and cardioplegia.

## ATP synthesis pathways

Given the critical need to maintain a constant level of ATP to support pump function, it is not surprising that the cell uses many reactions and pathways to synthesize ATP. In order of decreasing velocity (measured for the intact rat heart), the major ATP synthesizing pathways (Fig. 3.3) are the creatine kinase (CK) reaction (about 10 mM/s), oxidative phosphorylation (about 1 mM/s), and glycolysis (about 0.03 mM/s) (calculated from data given in refs 9 and 10). ATP concentration is kept essentially constant by the integration of these multiple pathways for ATP synthesis. Normally, ATP production by oxidative phosphorylation is sufficient to meet the constantly changing demands for energy. Under some conditions, the CK reaction uses the energy stored in the phosphoryl bond of phosphocreatine (PCr; structure shown in Fig. 3.1) to replete the ATP pool. PCr is present in heart in concentrations twice that of ATP. The reader should also be aware of a growing body of work from the Taegtmeyer laboratory on the role of glycogenolysis in supporting increased workloads [11].

## Capacity for ATP synthesis and contractile performance

Enzymes are catalysts. They do not determine whether a reaction takes place; instead, they determine how quickly it takes place. Biochemists have developed quantitative expressions allowing calculation of the speed of the reaction, called rate equations. One common feature of these rate equations is that the velocity of the reaction in linearly dependent on the amount of enzyme present. This is usually determined as the capacity of the reaction ($V_{max}$), i.e.

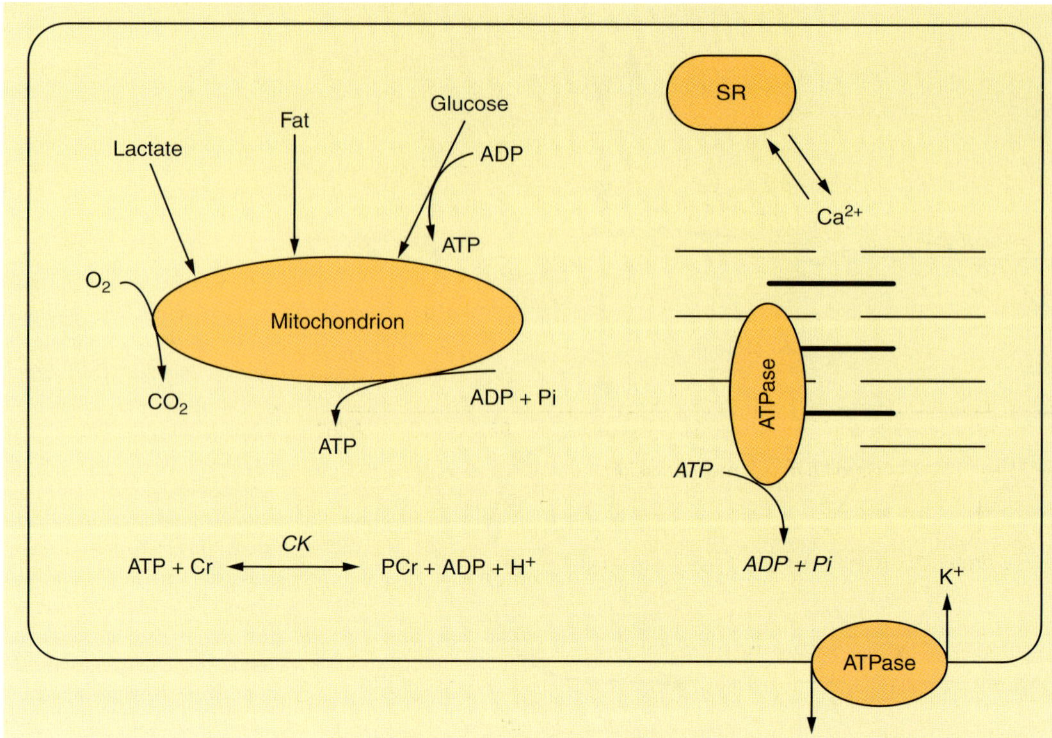


**Figure 3.3** *ATP synthesis and utilization pathways. (Drawn by Rong Tian, NMR Laboratory for Physiological Chemistry, Brigham and Woman's Hospital, Boston, MA, USA.)*

the activity measured under conditions when none of the substrates for the reaction is limiting. The velocity of the reaction also depends (but not always linearly or even monotonically) on the amount of substrate available to drive the reaction. A useful formula for estimating the velocity of a reaction is the product of $V_{max}$ and the concentration of its reactants.

It is important to emphasize that the velocity of a reaction in the intact cell is almost always a small fraction of the capacity for that reaction. For example, the velocity of the CK reaction determined in the intact beating rodent heart using [$^{31}$P]magnetization transfer is about one-tenth the capacity (maximal activity) for the CK reaction measured in tissue homogenates in a test-tube [9]. Another example is the observation that the glycolytic rate in the intact rat heart measured using [$^3$H]glucose and collecting $^3H_2O$ formed at the enolase step was unchanged in a heart in which glyceraldehyde phosphate dehydrogenase was inhibited by 70% [10]. Using a small and variable fraction of the total pool available is one solution to the problem of recruiting molecules for rapid use to respond to beat-to-beat changes in the needs of the organ.

***Example 1: The developing heart***

The developing heart is the quintessential example showing large changes in the capacity of reactions important for ATP synthesis. In the foetus and neonate, the increase in the fractional cell volume of mitochondria, a hallmark of development, occurs more or less in concert with the increase in myofibrillar protein mass and increased physical activity. One developmentally regulated muscle protein that has been studied in detail is CK [12]. Figure 3.4a shows values for the tissue activity of CK for foetal, neonatal, and adult mouse hearts as a function of heart weight and age. Figure 3.4b shows values for the creatine pool (the sum of free creatine and PCr). During the last trimester of development, the foetal heart rapidly accumulates both CK (here measured as activity) and its substrate creatine. Note that [ATP] stays constant throughout maturation, but PCr and creatine increase concomitantly. The rates of accumulation of both enzyme and substrate slow during neonatal development, but nonetheless both $V_{max}$ and the creatine pool continue to increase. Between 16 days' gestation and adulthood, $V_{max}$ increases about 30-fold, the creatine pool increases 50-fold, and the product of $V_{max}$ and

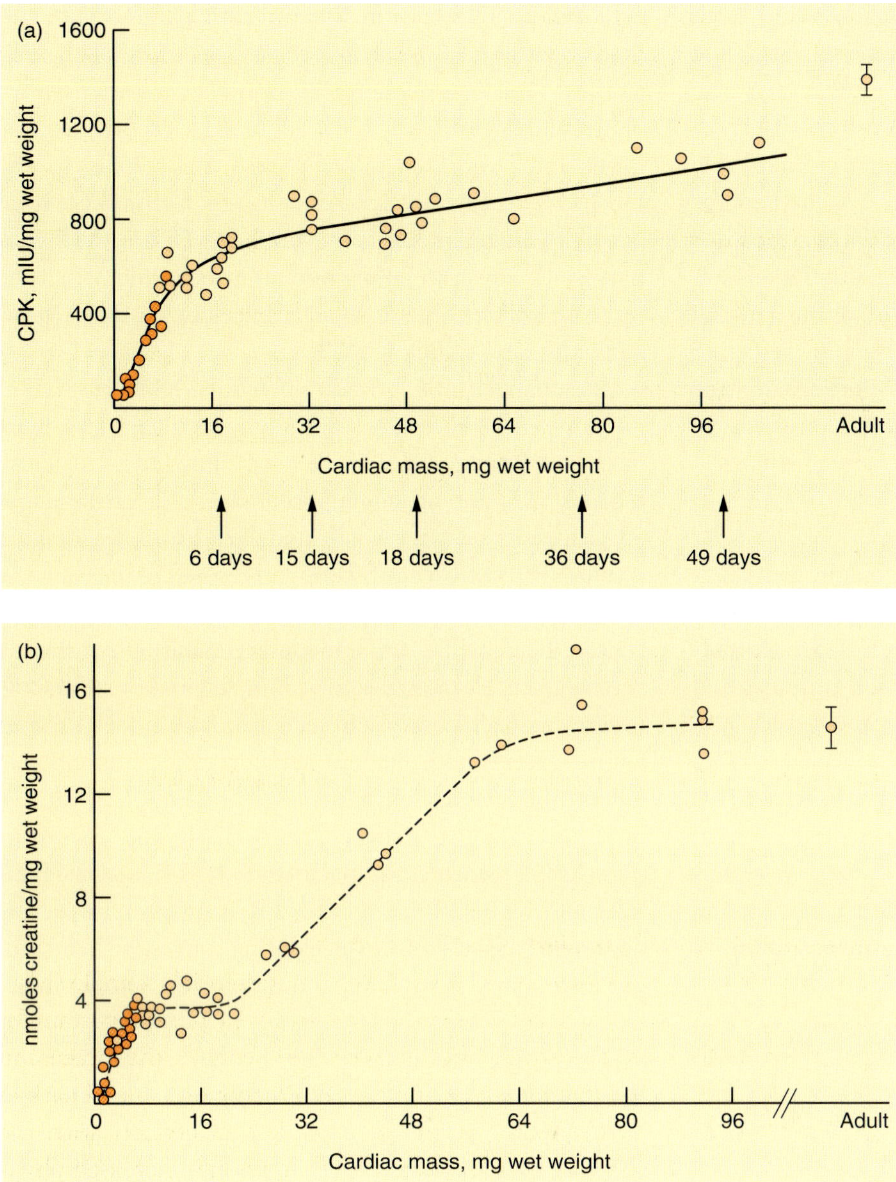


**Figure 3.4** *(a) Relationship between tissue concentration of creatine kinase expressed as milli-International Units (mIU)/mg wet weight and cardiac mass. (●) Values of hearts from 14–21-day-old fetuses; (○) values of hearts from newborn to 49 days postpartum. The average value for adult hearts (mean ± SEM for eight hearts) is also shown. Arrows indicate age of heart at various sizes. (b) Relationship between tissue creatine concentration (nmol/mg wet weight) in fetal (●), neonatal (○), and adult mouse hearts and cardiac mass. Creatine concentration is measured in total creatine, i.e. free creatine plus creatine phosphate. (Reprinted from ref. 12 with permission.)*

creatine increases about 1500-fold. This means that the capacity of this enzyme system increases about 1500-fold during this period of maturation and that, if needed to replete the ATP pool, the rate of repletion would be 1500 times faster in the adult heart than in the 16-day foetal heart.

### *Example 2: The Syrian hamster model of cardiomyopathy*

Contractile reserve is the ability of muscle to increase its contractile performance. By analogy, a useful term to describe the capacity for increased phosphoryl synthesis and supply is energy reserve. In this sense, CK is an energy reserve system because it functions to resynthesize ATP when other pathways are unable to meet demand. The relationship between contractile reserve and energy reserve has been defined in a longitudinal study of cardiomyopathy in the Syrian hamster (TO2 strain) [13]. In this study, contractile reserve was measured as the increase in isovolumic contractile performance elicited by increasing the extracellular calcium concentration in the perfusate of the intact hamster heart isolated from controls and myopathic animals at three ages. The ages corresponded to different stages of contractile dysfunction in this model of cardiomyopathy ranging from hypertrophy to severe failure. The capacity of the CK reaction was estimated as the product of $V_{max}$ of the

CK reaction times the total creatine concentration, both determined in tissue extracts made from these hearts. The relationship between the contractile reserve and the capacity is shown in Figure 3.5. The relationship for the normal heart covering the lifespan of the animal is remarkably linear. The indices for both contractile reserve and energy reserve cover a broad range of values. The data for the myopathic hearts follow the same relationship, but the range is very different. For the myopathic heart, all of the data fall in the lower left region of the graph. This result suggests that the myopathic heart has a lower capacity for regenerating ATP from PCr (and vice versa) and that the lower energy reserve correlates well with a lower contractile reserve.

*Example 3: The failing mammalian heart*

Evidence obtained using myocardium of patients with dilated cardiomyopathy also suggests that the capacity for ATP resynthesis via the CK reaction is compromised in the failing myocardium. This conclusion is based on measured decreases in both the tissue activity of CK (30–50% decrease in $V_{max}$) and the tissue content of total creatine, i.e. the sum of free creatine and PCr (60% decrease) [14, 15]. Consistent with the decrease in total creatine content, [$^{31}$P]NMR studies in the early 1990s by several groups [16–18] showed that PCr is decreased in the failing human myocardium compared with non-failing myocardium. A recent report using this technique showed that the PCr to ATP ratio is also lower in asymptomatic patients with cardiomyopathy [19]. Neubauer *et al.* suggested that the PCr to ATP ratio is a predictor of mortality in patients with dilated cardiomyopathy [20]. All of these reports describe lower ratios of PCr to ATP resonance areas in the [$^{31}$P]NMR spectrum (for example, see Figure 3.6). If, as occurs in animal models of severe heart failure, ATP content is also lower in failing human myocardium, then the decrease in PCr content would be even greater than reported by the ratio of PCr to ATP.

The changes in $V_{max}$ and the creatine pool observed in human heart failure are faithfully reproduced in animal models of heart failure. These results have been reviewed recently [21] and are summarized here. One of the major advantages of studying small animal models of heart failure is that [$^{31}$P]NMR spectroscopy can be used to measure the turnover rate of the phosphoryl group directly in the intact beating heart while simultaneously measuring contractile performance. Decreased cardiac function and/or contractile reserve has been observed in several animal models of heart failure, each with a different aetiology: the 18-month-old failing spontaneously hypertensive rat heart [22], the 10-month-old failing hamster heart [23], the rat heart 8 weeks following myocardial infarction [24], and the furazolidone-treated turkey poult [25]. Consistent with the depressed cardiac performance during congestive heart failure in humans, isovolumic contractile performance mea-

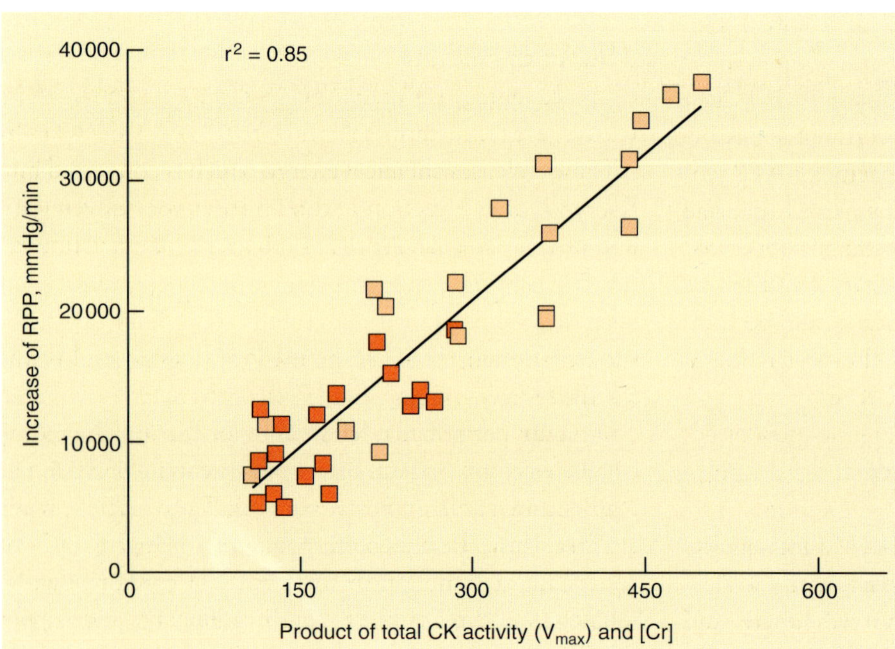


**Figure 3.5** *Relationship between predicted maximal creatine kinase (CK) reaction velocity* in vivo *and the isovolumic contractile reserve of the heart. The maximal CK reaction velocity was estimated as the product of $V_{max}$ of CK and the concentration of total creatine in the heart (x-axis). The contractile reserve is represented as the increase of the rate pressure product (RPP) in isolated isovolumic hearts by increasing total calcium concentration in the perfusate from 1.75 to 4.0 mM (y-axis). Each lightly coloured symbol stands for values obtained from one control hamster heart and each dark symbol stands for values from one cardiomyopathic hamster heart. Linear regression was performed using all data points from both control and cardiomyopathic hearts. (Reprinted from ref. 13 with permission.)*

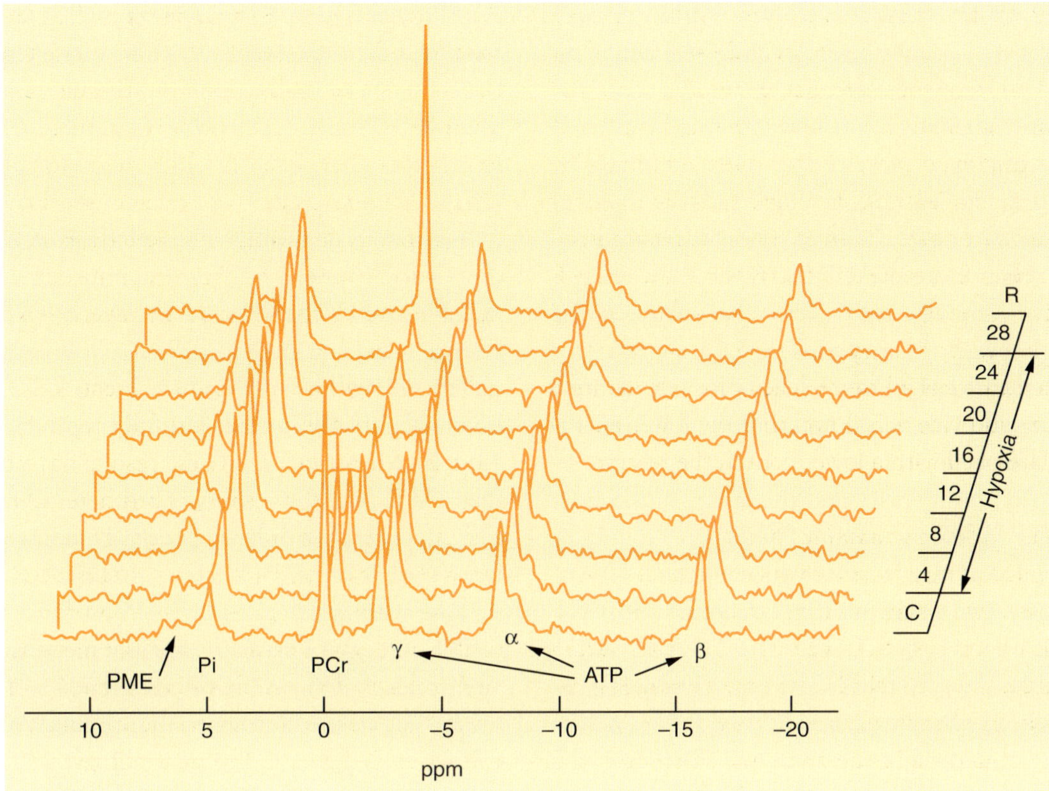


**Figure 3.6** *Representative stacks of [$^{31}$P] nuclear magnetic resonance (NMR) spectra from a rat heart subjected to hypoxic injury. Each spectrum represents 104 acquisitions obtained over a period of 4 min using a pulse angle of 45° and a recycle time of 2.18 s. The duration (min) of hypoxia is shown to the right of each panel. The first (C) and last (R) are spectra obtained from heart after 28 min of oxygenated perfusion and at the end of 30 min reoxygenation after a period of experimental injury. (Reprinted from ref. 8 with permission.)*

sured as the rate pressure product in hearts isolated from failing animals was much lower (typically 50–70% lower) than for hearts isolated from age-matched non-failing animals perfused under the same conditions of load and coronary flow. In concert with the decrease in contractile performance, the tissue content of PCr, the capacity for ATP synthesis via the CK reaction measured as tissue enzyme activity ($V_{max}$), and the rate of phosphoryl transfer measured as CK reaction velocity in the intact beating heart are all lower in the severely failing mammalian myocardium.

In conclusion, the phenotype of the failing myocardium includes large decreases in both total CK activity ($V_{max}$) and the creatine pool. These decreases are independent of species and aetiology, strongly suggesting that this is a property of failing myocardium. Decreased $V_{max}$ and PCr content combine to limit the velocity of the CK reaction and hence the capacity of the CK reaction to resynthesize ATP under conditions of severe mismatch in supply and demand.

## Defining the energetic state of the heart

### The fundamentals

Chemical energy is stored in the phosphoryl bonds of ATP. Cleavage of the terminal phosphoryl bond of ATP by ATPases releases chemical energy, which is converted into the work of contraction and relaxation, ion movements, and macromolecular synthesis (Fig. 3.1). The reaction is:

$$ATP + H_2O \rightarrow ADP + P_i + H^+$$

Chemical energy that can be used to do work in this way is called the free energy of ATP hydrolysis, ΔG.

An important principle essential for the understanding of bioenergetics is that the chemical reactions which use ATP are 'driven' by high ratios of [ATP] to [ADP], while ATP synthesis reactions are 'inhibited' by high [ATP] to [ADP] ratios. When the products of ATP hydrolysis accumulate as a result of a mismatch in demand and supply, ATPase activities are slowed and ATP synthesis pathways are stimulated. Quintessential examples of this principle are: (1) slowing of the cross-bridge cycling between actin and myosin by high concentrations of the products of ATP hydrolysis, ADP, and $P_i$ (see below for discussion); (2) inhibiting the glycolytic protein phosphofructokinase by high [ATP] and stimulation by high [ADP]; and (3) increasing the rate of oxidative phosphorylation by increasing concentrations of ADP and $P_i$. In this way, ATP and its hydrolysis products link the primary ATPases in the cell with the pathways for synthesis.

One way that the energy state of the cell can be defined is to determine the phosphorylation potential: [ATP]/[ADP $\times$ $P_i$]. This term reduces to one number the interplay between ATP availability and the ability of the end-products of ATP hydrolysis, namely ADP and $P_i$, to inhibit ATPase activities and simultaneously to stimulate ATP synthesis pathways. The phosphorylation potential in well-perfused myocardium is $> 300$ mM$^{-1}$ (ATP, ADP, and $P_i$ concentrations of about 10 mM, 30 μM, and 1 mM, respectively). Even a modest increase in ADP and $P_i$ (say, a doubling of each at essentially constant [ATP]) lowers the phosphorylation potential to about 80 mM$^{-1}$. Thus, the phosphorylation potential is a sensitive marker of the energy state of the cell. It is the critical component of the thermodynamic quantity representing the free energy of ATP hydrolysis, $\Delta G$.

The free energy of ATP hydrolysis defines the driving force for all reactions utilizing ATP in the cell for that set of conditions. It is calculated from the constant value for ATP hydrolysis under standard conditions of temperature and pressure for molar concentrations of reactants, $\Delta G°$, corrected for the actual concentrations of ATP, ADP, and $P_i$ in the cytosol. The expression is:

$$\Delta G = \Delta G° - RT \ln [\mathrm{ATP}]/[\mathrm{ADP}][\mathrm{P_i}],$$

where $\Delta G°$ is the standard free energy change of ATP hydrolysis ($-30.5$ kJ/mole under standard conditions of molarity, temperature, pH, and $Mg^{2+}$), $R$ is the gas constant (8.3 J/mol·K), and $T$ is the absolute temperature in Kelvin. The argument of the ln term is the phosphorylation potential. The value of $\Delta G$ for pyruvate or blood-perfused rodent heart is $-65$ kJ/mole; for a glucose-perfused heart working under the same load, $\Delta G$ becomes less negative, $-58$ kJ/mole, because the ADP and $P_i$ concentrations are higher. The less negative value means that the glucose-only perfused heart has a lower driving force for reactions utilizing ATP (the value is closer to zero). Notice that the values of the two terms in the equation ($\Delta G°$ and the ln term) are about the same; thus, to change $\Delta G$, there must be a large change in the ln term. Because it is often confusing to describe changes for a negative number, it is convenient to describe changes in $\Delta G$ in terms of its absolute value, $|\Delta G|$.

In order to determine whether there in a high enough driving force for the ATP-utilizing reactions, the values of $\Delta G$ obtained for the whole heart are compared with the literature values for $\Delta G$ for the actomyosin ATPase and the sodium and calcium pumps. Values of $|\Delta G|$ for the ATPases calculated under well-controlled conditions are about 52, 48, and 46 kJ/mole for the calcium, sodium, and the myofibrillar ATPases, respectively. Thus, even a heart perfused with glucose as its only exogenous carbon source for ATP synthesis has a $|\Delta G|$ (58 kJ/mole) sufficient to drive these ATPase reactions.

The concept of driving force is analogous to how a battery works. As long as the voltage is high enough to turn on the flashlight, the flashlight will turn on. With time, as the voltage runs down and becomes close to threshold, there is a brown-out. When the voltage falls below the threshold necessary to turn on the light, it will not turn on. Thus the sign (+, 0, or −) of $\Delta G$ determines the direction of the reaction or, in the case of the battery and of the ATPases, whether they function or not. One other point is instructive. New batteries have more voltage than batteries nearing the threshold value for turning on the flashlight. The flashlight turns on for both conditions, but the new batteries have more energy reserve. For biological studies, the difference between the $\Delta G$ for ATP hydrolysis measured for the tissue and the literature values for the $\Delta G$ needed to run the ATPase are referred to as the driving force for the reaction or the energy reserve. Evaluating the energy reserve of the heart can be useful for understanding metabolic events and ion movements in the cell.

## How does the cell maintain a high phosphorylation potential?

The answer comes from the integration of pathways for ATP synthesis with each other and also from the integration of the pathways for ATP utilization and synthesis. One of the major ways in which the myocyte maintains high values for the phosphorylation potential is via the CK reaction. While rapidly resynthesizing ATP by transferring a phosphoryl group from PCr to ADP, it functions to keep [ADP] low. Good examples of how the near ablation of CK activity leads to failure to keep [ADP] low are given both when CK activity was reduced by more than 95% acutely by inhibiting CK with sulfhydryl group modifiers [26] and when CK activity was reduced to less than 3% of normal by genetic manipulation [26].

Although the equilibrium position for the reaction is far to the right (i.e. in the direction of ATP synthesis), the CK reaction is reversible. The mitochondrial CK isoenzyme, in particular, functions in the reverse direction to synthesize PCr. In this way the reaction also keeps the $P_i$ concentration low. The coupling of the CK reaction and ATP hydrolysis can be formally written as:

$$\begin{array}{lcl} \mathrm{ATP} + \mathrm{H_2O} & \rightarrow & \mathrm{ADP} + \mathrm{P_i} + \mathrm{H^+} \\ \mathrm{PCr} + \mathrm{ADP} + \mathrm{H^+} & \rightarrow & \mathrm{Creatine} + \mathrm{ATP} \\ \hline \mathrm{Sum{:}\ PCr} & \rightarrow & \mathrm{Creatine} + \mathrm{P_i} \end{array}$$

The time-dependent changes in ATP, PCr, and $P_i$ during hypoxia illustrate this chemistry. The set of NMR spectra in Figure 3.7 show the fall in the PCr resonance area with the concomitant rise in $P_i$. The net transfer of the phosphoryl group from PCr to ATP in this case of profound mismatch in supply and demand is a classic example of using PCr to slow the rate of ATP depletion.

The CK reaction has more formal uses as well. Because [$^{31}$P]NMR spectroscopy provides values of PCr, ATP, and $H^+$ contents, rearranging the CK equilibrium expression provides a good estimate for the cytosolic or free ADP concentration. (Note that measurements using extracts of myocardial tissue, even those rapidly frozen and stored in liquid $N_2$, do not yield useful values for cytosolic [ADP] or [$P_i$]. In the case of ADP, this is because ADP is bound to each actin monomer as well as to other macromolecules. In the case of $P_i$, this is because it is difficult to prevent some hydrolysis of PCr while freezing tissue and extracting metabolites for biochemical assay.) In addition to values obtained from the [$^{31}$P]NMR spectrum, it is necessary to know the total (or free) creatine concentration and this is relatively easy to obtain in tissue samples:

$$[\mathrm{ADP}] = \frac{[\mathrm{ATP}][\mathrm{Free\ Cr}]}{[\mathrm{PCr}][\mathrm{H^+}]1.66 \times 10^9}$$

Thus, [$^{31}$P]NMR spectroscopy provides all of the critical input values for calculating $\Delta G$ and comparing it with known values for the primary ATPases in the cell. With this tool, one can at least begin to assess the relationships among [ATP], the products of ATP hydrolysis, ADP and $P_i$, $\Delta G$ and contractile function. Examples of some recent work in this area are summarized below.

***Example 1: Energy reserve and contractile performance***

The role of CK as an energy reserve system is clearly shown for the ATP supply–demand mismatch that occurs in hypoxia and ischaemia when phosphoryl transfer from PCr to ADP slows the rate of tissue ATP depletion (such as shown in Figure 3.7). Experiments conducted during the 1990s established a link between energy reserve and contractile reserve in the setting of contractile performance. The link has been shown in three types of experiment designed to perturb selectively the CK reaction in intact striated muscle. First, acute and selective chemical inhibition of CK activity in intact rat hearts with sulphydryl group modifiers, including iodoacetamide [27, 28] and an exogenously supplied NO donor [29], resulted in decreased contractile reserve when the heart was inotropically stressed with either high extracellular [$Ca^{2+}$] or norepinephrine. Secondly, in rat and turkey hearts in which the myocardial PCr pool was replaced with a poorly hydrolysable creatine analogue, β-guanidinopropionic, PCr content, CK reaction velocity, and heart function all decreased under high workload conditions [25, 30]. Thirdly, depleting muscle CK by transgenic technology reduced the ability of skeletal muscle to sustain burst work [31]. No comparable test of burst work has been made for the hearts of these animals (but see ref. 26).

Each of these experiments showed that decreasing energy reserve via the CK reaction limits the ability of striated muscle to recruit its contractile reserve. Moreover, the perturbations which result in chronic impairment of CK activity, such as the muscle CK knockout, can, depending on the muscle type, elicit compensatory changes in other pathways of ATP synthesis. Most notably, glycolytic capacity and the fractional cell volume of mitochondria increased in fast twitch skeletal muscle of the M-CK knockout mouse [31]. These results illustrate the important principle that ATP synthesis occurs by the integration of all ATP-synthesizing pathways. When one pathway is diminished or eliminated (in this case the CK reaction in fast twitch skeletal muscle), compensatory increases occur in the others. The biochemical remodelling of the skeletal muscle cell also emphasizes the importance of the CK reaction for phosphoryl transfer.

The characteristics of the relationship between energy reserve and contractile reserve for hearts with acutely inhibited CK provide several lessons in terms of energetics. The free energy of ATP hydrolysis using [$^{31}$P]NMR spectroscopy

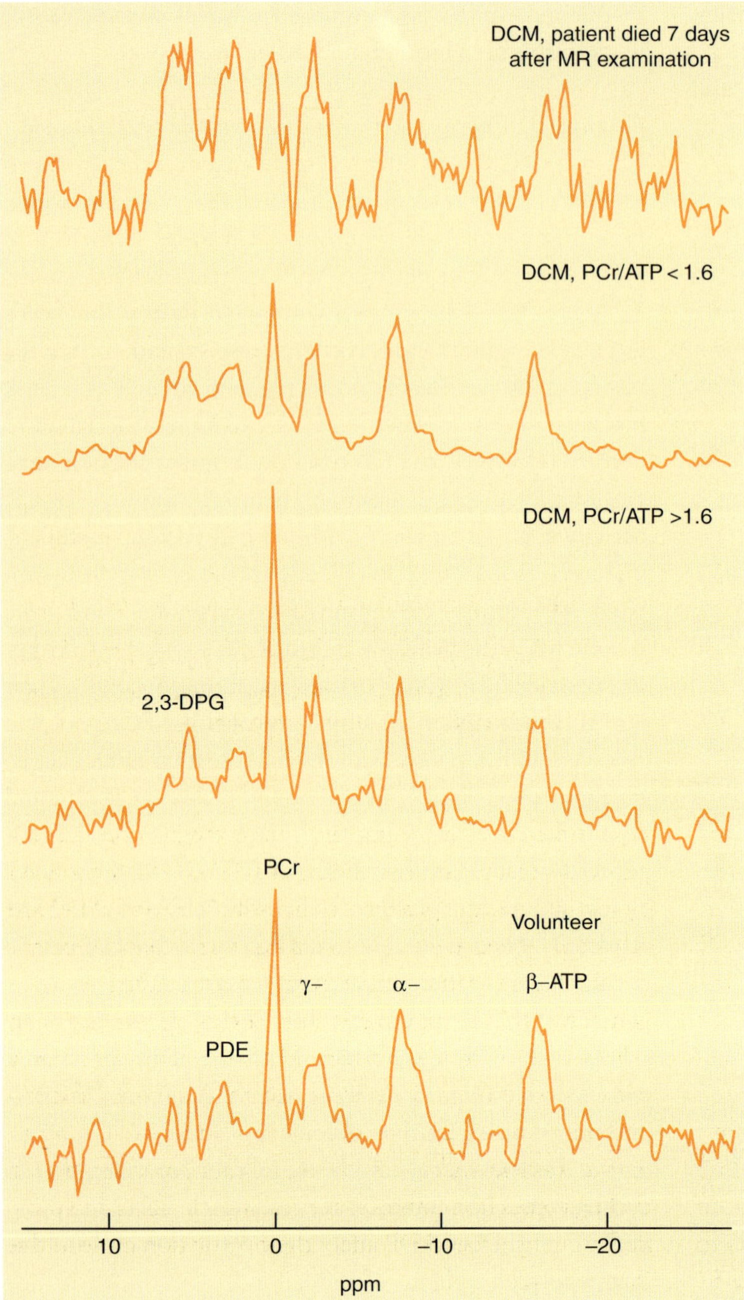


**Figure 3.7** *Cardiac [$^{31}$P]nuclear magnetic resonance (NMR) spectra of human hearts. From bottom to top: spectra from volunteer, patients with dilated cardiomyopathy (DCM) with normal phosphocreatine/ATP ratio, reduced phosphocreatine/ATP ratio, and severely reduced phosphocreatine/ATP ratio; the latter patient died 7 days after the NMR examination. PDE, phosphodiesters; PCr, phosphocreatine; and γ-, α-, and β-phosphates of ATP. (Reprinted from ref. 20 with permission.)*

and isovolumic contractile performance were measured in isolated rat hearts challenged to perform high work by increasing perfusate [$Ca^{2+}$] before and after supplying iodoacetamide to inhibit CK activity [27]. Figure 3.8 shows the linear fits of the relationship between isovolumic contractile performance assessed as the rate–pressure product (RPP) and $|\Delta G|$ for normal hearts with 100% CK activity and hearts with only about 1% CK activity. Also shown on the *x*-axis are literature values for $|\Delta G|$ determined for the primary ATPases of the cell, namely myosin, the sodium pump, and the calcium pump. Four points can be made. (1) At low workloads, CK-inhibited hearts operate at a lower $|\Delta G|$. This means that the CK-inhibited hearts have less free energy available for ATP hydrolysis. The difference between 59 kJ/mole for control hearts and 57 kJ/mole for CK-inhibited hearts is due to changes in the size of the metabolite pool: ATP levels fell from 11 to 10 mM, ADP increased from 60 to 110 μM, while $P_i$ remained about the same (about 6 mM). Thus, the ATP/ADP ratio fell from 192 to 90 and ATP/[ADP × $P_i$] fell from 32 to 15 $mM^{-1}$.

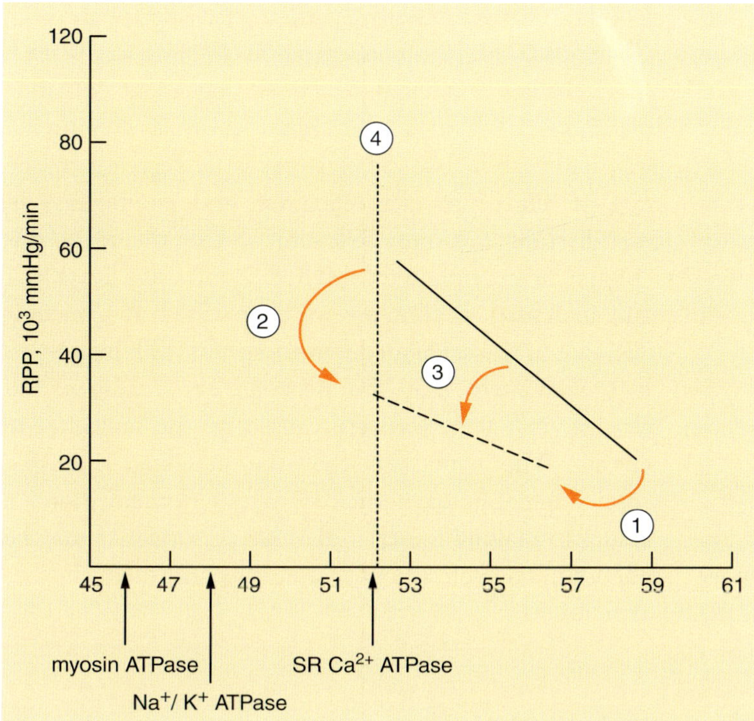


**Figure 3.8** *Relationship between rate pressure product (RPP) ($10^3$ mmHg/min) and the absolute value of the free energy release from ATP hydrolysis (kJ/mol) for hearts with 100% (solid line) and 1% (dashed line) creatine kinase activity. (Reprinted from ref. 21 with permission.)*

(2) The increase in RPP in CK-inhibited hearts for the equivalent challenge was much less than for normal hearts. Thus, reducing energy reserve by selectively inhibiting CK activity limits the contractile reserve of the heart. (3) The decrease in the slope of the RPP–ΔG relation for the CK-inhibited hearts compared with normal hearts shows that there is a large expenditure of free energy for a small change in RPP. There is less work output in CK-inhibited hearts for a similar energy expenditure. (4) For both normal and CK-inhibited hearts, essentially no data points fell beyond the value for $|\Delta G|$ for the calcium ATPase. At least under these conditions, there appears to be a limiting threshold. If the $|\Delta G|$ were to fall below 52 kJ/mole, the hearts would suffer calcium overload. If this interpretation is supported by other experiments, it would provide a rational basis for the link between energy starvation (or at least an energy limitation) and abnormal ion homoeostasis which would have significant implications for the failing heart.

### *Example 2: ADP and diastolic function*

Muscle contraction and relaxation are determined by the cyclic interaction between myosin and actin. The cross-bridge cycle is the story of protein–protein interaction and the hydrolysis of ATP. In the absence of ATP, actin and myosin form a strong complex. This protein–protein complex is dissociated by the binding of ATP. ATP is hydrolysed by myosin and the products of hydrolysis, $P_i$ and ADP, are released sequentially. $P_i$ is released when the conformational change in the actomyosin occurs, leading to force generation. ADP is released after the power stroke. The release of ADP from the purine-binding site on the myosin head allows ATP to bind, dissociating the actomyosin complex and allowing for subsequent cross-bridge cycling. Most of the understanding of the regulation of cross-bridge cycling comes from work on skeletal muscle fibers and purified proteins. Does ADP affect the contraction cycle in the intact heart?

Recently, Tian *et al.* devised strategies to manipulate free [ADP] in whole heart preparation without substantially altering any of the other known regulators of contraction, namely ATP, $P_i$, $H^+$ or $Ca^{2+}$, and the rate of glycolysis [10, 32]. In the normal heart, this was accomplished by inhibiting CK to varying degrees, thereby altering cytosolic [ADP]. In the hypertrophied/failing heart, the changes were the result of the adaptation (or maladaptation) in the CK system to hypertrophy. In both settings, a relationship between increased left ventricular end-diastolic pressure and increased [ADP] was found. The relationship is dose dependent (Fig. 3.9).

Taken together, these two studies demonstrate that increases in the average cytosolic ADP concentration in the absence of changes in any of the other known regulators of myofilament function are sufficient to slow cross-bridge cycling and impair diastolic function. In most settings, however, changes in [ADP] do not happen in isolation and many of the known regulators of cross-bridge cycling and responsiveness to the amplitude of the Ca transient change simultaneously. One of these will be described below.

***Example 3: Diastolic dysfunction and energetics in a mouse model of familial hypertrophic cardiomyopathy***

A mouse model of familial hypertrophic cardiomyopathy bearing the α-myosin heavy chain $(\alpha\text{-MHC})^{403/+}$ mutation has been successfully developed by the Seidman laboratory [33]. Mice homozygous for this mutation die in the first week of life, but the heterozygous mouse has a normal lifespan and can be studied. This single amino-acid replacement in the myosin head near to the actin binding loop is known to slow the rate of cross-bridge cycling. One important question is: what are the consequences of this mutation for the contractile properties of the intact heart? Using $[^{31}P]$NMR spectroscopy to study hearts isolated and perfused in the isovolumic mode, Spindler *et al.* [34] found no changes in systolic performance when hearts were challenged with high concentrations of calcium. Instead, these hearts exhibited workload-dependent diastolic dysfunction. Workload-dependent diastolic dysfunction was manifest in two different ways: a decrease in the rate of left ventricular relaxation and an increase in end-diastolic pressure. Relevant to the theme of this chapter, hearts from the $\alpha\text{-MHC}^{403/+}$ mice had lower PCr and increased $P_i$ contents which resulted in a modest decrease in the calculated free energy for ATP hydrolysis. It seems likely that the diastolic abnormalities and changes in energetics were caused by the mutation in myosin. The hypothesis that the increased energetic cost of maintaining normal systolic performance and a failure to maintain normal diastolic performance may be important characteristics of cardiomyopathy merits further exploration.

## Acknowledgements

The work summarized here from the author's laboratory had many contributors, four of whom merit particular acknowledgement: Drs Marianna Bak, Kurt Saupe, Matthias Spindler, and Rong Tian.

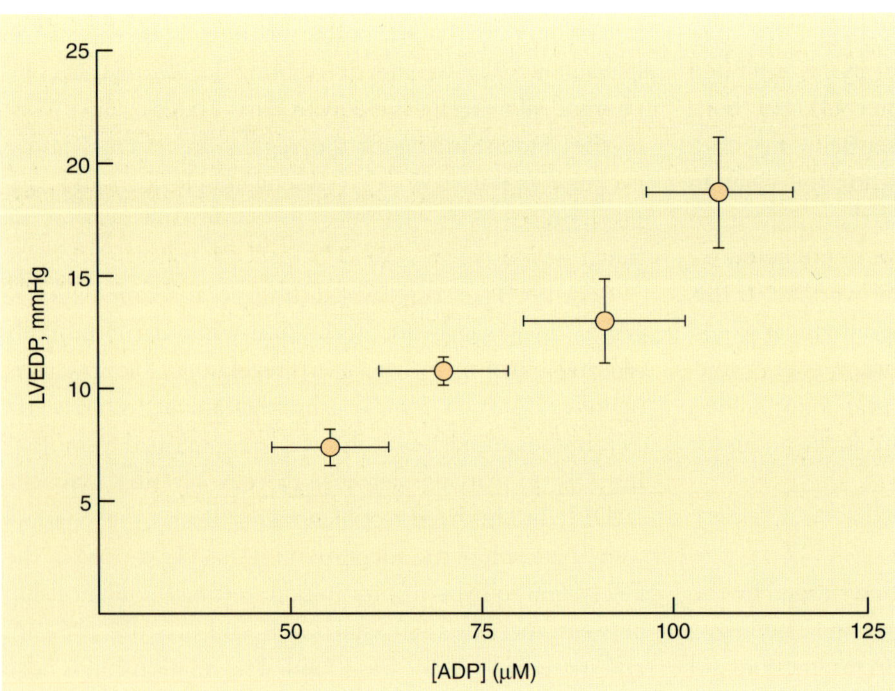


**Figure 3.9** *Relationship between the increase in [MgADP] and the increase in left ventricular end-diastolic pressure (LVEDP) using data collected from four groups of hearts treated with 0, 30, 90, or 120 mM iodo-acetamide. Data are shown as mean ± SEM. (Reprinted from ref. 10 with permission.)*

## References


1. Lewandowski ED, Ingwall JS. The physiological chemistry of energy production in the heart. In: Schlant RC, Alexander RW (eds) *The heart*. 8th edition. New York: McGraw-Hill, 1994, 153.
2. Bak MI, Ingwall JS. Regulation of cardiac AMP-specific 5′-nucleotidase during ischaemia mediates ATP resynthesis on reflow. *Am J Physiol* 1998; 274: C992–1001.
3. Zimmer H-G, Trendelenburg C, Kammermeier H, Gerlach E. *De novo* synthesis of myocardial adenine nucleotides in the rat. *Circ Res* 1973; 32: 635–42.
4. Skladanowski AC, Newby AC. Partial purification and properties of an AMP-specific soluble 5′-nucleotidase from pigeon heart. *Biochem J* 1990; 268: 117–22.
5. Truong LV, Collinson AR, Lowenstein JM. 5′-Nucleotidases in rat heart. *Biochem J* 1988; 253: 117–22.
6. Darvish A, Metting PJ. Purification and regulation of an AMP-specific cytosolic 5′-nucleotidase from dog heart. *Am J Physiol* 1993; 264: H1528–34.
7. Skladanowski AC, Smolenski RT, Tavenier M *et al.* Soluble forms of 5′-nucleotidase in rat and human heart. *Am J Physiol* 1996; 270: H1493–500.
8. Bak MI, Ingwall JS. Acidosis during ischaemia promotes adenosine triphosphate resynthesis in postischemic rat heart. *In vivo* regulation of 5′-nucleotidase. *J Clin Invest* 1994; 93: 40–9.
9. Bittl JA, Ingwall JS. Reaction rates of creatine kinase and ATP synthesis in the isolated rat heart: a $^{31}$P NMR magnetization transfer study. *J Biol Chem* 1985; 260: 3512–17.
10. Tian R, Christe ME, Spindler M *et al.* Role of MgADP in the development of diastolic dysfunction in the intact beating rat heart. *J Clin Invest* 1997; 99: 745–51.
11. Goodwin GW, Ahmad F, Taegtmeyer H. Preferential oxidation of glycogen in isolated working rat heart. *J Clin Invest* 1996; 97: 1409–16.
12. Ingwall JS. Developmental regulation of creatine kinase. In: Jacobus WE, Ingwall JS (eds) *Heart creatine kinase: the integration of isozymes for energy distribution*. Baltimore, MD: Williams and Wilkins, 1980.
13. Tian R, Nascimben L, Kaddurah-Daouck R, Ingwall JS. Depletion of energy reserve via the creatine kinase reaction during the evolution of heart failure in cardiomyopathic hamsters. *J Mol Cell Cardiol* 1996; 28: 755–65.
14. Ingwall JS, Kramer MF, Fifer MA *et al.* The creatine kinase system in normal and diseased human myocardium. *N Engl J Med* 1985; 313: 1050–4.
15. Nascimben L, Ingwall JS, Pauletto P *et al.* The creatine kinase system in failing and nonfailing human myocardium. *Circulation* 1996; 94: 1894–901.
16. Conway MA, Allis J, Ouwerkerk R *et al.* Detection of low phosphocreatine to ATP ratio in failing hypertrophied human myocardium by $^{31}$P magnetic resonance spectroscopy. *Lancet* 1991; 338: 973–6.
17. Hardy CJ, Weiss RG, Bottomley PA, Gerstenblith G. Altered myocardial high-energy phosphate metabolites in patients with dilated cardiomyopathy. *Am Heart J* 1991; 122: 795–801.
18. Neubauer S, Krahe T, Schindler R *et al.* $^{31}$P Magnetic resonance spectroscopy in dilated cardiomyopathy and coronary artery disease. Altered cardiac high energy phosphate metabolism in heart failure. *Circulation* 1992; 86: 1810–18.
19. Jung W-I, Sieverding L, Breuer J *et al.* $^{31}$P NMR spectroscopy detects metabolic abnormalities in asymptomatic patients with hypertrophic cardiomyopathy. *Circulation* 1998; 97: 2536–42.
20. Neubauer S, Horn M, Cramer M *et al.* Myocardial phosphocreatine to ATP ratio is a predictor of mortality in patients with dilated cardiomyopathy. *Circulation* 1997; 96: 2190–6.
21. Ingwall JS. Energetics of the normal and failing human heart: focus on the creatine kinase reaction. *Adv Organ Biol* 1998; 4A: 117–41.
22. Bittl JA, Ingwall JS. Intracellular high-energy phosphate transfer in normal and hypertrophied myocardium. *Circulation* 1987; 75 Suppl 1: I-96–101.
23. Nascimben L, Friedrich J, Liao R *et al.* Enalapril treatment increases cardiac performance and energy reserve via the creatine kinase reaction in myocardium of Syrian myopathic hamsters with advanced heart failure. *Circulation* 1995; 91: 1824–33.
24. Neubauer S, Horn M, Naumann A *et al.* Impairmant of energy metabolism in intact residual myocardium of rat hearts with chronic myocardial infarction. *J Clin Invest* 1995; 95: 1092–100.
25. Liao R, Nascimben L, Friedrich J *et al.* Decreased energy reserve in an animal model of dilated cardiomyopathy. Relationship to contractile performance. *Circ Res* 1996; 78: 893–902.
26. Saupe K, Spindler M, Tian R, Ingwall JS. Impaired cardiac energetics in mice lacking muscle-specific isoenzymes of creatine kinase. *Circ Res* 1998; 82: 898–907.
27. Tian R, Ingwall JS. Energetic basis for reduced contractile reserve in isolated rat hearts. *Am J Physiol* 1996; 270: H1207–16.
28. Hamman BL, Bittl JA, Jacobus WE *et al.* Inhibition of creatine kinase reaction decreases the contractile reserve of isolated rat hearts. *Am J Physiol* 1995; 269: H030–6.
29. Gross WL, Bak MI, Ingwall JS *et al.* Nitric oxide inhibits creatine kinase and regulates rat heart contractile reserve. *Proc Natl Acad Sci USA* 1996; 931: 5604–9.
30. Zwier JL, Jacobus WE, Korecky B, Brandeis-Barry Y. Bioenergetic consequences of cardiac phosphocreatine depletion induced by creatine analog deficiency. *J Biol Chem* 1991; 266: 20 296–304.
31. van Deursen J, Heerschap A, Oerlemans F *et al.* Skeletal muscles of mice deficient in muscle creatine kinase lack burst activity. *Cell* 1993; 74: 621–31.
32. Tian R, Nascimben L, Ingwall JS, Lorell BH. Failure to maintain a low ADP concentration impairs diastolic function in hypertrophied rat hearts. *Circulation* 1997; 96: 1313–19.
33. Geisterfer-Lowrance AAT, Christe M, Conner DA *et al.* A mouse model of familial hypertrophic cardiomyopathy. *Science* 1996; 272: 731–4.
34. Spindler M, Saupe KW, Christe ME *et al.* Diastolic dysfunction and altered energetics in the $\alpha MHC^{403/+}$ mouse model of familial hypertrophic cardiomyopathy. *J Clin Invest* 1998; 101: 1775–83.

# Transcriptional circuits mediating cardiac hypertrophy and heart failure 4

M. ABDELLATIF AND M. D. SCHNEIDER

## Introduction

In the context of the present volume on hypertrophy, heart failure, and cardiomyopathies, this chapter on transcription factors that govern heart muscle sets out to answer the following specific questions: What is meant by the 'hypertrophic phenotype', beyond just hypertrophic growth itself? How does the workload encountered by the heart lead to long-term changes in cardiac structure and performance? More precisely, what proteins within the cell relay a signal to the nucleus as a consequence of mechanical load, and what proteins within the nucleus provide the strongest explanations, at present, coupling load to growth and altered gene expression? Do proteins that control cardiac gene expression during normal heart formation also play a role in disease states by modulating the expression of cardiac structural genes?

Beginning in the late 1980s [1–6] and continuing to this day [7–9], the identification of specific changes in cardiac gene expression during hypertrophy and failure that might plausibly alter cardiac mechanical performance or the potential predisposition to arrhythmias has given rise to two fundamental questions, each with straightforward clinical implications. First, what are the *actual* consequences of altered cardiac gene expression, as measured by mechanical performance, susceptibility to sudden death, and other clinically pertinent endpoints? The emphasis here is to distinguish beneficial, homoeostatic responses from adverse, pathogenic ones (with recognition that some adaptations might prove to be a proverbial 'double-edged sword'). Secondly, what *gene-specific* or *hierarchical* mechanisms operate to create these individual alterations or the 'fetal/hypertrophic' phenotype more generally? The impetus here is a search for the signalling pathways that actually couple workload to long-term adaptations, both as an especially intriguing problem in its own right and as a source of novel targets for possible therapeutic interventions. In both instances, the overall strategy within the field has been by solving Koch's postulates, testing cause–effect relationships through a combination of physiological, pharmacological, and genetic methods. These genetic approaches are divided, in essence, between 'gain-of-function' mutations (increasing a protein's expression or activity) and their mirror image, 'loss-of-function' or 'dominant-negative' mutations (blocking a protein's expression or interfering with its activity, respectively).

## What responses comprise the 'hypertrophic phenotype'?

It is axiomatic that compensatory cardiac growth triggered by an increase in workload — systemic or pulmonary hypertension, aortic coarctation, outflow tract obstruction, aortic or pulmonic stenosis, or wall stress due, instead, to the loss of pump function following infarction — occurs predominantly through an increase in the size of cardiac myocytes (hypertrophy). Familial cardiac hypertrophy, while ultimately attributable to mutations in various sarcomeric proteins, results, more proximally, from an analogous increase in wall stress, owing to altered sarcomeric protein function [10–14].

Although claims exist for an increase in cardiac cell number (hyperplasia) as well, during load-induced cardiac growth such evidence is controversial [15, 16] and criteria to support these claims sometimes are used indiscriminately. For example, it has been long recognized that a parallel increase in DNA content per cell can accompany severe hypertrophy, but neither an increase in DNA synthesis, nor an increase in ploidy, nor nuclear division should be mistaken for cell proliferation. Indeed, the polyploid and multinucleated status of even normal adult ventricular myocytes distinguishes these from most other cell types. Likewise, chromatin condensation, potentially resembling that which takes place in the course of mitotic cell division, is a conspicuous hallmark of programmed cell death (apoptosis), a mechanism for cell demise which is recognized increasingly as a component of heart failure in animal models [17, 18] and humans [19, 20]. By contrast, at least thus far, there is little or no evidence to suggest that mitosis-specific cell-cycle regulators, or mitosis-specific protein phosphorylations — the biochemical signature of mitosis — reappear in failing hearts. Given this barrier to the creation of new daughter cells, regardless of whether the block is absolute or merely daunting, the mechanical performance of the myocardium in disease states is determined by modulatory changes in the intrinsic contractile properties of the existing cardiac myocytes, together with extrinsic mechanical factors such as chamber geometry and interstitial fibrosis. Moreover, given this constraint, ongoing cell loss via apoptosis, even at modest absolute rates, has been deemed likely to contribute, over time, to worsening pump function.

How might changes in intrinsic myocyte performance come about? Superimposed on the global increase in RNA and protein content per cell is a characteristic set of changes in levels of expression of particular cardiac genes,

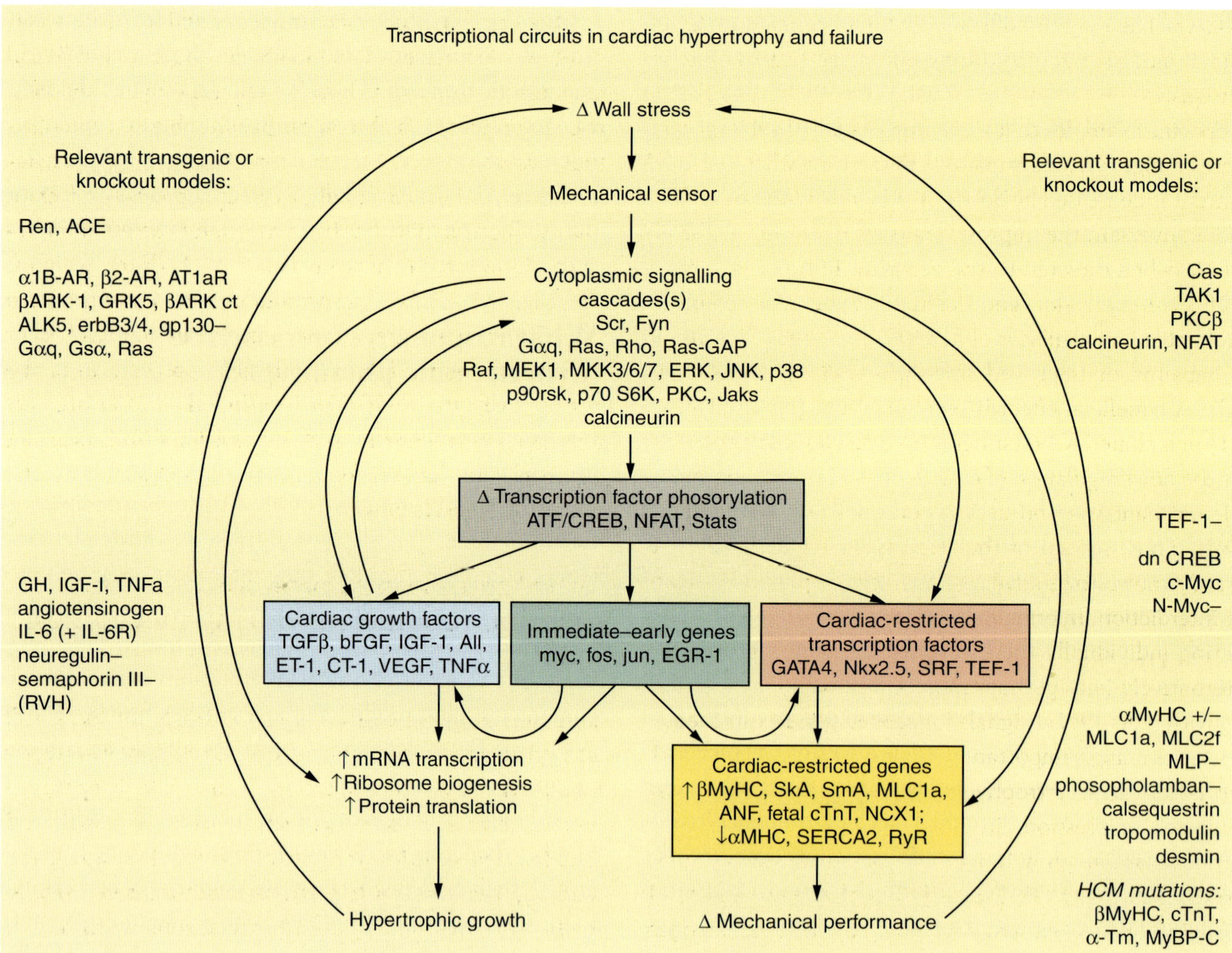


**Figure 4.1** *Schematic representation of signalling events in pressure-overload-induced hypertrophy. Hierarchical mechanisms that have been invoked to explain the regulation of multiple cardiac genes in tandem, by cardiac agonists, passive stretch, or load* in vivo *include at least four sets of transcriptional pathways: immediate-early gene induction, upregulation of cardiac-restricted transcription factors (or their coactivators), phosphorylation or dephosphorylation of transcription factors, and phosphorylation of RNA polymerase II itself. Relevant genetic models at each level of the signalling cascade are shown at the left- and right-hand margins of the figure.*

including sarcomeric proteins and regulators of calcium handling, often referred to, with some oversimplification, as a generalized 'fetal' phenotype (Fig. 4.1). This term derives from the fact that the best-known examples of the phenomenon encode proteins such as atrial natriuretic factor (ANF), and contractile protein isoforms that are highly expressed in the developing ventricle are expressed at lower (often negligible) levels in normal adult ventricles and are reinduced by a haemodynamic burden. Other examples include β-myosin heavy chains (β-MHC), the atrial isoform of myosin light chain-1 ($MLC_{1a}$), and the skeletal isoform of sarcomeric α-actin (SkA). Concurrently, several genes that are normally expressed at higher levels in adult than embryonic ventricles are downregulated, including α-MHC and the sarcoplasmic reticulum calcium 'pump', SRCA2. The majority of such changes occurs not only in animal models, but also during end-stage heart failure in humans.

Specific examples that assert the physiological impact of these changes include impaired contractility when α-MHC content is decreased by deleting one copy of the gene [21] and, conversely, the improved contractility resulting from $MLC_{1a}$ when directed to the ventricle in transgenic mice [22]. Overexpression and deletion of the gene for phospholamban, an inhibitor of SRCA2 pump function, result in impaired or improved calcium handling, respectively [23]. A beneficial effect is seen when exogenous SRCA2 [21] or a cloned $K^+$ channel [24] is delivered, to counteract the downregulation of endogenous proteins, improving calcium handling and action potential duration, respectively. Thus, several of the responses in hypertrophy are already known to be adverse, and might be plausible targets for interdiction. In principle, this might be achieved by correcting individually the levels of each gene's protein or, alternatively (and perhaps more attractively), by interfering with hierarchical signals for altered gene expression.

One seemingly important aspect to this plasticity of gene expression in hypertrophy and failure is the dramatically increased expression in the ventricle of numerous intramyocardial growth factors, including transforming growth factor-beta (TGF-β) [7], fibroblast growth factor-1 [25], insulin-like growth factor-1 [26], angiotensinogen [27] (along with increased expression of angiotensin-converting enzyme [28], enabling the formation of angiotensin-II), endothelin-1 [29], and cardiotropin-1 [30]. An early clue suggesting the operation of autocrine/paracrine mechanisms in myocardial hypertrophy was the finding that each of these can act on cardiac myocytes directly, most triggering the same changes in gene expression as does mechanical load itself [31–34; cf. 35]. As an illustration of the extensive cross-talk among these pathways, TGF-β is upregulated not only by aortic banding and passive mechanical stretch, but also by α-adrenergic agonists and angiotensin II. Some researchers have offered a contrasting interpretation of such cell-culture studies, indicating that some growth factor effects might be indirect, via the induction of a secondary factor in the cardiac fibroblasts [36, 37]. In either event, individual peptide growth factors initiate the array of responses in gene expression seen in hypertrophy, providing concrete evidence that simple signals can activate much, if not all, of the 'fetal' gene programme.

There are other potential modes of action. First, several of the factors cited immediately above (TGF-β and angiotensin II, most obviously) act not only on the ventricular myocyte but also on cardiac fibroblasts, promoting their proliferation, the production of excessive extracellular matrix, or both. Secondly, a direct depressant effect on myocyte contractility has been shown for the inflammatory cytokine tumour necrosis factor-α (TNF-α), which is upregulated in diseased myocardium [8] and is sufficient to cause heart failure after chronic infusion in humans [38] or in transgenic mice [18, 39]. Finally, upregulation of the angiogenic factor VEGF (Vascular Endothelial Growth Factor), as seen in hypertrophied myocardium [40], provides a possible mechanism for adjusting blood supply to the increase in muscle mass.

## What cytoplasmic proteins relay the signal to the nucleus during mechanical load?

The clinical evidence that argues strongly for local wall stress, rather than systemic factors, as the principal trigger for hypertrophy, is the exquisitely local, spatially appropriate, chamber-specific concordance between growth and load (e.g. left ventricular hypertrophy with left ventricular load, right ventricular hypertrophy with right ventricular load). This supposition has drawn vast support both from ingenious whole-animal experiments [41] and from the susceptibility of cardiac myocytes to passive mechanical stress when grown on stretchable membranes [42–44]. The nature of the actual mechanical sensor remains conjectural, although recent investigations point to the possibility of integrins, integrin-associated proteins, and functionally analogous proteins that mediate cell-to-cell attachments or cell-to-extracellular matrix attachments [45].

By comparison, a potentially bewildering array of intracellular signal-transducing proteins has been implicated in one or more aspects of hypertrophy, each, to varying degrees, depending on the particular candidate mediator. These include guanosine triphosphate (GTP)-binding proteins and their regulators [17, 46–54], as well as many protein kinases, especially serine/threonine kinases of the protein kinase C [55–57] and mitogen-activated protein kinase (MAPK) superfamilies, among them, in the latter case, ERK, JNK, and p38 [58–61]. More recently, src-like tyrosine kinases have been suggested to play a role in mechanical signalling as well [62–64]. Intriguing, albeit controversial, results have been reported for the calcium-dependent protein phosphatase, calcineurin [65–66]. Phosphatidylinositol-3-kinase has been implicated in cardiac signal transduction downstream of the Ras protein [46, 52, 67] as well as downstream of the cytokine receptor gp130 [68]. However, several lines of evidence indicate that distinguishable intracellular pathways mediate the global increase in myocyte mass versus upregulation of the characteristic fetal or hypertrophic programme [34, 47, 48], as will be detailed subsequently.

A detailed discussion of evidence regarding each of these would exceed the scope of the present chapter, and representative articles are cited. However, several of the mechanisms enumerated above act directly to phosphorylate or dephosphorylate particular transcription factors, as discussed below.

## What transcription factors mediate gene regulation in hypertrophy?

Perhaps the earliest transcriptional mechanism invoked to explain hypertrophic growth was the finding that immediate-early genes such as *fos*, *jun*, and *myc* — transcription factors that appear within minutes of adding a mitogen to cells — are also induced in cardiac cells by agonists causing hypertrophy, passive stretch in culture, or mechanical load *in vivo* [3, 6, 42, 69, 70]. As evidence favouring a causal relationship rather than mere correlation, forced expression of *fos* and *jun* suffices to upregulate the SkA promoter selectively [71, 72], as well as other hypertrophy-associated genes such as ANF [73] and TGF-β [74]. Several distinguishable mechanisms of action can mediate the effects of *fos* and *jun*, or other directly affected transcription factors, on any particular target gene: (1) direct binding to regulatory DNA sequences, as in the case of the promoter for TGF-$\beta_1$; (2) indirect binding to DNA-bound factors; or (3) induction of the DNA-bound factors. Only limited data exist, however, testing the putative functional role of load-inducible transcription factors as third messengers during cardiac hypertrophy *in vivo*. Indeed, forced expression of c-*myc* in the myocardium of transgenic mice resulted in mild hyperplasia (seemingly due to a modest delay in cell cycle exit), rather than in sustained hypertrophic growth [75].

Several cardiac-restricted transcription factors, the function of which is critical during normal heart formation, are also upregulated by hypertrophic signals, including Nkx2.5, a homologue of the *Drosophila* gene *tinman* [76]; the zinc-finger transcription factor, GATA-4 [77]; and one or more MEF2 'MADS box' transcription factors [78]. As mentioned for *fos* and *jun*, direct DNA binding by these factors to the promoters of hypertrophy-associated genes is only the most obvious potential mechanism of action. In the case of β-MHC, for example, the GATA-4 site is indispensable for induction of the gene by experimental aortic banding [79]. By contrast, both GATA-4 and Nkx2.5 can function as transcriptional adaptor proteins, or coactivators, tethered to DNA indirectly by other proteins such as serum response factor (SRF) [80] or even by one another [81–83].

Notwithstanding its name, and the resulting impression that it is ubiquitously and constitutively expressed, SRF is especially abundant in cardiac and skeletal muscle [84] and has been implicated in a variety of hypertrophic signalling pathways, including responses to $\alpha_1$-adrenergic agonists [85, 86], TGF-β [87], and forced expression of *fos*/*jun* [72]. For both adrenergic signalling [86] and for TGF-β signal transduction (present authors, unpublished date results), one key mechanism appears to be the p38-dependent phosphorylation of ATF6, a coactivator that is bound to the SRF transactivation domain and thus potentiates bound SRF.

Other examples of hypertrophic signals that alter transcription factor phosphorylation in cardiac cells include gp130 signalling to the signal transducer and activator of transcription proteins, STAT1 and STAT3 [88, 89], angiotensin II-induced STAT phosphorylation [90, 91], as well as STAT phosphorylation as an immediate-early response to mechanical load *in vivo* [92]. Phosphorylation results in translocation of STAT proteins to the nucleus, an obvious prerequisite for DNA binding. Illustrating the functional importance of such phosphorylations to signal transduction in hypertrophy, a non-phosphorylatable form of STAT3 blocked gp130-dependent induction of c-*fos* and ANF [89].

In one sense a mirror image of this pathway, the calcium-sensitive phosphatase, calcineurin, also controls the nuclear translocation of a target transcription factor (NFAT, the nuclear factor of activated T-cells), but does so by a dephosphorylation [65]. Among other possible mechanisms for its action in cardiac hypertrophy, NFAT serves as a coactivator for GATA-4 and thus can induce promoters that contain GATA-4 binding sites. Activated (calcium-independent) calcineurin and activated (nuclear-localized) NFAT each suffices to induce cardiac hypertrophy in transgenic mice. However, from initial attempts at pharmacological inhibition of this pathway, it seems clear that calcineurin-dependent and -independent mechanisms coexist [66, 93] and that no single transducer can yet be described as a universal, essential mediator of hypertrophy.

## A Ras-dependent pathway for phosphorylation of RNA polymerase II mediates global RNA and protein content

As explained earlier, cardiac hypertrophy can be dissected, both experimentally and conceptually, into the global increase in myocyte (and organ) size, with superimposition of the more recently identified selective changes in particular cardiac genes. Specific alterations in transcription factor abundance, intracellular trafficking, and activity readily account for at least some of the induction of hypertrophy-associated genes. However, this should not be mistaken for hypertrophy itself. Increasingly, a pharmacological and genetic dissection of hypertrophy into its constituent phenotypes is becoming possible, e.g. growth itself, the hypertrophic programme, and actin reorganization. Certain inhibitors of the global increase in RNA and protein content do not impair the selective upregulation of fetal cardiac genes [34, 46]; conversely, TGF-β induces the fetal programme but little or no change in protein content [31]. In short, for any chronic transgenic model leading to hypertrophy, it can be excessively speculative to conclude that a given component of the phenotype (including growth) is a direct consequence of the transgene, rather than an indirect effect of altered ventricular mechanics or autocrine/paracrine factors.

Recently, in a search for Ras protein dependent phosphorylation events that might help explain its requirement in hypertrophic growth, it was established that a Ras-dependent pathway controls the level of cyclin-dependent kinase-7 (Cdk7) in cardiac muscle cells and the extent of phosphorylation of RNA polymerase II (pol II), the major known substrate of Cdk7 [48]. Blocking endogenous Ras using a dominant-negative form of the protein reduced basal levels of uridine and phenylalanine incorporation into total RNA, mRNA, and protein, and likewise reduced cell size. Dominant-negative Ras markedly inhibited phosphorylation of the C-terminal domain of pol II, which is known to regulate transcript elongation. Conversely, $\alpha_1$-adrenergic stimulation enhanced pol II phosphorylation and Cdk7 expression, and both of these effects were blocked by dominant-negative Ras. Pressure overload *in vivo* led to an increase in both hyperphosphorylated and hypophosphorylated pol II, and to an increase in the pol II kinase, Cdk7. By cotransfecting Ras with wild-type pol II, versus pol II lacking the carboxy-terminal domain, in was shown that Ras activates transcription via this domain, and that phosphorylatable pol II ordinarily is limiting in cardiac muscle cells. One experimental priority is to learn whether this novel mechanism controlling the global increase in RNA and protein content also holds true for other, complementary cardiac agonists and for genetically determined hypertrophy *in vivo*.

## Implications and prospects for future directions

In summary, at least four sets of transcriptional pathways have been implicated in cardiac hypertrophy: immediate-early gene induction, upregulation of cardiac-restricted transcription factors (or their coactivators), phosphorylation or dephosphorylation of transcription factors, and phosphorylation of RNA polymerase II itself. The present review has emphasized the concept that myocardial hypertrophy encompasses an array of responses, specific as well as global, and that the multiple triggers and mediators for hypertrophy ultimately must be reconciled with one or more of these transcriptional mechanisms.

Several key questions remain unanswered at this point. Although hypertrophy- and failure-associated genes are now understood to include a number of overall categories (encoding sarcomeric proteins, ion pumps and channels, extracellular matrix components, intramyocardial growth factors, and transcription factors), other, unidentified targets are foreseeable, at least in principle. It is also unclear whether qualitative or merely quantitative differences in cardiac gene expression distinguish compensated hypertrophy from heart failure per se. Answers to these questions might be expected, in part, from newer technologies for high-throughput expression monitoring (gene-chip assays) and gene discovery (differential display or subtractive hybridization), in these complex pathophysiological settings.

Given the complex web of reported interactions summarized in Figure 4.1, and the multiple levels of the signalling cascade at which functional redundancy appears to exist, another fundamental challenge remains to define what protein (or proteins) are truly essential for hypertrophy. A related question concerns the possibly contrasting role of particular signalling proteins in transducing the immediate effect of a change in wall stress, versus their role in later aspects of this process, including secondary or tertiary signals involving autocrine and paracrine factors. Finally, the identity of mechanical sensors (which initiate this process) remains speculative.

To define a protein's indispensable role, here and in other aspects of hypertrophy, even greater reliance on genetic methods can be expected in order to exploit the specificity and efficacy of these manipulations (dominant-negative proteins or knockout mutations). For the immediate future, deletion of selected genes is feasible only in mice. Larger mammals are already accessible, however, to myocardial gene transfer *in vivo* (using viral vectors or 'naked' DNA) [94–96] and to the creation of genetically modified lines either by injecting the pronucleus of fertilized oocytes (the conventional transgenic approach) [97] or, more exotically, by fusion of somatic cells to enucleated oocytes (as done for cloned sheep and other species) [98]. Taken together, these technologies to map gene expression and pinpoint gene function should help to unravel the transcriptional circuits coupling mechanical stress to cardiac growth and dysfunction. Of at least equal importance, the knowledge obtained by this approach (often referred to as functional genomics) would create novel opportunities for pharamacological intervention, with the long-term hope of beneficial effects of alleviating or preventing the transition to heart failure. More speculatively, one might also point to the potential application of transcription factors to the problem of cardiac repair, either by overcoming the normal cell-cycle constraints that preclude effective regeneration following infarction [99], or by transdifferentiation, using cardiogenic factors discussed earlier in this chapter to recruit non-muscle cells to a cardiac fate [100].

## References


1. Schwartz K, de la Bastie D, Bouveret P *et al.* α-Skeletal muscle actin mRNAs accumulate in hypertrophied adult rat hearts. *Circ Res* 1986; 59: 551–5.
2. Izumo S, Lompré AM, Matsuoka R *et al.* Myosin heavy chain messenger RNA and protein isoform during cardiac hypertrophy: Interaction between hemodynamic and thyroid hormone-induced signals. *J Clin Invest* 1987; 79: 970–7.
3. Izumo S, Nadal-Ginard B, Mahdavi V. Proto-oncogene induction and reprogramming of cardiac gene expression produced by pressure overload. *Proc Natl Acad Sci USA* 1988; 85: 339–43.
4. Mercadier J-J, Samuel J-L, Michel J-B *et al.* Atrial natriuretic factor gene expression in rat ventricle during experimental hypertension. *Am J Physiol* 1989; 257: H979–87.
5. Mercadier J-J, Lompre A-M, Duc P *et al.* Altered sarcoplasmic reticulum $Ca^{2+}$-ATPase gene expression in the human ventricle during end-state heart failure. *J Clin Invest* 1990; 85: 305–9.
6. Mulvagh SL, Michael LH, Perryman MB *et al.* A hemodynamic load *in vivo* induces cardiac expression of the cellular oncogene, c-*myc* *Biochem Biophys Res Commun* 1987; 147: 627–36.
7. Takahashi N, Calderone A, Izzo NJ *et al.* Hypertrophic stimuli induce transforming growth factor-beta(1) expression in rat ventricular myocytes. *J Clin Invest* 1994; 94: 1470–6.
8. Torreamione G, Kapadia S, Lee J *et al.* Tumor necrosis factor-alpha and tumor necrosis factor receptors in the failing human heart. *Circulation* 1996; 93: 704–11.
9. Kaab S, Dixon J, Duc J *et al.* Molecular basis of transient outward potassium current downregulation in human heart failure: a decrease in Kv4.3 mRNA correlates with a reduction in current density. *Circulation* 1983; 98: 1383–93.
10. Cuda G, Fananapazir L, Zhu WS *et al.* Skeletal muscle expression and abnormal function of beta-myosin in hypertrophic cardiomyopathy. *J Clin Invest* 1993; 91: 2861–5.
11. Straceski AJ, Geisterfer-Lowrance A, Seidman CE *et al.* Functional analysis of myosin missense mutations in familial hypertrophic cardiomyopathy. *Proc Natl Acad Sci USA* 1994; 91: 589–93.
12. Sweeney HL, Straceski AJ, Leinwand LA *et al.* Heterologous expression of a cardiomyopathic myosin that is defective in its actin interaction. *J Biol Chem* 1994; 269: 1603–5.
13. Lankford EB, Epstein ND, Fananapazir L, Sweeney HL. Abnormal contractile properties of muscle fibers expressing beta-myosin heavy chain gene mutations in patients with hypertrophic cardiomyopathy. *J Clin Invest* 1995; 95: 1409–14.
14. Roopnarine O, Leinwand LA. Functional analysis of myosin mutations that cause familial hypertrophic cardiomyopathy. *Biophys J* 1998; 75: 3023–30.
15. Soonpaa MH, Field LJ. Survey of studies examining mammalian cardiomyocyte DNA synthesis. *Circ Res* 1998; 83: 15–26.

16. Anversa P, Kajstura J. Ventricular myocytes are not terminally differentiated in the adult mammalian heart. *Circ Res* 1998; 83: 1–14.
17. Adams JW, Sakata Y, Davis MG *et al.* Enhanced G alpha q signaling: a common pathway mediates cardiac hypertrophy and apoptotic heart failure. *Proc Natl Acad Sci USA* 1998; 95: 10 140–5.
18. Bryant D, Becker L, Richardson J *et al.* Cardiac failure in transgenic mice with myocardial expression of tumor necrosis factor-alpha. *Circulation* 1998; 97: 1375–81.
19. Narula J, Haider N, Virmani R *et al.* Apoptosis in myocytes in end-stage heart failure. *N Engl J Med* 1996; 335: 1182–9.
20. Olivetti G, Abbi R, Quaini F *et al.* Apoptosis in the failing human heart. *N Engl J Med* 1997; 336: 1131–41.
21. Jones WK, Grupp IL, Doetschman T *et al.* Ablation of the murine alpha myosin heavy chain gene leads to dosage effects and functional deficits in the heart. *J Clin Invest* 1996; 98: 1906–17.
22. Fewell JG, Hewett TE, Sanbe A *et al.* Functional significance of cardiac myosin essential light chain isoform switching in transgenic mice. *J Clin Invest* 1998; 101: 2630–9.
23. Kadambi VJ, Ponniah S, Harrer JM *et al.* Cardiac-specific overexpression of phospholamban alters calcium kinetics and resultant cardiomyocyte mechanics in transgenic mice. *J Clin Invest* 1996; 97: 533–9.
24. Nuss HB, Johns DC, Kaab S *et al.* Reversal of potassium channel deficiency in cells from failing hearts by adenoviral gene transfer: a prototype for gene therapy for disorders of cardiac excitability and contractility. *Gene Therapy* 1996; 3: 900–12.
25. Tomita Y, Kusama Y, Seino Y *et al.* Increased accumulation of acidic fibroblast growth factor in left ventricular myocytes of patients with idiopathic cardiomyopathy. *Am Heart J* 1997; 134: 779–86.
26. Donohue TJ, Dworkin LD, Ma JX *et al.* Antihypertensive agents that limit ventricular hypertrophy inhibit cardiac expression of insulin-like growth factor-I. *J Invest Med* 1997; 45: 584–91.
27. Baker KM, Chernin MI, Wixson SK, Aceto JF. Renin– angiotensin system involvement in pressure-overload cardiac hypertrophy in rats. *Am J Physiol* 1990; 259: H324–32.
28. Schunkert H, Dzau VJ, Tang SS *et al.* Increased rat cardiac angiotensin converting enzyme activity and mRNA expression in pressure overload left ventricular hypertrophy: effects on coronary resistance, contractility, and relaxation. *J Clin Invest* 1990; 86: 1913–20.
29. Yorikane R, Sakai S, Miyauchi T *et al.* Increased production of endothelin-1 in the hypertrophied rat heart due to pressure overload. *FEBS Lett* 1993; 332: 31–4.
30. Ishikawa M, Saito Y, Miyamoto Y *et al.* cDNA cloning of rat cardiotrophin-1 (CT-1): augmented expression of CT-1 gene in ventricle of genetically hypertensive rats. *Biochem Biophys Res Commun* 1996; 219: 377–81.
31. Parker TG, Packer SE, Schneider MD. Peptide growth factors can provoke 'fetal' contractile protein gene expression in rat cardiac myocytes. *J Clin Invest* 1990; 85: 507–14.
32. Parker TG, Chow K-L, Schwartz RJ, Schneider MD. Differential regulation of skeletal $\alpha$-actin transcription in cardiac muscle by two fibroblast growth factors. *Proc Natl Acad Sci USA* 1990; 87: 7066–70.
33. Shubeita HE, McDonough PM, Harris AN *et al.* Endothelin induction of inositol phospholipid hydrolysis, sarcomere assembly, and cardiac gene expression in ventricular myocytes: a paracrine mechanism for myocardial cell hypertrophy. *J Biol Chem* 1990; 265: 20 555–62.
34. Sadoshima J, Izumo S. Rapamycin selectively inhibits angiotensin II-induced increase in protein synthesis in cardiac myocytes *in vitro*: potential role of 70-kD S6 kinase in angiotensin II-induced cardiac hypertrophy. *Circ Res* 1995; 77: 1040–52.
35. Wollert KC, Taga T, Saito M *et al.* Cardiotrophin-1 activates a distinct form of cardiac muscle cell hypertrophy — assembly of sarcomeric units in series via gp130 leukemia inhibitory factor receptor-dependent pathways. *J Biol Chem* 1996; 271: 9535–45.
36. Harada M, Itoh H, Nakagawa O *et al.* Significance of ventricular myocytes and nonmyocytes interaction during cardiocyte hypertrophy: evidence for endothelin-1 as a paracrine hypertrophic factor from cardiac nonmyocytes. *Circulation* 1997; 96: 3737–44.
37. Harada M, Saito Y, Kuwahara K *et al.* Interaction of myocytes and nonmyocytes is necessary for mechanical stretch to induce ANP/BNP production in cardiocyte culture. *J Cardiovasc Pharmacol* 1998; 31: S357–9.
38. Bozkurt B, Kribbs SB, Clubb FJ, Jr *et al.* Pathophysiologically relevant concentrations of tumor necrosis factor-alpha promote progressive left ventricular dysfunction and remodeling in rats. *Circulation* 1998; 97: 1382–91.
39. Kubota T, McTiernan CF, Frye CS *et al.* Dilated cardiomyopathy in transgenic mice with cardiac-specific overexpression of tumor necrosis factor-alpha. *Circ Res* 1997; 81: 627–35.
40. Li J, Hampton T, Morgan JP, Simons M. Stretch-induced VEGF expression in the heart. *J Clin Invest* 1997; 100: 18–24.
41. Cooper G, Kent RL, Uboh CE *et al.* Hemodynamic versus adrenergic control of cat right ventricular hypertrophy. *J Clin Invest* 1985; 75: 1403–14.
42. Komuro I, Kaida T, Shibazaki Y *et al.* Stretching cardiac myocytes stimulates protooncogene expression. *J Biol Chem* 1990; 265: 3595–8.
43. Komuro I, Katoh Y, Kaida T *et al.* Mechanical loading stimulates cell hypertrophy and specific gene expression in cultured rat cardiac myocytes: possible role of protein kinase C activation. *J Biol Chem* 1991; 266: 1265–8.
44. Sadoshima J, Jahn L, Takahashi T *et al.* Molecular characterization of the stretch-induced adaptation of cultured cardiac cells: an *in vitro* model of load-induced cardiac hypertrophy. *J Biol Chem* 1992; 267: 10 551–60.
45. Ross RS, Pham C, Shai SY *et al.* Beta(1) integrins participate in the hypertrophic response of rat ventricular myocytes. *Circ Res* 1998; 82: 1160–72.
46. Abdellatif M, MacLellan WR, Schneider MD. p21 Ras as a governor of global gene expression. *J Biol Chem* 1994; 269: 15 423–6.
47. Abdellatif M, Schneider MD. An effector-like function of Ras GTPase-activating protein predominates in cardiac muscle cells. *J Biol Chem* 1997; 272: 525–33.
48. Abdellatif M, Packer SE, Michael LH *et al.* A Ras-dependent pathway regulates RNA polymerase II phosphorylation in cardiac myocytes: implications for cardiac hypertrophy. *Mol Cell Biol* 1998; 18: 6729–36.
49. Hunter JJ, Tanaka N, Rockman HA *et al.* Ventricular expression of a MLC-2v-ras fusion gene induces cardiac hypertrophy and selective diastolic dysfunction in transgenic mice. *J Biol Chem* 1995; 270: 23 173–8.
50. Hoshijima M, Sah VP, Wang YB *et al.* The low molecular weight GTPase rho regulates myofibril formation and organization in neonatal rat ventricular myocytes — involvement of Rho kinase. *J Biol Chem* 1998; 273: 7725–30.
51. Hines WA, Thorburn A. Ras and Rho are required for G alpha q-induced hypertrophic gene expression in neonatal rat cardiac myocytes. *J Mol Cell Cardiol* 1998; 30: 485–94.

52. Fuller SJ, Finn SG, Downward J, Sugden PH. Stimulation of gene expression in neonatal rat ventricular myocytes by ras is mediated by ral guanine nucleotide dissociation stimulator (Ral.GDS) and phosphatidylinositol 3-kinase in addition to Raf. *Biochem J* 1998; 335: 241–6.
53. Akhter SA, Luttrell LM, Rockman HA *et al*. Targeting the receptor-G(q) interface to inhibit *in vivo* pressure overload myocardial hypertrophy. *Science* 1998; 280: 574–7.
54. Aoki H, Izumo S, Sadoshima J. Angiotensin II activates RhoA in cardiac myocytes: a critical role of RhoA in angiotensin II-induced premyofibril formation. *Circ Res* 1998; 82: 666–76.
55. Kariya K, Karns LR, Simpson PC. Expression of a constitutively activated mutant of the beta isoenzyme of protein kinase C in cardiac myocytes stimulates the promoter of the beta myosin heavy chain isogene. *J Biol Chem* 1991; 266: 10 023–6.
56. Bowman JC, Steinberg SF, Jiang T *et al*. Expression of protein kinase C beta in the heart causes hypertrophy in adult mice and sudden death in neonates. *J Clin Invest* 1997; 100: 2189–95.
57. Wakasaki H, Koya D, Schoen FJ *et al*. Targeted overexpression of protein kinase C beta 2 isoform in myocardium causes cardiomyopathy. *Proc Natl Acad Sci USA* 1997; 94: 9320–5.
58. Sugden PH, Clerk A. 'Stress-responsive' mitogen-activated protein kinases (c-Jun N-terminal kinases and p38 mitogen-activated protein kinases) in the myocardium. *Circ Res* 1998; 83: 345–52.
59. Choukroun G, Hajjar R, Kyriakis JM *et al*. Role of the stress-activated protein kinases in endothelin-induced cardiomyocyte hypertrophy. *J Clin Invest* 1998; 102: 1311–20.
60. Wang YB, Huang SA, Sah VP *et al*. Cardiac muscle cell hypertrophy and apoptosis induced by distinct members of the p38 mitogen-activated protein kinase family. *J Biol Chem* 1998; 273: 2161–8.
61. Wang YB, Su B, Sah VP *et al*. Cardiac hypertrophy induced by mitogen-activated protein kinase kinase 7, a specific activator for c-jun NH2-terminal kinase in ventricular muscle cells. *J Biol Chem* 1998; 273: 5423–6.
62. Kuppuswamy D, Kerr C, Narishige T *et al*. Association of tyrosine-phosphorylated c-Src with the cytoskeleton of hypertrophying myocardium. *J Biol Chem* 1997; 272: 4500–8.
63. Laser M, Kasi VS, Hamawaki M *et al*. Differential activation of p70 and p85S6 kinase isoforms during cardiac hypertrophy in the adult mammal. *J Biol Chem* 1998; 273: 24 610–19.
64. Kovacic B, Dusko I, Damsky CH, Gardner DG. c-Src activation plays a role in endothelin-dependent hypertrophy of the cardiac myocyte. *J Biol Chem* 1998; 273: 35 185–93.
65. Molkentin JD, Lu JR, Antos CL *et al*. A calcineurin-dependent transcriptional pathway for cardiac hypertrophy. *Cell* 1998; 93: 215–28.
66. Sussman MA, Lim HW, Gude N *et al*. Prevention of cardiac hypertrophy in mice by calcineurin inhibition. *Science* 1998; 281: 1690–3.
67. Ho PD, Zechner DK, He HP *et al*. The Raf-MEK-ERK cascade represents a common pathway for alteration of intracellular calcium by Ras and protein kinase C in cardiac myocytes. *J Biol Chem* 1998; 273: 21 730–5.
68. Oh H, Fujio Y, Kunisada K *et al*. Activation of phosphatidylinositol 3-kinase through glycoprotein 130 induces protein kinase B and p70 S6 kinase phosphorylation in cardiac myocytes. *J Biol Chem* 1998; 273: 9703–10.
69. Starksen NF, Simpson PC, Bishopric N *et al*. Cardiac myocyte hypertrophy is associated with c-myc protooncogene expression. *Proc Natl Acad Sci USA* 1986; 83: 8348–50.
70. Komuro M, Kurabayashi M, Takaku F, Yazaki Y. Expression of cellular oncogenes in the myocardium during the developmental stage and pressure-overload hypertrophy of the rat heart. *Circ Res* 1988; 62: 1075–9.
71. Bishopric NH, Jayasena V, Webster KA. Positive regulation of the skeletal alpha-actin gene by fos and jun in cardiac myocytes. *J Biol Chem* 1992; 267: 25 535–40.
72. Paradis P, Maclellan WR, Belaguli NS *et al*. Serum response factor mediates AP-1-dependent induction of the skeletal alpha-actin promoter in ventricular myocytes. *J Biol Chem* 1996; 271: 10 827–33.
73. McDonough PM, Hanford DS, Sprenkle AB *et al*. Collaborative roles for c-Jun N-terminal kinase, c-Jun, serum response factor, and Sp1 in calcium-regulated myocardial gene expression. *J Biol Chem* 1997; 272: 24 046–53.
74. Kim SJ, Angel P, Lafyatis R *et al*. Autoinduction of transforming growth factor beta 1 is mediated by the AP-1 complex. *Mol Cell Biol* 1990; 10: 1492–7.
75. Jackson T, Allard MF, Sreenan CM *et al*. The c-*myc* protooncogene regulates cardiac development in transgenic mice. *Mol Cell Biol* 1990; 10: 3709–16.
76. Thompson JT, Rackley MS, OBrien TX. Upregulation of the cardiac homeobox gene Nkx2-5 (CSX) in feline right ventricular pressure overload. *Am J Physiol* 1998; 43: H1569–73.
77. Molkentin JD, Kalvakolanu DV, Markham BE. Transcription factor GATA-4 regulates cardiac muscle-specific expression of the alpha-myosin heavy-chain gene. *Mol Cell Biol* 1994; 14: 4947–57.
78. Molkentin JD, Markham BE. Myocyte-specific enhancer-binding factor (MEF-2) regulates alpha-cardiac myosin heavy chain gene expression *in vitro* and *in vivo*. *J Biol Chem* 1993; 268: 19 512–1920.
79. Hasegawa K, Lee SJ, Jobe SM *et al*. cis-acting sequences that mediate induction of beta-myosin heavy chain gene expression during left ventricular hypertrophy due to aortic constriction. *Circulation* 1997; 96: 3943–53.
80. Chen CY, Schwartz RJ. Recruitment of the tinman homolog nkx-2.5 by serum response factor activates cardiac alpha-actin gene transcription. *Mol Cell Biol* 1996; 16: 6372–84.
81. Durocher D, Charron F, Warren R *et al*. The cardiac transcription factors Nkx2-5 and GATA-4 are mutual cofactors. *EMBO J* 1997; 16: 5687–96.
82. Lee Y, Shioi T, Kasahara H *et al*. The cardiac tissue-restricted homeobox protein Csx/Nkx2.5 physically associates with the zinc finger protein GATA4 and cooperatively activates atrial natriuretic factor gene expression. *Mol Cell Biol* 1998; 18: 3120–9.
83. Sepulveda JL, Belaguli N, Nigam V *et al*. GATA-4 and Nkx-2.5 coactivate Nkx-2 DNA binding targets: role for regulating early cardiac gene expression. *Mol Cell Biol* 1998; 18: 3405–15.
84. Croissant JD, Kim JH, Eichele G *et al*. Avian serum response factor expression restricted primarily to muscle cell lineages is required for alpha-actin gene transcription. *Dev Biol* 1996; 177: 250–64.
85. Karns LR, Kariya K, Simpson PC. M-CAT, CArG, and Sp1 elements are required for alpha(1)-adrenergic induction of the skeletal alpha-actin promoter during cardiac myocyte hypertrophy — transcriptional enhancer factor-1 and protein kinase C as conserved transducers of the fetal program in cardiac growth. *J Biol Chem* 1995; 270: 410–17.
86. Thuerauf DJ, Arnold ND, Zechner D *et al*. p38 mitogen-activated protein kinase mediates the transcriptional induction of the atrial natriuretic factor gene through a serum response element. A poten-

tial role for the transcription factor ATF6. *J Biol Chem* 1998; 273: 20 636–43.

87. MacLellan WR, Lee TC, Schwartz RJ, Schneider MD. Transforming growth factor-beta response elements of the skeletal alpha-actin gene: combinatorial action of serum response factor, YY1, and the SV40 enhancer-binding protein, TEF-1. *J Biol Chem* 1994; 269: 16 754–60.
88. Kodama H, Fukuda K, Pan J *et al*. Leukemia inhibitory factor, a potent cardiac hypertrophic cytokine, activates the JAK/STAT pathway in rat cardiomyocytes. *Circ Res* 1997; 81: 656–63.
89. Kunisada K, Tone E, Fujio Y *et al*. Activation of gp130 transduces hypertrophic signals via STAT3 in cardiac myocytes. *Circulation* 1998; 98: 346–52.
90. Bhat GJ, Thekkumkara TJ, Thomas WG *et al*. Angiotensin II stimulates sis-inducing factor-like DNA binding activity — evidence that the AT(1A) receptor activates transcription factor-Stat91 and/or a related protein. *J Biol Chem* 1994; 269: 31443–9.
91. Mascareno E, Dhar M, Siddiqui MA. Signal transduction and activator of transcription (STAT) protein-dependent activation of angiotensinogen promoter: a cellular signal for hypertrophy in cardiac muscle. *Proc Natl Acad Sci USA* 1998; 95: 5590–4.
92. Pan J, Fukuda K, Kodama H *et al*. Role of angiotensin II in activation of the JAK/STAT pathway induced by acute pressure overload in the rat heart. *Circ Res* 1997; 81: 611–17.
93. Mende U, Kagen A, Cohen A *et al*. Transient cardiac expression of constitutively active galphaq leads to hypertrophy and dilated cardiomyopathy by calcineurin-dependent and independent pathways. *Proc Natl Acad Sci USA* 1998; 95: 13 893–8.
94. Von Harsdorf R, Schott RJ, Shen YT *et al*. Gene injection into canine myocardium as a useful model for studying gene expression in the heart of large mammals. *Circ Res* 1993; 72: 688–95.
95. Donahue JK, Kikkawa K, Johns DC *et al*. Ultrarapid, highly efficient viral gene transfer to the heart. *Proc Natl Acad Sci USA* 1997; 94: 4664–8.
96. Li Q, Bolli R, Qiu Y *et al*. Gene therapy with extracellular superoxide dismutase attenuates myocardial stunning in conscious rabbits. *Circulation* 1998; 98: 1438–48.
97. Cozzi E, White DJ. The generation of transgenic pigs as potential organ donors for humans. *Nat Med* 1995; 1: 964–6.
98. Wilmut I, Schnieke AE, McWhir J *et al*. Viable offspring derived from fetal and adult mammalian cells. *Nature* 1997; 385: 810–13.
99. Agah R, Kirshenbaum LA, Truong LD *et al*. Adenoviral delivery of E2F-1 directs cell cycle re-entry and p53-independent apoptosis in post-mitotic adult myocardium *in vivo*. *J Clin Invest* 1997; 100: 2722–8.
100. Murry CE, Kay MA, Bartosek T *et al*. Muscle differentiation during repair of myocardial necrosis in rats via gene transfer with MyoD. *J Clin Invest* 1996; 98: 2209–17.

# Histopathological basis of cardiomyopathic disorders 5

A. BURKE AND R. VIRMANI

## Introduction

The original definition by the World Health Organization (WHO) of cardiomyopathy was 'heart muscle disease of unknown cause'. Diseases that involved the myocardium but were of a known cause were considered separately and termed 'specific heart muscle diseases'. Since much progress has been made in understanding the aetiology and pathogenesis of heart disease, the distinction between cardiomyopathy and specific heart muscle disease has become less clear. The new 'Report of the 1995 World Health Organization/International Society and Federation of Cardiology Task Force on the definition and classification of cardiomyopathies' published in 1996 defines cardiomyopathies as diseases of the myocardium associated with cardiac dysfunction [1]. They are classified as follows:

(1) dilated cardiomyopathy
(2) hypertrophic cardiomyopathy
(3) right ventricular cardiomyopathy
(4) restrictive cardiomyopathy
    (a) idiopathic
    (b) secondary
        (i) amyloidosis
        (ii) Loeffler's eosinophilic endocardial fibrosis
        (iii) tropical endocardial fibrosis (Davies' disease).

## Hypertrophic cardiomyopathy

### Historical note

Teare [2] offered one of the first descriptions of hypertrophic cardiomyopathy in 1958, describing an autopsy case of sudden death. Using the term 'asymmetry of the heart in young adults', Teare hypothesized that the condition was likely to be a hamartoma that resulted in outflow tract obstruction. Further pathological characterization of the condition, later called idiopathic subaortic hypertrophic stenosis, followed [3]. It was gradually accepted that hypertrophic cardiomyopathy was a result of generalized ventricular dysfunction, and that significant outflow tract obstruction occurred in only 50–70% of patients [4]. The importance of myofibre disarray and its quantification by morphometric techniques occurred in the late 1970s [5–7]. Although an autosomal dominant mode of inheritance was described as early as 1960 [8, 9], the genetic basis for many of the inherited forms of the disease was established only in 1990, more than 30 years after the initial morphological description [10].

### Pathological studies

In the vast majority of individuals dying from hypertrophic cardiomyopathy, there is cardiomegaly, typically in the range of twice the normal heart weight. Heart weights of over 1000 g have been reported [11]; however, sudden death in hypertrophic cardiomyopathy may occur in the absence of left ventricular hypertrophy. The latter cases, although rare, have been documented on the basis of family studies and histological findings of myofibre disarray [12].

In contrast to dilated cardiomyopathy, the left ventricular cavity is small in early phases of the disease. The site of hypertrophy has been classified on the basis of echocardiographic criteria into four types [13] (Fig. 5.1): in type I, only the anterior ventricular septum is thickened; in type II, the entire septum is thick, with a normal free wall; in type III there is involvement of the free wall as well as the ventricular septum; and in type IV, the least common, the anterior septum is normal and the hypertrophy is found

The opinions or assertions contained herein are the private views of the authors and are not to be construed as official or reflecting the views of the Department of the Army, the Department of the Air Force, or the Department of Defense.

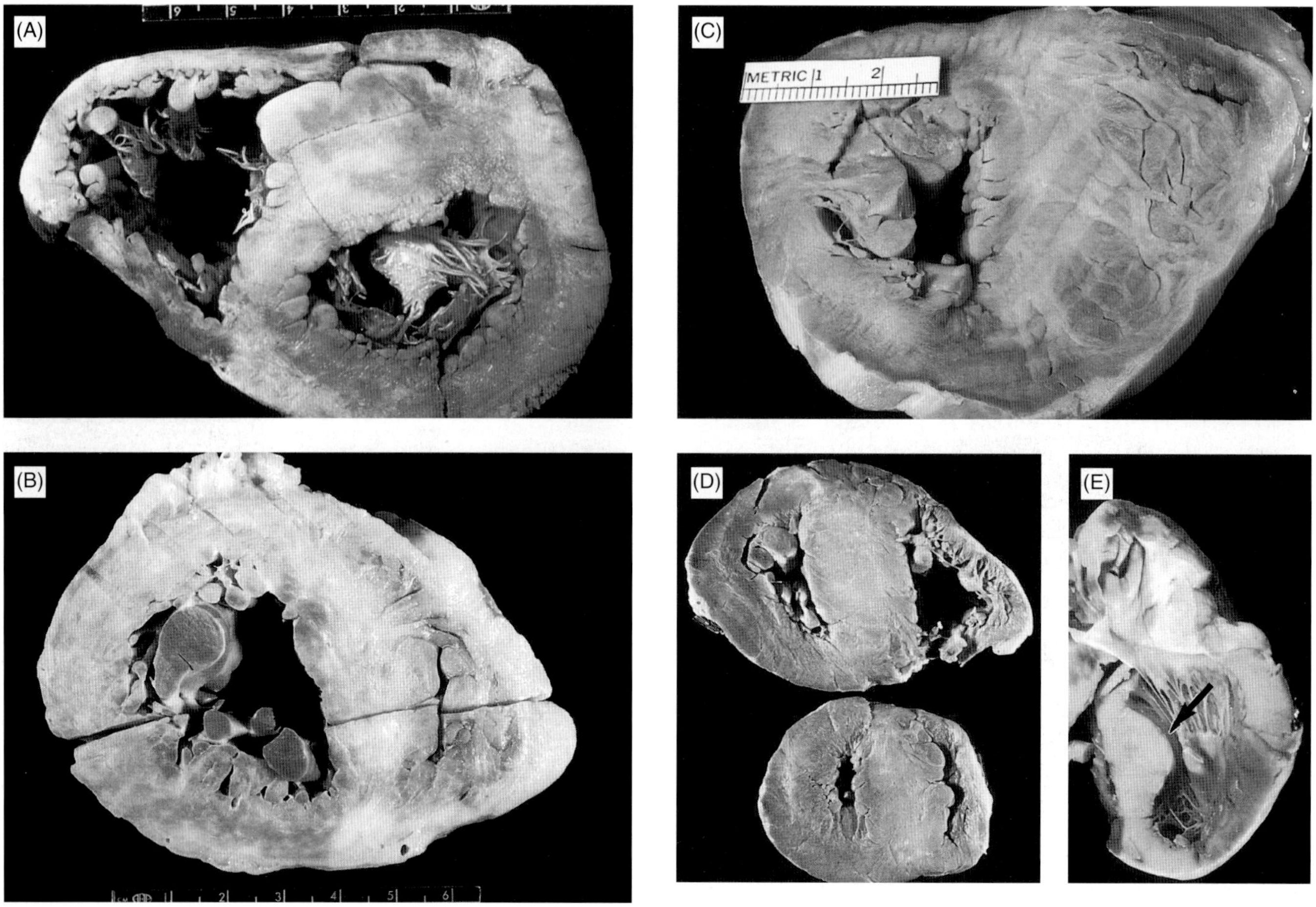


**Figure 5.1** *Patterns of septal hypertrophy in hypertrophic cardiomyopathy. (A) The typical form of septal asymmetry affects the anterior septum most markedly. The patient was a man in his 20s with previous episodes of syncope who died suddenly. (B) In another heart from a patient dying suddenly from hypertrophic cardiomyopathy, the anterior septum is especially thickened. (C) Occasionally, the entire septum is thickened to a similar degree. (D) A 34-year-old male without any significant medical history was found to be unresponsive. The heart weighed 480 g and the atria were mildly dilated. The predominant area of septal hypertrophy was towards the apex. Myofibre disarray can be appreciated grossly. (E) A 7-year-old male who died suddenly. At autopsy the left ventricle was hypertrophied and the left atrium was dilated. The septum was thicker than the free wall close to the base of the heart* (arrow) *at the level of the mitral valve. No discrete outflow tract plaque was present.*

in other locations of the septum or free wall. In 73% of hearts, there is a left ventricular outflow tract plaque, which correlates clinically with subaortic stenosis and systolic anterior motion of the anterior leaflet of the mitral valve [11]. Mitral valve thickening and elongation, with increased mass of the valve, is frequently observed (Fig. 5.2).

Histologically, myofibre disarray is a *sine qua non* for the diagnosis of hypertrophic cardiomyopathy (Fig. 5.3). Using an endpoint of 5% of the ventricular septum, a diagnostic sensitivity of 86% and a specificity of 90% are achieved [5]. The histological boundaries of myofibre disarray are not circumscribed, and the evaluation may be somewhat subjective. It must be kept in mind, in addition, that the evaluation of myofibre disarray is only possible if cross-sections (short-axis cuts) are taken for microscopic evaluation.

The ventricular septum in hypertrophic cardiomyopathy may also demonstrate interstitial and replacement fibrosis (Fig. 5.4), as well as foci of lymphocytic inflammation. The fibrosis is often most marked in areas of myofibre disarray. In patients with longstanding disease, there may be diffuse scarring throughout the ventricles and the free wall. In such cases, the distinction between hypertrophic cardiomyopathy and idiopathic restrictive cardiomyopathy may be difficult. It has been suggested that many cases of restrictive cardiomyopathy are, in fact, forms of hypertrophic cardiomyopathy [14]. In the dilated phase of hypertrophic

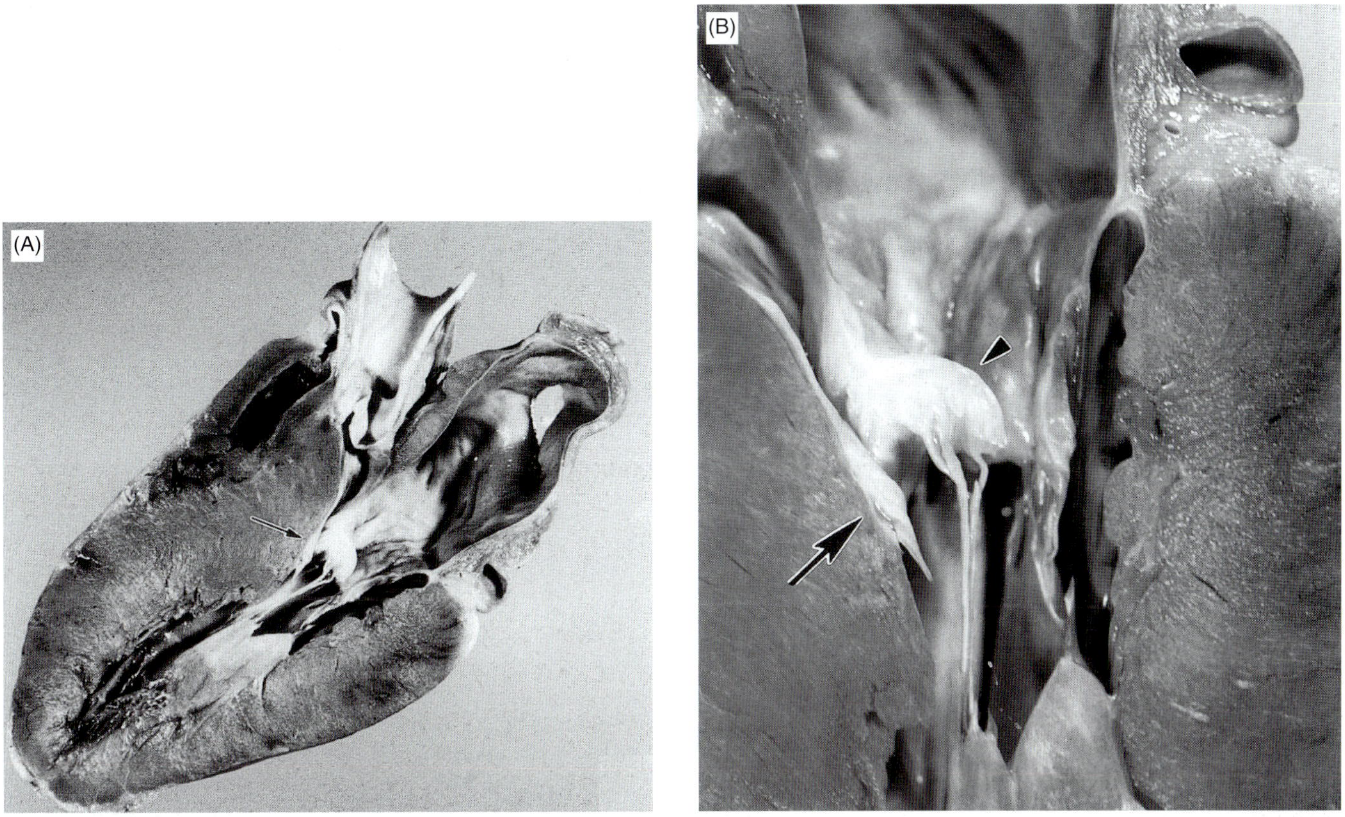


**Figure 5.2** *(A) A middle-aged patient with hypertrophic cardiomyopathy. The heart has been cut in the long-axis view of the left ventricular outflow tract. Note the dilated left atrium, the small left ventricular cavity, and the thick ventricular septum relative to the left ventricular free wall. There is a discrete outflow tract plaque* (arrow) *and a thickened anterior mitral leaflet. (B) Higher view of the heart to show the discrete outflow tract plaque and a thickened anterior mitral leaflet* (arrowhead).

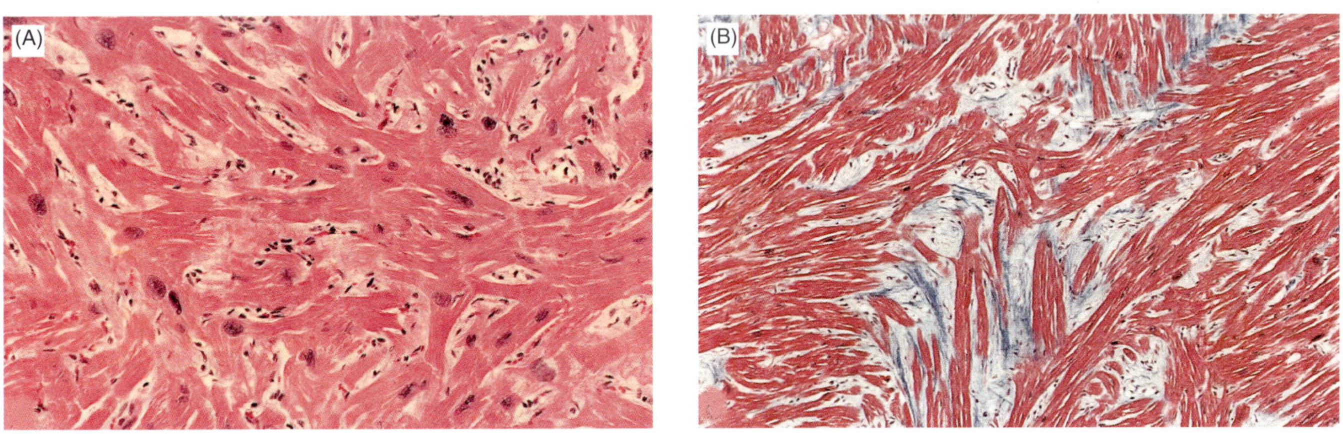


**Figure 5.3** *Fibromuscular disarray in hypertrophic cardiomyopathy. (A) Haematoxylin–eosin-stained section demonstrating hypertrophied myocytes with abnormal branching forms. (B) Masson trichrome stain demonstrating fibrosis in the area of myofibre disarray (blue-stained interstitial collagen).*

cardiomyopathy, extensive scarring may be present, but is predominantly found in the ventricular septum and the right ventricle [15].

Intramural coronary artery thickening is present in the ventricular septum in 83% of hypertrophic cardiomyopathy [16] (Fig. 5.5). It is debated whether the interstitial and replacement fibrosis are secondary to ischaemic insults or are an intrinsic part of the disease. It seems likely, although difficult to prove with certainty, that the majority of fibrosis is not related to ischaemia.

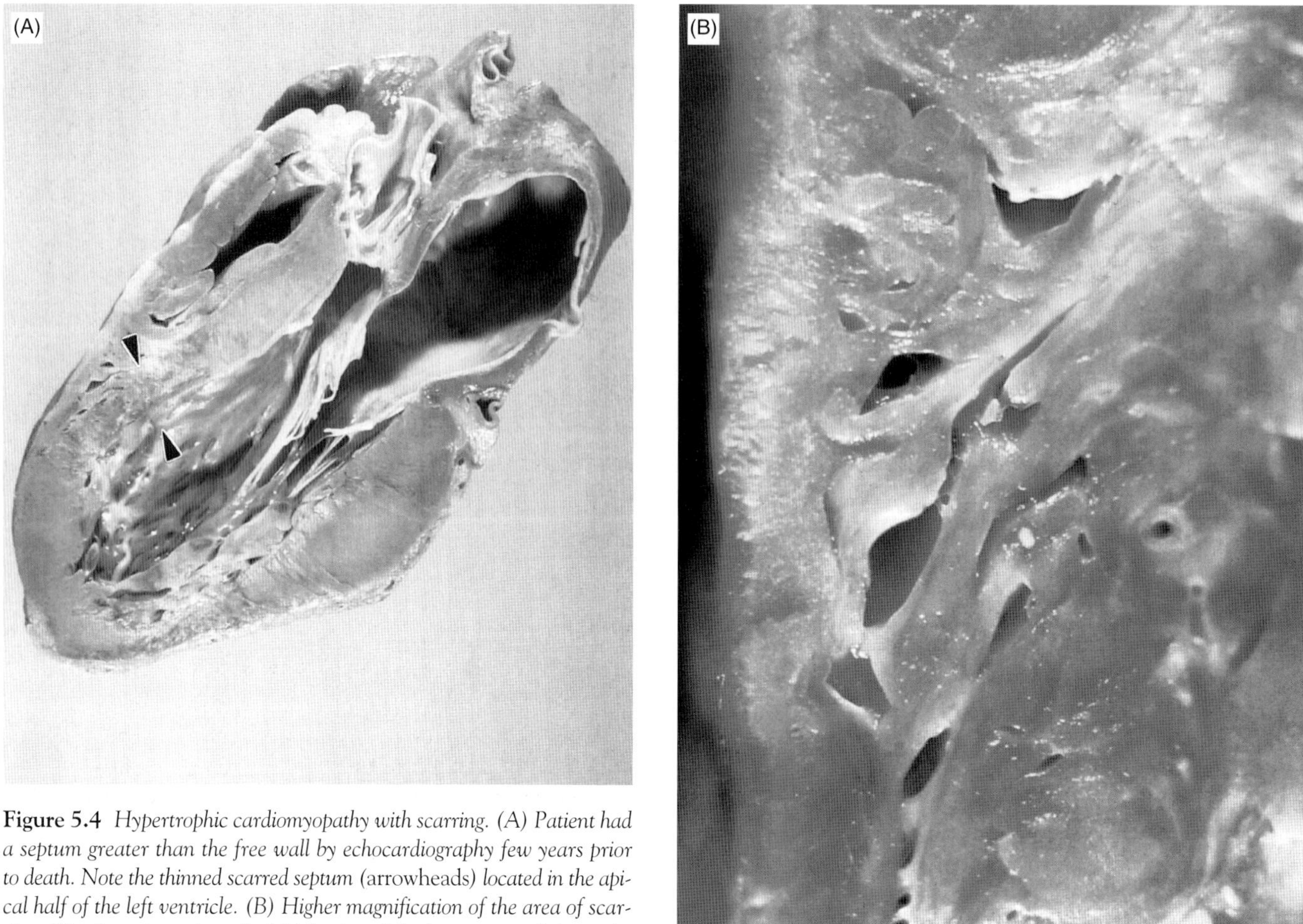


**Figure 5.4** *Hypertrophic cardiomyopathy with scarring. (A) Patient had a septum greater than the free wall by echocardiography few years prior to death. Note the thinned scarred septum* (arrowheads) *located in the apical half of the left ventricle. (B) Higher magnification of the area of scarring. Histology showed marked thickening of the intramyocardial arteries and surrounding fibrosis.*

A series of 57 hearts from 44 men and 13 women dying with hypertrophic cardiomyopathy was studied by the present authors. These patients were divided into four groups: those dying suddenly during exertion (mean age 22 years), those dying suddenly at rest (mean age 39 years), those dying from their disease not suddenly (mean age 58 years), and those dying of other causes (mean age 49 years). Those dying during exercise were significantly younger than the other groups. The mean heart weight was the greatest for the incidental group (730 g), but there were no significant differences among the other groups (range of means 579–680 g). Asymmetric hypertrophy with an outflow tract plaque was present more frequently in the exercise group (89%) than the incidental group (30%) or those dying of the disease at rest (58%). The degree of intramural coronary artery thickening was also greatest in the exertion group, being present in 100% of cases, compared with 60% of incidental cases and 75% of non-exertional deaths. These results suggest that there are morphological differences in hearts from patients with hypertrophic cardiomyopathy dying during exertion, in that there is a very high frequency of left ventricular outflow tract obstruction and intramural coronary artery thickening. Another large pathological study has shown greater myofibre disarray and intramural coronary artery disease in younger patients with asymmetric septal hypertrophy compared with elderly patients and younger patients with concentric hypertrophy [17].

## Clinical expression and epidemiology

The prevalence of hypertrophic cardiomyopathy in the USA has been estimated at 20–200 per 100 000 population [18, 19]. The variability in this range is probably due to study methodology, as the lower prevalence is based on patients presenting with symptomatic disease and the higher based on echocardiographic screening. There is a slight

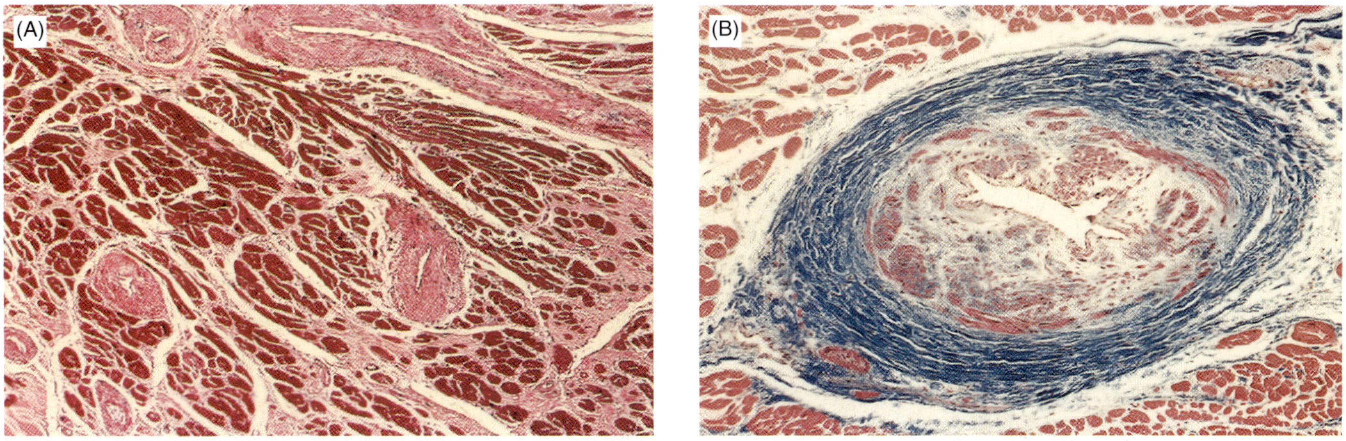


**Figure 5.5** *Intramural coronary artery thickening in hypertrophic cardiomyopathy. (A) Multiple intramural arteries in this section demonstrate significant thickening. (B) a Masson trichrome stain showing adventitial scarring (blue), with thickened and dysplastic media.*

**Table 5.1** Differential features of hypertrophic and dilated cardiomyopathy

| | Dilated cardiomyopathy | Hypertrophic cardiomyopathy |
|---|---|---|
| Incidence (yearly) | 6/100 000 | 2.5/100 000 |
| Mean age at diagnosis | 5th decade | 45 |
| Familial | 6–20% | 50–60% |
| Genetic basis | Unknown; rarely dystrophin gene abnormality | β-myocin heavy chain and others (see text) |
| Viral aetiology | 10–20% | None |
| Predominant functional defect | Systolic | Diastolic |
| LV chamber size | Increased | Decreased or normal |
| LV mass | Increased | Greatly increased |
| Left atrial size | Enlarged | Greatly enlarged |
| Sudden death | 20% | 40% |
| At presentation | 3% | 20% |
| Congestive heart failure | > 95% | 10% |
| Arrhythmias | Common | Common |
| 10 year survival | 15% | 60% |

male predominance. The mean age at presentation is approximately 45 years, and a bimodal distribution, with peaks in early and later adulthood, has been described (Table 5.1). The infantile form of the syndrome is probably a heterogeneous entity distinct from the adult disease. However, hereditary forms of the disease have been identified with expression of typical hypertrophic cardiomyopathy in infancy.

There are four major categories of presentation of hypertrophic cardiomyopathy. These are fairly equally distributed among syncopal episodes, chest pain, dyspnoea, and sudden cardiac death [18]. Because of the known familial nature of the illness, up to 25% of cases are identified incidentally because of an afflicted family member. However, the lack of efficacy of echocardiography as a screening tool for athletic programmes has been shown [20, 21].

The haemodynamic derangements in hypertrophic cardiomyopathy are caused by a small left ventricular cavity that restricts ventricular filling during diastole. The ejection fraction, in the initial phases of illness, is normal or increased. A subaortic pressure gradient is present in a little over half of patients, and is often variable and labile.

Echocardiographically, the hallmarks of hypertrophic cardiomyopathy include left ventricular hypertrophy, a small ventricular cavity, systolic anterior motion of the anterior leaflet of the mitral valve, and a characteristic ground-glass appearance of the myocardium. Asymmetric hypertrophy is typical, occurring in 80–98% of cases [13]. The distribution of left ventricular hypertrophy is heterogeneous, encompassing extensive and diffuse wall thickening to mild and segmental thickening. The anterior ventricular septum is thickening in 96% of patients, and in 83% is the predominant area of hypertrophy [13]. In the USA, the apical form of the disease is rare, accounting for only 1% of cases. True mitral valve prolapse occurs in 3% of patients, and is not considered increased in incidence over the general population. A greater extent of left ventricular hypertrophy is associated with younger age and more marked mitral valve systolic anterior motion and outflow obstruction but shows no relation to symptoms or gender [13].

In addition to echocardiography, magnetic resonance imaging (MRI) may help to assess the degree and extension of left ventricular hypertrophy. However, the amount and degree of hypertrophy bears little correlation with clinical findings in patients with hypertrophic cardiomyopathy [22, 23].

Sudden death is a common complication of hypertrophic cardiomyopathy, and is often precipitated by exercise. In series of athletes younger than age 30 years dying suddenly, hypertrophic cardiomyopathy is among the most common findings at autopsy [24]. Those features that most reliably identify high-risk patients include age younger than 30 years and a family history of hypertrophic cardiomyopathy with sudden death, genetic abnormalities associated with increased prevalence of sudden death, sustained ventricular or supraventricular tachyarrhythmias, recurrent syncope in the young, non-sustained ventricular tachycardias, and bradyarrhythmias.

The clinical course of patients with hypertrophic cardiomyopathy is highly variable. Overall, there is approximately 3% mortality per year in adults and a somewhat higher rate of mortality in children [25, 26]. In 10% of patients or more, there is a progression to dilated cardiomyopathy. Hearts from patients dying with the dilated form of hypertrophic cardiomyopathy may show diffuse scarring with myofibre disarray, and an absence of asymmetric hypertrophy or even thinning of the ventricular septum (Fig. 5.4). Hypertrophic cardiomyopathy appears to predispose to infective endocarditis. A few patients (2%) may develop severe mitral or aortic regurgitation, or both, requiring valve replacement secondary to infective endocarditis [27]. Therefore it has been recommended that patients with hypertrophic cardiomyopathy receive prophylactic antibiotic therapy during procedures that predispose to infective endocarditis.

Treatment for hypertrophic cardiomyopathy includes medical therapy, cardiac pacing and, in patients with outflow tract obstruction, surgical myectomy (Fig. 5.6). Atrioventricular synchronous pacing with appropriate placement of the lead in the right ventricular apex has been reported to reduce left ventricular outflow obstruction and symptoms in patients with hypertrophic obstructive cardiomyopathy [28]. However, treatment with pacing is controversial and some authorities do not support its use in patients with obstructive hypertrophic cardiomyopathy. A low perioperative mortality rate and a high late survival rate (72% at 15 years' follow-up) has been reported after surgical myectomy [29] (Fig. 5.6). Alternatives to surgical myectomy include a modified Konno procedure, with aortic valve replacement and left ventricular outflow reconstruction [30]. Non-surgical septal reduction has been attempted using selective coronary alcohol injection to induce localized septal infarcts, and one study has shown reduced symptoms and outflow gradient using this technique [31].

## Genetic findings and pathophysiology

If echocardiographic screening is performed on relatives of index cases of hypertrophic cardiomyopathy, up to 55% of families show at least one member with abnormalities suggestive of the disease. The genetic basis for hypertrophic cardiomyopathy is heterogeneous, but in all families studied, a mutation in sarcomeric proteins is found. A variety of mutations of the β-myosin heavy chain gene (the gene most frequently affected) have been identified, most of which are single-point missense mutations occurring in exons 9, 13, 14, 16, 19, 20, or 23 [32]. A subset of mutations, many of which occur in exons 13 and 14, is associated with an especially poor prognosis. The amino acid position 403 on exon 13, an apparent hotspot for the disease, may affect the myosin–actin dissociation in the contractile cycle [10, 32–34]. Mutant messenger ribonucleic acid (mRNA) has been identified in both cardiac and skeletal muscle, although symptoms related to skeletal muscle involvement are rare.

Between 10 and 15% of patients with familial hypertrophic cardiomyopathy possess mutations in the cardiac troponin T gene. In general, these patients have a relatively poor prognosis but only mild hypertrophy, especially those with a mutation at residue 340. Recently, a more benign mutation with a variable prognosis has been observed at residue 110 of the cardiac troponin T gene [35]. An

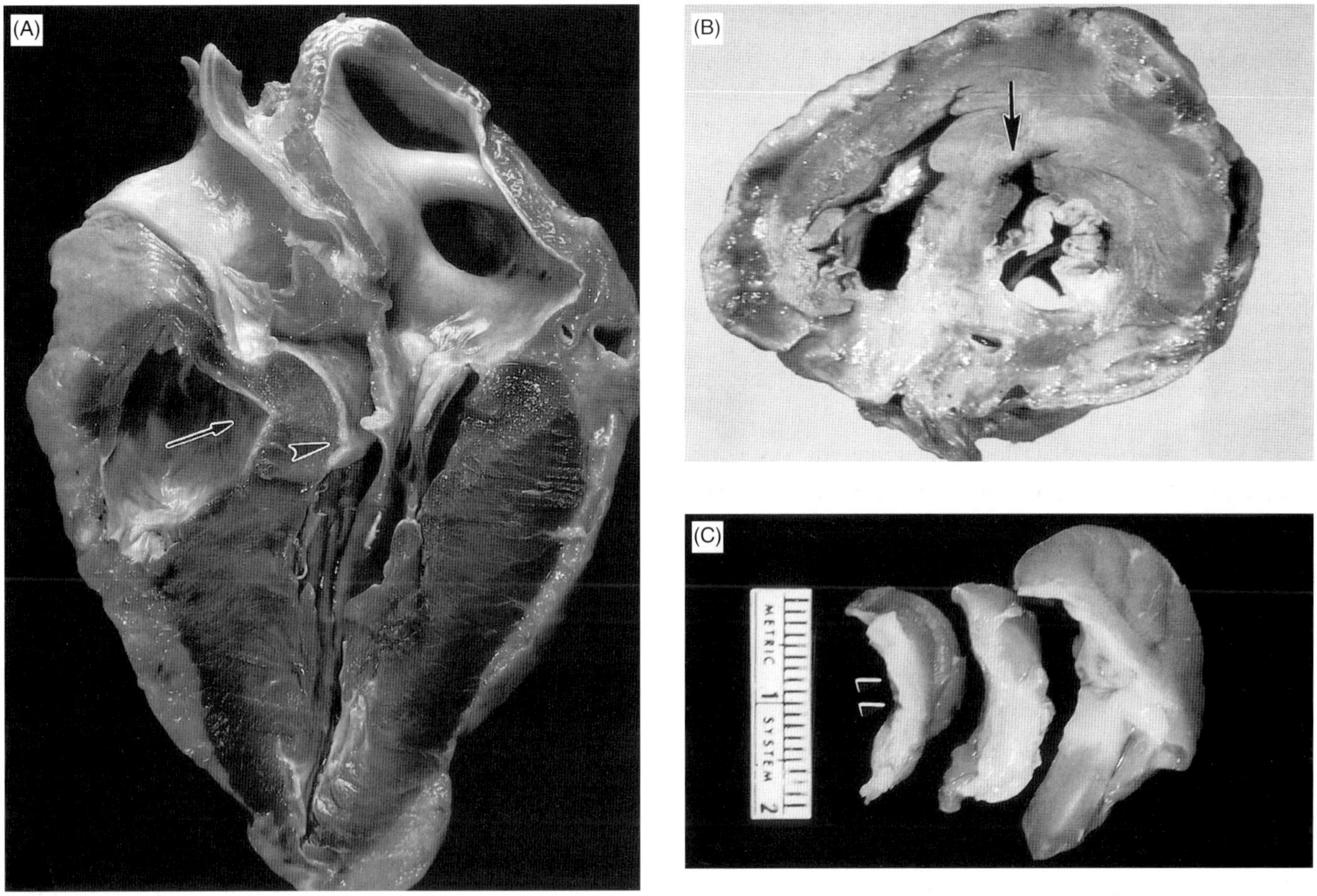


**Figure 5.6** *Surgical correction of hypertrophic cardiomyopathy. (A) The patient was a 62-year-old man with hypertrophic cardiomyopathy treated by myotomy and a myectomy performed from the right ventricle in the 1960s. He died in 1980 from metastatic carcinoma of the lung. Note the bulging ventricular septum close to the base of the heart at the myectomy site* (arrow) *and the discrete plaque in the left ventricular outflow tract* (arrowhead). *(B) Postoperative death in a patient who underwent a myotomy and myectomy from the left side of the heart (a more conventional method). Note that a wedge of the ventricular septum has been removed at surgery* (arrow). *(C) The myotomy specimen from the same patient illustrated in (B) showing three pieces of the myocardium with marked endocardial thickening* (arrowheads).

$Asp_{175}Asn$ $\alpha$-tropomyosin mutation has been identified which may result in a relatively benign disease expression [36]. Other sarcomeric proteins showing mutations in patients with familial hypertrophic cardiomyopathy include ventricular myosin essential light chain-1, ventricular myosin regulatory light chain-2, cardiac troponin-I, $\alpha$-tropomyosin, and cardiac myosin-binding protein C [37].

The mechanisms by which alterations in the cardiac contractile elements translate into the haemodynamic and pathological findings of hypertrophic cardiomyopathy are poorly understood [37]. Because the disease is inherited in an autosomal-dominant fashion, and most mutations are missense ones without a frameshift, the mutant proteins are believed to act as poison polypeptides that are incorporated in the sarcomere and change the function or assembly of the sarcomeric filaments. Mouse models and *in vitro* studies of myocyte cultures transfected with mutant proteins have provided preliminary data and have been recently reviewed [37]. The mechanisms leading to ischaemia and fibrosis have been debated. Septal hypertrophy has been associated with decreased coronary resistance reserve and changes in the coronary microcirculation [38]. Studies correlating blood flow and coronary vasodilator reserve with morphometric analysis of arterioles in endomyocardial biopsies have shown that preterminal subendocardial arterioles are reduced in total cross-sectional lumen areas, corresponding to an impaired coronary vasodilator capacity that may predispose to myocardial ischaemia [39].

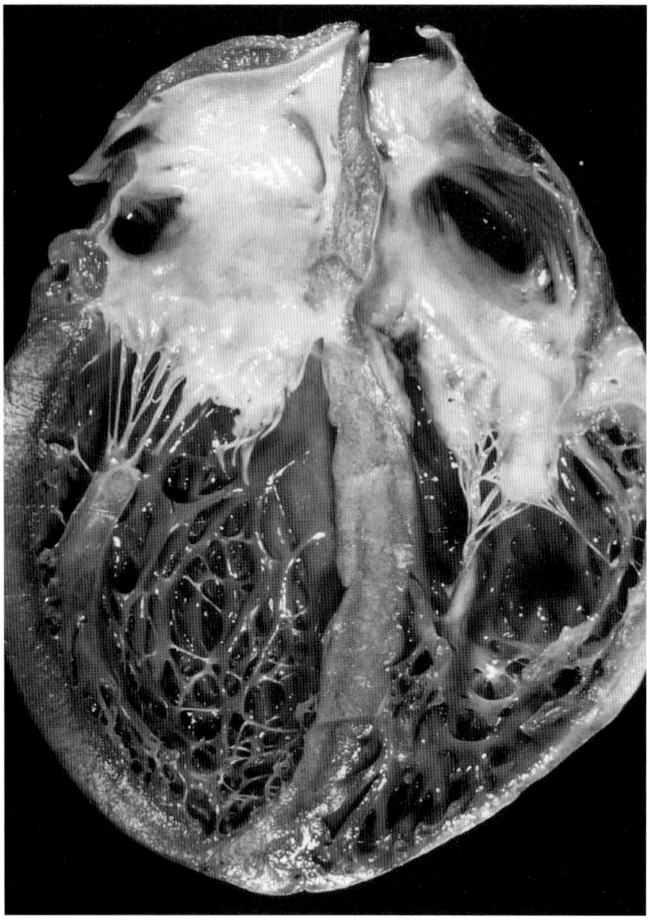

**Figure 5.7** *Idiopathic dilated cardiomyopathy. A 23-year-old man with a history of dilated cardiomyopathy for 2 years died with severe congestive heart failure. This four-chamber view of the heart shows marked dilatation of the ventricles and mild dilatation of the atria. The left ventricular wall is markedly thin and the septum is bowed towards the right ventricle. Despite the lack of ventricular hypertrophy, the heart weight was increased (500 g).*

It has long been postulated that in addition to ischaemia, arrhythmias in patients with hypertrophic cardiomyopathy may arise directly from disordered myocytes. Studies that localize desmosomes and tight junctions by using antibodies to desmoplakin and connexin have shown disorganization of the intercellular junctions and remodelling of gap junction distribution [40]. In general, possible mechanisms of ventricular arrhythmias in patients with hypertrophic cardiomyopathy include acute ischaemia secondary to subaortic stenosis, ventricular arrhythmias secondary to disordered muscle bundles in the ventricular septum, myocardial ischaemia secondary to small vessel coronary disease, and myocardial hypertrophy.

# Dilated cardiomyopathy

## Introduction and terminology

Idiopathic dilated cardiomyopathy denotes heart failure of undetermined aetiology and pathologically is a diagnosis essentially of exclusion. Because of a lack of understanding of the cellular mechanisms of the disease that unify it into a discrete entity, it is difficult to discern primary from secondary pathological and pathophysiological findings. Ongoing genetic and familial studies are gradually identifying specific causes of what is undoubtedly a heterogeneous disorder. At this time, the mechanisms of how some toxins and concomitant systemic disorders contribute causally to heart failure are incompletely understood. This chapter discusses some of the more common associated conditions linked with dilated cardiomyopathy. The reader is referred to Chapter 27 for a further discussion of the causes of heart failure in systemic disease, and Chapter 25 for an in-depth discussion of alcoholic cardiomyopathy.

## Pathological and anatomical findings

The typical pathological finding at autopsy is a four-chamber dilatation that is greater in the ventricles than the atria (Fig. 5.7). If there was a history of atrial fibrillation during life, atrial dilatation may be prominent. Using echocardiographic criteria, a left ventricular cavity diameter larger than 4 cm (excluding the papillary muscles) correlates loosely with the presence of congestive heart failure. Because of the confounding effects of autolysis and fixation, and the terminal state of the patient, cardiac failure must be corroborated by histological assessment of chronic congestion in the lungs and liver.

Cardiomegaly is nearly always a secondary manifestation of cardiac failure in idiopathic dilated cardiomyopathy [41]. The mean heart weight in a large series of such patients was 615 g (range 360–940 g) [11, 41, 42]. This increase in heart weight is often not accompanied by a significant increase in wall thickness, but the increase in muscle mass is due to global enlargement of the ventricles. In cases of dilated cardiomyopathy secondary to longstanding hypertension or obesity, wall thickness is often increased, in contrast to typical idiopathic forms of the disease [43]. However, in some patients with dilated cardiomyopathy there is very little cardiac enlargement. In these cases, there are few gross or histological changes in the heart despite the clinical diagnosis of congestive heart failure [43].

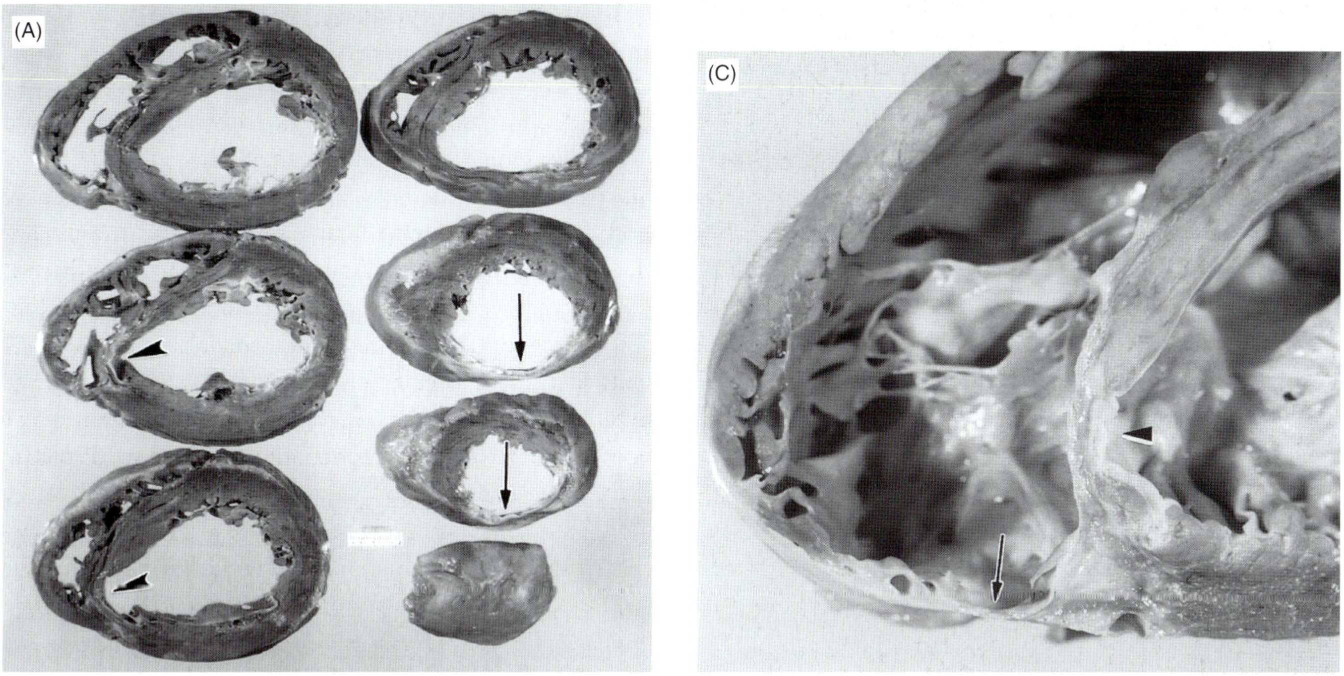


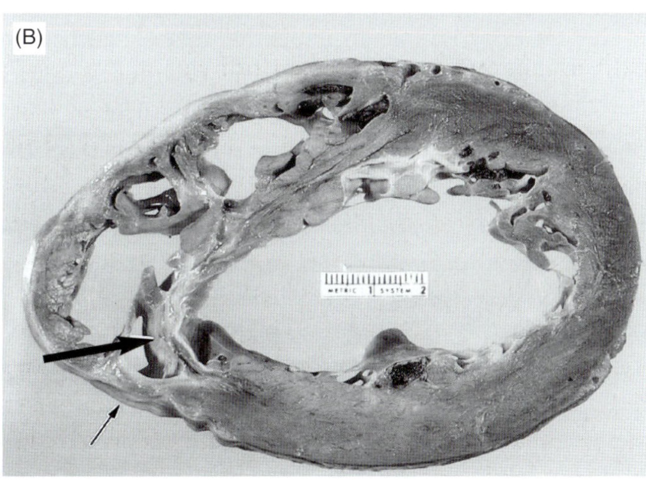


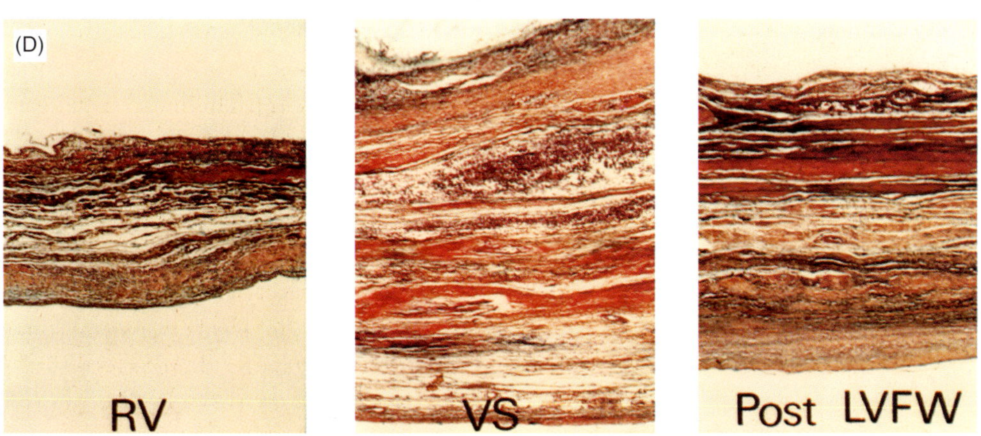


**Figure 5.8** *Idiopathic dilated cardiomyopathy with normal coronary arteries and transmural scarring of the posterior left ventricular wall and septum. The patient was a 62-year-old female with history of a 'heart murmur' and 'large heart' since the age of 53 years. She remained asymptomatic until the age of 60 years, when she developed exertional dyspnoea and pedal oedema. Nine months before her death an echocardiogram showed a poorly contracting dilated heart and worsening congestive heart failure. At autopsy the heart weighed 580 g and all four chambers were dilated. (A) Transmural scarring of the posterior wall of the left* (arrow) *and right ventricles and of the adjacent ventricular septum* (arrowheads). *(B) Slice of the midportion of the heart showing transmural scarring of the right ventricle* (arrow) *and ventricular septum* (large arrow). *(C) Transmural scarring of the posterior wall of the right ventricle* (arrow) *and septum* (arrowhead) *is seen in the base of the heart. (D) Photomicrographs of healed transmural scarring of the right ventricle (RV), ventricular septum (VS), and posterior (post) left ventricular free wall (LVFW).*

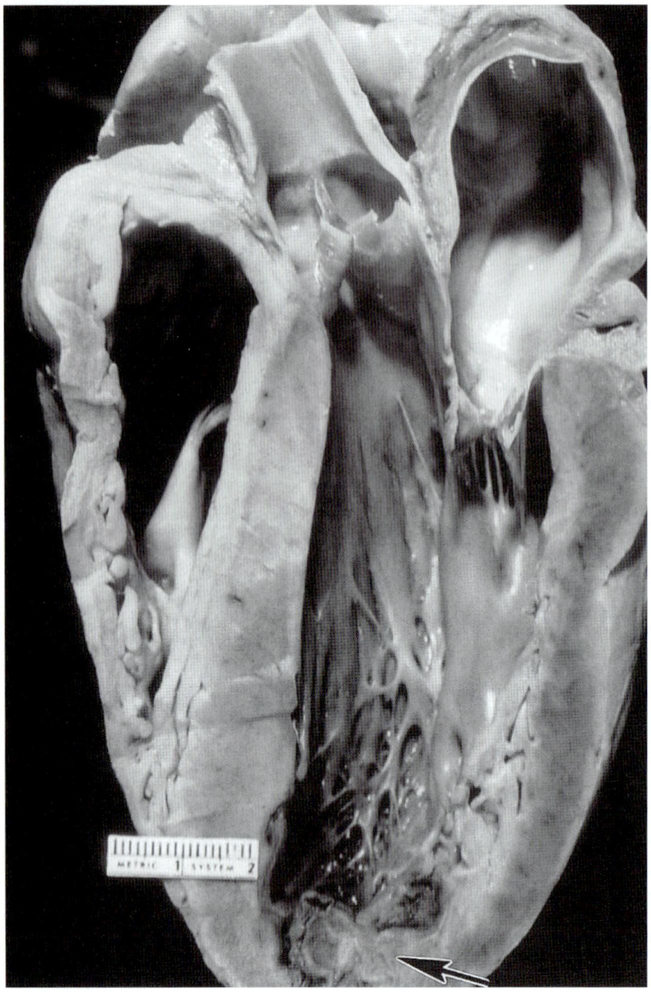


**Figure 5.9** *Long-axis view of the heart from a patient with idiopathic dilated cardiomyopathy. Note the dilated left ventricle. The dilatation is greater in the ventricle than in the atria. There is a thrombus present in the apex of the left ventricle* (arrow). *The autopsy showed renal and splenic infarcts.*

The myocardium in dilated cardiomyopathy is usually grossly unremarkable, but in about 15% of cases, gross subendocardial scars are present [11, 15, 41, 42]. Transmural scars with the appearance of ischaemic infarcts are less frequent [44] (Fig. 5.8). Mitral insufficiency is often a complication of cardiac dilatation, and in the majority of patients is believed to result from papillary muscle dysfunction secondary to ventricular dilatation and changes in ventricular wall shape [41]. In contrast, tricuspid regurgitation results from annular dilatation. In an autopsy series before the routine use of anticoagulation, right-sided mural thrombi were present in approximately one-third of hearts, and left-sided thrombi in nearly half [41] (Fig. 5.9). Endocardial fibrous plaques in the ventricles occur in about 10% of hearts, and are believed to be the result of organized thrombi. Mild diffuse or patchy endocardial fibrosis, especially towards the ventricular outflow tracts, is frequent and is probably a result of cardiac dilatation. The myocardium shows interstitial fibrosis and myocyte hypertrophy in most cases of idiopathic dilated cardiomyopathy (Fig. 5.10).

The coronary arteries in idiopathic dilated cardiomyopathy are by definition free of significant atherosclerotic disease. The term ischaemic cardiomyopathy has been used for patients with cardiac failure and a healed myocardial infarct due to stenosis of one or more coronary arteries (Fig. 5.11) [45]. Pathologists may encounter hearts from patients with severe cardiac failure, ventricular dilatation, and focally severe atherosclerosis in the absence of myocardial infarction. The possible contribution of ischaemia without infarct to heart failure in these patients is not fully understood.

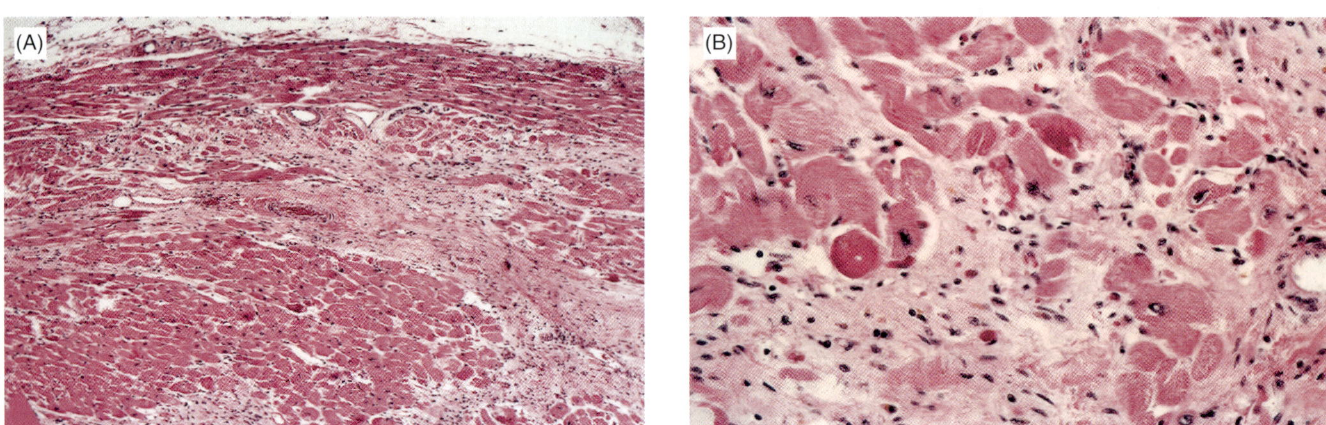


**Figure 5.10** *Idiopathic dilated cardiomyopathy. (A) Section of the left ventricle showing focal scarring and myocyte hypertrophy. (B) High-power view showing myocyte hypertrophy and focal scarring with interspersed fibroblasts and lymphocytes.*

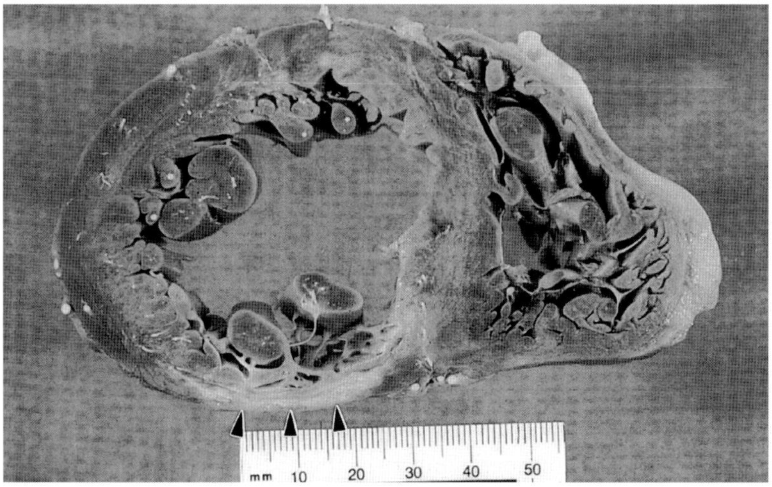


**Figure 5.11** *Ischaemic cardiomyopathy. Ventricular slice near the base of the heart showing a healed transmural myocardial infarction of the posterior left ventricular wall* (arrowheads) *and a markedly dilated left ventricular cavity in a man who died with severe congestive heart failure and had severe two-vessel coronary artery disease.*

The histological features of dilated cardiomyopathy are non-specific, and consist of myocyte hypertrophy, myocyte atrophy, and interstitial fibrosis [11, 41, 42, 46]. The degree of these changes is quite variable, however. Analogous to those cases with few gross findings, endomyocardial biopsies with normal histology have been described in patients with clinically diagnosed dilated cardiomyopathy [46]. Patients with clinical findings of cardiac failure but few if any pathological findings support the concept that the primary defect is at a subcellular metabolic level and that characteristic pathological changes are secondary.

Myocytes in hearts from patients with dilated cardiomyopathy have increased nuclear deoxyribonucleic acid (DNA) content, a mean increase in nuclear area, and irregularity of the nuclear outline [47]. Although the myocyte width may appear normal or reduced due to myocyte attenuation [48], the mean myocardial cell diameter in such patients has been calculated at 22 μm, compared with 17 μm in control subjects [49]. Heart biopsy studies have shown an association between per cent myofibre fraction and cardiac ejection fraction, suggesting that the degree of myofibre loss may have prognostic significance [50–52]. The degree of myofibrillar loss appears to be relatively small in patients with minimal cardiac dilatation [43]. Ultrastructural changes in dilated cardiomyopathy are numerous, and presumably secondary. These changes include increased transverse diameters of muscle cells, increased size of nuclei and Golgi complex, and increases in mitochondria, glycogen, and ribosomes [53]. Degenerative changes, such as cellular oedema, increased lipid droplets, lysosomes with autophagic vacuoles, lipofuscin, and T-tubular dilatation, are frequent [11]. Degenerative changes of the sarcomeres are frequent, and include disarray and dissolution of myofilaments, Z-band alterations including streaming and dense bodies, and myofibrillar loss [49, 54].

Chronic inflammation, primarily in the form of T-lymphocytes, is a frequent finding in dilated cardiomyopathy. The presence of inflammation may in some cases contribute to the myocyte damage, consistent with the progression of some patients with lymphocytic myocarditis to a clinical syndrome indistinguishable from dilated cardiomyopathy. In pathological studies, the degree of lymphocytic infiltrate has been a matter of debate, partly because of patient sampling differences, methodology of quantification, and the inflammatory foci of normal hearts [55]. Some reports show no increase in lymphocytes compared with a control population [42], whereas others show a wide range of inflammation in autopsy studies [46, 56]. When defined as inflammation with myocyte damage, myocarditis with adjacent myocyte necrosis is seen in fewer than 5% of cases of dilated cardiomyopathy [41]. In patients with recently diagnosed dilated cardiomyopathy, 13% of endomyocardial biopsies demonstrate myocarditis by the Dallas criteria, but these patients probably represent recent onset of heart failure after myocarditis [57]. There is evidence that there are increased numbers of T-cells in biopsies of patients with dilated cardiomyopathy in the absence of overt myocarditis [58].

Increased numbers of mature and developing collagen fibrils are present in the interstitial spaces in hearts with dilated cardiomyopathy [46]. Replacement fibrosis, with dropout of myocytes, may also occur, possibly due to previous sites of inflammation or ischaemia. Based on light-microscopic observations, the frequencies of patchy interstitial and focal replacement fibrosis are approximately 15% and 45%, respectively [41, 42], and are similar to those of cardiac fibrosis found in patients dying of other cardiovascular and neoplastic diseases [42]. The degree of fibrosis increases from the epicardium to the endocardium, probably because of the secondary effects of ischaemia, and is greater on the left side of the ventricular septum than the right [49]. The degree of interstitial fibrosis may be estimated by echocardiographic determination of the degree and cyclic variation of calibrated myocardial integrated backscatter [59]. Fibrosis in dilated cardiomyopathy may be accompanied by an alteration in isoforms of fibronectin, with a shift towards oncofoetal variants [60]. The increase in collagen is accompanied by a decrease in stable mature cross-links of pyridinoline, an increase in the activity of neutrophil-type collagenase and gelatinase, and a decrease in the activity of the tissue inhibitor of metalloproteinase, suggesting that normal collagen is degraded and replaced by fibrous intercellular deposits of poorly cross-linked collagen [61].

## Clinical expression and epidemiology

The most common symptoms of dilated cardiomyopathy are gradually increasing dyspnoea and fatigue related to heart failure. Chest pain occurs in one-quarter to half of patients and may be due to coronary microvascular disease [62], decreased coronary dilatory capacity [63], or pulmonary embolism. Systemic and pulmonary embolism occurs in the majority of patients during the course of the disease [41]. Ambulatory Holter monitoring will demonstrate unsustained ventricular tachycardia in about half of patients [64], complete bundle branch block in 50%, and atrial fibrillation in 25% [41]. Approximately 3% of patients die suddenly without previous symptoms [57], as a result of cardiac arrhythmias.

The main criteria for diagnosis are an ejection fraction of less than 45–55% and ventricular dilatation (left ventricular internal diastolic dimensions greater than 2.7 cm/m$^2$ of body surface area) [65]. Echocardiography typically demonstrates global hypokinesia.

The prevalence of dilated cardiomyopathy in the USA is about 37 per 100 000 individuals, with a yearly incidence rate of 6 per 100 000 [18, 66]. The age at presentation is typically between 20 and 60 years, with a mean in the fifth decade (Table 5.1). Men are two to three times more likely than women to develop the disease, and there is a slight predilection for blacks [66, 67].

Twenty per cent of patients with known dilated cardiomyopathy die suddenly secondary to arrhythmias, and in the majority of the remainder the cause of death is intractable heart failure [41]. The survival rate is about 35% at 5 years and 15% at 10 years. Most patients develop symptoms gradually, with a mean interval of approximately 50 months between onset and death. The most important risk factors for death are progressive ventricular dysfunction and significant arrhythmias [46]. Right ventricular dilatation has been shown to be an independent negative prognostic finding [68].

## Genetic findings and pathophysiology

The incidence of familial idiopathic dilated cardiomyopathy is unknown, but ranges from 2 to 56% [69, 70]. The incidence of a positive family history in patients with dilated cardiomyopathy was 7% and 20% in two carefully planned studies [71, 72]. The usual pattern of transmission is autosomal dominant with incomplete penetrance [72], although autosomal-recessive, X-linked, polygenic, and mitochondrial inheritance have been described [73]. With the exception of dystrophin-related dilated cardiomyopathy, which has an X-linked transmission, identification of the gene or genes involved has not yet been reported and there does not appear to be an association with human leucocyte antigen (HLA) type [69].

In less than 10% of males with familial dilated cardiomyopathy, there is an X-linked mutation in the 5′ region of the dystrophin gene [74]. In these patients, overt skeletal myopathy is absent. The absence of overt symptoms of Duchenne's muscular dystrophy may be due to the site of the mutation in cardiac-specific regulatory sequences [75]. Fifty per cent of men with typical or subclinical Duchenne's and Becker's muscular dystrophy eventually develop a mild or an overt form of dilated cardiomyopathy [76, 77]. The clinical and histological features of X-linked cardiomyopathy are similar to other forms of dilated cardiomyopathy. However, immunohistochemical studies on frozen sections show a decrease in dystrophin and there may be subtle changes of sarcolemmal membrane rupture on ultrastructural analysis.

It has recently been demonstrated that over 50% of female carriers of the Duchenne and Becker types of muscular dystrophy may develop clinical or echocardiographic signs of heart failure. Immunohistochemical studies of endomyocardial biopsies may be helpful in demonstrating decreased levels of dystrophin [78, 79].

The pathophysiology of sporadic idiopathic dilated cardiomyopathy is complicated by the fact that the disease is likely to be a heterogeneous group of disorders [46]. The mechanism of heart failure appears at least in part to be mediated by apoptosis of myocytes [80, 81]. A single case of dilated cardiomyopathy has been described secondary to a genetic deficiency of metavinculin, a cardiac isoform of the cytoskeletal protein vinculin, which connects actin microfilaments to the intercalated disk and membrane costameres of the heart [82]. The major associations and risk factors for dilated cardiomyopathy are viral myocarditis, diabetes mellitus, pregnancy, heredity, alcoholism, and autoimmunity. Cigarette smoking has been associated with dilated cardiomyopathy in some studies [83] but not others [84].

The proportion of cases of dilated cardiomyopathy secondary to a previous viral infection is difficult to ascertain and can be estimated by a variety of methods. About 13% of patients with unexplained heart failure demonstrate myocarditis [57, 85]. Enteroviral antibodies are usually found at a higher rate in patients with dilated cardiomyopathy than in controls [73], but the rate is generally less than 50%. Persistent immunoglobulin M (IgM) enteroviral antibodies in a small proportion of patients suggest the possibility of persistent, perhaps defective replication within the heart [73, 86]. Enteroviral RNA has been detected in a minority of biopsies from patients with dilated cardiomyopathy [87–90]. Prospective studies demonstrate that 15–50% of patients will develop cardiomyopathy. These studies may overestimate the true rate of the development of chronic disease, however, because of selection of patients with myocarditis who are especially ill [73, 91]. Recently, myocyte necrosis and myocarditis have been assessed in patients with dilated cardiomyopathy by antimyosin immunoscintigraphy. In this technique, antimyosin antibodies with high affinities affording sensitivity and specificity are radiolabelled with $^{111}$In. Most cases of biopsy-proven myocarditis are detected by this technique, as are nearly half of patients without myocarditis on biopsy. Whether the latter group represents false-negative biopsies or false-positive scans is unknown, although these cases appear to be more likely to resolve spontaneously, suggesting the former [92, 93].

There are several lines of evidence that point to an autoimmune mechanism in the pathogenesis of some forms of idiopathic dilated cardiomyopathy (see Chapter 24) [94]. Dilated cardiomyopathy has been reported in patients with systemic lupus erythematosus, serum sickness, polyarteritis nodosa, acquired immunodeficiency syndrome, and other immunological disorders including asthma [94, 95]. Serological studies have shown a host of circulating autoantibodies in acute myocarditis [94] as well as dilated cardiomyopathy. The antibodies include antimuscle-specific and heart-reactive antibodies, antilaminin, antimitochondrial antibodies, antimyosin heavy and light chain antibodies, and anti-β-adrenoceptor antibodies [96, 97]. The role of these antibodies in the pathogenesis of the disease and the role of viral infection in their elaboration are under investigation.

The mechanism of inflammatory-mediated damage in dilated cardiomyopathy has been assessed in endomyocardial biopsies by immunohistochemical localization of perforin and T-cell intracellular antigen-1, mediators of lymphocyte-mediated cytotoxicity. An association between the expression of these antigens and the presence of fibrosis was demonstrated, suggesting local activation of T-cells as a mediator of myocardial damage [98]. Antigen presentation of myocytes may be facilitated by antigens B7-1, B7-2, and CD40, as these are expressed in association with perforin-expressing cytotoxic lymphocytes and natural killer cells in the myocardial tissues of patients with dilated cardiomyopathy [99]. Interstitial and endothelial immune activation, as demonstrated by major histocompatibility complex (MHC) expression, has been associated with lymphocyte density, as well as upregulation of adhesion molecules in heart biopsies from patients with dilated cardiomyopathy, indicating that a chronic autoimmune process may persist [58]. Viral infection or autoimmune abnormalities may induce cytokines that increase nitric oxide, which has negative inotropic and cytotoxic effects on cardiac myocytes. Upregulation of inducible nitric oxide synthase and tumour necrosis factor-α has been observed in endomyocardial biopsies from patients with dilated cardiomyopathy, consistent with the hypothesis that myocardial damage in dilated cardiomyopathy may be mediated by cytokines [100].

Consumption of over 1 litre of ethanol weekly is associated with a 2.5 relative risk for the development of dilated cardiomyopathy [67]. The mechanism of alcohol toxicity may involve calcium binding and transport, mitochondrial respiration, myocardial lipid metabolism, myocardial protein synthesis, myofibrillar ATPase, or a combination of these cellular functions [101]. An in-depth discussion of the toxic effect of alcohol on the heart is found in Chapter 25. Gross and histological pathological features of hearts from alcoholics dying with cardiomyopathy have not shown specific changes [102, 103].

Diabetes mellitus is found in approximately 7% of patients with dilated cardiomyopathy [41]. The relative risk of dilated cardiomyopathy among diabetics is estimated at 1.6 that of the general population [84]. Small vessel disease may be involved in the pathogenesis of diabetic cardiomyopathy [46].

Approximately 10 in 100 000 peripartum women develop cardiomyopathy that is indistinguishable from idiopathic dilated cardiomyopathy (Fig. 5.12). Peripartum cardiomyopathy is defined as left ventricular dilatation and failure that first develops during the third trimester of pregnancy or in the first 6 months postpartum [105, 106]. The mortality is high, ranging from 25 to 60% [46]. Risk factors include advanced maternal age, multiparity, African descent, twinning, and long-term tocolysis, and there are occasional familial cases [104, 107, 108]. The pathophysiology of peripartum cardiomyopathy is unknown, but two studies suggest a high incidence of myocarditis [109, 110].

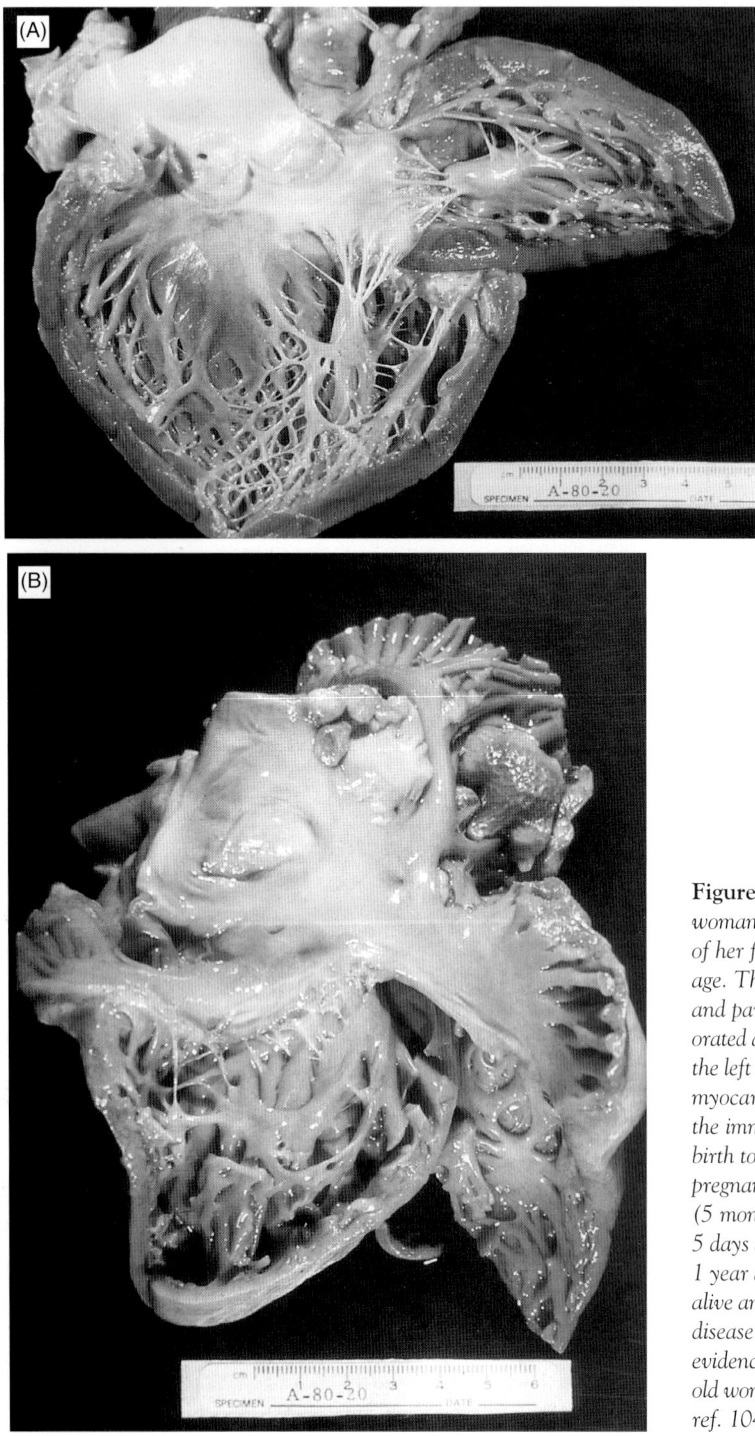


**Figure 5.12** *Familial postpartum cardiomyopathy in a 21-year-old woman with history of heart disease and irregular pulse in the 7th month of her first pregnancy. She delivered a baby girl who is well at 4 years of age. Three years later the mother presented with congestive heart failure and paroxysmal atrial tachyarrhythmias. Her condition gradually deteriorated and she died 5 months later. The heart was markedly dilated on both the left (A) and right (B) and there was extensive interstitial fibrosis of the myocardium. A family history revealed that there had been five deaths in the immediate family: her mother died at the age of 35 years after giving birth to the eighth child, and had evidence of heart disease at 7 months of pregnancy. The patient's eldest sister had died at the age of 23 years (5 months after giving birth to her first child). A 24-year-old sister died 5 days after the delivery of her third child. Two siblings died in infancy at 1 year and 2 years of age of unknown causes. Three sisters are currently alive and well: a 33-year-old unmarried female has asymptomatic cardiac disease characterized by atrial arrhythmias; a 29-year-old sibling has no evidence of heart disease and her three children are well; and a 26-year-old woman and her two daughters have no evidence of heart disease. (From ref. 104.)*

## Restrictive cardiomyopathy

### Haemodynamic findings and classification

The word 'restrictive' is used in cardiomyopathies to describe a stiff and rigid myocardium that results in abnormal diastolic function from defective ventricular filling. Contractile function is well maintained except in the terminal stages of the disease. A number of pathological states can lead to a restrictive cardiomyopathy: myocardial diseases, infiltrative diseases, storage diseases, and endomyocardial diseases (Table 5.2). By far the most common underlying cause of restrictive cardiomyopathy in the Western world is amyloidosis, whereas in the developing world the most common is endocardial fibrosis.

The clinical presentation of restrictive cardiomyopathy is similar to that of constrictive pericarditis. The laboratory tests that help to distinguish between the two are endomyocardial biopsy [111], computed tomographic (CT) scanning, MRI, and radionuclide angiography; currently, exploratory thoracotomy is rarely necessary. The haemodynamic features of restrictive disease are high systemic venous and pulmonary arterial pressures, with the left ventricular pressure higher than the right by at least 5 mmHg. The pressure discrepancy between the ventricles is accentuated by exercise, fluid challenge, and the Valsalva manoeuvre, and is not uniformly present in all patients. In contrast, constrictive pericarditis is not characterized by a significant (greater than 5 mmHg) difference between the right and left heart pressures. The systolic pulmonary artery pressure is usually more than 50 mmHg in restrictive cardiomyopathy, and is less than that in constrictive pericarditis. The plateau of the right ventricular diastolic pressure is usually at least one-third that of the peak right ventricular systolic pressure, and is less in constrictive pericarditis and restrictive cardiomyopathy. Despite these general distinctions, at least one-quarter of cases are not classified correctly by haemodynamic findings alone. CT and MRI scans can be helpful in demonstrating pericardial thickening and pericardial calcific deposits. Echocardiography may demonstrate a thickened left ventricular wall in patients with infiltrative disease; if this feature is pronounced, it may be helpful in distinguishing from constrictive pericardial disease.

Restrictive cardiomyopathies are classified by the site and nature of the process resulting in stiffening of the ventricular walls (Table 5.2).

**Table 5.2** Classification of the restrictive cardiomyopathies (data from ref. 111)

| Myocardial | Endomyocardial |
|---|---|
| Non-infiltrative | Endomyocardial fibrosis |
| Idiopathic | Hypereosinophilic syndrome |
| Scleroderma | Carcinoid |
| Infiltrative | Metastatic malignancies |
| Amyloid | Radiation |
| Sarcoid | Anthracycline toxicity |
| Gaucher's disease | |
| Hurler's disease | |
| Storage diseases | |
| Haemochromatosis | |
| Fabry's disease | |
| Glycogen storage diseases | |

### Amyloidosis

#### *Definition and morphological characteristics*

Since amyloidosis is the most frequent cause of restrictive cardiomyopathy in the Western world, it is important to characterize this disease in detail. Amyloidosis is a complex disease caused by the deposition of the unique β-pleated sheet fibril formed from various proteins by different mechanisms. In histological sections stained by haematoxylin and eosin it is recognized as a homogeneous flocculent eosinophilic deposit [113]. Despite morphological similarities in the accumulated proteins they are chemically different. The usual stains used to identify amyloid are the Congo Red stain (with or without potassium permanganate), which shows apple green (red–green) birefringence under polarized light, thioflavin T and S, the sulfated Alcian Blue stain, metachromatic stains (Crystal Violet stain, Methyl Violet, and Toluidine Blue), and Sirius Red [113]. However, none is specific for amyloid. Immunohistochemistry not only identifies amyloid specifically but can also help to identify the underlying protein [114, 115]. Transmission electron microscopy reveals that amyloid is a non-branching parallel array of 7–10 nm filaments or 2.5–5.5-nm-thick protofilaments, and demonstrates the exact location of the deposits within the myocardium [113], but does not identify the β-pleat, which is only shown by X-ray and infrared diffraction analyses. Staining with immunogold demonstrates the protein precursor of the amyloid. In addition to the protein responsible for the fibril structure, several other components are consistently present in amyloid. These include amyloid P component, perlecan, laminin, collagen IV, and fibronectin [113].

***Classification and nature of the protein composition***

Amyloid is classified according to the protein responsible for the fibril structure (Table 5.3). Primary amyloidosis is caused by a monoclonal population of plasma cells, often as a consequence of multiple myeloma [116]. The amyloid of primary amyloidosis is designated AL amyloid and is composed of portions of immunoglobulin light chain. Secondary amyloidosis is the result of production of non-immunoglobulin protein AA and is associated with chronic inflammatory diseases. Historically, these disease have been infections, specifically tuberculosis, chronic abscesses, and leprosy. Now, secondary amyloidosis is more commonly associated with various forms of arthritis, collagen vascular diseases, and subcutaneous drug use. Secondary amyloid may complicate neoplasms, such as Hodgkin's disease and renal cell carcinoma, in which inflammation is a prominent component. Senile systemic amyloidosis is due to the deposition of amyloid formed from transthyretin (prealbumin). Familial amyloidosis is inherited as an autosomal trait in young adults as a result of the production of a variant form of transthyretin. Over 50 separate mutations have been described. Families with this condition were first reported in Portugal, Japan, and Sweden. There are other forms of hereditary amyloidosis that may involve the heart but usually do not result in cardiomyopathy. The precursor protein in Finnish hereditary amyloidosis is gelsolin, an actin-binding protein, in Iowa type it is apolipoprotein A-I, and in Icelandic type cystatin C[15] [117–119]. It is not economically viable or necessary to identify these types by immunohistochemical testing. In the elderly, scattered amyloid deposits may be present in the aorta and atria. Isolated atrial amyloid occurs in most patients over 80 years of age, and is more frequent than aortic amyloid. Isolated atrial amyloid has previously been referred to as a form of senile amyloidosis, but is not related to systemic senile amyloidosis. The isolated atrial amyloid protein is related to atrial natriuretic factor and ventricular involvement is uncommon. Patients on chronic dialysis are also prone to amyloidosis. The principal component of haemodialysis-associated amyloid is $\beta_2$-microglobulin [120, 121]. Clinical symptoms result from the carpal tunnel syndrome, bone cyst, and spondyloarthropathy. The heart is the most frequent organ involved at autopsy, with effacement of small blood vessels, but symptomatic cardiac disease is not reported. Other amyloid types affect only certain organs or lesions, such as amyloid A$\beta$ in the brain, calcitonin in medullary carcinoma of the thyroid, and islet amyloid polypeptide in insulinomas.

In routine clinicopathological practice, the five different fibril proteins associated with the most common generalized amyloid syndromes are: amyloid A (AA), amyloid $\lambda$ (A$\lambda$)- and $\kappa$ (A$\kappa$)-light chain, transthyretin (ATTR), and $\beta_2$-microglobulin (A$\beta$2M) [122]. These are the most likely to be deposited in most tissues and organs and must be considered in the biopsy of any amyloidotic organ or tissue.

***Clinical findings***

Symptomatic cardiac involvement is common in systemic amyloidosis. The average age at presentation is approximately 60 years, and there is a male:female predominance of 2:1 to 4:1 [115, 116, 123–125]. The most common presentation is that of restrictive cardiomyopathy, with the dominant findings of peripheral oedema, jugular venous distension, and hepatomegaly in the absence of paroxysmal nocturnal dyspnoea and orthopnoea. Patients typically are normotensive or hypotensive. The left ventricle is stiff from the amyloid infiltration of the myocardium, producing the characteristic diastolic dip and plateau (square-root sign)

**Table 5.3** Nomenclature and classification of amyloidosis that may frequently involve the heart

| Amyloid protein | Protein precursor | Clinical syndrome | Age | Patients with symptomatic heart disease (%) |
|---|---|---|---|---|
| AA | apo SAA | Secondary (inflammation) | 50 | 0–5% |
| AL | Light chain $\kappa$ or $\lambda$ | Primary (idiopathic); myeloma | 60 | 20–30% |
| ATTR | Transthyretin (normal TTR) | Systemic senile amyloidosis | 70+ | Low |
| ATTR | Transthyretin (various mutations) | Familial amyloid with polyneuropathy, several types | 60 | 20–50% |
| AANF | Atrial natriuretic factor | Isolated atrial amyloid | 80+ | 0 |
| A$\beta$2M | $\beta_2$-Microglobulin | Chronic haemodialysis | — | 0 |

in the ventricular pulse. The second most common presentation of cardiac amyloidosis is congestive heart failure due to systolic dysfunction which results from atrial deposits with loss in atrial transport function. Patients with this presentation have a relentless clinical course that is complicated by anginal chest pain in the absence of epicardial coronary artery disease. Orthostatic hypotension occurs in about 10% of patients and is the result of amyloid infiltration of the autonomic nervous system or blood vessels. Conduction system involvement may result in arrhythmias and conduction disturbances but is the least common presentation. However, sudden death is relatively common, and is presumed to be arrhythmic in origin.

The chest roentgenogram usually shows cardiomegaly in patients with systolic dysfunction, but heart size may be normal. The electrocardiogram is usually abnormal and the most characteristic finding is diminished voltage. Atrial arrhythmias, especially atrial fibrillation, are common, and complex ventricular arrhythmias are also found frequently. Abnormalities of atrioventicular (AV) conduction are common in familial amyloidosis with polyneuropathy [117, 118]. The sinus node is frequently involved, resulting in sick sinus syndrome. Echocardiography usually shows normal ventricular wall thickness, except in advanced cases, when there is an increase in wall thickness. The ventricular cavities are typically small, with dilated atria. Although systolic function is usually normal, left ventricular diastolic dysfunction is often observed, providing prognostic information. A pericardial effusion is common, and the valves may be thickened. On echocardiography, the appearance of the amyloid is distinct, giving a granular sparkling texture to the cardiac walls [126]. In some cases, the left ventricular wall thickness is not uniform and resembles hypertrophic cardiomyopathy (Fig. 5.13). Scintigraphy with technetium-99m pyrophosphate is often strongly positive in cardiac amyloidosis, but false negatives have been

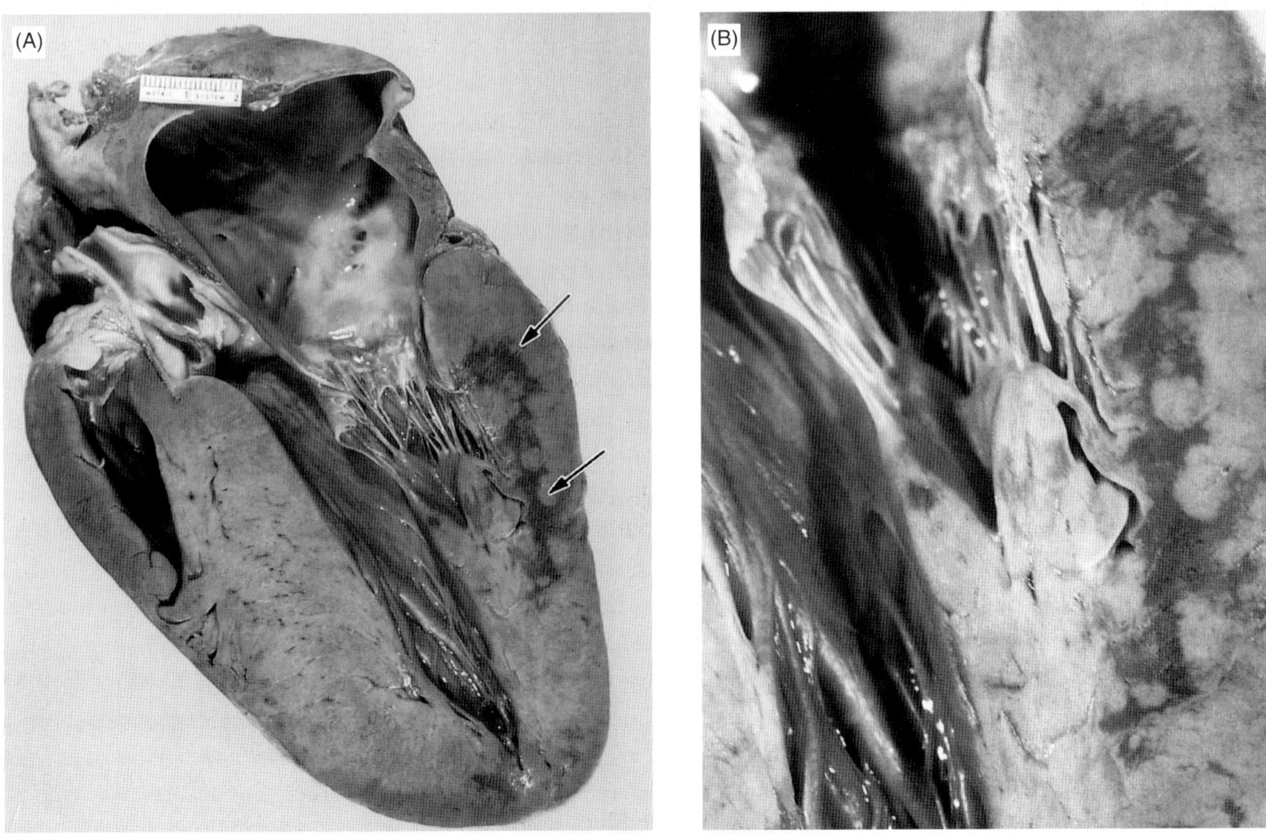


**Figure 5.13** *Restrictive cardiomyopathy: cardiac amyloidosis. (A) Long-axis view of the heart from a 46-year-old man who noted dyspnoea on walking 2 years before his death. At the age of 44 years, a diagnosis of hypertrophic cardiomyopathy was made based on the echocardiographic findings (septal:free wall ratio 1.7:1 and anterior systolic motion of the anterior mitral leaflet). Nine months before his death he had transient sudden left-sided weakness with slurred speech, worsening dyspnoea, transient chest pain, and a carpal-tunnel syndrome. The patient died in severe congestive heart failure, and a diagnosis of amyloidosis was never made during his life. At autopsy the heart weighed 780 g and deposits of amyloid were visible* (arrows) *in the left ventricular free wall. (From ref. 127.) (B) Close up of the left ventricular wall showing large amyloid deposits.*

reported [128]. Indium-labelled antimyosin antibody scanning can also detect amyloid involvement of the heart [129].

Senile cardiac amyloidosis is a frequent postmortem finding in individuals over 80 years of age and is generally regarded as a benign condition of no functional importance. However, at autopsy the amyloidosis has often been retrospectively associated with congestive heart failure and cardiac arrhythmias [11, 130], and endomyocardial biopsies have demonstrated senile cardiac amyloid deposits in patients with congestive heart failure [131]. In approximately 20% of symptomatic patients with a diagnosis of cardiac amyloidosis by endomyocardial biopsy, the amyloid type is ATTR; the majority of the remainder is AL [114]. The prognosis of patients with congestive heart failure and senile amyloidosis as demonstrated on biopsy is better than that of patients with primary amyloidosis. In addition, alkylating agents are not indicated for treatment of cardiac amyloidosis due to amyloid ATTR [132].

The familial form has three clinical presentations: progressive neuropathy, cardiomyopathy, or nephropathy. At the time of diagnosis, 83% of patients have peripheral neuropathy, 33% have autonomic neuropathy, and 27% have cardiomyopathy. Renal involvement is present in less than 10%, and liver involvement is rare. The median age at diagnosis is 64 years. Diagnosis can be established by subcutaneous fat aspirates (77% positive) or by rectal biopsy (78% positive), and in bone marrow specimens in 41% [118].

### *Gross and microscopic findings*

The heart weight in cardiac amyloidosis may range from mild to moderately increased. In an autopsy series of 54 symptomatic patients with cardiac amyloidosis, the mean heart weight was 554 g, with a range of 300–900 g; for women the mean heart weight was 484 g and for men 596 g. The myocardium is firm, rubbery, or waxy, which often allows for recognition on gross examination of the heart (Figs. 5.13–5.16). Atrial dilatation is almost always present, but the ventricles are usually normal in size, with dilatation being reported in 20% of cases. In patients with ventricular dilatation there are usually other conditions present that cause the dilatation, i.e. coronary artery disease with left ventricular transmural scarring or chronic lung disease. Symmetric left ventricular wall measurements are seen in 93% of patients and only 7% have a septum that is more than 1.3 times the thickness of the free wall. The amyloid imparts a focal, tan, granular, waxy appearance on the mural endocardium best appreciated in the atria. Valve involvement occurs in 80% of cases and is more common on the tricuspid and mitral valves (80%) than on the semilunar valves (50%). Focal transmural deposits in the left ventricle may be observed in less than 20% of cases.

Microscopically, amyloid may be present in large vessels, including the aorta, pulmonary arteries, venae cavae, and epicardial coronary arteries [114, 130]. In the heart, amyloid is located most frequently in the intramyocardial arteries and arterioles, the endocardium, and the myocardium, and less frequently in the pericardium. The myocardial involvement may be interstitial, pericellular, interstitial nodular, or a combination of these patterns (Figs. 5.13, 5.14). There have been few studies correlating histological findings with the type of amyloidosis. In a series of 47 hearts from 21 patients with primary amyloidosis and 26 patients with senile amyloidosis, Smith *et al.* [130] found that primary amyloidosis was associated with extensive infiltrates and a high frequency of interstitial and vascular amyloid. In contrast, senile amyloidosis was associated with less extensive infiltrates, which correlated with overall fewer cardiac symptoms, and a high incidence of nodular deposits. Pericardial deposits have been frequently reported. They are usually seen in cases of widespread cardiovascular involvement and are a predictor of severe myocardial disease. Conduction system involvement has been reported and is virtually always seen in conjunction with myocardial involvement. All conduction system components have been observed to be involved, including the sinoatrial node, AV node, bundle of His and its branches, the arteries to the nodes, and the peripheral ganglia and nerves. Although amyloid deposits in the conduction system may explain some of the conduction abnormalities, the same electrocardiographic abnormalities may be present in the absence of such deposits.

Endomyocardial biopsy is a safe and effective method for diagnosing cardiac amyloidosis. In diagnostic biopsies (non-transplant), amyloid is found in 4–8% of patients. In one study of patients with AL amyloid and cardiac symptoms, diagnosis by endomyocardial biopsy had a yield of 100%, whereas rectal and other biopsies were negative in as many as 25% of cases [125]. In the largest endomyocardial biopsy series reported from the Mayo clinic [114], the distribution of the amyloid type was as follows: 74% primary (AL), 22% senile (ATTR), and 4% familial (mutant TTR). The pattern of deposition in primary amyloidosis was more frequently pericellular (96%) and vascular (88%) than

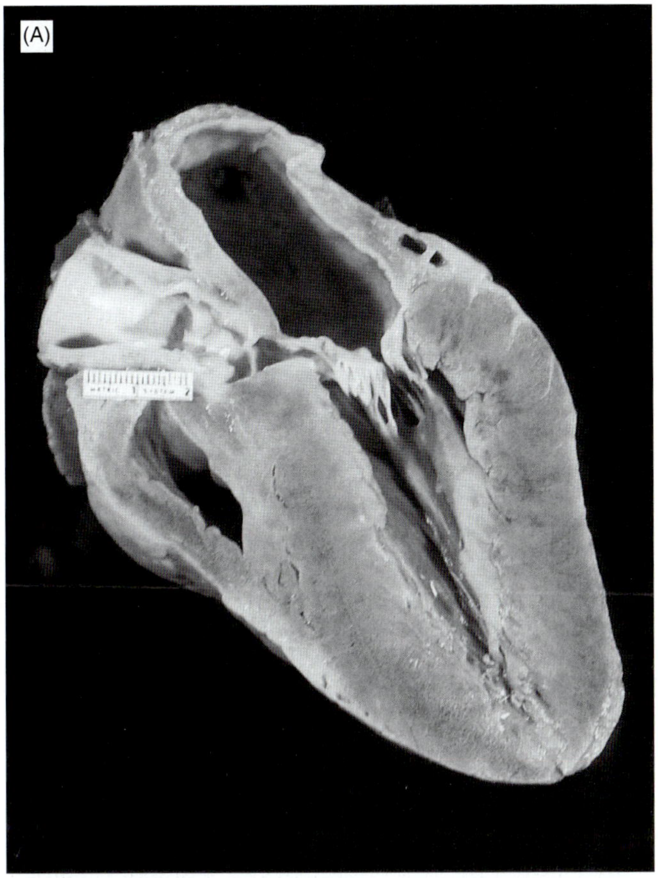


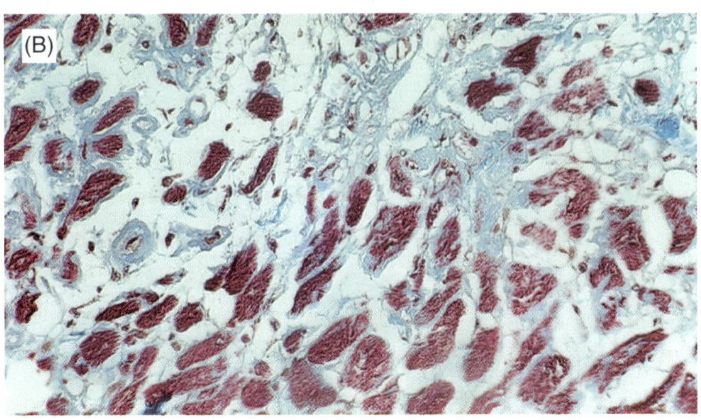


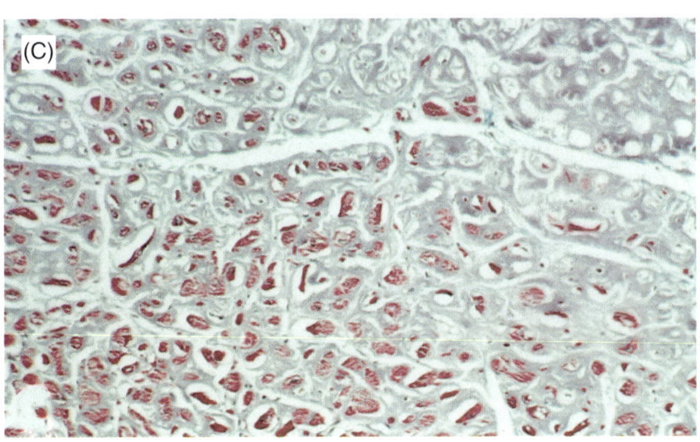


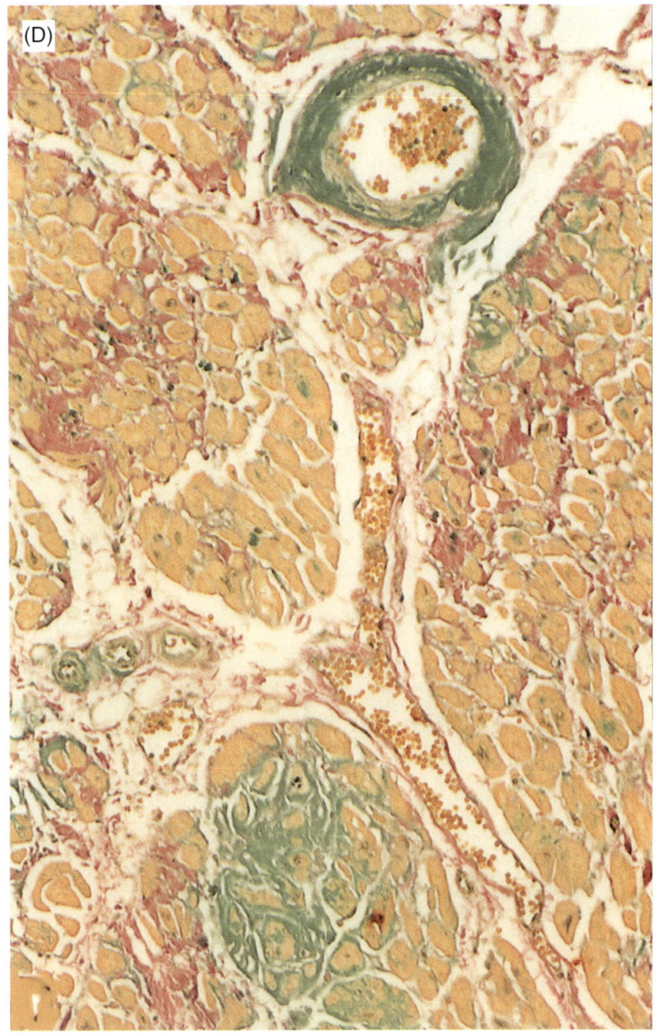


**Figure 5.14** *Cardiac amyloidosis secondary to multiple myeloma. Long-axis view of a heart in a 56-year-old woman who had been well 6 months prior to death when she developed periorbital purpura, pedal oedema, and right arm pain. She had syncope 1 month later and was found to have multiple myeloma. The electrocardiogram disclosed both atrial and ventricular arrhythmias and electrophysiological studies disclosed distal H-V block. The patient never had congestive heart failure and died at home suddenly. The heart weighed 430 g and had a firm, rubbery consistency. The long-axis view of the heart (A) shows mild dilatation of the left atrium and the left ventricular cavity is normal in size. (From ref. 127.) The septum appears thicker than the free wall. (B) Interstitial and focal amyloid deposits are present in the myocardium. (C) Trichrome stain showing interstitial amyloid deposits around individual myocytes. (D) Sulfated alcian blue stain demonstrating focal amyloid deposits in the interstitium and amyloid deposits in the intramyocardial vessels (amyloid appears green).*

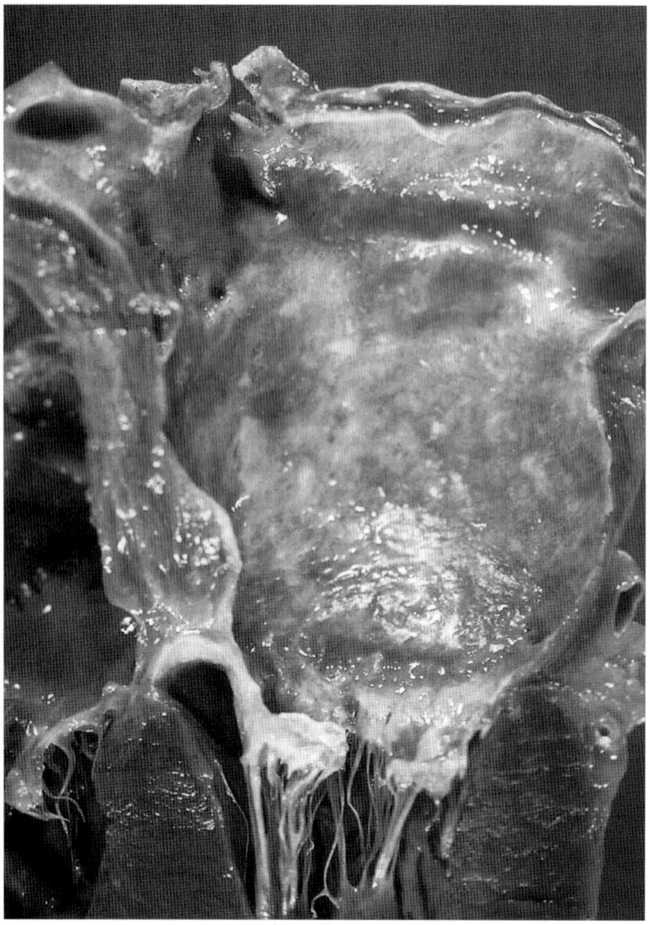

**Figure 5.15** *Senile cardiac amyloidosis. An 89-year-old man presented with shortness of breath, chest pain, and palpitations of 4 weeks' duration. He had pedal oedema for 2 years. The electrocardiogram showed atrial fibrillation with a ventricular response of 80–100 beats/min. A left anterior hemiblock had been present for 6 years. Chest X-ray showed cardiomegaly and echocardiography was technically difficult. The patient died in severe congestive heart failure. At autopsy the heart weighed 680 g, the atria were markedly dilated, and the ventricles were normal in size. The photograph demonstrates the posterior wall of the left atrium. The endocardial surface is glistening with waxy deposits. (From ref. 133.)*

nodular (50%) or endocardial (61%); in the senile form it was more often pericellular (95%) and nodular (82%) than vascular (26%) or endocardial (41%); and in the familial type it was always seen in the pericellular, nodular, and vascular distribution (100%) and was infrequent in the endocardium (25%). When amyloid was present, it was severe in extent, with more than 50% of the area affected [130].

### *Survival and treatment*

It is generally believed that treatment of cardiac amyloidosis is ineffective and unsatisfactory. However, some researchers report encouraging results in patients with primary amyloidosis treated with alkylating agents [116]. In general, the treatment is that of congestive heart failure, with diuretics and vasodilators, although hypotension may occur as a side-effect of these treatments. Digitalis glycosides and calcium channel blockers should generally be avoided. Cardiac pacing may be beneficial in the short term for patients with conduction system disease. A few patients have had cardiac transplantation with poor results, survival being 39% at 4 years [134].

## Endomyocardial disease

Endomyocardial disease occurs commonly in the tropical regions of the world, particularly in Africa, Asia, and South America. Major loci are Uganda and Nigeria in Africa, Kerala in southern India, Sri Lanka, and Brazil. Endomyocardial fibrosis (EMF), the typical sequela of tropical endomyocardial disease, is also known as Davies' disease after the detailed description given by J.N.P. Davies and his associates 50 years ago. Its prevalence is highest in Africa and accounts for 15–25% of deaths due to heart disease. EMF is equally frequent in men and women and is reported to occur in a wide age range of 4–70 years, with a mean of 30 years [135].

Loffler's endocarditis parietalis fibroplastica, or eosinophilic endomyocardial disease, is a disease that occurs in temperate climates, usually in men in the 4th decade, and is marked by hypereosinophilia of any cause (greater than 1500 eosinophils/mm$^3$ for at least 6 months) [136, 137]. Cardiac involvement occurs in three-quarters of the patients. The two diseases are now considered as one disease, with Loffler's endocarditis representing the early form and Davies' disease the late form.

### *Gross and microscopic pathology*

*Endomyocardial fibrosis (Davies' disease).* Davies' disease involves both the right and left ventricles in 50% of cases, in 40% of cases only the left ventricle is involved, and in 10% only the right ventricle [138–141]. With left ventricular involvement the posterior mitral valve leaflet is adherent to the left ventricular wall, with fibrosis and resultant mitral regurgitation (Fig. 5.17). The apex of the left ventricle also shows endocardial fibrosis which extends into the anterolateral papillary muscle. The outflow tract of the left ventricle is uninvolved. The right ventricle similarly shows abnormalities in the inflow portion of the ventricle. The right ventricular apex has dense endocardial fibrosis, which

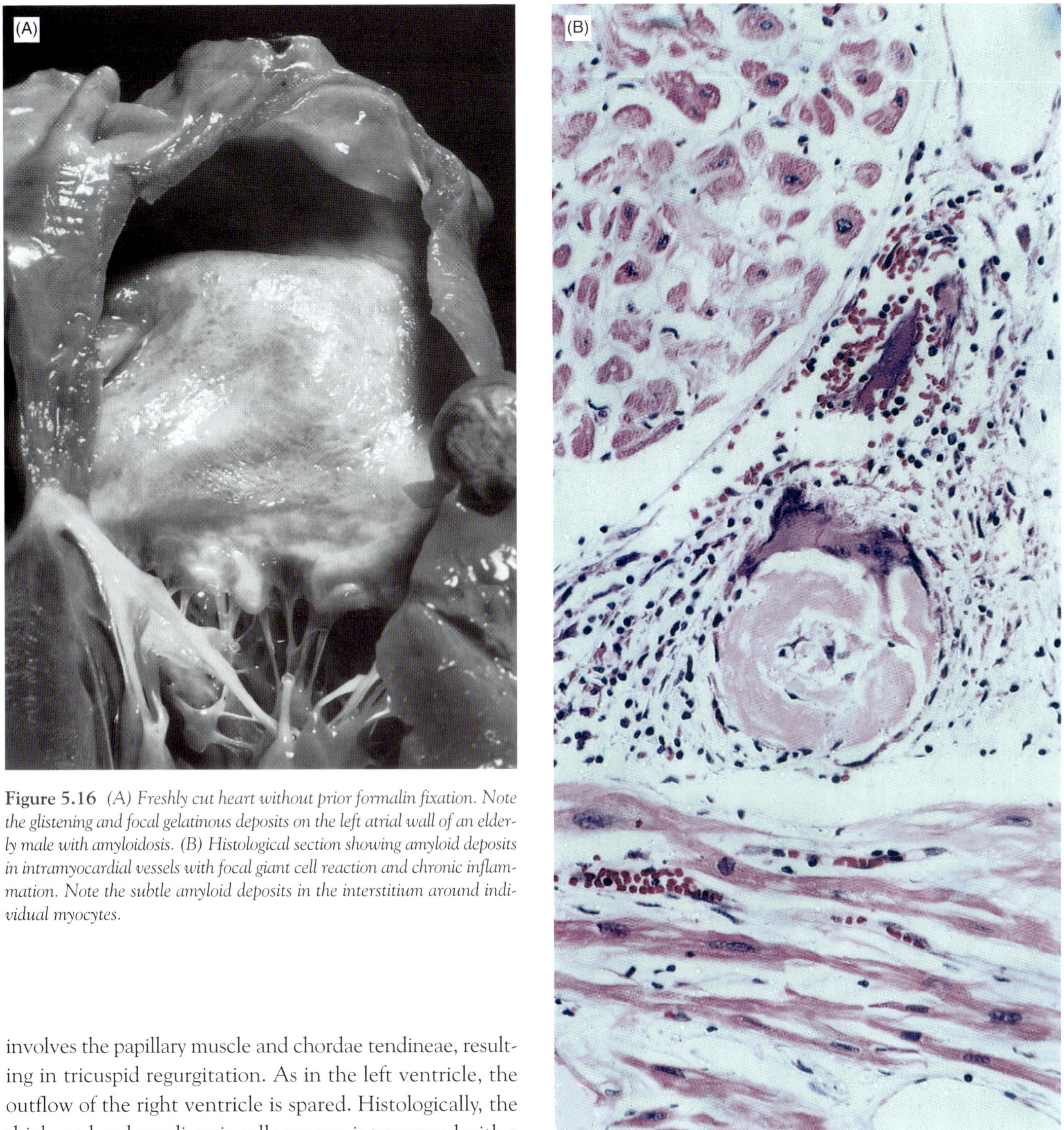


**Figure 5.16** *(A) Freshly cut heart without prior formalin fixation. Note the glistening and focal gelatinous deposits on the left atrial wall of an elderly male with amyloidosis. (B) Histological section showing amyloid deposits in intramyocardial vessels with focal giant cell reaction and chronic inflammation. Note the subtle amyloid deposits in the interstitium around individual myocytes.*

involves the papillary muscle and chordae tendineae, resulting in tricuspid regurgitation. As in the left ventricle, the outflow of the right ventricle is spared. Histologically, the thickened endocardium is collagenous, interspersed with a few elastic fibres (Table 5.4) [142]. Three zones can be identified: an inner layer of dense collagen, followed by a layer of loose connective tissue, and finally a layer of granulation tissue. The last zone consists of neocapillaries and inflammatory cells, which are comprised by lymphocytes, macrophages, plasma cells, and a few eosinophils and Anitschkow's cells. The cellularity of this layer is dependent on the activity of the disease.

*Hypereosinophilic syndrome (Loffler's endocarditis parietalis fibroplastica)* In temperate countries, the pathological findings of endomyocardial disease are similar to those of Davies' disease, except that early forms of the disease show much more thrombosis, are more rapidly progressive, affect

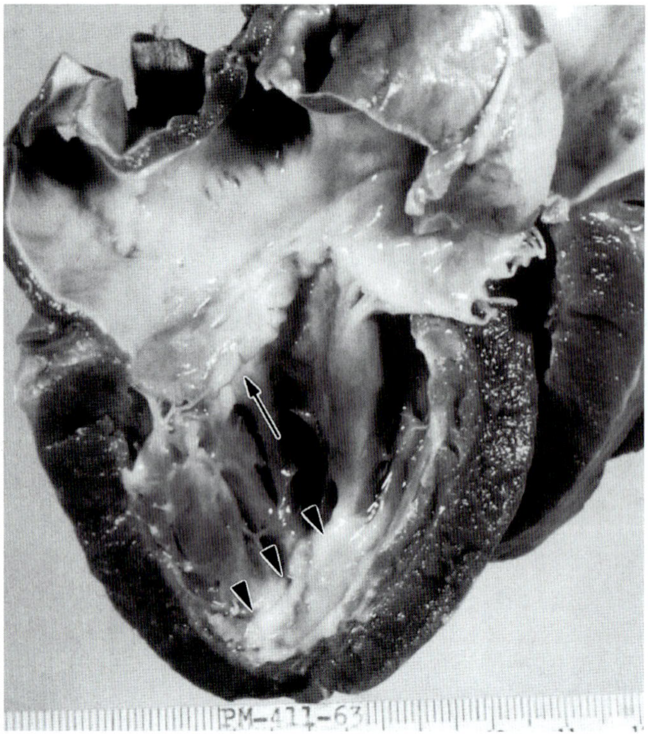

**Figure 5.17** *Davies' disease showing the left ventricle and atrium. Note endocardial fibrosis in the apex of the left ventricle* (arrowheads). *The posterior mitral leaflet is adherent to the left ventricular free wall* (arrow) *and the atrium is enlarged.*

principally males, and are associated with hypereosinophilia and arteritis. Until recently, the two entities were considered to be distinct. It is now well accepted, however, that Loffler's endocarditis and EMF are two phases of the same disease, with the former representing the early phase and the latter the late phase of the disease. In fact, three pathological stages of the disease are recognized: an acute necrotic stage, a thrombotic–necrotic stage, and a late fibrotic stage [143, 144]. In the necrotic stage there is peripheral hypereosinophilia, intense infiltration of the myocardium with eosinophils, and necrosis of the myocytes. An associated arteritis is also present. The acute necrotic stage is followed by the thrombotic stage, which usually occurs about a year following the myocarditis, when the inflammation begins to wane. The thrombus on the left side of the heart is seen beneath the posterior leaflet of the mitral valve and in the apex of the left ventricle, and may extend to envelop the posteromedial papillary muscle (Fig. 5.18). Similarly, thrombus is also present in the apex of the right ventricle, extending around the papillary muscles and involving the inferior surface of the tricuspid valve. The late stage of the disease is one of fibrosis. It is not clear whether the three stages are present in all patients during the course of illness, but all stages have been documented in patients with Loffler's endocarditis. In the tropical form of endemic EMF it has been impossible to document all three phases of the disease, and it has not been possible to confirm high levels of blood eosinophilia in the majority of patients.

## Clinical presentation

*Endomyocardial fibrosis (Davies' disease).* The most common symptoms are those of heart failure, although embolic symptoms may occur in up to one-third of patients. The majority of patients have bilateral cardiac involvement (50%) [143, 144]. With predominant left-sided involvement (40%) the symptoms are those of pulmonary congestion, and with predominant right-sided involvement (10%) the features of a restrictive cardiomyopathy are observed. Ventricular involvement is influenced by the geographical location. The majority of patients in Venezuela

**Table 5.4** Similarities and differences between hypereosinophilic syndrome and Davies' disease

| Characteristics | Hypereosinophilic syndrome | Davies' disease |
|---|---|---|
| Age at presentation (years) | 30–40 | 4–70 |
| Gender | Male > female | Both genders |
| Geographical distribution | Worldwide | Tropics |
| Tissue and peripheral eosinophilia | Present | Absent |
| Three phases of the disease: necrosis, thrombosis, and fibrosis | All three usually present | Only the fibrotic phase |
| Right and left ventricular involvement | Usually bilateral | 50% biventricular, 40% only left ventricle, 10% only right ventricle |

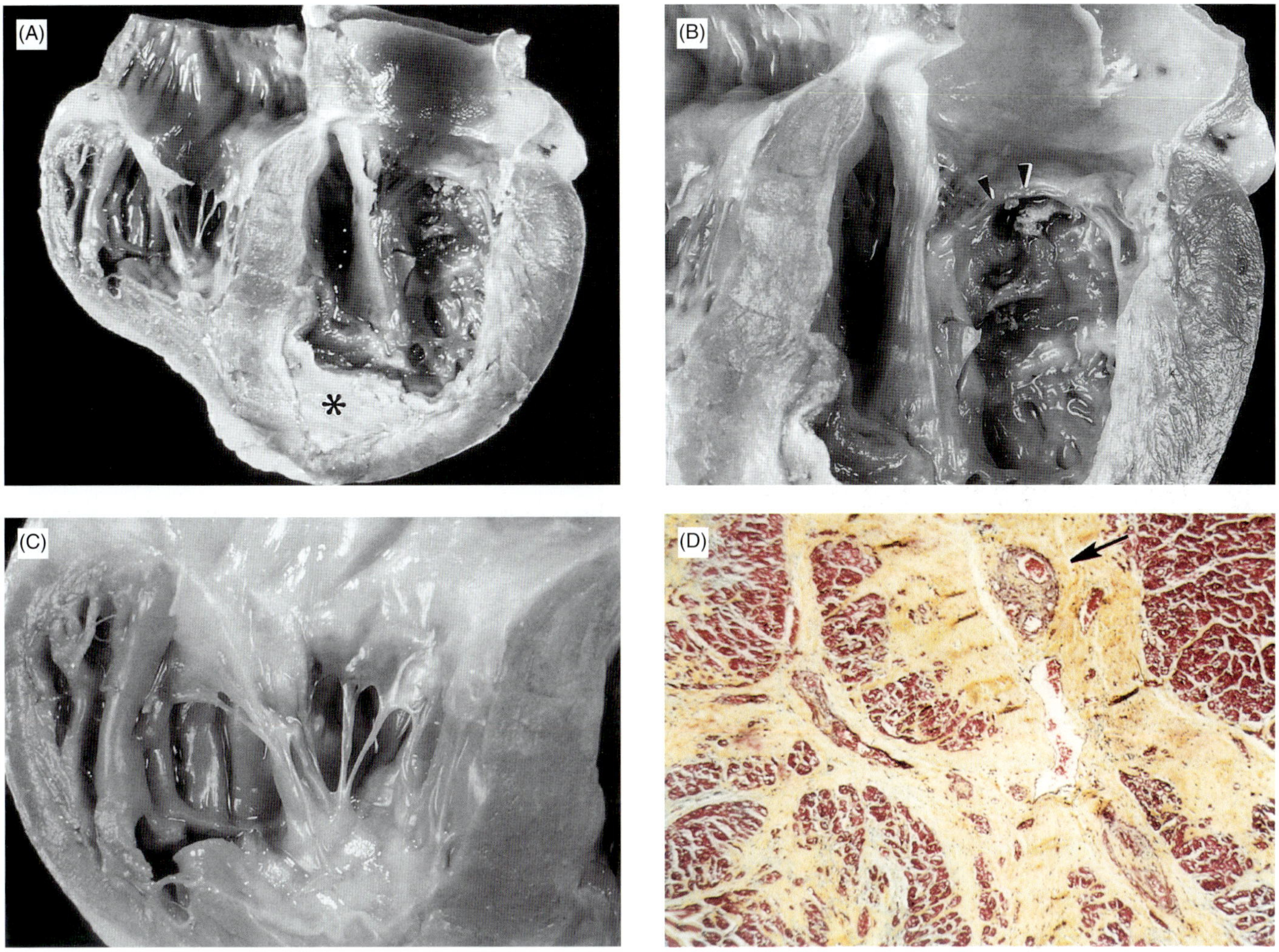


**Figure 5.18** *Hypereosinophilic syndrome in a 9-year-old boy who presented with increasing fatigue, anorexia, weight loss, fever, and absolute eosinophilia (48 000/μl). Pulmonary infiltrates occurred 3 months later. A murmur of mitral regurgitation was heard at 5 months after the onset of illness, and heart failure soon followed. Despite corticosteroid therapy the eosinophilia persisted intermittently until 1 month before death. The patient died within 9 months of the onset of illness. (A) The heart was enlarged and the atria and ventricles were dilated. Note the presence of a thrombus (*) in the left ventricular apex encircling the posteromedial papillary muscle. The right ventricle shows an area of apical endocardial fibrosis. (B) The posterior mitral leaflet* (arrowheads) *is adherent to the left ventricular free wall by a thrombus. (C) Close-up view of the right ventricular apex showing endocardial fibrosis surrounding the posterior papillary muscle. (D) Photomicrograph of the left ventricle. Note scarring and multiluminal channels in an intramyocardial coronary artery* (arrow). *(From ref. 145.)*

have left-sided involvement, whereas in Egypt, where there is a high rate of schistosomiasis, right ventricular involvement is the rule. In African cases, onset of the disease with fever, malaise, and at times itching and urticaria suggest an infectious/inflammatory aetiology. However, these features have not been noticed in cases from Kerala. The mean duration of clinical symptoms before death is approximately 7 months.

*Hypereosinophilic syndrome* The clinical features include an initial viral-like syndrome with fever, cough, and cutaneous rash, followed by congestive heart failure. Over 75% of patients with hypereosinophilic syndrome have severe heart failure, but many other organs, e.g. the lung, nervous system, skin, liver, and intestinal tract, show dysfunction. The common clinical manifestations include right and left ventricular failure with elevated pulmonary and systemic venous pressures, mitral and tricuspid regurgitation from the endocardial fibrotic involvement of the valve leaflets [146, 147], and systemic embolization [148, 149]. Endomyocardial biopsy shows endomyocardial thickening and fibrosis of varying degrees, and there may or may not be a thrombus infiltrated by eosinophils. Death is usually due to congestive heart failure, often associated with renal, hepatic, or respiratory failure.

### *Pathogenesis*

The causes of the eosinophilia in most patients of Loffler's endocarditis are unknown, but in some it may be the result of leukaemia or secondary to parasites, Churg–Strauss syndrome, granulomatous disorders, hypersensitivity, or neoplasms. Recently, eosinophilic endomyocardial disease has been described as a complication of eosinophilia–myalgia syndrome [150]. Eosinophilic endomyocardial disease is a result of the toxic effects of hypereosinophilia [151]. The mechanism of endocardial damage secondary to toxic products within the eosinophil granules is poorly understood but may involve tissue damage by major basic and cationic proteins. Because not all patients with eosinophilia have cardiac damage, it is possible that other processes may be involved in the damage to the endocardium. Intrinsic abnormalities in the eosinophils have been described, including cytoplasmic vacuolization, abnormal cytoplasmic granules, increased tendency for degranulation, phagocytosis of red blood cells, a prolonged half-life, an increase in receptors for C3 and IgG, and abnormal cellular kinetics.

### *Treatment*

Medical therapy such as corticosteroids and cytotoxic drugs (especially hydroxyurea) may improve the survival of patients with Loffler's endocarditis by reducing the number of circulating eosinophils and the resultant myocardial inflammation and damage. Some patients respond to interferon. In general, the treatment of congestive heart failure with digitalis, diuretics, afterload reduction, and anticoagulants is indicated. Surgical therapy for severe valve incompetence and endocardial stripping has had some clinical success.

# Arrhythmogenic right ventricular dysplasia

## Clinical findings

Arrhythmogenic right ventricular dysplasia–cardiomyopathy (ARVD) is defined clinically by abnormalities of conduction, repolarization and depolarization, ventricular arrhythmias, family history, and structural abnormalities of the right ventricle [152, 153]. Arrhythmias that characterize ARVD include idiopathic ventricular fibrillation, ventricular extrasystoles, and ventricular tachycardia of right ventricular origin (with a left bundle branch pattern) [154]. The ECG may show anterior precordial T-wave inversion and/or a QRS complex duration of $\geq$ 110 ms in the right precordial leads. Combining the time- and frequency-domain analyses of the signal-averaged ECG for the detection of late potentials (delayed myocardial activation) may be useful as a screening test to identify patients with ARVD in groups at high risk [155], although standard signal-average ECG techniques do not appear to be useful in diagnosing the minor forms of the disease [156].

### *Imaging studies*

Clinical identification of right ventricular structural abnormalities includes regional hypokinesia and segmental bulging, or global hypokinesia of the right ventricle during right ventricular angiography [157]. End-diastolic bulges with loss of trabecular structure and segmental contraction impairment of the right ventricle are the most valuable angiographic signs used to diagnose ARVD [158].

Contrast ventricular angiography remains the gold standard to establish the diagnosis but there are several additional techniques that may be helpful or that are under investigation. Fourier analysis of radionuclide angiography may be an additional tool for the diagnosis of ARVD [159]. Radionuclide angiography usually shows a moderately or markedly depressed right ventricular ejection fraction with normal or relatively well-preserved left ventricular function [160]. Cinemagnetic resonance imaging demonstrates abnormal fatty infiltration of the right ventricular myocardium and can show increased right ventricular dimensions as well as wall-motion abnormalities [161]. By ultrafast CT, the frequency of intramyocardial fatty components was 6% in ischaemic heart disease, 7% in Kawasaki's disease, 11% in hypertrophic cardiomyopathy, 18% in dilated cardiomyopathy, and 33% in ARVD [162, 163]. Transoesophageal echocardiography is a useful diagnostic tool and is more accurate than transthoracic echocardiography for the identification of ARVD [164]. Three-dimensional echocardiography is a promising approach for evaluating right ventricular wall-motion abnormalities as well as for demonstrating enlargement [165].

### *Epidemiology*

The highest reported incidence of ARVD is found in the Veneto Region of Italy, where it accounts for 20% of sudden cardiac deaths in young people under the age of 35 years [166]. In the USA, the most recent epidemiological data on the incidence of ARVD come from Olmsted County, Minnesota, where all residents aged 20–40 years who died suddenly and unexpectedly from 1960 to 1989 were autopsied and the medical records reviewed [167]. Of 54 autopsies, nine subjects (17%) died with morphological features suggestive of ARVD. The definition of ARVD was limited to the finding of 75% or greater infiltration of the right ventricular free wall by adipose tissue. Myocardial fibrosis was not mentioned, and no fatty infiltration was described in the left ventricle. Causes of death other than ARVD were established in six of the nine cases: one had acute aortic dissection, two had acute coronary syndromes secondary to coronary atherosclerosis, and three had a long history of recurrent seizures. Of the remaining autopsies, three deaths (5% of the total cases of sudden death) were attributed to ARVD. In the Minnesota study ARVD was a relatively frequent finding in young persons with sudden cardiac death, but not necessarily the primary cause of death. Of the nine individuals with ARVD, seven (78%) were women, which was substantially higher than in the Italian study (42%) [166]. A review of forensic autopsies performed in the state of Maryland found a much lower incidence (0.55%) of sudden cardiac death from ARVD in adults under 50 years old [168]. The differences in frequency of ARVD in the Maryland study compared with the report in Minnesota may be due to either a truly low incidence of ARVD in Maryland or the underdiagnosis of this entity at autopsy. Future studies, when pathologists have become more familiar with the anatomical features this entity, may more accurately establish its incidence in sudden death.

## Morphological studies

### *Autopsy studies*

There have been few pathological studies quantifying the degree of fat and fibrous tissue infiltrates in hearts from patients dying with ARVD. It has long been appreciated, and recently documented at autopsy, that fat infiltration occurs in greater than 50% of normal hearts [169]. In 1905, William Osler described 'parchment-like thinning of the [cardiac] walls with dilation of all chambers; in places in the right auricle and ventricle, only the epicardium remains' [170]. Since this early description, the nomenclature of this entity has changed from Uhl's anomaly (based on Uhl's description in 1952) [171] to right ventricular dysplasia-cardiomyopathy or arrhythmogenic right ventricle in 1979 [152]. There has been gradual greater understanding of the entity during the 1990s. It is possible that right ventricular dysplasia/cardiomyopathy encompasses a final pathway of multiple different entities. Thus far, the aetiology of this disorder remains unknown, but the disease is often familial with an autosomal dominant inheritance [172].

Basso *et al.* [173] described two morphological forms of ARVD, occurring with equal frequency, in 12 subjects in whom ARVD was the presumed cause of death. The lipomatous or fatty form of ARVD is characterized by partial or total replacement of the myocytes of the right ventricular free wall by adipose tissue, accompanied by necrosis in half of the cases. Fatty ARVD occurs mainly at the apex and infundibulum. No myocardial fibrosis is present, and the right ventricular wall thickness is normal (4–5 mm). The fibrous or fibrolipomatous type of ARVD is characterized by fibrosis, predominantly involving the right ventricular subepicardium, and most often seen in the posteroinferior wall. There is thinning of the involved right ventricular wall (2–3 mm), and lipomatous infiltration may be present or absent (Fig. 5.19). Inflammatory infiltration with necrosis of myocytes was frequently observed in the fibrous form [173].

The present authors described three cases of sudden death associated with ARVD [175] prior to their report of six more cases [168]. In the latter study, the age range was 19–28 years; five were males and one was female, and three were black. Three had previously documented episodes of ventricular tachycardia, and strenuous exercise preceded sudden death in five cases. Heart weights ranged from 280 to 530 g, all within normal limits when normalized for body size. Histological examination of the right ventricle showed a predominance of fatty infiltrates with focal interstitial fibrosis and interspersed myocytes in five cases; only one heart had fatty infiltration without fibrosis. Chronic inflammation with single-cell myocyte necrosis was identified in three cases, and only one had a family history of sudden death.

Lobo *et al.* [176] described 18 cases of ARVD, and emphasized that left ventricular involvement was present in seven hearts. These seven ranged in age from 24 to 60 years (mean 35 years); five were male, six died suddenly (three had previous arrhythmias), and one had undergone cardiac transplantation for heart failure. The heart weights ranged from 410 to 645 g, and all seven had fibro-

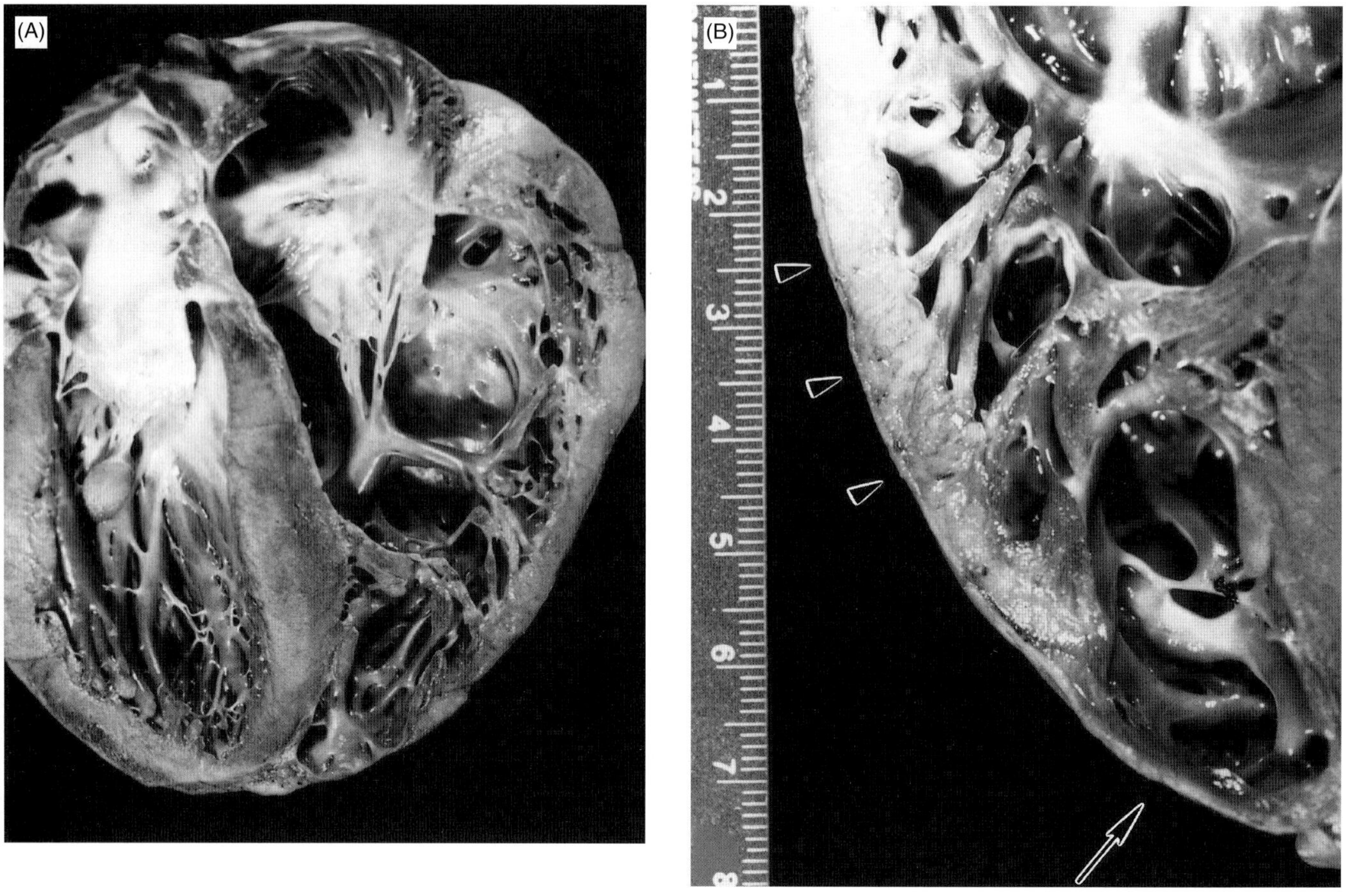


**Figure 5.19** *Arrhythmogenic right ventricular cardiomyopathy. (A) Marked right ventricular dilatation. The patient was a 13-year-old boy who died suddenly without a history of arrhythmia or a family history. (B) Higher magnification demonstrating apical aneurysm characterized by myocardial thinning* (arrow) *and gross fat infiltrates* (arrowheads)*. (C) Histologically, areas of fat infiltration with minimal myocardium are identified close to the endocardium. (D) Higher magnification of (C) demonstrating, in addition to fat, large amounts of fibrous tissue (grey areas). (From ref. 174 with permission.)*

fatty scars in the epicardial portion of the left ventricular free wall and in the right side of the ventricular septum (Fig. 5.20). The authors suggested that when left ventricular involvement is present, ARVD should be called arrhythmogenic ventricular dysplasia–cardiomyopathy rather than right ventricular dysplasia. This distinction, based on left ventricular pathology, may help to guide the search for the potential different aetiologies of ARVD.

The files of the Armed Forces Institute of Pathology were recently reviewed for all cases of ARVD and divided into two groups based on right ventricular morphology (similar to Basso *et al.* [173]), fibrofatty and fatty forms. Right and left ventricular intramural fat infiltration in ARVD hearts was quantitated morphometrically and compared with control obese and non-obese age-matched individuals dying of non-cardiac causes. Patients with fibrofatty type ARVD had maximal fat infiltration in the anterior wall of the right ventricle near the base, where it was significantly greater than in any of the other groups. Obese individuals had maximal fat infiltration in the right ventricular anterior wall near the apex which was more extensive than in non-obese controls, but which was similar in distribution and extent to both fatty and fibrofatty ARVD. Intramural fat was significantly greater in the fatty type of ARVD at the apex of the anterior and posterior right ventricular wall compared with control non-obese individuals. In cases of fibrofatty ARVD, inflammatory cell foci were present in 93% of hearts, and 80% had microscopic foci of left ventricular fibrosis and/or inflammation (Fig. 5.21). Vacuolated myocytes within scarred areas were typical (Fig. 5.22). Left ventricular fibrosis was predominately epicardially based

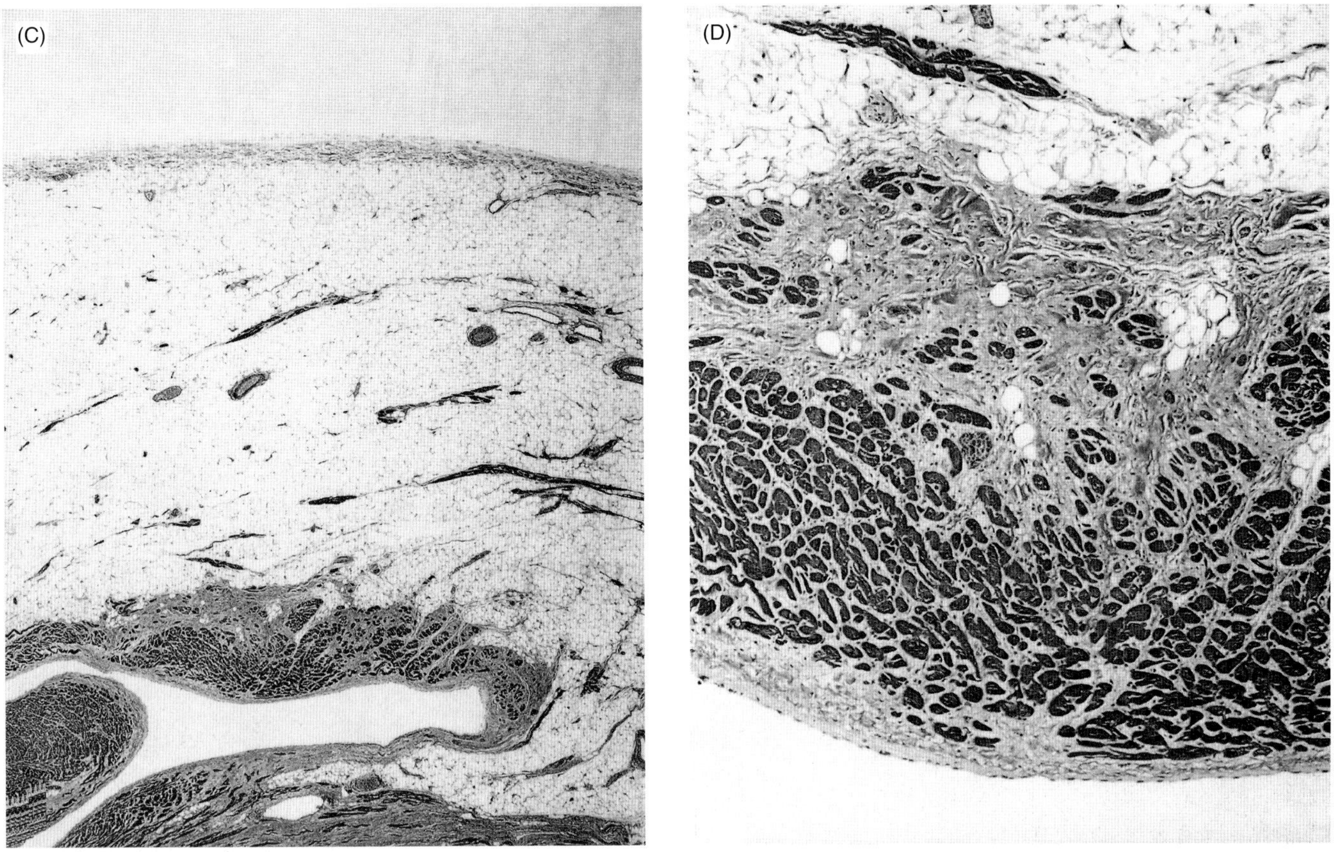


**Figure 5.19** *(Continued).*

and was greatest in the basal–lateral wall and least in the ventricular septum. Fibrosis was diffuse in the right ventricle without predilection for any particular wall in fibrofatty ARVD. No differences (between groups) in the degree of fibrosis or inflammation were noted with respect to family history, exercise at death, or history of arrhythmias. From a clinical standpoint, fibrofatty ARVD was frequently familial (27%), and associated with a clinical history of arrhythmias (40%) and with death during exercise (53%). In contrast, fatty ARVD was non-familial and not associated with a history of cardiac arrhythmias or death during exercise.

The conclusion of this study is that fibrofatty and fatty types of ARVD, both of which are associated with sudden unexpected death, are clinically and pathologically distinct. Fibrofatty ARVD is more common in the USA than the fatty variety, and is probably an inflammatory disease, which always involves the right ventricle diffusely, with a predilection for the outflow area. In 80% of fibrofatty ARVD cases presenting with sudden death, there is microscopic involvement of the left ventricle, predominantly the lateral wall, which may require multiple sections to detect. A familial pattern, clinical arrhythmias, and exercise-associated death are common. The other variety of ARVD, the fatty type, is relatively infrequent in the USA (13% in this series), occurs in slightly older individuals, is not usually familial, is associated with sudden death at rest, and has relatively non-specific pathological findings. The fatty ARVD is of unknown aetiology but does not appear to be inflammatory. Its aetiology may be related to abnormal right ventricular development or a derangement of metabolism, which results in partial fatty replacement of the right ventricular myocardium. The possibility that fatty ARVD is acquired is supported by the fact that it is seen in individuals in their 20s and 30s in the USA, with the exception of a single case report in a 7-year-old Italian–American boy [177]. The frequency of the two forms of ARVD in the authors' experience differs from Italian studies, which show that 40% of patients with ARVD have the fatty type, with a similar mean

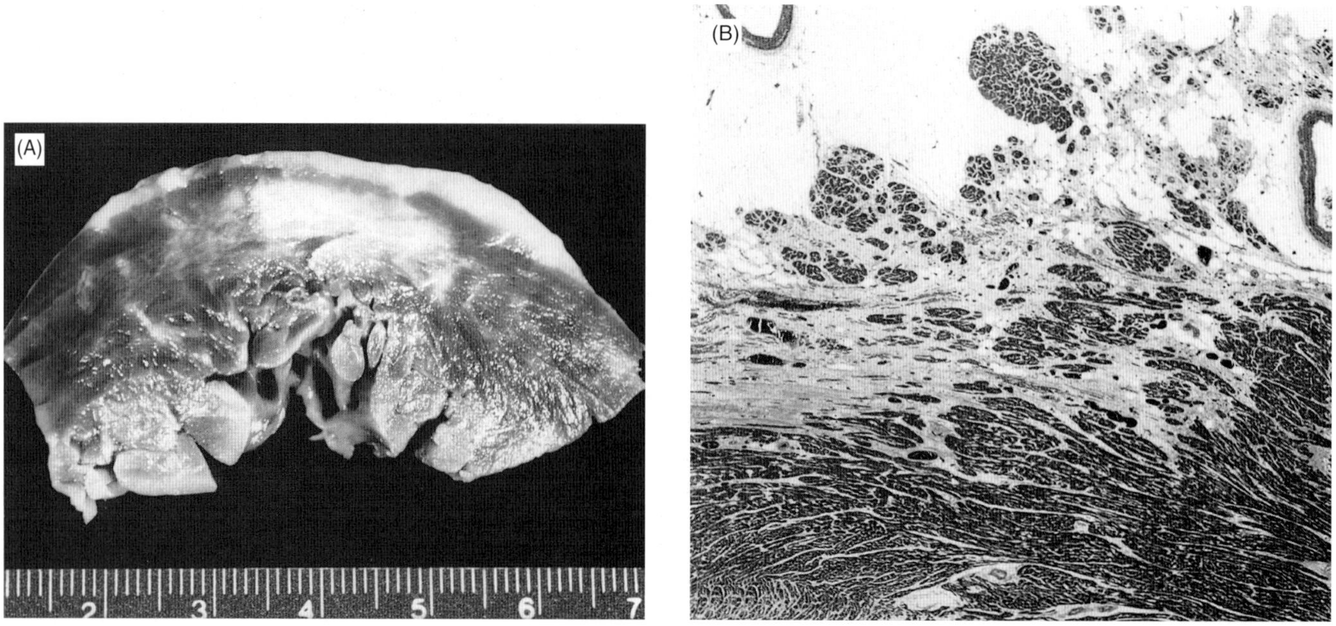


**Figure 5.20** *Arrhythmogenic right ventricular cardiomyopathy with left ventricular involvement, lateral wall. (A) Grossly evident pale area, which is a nearly transmural, subepicardial-based scar and fat (whitish area). (B) Histological section demonstrating subepicardial scarring and minimal subepicardial fat. (From ref. 174 with permission.)*

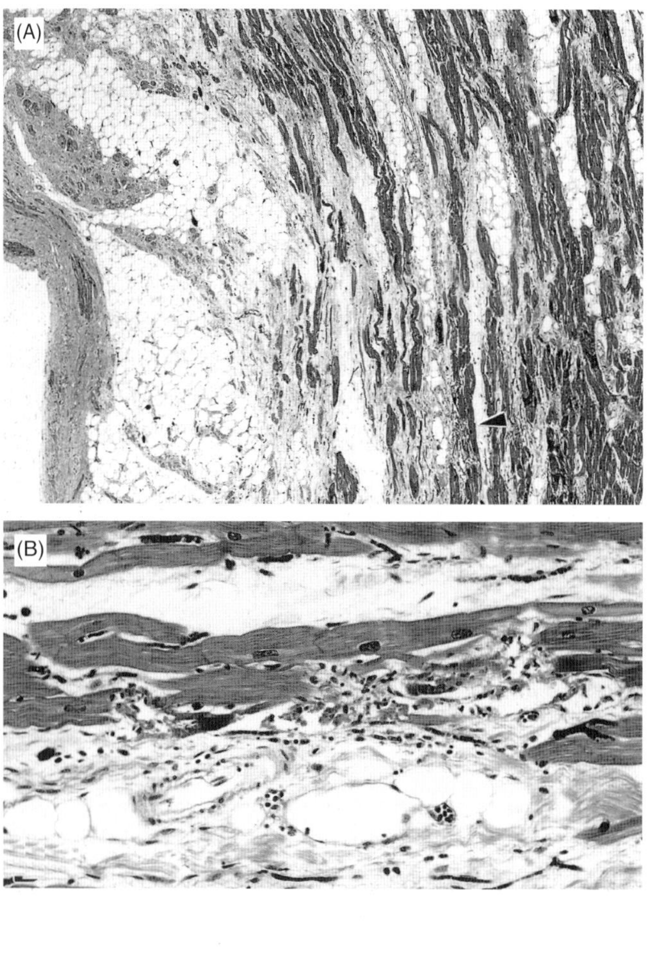


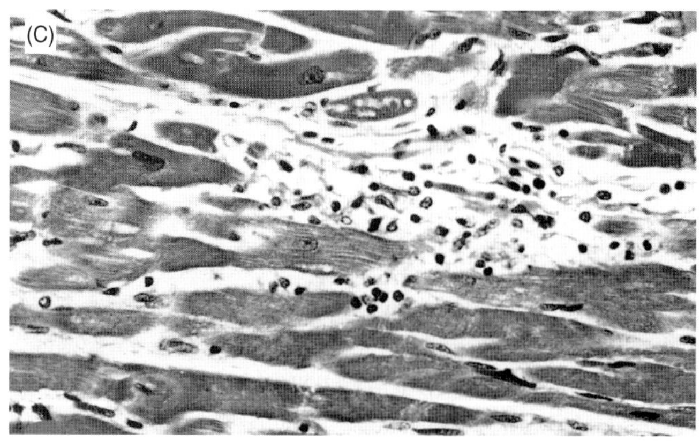


**Figure 5.21** *Arrhythmogenic right ventricular cardiomyopathy with inflammatory infiltrates. (A) Low-power view demonstrating rare foci of inflammation that are barely discernible* (arrowhead). *The epicardium is to the right and endocardium to the left. (B) Higher magnification of (A) demonstrating area of myocyte necrosis with lymphocytic infiltrates. (C) Area of lymphocytic infiltrate without myocyte necrosis. (From ref. 174 with permission.)*

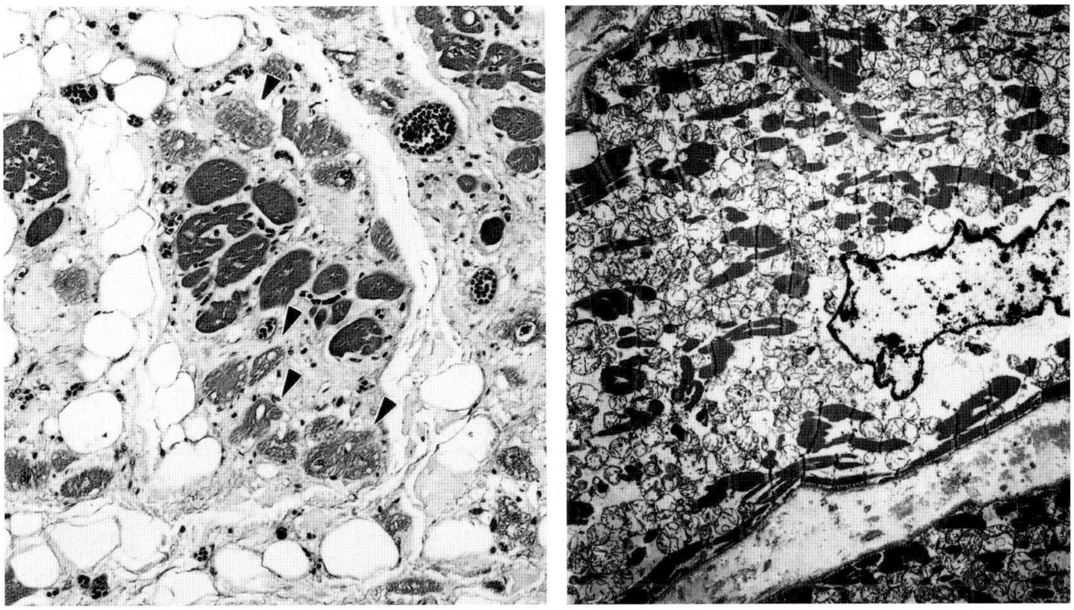

**Figure 5.22** *High-power view of an area of the right ventricular wall showing typical vacuolated myocytes* (arrowheads) *with surrounding fibrous tissue and fat. (From ref. 174 with permission). (B) Transmission electron microscopy of one of the vacuolated myocytes showing marked mitochondrial presence and only scattered myofibrils. Note the absence of fat in these vacuolated myocytes.*

age to those with the fibrofatty variety. A higher incidence of ventricular arrhythmias, myocarditis, and left ventricular involvement was seen in the fibrofatty variety of ARVD, and the right ventricular wall was thinner compared with the fatty type.

Finally, it has been suggested that Uhl's anomaly is a separate entity [173]. However, the two entities are similar, and Uhl's anomaly is probably an extreme form of ARVD with a parchment-like thinning of the right ventricle as originally described by Osler [175]. Both are causes of sudden death with or without prior congestive heart failure and may be associated with antemortem arrhythmias.

## Endomyocardial biopsy

Endomyocardial biopsy has been proven to be of value in cases of transplant rejection and for the monitoring of cardiac involvement in adriamycin-induced cytotoxicity, myocarditis, and other infiltrative processes. The value of endomyocardial biopsy in diagnosing ARVD is limited by sampling error, but has potential diagnostic use. Dembinski *et al.* [178] quantitated the surface area occupied by fat as well as the percentage of pieces in endomyocardial biopsies with fat from patients with a variety of cardiac diseases. Compared with controls, patients with ARVD had a greater area occupied by fat (19.8% vs 8.9%, $p < 0.0027$) and a greater number of pieces with adipose tissue (2.9 vs 1.0, $p < 0.0001$). There were no differences between men and women in the surface area of the fat or the percentage of pieces with fat. Older patients had more fat than younger patients (8.1% vs 4.8%, $p = 0.001$). Body mass index did not correlate with the percentage of biopsy tissue area occupied by fat. Larger biopsies were neither more frequently nor more involved by fat per area than were smaller biopsy specimens (6.4% vs 6.6% fat, respectively). In another biopsy study, Angelini *et al.* [179] compared not only the percentage area occupied by fat, but also the extent of fibrosis in patients with ARVD, dilated cardiomyopathy, and control patients. Fatty tissue was highest in ARVD (13.30 ± 17.30) compared with dilated cardiomyopathy (0.07 ± 0.31) and controls (0.33 ± 1.44, $p < 0.05$). The extent of fibrous tissue was not significantly different in ARVD (24.60 ± 11.37) compared with dilated cardiomyopathy (21.80 ± 9.29), but both had significantly more fibrous tissue than controls (8.10 ± 3.89, $p < 0.05$).

The precise structural abnormalities from a pathological standpoint have not been clarified, because right ventricular biopsy demonstrates abnormalities in as few as 40% of cases [180]. Fatty tissue and fibrous tissue exceeding 3.21 % and 40.38%, respectively, in right ventricular endomyocardial biopsy has been considered highly suspect for ARVD [179]. Morphometric analysis of biopsy sections showed a greater amount of fibrous tissue in the young patients ($p = 0.04$) and a prevalence of fatty tissue in the adults (odds ratio 12, $p = 0.005$).

In the authors' view, endomyocardial biopsy is of limited use in the diagnosis of ARVD. Autopsy studies have demonstrated that the fibrofatty changes diagnostic of the disease may be quite focal and found predominantly in the free wall of the right ventricle, which may not be sampled by the bioptome. Furthermore, fibrosis or fat in itself is not a specific diagnostic feature, and may be seen in dilated cardiomyopathy and other conditions. Only if a diagnostic area demonstrating fibrofatty change in association with vacuolization of myocytes is sampled can the biopsy be considered strongly suspicious for ARVD.

## References


1. Richardson P, McKenna W, Bristow M *et al.* Report of the 1995 World Health Organization/International Society and Federation of Cardiology Task Force on the definition and classification of cardiomyopathies. *Circulation* 1996; 93: 841–2.
2. Teare D. Asymmetrical hypertrophy of the heart in young adults. *Br Heart J* 1958; 20: 1–8.
3. Frank S, Braunwald E. Idiopathic hypertrophic subaortic stenosis. Clinical analysis of 126 patients with emphasis on the natural history. *Circulation* 1968; 37: 759–66.
4. Maron BJ, Roberts WC, Edwards JE *et al.* Sudden death in patients with hypertrophic cardiomyopathy: characterization of 26 patients with functional limitation. *Am J Cardiol* 1978; 41: 803–10.
5. Maron BJ, Roberts WC. Quantitative analysis of cardiac muscle disorganization in the ventricular septum of patients with hypertrophic cardiomyopathy. *Circulation* 1979; 4: 689–706.
6. Maron BJ, Epstein SE. Hypertrophic cardiomyopathy. Recent observations regarding the specificity of three hallmarks of the disease: asymmetric septal hypertrophy, septal disorganization and systolic anterior motion of the anterior mitral leaflet. *Am J Cardiol* 1980; 45: 141–54.
7. St John Sutton MG, Lie JT, Anderson KR *et al.* Histopathological specificity of hypertrophic obstructive cardiomyopathy. Myocardial fibre disarray and myocardial fibrosis. *Br Heart J* 1980; 44: 433–43.
8. Hollman A, Goodwin JF, Teare D, Renwick JW. A family with obstructive cardiomyopathy (asymmetrical hypertrophy). *Br Heart J* 1960; 22: 449–56.
9. Emanuel R, Withers R, O'Brien K. Dominant and recessive modes of inheritance in idiopathic cardiomyopathy. *Lancet* 1971; ii: 1065–7.
10. Geisterfer-Lowrance AA, Kass S, Tanigawa G *et al.* A molecular basis for familial hypertrophic cardiomyopathy: a beta cardiac myosin heavy chain gene missense mutation. *Cell* 1990: 999–1006.
11. Roberts WC, Ferrans VJ. Pathologic anatomy of the cardiomyopathies. Idiopathic dilated and hypertrophic types, infiltrative types, and endomyocardial disease with and without eosinophilia. *Hum Pathol* 1975; 6: 287–342.
12. Maron BJ, Kragel AH, Roberts WC. Sudden death in hypertrophic cardiomyopathy with normal left ventricular mass. *Br Heart J* 1990; 63: 308–10.
13. Klues HG, Schiffers A, Maron BJ. Phenotypic spectrum and patterns of left ventricular hypertrophy in hypertrophic cardiomyopathy: morphologic observations and significance as assessed by two-dimensional echocardiography in 600 patients. *J Am Coll Cardiol* 1995; 26: 1699–708.
14. Angelini A, Calzolari V, Thiene G *et al.* Morphologic spectrum of primary restrictive cardiomyopathy. *Am J Cardiol* 1997; 80: 1046–50.
15. Waller TA, Hiser WL, Capehart JE, Roberts WC. Comparison of clinical and morphologic cardiac findings in patients having cardiac transplantation for ischemic cardiomyopathy, idiopathic dilated cardiomyopathy, and dilated hypertrophic cardiomyopathy. *Am J Cardiol* 1998; 81: 884–94.
16. Maron BJ, Wolfson JK, Epstein SE, Roberts WC. Intramural ('small vessel') coronary artery disease in hypertrophic cardiomyopathy. *J Am Coll Cardiol* 1986; 8: 545–57.
17. Litovsky SH, Rose AG. Clinicopathologic heterogeneity in hypertrophic cardiomyopathy with regard to age, asymmetric septal hypertrophy, and concentric hypertrophy beyond the pediatric age group. *Arch Pathol Lab Med* 1998; 122: 434–41.
18. Codd MB, Sugrue DD, Gersh BJ, Melton LJD. Epidemiology of idiopathic dilated and hypertrophic cardiomyopathy. A population-based study in Olmsted County, Minnesota, 1975–1984. *Circulation* 1989; 80: 564–72.
19. Maron BJ, Gardin JM, Flack JM *et al.* Prevalence of hypertrophic cardiomyopathy in a general population of young adults. Echocardiographic analysis of 4111 subjects in the CARDIA study. *Circulation* 1995; 92: 785–89.
20. Maron BJ, Bodison SA, Wesley YE. Results of screening a large group of intercollegiate competitive atheletes for cardiovascular disease. *J Am Coll Cardiol* 1987; 10: 1214.
21. Lewis J, Maron B, Diggs J. Preparticipation echocardiographic screening for cardiovascular disease in a large, predominantly black population of collegiate athletes. *Am J Cardiol* 1989; 64: 1028.
22. Pons-Llado G, Carreras F, Borras X *et al.* Comparison of morphologic assessment of hypertrophic cardiomyopathy by magnetic resonance versus echocardiographic imaging. *Am J Cardiol* 1997; 79: 1651–6.
23. Posma JL, Blanksma PK, van der Wall EE, Hamer HP *et al.* Assessment of quantitative hypertrophy scores in hypertrophic cardiomyopathy: magnetic resonance imaging versus echocardiography. *Am Heart J* 1996; 132: 1020–7.
24. Maron BJ, Shirani J, Poliac LC *et al.* Sudden death in young competitive athletes. Clinical, demographic, and pathological profiles. *JAMA* 1996; 276: 199–204.
25. McKenna WJ. The natural history of hypertrophic cardiomyopathy. *Cardiovasc Clin* 1988; 19: 135–56.

26. Spirito P, Bellone P. Natural history of hypertrophic cardiomyopathy. *Br Heart J* 1994; 72: S10–12.
27. Roberts WC, Kishel JC, McIntosh CL *et al.* Severe mitral or aortic valve regurgitation, or both, requiring valve replacement for infective endocarditis complicating hypertrophic cardiomyopathy. *J Am Coll Cardiol* 1992; 19: 365–71.
28. Gadler F, Linde C, Juhlin-Dannfeldt A *et al.* Influence of right ventricular pacing site on left ventricular outflow tract obstruction in patients with hypertrophic obstructive cardiomyopathy. *J Am Coll Cardiol* 1996; 27: 1219–24.
29. Brunner-La Schonbeck MH, Rocca HP, Vogt PR *et al.* Long-term follow-up in hypertrophic obstructive cardiomyopathy after septal myectomy. *Ann Thorac Surg* 1998; 65: 1207–14.
30. Quinones JA, DeLeon SY, Vitullo DA *et al.* Regression of hypertrophic cardiomyopathy after modified Konno procedure. *Ann Thorac Surg* 1995; 60: 1250–4.
31. Knight C, Kurbaan AS, Seggewiss H *et al.* Nonsurgical septal reduction for hypertrophic obstructive cardiomyopathy: outcome in the first series of patients. *Circulation* 1997; 95: 2075–81.
32. Watkins H. Multiple disease genes cause hypertrophic cardiomyopathy. *Br Heart J* 1994; 72: S4–9.
33. Epstein MD, Cohn GM, Cyran F, Fananapazir L. Differences in clinical expression of hypertrophic cardiomyopathy associated with two distinct mutations in the beta-myosin heavy chain gene. A 908 Leu → Val mutation and a 403 Arg → Gln mutation. *Circulation* 1992; 1992: 345–52.
34. Vosberg HP. Myosin mutations in hypertrophic cardiomyopathy and functional implications. *Herz* 1994; 19: 75–83.
35. Anan R, Shono H, Kisanuki A *et al.* Patients with familial hypertrophic cardiomyopathy caused by a Phe110Ile missense mutation in the cardiac troponin T gene have variable cardiac morphologies and a favorable prognosis. *Circulation* 1998; 98: 391–7.
36. Coviello DA, Maron BJ, Spirito P *et al.* Clinical features of hypertrophic cardiomyopathy caused by mutation of a 'hot spot' in the alpha-tropomyosin gene. *J Am Coll Cardiol* 1997; 29: 635–40.
37. Bonne G, Carrier L, Richard P *et al.* Familial hypertrophic cardiomyopathy. From mutations to functional defects. *Circulation* 1998; 83: 580–93.
38. Krams R, Kofflard MJ, Duncker DJ *et al.* Decreased coronary flow reserve in hypertrophic cardiomyopathy is related to remodelling of the coronary microcirculation. *Circulation* 1998; 97: 230–3.
39. Schwartzkopff B, Mundhenke M, Strauer BE. Alterations of the architecture of subendocardial arterioles in patients with hypertrophic cardiomyopathy and impaired coronary vasodilator reserve: a possible cause for myocardial ischemia. *J Am Coll Cardiol* 1998; 31: 1089–96.
40. Sepp R, Severs NJ, Gourdie RG. Altered patterns of cardiac intercellular junction distribution in hypertrophic cardiomyopathy. *Heart* 1996; 76: 412–17.
41. Roberts WC, Siegel RJ, McManus BM. Idiopathic dilated cardiomyopathy: analysis of 152 necropsy patients. *Am J Cardiol* 1987; 60: 1340–55.
42. Rose AG, Beck W. Dilated (congestive) cardiomyopathy: a syndrome of severe cardiac dysfunction with remarkably few morphological features of myocardial damage. *Histopathology* 1985; 9: 367–79.
43. Keren A, Billingham ME, Popp RL. Features of mildly dilated congestive cardiomyopathy compared with idiopathic restrictive cardiomyopathy and typical dilated cardiomyopathy. *J Am Soc Echocardiogr* 1988; 1: 78–87.
44. Isner JM, Virmani R, Itscoitz SB, Roberts WC. Clinical pathologic conference. Left and right ventricular myocardial infarction in idiopathic dilated cardiomyopathy. *Am Heart J* 1980; 99: 235–42.
45. Atkinson JB, Virmani R. Congestive heart failure due to coronary artery disease without myocardial infarction: clinicopathologic description of an unusual cardiomyopathy. *Hum Pathol* 1989; 20: 1155–62.
46. Edwards WD. Cardiomyopathies. In: Virmani R, Atkinson JB, Fenoglio JJ (eds) *Cardiovascular pathology*. Philadelphia, PA: WB Saunders, 1991.
47. Rowan RA, Masek MA, Billingham ME. Ultrastructural morphometric analysis of endomyocardial biopsies. Idiopathic dilated cardiomyopathy, anthracycline cardiotoxicity, and normal myocardium. *Am J Cardiovasc Pathol* 1988; 2: 137–44.
48. Davies MJ, McKenna WJ. Dilated cardiomyopathy: an introduction to pathology and pathogenesis. *Br Heart J* 1994; 72: S24.
49. Unverferth DV, Baker PB, Swift SE *et al.* Extent of myocardial fibrosis and cellular hypertrophy in dilated cardiomyopathy. *Am J Cardiol* 1986; 57: 816–20.
50. Schwarz F, Mall G, Zebe H *et al.* Quantitative morphologic findings of the myocardium in idiopathic dilated cardiomyopathy. *Am J Cardiol* 1983; 51: 501–6.
51. Pelliccia F, d'Amati G, Cianfrocca C *et al.* Histomorphometric features predict 1-year outcome of patients with idiopathic dilated cardiomyopathy considered to be at low priority for cardiac transplantation. *Am Heart J* 1994; 128: 316–25.
52. Chopra P, Misra A, Talwar KK. Prognostic significance of pathological parameters of endomyocardial biopsy in clinical outcome of patients of dilated cardiomyopathy — I. Quantitative morphometric analysis. *Indian Heart J* 1991; 43: 415–20.
53. Ferrans VJ. Pathologic anatomy of the dilated cardiomyopathies. *Am J Cardiol* 1989; 64: 9–11C.
54. Schaper J, Froede R, Hein S *et al.* Impairment of the myocardial ultrastructure and changes of the cytoskeleton in dilated cardiomyopathy. *Circulation* 1991; 83: 504–14.
55. Anderson DW, Virmani R, Reilly JM *et al.* Prevalent myocarditis at necropsy in the acquired immunodeficiency syndrome. *J Am Coll Cardiol* 1988; 11: 792–9.
56. Tazelaar HD, Billingham ME. Leukocytic infiltrates in idiopathic dilated cardiomyopathy. *Am J Surg Pathol* 1986; 10: 405–12.
57. Latham RD, Mulrow JP, Virmani R *et al.* Recently diagnosed idiopathic dilated cardiomyopathy: incidence of myhocarditis and efficacy of prednisone therapy. *Am Heart J* 1989; 117: 876–82.
58. Kuhl U, Noutsias M, Seeberg B, Schultheiss HP. Immunohistological evidence for a chronic intramyocardial inflammatory process in dilated cardiomyopathy. *Heart* 1996; 75: 295–300.
59. Naito J, Masuyama T, Mano T *et al.* Ultrasonic myocardial tissue characterization in patients with dilated cardiomyopathy: value in noninvasive assessment of myocardial fibrosis. *Am Heart J* 1996; 131: 115–21.
60. Gabler U, Berndt A, Kosmehl H *et al.* Matrix remodelling in dilated cardiomyopathy entails the occurrence of oncofetal fibronectin molecular variants. *Heart* 1996; 75: 358–62.

61. Gunja-Smith Z, Morales AR, Romanelli R, Woessner JF, Jr. Remodelling of human myocardial collagen in idiopathic dilated cardiomyopathy. Role of metalloproteinases and pyridinoline cross-links. *Am J Pathol* 1996; 148: 1639–48.
62. Treasure CB, Vital JA, Cox DA *et al.* Endothelium-dependent dilation of the coronary microvasculature is impaired in dilated cardiomyopathy. *Circulation* 1990; 81: 772–9.
63. Opherk D, Schwarz F, Mall G *et al.* Coronary dilatory capacity in idiopathic dilated cardiomyopathy: analysis of 16 patients. *Am J Cardiol* 1983; 51: 1657–62.
64. Milechman G, Scheinman MM. Ventricular dysrhythmias and sudden death in dilated cardiomyopathy. In: Zipes DP, Rowlands DJ (eds) *Progress in cardiology*. Philadelphia, PA: Lea and Febiger, 1989; 85–94.
65. Manolio TA, Baughman KL, Rodeheffer R *et al.* Prevalence and etiology of idiopathic dilated cardiomyopathy. *Am J Cardiol* 1992; 69: 1458–66.
66. Gillum RF. Idiopathic cardiomyopathy in the United States 1970–1982. *Am Heart J* 1986; 111.
67. Coughlin SS, Szklo M, Baughman K, Pearson TA. The epidemiology of idiopathic dilated cardiomyopathy in a biracial community. *Am J Epidemiol* 1990; 131: 48–56.
68. Sun JP, James KB, Yang XS *et al.* Comparison of mortality rates and progression of left ventricular dysfunction in patients with idiopathic dilated cardiomyopathy and dilated versus nondilated right ventricular cavities. *Am J Cardiol* 1997; 80: 1583–7.
69. Mestroni L, Krajinovic M, Severini GM *et al.* Familial dilated cardiomyopathy. *Br Heart J* 1994; 72: S35–41.
70. Goerss JB, Michels VV, Burnett J *et al.* Frequency of familial dilated cardiomyopathy. *Eur heart J* 1995; 16 (Suppl O): 2–4.
71. Mestroni L, Miani D, Di Lenarda A *et al.* Clinical and pathologic study of familial dilated cardiomyopathy. *Am J Cardiol* 1990; 65: 1449–53.
72. Michels VV, Moll PP, Miller FA *et al.* The frequency of familial dilated cardiomyopathy in a series of patients with idiopathic dilated cardiomyopathy. *N Engl J Med* 1992; 326: 77–82.
73. Keeling PJ, McKenna WJ. Clinical genetics of dilated cardiomyopathy. *Herz* 1994; 19: 91–6.
74. Oldfors A, Eriksson BO, Kyllerman M *et al.* Dilated cardiomyopathy and the dystrophin gene: an illustrated review. *Br Heart J* 1994; 72: 344–8.
75. Muntoni F, Cau M, Ganau A *et al.* Brief report: deletion of the dystrophin muscle-promoter region associated with X-linked dilated cardiomyopathy. *N Engl J Med* 1993; 329: 921–5.
76. Angelini C, Fanin M, Pegoraro E *et al.* Clinical–molecular correlation in 104 mild X-linked muscular dystrophy patients: characterization of sub-clinical phenotypes. *Neuromusc Disord* 1994; 4: 349–58.
77. Melacini P, Fanin M, Danieli GA *et al.* Myocardial involvement is very frequent among patients affected with subclinical Becker's muscular dystrophy. *Circulation* 1996; 94: 3168–75.
78. Towbin JA, Hejtmancik JF, Brink P *et al.* X-linked dilated cardiomyopathy. Molecular genetic evidence of linkage to the Duchenne muscular dystrophy (dystrophin) gene at the Xp21 locus. *Circulation* 1993; 87: 1854–65.
79. Politano L, Nigro V, Nigro G *et al.* Development of cardiomyopathy in female carriers of Duchenne and Becker muscular dystrophies. *JAMA* 1996; 275: 1335–8.
80. Narula J, Haider N, Virmani R *et al.* Apoptosis in myocytes in end-stage heart failure. *N Engl J Med* 1996; 335: 1182–9.
81. Olivetti G, Abbi R, Quaini F *et al.* Apoptosis in the failing human heart. *N Engl J Med* 1997; 336: 1131–41.
82. Maeda M, Holder E, Lowes B *et al.* Dilated cardiomyopathy associated with deficiency of the cytoskeletal protein metavinculin. *Circulation* 1997; 95: 17–20.
83. Hartz AJ, Anderson AJ, Brooks HJ. The association of smoking and cardiomyopathy. *N Engl J Med* 1984; 311: 1201.
84. Coughlin SS, Szklo M, Baughman K, Pearson TA. Idiopathic dilated cardiomyopathy and atopic disease: epidemiologic evidence for an association with asthma. *Am Heart J* 1989; 118: 768–74.
85. Virmani R, Atkinson JB. Endomyocardial biopsy in the diagnosis of heart diseases. In: Virmani R, Atkinson JB, Fenoglio JJ, Jr (eds). *Cardiovascular pathology*. Volume 23. Philadelphia, PA: WB Saunders, 1991, 220–45.
86. Muir P, Nicholson F, Tilzey AJ *et al.* Chronic relapsing pericarditis and dilated cardiomyopathy: serological evidence of persistent enterovirus infection. *Lancet* 1989; i: 804–7.
87. Wiegand V, Tracy S, Chapman N, Wucherpfennig C. Enteroviral infection in end stage dilated cardiomyopathy. *Klin Wochenschr* 1990; 68: 914–20.
88. Archard LC, Bowles NE, Cunningham L. Molecular probes for detection of persisting enterovirus infection of human heart and their prognostic value. *Eur Heart J* 1991; 12: 56–9.
89. Easton AJ, Eglin RP. The detection of Coxsackievirus RNA in cardiac tissue by *in situ* hybridization. *J Gen Virol* 1988; 69: 285–91.
90. Giacca M, Severini GM, Mestroni L *et al.* Low frequency of detection by nested polymerase chain reaction of enterovirus ribonucleic acid in endomyocardial tissue of patients with idiopathic dilated cardiomyopathy. *J Am Coll Cardiol* 1994; 24: 1033–40.
91. Quigley PJ, Richardson PJ, Meany DT. Long term follow-up in biopsy proven myocarditis: progression to dilated cardiomyopathy. *Circulation* 1986; 74 (Suppl II): 142.
92. Dec GW, Palacios I, Yasuda T *et al.* Antimyosin antibody cardiac imaging: its role in the diagnosis of myocarditis. *J Am Coll Cardiol* 1990; 16: 97–104.
93. Khaw B-A, Narula J. Non-invasive detection of myocyte necrosis in myocarditis and dilated cardiomyopathy with radiolabelled antimyosin. *Eur Heart J* 1995; 16(Suppl O): 119–23.
94. Caforio ALP. Role of autoimmunity in dilated cardiomyopathy. *Br Heart J* 1994; 72: S30–4.
95. Calforio ALP, Goldman JH, Baig MK *et al.* Organ-specific cardiac autoantibodies in dilated cardiomyopathy — an update. *Eur Heart J* 1995; 16 (Suppl O): 64–7.
96. Ansari AA, Wang YC, Danner DJ *et al.* Abnormal expression of histocompatibility and mitochondrial antigens by cardiac tissue from patients with myocarditis and dilated cardiomyopathy. *Am J Pathol* 1991; 139: 337–54.
97. Limas CJ, Goldenberg IF, Limas C. Autoantibodies against beta-adrenoceptors in human idiopathic dilated cardiomyopathy. *Circ Res* 1989; 64: 97–103.
98. Badorff C, Noutsias M, Kuhl U, Schultheiss HP. Cell-mediated cytotoxicity in hearts will dilated cardiomyopathy: correlation with interstitial fibrosis and foci of activated T lymphocytes. *J Am Coll Cardiol* 1997; 29: 429–34.

99. Seko Y, Takahashi N, Ishiyama S *et al.* Expression of costimulatory molecules B7-1, B7-2, and CD40 in the heart of patients with acute myocarditis and dilated cardiomyopathy. *Circulation* 1998; 97: 637–9.
100. Satoh M, Nakamura M, Tamura G *et al.* Inducible nitric oxide synthase and tumor necrosis factor-alpha in myocardium in human dilated cardiomyopathy. *J Am Coll Cardiol* 1997; 29: 716–24.
101. Wynne J, Braunwald E. The cardiomyopathies and myocarditides: toxic, chemical, and physical damage to the heart. In: Braunwald E (ed.) *Heart disease*. Philadelphia, PA: WB Saunders, 1992.
102. Rubin E, Urbano-Marquez A. Alcoholic cardiomyopathy. *Alcohol Clin Exp Res* 1994; 18: 111–14.
103. Hibbs RG, Ferrans VJ, Black WC *et al.* Alcoholic cardiomyopathy. An electron microscopic study. *Am Heart J* 1963; 69: 766–79.
104. Voss EG, Reddy CVR, Detrano R *et al.* Familial dilated cardiomyopathy. *Am J Cardiol* 1984; 54: 456–7.
105. Homans DC. Peripartum cardiomyopathy. *N Engl J Med* 1985; 312: 1432–7.
106. Cunningham FG, Pritchard JA, Hankins GD *et al.* Peripartum heart failure: idiopathic cardiomyopathy or compounding cardiovascular events? *Obstet Gynecol* 1986; 67: 157–68.
107. Lampert MB, Weinert L, Hibbard J *et al.* Contractile reserve in patients with peripartum cardiomyopathy and recovered left ventricular function. *Am J Obstet Gynecol* 1997; 176: 189–95.
108. Pearl W. Familial occurrence of peripartum cardiomyopathy. *Am Heart J* 1995; 129: 421–2.
109. Midei MG, DeMent SH, Feldman AM *et al.* Peripartum myocarditis and cardiomyopathy. *Circulation* 1990; 81: 922–8.
110. O'Connell JB, Costanzo-Nordin MR, Subramanian R *et al.* Peripartum cardiomyopathy: clinical, hemodynamic, histologic and prognostic characteristics. *J Am Coll Cardiol* 1986; 8: 52–6.
111. Wynne J, Braunwald E. The cardiomyopathies and myocarditis. In: Braunwald E (ed.) *Heart disease: a textbook of cardiovascular medicine*. Philadelphia, PA: WB Saunders, 1997: 1404–63.
112. Schoenfeld MH, Supple EW, Dec GW, Jr *et al.* Restrictive cardiomyopathy versus constrictive pericarditis: role of endomyocardial biopsy in avoiding unnecessary thoracotomy. *Circulation* 1987; 75: 1012–17.
113. Walley VM, Kisilevsky R, Young ID. Amyloid and the cardiovascular system: a review of pathogenesis and pathology with clinical correlations. *Cardiovasc Pathol* 1995; 4: 79–102.
114. Crotty TB, Li C-Y, Edwards WD, Suman VJ. Amyloidosis and endomyocardial biopsy: correlation of extent and pattern of deposition with amyloid immunophenotype in 100 cases. *Cardiovasc Pathol* 1995; 4: 39–42.
115. Arbustini E, Merlini G, Gavazzi A *et al.* Cardiac immunocyte-derived (AL) amyloidosis: an endomyocardial biopsy study in 11 patients. *Am Heart J* 1995; 130: 528–36.
116. Gertz MA, Kyle RA, Greipp PR. Response rates and survival in primary systemic amyloidosis. *Blood* 1991; 77: 257–62.
117. Maury CP. Gelsolin-related amyloidosis. Identification of the amyloid protein in Finnish hereditary amyloidosis as a fragment of variant gelsolin. *J Clin Invest* 1991; 87: 1195–9.
118. Gertz MA, Kyle RA, Thibodeau SN. Familial amyloidosis: a study of 52 North American-born patients examined during a 30-year period. *Mayo Clin Proc* 1992; 67: 428–40.
119. Adams D, Said G. Ultrastructural immunolabelling of amyloid fibrils in acquired and hereditary amyloid neuropathies. *J Neurol* 1996; 243: 63–7.
120. Campistol JM, Argiles A. Dialysis-related amyloidosis: visceral involvement and protein constituents. *Nephrol Dial Transplant* 1996; 11 (Suppl 3): 142–5.
121. Gal R, Korzets A, Schwartz A *et al.* Systemic distribution of beta 2-microglobulin-derived amyloidosis in patients who undergo long-term hemodialysis. Report of seven cases and review of the literature. *Arch Pathol Lab Med* 1994; 118: 718–21.
122. Rocken C, Schwotzer EB, Linke RP, Saeger W. The classification of amyloid deposits in clinicopathological practice. *Histopathology* 1996; 29: 325–35.
123. Frenzel H, Schwartzkopff B, Kuhn H *et al.* Cardiac amyloid deposits in endomyocardial biopsies. Light microscopic, ultrastructural, and immunohistochemical studies. *Am J Clin Pathol* 1986; 85: 674–80.
124. Hamer JP, Janssen S, van Rijswijk MH, Lie KL. Amyloid cardiomyopathy in systemic non-hereditary amyloidosis. Clinical, echocardiographic and electrocardiographic findings in 30 patients with AA and 24 patients with AL amyloidosis. *Eur Heart J* 1992; 13: 623–7.
125. Pellikka PA, Holmes DR, Jr, Edwards WD *et al.* Endomyocardial biopsy in 30 patients with primary amyloidosis and suspected cardiac involvement. *Arch Intern Med* 1988; 148: 662–6.
126. Cueto-Garcia L, Reeder GS, Kyle RA *et al.* Echocardiographic findings in systemic amyloidosis: spectrum of cardiac involvement and relation to survival. *J Am Coll Cardiol* 1985; 6: 737–43.
127. Roberts WC, Waller BF. Cardiac amyloidosis causing cardiac dysfunction: analysis of 54 necropsy patients. *Am J Cardiol* 1983; 52: 137–46.
128. Hawkins PN, Lavender JP, Pepys MB. Evaluation of systemic amyloidosis by scintigraphy with $^{123}$-labeled serum amyloid P component. *N Engl J Med* 1990; 323: 508–13.
129. Lekakis J *et al.* Cardiac amyloidosis detected by indium-111 antimyosin imaging. *Am Heart J* 1992; 124: 1630–1.
130. Smith TJ, Kyle RA, Lie JT. Clinical significance of histopathologic patterns of cardiac amyloidosis. *Mayo Clin Proc* 1984; 59: 547–55.
131. Olson LJ, Gertz MA, Edwards WD *et al.* Senile cardiac amyloidosis with myocardial dysfunction. Diagnosis by endomyocardial biopsy and immunohistochemistry. *N Engl J Med* 1987; 317: 738–42.
132. Kyle RA, Spittell PC, Gertz MA *et al.* The permortem recognition of systemic senile amyloidosis with cardiac involvement. *Am J Med* 1996; 101: 395–400.
133. Fogo A, Virmani R. Cardiac amyloidosis. *Primary Cardiol* 1984; 10: 54–67.
134. Hosenpud JD, DeMarco T, Frazier OH *et al.* Progression of systemic disease and reduced long-term survival in patients with cardiac amyloidosis undergoing heart transplantation. Follow-up results of a multicenter survey. *Circulation* 1991; 84: III338–43.

135. Goodwin JF. Endomyocardial disease — clinical features. *Postgrad Med J* 1983; 59: 154–6.
136. Chew CY, Ziady GM, Raphael MJ *et al.* Primary restrictive cardiomyopathy. Non-tropical endomyocardial fibrosis and hypereosinophilic heart disease. *Br Heart J* 1977; 39: 399–413.
137. Child JS, Perloff JK. The restrictive cardiomyopathies. *Cardiol Clin* 1988; 6: 289–316.
138. Falase AO. Endomyocardial fibrosis in Africa. *Postgrad Med J* 1983; 59: 170–8.
139. Fawzy ME, Ziady G, Halim M *et al.* Endomyocardial fibrosis: report of eight cases. *J Am Coll Cardiol* 1985; 5: 983–8.
140. Rashwan MA, Ayman M, Ashour S *et al.* Endomyocardial fibrosis in Egypt: an illustrated review. *Br Heart J* 1995; 73: 284–9.
141. Waller BF. Pathology of the cardiomyopathies. *J Am Soc Echocardiogr* 1988; 1: 4–19.
142. Chopra P, Narula J, Talwar KK *et al.* Endomyocardial fibrosis: an endomyocardial biopsy study. *Hum Pathol* 1990; 21: 613–21.
143. Davies J, Spry CJ, Vijayaraghavan G, De Souza JA. A comparison of the clinical and cardiological features of endomyocardial disease in temperate and tropical regions. *Postgrad Med J* 1983; 59: 179–85.
144. Davies J, Spry CJ, Sapsford R *et al.* Cardiovascular features of 11 patients with eosinophilic endomyocardial disease. *Q J Med* 1983; 52: 23–39.
145. Olson T *et al. Pediatr Cardiol* 1982; 3: 161–9.
146. Hendren WG, Jones EL, Smith MD. Aortic and mitral valve replacement in idiopathic hypereosinophilic syndrome. *Ann Thorac Surg* 1988; 46: 570–1.
147. Tanino M, Kitamura K, Ohta G. *et al.* Hypereosinophilic syndrome with extensive myocardial involvement and mitral valve thrombus instead of mural thrombi. *Acta Pathol Jpn* 1983; 33: 1233–42.
148. Arnold M, McGuire L, Lee JC. Loeffler's fibroplastic endocarditis. *Pathology* 1988; 20: 79–82.
149. Parrillo JE, Borer JS, Henry WL *et al.* The cardiovascular manifestations of the hypereosinophilic syndrome. Prospective study of 26 patients, with review of the literature. *Am J Med* 1979; 67: 572–82.
150. Berger PB, Duffy J, Reeder GS *et al.* Restrictive cardiomyopathy associated with the eosinophilia–myalgia syndrome. *Mayo Clin Proc* 1994; 69: 162–5.
151. Sasano H, Virmani R, Patterson RH *et al.* Eosinophilic products lead to myocardial damage. *Hum Pathol* 1989; 20: 850–7.
152. Fontaine G, Guirandon G, Frank R *et al.* Arrhythmogenic right ventricular dyspalsia: a previously unrecognized syndrome. *Circulation* 1979; 60 (Suppl 2) 65–75.
153. McKenna WJ, Thiene G, Nava A *et al.* Diagnosis of arrhythmogenic right ventricular dysplasia/cardiomyopathy. Task Force of the Working Group Myocardial and Pericardial Disease of the European Society of Cardiology and of the Scientific Council on Cardiomyopathies of the International Society and Federation of Cardiology. *Br Heart J* 1994; 71: 215–18.
154. Marcus FI, Fontaine GH, Guiraudon G *et al.* Right ventricular dysplasia: a report of 24 adult cases. *Circulation* 1982; 65: 384–98.
155. Kinoshita O, Fontaine G, Rosas F *et al.* Time- and frequency-domain analyses of the signal-averaged ECG in patients with arrhythmogenic right ventricular dysplasia. *Circulation* 1995; 91: 715–21.
156. Oselladore L, Nava A, Buja G *et al.* Signal-averaged electrocardiography in familial form of arrhythmogenic right ventricular cardiomyopathy. *Am J Cardiol* 1995; 75: 1038–41.
157. Peters S, Troster J, Hartwig CA, Reil GH. Selective right ventricular angiography in apparently idiopathic ventricular fibrillation. *Heart Vessels* 1995; 10: 211–13.
158. Breithardt G, Wichter T, Haverkamp W *et al.* Implantable cardioverter defibrillator therapy in patients with arrhythmogenic right ventricular cardiomyopathy, long QT syndrome, or no structural heart disease. *Am Heart J* 1994; 127: 1151–8.
159. Le Guludec D, Slama MS, Frank R *et al.* Evaluation of radionuclide angiography in diagnosis of arrhythmogenic right ventricular cardiomyopathy. *J Am Coll Cardiol* 1995; 26: 1476–83.
160. Daliento L, Rizzoli G, Thiene G *et al.* Diagnostic accuracy of right ventriculography in arrhythmogenic right ventricular cardiomyopathy. *Am J Cardiol* 1990; 66: 741–5.
161. Molinari G, Sardanelli F, Gaita F *et al.* Right ventricular dysplasia as a generalised cardiomyopathy? Findings on magnetic resonance imaging. *Eur Heart J* 1995; 16: 1619–24.
162. Marcus FI, Fontaine G. Arrhythmogenic right ventricular dysplasia/cardiomyopathy: a review. *Pacing Clin Electrophysiol* 1995; 18: 1298–314.
163. Hamada S, Takamiya M, Ohe T, Ueda H. Arrhythmogenic right ventricular dysplasia: evaluation with electron-beam CT. *Radiology* 1993; 187: 723–7.
164. Piccoli BD, Rigo F, Caprioglio F *et al.* Comparison between transoesophageal and transthoracic echocardiographic investigation in arrhythmogenic right ventricular dysplasia. *J Am Coll Cardiol* 1992; (Abstract) 19: 236A: 941–71.
165. Zachara E, Greco C, Salustri A *et al.* Three dimensional echocardiography in right ventricular dysplasia. First International Symposium of Arrhythmogenic Right Ventricular Dysplasia–Cardiomyopathy, Paris, France, 1996.
166. Thiene G, Nava A, Corrado D *et al.* Right ventricular cardiomyopathy and sudden death in young people. *N Engl J Med* 1988; 318: 129–33.
167. Shen W-K, Edwards WD, Hammill SC *et al.* Sudden unexpected non-traumatic death in 54 young adults: A 30 year population-based study. *Am J Cardiol* 1995; 76: 148–52.
168. Goodin JC, Farb A, Smialek JE *et al.* Right ventricular dysplasia associated with sudden death in young adults. *Mod Pathol* 1991; 4: 702–6.
169. Fontaliran F, Fontaine G, Fillette F *et al.* Nosologic frontiers of arrhythmogenic dysplasia. Quantitative variations of normal adipose tissue of the right heart ventricle. *Arch Mal Coeur Vaiss* 1991; 84: 33–8.
170. Osler W. *The principles and practice of medicine*. New York: Appleton-Century-Crofts, 1905.
171. Uhl HS. A previously undescribed congenital malformation of the heart: almost total absence of the myocardium of the right ventricle. *Bull Johns Hopkins Hosp* 1952; 91: 197–209.
172. Laurent M, Descaves C, Biron Y *et al.* Familial form of arrhythmogenic right ventricular dysplasia. *Am Heart J* 1987; 113: 1222–8.

173. Basso C, Thiene G, Corrado D *et al*. Arrhythmogenic right ventricular cardiomyopathy. Dysplasia, dystrophy, or myocarditis? *Circulation* 1996; 94: 983–91.
174. Burke AP, Farb A, Tashko G, Virmani R. Arrhythmogenic right ventricular cardiomyopathy and fatty replacement of the right ventricular myocardium: are they different diseases? *Circulation* 1997; 97: 1571–80.
175. Virmani R, Robinowitz M, Clark M, McAllister H. Sudden death and partial absence of the right ventricular myocardium: a report of three cases and a review of the literature. *Arch Pathol Lab Med* 1982; 106: 163–7.
176. Lobo FV, Heggtveit HA, Butany *et al*. Right ventricular dysplasia: morphological findings in 13 cases. *Can J Cardiol* 1992; 8: 261–8.
177. Pawel BR, de Chadarevian JP, Wolk JH *et al*. Sudden death in childhood due to right ventricular dysplasia: report of two cases. *Pediatr Pathol* 1994; 14: 987–95.
178. Dembinski AS, Dobson JR, Wilson JE *et al*. Frequency, extent, and distribution of endomyocardial adipose tissue: morphometric analysis of endomyocardial biopsy specimens from 241 patients. *Cardiovasc Pathol* 1994; 3: 33–41.
179. Angelini A, Thiene G, Boffa G *et al*. Endomyocardial biopsy in right ventricular cardiomyopathy. *Int J Cardiol* 1993; 40: 273–82.
180. Mehta D, Davies MJ, Ward DE, Camm AJ. Ventricular tachycardias of right ventricular origin: markers of subclinical right ventricular disease. *Am Heart J* 1994; 127: 360–6.

# Classification and nomenclature of cardiomyopathic disorders 6

B. MAISCH

## Introduction

The World Health Organization (WHO) International Society and Federation of Cardiology (ISFC) classification of 1995, published in 1996 [1], defines cardiomyopathy as a disease of the heart muscle with a demonstrable disturbance of cardiac function. Accordingly, five forms of cardiomyopathy are described: dilated cardiomyopathy (DCM), hypertrophic cardiomyopathy (HCM), restrictive cardiomyopathy (RCM), arrhythmogenic right ventricular cardiomyopathy (ARVCM), and non-classified cardiomyopathies (NCCM) (Fig. 6.1, Table 6.1).

The distinctive features of the first four forms of cardiomyopathy are primarily haemodynamic. The left ventricle is primarily affected in dilated, hypertrophic and restrictive cardiomyopathies and the right ventricle predominantly in ARVCM. In contrast to the previous WHO/ISFC classification of 1980 [2], the new definition has made some important changes. The term cardiomyopathy is no longer reserved for idiopathic forms of heart muscle disease. It can now also be used for specific cardiomyopathies, which were previously defined according to their aetiology and/or pathogenesis (Table 6.2). The specific forms of dilated heart muscle disease include familial or genetically determined, inflammatory, viral or immunologically mediated, alcoholic and toxic, ischaemic, valvular or hypertensive, or metabolic cardiomyopathies, as well as cardiomyopathy in the context of systemic diseases such as lupus erythematosus (SLE), primary chronic polyarthritis (PCP), periarteriitis nodosa, dermatomyositis, sarcoidosis, or the leukaemias (Table 6.2). This broader definition of cardiomyopathy is unavoidable, since in the English literature the term ischaemic cardiomyopathy is the most frequently quoted form of cardiomyopathy, although

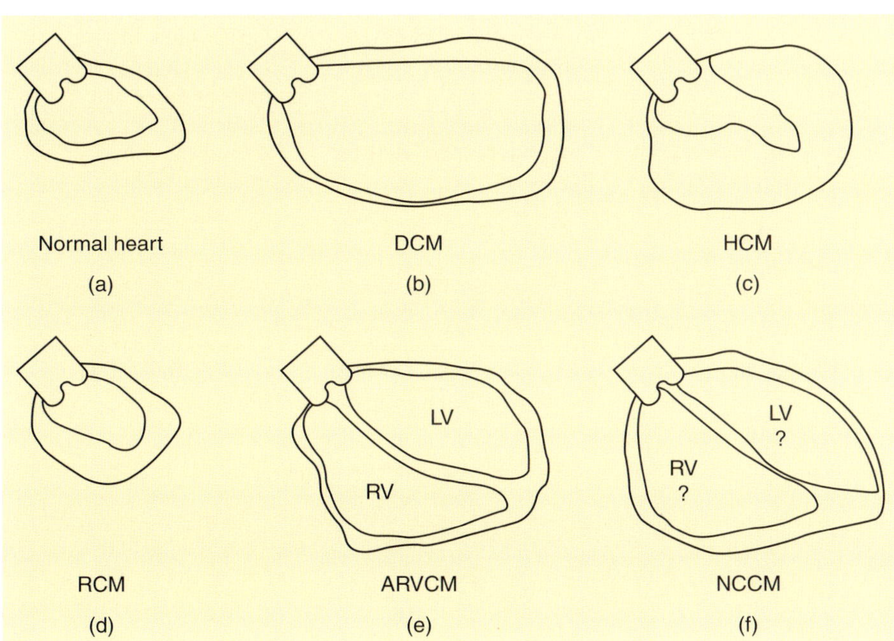


**Figure 6.1** *Classification of cardiomyopathies according to haemodynamic and macroscopic criteria: (a) normal heart; (b) dilated cardiomyopathy (DCM; systolic pump defect with associated diastolic compliance disturbance; (c) hypertrophic cardiomyopathy (HCM; with subvalvular, midventricular, or apical manifestation); (d) restrictive cardiomyopathy (RCM); (e) arrhythmic right ventricular cardiomyopathy (ARVC; dysplasia); (f) non-classified cardiomyopathies (NCCM).*

**Table 6.1** Classification of the cardiomyopathies (WHO/ISFC, 1995) [1]

| Name | Abbreviation | Characteristics |
|---|---|---|
| 1. Dilated cardiomyopathy | DCM | Systolic pump failure |
| 2. Hypertrophic cardiomyopathy with and without obstruction | HOCM or HCM IHSS[a] | Diastolic compliance failure (= disturbance of the elasticity of the heart muscle in diastole = increased stiffness) |
| 3. Restrictive cardiomyopathy | RCM | Endomyocardial fibrosis (with or without eosinophilia), diastolic compliance failure |
| 4. Arrhythmic right ventricular cardiomyopathy | ARVCM | Mainly right ventricular combined pump failure with ventricular tachycardia |
| 5. Non-classified cardiomyopathies | NCCM | e.g. fibroelastosis, minimal cardiomyopathy, mitochondrial cardiomyopathy, carcinoid heart, atrial arrhythmogenic forms |

[a]IHSS = infundibular hypertrophic subaortic stenosis as named in childhood.

**Table 6.2** Classification of dilated cardiomyopathies based on aetiological and pathogenetic aspects

| Type and aetiology | Haemodynamics | Specific diagnosis | Treatment |
|---|---|---|---|
| 1. Unknown aetiology and pathogenesis idiopathic unclear | DCM, SCD | Echocardiography LV angiography, myocardial biopsy | |
| 2. Known or probable aetiology and pathogenesis (specific cardiomyopathies) | | | |
| Familial genetic | DCM | Genealogical tree | According to heart insufficiency |
| Ischaemic cardiomyopathopy: Remodelling after infarction | DCM | Echocardiography, LV angiocardiography | According to heart insufficiency |
| Valvular cardiomyopathy: Remodelling with vitium | DCM | Echocardiography, LV angiography | Valvular replacement and heart failure therapy |
| Hypertensive cardiomyopathy: Left ventricular hypertrophy with high pressure | DCM/HCM | Echocardiography, LV angiography | Antihypertensive therapy |
| Inflammatory cardiomyopathy: (acute and chronic myocarditis) | DCM, SCD | Endomyocardial biopsy, polymerase chain reaction | Heart failure therapy, causal therapy, microbles (see Table 7.5) |
| Collagenosis:<br>Rheumatic carditis<br>Lupus erythematodes disseminatus<br>Dermatomyositis<br>Sclerodernia (systemic sclerosis)<br>Spondylarthritis ankylopoetica<br>Rheumatic heart failure (Bechterew) | DCM or SCD, often with PE | Diagnosis of the underlying disease | Treatment of the underlying disease |
| Toxic cardiomyopathies:<br>Alcohol (+ acetylaldehyde)<br>Drugs<br>• cytostatic adriamycin<br>• tricyclic antidepressants<br>• other drugs | DCM | Echocardiography, possibly endomyocardial biopsy | Abstention from the noxa |
| Uraemic | PE | | |
| CO poisoning | | | |
| Cobalt ('Quebec beerdrinker's disease') | | | |

**Table 6.2** (*Continued*)

| Type and aetiology | Haemodynamics | Specific diagnosis | Treatment |
|---|---|---|---|
| Metabolic and endocine illness | DCM | Echocardiography, possibly endomyocardial biopsy | Removal of the metabolic disturbance, myocardial treatment of the underlying disease |
| Hyperthyroidism (high output failure) | | | |
| Hypothyroidism (myxoedemic heart) | HCM | | |
| Acromegaly | HCM | | |
| Pheochromocytoma | HCM | | |
| Diabetes mellitus DCM | | | |
| Haemochromatosis | HCM | | |
| Amyloidosis: primary | HCM | | |
| secondary | HCM | | |
| Infiltrative illnesses, e.g. Refsum, Fabry, mucopolysaccharidosis, lipidoses, glycogen storage illness, porphyria, gout, oxalosis, mucoviscidosis | | | |
| Hyperergic cardiomyopathies | | | |
| Drugs, e.g. penicillin, phenylbutazone, aureomycin, tuberculostatics, reserpine | DCM, SCD, often with pericarditis | Echocardiography or immunserology, probably antiphlogistics and anticardiac antibodies | Elimination or avoidance of the noxa, probably prednisone or immunosuppressive therapy |
| Postvaccination | | | |
| illness of the serum | | | |
| postcardiotomy syndrome | | | |
| (Dressler syndrome) postinfarct syndrome | | | |
| Neuromuscular illnesses | DCM, SCD | | |
| Friedreich's ataxia | | Echocardiography, probably endomyocardial biopsy, coronary angiography | Treatment of the basic illness |
| Myotonic muscle dystrophy | | | |
| Progressive muscle dystrophy | | | |
| Myasthenia gravis | | | |
| Neoplastic cardiomyopathies | | | |
| Primary and metastatic neoplasma | DCM | Echocardiography, probably endomyocardial biopsy, pericardial puncture | Treatment of the basic illness, surgery if possible |
| Lymphatic myeloic leukaemia | SCD with PE | | |
| Granulomatosus cardiomyopathy | DCM or SCD | Echocardiography, probably thallium-scintigraphy, probably biopsy, angiotensin-converting enzyme determination | Treatment in the range of the underlying illness<br>Probably prednisone |
| Sarcoidosis | | | |
| Cardiomyopathies from physical causes | DCM | Echocardiography, sometimes with PE, probably invasive diagnosis and biopsy | Symptomatic |
| Therapy with ionized radiation | | | |
| Electric shock | | | |
| Heat stroke | | | |
| Cardiac trauma | | | |
| Peripartum cardiomyopathy | DCM or SCD | Echocardiography, endomyocardial biopsy, serology on cardiotropic viruses | Symptomatic, no salt |
| Nutritional disturbances | | | |
| Beriberi (vitamin B[1] deficiency) | DCM or SCD | Echocardiography, diagnosis of nutritional disturbance | Treatment of the nutritional disturbance or avitaminosis |
| Kwashiorkor | | | |
| Pellagra | | | |
| Scurvy (vitamin C deficiency) | | | |

DCM = dilated cardiomyopathy; SCD = segmental cardiac dysfunction; PE = pericardial effusion; HCM = hypertropic cardiomyopathy.

it should be referred to as a specific heart muscle disease. Similarly, in the European scientific cardiac community, commonly used terms such as 'alcoholic cardiomyopathy' or 'adriamycin cardiomyopathy' should be named secondary heart muscle diseases, according to the previous definition.

Cardiomyopathy is no longer defined as a heart muscle disease of unknown cause alone, but also as a disease of known causes. This is exemplified by hypertrophic cardiomyopathy, which nowadays is defined by molecular genetics in about 50% of the cases. Similarly, familial dilated cardiomyopathy can now be defined in a sizeable number of cases by molecular genetics (Table 6.3).

Within the realm of dilated cardiomyopathies, new terms have been introduced, such as ischaemic cardiomyopathy. This condition has been reserved for the remodelling process of the non-infarcted myocardium. Ischaemic cardiomyopathy does not refer to the haemodynamic disturbance resulting directly from the infarct-associated aneurysm or from the wall motion abnormality in hibernating or stunned myocardium. It is reserved solely for the remodelling process of the non-infarcted, non-ischaemic myocardium. For this reason, the term 'ischaemic' is somewhat misleading.

Hypertensive cardiomyopathy includes hypertrophy of myocytes, disproportional fibrosis, and microangiopathy by medial hypertrophy of small arteries. Valvular cardiomyopathy is defined as cardiac dysfunction which cannot be sufficiently explained by the valvular process of regurgitation or stenosis. In addition, the term inflammatory cardiomyopathy has been defined for the first time as acute and chronic myocarditis associated with cardiac dysfunction.

It was more than appropriate to include right ventricular arrhythmogenic cardiomyopathy as the fourth form of cardiomyopathy. The previous term, dysplasia, is replaced by cardiomyopathy of the right ventricle.

**Table 6.3** Genotypes and phenotypes of familial cardiomyopathy

| Type and author | Code | Genotype | Phenotype |
|---|---|---|---|
| 1. Autosomal–dominant cardiomyopathies<br>X-chromosomal dystrophinopathies | | | |
| (a) Juvenile X-chromosomal cardiomyopathy | XLCM | xp21 + variation | Without participation of skeletal muscle, age < 25 years |
| (b) Duchenne's muscular dystrophy (DMD) | XLCM | xp21 + variation | With participation of skeletal muscle |
| (c) Becker's muscle dystrophy (BMD) | XLCM | xp21 + variation | With direct participation of skeletal muscle |
| DCM with disturbance of electrical conduction and dysfunction of the sinus node (SSS) | | | |
| (a) Kass *et al.* (1994) [3] | CMD1A | 1p1-q1 | Disturbance of AV conduction associated with connexin 40<br>Disturbance of AV conduction, SSS |
| (b) Olson and Keating (1996) [4] | CDCD2 | 3p22-3p55 | Disturbance of AV conduction, SSS, SV tachycardia |
| (c) Messina *et al.* (1997) [5] | FDC–CDM | 6q23 | Disturbance of electrical conduction, SSS, |
| Other non-X-chromosomal DCM forms in families | | | |
| (a) Bowles *et al.* (1996) [6]: Familial DCM (+ MPS) | CMPD3 | 10q21-q23 | DCM partial with mitral valve prolapse |
| (b) Krajinovic *et al.* (1995) [7]: Familial DCM | CMPD1 | 9q13 | Familial DCM without participation of skeletal muscle |
| (c) Durand *et al.* (1995) [8]: Familial DCM | CMPD2 | 1q32 | Familial DCM without participation of skeletal muscle |
| 2. Autosomal–recessive DCM<br>Mutation of the gene of fat oxidation | | | e.g. disturbance of carnitin metabolism |
| 3. Mitochondrial cardiomyopathies<br>Ozawa *et al.* (1990) [9]<br>Wallace (1992, 1994) [10, 11]<br>Li *et al.* (1995, 1997) [12, 13] | | | Deletion and point mutation of the mitochondrial DNA (maternal), pathogenesis of discussed relevance, often with neuromuscular manifestations (histology: ragged red fibres) |

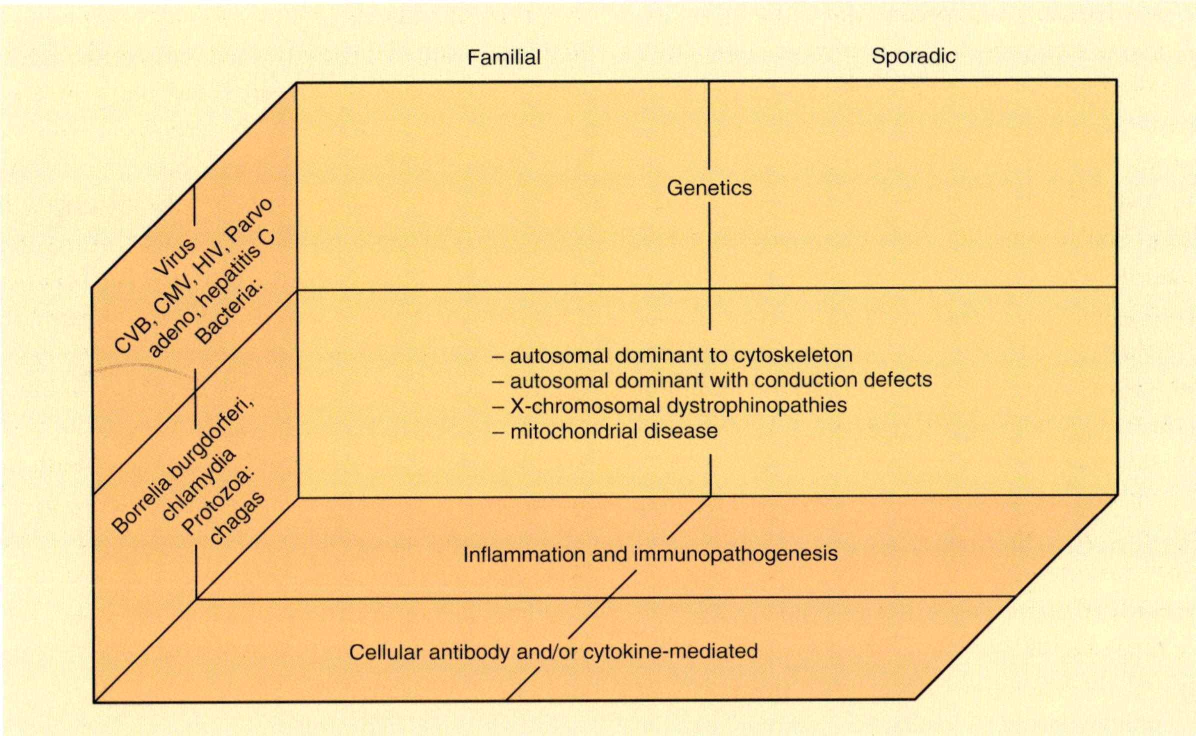


**Figure 6.2** *Diagnostic matrix of dilated cardiomyopathy (DCM). The coordinates show the importance of familial predisposition (genotype), microbiotic aetiology, inflammatory, and immunological pathogenesis for the phenotype of DCM.*

## Dilated cardiomyopathy

Dilated cardiomyopathy (DCM) is defined haemodynamically as systolic pump failure with cardiomegaly and decreased ejection fraction [1]. The reduction in systolic indices is often associated with an altered diastolic compliance or dysfunction. The structural correlates of diastolic dysfunction include interstitial fibrosis and quantitative alterations of the extracellular matrix (Fig. 6.2), which are followed by lusitropic (or relaxation) changes.

Idiopathic dilated cardiomyopathy is more common in men than women (ratio 2:1), prevalence is 36 per 100 000, and the incidence 6 per 100 000. Familial forms are observed in 15–20% of patients [14]. Table 6.3 lists the genotypes and phenotypes of familial cardiomyopathy identified so far. Key symptoms include those of heart failure (such as dyspnoea), which are graded according to the New York Heart Association classification. Precordial discomfort can be secondary to increased wall tension and relative coronary underperfusion of the small vessels. Atypical angina may also exist with pericardial involvement. Severe rhythm disturbances are more common with a reduction in left ventricular ejection fraction.

A haemodynamic classification according to ejection fraction has been suggested previously as the Tokyo classification, wherein the incidence of sudden cardiac death increases proportionally to the decrease in ejection fraction (Table 6.4). Treatment follows the concept of heart failure, including restriction of physical activity, in severe cases bed-rest, angiotensin-converting enzyme (ACE) inhibitors or

**Table 6.4** Haemodynamic classification of dilated cardiomyopathy (Tokyo classification)

| Stage | Ejection fraction (%) | Characteristics |
|---|---|---|
| I | > 55 | Only segmental wall motion abnormality |
| II | 40–54 | Global and segmental contraction abnormality is mild heart failure |
| III | 25–40 | Moderate global heart failure |
| IV | < 25 | Severe disturbance<br>State of (pre)transplantation |

antithrombin-II (AT-II) antagonists, digitalis especially in atrial fibrillation or with tachycardia, diuretics for oedema and a trial of low-dose β-blockaders (e.g. Carvedilol or metropolol). Surgical treatment is necessary in the terminal stage only and includes heart transplantation, implantation of assist devices, or in selected cases dynamic cardiomyoplasty. In severe valvular regurgitation, valve replacement is helpful. Recently, the Batista procedure of partial ventriculectomy has been introduced into the therapeutic repertoire, a procedure which awaits further confirmation in controlled clinical trials. More promising appears ventricular resynchronization through biventricular stimulation in patients with LBBB.

## Specific cardiomyopathies

In contrast to the aetiologically unclear idiopathic forms, specific cardiomyopathy is a muscle disease in which the aetiology or pathogenesis is well established (Fig. 6.2). The specific cardiomyopathies, which are enumerated in Table 6.2, demonstrate the haemodynamic characteristics of dilated cardiomyopathy.

### Ischaemic cardiomyopathy

Ischaemic cardiomyopathy is defined as cardiac dysfunction of the non-ischaemic and non-infarcted myocardial segment and is the consequence of the remodelling process.

### Valvular cardiomyopathy

This is defined as myocardial dysfunction which is disproportionate to the valvular disease.

### Hypertensive cardiomyopathy

Structurally, hypertensive cardiomyopathy is characterized by left ventricular hypertrophy and microangiopathy which lead to symptoms, diastolic dysfunction, or in the late stages systolic dysfunction.

### Alcoholic cardiomyopathy

The clinical diagnosis is often established by suspicion and exclusion. The exact daily amount of alcohol that needs to be consumed and for what period for alcoholic cardiomyopathy to occur are unknown. To ascertain chronic abuse determination of CDT and gamma-GT as respective trade and state markers are recommended. The muscle disorder is caused by alcohol and its first metabolite, acetaldehyde. A specific disposition appears to be a prerequisite for this cardiomyopathy. In the beginning supraventricular arrhythmias such as paroxysmal atrial fibrillation, can occur frequently. Since these rhythm disturbances frequently occur after alcoholic consumption during the holidays and the weekends they have been called the 'holiday heart syndrome'. In end-stage disease irreversible heart failure sets in. Progression can be interrupted successfully in the early stages by abstinence from alcohol consumption and the cardiomyopathy remains reversible as long as severe structural alterations in the myocardium are not present.

The rare beriberi heart disease is a consequence of a vitamin $B_1$ (thiamine) deficiency. This deficiency can also occur in alcoholics as a result of malnutrition. In contrast to low-output alcoholic cardiomyopathy, beriberi cardiomyopathy is a hyperkinetic heart syndrome with high output failure. The therapeutic administration of vitamin $B_1$ results in prompt amelioration of the symptoms and normalization of haemodynamics.

Cobalt-associated cardiomyopathy was first described in Quebec. It is a form of alcohol-related cardiomyopathy that no longer occurs, since the use of cobalt as a stabilizer of the foam of beer was discontinued.

### Toxic cardiomyopathy

These are heart muscle diseases induced by drugs such as phenothiazine, tricyclic antidepressants, and lithium carbonate. Use of these drugs can lead to functional disturbances, arrhythmias, and alterations of electrocardiographic repolarization. Sudden cardiac death has been described. Similarly, drug abuse, as with cocaine, can lead to cardiomyopathy. The most prominent drug to induce cardiomyopathy is adriamycin. For this reason the dose of adriamycin is limited to 500 $mg/m^2$ of body surface area. Adriamycin given beyond this limit often causes irreversible heart muscle disease with 'Swiss cheese-like lesions' in myocardial cells and subacute forms of cardiac damage, such as pericardial effusions, rhythm disturbances, and irreversible disturbances of pump function.

Treatment of mediastinal disease with ionized radiation can cause a cardiomyopathy that is often associated with chronic pericardial effusion and constriction.

### Cardiomyopathies associated with endocrine diseases

The manifestations of heart muscle diseases associated with endocrine diseases depend on the severity of the underly-

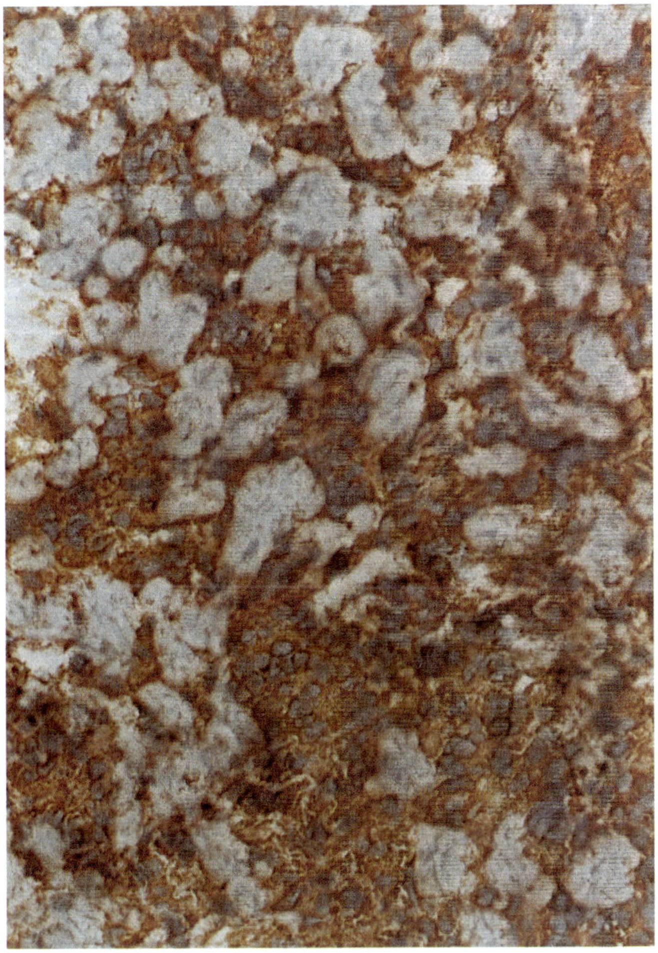

**Figure 6.3** *Enhanced major histocompatibility complex (MHC) class II expression in an endomyocardial biopsy of a patient with chronic myocarditis.*

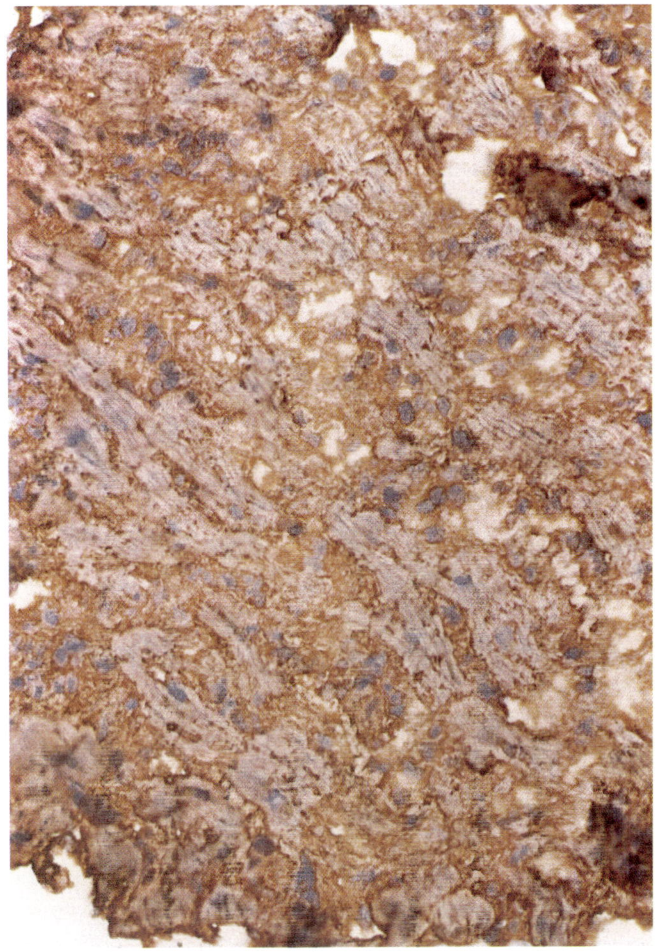

**Figure 6.4** *Acute myocarditis with myocytolysis. Demonstration of CD3-positive cells located adjacent to myocardial tissues.*

ing endocrine disorder. Diagnosis is easy when the endocrine disease is known, such as myxoedema or thyreotoxicosis.

## Inflammatory cardiomyopathy (myocarditis and perimyocarditis)

In comparison to the previous classification, inflammatory cardiomyopathy is now specifically categorized [1]. It is defined as acute or chronic myocarditis with cardiac dysfunction. Viral myocarditis and immunologically mediated cardiomyopathy are also included in this subgroup.

Heretofore, the different forms of myocarditis were assessed histologically according to the Dallas classification [15]. However, integrate viral heart disease and autoimmune myocarditis into the WHO/ISFC classification, two ISFC task forces have defined inflammatory cardiomyopathy more precisely and also identified the associated microbial aetiology. In a consensus conference, the specific methods needed to uncover viral RNA have been outlined by an international expert committee [16, 17].

The diagnostic matrix of dilated cardiomyopathy in Figure 6.3 demonstrates all aspects relevant to the description of aetiology and pathogenesis, in addition to the well-known haemodynamic changes.

### New pathohistological and immunological diagnostic criteria of myocarditis or inflammatory cardiomyopathy

The diagnosis of myocarditis or dilated myocardiopathy with inflammation cannot be certain without the use of endomyocardial biopsy and histological, immunohistological, molecular biological, and virological analyses. The

Dallas classification [15] defined active myocarditis as an infiltrate with necrosis of myocytes (Fig. 6.4). The persisting myocarditis was diagnosed when the identical criteria were fulfilled in a second biopsy. Healing or resolving myocarditis was considered when a sparse infiltrate, and no or little myocytolosis and fibrosis was observed in the consecutive biopsy. Healed or resolved myocarditis was defined as focal or diffuse fibrosis after a positive first biopsy. The histological criteria of healed myocarditis were identical to the histological findings in idiopathic dilated cardiomyopathy. Borderline myocarditis in the Dallas criteria is defined as the presence of lymphocytes or focal nests of lymphocytes in the absence of myocyte necrosis. Another biopsy was recommended if the diagnosis of borderline myocarditis was made.

This Dallas classification lacks a description of 'chronic' myocarditis and a discrimination from 'borderline' myocarditis. Therefore, two expert groups of the World Heart Federation (former ISFC) have defined the immunhistological criteria of inflammatory cardiomyopathy (DCMi) as more than 14 lymphocytes or macrophages/mm$^3$ [16]. They also defined, in a second consensus document, the methodical standards for the demonstration of viral RNA and DNA in the myocardium [17]. For chronic myocarditis or dilated myocardiopathy with inflammation, necrosis and apoptosis are non-obligatory criteria, although they can be present (Table 6.5). As signs of immune activation, an increased expression of major histocompatibility (MHC) class I and II antigens or of adhesion molecules can be found (Fig. 6.3).

The perimyocarditis as per the new classification is a combination of histologically defined myocarditis and an inflammatory exudative pericardial reaction. To make the diagnosis of perimyocarditis, endomyocardial biopsy is helpful but not obligatory. The assumption that the inflammatory reaction of the pericardium (in the form of pericardial effusion) would also affect the myocardium is justified when a segmental wall motion abnormality or transient or permanent cardiomegaly is coexistent. For the demonstration of the microbial agent in the epicardium or in the pericardial effusion, however, analysis of the effusion or of the endomyocardial or epicardial biopsy is obligatory.

An aetiopathogenetic classification of inflammatory cardiomyopathy/myocarditis depends on the pathogenetic microbial agent, which can include cardiotropic viruses [7, 18–24], bacteria such as *Borrelia burgdorferi* or *Chlamydia pneumoniae*, or protozoa. This is best accomplished by polymerase chain reaction or *in situ* hybridization in cardiac tissue (Table 6.6). A detailed description on the incidence of DNA and RNA viruses in cardiomyopathy is found in Table 6. Remarkably, hepatitis C viruses are also associated with myocarditis, and described in up to 15% of cardiomyopathies by Matsumori *et al.* [22]. Parvo B19 appears to be a new, under-diagnosed DNA-virus in this context.

**Table 6.5** Histological and immunohistological definition of myocarditis after the Dallas classification [15] and the ISFC/WHO criteria [17]

| Diagnosis | Conventional histology (Dallas criteria, 1987) | Histological and immuhistological criteria (ISFC classification, 1998) |
|---|---|---|
| 1. Active/acute myocarditis | Infiltrate, myocytolysis oedema | 1–3 identical infiltrate, characterized by monoclonal antibodies, immunoglobulin and complement fixation, *de novo* expression of MHC-I and II, antigens and adhesion molecules |
| 2. Continuous myocarditis | As 1 but in follow-up biopsy by continuous observation | |
| 3. Healing myocarditis | Sparse infiltrate, facultative myocytolysis, reparative fibrosis | |
| 4. Borderline myocarditis | Dispersed, rare lymphocytes without myocytolysis | Borderline diagnosis to myocarditis with 1–13 lymphocytes/mm$^3$ |
| 5. Chronic myocarditis (dilated cardiomyopathy with immunohistological inflammation) | Not defined | $\geq$ 14 lymphocytes (+ macrophages)/mm$^3$, facultative criteria, see above |

**Table 6.6** Aetiological, pathogenetic and haemodynamic determinations of inflammatory cardiomyopathy (myocarditis)

| Aetiology and pathogenesis | | | Haemodynamics | Specific diagnosis | Therapy |
|---|---|---|---|---|---|
| 1. Microbial | | | Dilated cardiomyopathy (DCM) Segmental cardial dysfunction (SCD) Pericardial effusion (PE) | Echocardiography, endomyocardial biopsy with histology, immunohistology of an infiltrate and immunglobulin or complement fixation and demonstration of the microbial agent (*in situ* hybridization, polymerase chain reaction) Serology against cardiac antigens and viral or microbial agent Endomyocardial biopsy with histology and immunhistology (biopsy > 14 infiltrative cells/mm$^3$; negative proof of viruses or bacteria) | Restriction of physical activity, symptomatic heart failure therapy, immunomodulative antiviral, antimicrobial, immunosuppressive therapy (in clinical trials) |
| | Viruses | RNA viruses: Picorna (coxsackie A, B, echo, polio) Orthomyxo (influenza A, B) Paramyxo (rubella, mumps) Toga (Chikunguna, dengue, yellow fever, rubella) Rhabdo (rabies) Arena (lymphocytic choriomeningitis) | | | |
| | | DNA viruses: Smallpox (variola, vaccinia) Herpes (varicella-zoster, cytomegalo, Epstein–Barr, herpes human 6 Adenovirus Parvo B19 | | | |
| | Bacteria | Diphtheria, sepsis | | | |
| | Spirochetes | (Syphilis, leptospirosis, *Borrelia burgdorferi*), *Chlamydia pneumoniae* | | | |
| | Others | *Rickettsia burnetii* (Q-fever) | | | |
| | Protozoa | *Trypanosoma cruzi* (Chagas' disease) Toxoplasmosis, amoebiasis, malaria, leishmaniosis | | | |
| | Parasites | Trichinae, echinococci , ascaridae | | | |
| 2. Autoreactive | | Lymphocyte and/or humoral cause, primary or secondary immunpathogenesis | | | |

## Pathogenesis and immunopathogenesis

The microbial infection first induces an antimicrobial immune response by means of humoral and cellular effector and regulator mechanisms (Fig. 6.5). Both the lytic viral cytopathology alone and the antiviral immune response can cause inflammation in the myocardium and myocyte necrosis [18–21, 23–25] or apoptosis (Schaper *et al.*, 1998; Kruse *et al.*, 1998; Pankuweit *et al.*, 1998, personal communications and in press). A second immune response to the myocardium by cross-reactivity of viral and cardiac epitopes has been postulated [16, 19, 24, 26–32]. Antigenic or molecular mimicry may be the most important pathogenetic principle that leads to anticardiac autoreactivity [23, 26, 28–32].

Cytotoxic T-lymphocytes, natural killer cells, and mediators as well as cross-reactive antiviral and other anticardiac antibodies may cause myocyte necrosis. Cytokine-mediated cardiodepression plays a yet underestimated role. A vast spectrum of potentially pathogenetic relevant anticardiac antibodies has been described. Of particular interest are antibodies directed against epitopes on the sarcolemma (e.g. the myolemma; Fig. 6.6, the calcium channel, receptors such as the β- and α-receptor), contractile proteins (myosin, actin, and tropomyosin), the extracellular matrix (desmin, laminin), and mitochondria (ANT, M7, mitochondrial enzymes) and sarcoplasmic reticular antigens (Fig. 6.7). The assumption of a secondary immunopathogenesis is also based on the fact that the complement, immunoglobulin G IgG, IgA, and IgM antibodies are bound to the sarcolemma, the interstitial connective tissue, and the capillaries in the endomyocardial biopsies [28, 29]. Apart from pathogenetically relevant antibodies, polyclonal stimulation of the

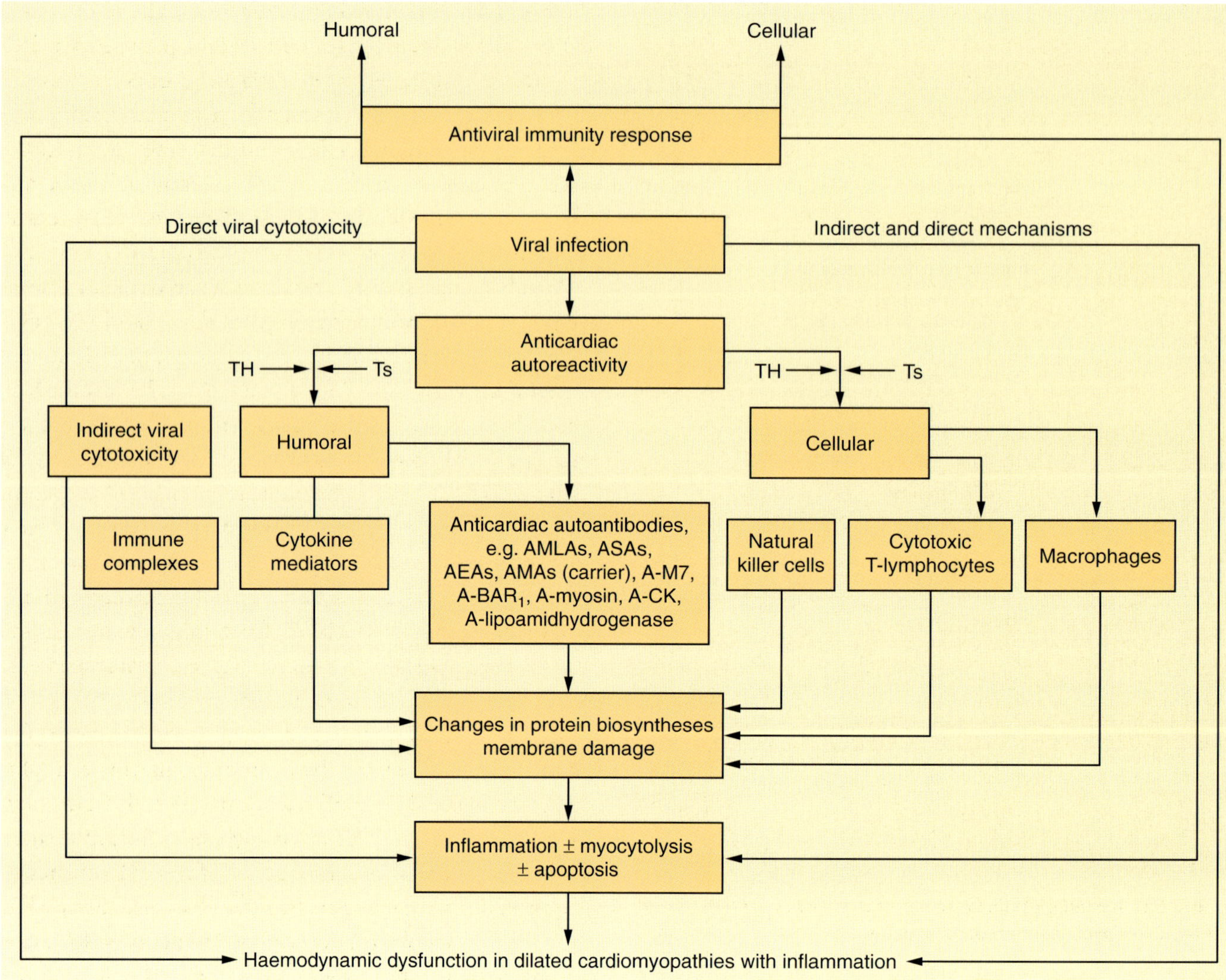


**Figure 6.5** *Immunological response to a viral infection of cardiotropic viruses. There is always an antiviral immune response, often followed by an anticardiac autoreactivity. With cardiotropic viruses these mechanisms can contribute to the clinical symptoms of myocarditis and dilated cardiomyopathy, respectively.*

immunoglobulin production against cardiac epitopes can occur, which in turn could be an epiphenomenon. Most antibodies that can be found in the biopsy can also be demonstrated in the peripheral blood [28, 29].

## Pathophysiology

The causes of the disturbed haemodynamics in dilated cardiomyopathy can be as variable as the clinical manifestations of the myocardiopathy itself. This may be due to the underlying aetiological and pathophysiological factors: viral or bacterial cytotoxocity, influence of the secondary immunopathogenesis with cytotoxic T-cells, negative inotropic cytokines, cardiodepressive membrane against the sarcolemma (ASA) or the myolemma (AMLA), antimitochondrial antibodies, negatively chronotropic anti-$\beta_1$-receptor or acetylcholine receptor antibodies [28], and many other factors such as antimyosin antibodies. In addition, structural alterations such as fibrosis, myocytolosis and hypertrophy, metabolic disturbances of the cell organelles, altered geometric conditions of contraction (dilatation, inotropy, and stiffness), an altered coronary reserve, the vasospasm of small coronary arteries, or the true angiitis of small vessels can lead to disturbed contraction and relaxation. A marked fibrosis can by itself impair the contraction of virtually intact muscle fibres (the strangulation theory of K. T. Weber). Toxins or cytokines can change the mem-

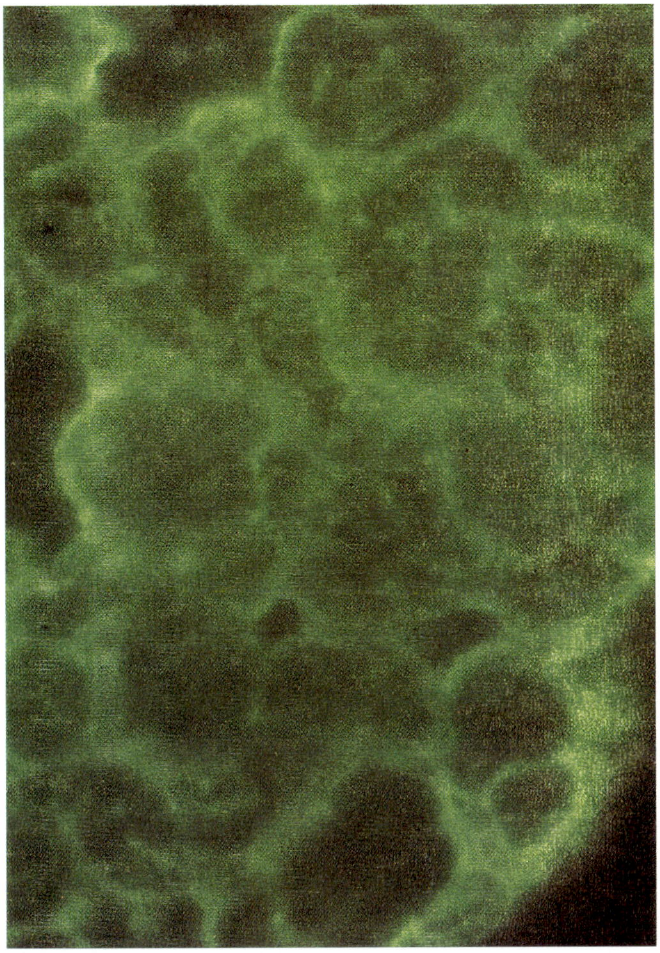

**Figure 6.6** *Immunoglobulin G fixation in an endomyocardial biopsy of a 29-year-old man with chronic myocarditis.*

brane transportation of ions or substrates during cardiac inflammation. In a number of patients, genetic predisposition as exemplified by dystrophin deficiency can be found [14]. A loss of matrix proteins such as dystrophin or an increase in mitochondrial DNA deletions [9, 10, 12, 33] or point mutations [13, 24] as mitochondrial cardiomyopathy can contribute to the phenotype of cardiomyopathy in an individual patient.

## Hypertrophic cardiomyopathy

Haemodynamically, hypertrophic cardiomyopathy is a prominent disturbance of cardiac compliance. It accompanies an increased filling pressure of the left and sometimes also the right ventricle, when excessive hypertrophy of the septal wall occurs (Figs. 6.1, 6.5). Hypertrophic cardiomyopathy occurs less frequently than dilated cardiomyopathy. It is more common in men, the annual incidence is 2.5 patients per 100 000, and the prevalence is 19.7 per 100 000. More recent investigations indicate an even higher incidence and prevalence. The manifestation of hypertrophic cardiomyopathy and the observation of the clinical phenotype can be observed in early childhood and also in the third to seventh decades. The disease may remain asymptomatic in many patients for their entire lifetime.

Family members very often have a similar heart disease or symptoms. About 50% of cases demonstrate familial hypertrophic cardiomyopathy. An autosomal dominant inheritance with variable penetrance can be assumed. In about 50% of the families investigated, a defect of chromosome 14 has been identified for a gene which codes for β-myosin (14q1). From this gene, more than 50 mutations have now been identified. Other familial gene defects have been found on chromosome 1 (1q3) for troponin T, on chromosome 11 (11q13) for the myosin binding protein, and on chromosome 15 (15q2) for α-tropomyosin. At present, hypertrophic cardiomyopathy is one of the most well-characterized diseases in molecular genetics.

Under haemodynamic considerations, hypertrophic obstructive cardiomyopathy or infundibular hypertrophic subaortic stenosis (IHSS) is distinguished from non-obstructive hypertrophic cardiomyopathy. Mitral regurgitation can occur as a consequence of altered ventricular geometry due to asymmetric hypertrophy, particularly when an outflow tract obstruction can be found. By echocardiography, hypertrophy of the septum and of the free inferior wall is easily identified. Two-dimensional echocardiography shows the small end-systolic ventricular volume, the outflow tract obstruction, and the systolic anterior movement (SAM) of the anterior mitral valve leaflet, and a mesosystolic retraction of the opening of the aortic valve. The intracavitary gradient can be assessed by colour flow Doppler echocardiography, and mitral regurgitation can be quantified. The disturbance of diastolic compliance can be assessed by altered diastolic intervals and the pathological E/A ratio in endocardiography. The diagnostic matrix of hypertrophic cardiomyopathy is presented in Figure 6.7.

To diagnose hypertrophic obstructive or non-obstructive cardiomyopathy, cardiac catheterization is helpful in many cases but not obligatory. Coronary angiography may occasionally demonstrate muscle bridges, but these are of no therapeutic consequence.

In endomyocardial biopsies of non-obstructive forms, exclusion of secondary heart muscle diseases is most

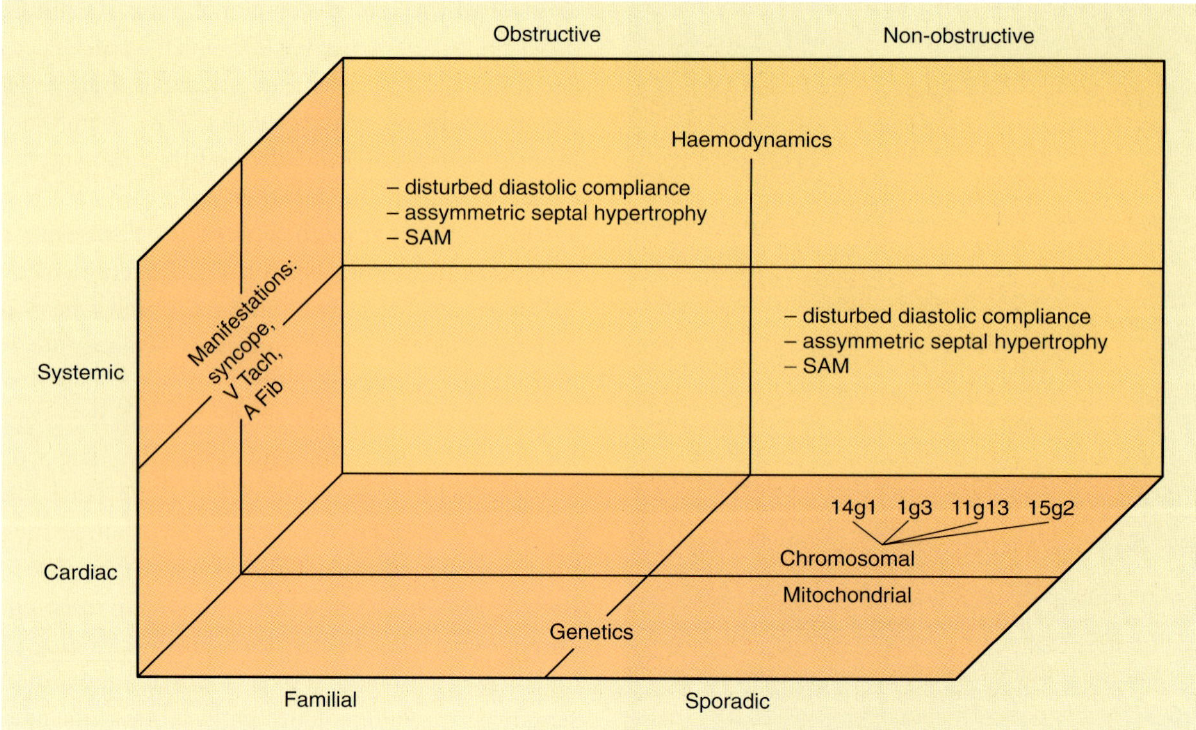


**Figure 6.7** *Diagnostic matrix of hypertrophic cardiomyopathy, showing genotype, haemodynamics, and cardiac manifestations.*

important, since amyloidosis, storage diseases such as glycogenosis, or Fabry's disease can mimic the echocardiographic appearance of non-obstructive hypertrophic cardiomyopathy.

It is important to avoid all measures which may cause or provoke obstruction, such as administration of positive inotropes, digitalis, sympathaticomimetics, calcium, or nitroglycerin and isometric physical activity. Therapeutic approaches with calcium antagonists of the verapamil-type or by β-blockade have been often disappointing. If severe obstruction is present, surgical intervention such as myectomy or myotomy, percutaneous transluminal septal myocardial ablation (PTSMA), or transcoronary ablation of septal hypertrophy (TASH) by instillation of 100% alcohol into a coronary septal artery are the present treatments of choice. The implantation of a universal DDD pacemaker with a short, programmable PQ-interval has been attempted, with some symptomatic benefit. Pacemaker therapy is not superior, however, to myectomy or PTSMA for symptomatic relief. If severely complex ventricular arrhythmias occur, amiodarone or an automatic implantable cardioverter–defibrillator can improve prognosis.

## Restrictive or obliterative cardiomyopathy

Restrictive cardiomyopathy is rare in Europe and, if present, is encountered as Loeffler's endocarditis. It occurs more frequently in tropical countries as endomyocardial fibrosis. Therefore, one distinguishes between endomyocardial fibrosis with (former) and without (latter) eosinophils. In the pathogenesis of eosinophilic endocardial fibrosis cationic proteins released by eosinophils play an important role. Three histological stages can be identified in Loeffler's endocarditis:

- stage I, eosinophilic endomyocarditis
- stage II, partial formation of thrombosis
- stage III, fibrosis.

The diagnostic matrix of the restrictive cardiomyopathy is provided in Figure 6.8.

In haemodynamic terms, the left ventricle is of normal size but has an abrupt disturbance of diastolic elasticity. Intravcavitary thrombosis is often associated. At the early stages, a third heart sound is characteristic. In the apex cardiogram a rapid early filling wave is seen. In contrast to

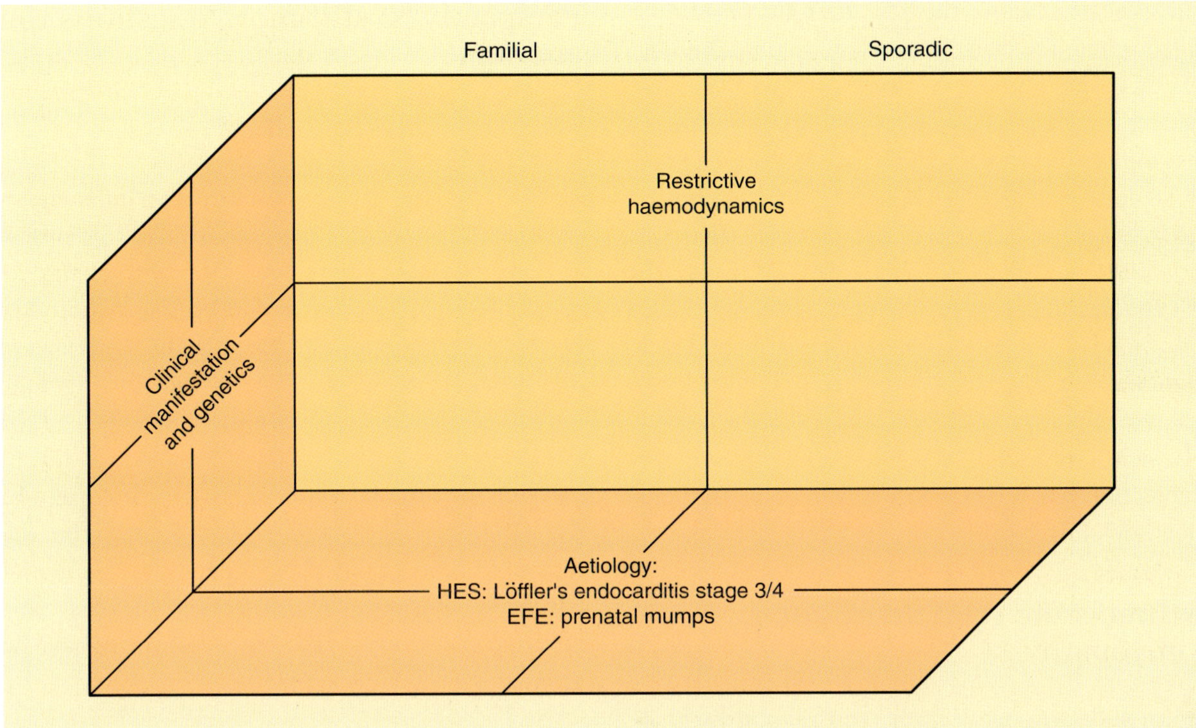


**Figure 6.8** *Diagnostic matrix of restrictive cardiomyopathy: restrictive haemodynamics, aetiological evidence of an eosinophilic endocarditis, Loeffler, or endocardial fibroelastosis (EFE) due to a prenatal mumps infection must be checked.*

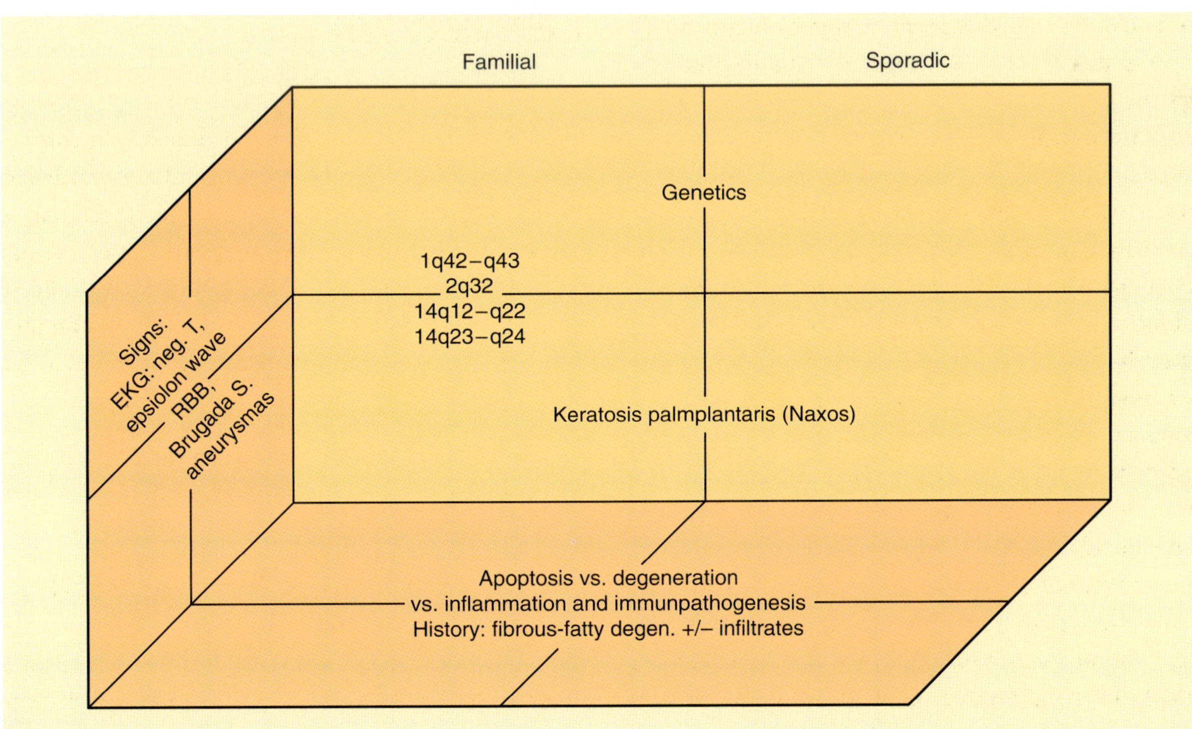


**Figure 6.9** *Diagnostic matrix of arrhythmogenic right ventricular dysplasia (AVRCM): morphological, electrophysiological, and genetic findings are diagnostic and pathogenetic features.*

constrictive heart disease, the left diastolic pressure is always higher than the diastolic pressure on the right side. Electrocardiogram and chest X-ray are not characteristic.

Secondary cardiomyopathies such as amyloidosis and other infiltrative diseases of the myocardium can present as a restrictive cardiomyopathy and should be excluded by endomyocardial biopsy. A causative therapy is often not possible and anticoagulation is advisable. In Loeffler's endocarditis steroids and azathioprine may be of help. The number of eosinophils should be kept below 100 000/mm$^3$.

For the aetiology of the rare endocardial fibroelastosis, which is also a restrictive cardiomyopathy, a prenatal mumps infection has been identified with molecular biological methods (Fig. 6.8).

## Arrhythmogenic right ventricular cardiomyopathy

Pathological and anatomical characteristics of arrhythmogenic right ventricular cardiomyopathy (ARVCM) include segmental thinning of the right ventricular muscle with replacement by fibrosis and fat. The left ventricle may be involved in up to 50% of cases. In a clinical setting, complex rhythm disturbances may be lethal. The characteristic electrocardiographic epsilon wave may often be observed in leads V1 and V2. Right ventricular outflow tract tachycardia is observed frequently. The aetiology or ARVCM is unclear. Hereditary factors (e.g. in genetically transmitted keratosis pedoplantaris naxos) have been suspected in a number of patients. Genetic mutations have been shown at 1q42-q43, 2q32, 14q23-24 and 14q12-22 loci. For the remaining patients, including the sporadic cases, an intrauterine myocarditis of the foetus with a typical healing by reparative fibrosis and fat replacement have been discussed, which may also be supported by a familiar predisposition.

The clinical diagnosis is based on echocardiography, magnetic resonance imaging for recognition of fat, and characteristic electrocardiographic changes (epsilon wave and right ventricular outflow tract tachycardia). The histological diagnosis of degenerative changes, e.g. fibrous tissue and fat, and the demonstration of viral persistence can only be made by right ventricular endomyocardial biopsy or post mortem. Figure 6.9 shows the diagnostic matrix of ARVCM under genetic, haemodynamic, clinical, and aetiological considerations.

## Perspectives: still more questions than answers

The new classification of the WHO/ISFC Task Force of 1995 and the consensus conferences of the two World Heart Federation expert committees on inflammatory cardiomyopathy (myocarditis) and viral cardiomyopathy in 1997/1998 upgraded the understanding of the complex clinical, molecular, viral, immunopathogenetic, and pathophysiological processes involved in the cardiomyopathies. Molecular genetics, molecular biology, virology, and immunology have provided new answers to the old questions of the aetiopathogenesis of cardiomyopathies. Development of a new classification is the current basis for the clinical work, study protocols, and the scientific research. The molecular genetics of immunological advances only 'bridge the gap between knowledge and ignorance' (J. F. Goodwin). The recent advances have not only given answers but also posed new questions.

## References


1. Richardson P, McKenna W, Bristow M *et al.* for the WHO/ISFC Task Force. Report of the 1995 World Health Organization/International Society and Federation of Cardiology Task Force on the Definition and Classification of Cardiomyopathies. *Circulation* 1996; 93: 841–2.
2. Report of the WHO/ISFC Task Force on the Definition and Classification of Cardiomyopathies. *Br Heart J* 1980; 44: 672–3.
3. Kass S, MacRae C, Graber HL *et al.* A gene defect that causes conduction sysem disease and dilated cardiomyopathy maps to chromosome 1p1-1q1. *Nat Genet* 1994; 7: 546–51.
4. Olson TM, Keating MT. Mapping a cardiomyopathy locus to chromosome 3p22-p25. *J Clin Invest* 1996; 97: 528–32.
5. Messina DN, Speer MC, Pericak Vance MA *et al.* Linkage of familial dilated cardiomyopathy with conduction defect and muscular dystrophy to chromosome 6q23. *Am J Hum Genet* 1997; 61: 909–17.
6. Bowles KR, Gajarski R, Porter P *et al.* Gene mapping of familial autosomal dominant dilated cardiomyopathy to chromosome 10q21-23. *J Clin Invest* 1996; 98: 1355–60.
7. Krajinovic M, Pinamonti B, Sinagra G *et al.* Linkage of familial dilated cardiomyopathy to chromosome 9. Heart Muscle Disease Study Group. *Am J Hum Genet* 1995; 507: 846–52.
8. Durand JB, Bachinski LL, Bieling LC *et al.* Localization of a gene responsible for familial dilated cardiomyopathy to chromosome 1q32. *Circulation* 1995; 92: 387–9.
9. Ozawa T, Tanaka M, Sugyama S *et al.* Multiple mitochondrial DNA deletions exist in cardiomyocytes of patients with hypertrophic or dilated cardiomyopathy. *Biochem Biophys Res Commun* 1990; 170: 830–6.
10. Wallace DC. Diseases of the mitochondrial DNA. *Annu Rev Biochem* 1992; 61: 1175–212.

11. Wallace DC. Mitochondrial DNA mutations in diseases of energy metabolism. *J Bioenerg Biomembr* 1994; 26: 241–50.
12. Li YY, Hengstenberg C, Maisch B. Whole mitochondrial genome amplification reveals basal level multiple deletions in mtDNA of patients with dilated cardiomyopathy. *Biochem Biophys Res Commun* 1995; 210: 211–18.
13. Li YY, Maisch B, Rose ML, Hengstenberg C. Point mutations in mitochondrial DANN of patients with dilated cardiomyopathy. *J Mol Cell Cardiol* 1997; 29, 2699–709.
14. Towbin JA, Hejtmancik JF, Brink P *et al.* X-linked dilated cardiomyopathy. Molecular genetic evidence of linkage to the Duchenne muscular dystrophy (dystophin) gene at the Xp21 locus. *Circulation* 1993; 87: 1854–65.
15. Aretz H, Billingham M, Edwards W *et al.* Myocarditis: a histopathologic definition and classification. *Am J Cardiovascular Pathol* 1986; 1: 3–14.
16. Maisch B, Factor S, Gröne F *et al.* Report of the 1997 World Health Organisation and International Society and Federation of Cardiology Expert Committee on the definition of inflammatory cardiomyopathy (myocarditis). 2000 (submitted).
17. Maisch B, Aepinius C, Aitken K *et al.* Consensus-Report of the 1997 International Society and Federation of Cardiology Expert Committee on the Definition of Viral Cardiomyopathy. 2000 (submitted).
18. Banatvala JE (ed.) *Viral infections of the heart*. London: Hodder & Stoughton, 1990.
19. Bowles N, Towbin J. Viral heart muscle disease in children. *Newslett Scient Council Cardiomyopath* 1996; 11: 4–5.
20. Maisch B, Schönian U, Crombach M *et al.* Cytomegalovirus associated inflammatory heart muscle disease. *Scand J Infect Dis* 1993; Suppl 88: 135–48.
21. Martin AB, Webber S, Fricker J *et al.* Acute myocarditis: rapid diagnosis in children. *Circulation* 1994; 90: 330–9.
22. Matsumori A, Matoba Y, Sasayama S. Dilated cardiomyopathy associated with hepatitis C infection. *Circulation* 1995; 92: 2519–25.
23. Schönian U, Crombach M, Maisch B. Assessment of cytomegalovirus DNA and protein expression in patients with myocarditis. *Clin Immun Immunopathol* 1993; 68: 229–33.
24. Woodruff JF. Viral myocarditis: a review. *Am J Pathol* 1980; 101: 427–84.
25. Kandolf R, Ameis D, Kirschner P *et al. In situ* detection of enteroviral genomes in myocardial cells by nucleic acid hybridization: an approach to the diagnosis of viral heart disease. *Proc Natl Acad Sci USA* 1987; 84: 6272–6.
26. Hengstenberg C, Rose ML, Olsen EGJ, Maisch B. Immune response of the endothelium in myocarditis, dilated cardiomyopathy and rejection after heart transplantation. *Eur Heart J* 1991; 12 (Suppl D): 147–51.
27. Kühl U, Daun B, Seeberg B *et al.* Dilatative Kardiomyopathie — eine chronische Myokarditis? Immunhistologische Charakterisierung lymphozytärer Infiltrate. *Herz* 1992; 17: 97–106.
28. Maisch B. Immunologic regulator and effector functions in perimyocarditis, postmyocarditic heart muscle disease and dilated cardiomyopathy. *Basic Res Cardiol* 1986; 81: 217–42.
29. Maisch B, Bauer, Cirsi M, Kochsiek K. Cytolytic cross-reactive antibodies directed against the cardiac membrane and viral proteins in coxsackievirus B3 and B4 myocarditis. Characterization and pathogenetic relevance. *Circulation* 1993; 87 (Suppl IV): 49–65.
30. Pankuweit S, Portig I, Lottspeich F, Maisch B. Autoantibodies in sera of patients with myocarditis: characterization of the corresponding proteins by isoelectric focusing and N-terminal sequence analysis. *J Mol Cell Cardiol* 1997; 29: 77–84.
31. Pohlner K, Portig I, Pankuweit S *et al.* Identification of mitochondrial antigens recognized by antibodies in sera of patients with idiopathic dilated cardiomyopathy by two-dimensional gel electrophoresis and protein sequencing. *Am J Cardiol* 1997; 80: 1040–5.
32. Schultheiss HP. Disturbance of the myocardial energy metabolism in dilated cardiomyopathy due to autoimmunological mechanisms. *Circulation* 1993; 87 (Suppl IV): 43–8.
33. Maisch B. Alcohol and the heart. *Herz* 1996; 21: 207–12.

# SECTION II

# Pathogenetic mechanisms on evolution of cardiomyopathic disorders

# Gene mutations that cause hypertrophic cardiomyopathy 7

C. E. SEIDMAN, D. FATKIN AND J. G. SEIDMAN

## Introduction

Hypertrophic cardiomyopathy is a common disease of heart muscle characterized by unexplained cardiac hypertrophy and myocyte disarray. The initial clinical description of the disease appeared in 1869 [1]. Since then, studies of this intriguing pathology have labelled the condition as hypertrophic obstructive cardiomyopathy, asymmetric septal hypertrophy, and, most commonly, idiopathic hypertrophic subaortic stenosis (IHSS). However, molecular genetic investigations have provided substantial insights into the pathogenesis of the disease, and today the disease should no longer be considered idiopathic. Hypertrophic cardiomyopathy is recognized as a disease of the sarcomere. This chapter will review the biomedical research that elucidated the pathogenesis of this disorder and indicate how these findings impact on the contemporary diagnosis and management of affected individuals.

## Clinical features of hypertrophic cardiomyopathy

Hypertrophic cardiomyopathy is diagnosed based on the finding of unexplained cardiac hypertrophy, a finding that occurs commonly in the general population. Echocardiography studies of healthy young adults recently identified unexplained cardiac hypertrophy in 1 of 500 individuals [2]. Patient histories further demonstrate that hypertrophic cardiomyopathy occurs as either sporadic or familial disease, which is inherited as an autosomal dominant trait. Estimates of familial versus sporadic disease vary, but at least 50% of affected individuals have inherited hypertrophic cardiomyopathy from an affected parent [3, 4]. Analyses of the disorder in many large pedigrees typically demonstrate a high degree of disease penetrance. That is, approximately half of the first-degree adult relatives of an affected individual will develop the disorder (Fig. 7.1). Disease manifestations that are common between affected family members probably reflect the influence of the shared causal gene mutation, whereas differences in phenotype between family members may reflect unique background genes, lifestyles, and environment.

In both familial and sporadic hypertrophic cardiomyopathy, the spectrum of clinical manifestations is broad [5, 6]. Disease symptoms may be absent, and when present can be mild or debilitating, stable or progressive. The discovery of genetic aetiologies for the disorder has both provided the opportunity for complete assessment of the natural history of the disease and indicated the important contribution that genotype has over disease phenotype. Age of onset of cardiac hypertrophy, severity of the hypertrophic response, and survival are all influenced in part by the causal sarcomere protein defect in an affected individual. While a general review of the clinical manifestations of disease follows, the unique influence of particular genotypes is discussed in subsequent sections.

Dyspnoea and angina are common presenting complaints and may be associated with palpitations that are transient or protracted, resulting in dizziness and even syncope. Sudden death occurs in both clinically symptomatic and asymptomatic patients and may be the presenting sign of the disease. Although no single factor correlates with the presence or severity of symptoms, the pathophysiology of hypertrophic cardiomyopathy appears to account for some manifestations of the disease [7]. Dyspnoea and angina are often prominent when left ventricular hypertrophy and diastolic dysfunction are severe [8, 9]. Palpitations, particularly those due to supraventricular tachyarrhythmias, are common, with progressive left atrial enlargement; this finding also increases the risk for thromboembolic events. Late stages of disease can be associated with paroxysmal nocturnal dyspnea, orthopnoea, and peripheral oedema,

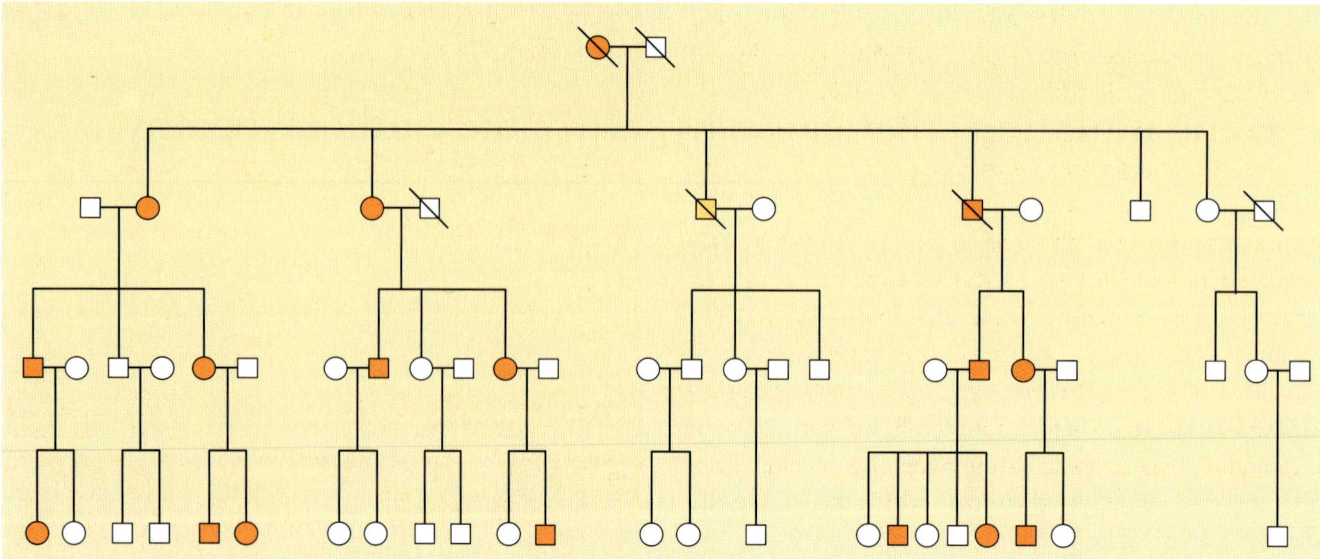

**Figure 7.1** *Autosomal–dominant inheritance in a pedigree with hypertrophic cardiomyopathy. Male and female are represented by squares and circles, respectively. Disease status is indicated: solid symbols, affected; clear symbols, unaffected; grey symbols, affection status unknown. Diagonal slashes denote deceased family members. Note that affected individuals transmit hypertrophic cardiomyopathy to half of their offspring. In contrast, no offspring of unaffected individuals develop the disease.*

symptoms that can herald the onset of congestive cardiac failure. In contrast, the presence or severity of left ventricular outflow tract obstruction does not consistently produce symptoms.

Clinical diagnosis of hypertrophic cardiomyopathy depends on physical examination, electrocardiography, and two-dimensional echocardiography. The cardiac examination may be unremarkable. When ventricular hypertrophy perturbs diastolic filling a loud fourth heart sound is often heard. Murmurs from turbulent blood flow through a narrowed outflow tract or mitral regurgitation are often found. The former is a systolic crescendo–decrescendo ejection murmur, prominent at the left sternal border and the apex, which characteristically increases with the Valsalva manoeuvre or on standing from a squatting position. A pansystolic, blowing murmur that radiates to the axilla may indicate mitral regurgitation.

The electrocardiogram is an important component of diagnostic studies in hypertrophic cardiomyopathy. Electrocardiographic abnormalities are present in the majority of affected individuals [10] and may precede the development of echocardiographic evidence of hypertrophy [11]. Typical findings include voltage criteria left ventricular hypertrophy, atrial enlargement, and ST-segment and T-wave repolarization abnormalities [12]. Giant negative T-waves in leads V4–V6 are characteristically found with the apical pattern of left ventricular hypertrophy that has been reported predominantly in Japanese patients with hypertrophic cardiomyopathy [13]. A pseudoinfarction pattern with prominent Q-waves may be present in the inferior (II, III, aVF) and precordial (V2–V6) leads [14, 15]. Rhythm disturbances become more prominent with disease duration and include atrial tachycardias (fibrillation or flutter) and ventricular arrhythmias. Hypertrophic cardiomyopathy associated with accessory pathways (Wolff–Parkinson–White syndrome) may indicate a distinct and as yet unknown genetic aetiology (chromosome 7, locus) [16].

Transthoracic echocardiography is the primary modality for diagnosing individuals with hypertrophic cardiomyopathy. Although the hallmark of disease is considered asymmetric hypertrophy (interventricular septum greater than left ventricular free wall hypertrophy), echocardiographic studies of large affected populations indicate that no single morphological pattern is pathognomonic for disease diagnosis [17, 18]. Hypertrophy can be extensive and diffuse or mild and segmental, and diagnosis depends only on finding unexplained hypertrophy (ventricular wall thickness 1.3 cm or greater) in any ventricular location. Additional echocardiographic findings [19, 20] typically include enlargement of the left atrial chamber, mitral regurgitation (due to abnormal coaptation of the mitral valve leaflets), and altered systolic contractile function. Structural abnormalities of the mitral valve and subvalvular apparatus may be present [21], including increased leaflet area, elongation and prolapse of leaflets, and direct papillary muscle insertion into the anterior leaflet. Colour-flow Doppler studies are useful in defining the left ventricular outflow tract gradient and diastolic dysfunction [20]. Significant subaortic gradients are evident in fewer than 25% of affected individuals and result from impediment to ventricular outflow caused by asymmetric hypertrophy of the proximal interventricular septum in combinations with systolic anterior motion (SAM) of the mitral valve with subsequent mitral leaflet–septal contact. Some patients with longstanding hypertrophic cardiomyopathy develop atrial and ventricular chamber dilatation with reduced systolic function; the echocardiographic features of this 'burnt out' phase mimic those of dilated cardiomyopathy [22, 23].

The gross pathology of hypertrophic cardiomyopathy is variable. Myocardial hypertrophy remains the anatomical hallmark of disease, but a normal ventricular mass does not exclude the diagnosis [24]. Hypertrophy is most often asymmetric, with septal involvement greater than ventricular free wall, but can also be concentric (Fig. 7.2A) or focal (particularly involving the apex). Isolated right ventricular hypertrophy can occur, but typically right chamber involvement is found with substantial left ventricular disease. Left atrial enlargement is common and may be associated with morphological abnormalities of the mitral valve [21]. Discoloration of the subaortic endocardial septal surface is found in patients with outflow tract obstruction and SAM.

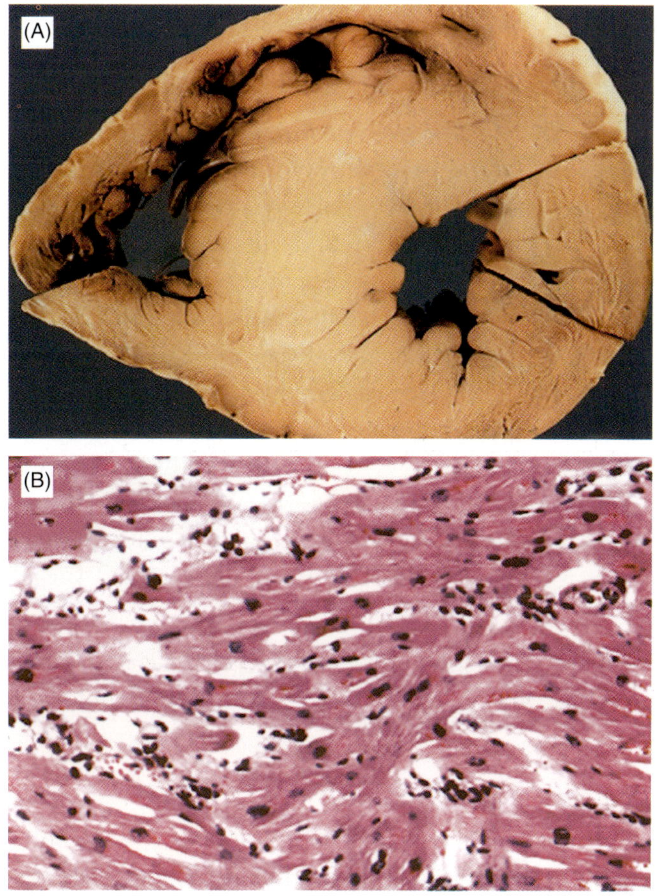


**Figure 7.2** *Pathological features of hypertrophic cardiomyopathy. (A) Gross morphology showing massive left and moderate right ventricular hypertrophy. (B) Myocyte and myofibrillar disarray is evident by hematoxylin and eosin staining of left ventricular tissue section. Note the marked interstitial fibrosis (pale pink cytoplasm with dense nuclei).*

Disorganization of the myocardial architecture (Fig. 7.2B) is the *sine qua non* of histopathology in hypertrophic cardiomyopathy [24–27] and such findings can be evident in affected individuals with normal ventricular mass. Enlarged myocytes may contain large, bizarrely shaped nuclei. The fibre orientation of the myocardium can be haphazard, interwoven (herringbone pattern), or whirled. Myocyte disarray is often accompanied by interstitial fibrosis [28], due to the premature death of myocyte populations. Inflammatory cells are absent. Intimal proliferation of intramural coronary arteries [29] is most evident when hypertrophy is severe.

## Molecular genetics of hypertrophic cardiomyopathy

Neither a unifying pathogenic mechanism nor a biochemical defect for hypertrophic cardiomyopathy was understood prior to the application of human molecular genetic studies. Recognition that the disease was transmitted in an autosomal–dominant mode allowed cosegration or linkage analysis, in which the chromosome location of disease genes could be ascertained. Such studies involve the clinical evaluation of affected families to ascertain disease status in combination with genetic analyses to identify a DNA marker that is coinherited with affected, but not with unaffected disease status. DNA markers used in such studies are polymorphisms, or variations in nucleotide sequence that are known to occur at a precise region of the genome. Thus, the identification of a polymorphism that segregates with disease status defines the chromosome location of a disease gene.

Once the chromosome location for a disease gene is known, candidate genes can be evaluated for potential disease-causing mutations. Candidate genes are defined as those that map to the disease locus and are expressed in the tissue that manifests the disease phenotype. Alternatively, positional cloning techniques are used to identify novel genes that may be involved in the pathology. Disease-causing mutations in hypertrophic cardiomyopathy comprise missense mutations (single nucleotide changes that alter the encoded amino acid) or small insertions or deletions. Large gene rearrangements (translocations or inversions) have not been found to cause disease.

Linkage analyses in familial hypertrophic cardiomyopathy and candidate gene analyses have defined disease loci (Fig. 7.3) on chromosomes 1q31 [30], 3p [31], 7 [16], 11p11.2 [32], 12q2 [31], 14q1 [33] and 15q2 [34], and 19p13.2-q13.2 [35]. Except for the chromosome 7 locus, where the disease gene remains unknown, mutations in a contractile protein gene [cardiac troponin T and I, ventricular regulatory light chain, cardiac myosin binding protein-C, essential light chain, β-cardiac myosin heavy chain (MHC), and α-tropomyosin] have been identified at each disease locus. Collectively, these genetic studies have demonstrated that hypertrophic cardiomyopathy is a disorder of the sarcomere.

### β-Cardiac myosin heavy chain gene mutations

Of the more than 20 genes which encode MHC in the human genome, only α- and β-MHC are expressed at high levels within the myocardium of the heart. The α- and β-MHC genes reside on chromosome 14q1, span approximately 30 000 base pairs, and are organized into 40 exons [36]. During development, α-MHC is abundant, but after birth, β-MHC expression predominates in the ventricular myocardium. Mutations in the β-MHC gene account for a

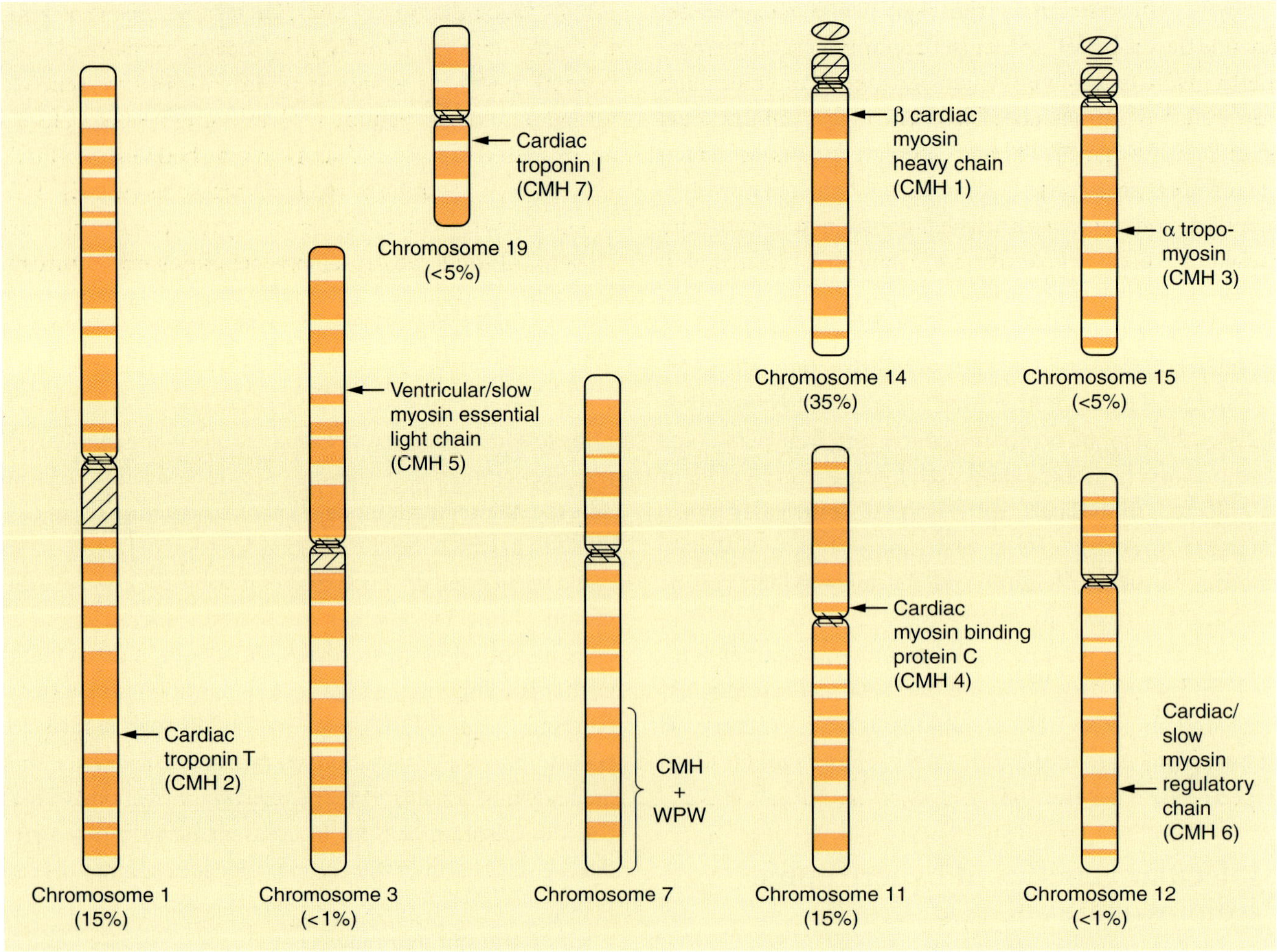


**Figure 7.3** *Hypertrophic cardiomyopathy is a genetically heterogeneous disorder, caused by mutations in sarcomere genes. The chromosome locations of hypertrophic cardiomyopathy disease genes are shown with estimates (inparentheses) of the amount of disease caused by mutations in each gene.*

substantial fraction of hypertrophic cardiomyopathy, whereas no disease-causing mutations have been identified in the α-MHC gene.

Mutations in the β-cardiac MHC account for 30–35% of all hypertrophic cardiomyopathies [37]. More than 40 different mutations have been identified, all of which are missense, and are predicted to alter one encoded amino acid in the head or head-rod junction of the protein. Figure 7.4 provides an example of DNA sequence analyses of one β-cardiac MHC missense mutation. To date, no mutations have been identified in sequences encoding the rod region. These mutations are typically family specific [38–40], and unique defects are found in different families (termed allelic or intragenic heterogeneity).

Mutations in β-cardiac MHC are expressed with nearly complete disease penetrance in the adult. Although children with these mutations may not have evidence of disease, β-cardiac MHC mutations typically produce clinically demonstrable pathology by late adolescence. These defects typically produce substantial cardiac hypertrophy: two-dimensional echocardiographic studies have demonstrated mean maximal left ventricular wall thickness of 23.7 ± 7.7 mm in affected individuals with different myosin mutations [37].

Life expectancy with hypertrophic cardiomyopathy caused by a β-cardiac MHC mutation varies considerably and survival appears to be influenced by the specific disease-causing mutation [37, 39, 40]. Individuals with the $Arg_{719}$Trp or $Arg_{403}$Gln mutation have markedly shortened life expectancies (average age of death, 38 and 45 years, respectively), whereas survival is near normal in individuals with the $Val_{606}$Met mutation. Although the location of mutations within the β-cardiac MHC polypeptide does not predict those with a benign versus a malignant clinical phenotype, non-conservative mutations (those which alter the charge of the amino acid) appear to have a more adverse outcome on survival. These data, while still incomplete, indicate that genotype may assist in risk stratification of sudden and premature death in hypertrophic cardiomyopathy.

## Cardiac myosin-binding protein C gene mutations

A prevalent cause of hypertrophic cardiomyopathy is mutation in the cardiac myosin-binding protein C gene, encoded on chromosome 11p11.2 [32]. This gene spans 24 kb of genomic DNA and is organized into 37 exons that encode a 1274 amino acid peptide [41]. Although other isoforms are expressed in muscles throughout the body, myosin-binding protein C is expressed solely in cardiac tissue [42]. This protein has structural and regulatory functions in the sarcomere. During cardiac embryogenesis, cardiac myosin

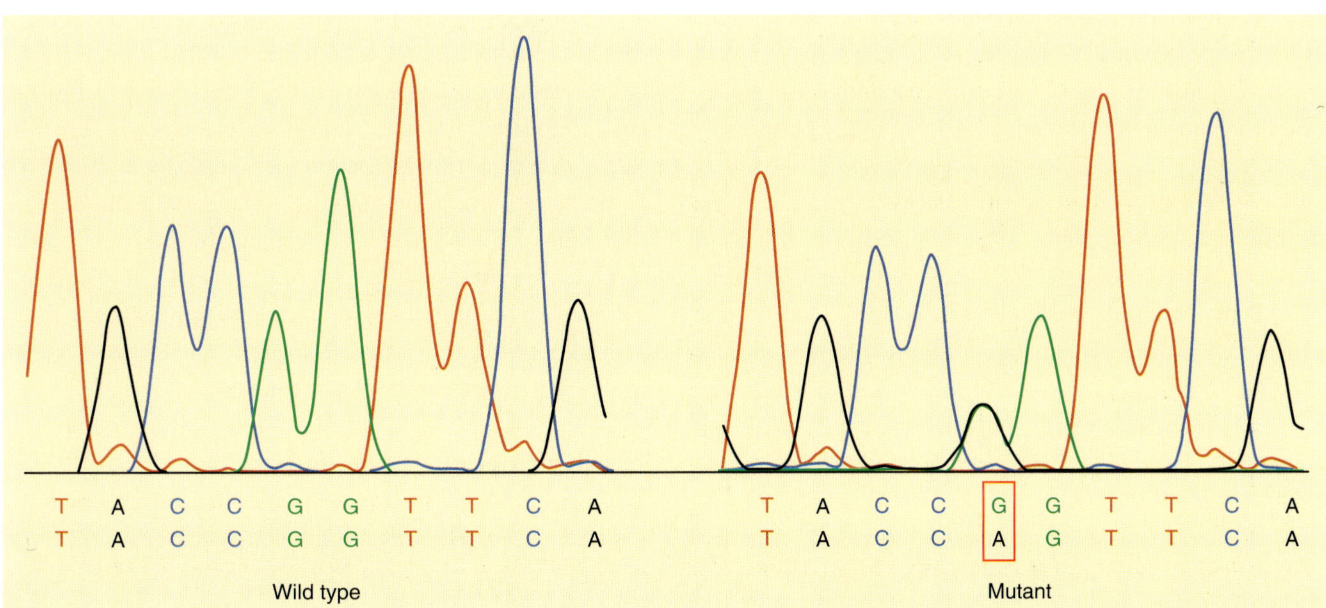


**Figure 7.4** *DNA sequence trace defining a mutation in the β-myosin heavy chain gene. Note that the sample is heterozygous for a G → A mutation, which alters a conserved arginine at residue 403 to glutamine.*

binding protein C is thought to participate in the alignment of thick filaments by binding MHC and titin [43, 44]. In the adult myocardium, phosphorylation of cardiac myosin-binding protein C by a catecholamine-sensitive pathway may provide dynamic regulation of cardiac contraction in response to adrenergic stimuli. Whether these or other unknown functions are perturbed by mutations that cause hypertrophic cardiomyopathy remains unknown.

Although initial studies suggested that these defects accounted for approximately 15% of cases, the delayed expression of myosin-binding protein C mutations appears to have underestimated their incidence [45]. A broad range of gene defects, including missense and splice signal mutations, insertions, and deletions in cardiac myosin-binding protein C has been reported [45, 46]. Many of these mutations are predicted to truncate the encoded protein with loss of the myosin- and titin-binding domains [41, 47].

Hypertrophic cardiomyopathy caused by cardiac myosin-binding protein C mutations is often quiescent until late in adult life [45]. Clinical evaluations of adults, aged 50 years or younger, with cardiac myosin-binding protein C defects showed cardiac hypertrophy only in 58%. Disease penetrance was found to remain incomplete until the age of 60 years. Survival is generally better than that observed among patients with hypertrophic cardiomyopathy caused by mutations in other sarcomere protein genes. Although the risk of premature sudden death is substantially increased in one cardiac myosin-binding protein C mutation, the findings of good survival and reduced disease penetrance associated with most defects indicate that cardiac myosin-binding protein C mutations account for a milder form of hypertrophic cardiomyopathy in many patients.

### Cardiac troponin T gene mutations

Mutations in the troponin T gene encoded in 17 kb of DNA on chromosome 1q31 [30] account for approximately 15% of hypertrophic cardiomyopathy [48]. Alternative splicing of 17 exons gives rise to multiple different protein isoforms. Only the cardiac troponin T isoform is expressed in the foetal and adult heart [42], where it functions with components I and C of the troponin complex to modulate tropomyosin binding.

In addition to missense mutations, defects in splice signals and small deletions of the cardiac troponin T gene have been reported to cause hypertrophic cardiomyopathy [48–50]. The disease phenotype caused by these defects is characterized by substantially less hypertrophy than that observed with myosin mutations. The mean maximal left ventricular wall thickness resulting from six different cardiac troponin T mutations was $16.7 \pm 5.5$ mm [48], and some adults with these mutations had normal cardiac wall thickness. In addition, cardiac troponin T mutations have been identified in individuals who do not fulfil standard diagnostic criteria (unexplained cardiac hypertrophy of greater than 13 mm). Despite this reduced penetrance, many cardiac troponin T mutations are associated with markedly reduced survival [48, 50], and sudden death has occurred in genetically affected individuals with normal clinical studies. Gene-based diagnosis may therefore be particularly important in the risk stratification of this aetiology of hypertrophic cardiomyopathy.

### α-Tropomyosin gene mutations

Tropomyosin is a rigid, rod-shaped protein that binds actin and functions both to stabilize and to stiffen thin filaments of the sarcomere [42]. The α-tropomyosin gene is located on chromosome 15q2 and consists of 15 exons, of which ten are transcribed in a tissue-specific manner [34]. Within the ventricular myocardium, α-tropomyosin contains 284 amino acids and has two troponin T-binding domains.

Mutations in the α-tropomyosin gene account for less than 3% of hypertrophic cardiomyopathy [48]. All disease-causing mutations are missense and alter residues in the troponin T-binding domains. Because the α-tropomyosin isoform found in cardiac tissue is also abundant in other striated muscle, the cardiac-specific phenotype produced by these mutations may reflect interactions that are specific for cardiac troponin T. Amino acid 175 in the α-tropomyosin gene appears to be a mutational hotspot [51]. The $Asp_{175}Asn$ mutation has arisen in multiple families and the flanking haplotypes found in these families are unique, thus indicating *de novo* mutation. Intriguingly, the hypertrophic response to the $Asp_{175}Asn$ mutation varies considerably between different families, providing evidence for the interactions between genotype, other genes, and environment in producing the morphological expression of disease.

### Cardiac troponin I gene mutations

The cardiac troponin I gene is encoded on chromosome 19p13.2-q13.2 [52] and organized into eight exons that span 6.2 kb. Cardiac troponin I, a 210 amino acid protein, is expressed exclusively in cardiac tissue [42] and functions to inhibit muscle contraction in the absence of calcium [45, 53]. Only six troponin I defects that cause hypertrophic cardiomyopathy have been reported [35], five of which are missense. There have been few clinical data regarding the clinical manifestations of these defects, but two mutations were reported to produce a predominance of apical hypertrophy and electrocardiographic findings of negative T-waves.

### Myosin light chain gene mutations

The myosin regulatory light chains and myosin essential light chains are encoded on chromosomes 12q and 3p, respectively [54]. These small molecules are associated with the neck region of the MHC and although an exact role of these light chains in muscle physiology is not understood they may regulate biophysical properties of myosin through interactions with calcium [42]. It has been proposed that light chain molecules play a particularly important role in the stretch activation response of the cardiac papillary muscles. There are atrial and ventricular isoforms of regulatory light chain molecules; the ventricular isoform is 166 amino acids and undergoes reversible phosphorylation. Two of five essential light chain isoforms are expressed in heart tissues; the myosin light chain-1 slow/ventricular isoform is a 195 amino acid peptide found in the ventricular myocardium.

Mutations in the ventricular isoform of the regulatory light chain and myosin light chain-1 slow/ventricular isoform of the essential light chain are rare causes of hypertrophic cardiomyopathy. Despite large screening studies [31, 55], fewer than ten gene defects have been reported, most of which are missense mutations. Surprisingly, the cardiac phenotype-associated defect in either regulatory protein is ventricular hypertrophy with midchamber thickening that can be severe and result in haemodynamic obstruction, apparent as an hourglass morphology during ventriculography.

### Cardiac actin gene mutations

The most recent gene to be implicated in hypertrophic cardiomyopathy is cardiac actin. Surprisingly, mutations in cardiac actin can also cause familial dilated cardiomyopathy. Located on chromosome 15q, human cardiac actin has six exons that encode a 375 amino acid protein [56] with two functional domains. The amino-terminus of actin filaments forms cross-bridges with myosin. The carboxyl-terminus of the actin filament binds Z-band proteins and dystrophin, a cytoskeletal molecule that links myofibrils to the extracellular matrix [42].

Missense mutations in cardiac actin have recently been identified as causing hypertrophic cardiomyopathy [57]. Based on their location near a putative myosin binding site, force generation may be perturbed by these defects. In contrast, mutations that result in cardiac dilatation are located in actin domains implicated in force transmission to adjacent sarcomeres and the extracellular matrix. Because of the rarity of these gene defects, the clinical phenotypes of hypertrophic cardiomyopathy caused by actin mutations are not well defined.

### Chromosome 7 disease locus

The disease gene located on chromosome 7, which can be mutated in hypertrophic cardiomyopathy, remains unknown. Affected individuals with mutations in the gene typically exhibit Wolff–Parkinson–White syndrome [16] and atrioventricular node dysfunction in addition to typical morphological features of cardiac hypertrophy. Identification of this gene may elucidate previously unrecognized links between the sarcomere and cardiac conduction system or alternatively indicate that mutations in other cardiac proteins can also produce a hypertrophic phenotype.

## Implications of genetic research on clinical care

Definition of the molecular aetiologies for human disease has the potential to improve diagnosis and provide insights into pathophysiology and the diversity of clinical course and outcome. Although still in its infancy, the science of gene mutations causing hypertrophic cardiomyopathy has begun to address some of these issues.

Family history in hypertrophic cardiomyopathy often provides the most important clues for appropriate diagnosis. However, when unexplained cardiac hypertrophy is found without evidence for a heritable trait, diagnosis can be difficult. Definition of the molecular basis for familial hypertrophic cardiomyopathy has prompted genetic analyses of these same genes in sporadic cases of disease. Analyses of β-MHC and α-tropomyosin gene sequences [58, 59] in DNA samples derived from individuals with sporadic disease indicate that *de novo* mutations can account for isolated cases of hypertrophic cardiomyopathy. Moreover, these defects can be transmitted to offspring, thereby initiating familial patterns in subsequent generations.

The pattern of transmission of gene mutations in familial and sporadic hypertrophic cardiomyopathy indicates that half of all offspring of an affected individual will develop the disorder (Fig. 7.1). Unfortunately, accurate assessment of clinical status is complicated by the age-related penetrance of hypertrophic cardiomyopathy. That is, an individual who has inherited a disease-causing β-cardiac myosin mutation may not develop signs or symptoms of disease until after puberty, or late in middle age, if the aetiology is a cardiac myosin-binding protein C mutation [45]. Gene-based diagnosis can therefore selectively target by longitudinal evaluation those individuals at risk for disease [11, 60]. In addition to excluding the unnecessary screening of genetically unaffected individuals, gene-based diagnosis may someday allow intervention in advance of the development of cardiac hypertrophy.

Perhaps the most important role of gene-based diagnosis in hypertrophic cardiomyopathy relates to the potential to identify individuals at high risk for the most serious complication of the disease, sudden death. While clinical and anatomical features of disease do not appear to discriminate between individuals at risk for premature death, genotype has provided some insight. For example, mutations $Arg_{403}Gln$ or $Arg_{453}Cys$ in the β-cardiac MHC gene [39] and several cardiac troponin T defects [48] portend poor survival. In contrast, the β-cardiac MHC gene defect $Val_{606}Met$ and most cardiac myosin-binding protein C mutations are associated with normal life expectancies [45].

With the potential clinical value of defining the natural history of hypertrophic cardiomyopathy by genotype, why is such information limited to only a few gene defects? The answer lies in the complexity of defining a mutation for an autosomal–dominant disorder that exhibits substantial genetic heterogeneity (Fig. 7.3). There is little evidence of a strong founder effect and a different mutation is found in nearly all families. Hence, identification of a disease-causing mutation requires analysis of each of the eight sarcomere genes and the unknown gene encoded on chromosome 7. Furthermore, because a single nucleotide substitution in one of the two genomic copies of any of the sarcomere genes is sufficient to cause disease, genetic analyses must be completely accurate. Automated DNA sequence analyses (Fig. 7.4) in combination with other laboratory robotics has increased the capacity for definition of mutations, and may allow both the speed and accuracy necessary for clinical use. Progress in chip technology also provides promise, particularly for analysis of missense mutations. The continued evolution of these methodologies has great potential for defining the full spectrum of gene mutations that cause hypertrophic cardiomyopathy and this information ultimately should improve diagnosis and management.

## References


1. Hallopeau M. Retrecissement ventriculo-aortique. *Gazette Med Paris* 1869; 24: 683.
2. Maron BJ, Gardin JM, Flack JM *et al.* Prevalence of hypertrophic cardiomyopathy in a general population of young adults: echocardiographic analysis of 4111 subjects in the CARDIA study: Coronary Artery Risk Development in (Young) Adults. *Circulation* 1995; 92: 785–9.
3. Greaves S, Roche AH, Neutze JM *et al.* Inheritance of hypertrophic cardiomyopathy: a cross sectional and M mode echocardiographic study of 50 families. *Br Heart J* 1987; 58: 259–66.
4. Kimura A, Harada H, Park JE *et al.* Mutations in the cardiac troponin I gene associated with hypertrophic cardiomyopathy. *Nat Genet* 1997; 16: 379–82.
5. Maron BJ, Bonow RO, Cannon RO *et al.* Hypertrophic cardiomyopathy. Interrelations of clinical manifestations, pathophysiology and therapy. *N Engl J Med* 1987; 316: 780, 844–52.
6. Wigle Ed, Rakowski H, Kimball BP *et al.* Hypertrophic cardiomyopathy. Clinical spectrum and treatment. *Circulation* 1995; 92: 1680–92.
7. Spirito P, Seidman CE, McKenna WJ *et al.* The management of hypertrophic cardiomyopathy. *N Engl J Med* 1997; 336: 775–85.
8. Ten Cate FJ, Serruys PW, Mey S *et al.* Effects of short-term administration of verapamil on left ventricular relaxation and filling dynamics measured by a combined hemodynamic–ultrasonic technique in patients with hypertrophic cardiomyopathy. *Circulation* 1983; 68: 1274–9.
9. Lorell BH, Paulus WJ, Grossman W *et al.* Modification of abnormal left ventricular diastolic properties by nifedipine in patients with hypertrophic cardiomyopathy. *Circulation* 1982; 65: 499–507.
10. Maron BJ, Wolfson JK, Ciro E *et al.* Relation of electrocardiographic abnormalities and patterns of left ventricular hypertrophy identified by 2-dimensional echocardiography in patients with hypertrophic cardiomyopathy. *Am J Cardiol* 1983; 51: 189–194.
11. Rosenzweig A, Watkins H, Hwang D-S *et al.* Preclinical diagnosis of familial hypertrophic cardiomyopathy by genetic analysis of blood lymphocytes. *N Engl J Med* 1991; 325: 1753–60.
12. Schamroth L. Ventricular hypertrophy. In: *An introduction to electrocardiography*. 5th edition. Oxford: Blackwell Scientific Publications, 1976, 68.
13. Yamaguchi H, Ishimura T, Nishiyama S *et al.* Hypertrophic nonobstructive cardiomyopathy with giant negative T-waves (apical hypertrophy): ventriculographic and echocardiographic features in 30 patients. *Am J Cardiol* 1979; 44: 401–12.
14. Lemery R, Kleinebenne A, Nihoyannopoulos P *et al.* Q waves in hypertrophic cardiomyopathy in relation to the distribution and severity of right and left ventricular hypertrophy. *J Am Coll Cardiol* 1990; 16: 368–74.
15. Maron BJ. Q waves in hypertrophic cardiomyopathy: a reassessment. *J Am Coll Cardiol* 1990; 16: 375–6.
16. MacRae CA, Ghaisas N, Kass S *et al.* Familial hypertrophic cardiomyopathy with Wolff–Parkinson–White syndrome maps to a locus on chromosome 7q3. *J Clin Invest* 1995; 96: 1216–20.
17. Maron BJ, Wolfson JK, Ciro E *et al.* Relation of electrocardiographic abnormalities and patterns of left ventricular hypertrophy identified by 2-dimensional echocardiography in patients with hypertrophic cardiomyopathy. *Am J Cardiol* 1983; 51: 189–94.

18. Klues HG, Schiffers A, Maron BJ. Phenotypic spectrum and patterns of left ventricular hypertrophy in hypertrophic cardiomyopathy: morphologic observations and significance as assessed by two-dimensional echocardiography in 600 patients. *J Am Coll Cardiol* 1995; 26: 1699–1708.
19. Schwammenthal E, Nakatani S, He S *et al*. Mechanism of mitral regurgitation in hypertrophic cardiomyopathy. Mismatch of posterior to anterior leaflet length and mobility. *Circulation* 1998; 98: 856–65.
20. Grigg LE, Wigle ED, Williams WG *et al*. Transesophageal Doppler echocardiography in obstructive hypertrophic cardiomyopathy: clarification of pathophysiology and importance in intraoperative decision making. *J Am Coll Cardiol* 1992; 20: 42–52.
21. Klues HG, Maron BJ, Dollar AL *et al*. Diversity of structural mitral valve alterations in hypertrophic cardiomyopathy. *Circulation* 1992; 85: 1651–60.
22. Frank S, Braunwald E. Idiopathic hypertrophic subaortic stenosis: clinical analysis of 126 patients with emphasis on the natural history. *Circulation* 1968; 37: 759–88.
23. Shah PM, Adelman AG, Wigle ED *et al*. The natural (and unnatural) history of hypertrophic obstructive cardiomyopathy. *Circ Res* 1974; 35 (Suppl 2): 179–95.
24. McKenna WJ, Stewart JT, Nihoyannopoulos P *et al*. Hypertrophic cardiomyopathy without hypertrophy: two families with myocardial disarray in the absence of increased myocardial mass. *Br Heart J* 1990; 63: 287–90.
25. Ferrans VJ, Morrow AG, Roberts WC. Myocardial ultrastructure in idiopathic hypertrophic subaortic stenosis. A study of operatively excised left ventricular outflow tract muscle in 14 patients. *Circulation* 1972; 45: 769–92.
26. Dingemans KP, Becker AE. Specificity of cellular and myofibrillar disoreintation in hypertrophic obstructive cardiomyopathy. *Arch Pathol Lab Med* 1977; 101: 493–9.
27. Maron BJ, Roberts WC. Quantitative analysis of cardiac muscle cell disorganization in the ventricular septum of patients with hypertrophic cardiomyopathy. *Circulation* 1979; 59: 689–706.
28. St. John Sutton MG, Lee JT, Anderson KR *et al*. Histopathological specificity of hypertrophic obstructive cardiomyopathy. Myocardial fiber disarray and myocardial fibrosis. *Br Heart J* 1980; 44: 433–43.
29. Maron BJ, Epstein SE, Roberts WC. Hypertrophic cardiomyopathy and transmural myocardial infarction without significant atherosclerosis of the extramural coronary arteries. *Am J Cardiol* 1979; 43: 1086–1102.
30. Watkins H, MacRae C, Thierfelder L *et al*. A disease locus for familial hypertrophic cardiomyopathy maps to chromosome 1q3. *Nat Genet* 1993; 3: 333–37.
31. Poetter K, Jiang H, Hassanzadeh S *et al*. Mutations in either the essential or regulatory light chains of myosin are associated with a rare myopathy in human heart and skeletal muscle. *Nat Genet* 1996; 13: 63–69.
32. Carrier L, Hengstenberg C, Beckmann JS *et al*. Mapping of a novel gene for familial hypertrophic cardiomyopathy to chromosome 11. *Nat Genet* 1993; 4: 311–13.
33. Jarcho JA, McKenna W, Pare JAP *et al*. Mapping a gene for familial hypertrophic cardiomyopathy to chromosome 14ql. *N Engl J Med* 1989; 321: 1372–8.
34. Thierfelder L, MacRae C, Watkins H *et al*. A familial hypertrophic cardiomyopathy locus maps to chromosome 15q2. *Proc Natl Acad Sci USA* 1993; 90: 6270–9.
35. Kimura A, Harada H, Park JE *et al*. Mutations in the cardiac troponin I gene associated with hypertrophic cardiomyopathy. *Nat Genet* 1997; 16: 379–82.
36. Saez LJ, Gianola KM, McNally EM *et al*. Human cardiac myosin heavy chain genes and their linkage in the genome. *Nucl Acids Res* 1987; 15: 5443–59.
37. Watkins H, Rosenzweig A, Hwang *et al*. Characteristics and prognostic implications of myosin missense mutations in familial hypertrophic cardiomyopathy. *N Engl J Med* 1992; 326: 1108–14.
38. Dausse E, Komajda M, Dubourg O *et al*. Familial hypertrophic cardiomyopathy: microsatellite haplotyping and identification of a hotspot for mutations in the β-myosin heavy chain gene. *J Clin Invest* 1993; 92: 2807–13.
39. Anan R, Greve G, Thierfelder L *et al*. Prognostic implications of novel β-myosin heavy chain gene mutations that cause familial hypertrophic cardiomyopathy. *J Clin Invest* 1994: 93: 280–5.
40. Fananapazir L, Dalakas MC, Cyran F *et al*. Missense mutations in the β-myosin heavy chain gene cause central core disease in hypertrophic cardiomyopathy. *Proc Natl Acad Sci USA* 1993; 90: 3993–7.
41. Carrier L, Bonne G, Bahrend E *et al*. Organization and sequence of human cardiac myosin binding protein C gene (MYBPC3) and identification of mutations predicted to produce truncated proteins in familial hypertrophic cardiomyopathy. *Circ Res* 1997; 80: 427–34.
42. Schiaffino S, Reggiani C. Molecular diversity of myofibrillar proteins: gene regulation and functional significance. *Physiol Rev* 1996; 76: 371–423.
43. Hofmann PA, Hartzell HC, Moss RL. Alterations in $Ca^{2+}$ sensitive tension due to partial extraction of C-protein from rat skinned cardiac myocytes and rabbit skeletal muscle fibers $Ca^{2+}$ activation. *J Gen Physiol* 1991; 97: 1141–63.
44. Gautel M, Suffardi O, Freiburg A *et al*. Phosphorylation switches specific for the cardiac isoform of myosin binding protein C: a modulator of cardiac contraction? *EMBO J* 1995; 14: 1952–60.
45. Niimura H, Bachinski LL, Sangwatanaroj S *et al*. Mutations in the gene for cardiac myosin-binding protein C and late-onset familial hypertrophic cardiomyopathy. *N Engl J Med* 1998; 338: 1248–57.
46. Yu B, French JA, Carrier L *et al*. Molecular pathology of familial hypertrophic cardiomyopathy caused by mutations in the myosin binding protein C gene. *J Med Genet* 1998; 35: 205–10.
47. Rottbauer W, Gautel M, Zehelein J *et al*. Novel splice donor site mutation in the cardiac myosin binding protein C gene in familial hypertrophic cardiomyopathy: characterization of cardiac transcript and protein. *J Clin Invest* 1997: 100: 475–82.
48. Watkins H, McKenna WJ, Thierfelder L *et al*. Mutations in the genes for cardiac troponin T and α-tropomyosin in hypertrophic cardiomyopathy. *N Engl J Med* 1995; 332: 1058–64.
49. Forissier JF, Carrier L, Farza H *et al*. Codon 102 of the cardiac troponin T gene is a putative hot spot for mutations in familial hypertrophic cardiomyopathy. *Circulation* 1996; 94: 3069–73.
50. Moolman JC, Corfield VA, Posen B *et al*. Sudden death due to troponin T mutations. *J Am Coll Cardiol* 1997; 29: 549–55.
51. Coviello DA, Maron BJ, Spirito P *et al*. Clinical features of hypertrophic cardiomyopathy caused by mutation of a "hot spot" in the α-tropomyosin gene. *J Am Coll Cardiol* 1997; 29: 635–40.

52. Nakajima-Taniguchi C, Matsui H, Fujio Y *et al*. Novel missense mutation in cardiac troponin T gene found in Japanese patient with hypertrophic cardiomyopathy. *J Mol Cell Cardiol* 1997; 29: 839–43.
53. Tobacman LS. Thin filament-mediated regulation of cardiac contraction. *Annu Rev Physiol* 1996; 58: 447–81.
54. Fodor WL, Darras B, Seharaseyon J *et al*. Human ventricular/slow twitch myosin alkali light chain gene: characterization, sequence, and chromosomal location. *J Biol Chem* 1989; 264: 2143–9.
55. Flavigny J, Richard P, Isnard R *et al*. Identification of two novel mutations in the ventricular regulatory myosin light chain gene (MYL2) associated with familial and classical forms of hypertrophic cardiomyopathy. *J Mol Med* 1998; 76: 208–14.
56. Hamada H, Petrino MG, Kakunaga T. Molecular structure and evolutionary origin of human cardiac muscle actin gene. *Proc Natl Acad Sci USA* 1982; 79: 5901–5.
57. Mogensen J, Klausen IC, Pedersen AK *et al*. β-Cardiac actin is a novel disease gene in familial hypertrophic cardiomyopathy. *J Clin Invest* 1999; 103: R39–43.
58. Greve G, Bachinski L, Friedman DL *et al*. Isolation of a *de novo* mutant myocardial β-MHC protein in a pedigree with hypertrophic cardiomyopathy. *Hum Mol Genet* 1994; 3: 2073–75.
59. Watkins H, Anan R, Coviello DA *et al*. A *de novo* mutation in α-tropomyosin that causes hypertrophic cardiomyopathy. *Circulation* 1995; 91: 2302–5.
60. Maron BJ, Moller JH, Seidman CE *et al*. Impact of laboratory molecular diagnosis on contemporary diagnostic criteria for genetically transmitted cardiovascular diseases: hypertrophic cardiomyopathy, long-QT syndrome, and Marfan syndrome. *Circulation* 1998; 98: 1460–71.

# Abnormalities of calcium homoeostasis and defective excitation–contraction coupling in cardiomyopathy

8

J. K. GWATHMEY, F. DEL MONTE, R. KAPRIELIAN AND R. J. HAJJAR

## Introduction

In the myopathic heart, several abnormalities have been characterized at the cellular level [1–15]. These include changes at the level of the sarcolemma, sarcoplasmic reticulum, myofilaments, and mitochondria, all of which contribute to depressed contractile function and reserve [1–25] (Fig. 8.1). Identifying the mechanisms by which these changes contribute to the observed pathology is frequently confounded by simultaneous alterations in multiple signalling pathways in the complex milieu of the failing or myopathic heart. In this chapter the abnormalities that lead to the abnormal regulation of intracellular calcium and myofilament function are considered.

## Excitation–contraction coupling

In the mammalian heart the intracellular calcium ($Ca^{2+}$) movements are tightly regulated at various levels within the cell. Release of calcium is at a rate that allows binding to the contractile apparatus, as well as the removal of calcium at a rate that allows dissociation of calcium from the

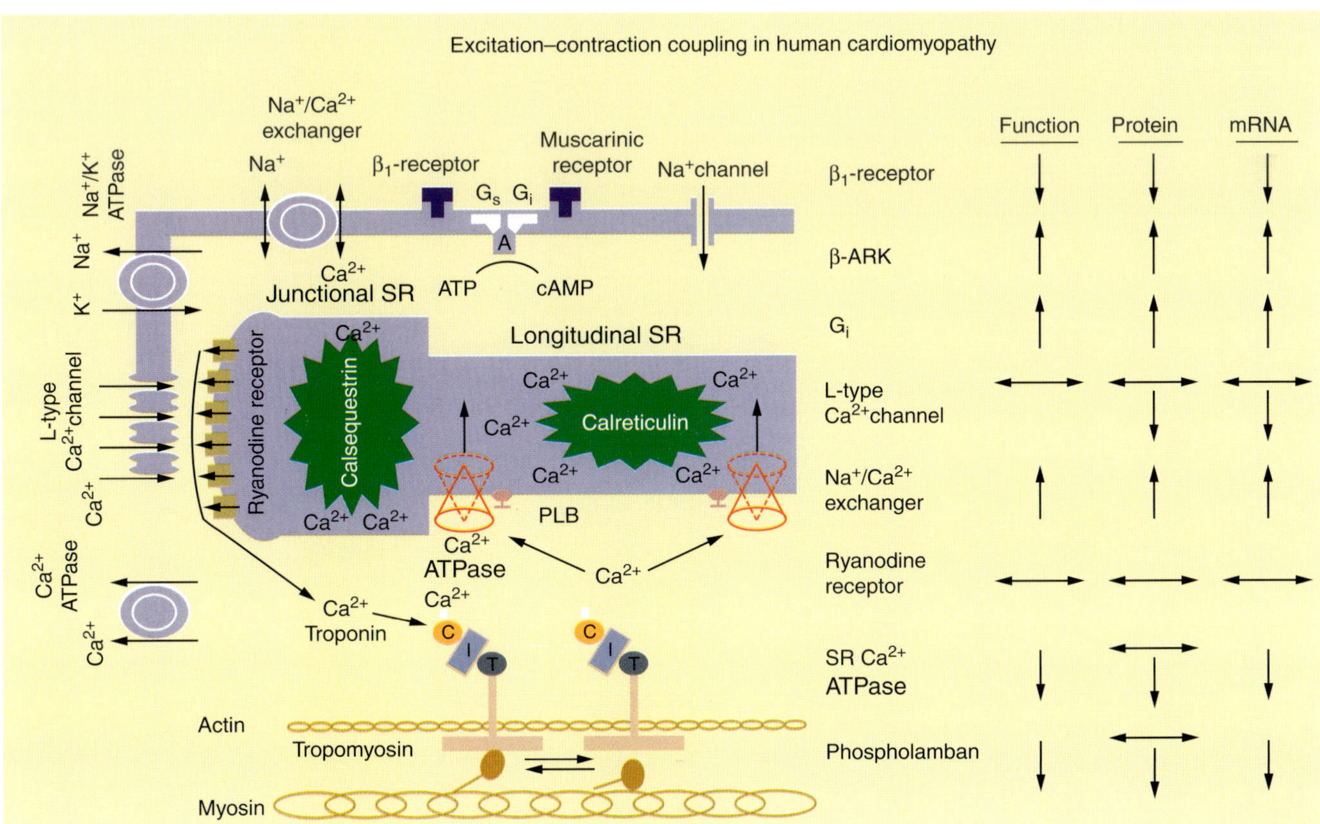


**Figure 8.1** *Excitation–contraction coupling abnormalities in human cardiomyopathy.*

myofilaments and muscle relaxation [26–28]. This concordant regulation must be intimately associated with the rate of electrical–mechanical coupling, i.e. heart rate, and change in a dynamic manner in response to changes in the frequency and/or intensity of muscle contraction (inotropy). Excitation leading to contraction and relaxation occurs through a series of co-ordinated steps whereby electrical excitation across the sarcolemma results in the opening of voltage-gated calcium channels, allowing the entry of a small amount of calcium into the cell (Fig. 8.2). This triggers the release of a larger amount of calcium (approx. 1–10 μM) from the sarcoplasmic reticulum (SR) stores through the calcium-release channels or ryanodine receptors. This increase in intracellular calcium concentration activates the myofilaments, leading to contraction. Myocardial relaxation occurs when the cytosolic calcium concentration is lowered to diastolic or resting concentrations (approx. 100–300 nM). The calcium-removal activity of the SR is via SERCA2a with maximal activity ($V_{max}$) regulated by phospholamban [26]. In the unphosphorylated state, phospholamban inhibits the SR $Ca^{2+}$-adenosine triphosphatase (ATPase) (SERCA2a), whereas phosphorylation of phospholamban by cyclic adenosine monophosphate (cAMP)-dependent protein kinase or by $Ca^{2+}$-calmodulin-dependent protein kinase reverses this inhibition [26–31] and increases $V_{max}$ without a change in calcium affinity ($K_a$).

## Calcium-induced calcium release

Calcium-induced calcium release has been refined to the level of understanding of microdomains by recent data using confocal microscopy. The presence of intracellular calcium sparks arises from a cluster of ryanodine receptors in close proximity to voltage-dependent calcium channels [26]. In local control, the coupling of a calcium channel with a cluster of ryanodine receptors allows calcium influx through a single calcium channel to increase the local concentration of calcium in the vicinity of a ryanodine receptor, producing a $Ca^{2+}$ spark. When a large number of calcium channels is activated, multiple $Ca^{2+}$ sparks or calcium releases from the SR combine to increase cytosolic calcium, which then leads to myofilament activation [26]. The local control phenomenon in cardiac muscles is based on the observation made in the early 1980s by Alexandre Fabiato [27, 28] that SR calcium release is controlled by

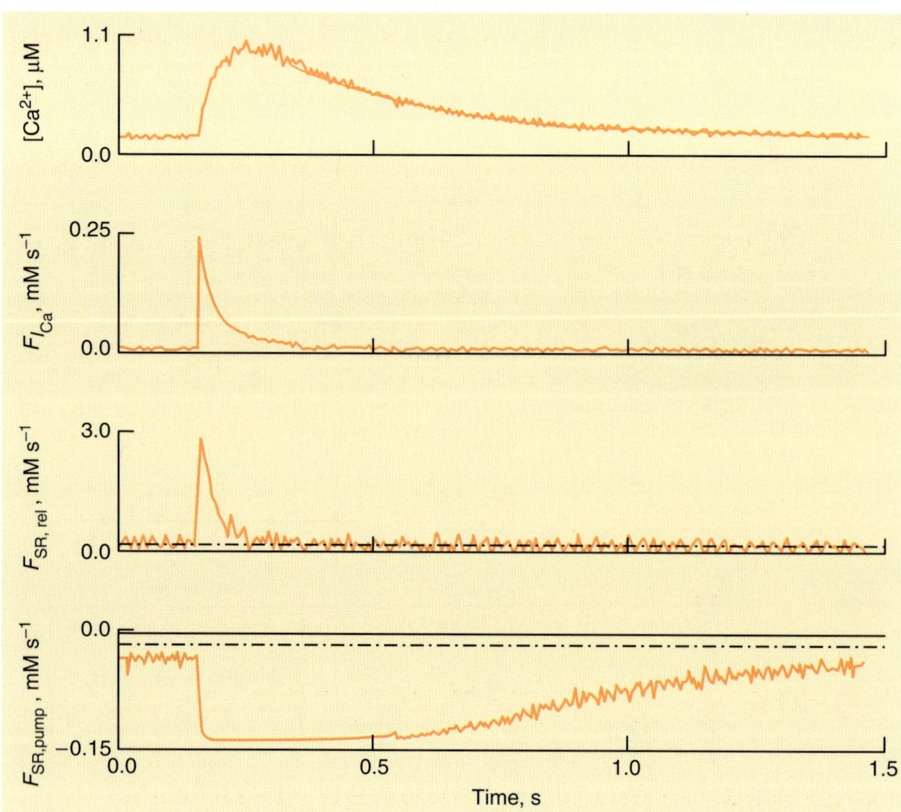


**Figure 8.2** *Recordings from a cardiomyocyte of $[Ca^{2+}]_i$, flux through L-type $Ca^{2+}$ channels, sarcoplasmic reticulum (SR) $Ca^{2+}$ release and uptake [16].*

calcium entry through L-type voltage-dependent calcium channels, which has been reconfirmed using confocal microscopy. Spontaneous SR calcium release is thought to be independent events that can be recruited by the calcium entering through single L-type calcium channels.

The structural basis for the local control theory is that the ryanodine receptors are juxtaposed to the L-type calcium channels in transverse tubules. These ryanodine receptors can therefore be activated by the calcium within the microdomain, thereby triggering release of calcium through the ryanodine channels, and are viewed as calcium sparks. Intracellular calcium transients as detected with intracellular calcium indicators may therefore be thought of as the spatial and temporal summation of calcium sparks when a large number of L-type calcium channels is activated, inducing calcium release from the SR.

## Calcium-handling myopathic hearts

The myopathic heart exhibits abnormalities in both the systolic and diastolic phase. Changes in diastolic function often appear earlier than systolic dysfunction. In fact, compensated hypertrophy phenotypically demonstrates impaired relaxation parameters in the presence of normal or increased systolic function [32–36]. The same feature can be recognized both *in vitro* at the tissue level [34, 36] and at the isolated myocyte level.

Muscle strips and single cardiomyocytes from myopathic hearts show a reduced systolic force when stimulated at higher frequencies, an elevated diastolic force, and a slowed relaxation [5, 7, 37–39]. The first report of abnormalities in calcium handling was made in 1987, when calcium transients recorded with the calcium indicator aequorin from trabeculae from myopathic human hearts removed at the time of cardiac transplantation revealed a significantly prolonged calcium transient with an elevated end-diastolic intracellular calcium [38] (Fig. 8.3). This report was followed in 1992 by recordings in single isolated cardiomyocytes loaded with the fluorescent indicator Fura-2 from myopathic hearts [39]. The calcium transients were characterized as having elevated diastolic calcium levels, a decreased systolic calcium, and prolonged relaxation phase (Fig. 8.4). Studies using the bioluminescent protein aequorin on isolated myocardium from patients with cardiomyopathy [7, 38, 41] found that systolic calcium concentration was unaltered at lower stimulation rates when forces were similar between non-failing and myopathic human myocardium, while the diastolic calcium concentration was either unchanged or elevated [24, 37, 41]; however, at higher stimulation rates there was a decrease in the peak of the calcium transient [40]. The uncertainties regarding the details of alterations in calcium in isolated muscle or myocytes from myopathic myocardium may be due to the fact that investigators are not studying

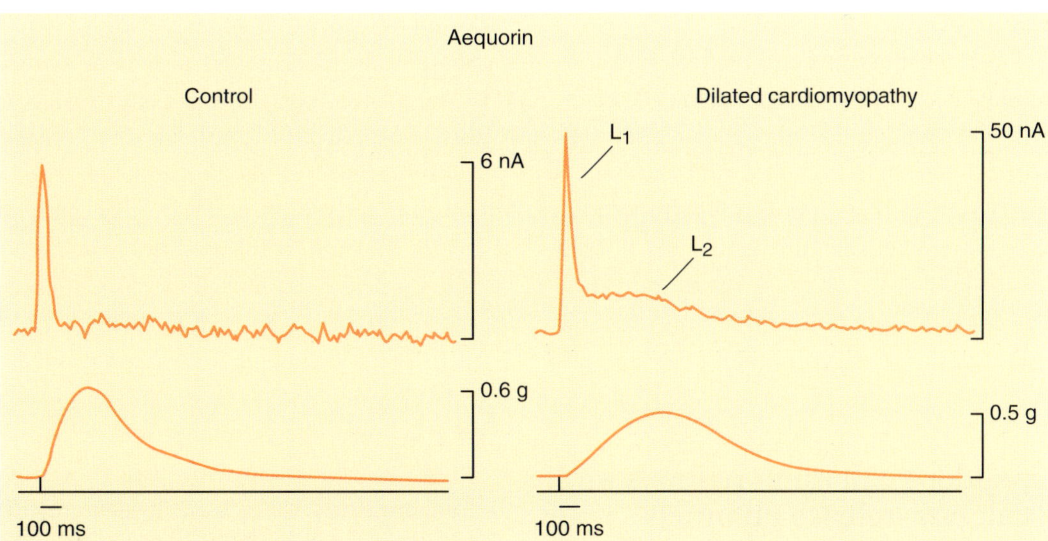


**Figure 8.3** *Abnormal calcium handling in trabeculae from the left ventricles of patients with end-stage heart failure compared with control patients. (From ref. 38 with permission.)*

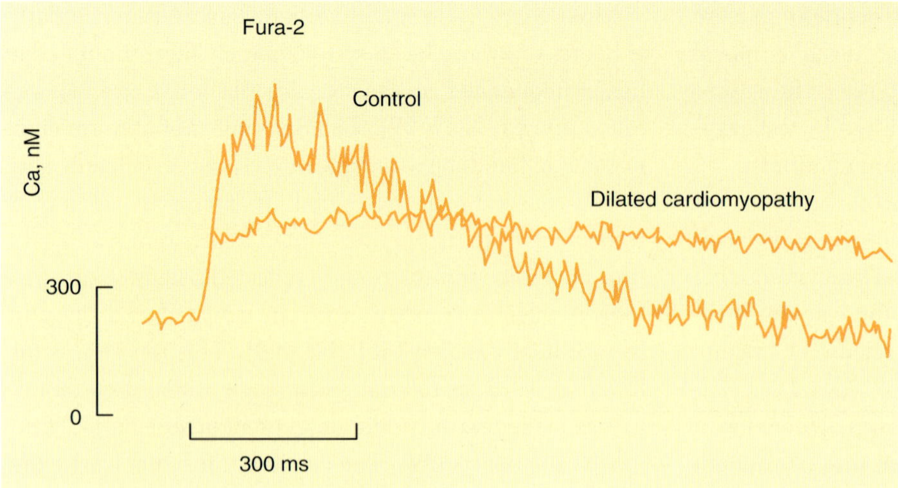


**Figure 8.4** *Fura-2 calcium signal from isolated myocytes from myopathic and non-failing human hearts. (From ref. 39 with permission.)*

identical patients or sharing human tissue resources. Sarcomere shortening can significantly alter the intracellular calcium transient [41]. Measurement of tension from intact single isolated myocytes is now possible. Furthermore, calibration of a fluorescent calcium indicator is only possible when the indicator is present exclusively in the cytosol and the *in situ* dissociation constant is accurately known. None of the studies regarding calcium reported to date that used fluorescent indicators has fulfilled these conditions when studying human myocardium. Hence, whether the peak amplitude of the calcium transient is altered remains a controversial issue. However, it is interesting that at higher levels of stimulation, the amount of calcium released from the SR as detected with aequorin has also been found to be decreased in myopathic human hearts [40] and is associated with a decrease in peak twitch force.

Since intracellular calcium transients and calcium concentrations are regulated by the voltage-dependent calcium channel, the SR ryanodine calcium-release channels, the SERCA2a/phospholamban complex, and the Na/Ca exchanger, several studies have focused on the relative changes in these proteins between myopathic and normal hearts. The present knowledge on these key steps in excitation–contraction coupling in the myopathic heart is reported here, as well as speculation on functional implications.

## Voltage-dependent calcium channels and ryanodine calcium-release channels

Calcium channels measured with radioligand-binding assays have reported conflicting findings. One group has reported a 20–30% reduction in mRNA and $B_{max}$ for dihydropyridine binding [42, 43]. However, two other groups found no difference in the number of calcium channels as measured with radioligand binding [44, 45, 47, 48]. Despite these conflicting reports it is appreciated that radioligand-binding can detect nascent channels and is only a surrogate marker of the number of active calcium channels [43].

Interestingly, calcium current density measured using electrophysiological techniques and the whole-cell patch-clamp technique supported the conclusions that calcium channel number is not changed as no difference was noted in current–voltage relationship or peak calcium current in non-failing and myopathic hearts ($-3.8 \pm 1.2$ pA/pF vs $-4.7 \pm 2.4$ pA/pF) (Fig. 8.5). The use of confocal microscopy and the measurement of sparks has not yet been reported in myopathic and non-failing human hearts.

Some studies suggest that altered myocyte calcium handling plays an important role in the development of heart failure in humans [5, 7, 46]. This hypothesis is consistent with alterations found in some of the key proteins involved in the uptake and release of calcium in myopathic hearts. Calcium is released from the SR via a calcium-sensitive release channel, the ryanodine receptor (RYR). Investigators have shown RYR mRNA to be reduced in both myopathic human hearts and animal models [47]. Inconsistent reports on RYR protein levels in myopathic human myocardium have appeared in the literature [48]. Research has shown altered gating mechanisms [49] and altered responses to caffeine [50] in myopathic human myocardium, while others [51] have found normal basic properties. Thus, although gene expression of the RYR may be unchanged, its gating behaviour, i.e. activity, might be

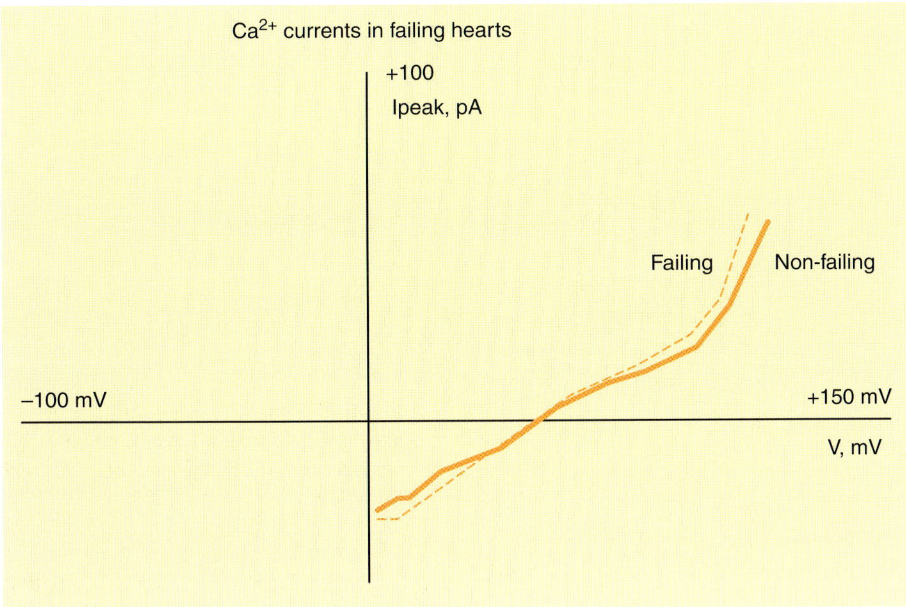


**Figure 8.5** *Calcium current–voltage relationship from patch-clamped isolated myocytes from non-failing and myopathic human hearts. (From ref. 39 with permission.)*

impaired in failing myocardium. This concept was first reported by O'Brien and Gwathmey, who found that the release of calcium through the ryanodine receptor was changed in myopathic human myocardium [3]. The rate constants for SR calcium pumping and calcium release channel activity have been reported to be decreased by 64% and 75%, respectively. The calcium-release channel was found to be in the more open state for myopathic hearts than for non-failing hearts. Longer opening times of the calcium-release channel occur with oxidative injury, partial proteolysis, or increases in adrenergic-mediated phosphorylation. The idea of abnormal channel function in myopathic human myocardium was also supported by the finding that diseased myocardium had a seven-fold increase in resistance to caffeine effects (agonist) [50]. Surprisingly, however, studies of single calcium-release channels isolated from myopathic human myocardium and embedded in artificial lipid bilayers revealed no abnormalities [51].

The activities of both the L-type calcium channels and the ryanodine-release channels from patients with cardiomyopathy, recorded under voltage-clamp conditions, are essentially the same as in normal hearts. However, even though the L-type calcium channels and the ryanodine-release channels may be expressed in normal amounts, their function may be abnormal in failing hearts. It has been shown recently that in failing myocardial cells, L-type calcium channels have a reduced ability to activate adjacent ryanodine receptors [52]. These results would point towards impaired coupling between L-type calcium channels and adjacent ryanodine receptors. It is still unclear whether all forms of heart failure have this type of coupling abnormality, but it would seem that this type of defect in the microenvironment of adjacent channels might be the basis for dysfunction at the level of excitation–contraction coupling, especially at high frequencies of contraction.

## Sarcoplasmic reticulum $Ca^{2+}$ ATPase activity and the $Na^+/Ca^{2+}$ exchanger

Calcium transport into the SR occurs via the SR ATPase calcium pump (SERCA). Although reports consistently find decreased SERCA mRNA levels in myopathic human hearts, several reports found no change in SERCA protein levels [53]. The reduction in β-adrenergic responsiveness seen in myopathic human hearts could result in a decreased level of phospholamban phosphorylation *in vivo*, thus resulting in depressed SERCA activity, even in the presence of normal levels of the protein in the failing heart [2, 31, 54–56, 53]. Nevertheless, myopathic human myocardium has demonstrated some defect in SR function [2, 7, 55–57]. Specifically, 'relaxation abnormalities' correlated with deficient SR calcium uptake have been associated with a decreased expression level of SR $Ca^{2+}$-ATPase and reduction in SR $Ca^{2+}$-ATPase activity [56] (Fig. 8.6).

Calcium is removed from the cytosol by the sarcolemmal $Na^+/Ca^{2+}$ exchanger, which has high capacity but low affinity and is the major calcium extrusion mechanism of the

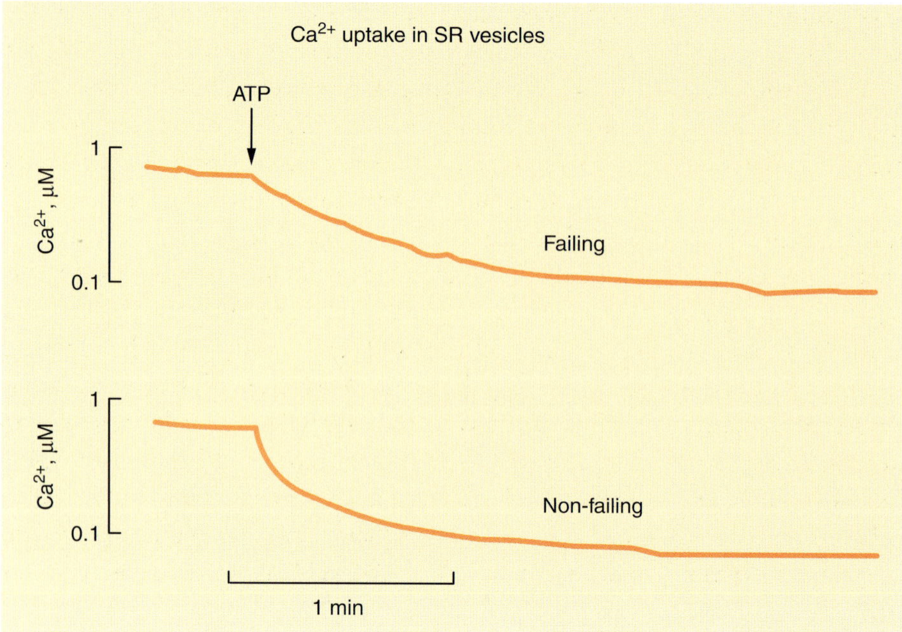


**Figure 8.6** *Sarcoplasmic reticulum (SR) vesicles isolated from a failing and non-failing heart were activated with ATP. $Ca^{2+}$ was monitored by Fura-2 and once the reaction had started by the addition of ATP, $Ca^{2+}$ levels decreased more rapidly in the non-failing versus failing tissues [3].*

cardiac myocyte. This system returns calcium concentrations to diastolic levels (100–300 nM) and may, therefore, contribute significantly to myocardial relaxation. Most studies indicate that mRNA and protein levels of the $Na^+/Ca^{2+}$ exchanger are increased in human myopathic hearts, but not in all preparations [6]. Likewise, the functional capacity of the $Na^+/Ca^{2+}$ exchanger to transport calcium is increased [6, 58]. The consequence of an increased activity of the $Na^+/Ca^{2+}$ exchanger in failing hearts may be to compensate for the reduction in SR $Ca^{2+}$-ATPase activity. Increased activity of the $Na^+/Ca^{2+}$ exchanger should aid in myocardial relaxation, albeit at the cost of reduced calcium release from the SR during systole. This would be particularly evident at higher rates of stimulation, and thus lead to a blunted frequency response as is commonly seen in myopathic human myocardium [55, 57].

The $Na^+/Ca^{2+}$ exchanger can operate to bring calcium into the cell or extrude calcium out from the cell. It would be predicted that a transfer of calcium removal from the SR to sodium-mediated calcium extrusion should impact sodium homoeostasis within the cell. Several observations are consistent with a change in sodium control in failing human myocardium. There is an increase in sensitivity to compounds which produce positive inotropic effects through raised intracellular sodium, either by inhibiting the $Na^+/K^+$-ATPase or by opening $Na^+$ channels, in muscle strips from failing human hearts [46, 47]. It has been suggested that the relaxation abnormalities produced by the loss of SERCA2a activity could be, at least partially, compensated for by an increase in the activity of the $Na^+/Ca^{2+}$ exchanger [55, 57].

Studies have found two groups of patients with heart failure with distinct changes in myocardial calcium handling [7]. Whereas SERCA2a activity is decreased in many patients, the $Na^+/Ca^{2+}$ exchanger is upregulated in only one subset. Ventricular muscle strips from the group without an increase in the $Na^+/Ca^{2+}$ exchanger revealed far poorer function, particularly with respect to diastolic parameters. Moreover, the increase in the $Na^+/Ca^{2+}$ exchanger corresponded to a flat or positive frequency response, whereas the observed picture of a negative frequency response was not accompanied by an increase in expression of the $Na^+/Ca^{2+}$ exchanger. This provides a basis for the hypothesis that the relaxation dysfunction produced by the loss of SERCA2a might, at least partially, be compensated for by an increase in the $Na^+/Ca^{2+}$ exchanger activity.

Recently, in a very elegant study in failing human myocytes, $Ca^{2+}$ transients and contractions exhibit an SR-related, phasic component and a slow, reverse-mode $Na^+/Ca^{2+}$ exchange–related tonic component. These findings showed that calcium influx via reverse-mode $Na^+/Ca^{2+}$ exchange during the action potential may contribute to the slow decay of the calcium transient in failing human myocytes [58].

The slow relaxation and abnormal force–frequency relationship observed in isolated muscles, as well as in isolated myocytes from failing hearts, indicate a deficiency in calcium reuptake by the SR. With a pharmacological approach, the failing phenotype can be potentially reproduced in normal cardiomyocytes from both human and animal models of heart failure by exposing contracting cardiac muscle cells to the SERCA inhibitor thapsigargin for a period sufficient to block calcium uptake and allow emptying of SR stores [55]. Biochemical measurements also support the idea that calcium cycling abnormalities contribute at least in part to the functional observations [2, 38, 56, 59]. As described by several investigators, quantification of the steady-state levels of SERCA2a mRNA levels has revealed that they are markedly reduced in both failing human hearts and experimental models of heart failure [7, 47]. Associated with a decrease in mRNA, there is a decrease in SR $Ca^{2+}$-ATPase activity and SR calcium uptake from SR vesicles and membranes isolated from failing human heart [2, 7, 56]. Indeed, in experiments where the SR vesicles were isolated from human hearts, vesicles from failing human hearts had decreased rates of calcium uptake compared with normal hearts (Fig. 8.6). The protein levels of SR $Ca^{2+}$-ATPase of failing human hearts have been shown to be significantly reduced by certain investigators, while other studies have failed to show significant changes between protein levels of SR $Ca^{2+}$-ATPase in non-failing and failing human myocardium [7, 53, 56]. The reason for this discrepancy is not clear; however, human heart tissue is very heterogeneous among different cardiac transplantation centres and donor hearts have also a number of abnormalities. In addition, the changes that have been observed in the more homogeneous models of heart failure have been small (30–40%), therefore the inhomogeneities that are present in human hearts may mask these small differences.

## Phospholamban

As detailed earlier, phospholamban is an integral protein of the sarcoplasmic reticulum of mammalian myocardium and it regulates SR $Ca^{2+}$-ATPase activity. Oligomeric phospholamban is a pentamer of five identical subunits, each containing 42 amino acids. Phospholamban is highly conserved and present in a single copy in the genome of mammalian and avian species. Phospholamban in its unphosphorylated state inhibits SR $Ca^{2+}$-ATPase activity. Protein phosphatases reverse this process and dephosphorylate phospholamban. The myocardium contains type 1 and type 2 phosphatases. The type 1 enzyme is mainly responsible for the dephosphorylation of phospholamban. Protein phosphatase inhibitor 1 has been shown to be present in cardiac tissue. Phosphorylation of protein phosphatase inhibitor 1 causes a decrease in phosphatase activity.

A decrease in SR $Ca^{2+}$-ATPase activity is one of the hallmarks of human heart failure. It is associated with impaired relaxation and prolonged calcium transients. The decrease in SR $Ca^{2+}$-ATPase activity has been attributed to a change in the relative expression of phospholamban to SERCA2a. This ratio is changed in failing human myocardium as well as in animal models of heart failure [47]. Recent studies using adenoviral gene transfer of phospholamban demonstrated that an increase in the ratio of phospholamban to SERCA2a could mimic heart failure *in vitro* and *in vivo*.

More recently, investigators have concentrated on the regulation of phospholamban in heart failure. Studies have demonstrated a decreased phosphorylation state of phospholamban in heart failure [2] which may contribute to the decrease in SR $Ca^{2+}$-ATPase activity. It is possible that the decreased phosphorylation of phospholamban is caused by an increase in phosphatase activity in heart failure. An increase in cardiac phosphatase activity has been reported in myopathic human myocardium as well as in animal models of heart failure [60].

## Targeting genes to the heart

As discussed elsewhere in this book, various viral vectors have been used for research purposes [61, 62]. Among them, retroviruses have been the most extensively studied and used clinically [62]. Recombinant adenoviral vectors, in contrast, offer several significant advantages [61]. The viruses can be prepared at extremely high titre, infect non-replicating cells, and allow incorporation of relatively large or even multiple cDNAs. They offer the opportunity to investigate the role of local signal transduction pathways in both *in vitro* and *in vivo* model systems. Adenoviral vectors confer high-efficiency and high-level transduction of cardiomyocytes *in vitro* [61] (Fig. 8.7). *In vivo* cardiac gene transfer has also been achieved using recombinant adenoviral vectors [63]. Using an *in vivo* perfusion approach, the feasibility of modulating ventricular function has been demonstrated recently [63]. In this approach, the viral solution is injected above the aortic valve while the aorta and

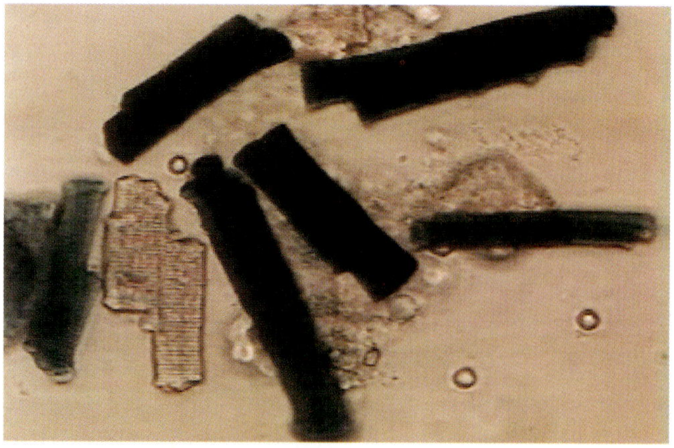

**Figure 8.7** *Isolated human cardiomyocytes infected with adenovirus carrying β-galactosidase [64].*

pulmonary artery are transiently cross-clamped. The virus is then forced down the coronaries, resulting in relatively diffuse transduction of the myocardium. Alternative approaches, such as direct myocardial injection and selective coronary cannulation, are also actively being pursued, but result in focal transgene expression and may be more applicable to focal diseases such as ischaemic heart disease rather than cardiomyopathies which often affect the heart more globally. Nevertheless, these early animal studies establish that *in vivo* adenoviral gene transfer can not only achieve transgene expression in the myocardium, but also modulate intrinsic functional properties of the intact heart. While expression and functional effects will need to be assessed for each application individually, these data encouragingly suggest that recombinant adenoviral vectors with this transduction technique produce important expression in a substantial proportion of the myocardium [64].

## Altering the sarcoplasmic reticulum $Ca^{2+}$-ATPase pump/phospholamban ratio by gene transfer

Three different genes (*SERCA1*, *2*, and *3*) encode for five distinct SERCA isoforms in the mammalian skeletal, smooth and cardiac muscle. The *SERCA2* gene encodes for two distinct isoforms for the cardiac (*SERCA2a*) or the smooth muscle (*SERCA2b*), both being modulated by the phosphoprotein phospholamban. The relative ratio of phospholamban/SERCA2a is an important determinant of SR function in cardiac myocytes and an increased ratio of phospholamban/SERCA2a is characteristic of heart failure in animal models and particularly in human myocytes, which mainly rely on the SERCA2a calcium pump for the removal of calcium from the cytoplasm [64, 65].

Increasing levels of phospholamban relative to SERCA2a in isolated cardiac myocytes significantly altered intracellular calcium handling by prolonging the relaxation phase of the calcium transient, decreasing calcium release, and increasing resting calcium [66]. These results support the hypothesis that altering the relative ratio of phospholamban to SERCA2a can account for the abnormalities in calcium handling observed in failing ventricular myocardium. Overexpressing SERCA2a can largely 'rescue' the phenotype created by higher phospholamban to SERCA2a ratios. These results can be reproduced *in vitro* and *in vivo* in animal models of heart failure as well as in myocytes from failing human hearts, where cells overexpressing SERCA2a recover the functional characteristics of normal cardiac myocytes (Fig. 8.8). Dilmann *et al.* have shown that adenovirus-mediated expression of SERCA2 transgene cultured neonatal myocytes treated with phorbol-12-myristate-13-acetate (PMA), a compound that decreases endogenous SERCA2 expression and results in prolongation of calcium transients, can reconstitute depressed endogenous SERCA2 levels, shorten prolonged calcium transients, and augment SR calcium uptake [67]. In animal models of pressure overload hypertrophy and heart failure *in vivo* overexpression of SERCA2a improves LV systolic and diastolic function, indicating that enhancing contractility at the cellular level can be translated into improved ventricular function [65]. It is conceivable that such an approach might be used *in vivo* to normalize altered calcium regulation in human heart failure. It is also conceivable that by decreasing the levels of phospholamban using antisense strategies, the SERCA2a/phospholamban ratio can be reconstituted towards normal.

The rescue effect by SERCA2a is especially encouraging since it suggests that restoring the normal phospholamban/SERCA2a ratio through somatic gene transfer might correct the abnormalities of calcium handling and contraction seen in failing hearts.

## Contractile proteins in myopathic myocardium

Impairment of myocardial contractility at the level of the myocyte in the failed human heart remains controversial.

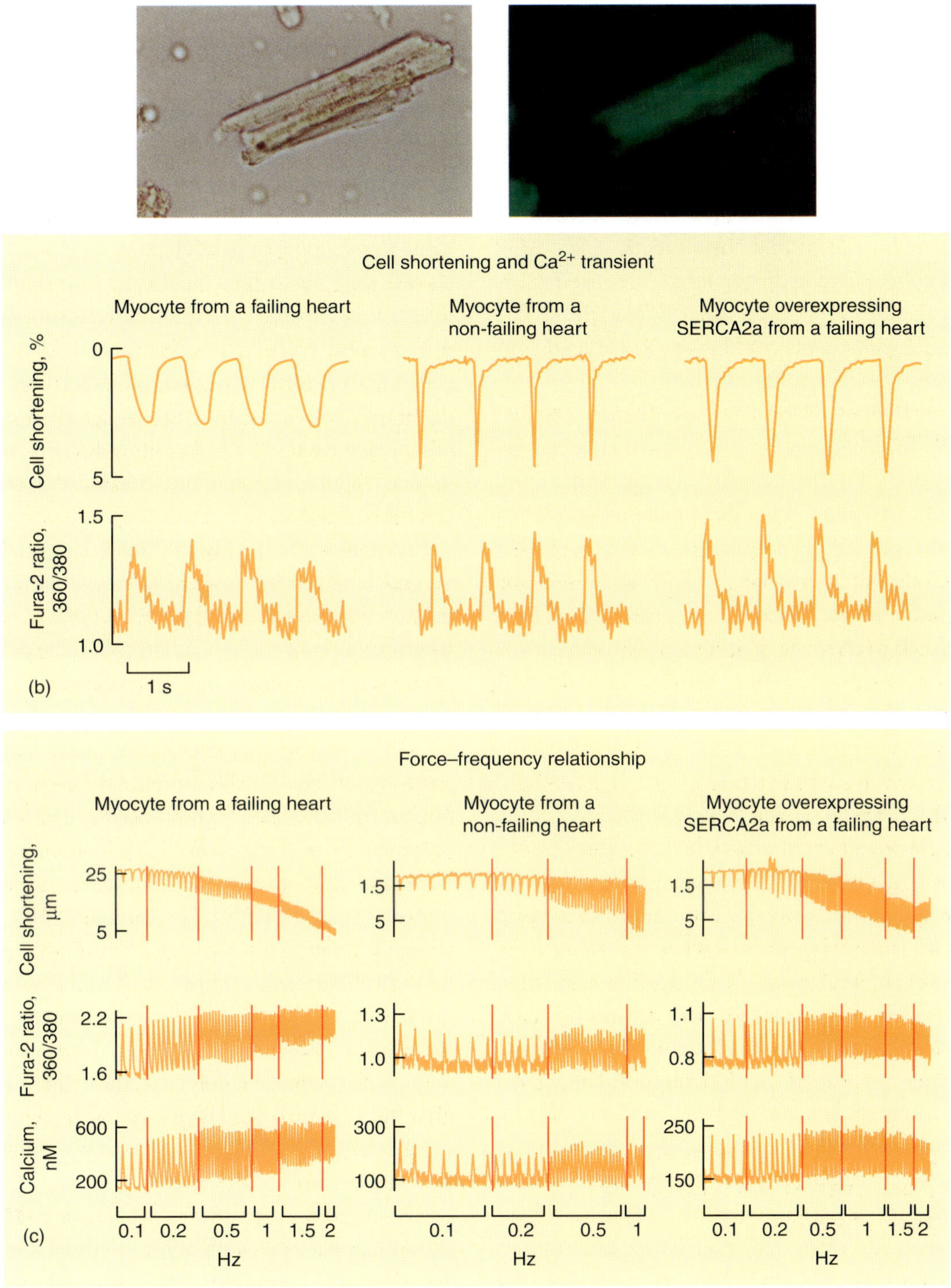


**Figure 8.8** *(a) Following isolation, failing human cardiomyocytes were infected with Ad.SERCA2a. Twenty-four hours after infection a cardiomyocyte is visualized with white light (a) and at 510 nm with a single excitation peak at 490 nm of blue light. Coexpression of GFP demonstrates visually that SERCA2a is being expressed in the cell. (b) Recordings from cardiomyocytes isolated from a donor non-failing heart and from a failing heart infected with either Ad.GFP or Ad.SERCA2a, stimulated at 1 Hz at 37°C. The failing cell had a characteristic decrease in contraction and prolonged relaxation along with a prolonged $Ca^{2+}$ transient. Overexpression of SERCA2a in the failing cardiomyocyte normalized these parameters. (c) Recordings from the same cardiomyocytes as in (b) stimulated at increasing frequencies. The failing cardiomyocyte demonstrated a decrease in contraction amplitude and an increase in diastolic tone and $Ca^{2+}$. Overexpression of SERCA2a restored the frequency-dependent increase in contraction amplitude and mitigated the increase in diastolic $Ca^{2+}$ and length [64]; (GFP = green fluorescent protein).*

A hypothesis with regard to the negative force–interval relationship seen at higher frequencies of contraction is a change in the coupling between transsarcolemmal calcium influx and ryanodine release channels [37, 40, 55]. Another hypothesis to explain the depressed contractility seen in heart failure is a change in the myofilament calcium responsiveness [1, 11–13, 48–77] as a result of the accumulation of metabolites and byproducts, e.g. ADP, inorganic phosphate, and hydrogen ions. A reduced calcium sensitivity and/or a decrease in co-operativity of the thick and thin myofilaments could result in reduced contractile activation and force development.

In myopathic human myocardium, myofilament calcium responsiveness has been reported to be both changed [1] and unchanged [9, 11, 78]. Nevertheless, in human and experimental heart failure, a number of changes has been reported to occur at the contractile elements. These include an isoform shift in troponin T (TnT) and a decrease in myosin light chain kinase-2 [79, 80–82]. These changes are believed to be partially responsible for a decrease in myofibrillar ATPase activity [13, 83–85], a decreased cross-bridge cycling rate [86], and an altered responsiveness to agents acting on the myofilaments [11, 87].

Questions on the remodelling process at the level of the contractile elements are centred on the functional significance of a particular isoform population and altered distribution. Although changes in the distribution of myosin isoforms occur with changes in cardiac workload (e.g. increased α-myosin heavy chain), the myosin isoenzyme population does not always correlate with function [12, 13, 81]. The question arises as to whether thin filament functional properties are altered during long-term changes in myocardial activity and haemodynamic load.

Heart failure is associated with changes in the distribution and content of contractile proteins. Investigators have found decreased myocardial myofibrillar ATPase activity in the failing human heart [84]. However, a large isoform shift of V1 myosin to V3 myosin is not seen in diseased myocardium of humans with cardiomyopathy, since cardiac myosin is mostly (>70%) in the V3 form. However, there is a significant increase in α-heavy myosin heavy chain in myopathic human hearts. Hence, alterations in other contractile proteins play a role in determining the contractile properties of failing myocardium. Several observations support this hypothesis. Research shows increased expression of a foetal cardiac isoform of TnT in myopathic human myocardium [80] and shifts in TnT isoform expression correlate with changes in the calcium responsiveness of the myofilaments.

Margossian *et al.* [82] reported a marked decrease in the myosin light chain content in myopathic human hearts, apparently due to increased levels of protease in these hearts, while others have demonstrated an increase in the atrial form of myosin light chain-1. Morano *et al.* [72] have shown that alterations in the myosin light chain–actin interaction can have a profound effect on tension development and calcium responsiveness. Likewise, research shows that myosin light chain-2 extraction can result in decreased velocity of shortening as well as decreased calcium responsiveness. Thus, changes in myosin light chain in heart failure may be of functional consequence for contractile activation.

Previous studies using multicellular preparations from several laboratories have indicated unaltered maximum tension development in human myopathic hearts [9, 88]. Interpretation of these mechanical studies is questionable since sarcomere length was not measured during contractile activation. Kentish *et al.* [41] showed that control of sarcomere length is essential in the study of myofibrillar calcium responsiveness. However, when sarcomere length is not controlled during activation, ambiguous data are often obtained.

Studies employing multicellular preparations are further limited by the difficulty in excluding the influence of changes in the extracellular matrix. Therefore, single isolated myocytes are starting to be used for the study of myofilament function in myopathic human myocardium. Myocardium from failing human hearts may also have depressed contractile force at the level of the isolated myocyte that may or may not be solely due to availability of intracellular calcium and/or intrinsic changes in the regulatory contractile elements.

The failure to demonstrate differences in contractile activation in myopathic human myocardium might reflect the experimental conditions and substrate concentrations under which the experiments were performed. A recent study compared and examined the effects of cAMP and protein kinase A, cGMP, acidosis, and inorganic phosphate in both non-failing and myopathic human myocardial fibres.

In myopathic human hearts, β-myosin heavy chain and the levels of β-myosin heavy chain mRNA are unchanged [81], a finding consistent with the results of

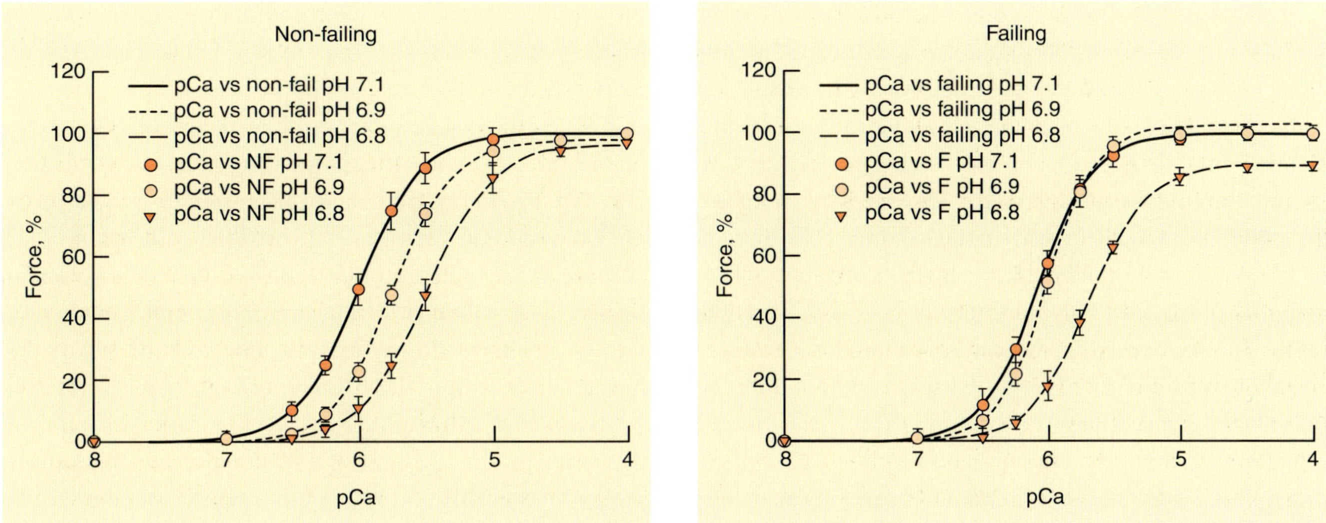


**Figure 8.9** *Calcium–force relationship in non-failing (A) and myopathic (B) human myocardium to changes in intracellular pH. All calcium–force relationships have been combined to varying intracellular pHs for ease of comparison. Notice that there is no difference in the calcium–force relationship at pH 7.1. There was a significant difference in myofilament calcium sensitivity seen at pH 6.9 and 6.8 between non-failing and myopathic human myocardium. For myopathic human myocardium, the calcium–force relationship was shifted to the left on the calcium axis, indicating an increase in myofilament calcium sensitivity compared with non-failing myocardium at the same intracellular pH.* —●— = *pH 7,1;* ···●··· = *pH 6.9;* —▲— = *pH 6.8 [1].*

similar maximum calcium-activated force (0.30 ± 0.09 vs 0.34 ± 0.08 g/mm$^2$ for non-failing and myopathic skinned fibres and 1.23 ± 0.49 vs 1.84 ± 0.74 g/mm$^2$ for intact muscle preparations) [9, 11]. Hence, alterations in other contractile proteins are likely to play a role in determining the contractile properties of myopathic human myocardium. Several observations support this hypothesis.

Changes in myofilament calcium sensitivity have been observed in response to pH, inorganic phosphate, cAMP, and cGMP, which are probably achieved through different mechanisms. Findings at pH 7.1 are also similar to most models of hypertrophy studied, which demonstrate similar calcium–force relationships [1, 35, 78] (Fig. 8.9). These experiments showed that reducing pH from 7.1 to 6.8 decreased sensitivity to $[Ca^{2+}]_i$ without effecting maximal calcium-activated force. However, at the lower pH of 6.8, fibres from failing hearts demonstrated a significant decrease. At more acidic pH, the calcium–force relationship for myopathic myocardium was shifted to the left on the calcium axis, indicating an increased sensitivity of the myofilaments to calcium [1].

Hydrogen ion concentration decreases the affinity of troponin C (TnC) for calcium. The decrease in maximal calcium-activated force seen in myopathic myocardium at pH 6.8 and the smaller shifts in myofilament calcium sensitivity may therefore suggest adaptive changes at the level of TnC. Two missense point mutations in TnC in failing myocardium have been shown to result in a decrease in myofilament calcium sensitivity [10]. This suggests that the differences in calcium activation may reside at the level of TnC.

Inorganic phosphate greatly inhibits the maximum calcium-regulated force in skinned fibres and directly inhibits myosin [1, 74–76]. Kentish [74] reported both depressant effects and desensitization of the myofilaments in the presence of inorganic phosphate (Fig. 8.10). In myopathic human myocardium a decrease in $F_{max}$ (maximal force at saturating calcium concentrations) and decreased sensitivity of the myofilaments to calcium were shown in response to 15 mM phosphate. A decrease in $F_{max}$ can be the result of uncoupling of cross-bridges [70].

Inorganic phosphate increases the population of weak cross-bridges and results in a decrease in maximal calcium-activated force and a rightward shift on the calcium axis. In myopathic hearts, it would be expected that a greater inhibition and reduction in force would be present. However, in myocardium from myopathic hearts with reduced myofibrillar ATPase activity, the inhibitory effects might be overridden under conditions of prolonged cross-bridge attachment. Therefore, under these conditions, the effect of inorganic phosphate should be reduced, which supports the experimental observations (Fig. 8.10).

Changes in cross-bridge cycling rate have been shown to shift the calcium–force relationship [75]. Myocardium from failing hearts has a slower cross-bridge cycling rate [86] (Fig. 8.11). Slowing of the cross-bridge cycling rate results in a leftward shift in the calcium-axis owing to longer TnC calcium interactions. This might explain why inorganic phosphate had a smaller effect on the maximal calcium-activated force and a smaller shift to higher calcium concentrations in myopathic myocardium. Longer TnC–calcium interactions in myopathic myocardium should also result in a smaller shift to higher $[Ca^{2+}]_i$ with lowering of intracellular pH, which supports the experimental observations.

It remains unknown whether contractile protein phosphorylation is altered *in vivo* in human heart failure, as suggested for other regulatory proteins, e.g. phospholamban [2, 89–91]. To account for varying levels of contractile protein phosphorylation, protein kinase was applied to phosphorylate maximally the contractile proteins. It is, however, possible that maximal phosphorylation masks (by saturation) potential intrinsic alterations in contractile function induced by heart failure. An attempt was made to resolve this issue by studying both the native state and saturated levels.

The presence of cAMP caused a decrease in the sensitivity of the myofilaments in both non-failing and myopathic fibres (Fig. 8.12). One explanation is that cAMP, in the presence of native protein kinase A (PKA), induced phosphorylation of troponin I (TnI). In the presence of cAMP, muscles from myopathic hearts exhibited a greater shift to higher $[Ca^{2+}]_i$ than that seen in non-failing myocardium. This indicates either changes in the composition/activation of TnI or differing amounts of PKA. However, no isoforms of TnI have been identified in failing human myocardium [89, 90]. PKA content has not been reported to be different between non-failing and myopathic myocardium [31]. A more likely explanation is that the level of phosphorylation in failing fibres is lower than in non-failing myocardium, as similarly shown for phospholamban. Myopathic human myocardium has been reported to have lower concentrations of intracellular cAMP [31, 54]. In support of this concept, the addition of cAMP-dependent PKA in the presence of cAMP did not cause a significant shift to the right on the calcium axis in myocardium from failing hearts. The shifts seen in non-failing myocardium in the presence of both cAMP and PKA were similar to the shift seen in myopathic fibres with cAMP alone.

Although the experimental conditions were the same between non-failing and myopathic tissues, differences in the activation of TnI remain a possible explanation. If there were different phosphorylation levels, the addition of cAMP-dependent PKA in the non-failing muscles should have shifted the calcium–force relationship to the right by as much as in the failing fibres, unless there were changes in the structure and/or function of TnI. This is concurrent with the experimental results.

TnT populations have been shown to affect myofilament

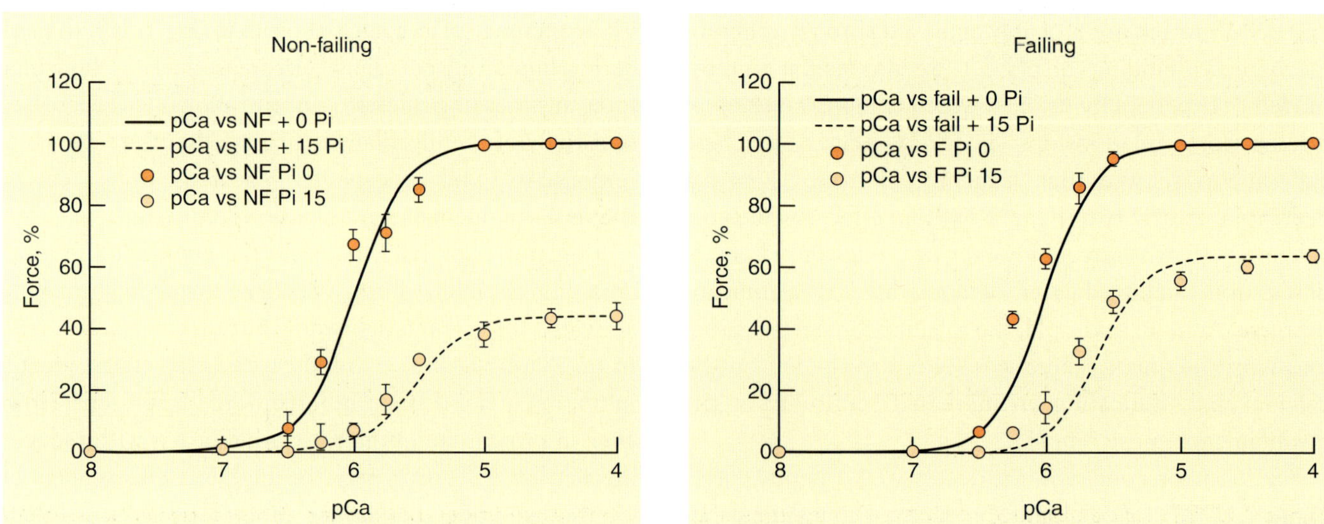


**Figure 8.10** *Effects of increasing inorganic phosphate on myofilament calcium activation in non-failing (A) and failing (B) human myocardium. Notice the greater depresent effects of inorganic phosphate on the maximum calcium-activated force in non-failing human myocardium. —●— = control; ···●··· = 15 mM inorganic phosphate.*

calcium responsiveness. However, PKA has a higher affinity to TnI than to TnT. Current concepts indicate that TnI promotes a closed state in which cross-bridges interact with the thin filament but in a weak non-force generating reaction. Phosphorylation at the PKA sites of TnI appears to reduce the affinity of cross-bridges for the thin filament. The reduced phosphorylation may reflect differences in the amount of light chain-2 that result in stiffer cross-bridges

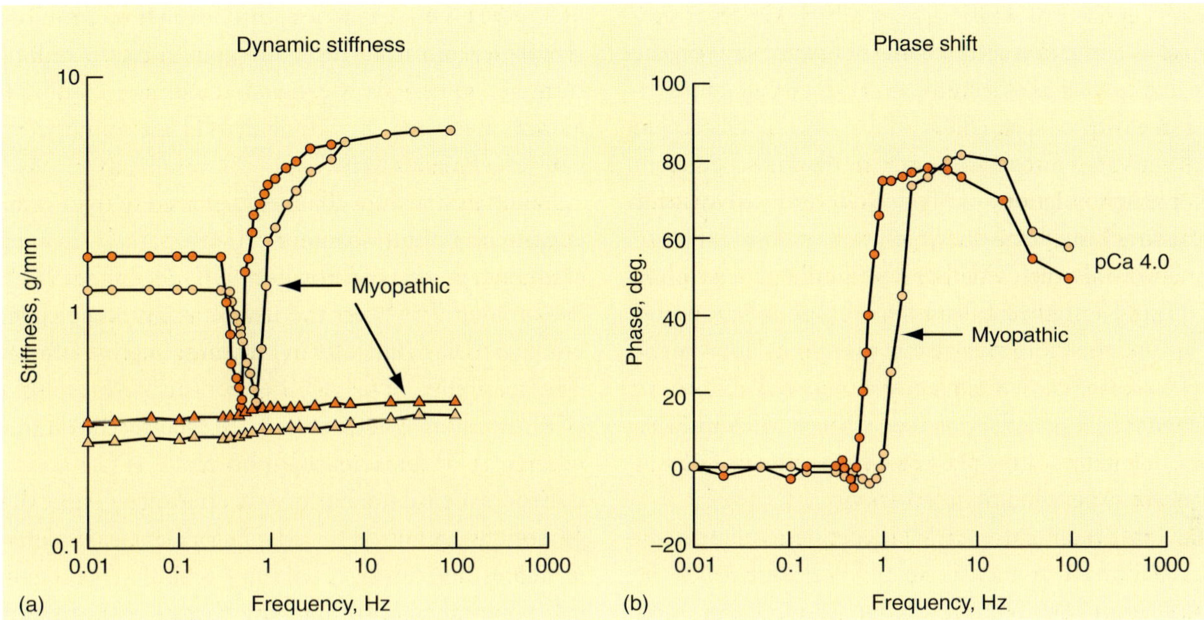


**Figure 8.11** *Dynamic stiffness curves and phase shift curves of skinned fibre preparations from normal (●) and myopathic muscles maximally activated at a pCa of 4.0 (●). Note in the myopathic hearts (▲) the frequency of minimal stiffness a reflection of cross-bridge cycling is lower than normal hearts (▲) [86].*

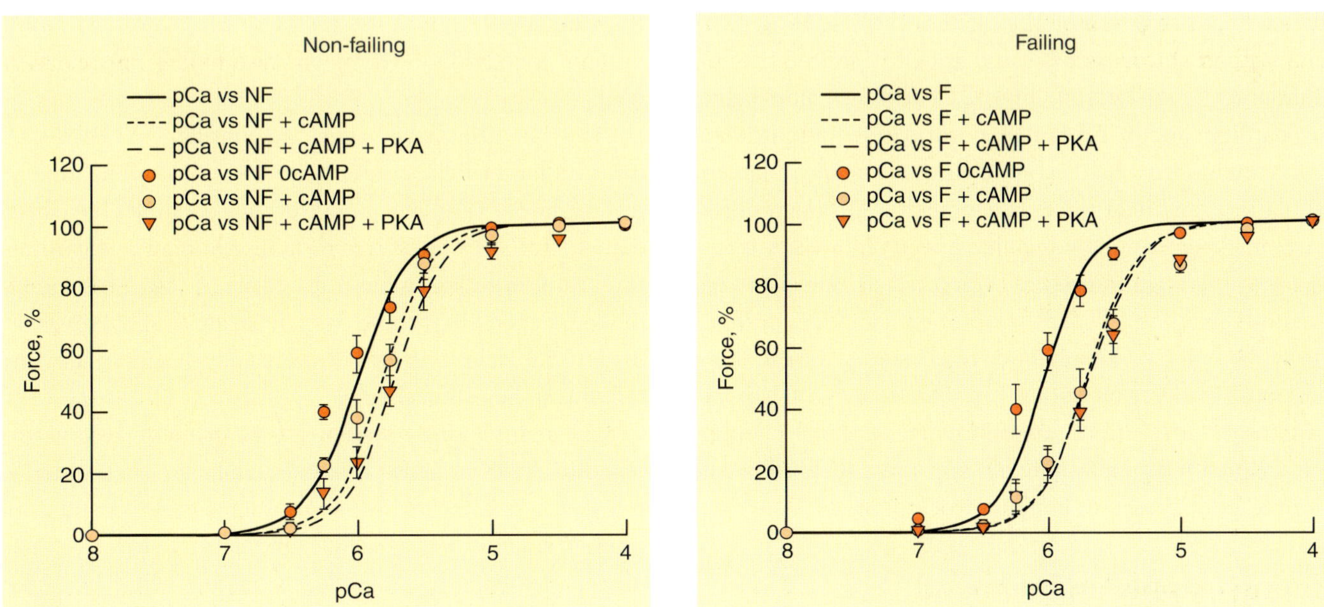


**Figure 8.12** *Effect of the addition of 10 μM D-cAMP and protein kinase A (PKA) to non-failing (A) and failing (B) human myocardium. D-cAMP caused a greater shift to higher intracellular calcium concentrations in failing compared with that seen in non-failing human myocardium. The addition of PKA in the presence of D-cAMP did not result in a further shift on the calcium axis in fibres from failing hearts. In non-failing human myocardium, D-cAMP caused a lesser shift to higher intracellular calcium concentrations. A further significant shift was observed with the addition of PKA. ——●—— = control; ···●··· = with 10 μM D-cAMP; ---▲--- = with 10 mM D-cAMP and 1 mg/ml PKA [1].*

and/or a stronger calcium-regulated binding state in myopathic myocardium. This would explain the reduced myofilament responsiveness to changes in pH and inorganic phosphate.

Protein kinase C is the only kinase known to phosphorylate both cardiac TnI and TnT *in vitro* [91]. However, protein kinase C activation resulted in a rightward shift on the calcium axis as well as a decrease in maximal calcium-activated force [87] (Fig. 8.13, Table 8.1). Decreased maximal activated force and change in the Hill coefficient suggest phosphorylation of TnT [87, 91]. Myopathic human tissues have been shown to express two TnT isoforms and were less affected by protein kinase C activation. Both TnT and TnI have at least two phosphorylation sites [91]. The data therefore suggest that phosphorylation of the two TnT isoforms cannot explain the observed changes in myofilament calcium activation seen with cAMP and PKA. However, differences at the phosphorylation sites of TnI may explain these experimental observations.

Cyclic GMP stimulates cAMP-dependent phosphodiesterase, resulting in an increase in cAMP hydrolysis. Cyclic GMP activation of cGMP protein kinase results in phosphorylation of TnI and should result in a decrease in myofilament calcium responsiveness. If, as proposed, failing myocardium has significantly less cAMP, then a smaller inhibitory effect would have been expected for the cGMP-induced rightward shift on the calcium axis (Fig. 8.14). The data support this hypothesis in that cGMP shifted the calcium–force relationship by $\Delta 0.2$ μM in non-failing myocardium and by $\Delta 0.45$ μM in myopathic myocardium.

In conclusion, it has become clear that thin myofilament regulation can affect force development. Although differences in experimental findings have been reported by investigators investigating agents targeted at myofilament calcium sensitivity [11, 78], adaptational changes may not always be detected by standard steady-state calcium–force relationship determinations [9]. Differences in isotype, structural interaction, phosphorylation level, and/or intracellular milieu may alter the apparent myofibrillar calcium responsiveness in human myocardium.

## Energy supply and demand

All cellular processes, maintaining membrane stability, ion homoeostasis, macromolecular synthesis, as well as external work, depend on the availability of ATP. When considering the potential role of myocardial energetics one must consider ATP supply as well as demand (Fig. 8.15). Another hypothesis that explains heart failure is that there is an inadequate energy supply. The estimates of energy supply have been made from activities (maximum velocity, $V_{max}$) of key enzymes involved in ATP-producing pathways, i.e. creatine kinase reaction, oxidative phosphorylation, and glycolysis, and from high-energy phosphate content and turnover rates. On the demand side are cardiac performance measures, myofibrillar ATPase activity, and SR $Ca^{2+}$-ATPase activity.

Whether there are changes in enzyme activity or in high-energy phosphate content in myopathic human myocardium has been controversial [16–18, 23–25, 92]. Part of the problem has been the use of biopsy samples and, for human studies, difficulty in obtaining appropriate controls. The feasibility of using the non-invasive technique of [$^{31}$P]nuclear magnetic resonance spectroscopy to measure relative ATP and creatine phosphate (PCr) contents in human myocardium has now been shown. Three different groups have reported that the PCr/ATP ratio is diminished in failing human myocardium [20–22]. Direct measurement of total creatine in failing human myocardium shows that the guanidine pool is lower [86]. The majority of the evidence shows that the primary energy reserve molecule, PCr, is diminished in failing human myocardium. The tissue content of creatine kinase that catalysed phosphoryl transfer between ATP and PCr is also lower in failing human myocardium than in non-failing myocardium [20].

On the utilization side, myofibrillar ATPase and myofibrillar protein content are lower in failing human myocardium [84]. Cross-bridge cycling dynamics have been demonstrated to be slower in failing human myocardium than in non-failing human myocardium [86]. It is tempting to speculate that these two effects are adaptive responses, but the relationship between energy supply and use remains to be established.

The creatine kinase system acts as an energy reserve system during high workloads or increased force of contraction (inotrophy). The link between energy reserve and contractile reserve was clearly demonstrated in an animal model of myopathy that closely mimics what has been shown in human myocardium [23]. Mekhfi *et al.* demonstrated that creatine-depleted hearts also have slower cross-bridge cycling rates and a decrease in the fast (α) myosin isoform [24]. All of these data indicate that creatine-deficient hearts have decreased contractile reserve. The blunt-

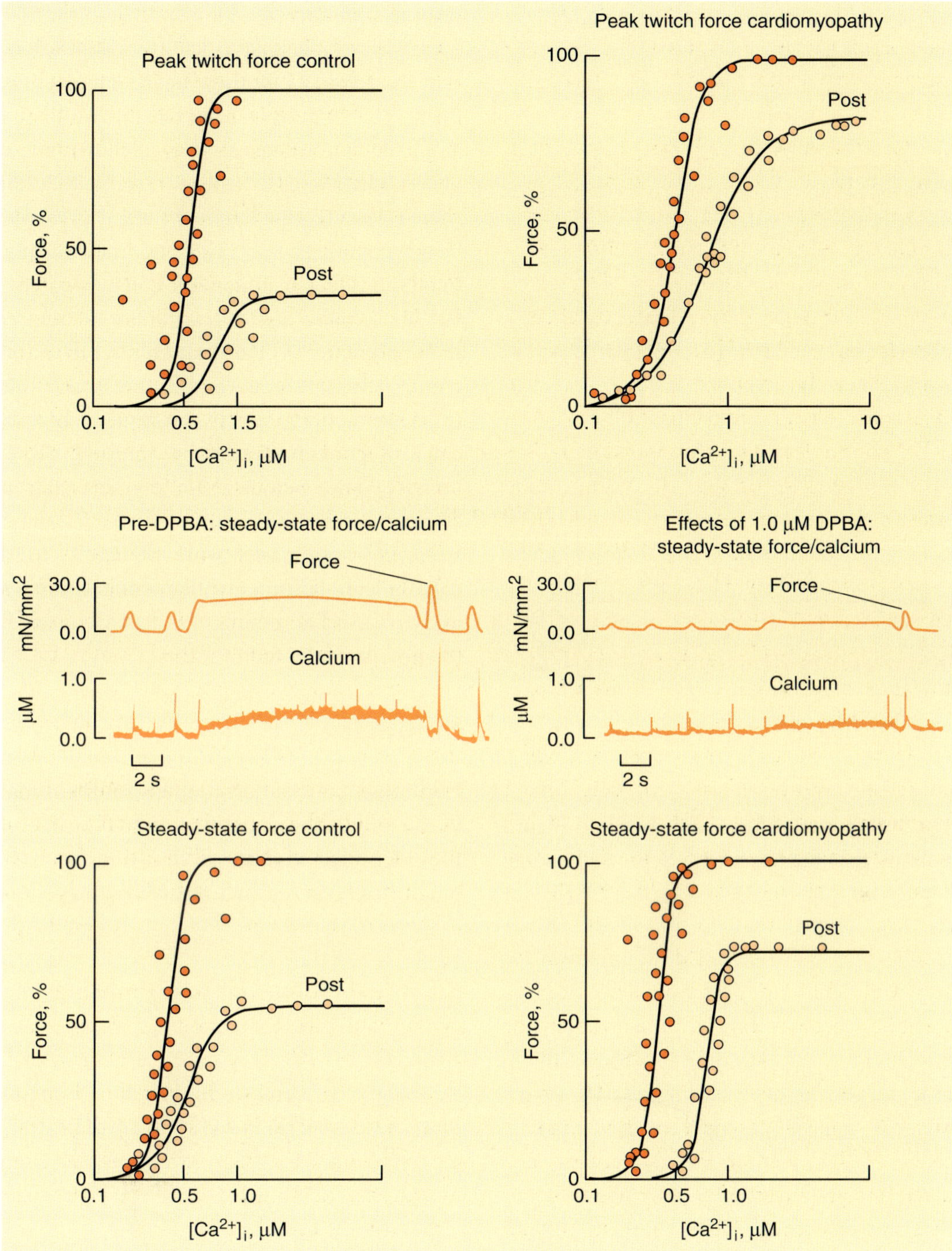


**Figure 8.13** *Relations of twitch force and twitch intracellular calcium concentration are shown in the presence of 12-deoxyphorbol-13-isobutyrate-20-acetate (DPBA) in both non-failing and myopathic muscles. The effect of DPBA on the steady-state calcium–force is depicted in control* (n = 5) *and myopathic* (n = 8) *muscles. Arrows denote post-tetanic potentiation.* ● = *Pre-DPBA;* ● = *post-DPBA. (From ref. 87 with permission.)*

ed or negative force frequency response may therefore be due in part to decreased contractile reserve in response to diminished myocardial energetics [88, 94]. One consequence of decreased energy reserve may be a lower calcium gradient across the SR and/or sarcolemma. Creatine kinase functions to maintain high ATP and low ADP and inorganic phosphate. The minimum values for the free energy needed to drive the SR $Ca^{2+}$-ATPase,

**Table 8.1** Hill coefficients and $[Ca^{2}+]_{50\%}$ from relations between force and $[Ca^{2}+]i$

| Group | $[Ca^{2+}]_{50\%}$ (µM) | $n_h$ | $n$ |
|---|---|---|---|
| *Steady-state force–$[Ca^{2+}]_i$* | | | |
| Control | | | |
| Pre-DPBA | 0.58 ± 0.01 | 5.00 ± 0.02 | 5 |
| + DPBA | 0.70 ± 0.02* | 2.60 ± 0.10* | 5 |
| Myopathic | | | |
| Pre-DPBA | 0.60 ± 0.04 | 5.60 ± 0.23 | 8 |
| + DPBA | 0.97 ± 0.06* | 6.00 ± 0.15* | 8 |
| *Peak twitch force–peak $[Ca^{2}+]i$* | | | |
| Control | | | |
| Pre-DPBA | 1.00 ± 0.02 | 5.20 ± 0.08 | 5 |
| + DPBA | 1.30 ± 0.05* | 3.20 ± 0.10* | 5 |
| Myopathic | | | |
| Pre-DPBA | 0.72 ± 0.13 | 4.57 ± 0.21 | 3 |
| + DPBA | 0.98 ± 0.11* | 3.76 ± 0.33* | 3 |

All results are expressed as mean ± SEM. The mean values of the Hill parameters were derived from curves fitted individually to the data of each experiment. Differences between means of $[Ca^{2+}]50\%$ of two groups were tested for significance by analysis of variance. *nh*, Hill coefficient; *n*, number of samples. *$p < 0.01$ vs. pre-DPBA (analysis of variance).

$Na^+/K^+$-ATPase and myosin ATPase are shown in Figure 8.16. The plot shows that the heart with depressed energy reserve has a reduced rate–pressure product (RPP) in response to increased force of contraction induced by increasing intracellular calcium concentration. It also shows that the value ΔG for these hearts approaches the free energy of ATP hydrolysis required for the SR calcium pump. This calculation suggests that calcium homoeostasis can be affected by decreased energy reserve. In addition, because there is less creatine kinase driving the reaction there might be an accumulation of ADP and inorganic phosphate, both of which affect myofilament calcium–force relationships. An abnormally high intracellular calcium concentration requires greater ATP utilization rates to restore normal calcium gradients across the SR and sarcolemma. Conversely, reduced energy supply can result in higher intracellular calcium concentrations by limiting SR $Ca^{2+}$-ATPase activity. The vicious cycle predicts that patients with compensated heart failure can decompensate when stressed by increased work demands. In this scenario, calcium metabolism, myofilament calcium responsiveness, and myocardial energetics are all interrelated in the phenotype of the failing heart.

## Summary

Excitation–contraction coupling mechanisms are abnormal in the failing or myopathic heart. The different abnormalities identified to date are shown in Figure 8.1. Although much has been learned regarding the cellular markers of

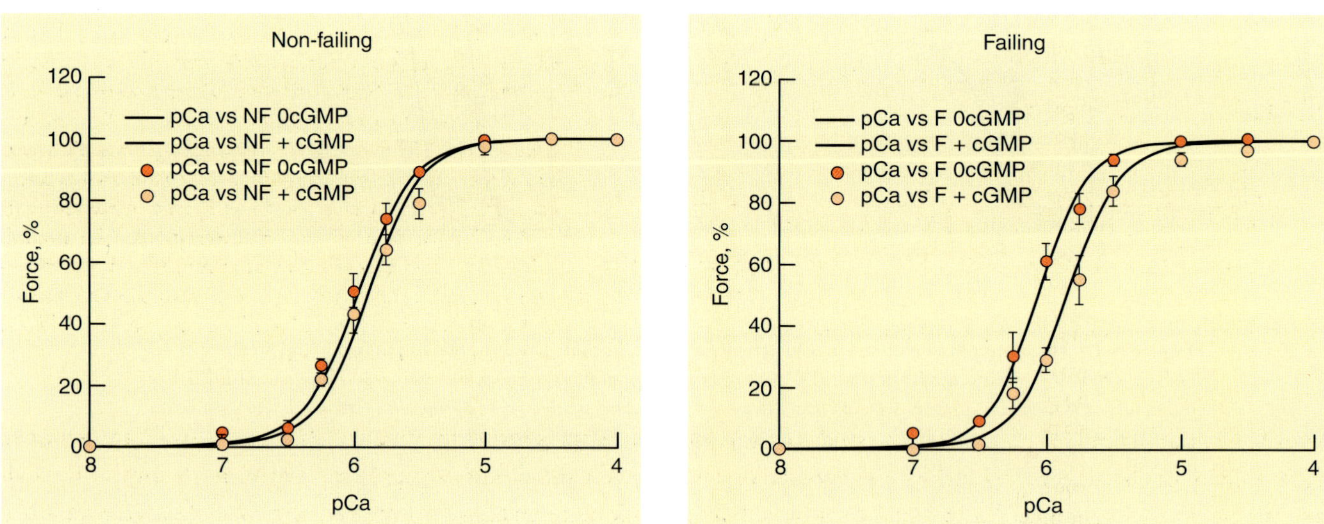


**Figure 8.14** *Effect of the addition of 10 µM 8-bromo-cGMP on the calcium–force relationship to non-failing (A) and failing (B) human myocardium. 8-Bromo-cGMP caused a Δ0.2 µM shift on the calcium axis for non-failing and a Δ0.45 µM shift for failing human myocardium. The calcium–force relationships were combined in C for ease of comparison.* —●— = *control, non-failing myocardium;* ···●··· = *10 µM 8-bromo-cGMP in non-failing myocardium;* —▲— = *control, failing myocardium;* ···▲··· = *10 µM 8-bromo-cGMP in failing.*

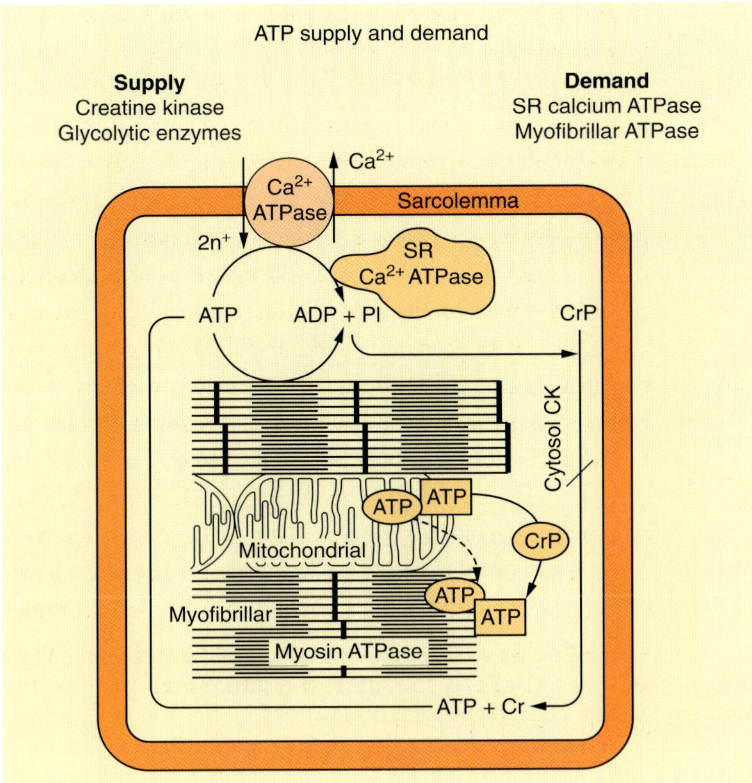


**Figure 8.15** *Scheme of energy supply and demand. CrP, creatine phosphate; Mito CK, mitochondrial creatine kinase; MM-CK, muscle isoform of CK. (From ref. 92 with permission.)*

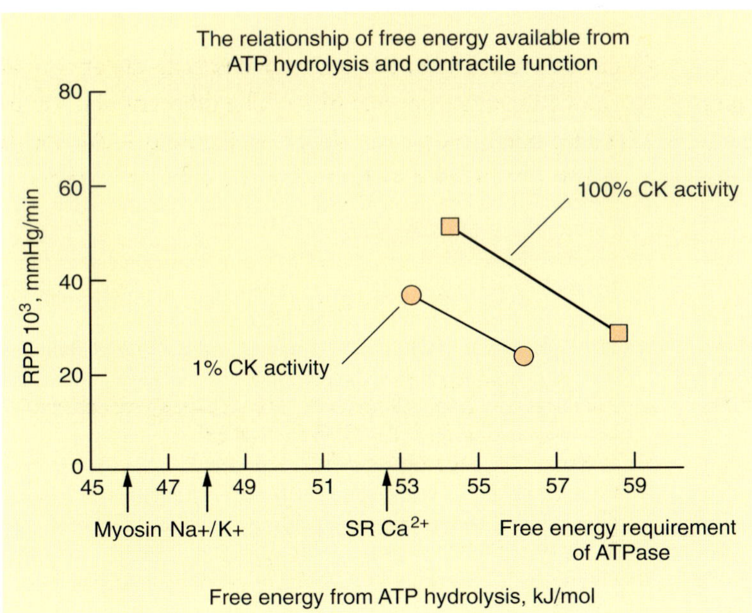


**Figure 8.16** *Plots of the rate–pressure product (RPP) vs absolute value of free energy available from ATP hydrolysis for a rat heart with 100% creatine kinase (CK) activity and one in which CK activity was chemically inhibited to 1% of control. Changes in the RPP were made by increasing extracellular calcium concentration. Free energy for ATP hydrolysis was calculated. ATP and inorganic phosphate $P_i$ were measured using [$^{31}$P]nuclear magnetic resonance spectroscopy and ADP was calculated using the CK equilibrium expression. Also shown are values for the free energy requirement for the sarcoplasmic reticulum $Ca^{2+}$ ATPase and $Na^+/K^+$-ATPase and myosin ATPase. (From ref. 92 with permission.)*

heart failure much remains unknown. The study of the contractile elements has lagged behind studies centred on the calcium regulatory proteins. An integrative approach and mechanistic thinking combining calcium regulation, myofilament calcium activation, and myocardial energetics is most likely to provide key new insights into the mechanisms of heart failure and direct the development of new therapies for its treatment. Changes in ADP and reduced myocardial energy supply can significantly impact the calcium–force relationship in the absence of changes in intracellular calcium concentrations. It is likely that the outcomes, force or pressure development, as well as relaxation parameters are intimately related to all of these cellular events.

## Acknowledgements

This work was supported in part by grants from NIH: HL-60323 and HL-49574 (JKG); HL-50361 and HL-57623 (RJH), a Doris Duke Charitable Foundation Clinician Scientist Award, and an American Federation of Aging Research Grant (RJH).

## References


1. Hajjar RJ, Schwinger RHG, Schmidt U *et al.* Myofilament calcium regulation in human myocardium: effects of pH and inorganic phosphate. *Circulation* 2000; 101 1679–1685.
2. Schmidt U, Hajjar RJ, Kim CS *et al.* Human heart failure: cAMP stimulation of SR $Ca^{2+}$-ATPase activity and phosphorylation level of phospholamban. *Am J Physiol* 1999; 277: H474–80.
3. O'Brien PJ, Gwathmey JK. Myocardial Ca(2+)- and ATP-cycling imbalances in end-stage dilated and ischaemic cardiomyopathies. *Cardiovasc Res* 1995; 30: 394–404.
4. Holmberg S, Williams A. Single channel recordings from human cardiac sarcoplasmic reticulum. *Circ Res* 1989; 65: 1445–9.
5. Mulieri LA, Leavitt BJ, Martin BJ *et al.* Myocardial force–frequency defect in mitral regurgitation heart failure is reversed by forskolin. *Circulation* 1993; 88: 2700–4.
6. Hasenfuss G, Schillinger W, Lehnart SE *et al.* Relationship between $Na^{+}$–$Ca^{2+}$-exchanger protein levels and diastolic function of failing human myocardium. *Circulation* 1999; 99: 641–8.
7. Hasenfuss G, Reinecke H, Studer R *et al.* Relation between myocardial function and expression of sarcoplasmic reticulum Ca(2+)-ATPase in failing and nonfailing human myocardium. *Circ Res* 1994; 75: 434–42.
8. Perez NG, Hashimoto K, McCune S *et al.* Origin of contractile dysfunction in heart failure: calcium cycling versus myofilaments. *Circulation* 1999; 99: 1077–83.
9. Gwathmey JK, Hajjar RJ. Relation between steady-state force and intracellular calcium in intact human myocardium: index of myofibrillar responsiveness to $Ca^{2+}$. *Circulation* 1996; 82: 1266–78.
10. Liao R, Gwathmey JK, Wang CK. Functional significance of two missense mutations in troponin C found in human myocardium with idiopathic dilated cardiomyopathy. *Circulation* 1998; 98: I–625.
11. Hajjar RJ, Gwathmey JK, Briggs GM, Morgan JP. Differential effect of DPI 201–106 on the sensitivity of the myofilaments to $Ca^{2+}$ in intact and skinned trabeculae from control and myopathic human hearts. *J Clin Invest* 1988; 82: 1578–84.
12. Solaro RJ. Myosin and why hearts fail. *Circulation* 1992; 85: 1945–7.
13. Solaro RJ, Gao L, Olson CC, Gwathmey JK. Control of myofilment activation in heart failure. *Circulation* 1993; 87: VII-38–43.
14. Anderson PAW, Greig A, Mark TM *et al.* Molecular basis of human cardiac troponin T isoforms expressed in the developing, adult, and failing heart. *Circ Res* 1995; 76: 681–6.
15. Margossian SS, White HD, Caulfied JD *et al.* Light chain 2 profile and activity of human ventricular myosin during dilated cardiomyopathy: identification of a causal agent for impaired myocardial function. *Circulation* 1992; 85: 1720–33.
16. Nascimben L, Ingwall JS, Pauletto P *et al.* Creatine kinase system in failing and nonfailing human myocardium. *Circulation* 1996; 94: 1894–901.
17. Ingwall JS. Is the failing myocardium energy starved? The role of the creatine kinase system. *Heart Failure* 1994; 10: 128–36.
18. Katz AM. Changing strategies in the management of heart failure. *J Am Coll Cardiol* 1989; 13: 513–23.
19. Regitz V, Fleck E. Myocardial adenosine nucleotide concentrations and myocardial norepinephrine content in patients with heart failure secondary to idiopathic dilated cardiomyopathy or ischaemic cardiomyopathy. *Am J Cardiol* 1992; 69: 1574–80.
20. Hardy CJ, Weiss RG, Bottomley PA, Gerstenblith G. Altered myocardial high-energy phosphate metabolites in patients with dilated cardiomyopathy. *Am Heart J* 1991; 122: 795–801.
21. Conway MA, Attis J, Ouwerkerk R *et al.* Detection of low PCr to ATP ratio in failing hypertrophied human myocardium by $^{31}P$ NMR. *Lancet* 1991; 338: 973–976.
22. Neubauer S, Krabe T, Schindler R *et al.* $^{31}P$ magnetic resonance spectroscopy in dilated cardiomyopathy and coronary artery disease. Altered high-energy phosphate metabolism in heart failure. *Circulation* 1992; 86: 1810–18.
23. Liao R, Nascimben L, Friedrich J *et al.* Decreased energy reserve in an animal model of dilated cardiomyopathy. Relationship to contractile performance. *Circ Res* 1996; 78: 893–902.
24. Mekhfi H, Hoerter J, Lauer C *et al.* Myocardial adaptation to creatine deficiency in rats fed with beta-guanidinopropionic acid, a creatine analogue. *Am J Physiol* 1990; 258: H1151–8.
25. Ingwall JS, Nascimben L, Gwathmey JK. Heart failure: is the pathology due to calcium overload or to mismatch in energy supply and demand? In: JK Gwathmey, GM Briggs, PD Allen (eds) *Heart failure, basic science and clinical aspects*. New York: Marcel Dekker, 1993, 667–700.
26. Wier WG, Egan TM, Lopez-Lopez JR, Balke CW. Local control of excitation–contraction coupling in rat heart cells. *J Physiol* 1994; 474: 463–71.
27. Fabiato A. Calcium release in skinned cardiac cells: variations with species, tissues, and development. *Fed Proc* 1982; 41: 2238–44.
28. Fabiato A. Calcium-induced release of calcium from the cardiac sarcoplasmic reticulum. *Am J Physiol* 1983; 245: C1–14.
29. Davia K, Hajjar RJ, Terracciano CMN *et al.* Functional alterations in adult rat myocytes following overexpression of phospholamban using adenovirus. *Physiol Genomics* 1999; 1: 41–50.
30. Huang B, Wang S, Qin D *et al.* Diminished basal phosphorylation level of phospholamban in the postinfarction remodeled rat ventricle: role of beta-adrenergic pathway, G(i) protein, phosphodiesterase, and phosphatases. *Circ Res* 1999; 85: 848–55.
31. Bohm M, Reiger B, Schwinger RH, Erdmann E. cAMP concentrations, cAMP dependent protein kinase activity, and phospholamban in nonfailing and failing myocardium. *Cardiovasc Res* 1994; 28: 1713–19.
32. Gwathmey JK, Bentivegna LA, Ransil BJ *et al.* Relationship of abnormal intracellular calcium mobilisation to myocyte hypertrophy in human ventricular myocardium. *Cardiovasc Res* 1993; 27: 199–203.
33. Gwathmey JK, Liao R, Hajjar RJ. *Intracellular free calcium in hypertrophy and failure*. 2nd edition. Norwell, MA: Kluwer Academic Publishers, 1994.
34. Gwathmey JK, Morgan JP. Sarcoplasmic reticulum calcium mobilization in the right ventricular pressure-overload hypertrophy in the ferret: relationships to diastolic dysfunction and a negative treppe. *Pflugers Arch* 1993; 422: 599–608.
35. Perreault CL, Bing OHL, Brooks WW *et al.* Differential effects of cardiac hypertrophy and failure on right versus left ventricular calcium activation. *Circ Res* 1990; 67: 707–12.

36. Gwathmey JK, Morgan JP. Altered calcium handling in experimental pressure-overload hypertrophy in the ferret. *Circ Res* 1985; 57: 836–43.
37. Gwathmey JK, Slawsky MT, Hajjar RJ *et al.* Role of intracellular calcium handling in force-interval relationships of human ventricular myocardium. *J Clin Invest* 1990; 85: 1599–613.
38. Gwathmey JK, Copelas L, MacKinnon R *et al.* Abnormal intracellular calcium handling in myocardium from patients with end-stage heart failure. *Circ Res* 1987; 61: 70–6.
39. Beuckelmann DJ, Nabauer M, Erdmann E. Intracellular calcium handling in isolated ventricular myocytes from patients with terminal heart failure. *Circulation* 1992; 85: 1046–55.
40. Liao R, Helm PA, Hajjar RJ *et al.* [$Ca^{2+}$]*i* in human heart failure: A review and discussion of current controversy. *Yale Journal of Biology and Medicine* 1994; 67247–264.
41. Kentish JC, ter Keurs HEDJ, Ricciardi L *et al.* Comparison between the sarcomere length–force relations of intact and skinned trabeculae from rat right ventricle: influence of calcium concentrations on these relations. *Circ Res* 1986; 58: 755–68.
42. Takahashi T, Allen PD, Lacro RV *et al.* Expression of dihydropyridine receptor ($Ca^{2+}$ channel) and calsequestrin genes in the myocardium of patients with end-stage heart failure. *J Clin Invest* 1992; 90: 927–35.
43. Gruver EJ, Glass MG, Marsh JD, Gwathmey JK. An animal model of dilated cardiomyopathy: characterization of dihydropyridine receptors and contractile performance. *Am J Physiol* 1993; 265: H1704–11.
44. Rasmussen RP, Minobe W, Bristow MR. Calcium antagonist binding sites in failing and nonfailing human ventricular myocardium. *Biochem Pharmacol* 1990; 39: 691–6.
45. Gruver EJ, Morgan JP, Stambler BS, Gwathmey JK. Uniformity of calcium channel number and isometric contraction in human right and left ventricular myocardium. *Basic Res Cardiol* 1994; 89: 139–48.
46. Gwathmey JK, Warren SE, Briggs GM *et al.* Diastolic dysfunction in hypertrophic cardiomyopathy. Effect on active force generation during systole. *J Clin Invest* 1991; 87: 1023–31.
47. Davidoff AJ, Gwathmey JK. Pathophysiology of cardiomyopathies: Part I. Animal Models and Humans. *Curr Opin Cardiol* 9(3): 357–368.
48. Go LO, Moschella MC, Watras J *et al.* Differential regulation of two types of intracellular calcium release channels during end-stage heart failure. *J Clin Invest* 1995; 95: 888–94.
49. Brillantes AM, Allen PD, Takahashi T *et al.* Differences in cardiac calcium release channel (ryanodine receptor) expression in myocardium from patients with end-stage heart failure caused by ischaemic vs. dilated cardiomyopathy. *Circ Res* 1992; 1: 18–26.
50. D'Agnolo A, Luciani GB, Mazzucco A *et al.* Contractile properties and $Ca^{2+}$ release activity of the sarcoplasmic reticulum in dilated cardiomyopathy. *Circulation* 1992; 85: 518–25.
51. Holmberg SRM, Williams AJ. Single channel recordings from human cardiac sarcoplasmic reticulum. *Circ Res* 1989; 65: 145–9.
52. Litwin SE, Zhang D, Bridge JH. Dyssynchronous $Ca^{2+}$ sparks in myocytes from infracted hearts. *Circ Res* 2000; 87: 1040–7.
53. Movsesian MA, Karimi M, Green K *et al.* $Ca^{2+}$-transporting ATPase, phospholamban, and calsequestrin levels in nonfailing and failing human myocardium. *Circulation* 1994; 90: 653–657.
54. Feldman MD, Copelas L, Gwathmey JK *et al.* Deficient production of cyclic AMP: pharmacologic evidence of an important cause of contractile dysfunction in patients with end-stage heart failure. *Circulation* 1987; 75: 331–9.
55. Schmidt U, Hajjar RJ, Carles M, Gwathmey JK. Calcium homeostasis in human heart failure. In: Bittar EE, Altshuld RA, Haworth RA (eds) *Advances in organ biology*. JAI Press Inc: Stamford, Connecticut, USA and London, England, 1998; 63–80.
56. Schmidt U, Hajjar RJ, Helm PA *et al.* Contribution of abnormal sarcoplasmic reticulum ATPase activity to systolic and diastolic dysfunction in human heart failure. *J Molec Cell Cardiol* 1998; 30: 1929–37.
57. Schmidt U, Hajjar RJ, Gwathmey JK. The force-interval relationship in human myocardium. *J Cardiac Failure* 1995; 1: 311–21.
58. Dipla K, Mattiello JA, Margulies KB *et al.* The sarcoplasmic reticulum and the $Na^{+}/Ca^{2+}$ exchanger both contribute to the $Ca^{2+}$ transient of failing human ventricular myocytes. *Circ Res* 1999; 84: 435–444.
59. Hajjar RJ, Schmidt U, Helm P, Gwathmey JK. $Ca^{++}$ sensitizers impair cardiac relaxation in failing human myocardium. *J Pharmacol Exp Ther* 1997; 280: 247–54.
60. Neumann J, Eschenhagen T, Jones LR *et al.* Increased expression of cardiac phosphatases in patients with end-stage heart failure. *J Mol Cell Cardiol* 1997; 29: 265–72.
61. Graham FL, Prevec L. Methods for construction of adenovirus vectors. *Mol Biotechnol* 1995; 3: 207–20.
62. Askari F, Hitomi E, Thiney M, Wilson JM. Retrovirus-mediated expression of HUG Brl in Crigler–Najjar syndrome type I human fibroblasts and correction of the genetic defect in Gunn rat hepatocytes. *Gene Ther* 1995; 2: 203–8.63. Hajjar RJ, Schmidt U, Matsui T *et al.* Modulation of ventricular function through gene transfer *in vivo*. *Proc Natl Acad Sci* 1998; 95: 5251–6.
63. Hajjar TJ, Schmidt U, Matsui T *et al.* Modulation of ventricular function through gene transfer *in vivo*. *Proc Natl Acad Sci* 1998; 95 5251–6.
64. del Monte F, Harding SE, Schmidt U *et al.* Restoration of contractile function in isolated cardiomyocytes from failing human hearts by gene transfer of SERCA2a. *Circulation* 1999; 100: 2308–2311.
65. Miyamoto MI, del Monte F, Schmidt U *et al.* Adenoviral gene transfer of SERCA2a improves left-ventricular function in aortic-banded rats in transition to heart failure. *Proceed Nat Acad Sci USA* 2000; 97(2): 793–8.
66. Hajjar RJ, Schmidt U, Kang JX *et al.* Adenoviral gene transfer of phospholamban in isolated rat cardiomyocytes: rescue effects by concomitant gene transfer of sarcoplasmic reticulum $Ca^{2+}$ ATPase. *Circ Res* 1997; 81: 145–53.
67. Yao A, Su Z, Dillmann WH *et al.* Sarcoplasmic reticulum function in murine ventricular myocytes overexpressing SR CaATPase. *Journal of Molecular and Cellular Cardiology* 1998; 30(12): 2711–18.
68. Morano I, Bletz C, Wojciechowski, Ruegg JG. Modulation of cross-bridge kinetics by myosin isoenzymes in skinned human heart fibres. *Circ Res* 1991; 68: 614–18.
69. Brandt PW, Cox RN, Kawai M, Robinson T. Regulation of tension in skinned muscle fibres: effect of cross-bridge kinetics on apparent $Ca^{2+}$ sensitivity. *J Gen Physiol* 1982; 79: 997–1016.
70. Gwathmey JK, Hajjar RJ, Solaro RJ. Contractile deactivation and uncoupling of cross-bridges. Effects of 2,3-butanedione monoxime on mammalian myocardium. *Circ Res* 1991; 69: 1280–92.
71. de Tombe PP, Wannenburg T, Fan D, Little WC. Right ventricular contractile protein function in rats with left ventricular myocardial infarction. *Am J Physiol* 1996; 217: H73–9.
72. Morano I, Ritter O, Bonz A *et al.* Myosin light chain-actin interaction regulates cardiac contractility. *Circ Res* 1995; 76: 720–5.

73. Anderson PAW, Moore GE, Nassar RN. Developmental changes in the expression of rabbit left ventricular troponin T. *Circ Res* 1988; 63: 742–7.
74. Kentish JC. The effects of inorganic phosphate and creatine phosphate on force production in skinned muscles from rat ventricle. *J Physiol Lond* 1986; 370: 584–604.
75. Herzig J, Peterson JW, Ruegg JC, Solaro RJ. Vanadate and phosphate ions reduce tension and increase cross-bridge kinetics in chemically skinned heart muscle. *Biochim Biophys Acta* 1981; 672: 191–6.
76. Solaro RJ, Holroyde MJ, Herzig JW, Peterson J. Cardiac relaxation and myofibrillar interactions with phosphate and vanadate. *Eur Heart J* 1980; 1: 21–7.
77. Veksler VI, Ventura-Clapier R, Lechene P, Vassort G. Functional state of myofibrils, mitochondria, and bound creatine kinase in skinned ventricular fibres of cardiomyopathic hamsters. *J Mol Cell Cardiol* 1988; 20: 329–42.
78. Bohm M, Diet F, Kemkes B *et al.* Inotropic response to DPI-201-106 in the failing human heart. *Br J Pharmacol* 1989; 98: 275–83.
79. Anderson PAW, Malouf NN, Oakeley AE *et al.* Troponin T isoform expression in humans. *Circ Res* 1991; 69: 1226–33.
80. Anderson PAW, Oakley A, Allen PD. Human troponin T expression in normal and end-stage heart failure patients. *Circulation* 1989; 80: 503 (Abstract).
81. Mercadier JJ, Bouveret P, Gorga L *et al.* Myosin isoenzymes in normal and hypertrophied human ventricular myocardium. *Circ Res* 1983; 53: 52–62.
82. Margossian SS, White HD, Caulfield JB *et al.* Light chain 2 profile and activity of human ventricular myosin during dilated cardiomyopathy: identification of a causal agent for impaired myocardial function. *Circulation* 1992; 85: 1720–33.
83. Alpert NR, Gordon MS. Myofibrillar adenosine triphosphatase activity in congestive heart failure. *Am J Physiol* 1962; 202: 940–6.
84. Pagani ED, Alousi AA, Grant AM *et al.* Changes in myofibrillar content and Mg-ATPase activity in ventricular tissue from patients with heart failure caused by coronary artery disease, cardiomyopathy, or mitral valve insufficiency. *Circ Res* 1988; 63: 380–5.
85. Boheler KR, Carrier L, de la Bastie D *et al.* Skeletal actin mRNA increases in the human heart during ontogenic development and is the major isoform of control and failing adult hearts. *J Clin Invest* 1991; 88: 323–30.
86. Hajjar RJ, Gwathmey JK. Cross-bridge dynamics in human ventricular myocardium: regulatory properties of contractility in the failing heart. *Circulation* 1992; 86: 1819–26.
87. Gwathmey JK, Hajjar RJ. Effect of protein kinase C activation on sarcoplasmic reticulum function and apparent myofibrillar $Ca^{2+}$ sensitivity in intact and skinned muscles from normal and diseased human myocardium. *Circ Res* 1990; 67: 744–52.
88. Hasenfuss G, Holubarsch C, Hermann HP *et al.* Influence of the force–frequency relationship on haemodynamics and left ventricular function in patients with non-failing hearts and in patients with dilated cardiomyopathy. *Eur Heart J* 1994; 15: 164–70.
89. Sasse S, Brand NJ, Kyprianou P *et al.* Troponin I gene expression during human cardiac development and end-stage heart failure. *Circ Res* 1993; 72: 932–8.
90. Hunkeler NM, Kullman J, Murphy AM. Troponin I isoform expression in human heart. *Circ Res* 1991; 69: 1409–14.
91. Katoh N, Wise BC, Kuo JF. Phosphorylation of cardiac troponin inhibitory subunit (troponin I) and tropomyosin-binding subunit (troponin T) by cardiac phospholipid-sensitive $Ca^{2+}$-dependent protein kinase. *Biochemistry* 1983; 209: 189–95.
92. Gwathmey JK, Ingwall JS. Basic pathophysiology of congestive heart failure. *Cardiol Rev* 1995; 3(5): 282–91.
93. Haber HL, Simek CL, Gimple LW *et al.* Why do patients with congestive heart failure tolerate the initiation of β-blocker therapy? *Circulation* 1993; 88: 1610–19.
94. Gwathmey JK, Kim CS, Hajjar RJ *et al.* Cellular and molecular remodeling in a heart failure model treated with the beta-blocker carteolol. *Am J Physiol* 1999; 276: H1678–H1690.

# Local hormonal adaptations in myopathic hearts 9

J. SADOSHIMA

## Introduction

Although it is well known that mechanical forces have a variety of effects on the structure and function of cells, little is known about how such forces are converted into the intracellular signals of gene regulation [1–3]. External load plays a critical role in determining muscle mass and its phenotype in both cardiac and skeletal muscle *in vivo* [4]. In cultured primary skeletal muscle cells grown on an elastic substrate, protein synthesis increases in response to the static stretch of the substrate [5]. Similarly, stretching cardiac myocytes cultured in serum-free media by 10–20% above resting length causes an increase in protein synthesis without DNA synthesis (hypertrophy) [6–8]. This indicates that individual skeletal and cardiac myocytes are able to sense external load. Mechanical stimuli also cause a rapid change in gene expression [6, 8]. Linear stretch of cardiac myocytes *in vitro* causes transcriptional activation of immediate-early genes followed by an induction of 'foetal' genes, such as atrial natriuretic factor (ANF), skeletal α-actin, and β-myosin heavy chain (MHC) [6, 8]. The phenotypic feature of stretched myocytes *in vitro* is similar to that of pressure overload-induced hypertrophy *in vivo* [9]. Analysis of cell signalling mechanisms has indicated that stretch activates multiple signal transduction pathways, similar to growth factor-induced cell signalling [10, 11]. Mechanical stretch activates autocrine/paracrine growth factors in the heart, such as the tissue (cardiac) renin–angiotensin system [12, 13]. Locally produced hormonal factors directly stimulate the growth response of cardiac cells, independent of their effects on haemodynamics.

Studies on the mechanism of load-induced cardiac hypertrophy have focused on the following three subjects: the mechanosensing mechanisms, the role of autocrine/paracrine factors, and the growth factor-mediated signal transduction mechanisms. The past few years have seen dramatic progress in the elucidation of the intracellular signalling mechanism of cardiac hypertrophy [3, 14–16]. This review discusses the role of autocrine/paracrine factors in the pathogenesis of cardiac hypertrophy, emphasizing the link between mechanical forces and autocrine/paracrine factors.

## Mechanosensing mechanisms

One of the most difficult questions regarding the mechanism of load-induced cardiac hypertrophy concerns how cardiac myocytes initially sense mechanical stresses. It is unlikely that cardiac myocytes possess specialized mechanosensing, molecules, such as those in the inner ear hair cells and touch sensors in the skin. Although mechanical stretch activates multiple second messenger systems in cardiac myocytes [10, 11], it is unknown which molecules are directly activated by stretch and which are indirectly activated by other upstream modulators. The mechanosensitive molecule is assumed to have some interaction with the plasma membrane in order to be regulated by membrane tension. Tension has long been recognized as a regulator of biochemical activities in skeletal muscle [17], and even the subtle force generated by membrane tension seems sufficient to alter the activity of various enzymes [18]. Accumulating evidence suggests that various mechanical forces affect the activities of several membrane-associated molecules in mammalian cells. Among them, heterotrimeric G proteins, integrins, ion channels and transporters, tyrosine kinases, and proteases are likely to play an important role in stretch-induced cellular responses in cardiac myocytes (Fig. 9.1). Promoter analysis of genes regulated by mechanical forces has indicated that mechanical forces may stimulate unique signalling mechanisms distinct from those activated by growth

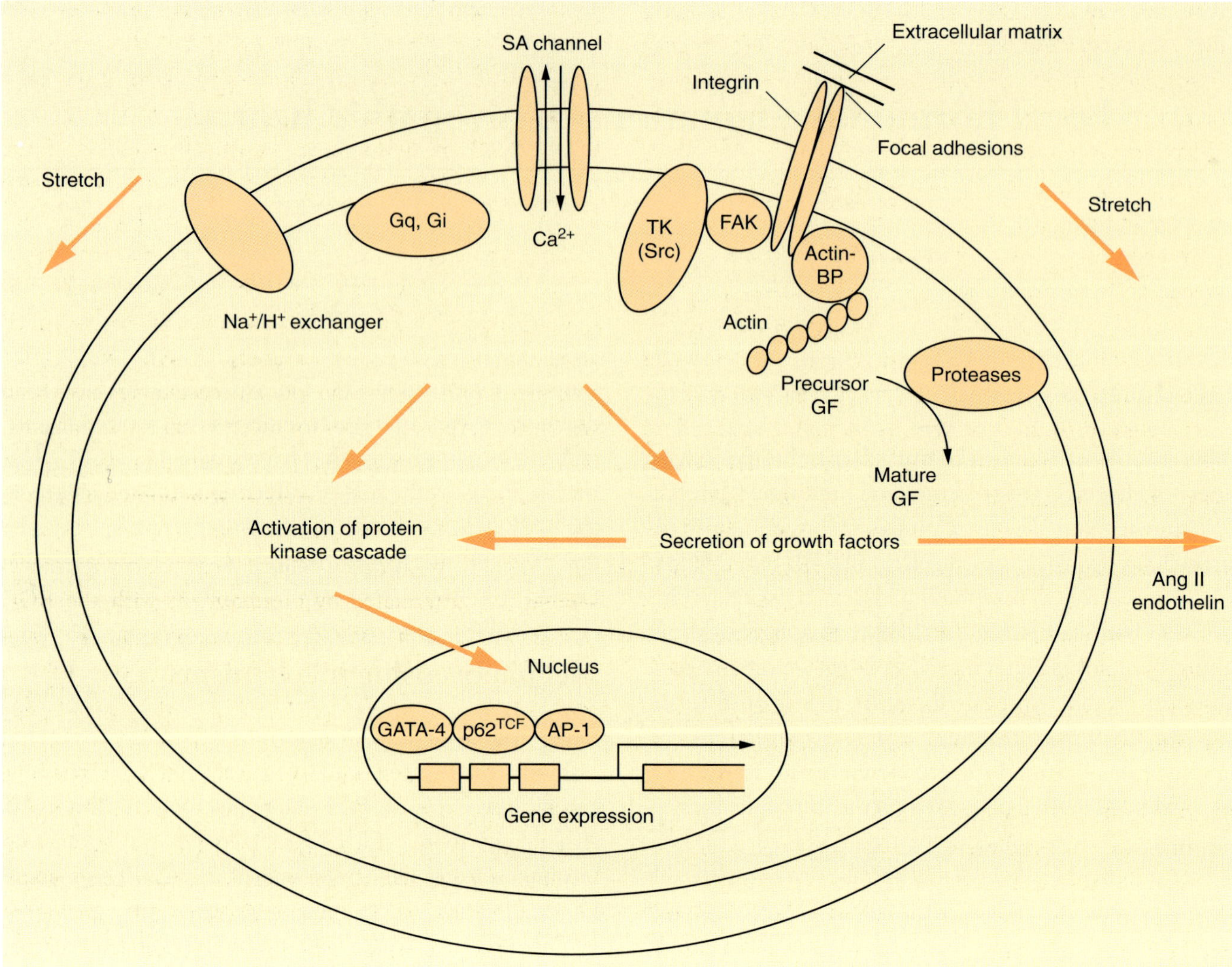


**Figure 9.1** *Putative mechano-sensors and their roles in stretch-induced cardiac hypertrophy. SA channel: stretch-activated ion channel; TK: tyrosine kinase; FAK: focal adhesion kinase; actin-BP: actin-binging protein; GF: growth factor.*

factors (see below). Understanding the mechanosensing mechanism is important because activation of these mechanosensors or mechanotransducers leads to stretch-induced secretion/production of autocrine/paracrine factors and/or directly causes hypertrophic responses through activation of the protein kinase cascade.

## Heterotrimeric G proteins

The heterotrimeric GTP binding protein (G protein) is localized at the plasma membrane and works as an interface between the seven membrane-spanning G protein-coupled receptors (GPCR) and their downstream effector molecules. Ligand binding to the GPCR causes GTP to bind to the Gα-subunit and Gβγ to dissociate from the Gα-subunit. Gα and Gβγ activate distinct downstream effector molecules. Although it is generally assumed that ligand binding to the GPCR is the primary stimulus for G protein activation, recent evidence suggests that mechanical strain also causes rapid activation of heterotrimeric G proteins, namely Gαq and Gαi, in cardiac fibroblasts [19]. Similarly, membrane swelling caused by hypotonicity activates Gαi, thereby inhibiting isoproterenol-stimulated cyclic adenosine monophosphate (cAMP) accumulation in cardiac myocytes [20]. Stretch-induced prostaglandin F2α production, cyclooxygenase activity, and cell growth in skeletal muscle are inhibited in the presence of pertussis toxin, suggesting that stretch may activate Gαi in skeletal muscle [21]. Agonists for the GPCR, such as bradykinin and angiotensin II (AngII), and strain cause GTP loading of different sets of G proteins, suggesting that GTP loading by mechanical strain may not be mediated by autocrine/paracrine production of growth factors. Since heterotrimeric G proteins are localized at least in part at focal adhesions, the sites for the transmission of mechanical force, it is possible that mechanical forces are directly transmitted to the heterotrimeric G protein. This hypothesis is supported by the evidence that the fluid shear stress, another mechanical stress, stimulates GTP loading of the purified G protein reconstituted into phospholipid vesicles [22]. To determine whether increases in the membrane tension (strain) similarly affects heterotrimeric G protein as increases in the fluid shear stress would require the development of a lipid bilayer system, in which the intrinsic tension of the membrane could be precisely controlled. Since the mammalian heterotrimeric G proteins possess well-conserved amino acid sequences, it is interesting that mechanical strain activates $G\alpha q$ and $G\alpha i_1$ but not $G\alpha i_3$ in cardiac fibroblasts. Identifying the unique sequence that confers the mechanosensitivity to the heterotrimeric G protein would help to explain how G proteins are activated by mechanical forces.

## Integrins and focal adhesions

Integrins are heterodimeric transmembrane receptors that couple the extracellular matrix with the actin cytoskeleton at the site of focal adhesion [23]. Integrins have been shown to be an important determinant of the morphology of cardiac myocytes *in vitro* [24]. They play a pivotal role in early cardiac development, providing positional information for migration and differentiation of cardiac cells [25]. Since the cytoplasmic domain of the integrin physically associates with cytoskeletal elements [23, 26], integrins transmit mechanical signals to the cytoskeleton [27]. The cytoplasmic domain of the β-integrin also interacts with the amino-terminal domain of focal adhesion tyrosine kinase (FAK). FAK further interacts with various signalling molecules, such as Src, Fyn, $p130^{Cas}$, Graf (GTPase regulator associated with FAK), Grb2, and PI-3 kinase [23, 26]. These signalling molecules further activate various downstream protein kinase cascades, including $p21^{ras}$, mitogen-activated protein (MAP) kinases, Rho/Cdc42, PIP-5 kinase, protein kinase C (PKC), and $p70^{S6K}$ [23, 26]. Integrins are therefore very attractive candidates for being mechanotransducers, which convert mechanical signals into the intracellular second messenger signalling. Although cell adhesion and spread through integrins are sufficient to stimulate signalling molecules, cells may undergo apoptosis if the mechanical forces transmitted across integrins are not large enough [28]. It has been shown that tension exposes a cryptic site in the fibronectin molecule and promotes self-assembly of the fibronectin matrix [29]. This indicates that mechanical forces actively generate cell signals involving both integrins and extracellular matrices for cell survival and growth.

Cardiac myocytes not only have focal adhesions at their distal ends but also form cytoskeletal–sarcolemmal attachments along the Z-lines, which are called costameres [30]. Focal adhesions and costameres have been shown to serve as the sites for mechanical force transmission in cardiac myocytes [31]. The signalling mechanism generated at the site of the focal adhesions is not fully understood. The tyrosine phosphorylation of FAK and paxillin caused by hypotonic swelling of cardiac myocytes was significantly attenuated by pretreatment with the RGD peptide, a specific ligand for some integrins [32]. This suggests that RGD-sensitive integrins may play a role in swelling-induced tyrosine kinase activation. In cardiac fibroblasts, static biaxial stretch activates MAP kinases, including ERK-2 and C-Jun N-terminal kinase-1 (JNK-1), and inhibitors for specific integrins block the activation of these protein kinases. ERK and JNK require different extracellular matrices as well as distinct isoforms of integrins for their activation by stretch [33]. These results suggest that integrins mediate mechano chemical transduction and that the integrin–extracellular matrix confers specificity and versatility to the signalling mechanism by stretch. Expression of integrin and focal adhesions, such as costameres, are upregulated by mechanical stretch [34], suggesting that mechanical stresses initiate positive feedback mechanisms in integrin-mediated cell signalling. Recently, integrins have been shown to play an essential role in cardiac hypertrophy caused by a humoral factor, phenylephrine [35]. Pretreatment of neonatal rat cardiac myocytes with the RGD peptide did not inhibit stretch-induced c-*fos* gene induction. This suggests that RGD-sensitive integrins are not essential for stretch-induced c-*fos* expression [36]. The role of RGD-insensitive integrins in stretch-induced hypertrophic responses remains to be demonstrated.

## Ion channels and ionic transporters

Stretching of the ventricular wall by increased end-diastolic volume accelerates the rate of repolarization and shortens the duration of the action potential, resulting in depolarization of the resting membrane potential [37]. It is therefore likely that mechanical stress affects ion channels in the heart. There are several kinds of stretch-activated ion channels in the heart, including non-selective cation channels and $K^+$ channels with different ionic conductances [38, 39]. These cardiac stretch-activated channels are sensitive to $Gd^{3+}$ [38, 39], a known inhibitor of such channels. Besides these typical $Gd^{3+}$-sensitive channels, mechanical stress affects a wide variety of ionic channels/currents in the heart, such as the $K^+_{ATP}$ channel [40], delayed $K^+$-rectifier channel [41], $Cl^-$channel [42], L-type $Ca^{2+}$ channel [43], $Na^+/K^+$ pump [44], $Ca^{2+}$-activated nonselective cation channel, and $Na^+/Ca^{2+}$ exchanger [41]. Stretch also activates the $Na^+/H^+$ exchanger in cardiac myocytes [45], thereby causing intracellular alkalinization, which often couples to cell growth responses.

Opening the typical cationic stretch-activated channels causes increases in intracellular $Ca^{2+}$ because some of these channels are permeable to $Ca^{2+}$, and the influx causes $Ca^{2+}$-induced $Ca^{2+}$ release [38, 39]. Opening the non-selective cation channels at resting membrane potentials causes an inward current, thereby depolarizing the membrane and increasing membrane excitability [46]. A swelling-activated $Gd^{3+}$-sensitive cation current ($I_{Cir,swell}$) is persistently activated in cardiac myocytes isolated from dogs with rapid pacing-induced heart failure. Blocking $I_{Cir,swell}$ by $Gd^{3+}$ in myocytes isolated from failing hearts decreased cell volume. These observations are consistent with the belief that myocytes in the failing heart behave as if they are stretched. Thus, activation of the mechanosensitive channel may contribute to cell hypertrophy, dysrhythmias, and contractile dysfunction [47]. Since the treatment of myocytes with $Gd^{3+}$ does not affect stretch-induced c-*fos* expression or stretch-induced increases in the rate of protein synthesis, $Gd^{3+}$-sensitive stretch-activated channels may not be involved in all stretch-induced hypertrophic responses [36]. However, this does not exclude the possible involvement of $Gd^{3+}$-insensitive mechanosensitive ion channels in stretch-induced hypertrophic responses.

Whether stretch-activated channels are the initial mechanosensors of stretch-induced cardiac hypertrophy remains to be determined. It has been suggested that these channels directly interact with the cytoskeleton, and thus have an intrinsic ability to sense the cell stretch [48, 49]. In vascular endothelial cells these channels are activated within a few milliseconds by negative pressure applied by a suction patch pipette [50]. A cloned renal epithelial $Na^+$, channel, whose mRNA expression is also observed in the heart, has been shown to display stretch-induced activation in planar lipid bilayers [51]. Thus, some stretch-activated channels are directly activated by increases in membrane tension; on other occasions, they are activated secondarily by second messengers such as increased $[Ca^{2+}]_i$ [41]. Fatty acids, generated by mechanically activated phospholipases, may be the intermediaries in the activation of stretch-activated channels in toad smooth muscle cells [52]. Isolation of stretch-activated channel genes [48], determination of their mechanosensitivity in the lipid bilayer system, and the subsequent genetic approaches such as gene disruption [53] are essential for determining whether the such channels are the true mechanosensors in stretch-induced hypertrophy. Mechanical stress caused by direct uniaxial stretch and that by hypo-osmotic cell inflation affects different ionic currents in guinea-pig ventricular myocytes [44], indicating that the nature of mechanical stimuli greatly influences their electrophysiological effects. Stimulus-specific activation of distinct mechanosensitive ion channels may potentially explain differences in the phenotype of the hypertrophy by different types of mechanical stimuli.

## Tyrosine kinases

Receptor-type tyrosine kinases have transmembrane segments and some of the non-receptor-type tyrosine kinases, such as the Src family tyrosine kinases, are anchored to the inner surface of cell membranes through their N-terminal myristoylation site. Thus, stretch may directly cause conformational changes of tyrosine kinases, thereby activating them. In support of this hypothesis, mechanical stretch of cardiac myocytes causes a rapid increase in the phosphotyrosine content of multiple proteins within 1 min [10]. Hypotonic cell swelling of cardiac myocytes also causes rapid activation of tyrosine kinases [54]. Hypotonic swelling-induced c-*fos* gene expression was abolished by typrosine kinase inhibitors but not by inhibitors of PKC, phospholipase C (PLC), or AngII antagonists [54]. In contrast, stretch-induced c-*fos* gene induction was inhibited by inhibitors of tyrosine kinases, PKC, and PLC, as well as AngII antagonists [10]. These results suggest that hypotonic cell swelling and linear stretch activate separate signalling mechanisms. The identity of the tyrosine kinases that are activated by stretch in cardiac myocytes is poorly characterized. Hypotonic cell swelling rapidly activates Src in cardiac myocytes [55]. Similarly, c-Src and FAK were found to be associated with the cytoskeleton (and possibly activated) in the pressure-overloaded cat heart [56]. Hypotonic swelling caused increases in tyrosine phosphorylation of FAK, which is localized at the focal adhesions through its interaction with β-integrin [55]. Stretch-induced activation of tyrosine kinase is responsible for several stretch-induced cellular responses. The tyrosine kinase inhibitor abolished upregulation of the angiotensin II type 1a(AT1a) receptor caused by stretch [57] and swelling-induced activation of the chloride current [58].

The mechanism of tyrosine kinase activation by mechanical stress is unclear. However, mechanical stress activates tyrosine kinase very rapidly. In cardiac myocytes, hypotonic stress causes cell swelling within a few seconds. A significant increase in tyrosine phosphorylation can be observed in 5 s, the earliest time interval examined [54]. In the same preparation, hypotonic stress caused an increase in $[Ca^{2+}]_i$, but the onset of increase in $[Ca^{2+}]_i$ was much slower compared with that of tyrosine phosphorylation [54]. Thus, activation of the tyrosine kinases is one of the earliest cellular responses observed at the whole cell level in response to cell swelling. It is possible, however, that an activator of tyrosine kinases may exist and can be activated by mechanical stress much earlier. Further studies are necessary to elucidate how tyrosine kinase is activated by mechanical stress.

## Proteases

Mechanical stretch of cardiac cells has been shown to affect the activities of proteases, which are localized at the plasma membrane. Stretching neonatal rat cardiac myocytes stimulates proprotein-processing endopeptidase furin, which cleaves the RXXR motif found in brain natriuretic factor precursor [59]. The furin-specific protease inhibitors block both stretch-induced hypertrophic growth of cardiac myocytes and the processing of brain natriuretic protein (BNP), while other serine protease inhibitors affect neither. Furin plays an important role in cell proliferation by cleaving the RXXR motif on growth-related precursor peptides. Cardiac myocytes produce peptides with the furin-cleavable motif, including BNP, transforming growth factor-β (TGF-β), endothelin-1 (ET-1), and PTHrP, some of which could cause cardiac hypertrophy. Stretch-induced activation of proteases may be an important mechanism underlying the secretion of growth factor. In fibroblasts, stretch activates transmembrane matrix metalloproteinase and tissue plasminogen activator, which may play a role in remodelling the extracellular matrix [60]. Although the mechanism of protease activation by stretch is unknown, one attractive hypothesis is that membrane tension might directly affect the activities of the enzyme localized at the plasma membrane. Stretch has been shown to stimulate apoptotic cell death of cardiac myocytes [61]. It is likely that caspases, proteases that promote apoptosis, are activated by mechanical stress. Mechanical forces also affect the proteolytic susceptibility of the myofibrillar proteins [62]. It is speculated that the muscle-loading condition may affect myofibrillar assembly and stability through the extracellular matrix–integrin–cytoskeletal complex. It is likely that many other mechanisms also contribute to changes in protein susceptibility to proteolysis in response to mechanical stress.

## Transcriptional regulation

Evidence suggests that transcription of some hypertrophic genes by mechanical forces may be mediated by transcription factors and *cis* elements that are distinct from those responsible for gene expression by known hypertrophic humoral factors. In cultured neonatal rat ventricular myocytes, the *cis* elements responsible for ET-1 or $\alpha_1$-adrenergic receptor stimulation-induced ANF gene expression have been identified within 638 bp of the rat ANF 5′ flanking sequence. However, these *cis* elements are not sufficient for stretch-induced ANF expression *in vitro* [8] and ANF expression by pressure overload *in vivo* [63]. Although transcriptional regulation is the last step of cell signalling and far from the initial sensing mechanism, elucidation of its mechanism should provide useful information about the upstream mechanosensing mechanism. Thus, a brief discussion of the mechanism of gene transcription by mechanical stress follows. Several *cis*-regulatory elements, which are activated by mechanical stress/pressure overload, have been identified in cardiac myocytes. These include the serum response element (SRE) as well as the binding sites for AP-1 and GATA-4.

Transfection of cultured neonatal cardiac myocytes with *c-fos* promoter–reporter gene constructs indicated that the SRE is both necessary and sufficient to confer stretch responsiveness to the *c-fos* promoter and that the Ets domain adjacent to the SRE core, a binding site of the ternary complex factor $p62^{TCF}$, is essential for transcriptional activation [10]. This suggests that the signal generated by mechanical stretch activates the serum response factor (SRF)–p62$^{TCF}$ complex via the SRE, causing induction of c-*fos*. A similar finding was obtained by direct injection of the c-*fos* promoter reporter gene constructs into the intact adult rat heart, which were then subjected to pressure overload in Langendorff (perfused) preparation [64]. Furthermore, c-*fos* induction by hypotonic cell swelling, another type of mechanical stress that increases membrane tension, is also mediated by activation of SRF-p62$^{TCF}$ in cardiac myocytes [54]. Thus, activation of SRF–p62$^{TCF}$ may be the general mechanism of c-*fos* activation in response to increased membrane tension in cardiac myocytes.

A unique element similar to AP-1 has been shown to be necessary to cause transcriptional activation of ANF by acute pressure overload in the dog ascending aortic stenosis model [65]. The gel mobility shift assay indicated that an AP-1-like element is recognized predominantly by a yet unknown factor, whose concentration appears uninfluenced by banding, and also by authentic AP-1. The role of these proteins in ANF gene expression by pressure overload remains to be demonstrated [65]. In transgenic mice harboring up to −3003 bp of the rat ANF 5′ flanking region ligated upstream from a luciferase promoter, transverse aortic constriction failed to stimulate reporter activities in the ventricle [63]. Thus, the *cis*-regulatory element responsible for pressure overload-induced ANF expression may be different from species to species.

In the *in vivo* rat, the GATA-4 binding site in the β-MHC promoter sequence plays an essential role in transcriptional activation of β-MHC by aortic constriction [66]. Both AP-1 and GATA-4 binding sites are also essential for pressure overload-induced transcriptional activation of AT1a receptor gene expression [67]. Pressure overload increases expression of immediate-early genes, Fos and Jun B, thereby causing the strong binding of these proteins to the AP-1 element. Similarly, the binding of GATA-4, but not GATA-6, to the GATA-4 element, is stimulated by pressure overload [67]. Captopril treatment blocked pressure overload-induced transcriptional activation of the AT1a receptor and AngII caused transcriptional activation of the AT1 receptor promoter [67]. It should be noted, however, AngII has been shown to cause downregulation of the AT1 receptor expression in many other cell types. It is therefore unclear whether AngII mediates activation of AP-1 and GATA-4. It is not known whether activation of these elements is directly caused by mechanical stress or mediated by growth factors whose production is stimulated by mechanical stress. Further studies are required to identify the link between the mechanosensing molecules and these transcription factors/*cis* elements.

## Autocrine and paracrine mechanisms

### Mechanical forces and growth factor secretion and production

One of the most important characteristics of the cell signalling mechanism that is initiated by the mechanical stretch of cardiac and skeletal myocytes is the activation of multiple second messenger systems [2, 10, 11, 68, 69], which is highly reminiscent of growth factor-induced intracellular signaling [70]. The presence of autocrine/paracrine growth factors has been proposed as one of the important mechanisms in the pathogenesis of stretch-induced organ hypertrophy [2]. Mechanical stress causes local production and/or secretion of growth factor(s), which in turn mediates cellular responses in the heart. Culture media conditioned by stretched rat ventricular myocytes contain a soluble factor, which causes c-*fos* expression and ERK activation in non-stretched cardiac myocytes [10, 71]. The factor has been subsequently identified as AngII (see below). Stretch-induced secretion of AngII and ET-1 mediates hypertrophy in neonatal rat cardiac myocytes [10, 71]. Coronary venous effluent collected from a perfused Langendorff heart subjected to stretch was able to induce vascular endothelial cell growth factor (VEGF) expression in non-stretched hearts, which was identified to be mediated by stretch-induced secretion of TGF-β [72]. Thus, many, if not all, effects of mechanical stretch seem to be mediated by the production and secretion of soluble factor(s) in and from cardiac myocytes. For this reason, identifying which and how growth factors are modulated by mechanical stress is important to understand the mechanism of load-induced cardiac hypertrophy.

Different types of mechanical stresses, such as pressure versus volume overloading, may stimulate different growth factors, thereby causing hypertrophy with different phenotypes. For example, the hypertrophic response induced by cytokines, including cardiotrophin-1 (CT-1) and leukaemia inhibitory factor (LIF), signalling through gp130, is distinct from that induced by AngII. AngII induces a uniform increase in the myocyte size, resulting from the addition of myofibrils in parallel, reminiscent of the changes observed in myocytes from the pressure-overloaded heart. In contrast, CT-1 and LIF induce a predominant increase in cell length with the addition of new sarcomeric units in series but no concomitant increase in cell width [73]. This morphology is reminiscent of changes observed in myocytes from the volume-overloaded heart. Since stretch causes activation of gp130 and downstream JAK/STAT signalling pathways [74, 75], it is possible that stretch causes the secretion of cytokines. Increased expression of interleukin-1β and monocyte chemoattachment protein-1 has been demonstrated recently in the pressure-overloaded heart [76]. However, stimulus- (load-)specific production of growth factors has not been demonstrated.

## Importance of the Gq protein-coupled receptors in cardiac hypertrophy

One of the important characteristics of the growth response in cardiac muscle is that agonists for the Gq protein-coupled receptor (GqPCR) play a critical role in cardiac growth and development. Agonists for the GqPCR have been shown to be both necessary and sufficient for the growth response of cardiac muscle. Mice lacking both Gαq and Gα11 die at day 11 owing to cardiac myocyte hypoplasia [77]. One intact allele of the Gαq or Gα11 gene was sufficient to overcome the early block in heart development resulting from the complete absence of Gαq/Gα11, suggesting that there is overlap in Gαq and Gα11 gene functions. Since neither angiotensinogen nor endothelin-knockout mice showed a cardiac phenotype similar to the Gαq/Gα11-deficient mice, either multiple factors which signal through both Gαq and Gα11 or an unidentified factor which couples to Gαq/Gα11 critically mediates cardiac growth. The Gαq signalling pathway continues to play an important role in cardiac muscle growth after birth, in which cardiac hypertrophy is the predominant form of cell growth. In mice with heart-specific expression of a minigene encoding the carboxyl-terminal Gαq, which selectively blocks coupling between GqPCR and Gαq, cardiac hypertrophy by pressure overload is effectively, if not completely, suppressed [78]. This not only suggests the importance of Gαq in mediating cardiac hypertrophy but also indicates that pressure overload activates Gαq via receptor–Gαq interaction. It is possible, however, that both Gαq-coupled receptor and mechanical forces require the same amino-acid sequence in the carboxyl-terminal of Gαq for interaction and activation. Overexpression of Gαq in neonatal rat cardiac myocytes and transgenic mice causes cardiac hypertrophy, suggesting that Gαq is sufficient to stimulate cardiac hypertrophy [79, 80]. Cardiac myocytes isolated from Gαq transgenic mice develop the changes of congestive heart failure significantly more quickly than those from non-transgenic mice [81]. Whether such contractile dysfunction is specifically caused by Gq-mediated cell signals or is secondary to any type of cardiac hypertrophy has not yet been determined. Transgenic mice with cardiac-specific overexpression of Ras oncogene, which also develop cardiac hypertrophy, have normal systolic function and selective diastolic dysfunction [82]. In this regard, signalling molecules downstream of Gαq may specifically induce hypertrophy with contractile dysfunction.

Why is Gαq-mediated cell signalling so important in the growth of cardiac muscle? One possible explanation may be that PLC-mediated signals, including $Ca^{2+}$ and PKC, are essential for cardiac myocyte growth [83, 84]. Gq protein-coupled receptors, such as AngII, activate a plethora of signalling molecules, including tyrosine kinases. Such versatile functions of the Gq-coupled receptor may be required for cardiac muscle growth [85]. Both Gq-agonists and serum growth factors activate very similar signalling molecules and cause hypertrophy and hyperplasia in cardiac myocytes and fibroblasts, respectively. However, the long-term signalling mechanisms, such as regulation of the cell cycle machinery, are substantially different between Gq-agonists and serum [86]. Further characterization of Gq-mediated cell signalling will help to reveal its unique and important aspects in cardiac myocytes.

## Role of angiotensin II in cardiac hypertrophy

Among the agonists of GqPCR, accumulating evidence suggests that AngII may be a critical factor mediating many types of load-induced hypertrophy *in vivo*. Treating rats that have abdominal aortic coarctation with an angiotensin-converting enzyme (ACE) inhibitor or with AngII type I receptor antagonists (losartan and TCV 116) prevented (or caused regression of) left ventricular hypertrophy [87–90]. The ACE inhibitor fosinopril prolonged survival of rats with pressure overload [91]. Similarly, treating rats that have aortocaval shunt with losartan or the ACE inhibitor quinapril prevented cardiac hypertrophy [92]. Treating animals or patients with myocardial infarction with ACE inhibitors prevented cardiac remodelling and reduced mortality [93, 94]. The recent ELITE (Evaluation of Losartan in the Elderly) trial also demonstrated that AT1 receptor blockade is efficient in treating patients with heart failure [95]. All of these phenomena are consistent with the involvement of the renin–angiotensin system in the heart and its activation by haemodynamic loading. In support of this, there is now clear evidence for the existence of the cardiac renin–angiotensin system.

The role of AngII as a critical mediator of stretch-induced hypertrophy has been also shown in cultured neonatal rat cardiac myocytes *in vitro*. AngII receptor antagonists, such as [$Sar^1$ $Ile^8$]AngII (antagonist for the AngII type I and II receptors), losartan, and TCV11974 (antagonists for the AngII type I receptor), inhibit major markers of stretch-induced hypertrophy, such as c-*fos* gene expression, MAP kinase activation, increases in the rate of protein synthesis, and induction of foetal type genes, such as ANF and skeletal α-actin, suggesting that AngII plays a critical role in stretch-induced hypertrophy in the neonatal rat myocyte culture system [13, 71].

The evidence described above clearly indicates that AngII is an important mediator of many types of load-induced cardiac hypertrophy. However, it is important to note that AT1 receptor antagonists and ACE inhibitors are not effective in suppressing all types of load-induced cardiac hypertrophy *in vivo*. Accumulating evidence suggests that some stretch-induced hypertrophic effects are also mediated by AngII-independent mechanisms. Part of the stretch-induced hypertrophic response may be mediated by other autocrine/paracrine growth factors, such as ET-1 [96], or by the signalling mechanism directly activated by stretch. AngII-independent and -independent components of cardiac hypertrophy are discussed further below.

## Characteristics of angiotensin II-induced cardiac hypertrophy

AngII can cause cardiac hypertrophy both *in vivo* and *in vitro*. It increases protein synthesis and gene expression characteristic of hypertrophy in the adult rat heart *in vivo* or the isolated perfused heart [97–99]. Myocardial injection of a plasmid encoding an engineered AngII-fusion protein, in which AngII is made and processed intracellularly and released within a highly localized area of cardiac muscle, caused localized expression of ANF in the rat heart without systemic effects of AngII [100]. Cardiac myocyte-specific overexpression of the AT1a receptor under the control of the α-MHC promoter in the transgenic mouse caused massive atrial enlargement with myocyte hyperplasia at birth [101]. The disproportionate effect of the transgene on atrial enlargement without a clear ventricular phenotype is thought to be due to expression of α-MHC in the inflow tract of the developing heart. Thus, locally produced AngII can promote cardiac myocyte growth in the heart, probably independently of its haemodynamic effects. Signalling mechanisms activated by the AT1 receptor are capable of initiating cell growth responses in cardiac myocytes.

In cultured neonatal rat cardiac myocytes, exogenously applied AngII causes hypertrophy of cardiac myocytes and mitogenic responses of cardiac fibroblasts [102, 103]. The characteristic hypertrophic responses caused by AngII stimulation in neonatal rat cardiac myocytes are summarized as follows [71, 99, 102–109]:

- increase in the rate of protein synthesis without affecting the rate of protein degradation
- increase in the total protein content
- induction of immediate-early genes (c-*fos* c-*jun*, c-*myc*, *jun* B and *Egr*-1)
- induction of foetal type genes (ANF, skeletal α-actin, and β-MHC)
- sarcomeric reorganization of actin filament
- induction of growth factor genes (angiotensinogen, TGF-b1, endothelin-1)
- hyperplasia of cardiac fibroblasts
- induction of extracellular matrix (fibronectin, collagen I and collagen III)
- upregulation of integrin receptors (integrin β1)
- stimulation of apoptosis.

Importantly, the phenotypes of hypertrophy as well as the magnitude of the responses of cardiac myocytes to AngII are very similar, if not identical, to those to mechanical stretch, indicating that locally produced and secreted AngII is sufficient to cause cardiac hypertrophy *in vitro*. Using confocal microscopy, Liu *et al.* [110] demonstrated that AngII significantly increases the volume and protein content of adult rat ventricular myocytes, suggesting that adult cardiac myocytes also possess the AT1 receptor and undergo hypertrophy in response to AngII stimulation *in vitro*. It should be noted, however, that the hypertrophic effects of AngII on cardiac myocytes have been challenged by several investigators, who reported the lack of increased protein synthesis (hypertrophic effects) by AngII treatment either in cultured neonatal or in adult cardiac myocytes [111, 112]. Several possibilities may explain this discrepancy. First, the hypertrophic effect of AngII depends on the AT1 receptor density in cardiac myocytes. AngII exhibits stronger hypertrophic effects on cardiac myocytes isolated from the postinfarcted heart, which have a higher density of the AT1 receptor compared with normal myocytes [110]. Although the *in situ* reverse transcription–polymerase chain reaction has shown that mRNA of the AT1 receptor is present in cardiac myocytes in sections of the left ventricle [113], the density of the AT1 receptor in cardiac myocytes is reported to be lower than in cardiac fibroblasts [114, 115]. It is possible that expression of the AT1 receptor may be downregulated in some culture conditions. Secondly, AT2 receptor-mediated signalling has been shown to counteract the hypertrophic effects mediated by the AT1 receptor [116, 117]. The hypertrophic effects of AngII are less obvious when there are more AT2 receptors than AT1 receptors. The level of AT2 receptor expression in cultured cardiac myocytes seems variable among several reports [104, 114]. Thirdly, AngII stimulates either necrosis or apoptosis of cardiac myocytes through AT1 receptor-dependent mechanisms [118–120]. Although it is unclear how and when myocytes will undergo cell death instead of hypertrophy, these cell death mechanisms should negatively affect the hypertrophic effects of AngII. Fourthly, the ability of AngII to stimulate protein synthesis *in vitro* is less prominent compared with that of other Gq agonists, such as ET-1 and phenylephrine, although the magnitude of the cardiac hypertrophy caused by AngII more closely resembles that by mechanical stress *in vitro*. Thus, documenting such modest hypertrophic effects is sometimes difficult *in vitro*, where the net balance of protein synthesis is often negative (atrophic) in serum-free cultures [110]. Preliminary studies indicate that AngII causes less prominent activation of p38, a member of the MAP kinase family that has strong hypertrophic effects [121], compared with phenylephrine, while both AngII and phenylephrine strongly activate ERK (unpublished observation). Although it is generally assumed that agonists for the GqPCR activate similar downstream signalling molecules, such agonist-specific signalling mechanisms may explain the subtle difference in phenotypes of cardiac hypertrophy caused by various GqPCR agonists [85, 122, 123].

## Production of angiotensin II and existence of the local renin–angiotensin system in the heart

The heart expresses all components of the renin–angiotensin system (RAS) in both mRNA and proteins that allow local production of AngII [124, 125]. However, the level of angiotensinogen, renin, and ACE mRNA expression in the heart under control conditions is low compared with other organs and tissues, such as the kidney and vascular smooth muscle [126]. Although conflicting results have been reported as to whether cardiac myocytes can produce a significant amount of renin [124, 127], significant levels of renin do exist (whether made in the heart or taken up from the systemic circulation) and contribute to the local synthesis of AngII. Several lines of evidence support the notion that the heart apparently has the ability to produce AngII locally, and this is sufficient to work as an autocrine growth factor. First, using radiolabelled angiotensin infusions, it has been shown that AngII is produced at tissue sites by conversion of *in situ* synthesized rather than blood-derived AngI in pigs. Cardiac AngII production can be observed even when the production of cirulating AngII is effectively suppressed by captopril treatment [128]. Secondly, AngI and AngII levels of the interstitial fluid space of the heart are more than 100-fold higher than those of the plasma and are not affected by application of AngI or captopril in the systemic circulation. This suggests that AngII production in heart tissue is substantial and is mediated by different mechanisms between the interstitial and intravascular spaces. Since captopril is shown to enter the interstitial space and inhibit ACE, enzymes other than ACE, such as chymase, should be available in this space [129]. This observation potentially explains why cardiac myocytes secrete significant amounts of AngII in response to stretch, despite the fact that the basal mRNA expression of renin and ACE is low. Thirdly, various stresses, including mechanical stretch and ischaemia, cause upregulation of renin–angiotensin system genes, including angiotensinogen, renin, ACE, and AT1 receptor, in cultured cardiac myocytes *in vitro* [104], possibly leading to increased AngII production and higher sensitivity to AngII in cardiac myocytes under mechanical overload.

It has been shown that mechanical stretch of neonatal rat cardiac myocytes in serum-free culture caused a more than 100-fold increase in AngII concentrations in culture media (approximately 500 pM), peaking at 10 min [13]. Such stretch-induced secretion of AngII from neonatal rat cardiac myocytes has been subsequently confirmed by multiple investigators [61, 71, 130–132]. A 30-min stretch of cardiac myocytes did not change the activity of renin and ACE but significantly reduced the intracellular AngII content, suggesting that mechanical stretch causes secretion of preformed AngII rather than acutely stimulating *de novo* synthesis of AngII through the authentic

RAS. Alternatively, stretch may in part increase AngII synthesis by activating proteases (other than renin or ACE), which cleave the angiotensin precursor peptides. AngII was found to be stored at least in part in the secretory granule-like structure in ventricular myocytes [13]. It is likely that ventricular myocytes, like atrial myocytes, use the regulated type of secretion for stretch-induced secretion of AngII. It has been recently shown that ventricular myocytes possess the capacity for regulated secretion of ANF in response to ET or high KCl stimulation [133].

The signal transduction mechanism that causes stretch-induced secretion of AngII from cardiac myocytes is unknown. Mechanical stretch-induced growth factor secretion in some other cell systems showed a transient secretion, peaking at about 10–120 min [134], suggesting the presence of growth factor stores that are released acutely by mechanical stress. In atrial myocytes, stretch causes secretion of ANF from stretch-sensitive, rapidly depletable pools that consist of newly synthesized ANF [135]. Several possibilities can be considered as the mechanism of AngII secretion. First, mechanical stretch activates PKC, $Ca^{2+}$, and small GTP-binding proteins, such as Rab, or other signalling mechanisms, which in turn may stimulate growth factor secretion [136, 137]. Secondly, mechanical stress transiently causes an alteration in the sarcolemmal permeability that allows release of cytosolic growth factors, which has been shown in pacing-induced basic fibroblast growth factor (bFGF) release from adult rat ventricular cardiac myocytes [138]. Finally, membrane tension may directly regulate membrane traffic and stimulate exocytosis and secretion [18].

Several lines of *in vivo* evidence suggest that the cardiac RAS is upregulated chronically in load-induced hypertrophy. Messenger RNA expression of angiotensinogen, renin, ACE, and the AngII receptor is upregulated in cardiac hypertrophy caused by pressure overload and myocardial infarction *in vivo* [12, 139–143]. At the protein level, upregulation of ACE activity and AngII receptor binding were demonstrated [139, 140], and the percentage of myocytes containing renin. AngI, and AngII was significantly increased in hypertrophied hearts [141]. The upregulation of the cardiac RAS was also observed in the mechanical stretch of neonatal rat cardiac myocytes *in vitro* [104, 144]. Treatment of cultured cardiac myocytes with exogenous AngII also upregulates mRNA expression of angiotensinogen, renin, and ACE, but not the AngII receptor [102, 104]. This suggests that mechanical stretch initially causes acute secretion of AngII, and secreted AngII initiates a positive feedback mechanism, thereby upregulating the local RAS over a long period. Interestingly, however, AngII seems dispensable for upregulation of RAS system genes by mechanical stretch. Stretch-induced upregulation of mRNA of angiotensinogen, renin, and ACE in neonatal rat cardiac myocytes was observed even in the presence of AngII receptor antagonists. In dogs with chronic volume-overload hypertrophy, upregulation of the AT1 receptor mRNA was not prevented by normalization of the left ventricular AngII content by ACE inhibitor treatment [145]. It is therefore likely that upregulation of the AT1 receptor in volume overload is mediated by stretch-rather than AngII-mediated signalling mechanisms. Stretch-induced upregulation of the AT1 receptor in the neonatal rat cardiac myocyte is inhibited by the tyrosine kinase inhibitor genistein. Involvement of AP-1, GATA-4, and p53 transcription factors has been suggested for pressure overload- or mechanical stretch-induced upregulation of the RAS genes, such as angiotensinogen and the AT1 receptor [61, 67, 146]. Further investigations are required to demonstrate how mechanical stress regulates the expression of these genes via Ang II-independent mechanisms in cardiac myocytes.

Upregulation of the RAS genes by stretch seems to be cell-type specific. Stretch upregulates the RAS only in cardiac myocyte cultures, not in cardiac fibroblast cultures, despite the fact that cardiac fibroblasts express immediate-early genes, including c-*fos* and Egr-1, and prolifenate in response to stretch [104]. In support of this observation, both the intracellular $Ca^{2+}$ response to AngII and the AT1 receptor densities were elevated in cardiac myocytes, but not in cardiac fibroblasts, isolated from volume-overloaded rat hearts [147]. It has been shown that stretch causes secretion of AngII from cardiac myocytes but not from cardiac fibroblasts in culture [13]. Taken together, it is possible that some stretch-sensitive signalling mechanisms may be missing in fibroblasts. The above evidence does not exclude the role of cardiac fibroblasts in stretch-induced cell responses, however, since cardiac myocyte cultures used in *in vitro* experiments are not pure myocyte cultures. It is possible that both basal and stretch-induced secretion of 'paracrine' factors from the cardiac fibroblasts may modulate stretch-induced cell responses in cardiac myocytes. A possible role of ET-1 secreted from cardiac non-myocytes in modulating stretch-induced ANF/BNP production has been suggested recently [148].

The level of angiotensin receptor expression is affected by the presence of heart failure. Although expression of the AT1 receptor is upregulated in compensated left ventricular hypertrophy, it eventually decreases in the human decompensated ventricle with idiopathic dilated cardiomyopathy. In contrast, the level of the AT2 receptor is not affected significantly [113]. In a dog model of right ventricular hypertrophy and failure, mRNA expression of ACE and the AT2 receptor is upregulated, while that of chymase and the AT1 receptor is downregulated [149]. The resultant increases in the ratio of the AT2 to AT1 receptor may either inhibit cellular growth (myocyte hypertrophy) or promote apoptosis, thereby affecting the progression of heart failure. Recent *in vivo* data suggest that AT2 receptor-specific stimulation (in the presence of the AT1 receptor antagonist) has cardioprotective effects in rats with heart failure [150].

In summary, available evidence suggests that stretch efficiently stimulates the RAS in cardiac myocytes in multiple ways. First, mechanical stress causes acute secretion of AngII. Subsequently, both AngII and mechanical stress stimulate expression of the cardiac RAS genes through distinct mechanisms, thereby increasing chronic cardiac (local) production of AngII. Cardiac production of AngII initiates positive feedback mechanisms for enhanced AngII production. Stretch also stimulates expression of the AT1 receptor. Thus, stretch increases both production of AngII and the sensitivity of cardiac myocytes to AngII, thereby causing cardiac hypertrophy more efficiently than AngII alone in unstretched cardiac myocytes. As an example of increased sensitivity to AngII, it has been shown that the effect of AngII on impairing myocardial contraction and relaxation is enhanced in hypertrophic compared with normal myocardium [139].

## Angiotensin II-dependent and -independent mechanisms in stretch-induced activation of signalling molecules

AngII and stretch activate very similar sets of second messengers in neonatal rat cardiac myocytes *in vitro*. Since stretch causes secretion of AngII from neonatal rat cardiac myocytes, stretch-induced activation of second messengers could be mediated by AngII rather than by stretch itself. It has been shown that stretch-induced activation of ERK1/2 is markedly attenuated in the presence of the AT1 receptor antagonist [71]. Accumulation of inositol phosphates by elevated left ventricular pressure in the rat heart [151] and stretch-induced activation of the $Na^+/H^+$ exchanger in cat papillary muscle are abolished by AT1 receptor blockade [45]. These results indicate that AngII mediates stretch-induced activation of some second messengers.

Recent evidence suggests, however, that stretch-induced activation of several signalling molecules is mediated by both AngII-dependent and -independent mechanisms. These include JNKs [152], PKCE [151], and the JAK family of tyrosine kinases [75]. Since stretch-induced secretion of AngII peaks at 10 min, the activation of second messengers with earlier peaks could be directly stimulated by mechanical stress or mediated by stretch-induced secretion of other autocrine/paracrine factors. Identification of the AngII-independent components in stretch-induced cell signalling may potentially lead to elucidation of the mechanosensing as well as novel autocrine/paracrine mechanisms. Systematic examination of stretch-induced cell signaling in the presence of the AT1 blockade is essential to address this issue.

## Angiotensin II-dependent and -independent mechanisms in stretch-induced cardiac hypertrophy

Initial reports suggested that major hypertrophic responses caused by stretch have been effectively suppressed by the AT1 receptor antagonists in cultured neonatal rat cardiac myocytes [13]. However, accumulating evidence suggests that AngII does not mediate all of the hypertrophic responses in various animal models of cardiac hypertrophy both *in vivo* and *in vitro*. As discussed above, since stretch-induced activation of some second messengers occurs in an AngII-independent manner, hypertrophic responses predominantly mediated by those signalling molecules may also be AngII independent. Another important consideration is the availability of autocrine/paracrine growth factors as well as the abundance of their receptors in each hypertrophy model. Expression of autocrine/paracrine mechanisms is affected by various factors, such as age and species or strain of animal, type of mechanical stress, and cell culture conditions (cell density, types of extracellular matrix, culture medium, etc.). Finally, different types of mechanical stress may use different autocrine/paracrine factors or stimulate hypertrophy directly. For example, in rats with severe ascending aortic stenosis or pulmonary artery constriction, the AT1 receptor antagonist or ACE inhibitor failed to prevent or diminish cardiac hypertrophy [153, 154].

Among major hypertrophic responses commonly seen in various models of hypertrophy, stretch-induced c-*fos* immediate-early gene expression is consistently blocked in the presence of the AT1 receptor antagonist [13, 71, 111]. Since the c-*fos* gene is induced within 30 min of stretch, the factor (or factors) that is rapidly secreted by stretch mediates this response [6, 8]. This indicates that AngII may be the predominant factor, and is secreted in the early phase of stretch. The peak of stretch-induced secretion of AngII is observed around 10 min [13].

Wiesner *et al.* [155] compared β-MHC gene expression in rats with ascending and abdominal aortic stenosis. The left ventricular weight and peak systolic pressure were significantly elevated in both types of aortic stenosis compared with sham-operated animals. However, significant increases in β-MHC expression were observed only in rats with abdominal aortic coarctation, which is accompanied by significant increases in plasma renin. This indicates that mechanical stretch alone is not sufficient for expression of β-MHC mRNA and that other factors, including activation of the RAS, are required for development of a specific hypertrophic phenotype.

Mechanical stretch not only stimulates hypertrophy but also promotes apoptosis of adult cardiac myocytes *in vitro*. Stretch-induced apoptosis may cause substantial loss of cardiac myocytes and therefore has been suggested to play an important role in the development of congestive heart failure. Stretch-induced apoptosis is accompanied by phosphorylation and activation of p53, which in turn increases the Bax/Bcl-2 ratio as well as mRNA expression of angiotensinogen and the AT1 receptor. Stretch-induced apoptosis and transcriptional activation of p53 are mediated by the AT1 receptor-dependent mechanism [61]. Thus, stretch seems to initiate a positive feedback loop, which consists of secretion of AngII, activation of p53, and upregulation of RAS genes.

Other aspects of stretch-induced hypertrophy may be mediated by both AngII and other mechanisms. Kent and McDermott [111] reported that stretch-induced increases in protein synthesis and expression of the $Na^+/Ca^{2+}$ exchanger in adult cardiac myocytes are not affected by the non-selective AngII receptor antagonist [$Sar^1$, $Ile^8$] AngII. Stretch-induced expression of c-*fos* was completely abolished by [$Sar^1$, $Ile^8$] AngII in the same preparation, suggesting that AngII plays only a limited role in the stretch-induced hypertrophy of adult cardiac myocytes. It should be noted, however, that these experiments were conducted in a condition of low cell density and the authors did not detect increases in protein synthesis in response to AngII stimulation. Thus, the possibility exists that the results reflect the difference in the level of the AT1 receptor expression, rather than the difference in the signalling mechanisms of hypertrophy between adult and neonatal cardiac myocytes. ANF secretion in response to acute volume overload in conscious rats is more effectively suppressed by inhibition of the ET A/B receptor than by the AT1 receptor. Combined inhibition of the ETA/B and AT1 receptors completely blocks the ANF response to acute volume overload, suggesting the predominant role of the autocrine/paracrine factors, especially of ET1, in stretch-induced secretion of ANF [156]. ETA/B or AT1 receptor blockade suppresses stretch-induced BNP production by no more than 50–60% in neonatal rat cardiac myocytes *in vitro*. The rest may be mediated independently of autocrine/paracrine activity [132].

## Pressure overload causes cardiac hypertrophy in AT1a receptor knockout mice

Whether the AT1 receptor is essential for load-induced cardiac hypertrophy was tested using the AT1a receptor knockout mouse. Coarctation of the abdominal aorta in these mice caused increases in the left ventricle/body weight ratio, a hallmark of cardiac hypertrophy, and increased gene expression, including c-*fos* and BNP [157]. The results suggest that AngII-independent mechanisms mediate load-induced cardiac hypertrophy in the absence of the AT1a receptor. Several theories may explain the apparent discrepancies between this observation and previous observations, which suggest an essential role for AngII in load-induced hypertrophy *in vivo*. First, since two distinct genes (AT1a and AT1b receptors) encode the AT1 receptor in the rodent, the AT1b receptor still exists in AT1a receptor knockout mice, where it plays an important role in maintaining the blood pressure [158]. Since expression of the AT1 receptor in cardiac myocytes is upregulated on stretch, the level of expression of the AT1b receptor after abdominal coarctation in AT1a knockout mice remains to be determined. In addition, AT1a receptor knockout mice have markedly elevated plasma renin levels due to liberation from the negative feedback by the AT1 receptor, suggesting that the RAS is stimulated in this model [159]. This involvement cannot be completely eliminated in this animal model. Secondly, some compensatory mechanisms are clearly activated in AT1a knockout mice. It has been shown that ERK activity is elevated both in control and stretched cardiac myocytes obtained from AT1a knockout mice [157]. Hyperactivation of ERK in both control and stretched myocytes has also been reported in angiotensinogen knockout mice [160]. Although the mechanism of increased ERK in these animals is unknown, it is possible that some growth factors are upregulated to compensate for the loss of AngII signals. Stretch-induced activation of ERK is abolished by losartan in cardiac myocytes obtained from control mice but not from angiotensinogen knockout mice [160]. If any non-specific effects of losartan inhibit ERK activity, such inhibition should have been observed in myocytes obtained from angiotensinogen knockout mice. These results indicate that compensatory mechanisms are activated in the knockout mice. To overcome these problems and correctly determine the role of AngII in stretch-induced cardiac hypertrophy, conditional knockout of both AT1a and AT1b receptors or angiotensinogen seems necessary. Regardless of these limitations, however, the results of knockout studies indicate that the heart can prepare alternative (AngII-independent) mechanisms that convert mechanical stretch into hypertrophic responses under certain conditions.

### Interaction among growth factors

The expression and secretion of one growth factor is affected by that of other growth factors. Thus, secretion of one growth factor by mechanical stress upregulates another growth factor, which may further affect expression of many other growth factors. For example, stretch-induced upregulation of VEGF is mediated at least in part by TGF-β [72]. AngII upregulates mRNA expression of various growth fac tors, such as TGF-$\beta_1$, PDGF, BFGF, ET-1, and insulin-like growth factor, in the heart and vascular smooth muscle [161–164]. AngII and other growth factors, such as PDGF and ET-1, potentiate each other's growth-promoting effects [96]. Accumulating evidence suggests that ET-1 mediates many AngII-induced cardiovascular responses [67, 163]. For example, the ET type A receptor antagonist diminishes the hypertensive response to AngII [165]. The receptor antagonist for ET-1 blocks AngII-induced activation of the $Na^+/H^+$ exchanger and the hBNP promoter. ET-1-induced activation of $Na^+/H^+$ exchanger and hBNP was not inhibited by losartan [45, 132], suggesting that the effect of AngII can be mediated by ET-1, but the reverse is unlikely. Stretch-induced activation of the $Na^+/H^+$ exchanger and hBNP is blocked by receptor antagonists for AngII and ET-1 [45, 132]. Stretch-induced activation of the preproendothelin-1 gene is mediated by AngII-dependent mechanisms [132]. Stretch causes secretion of ET-1 from neonatal rat cardiac myocytes, and the secreted ET-1, even at very low concentrations, potentiates AngII-induced Raf-1 and ERK activation [96]. Recently, a novel single membrane-spanning receptor with both ET-1- and AngII-specific binding has been cloned. This receptor is expressed abundantly in the heart [166]. Although its functional significance is unknown, the existence of such a receptor may explain the molecular link between AngII and ET-1. Thus, AngII may commonly use ET to mediate some of its effects. It is likely that cardiac myocytes use these hierarchical and/or synergistic interactions among growth factors to co-ordinate finely stimulus-specific phenotypes of cardiac hypertrophy. Although AngII seems to be a primary mediator of stretch-induced hypertrophy in neonatal rat cardiac myocytes, other growth factors, the expression of which is modulated by AngII, may in concert mediate such hypertrophy (Fig. 9.2).

## Future directions

The recent progress made in defining the key steps of the signalling mechanism of load-induced cardiac hypertrophy has been described here. Although the involvement of autocrine/paracrine factors, including AngII and ET-1, has become more evident during the past few years, many questions remain unanswered in each step of the cell signalling process in load-induced cardiac hypertrophy. For example, whether or not distinct growth factors are produced in response to different types of mechanical stress, such as pressure overload, volume overload, and cardiac dysfunction due to myocardial infarction, is still unknown. Development of *in vitro* models that can precisely reproduce defined mechanical stresses is required to determine how different types of mechanical stresses cause the secretion and production of distinct signalling molecules. Since signalling molecules directly activated by mechanical forces may cause secretion and production of growth factors or directly contribute to formation of different hypertrophic phenotypes, identification of mechanosensitive molecules for each mechanical stress is important. Since the mechanism of hypertrophy is affected by the availability of the autocrine/paracrine factors and their receptors in the myocardium, the contribution of distinct growth factors must be determined in each type of load-induced

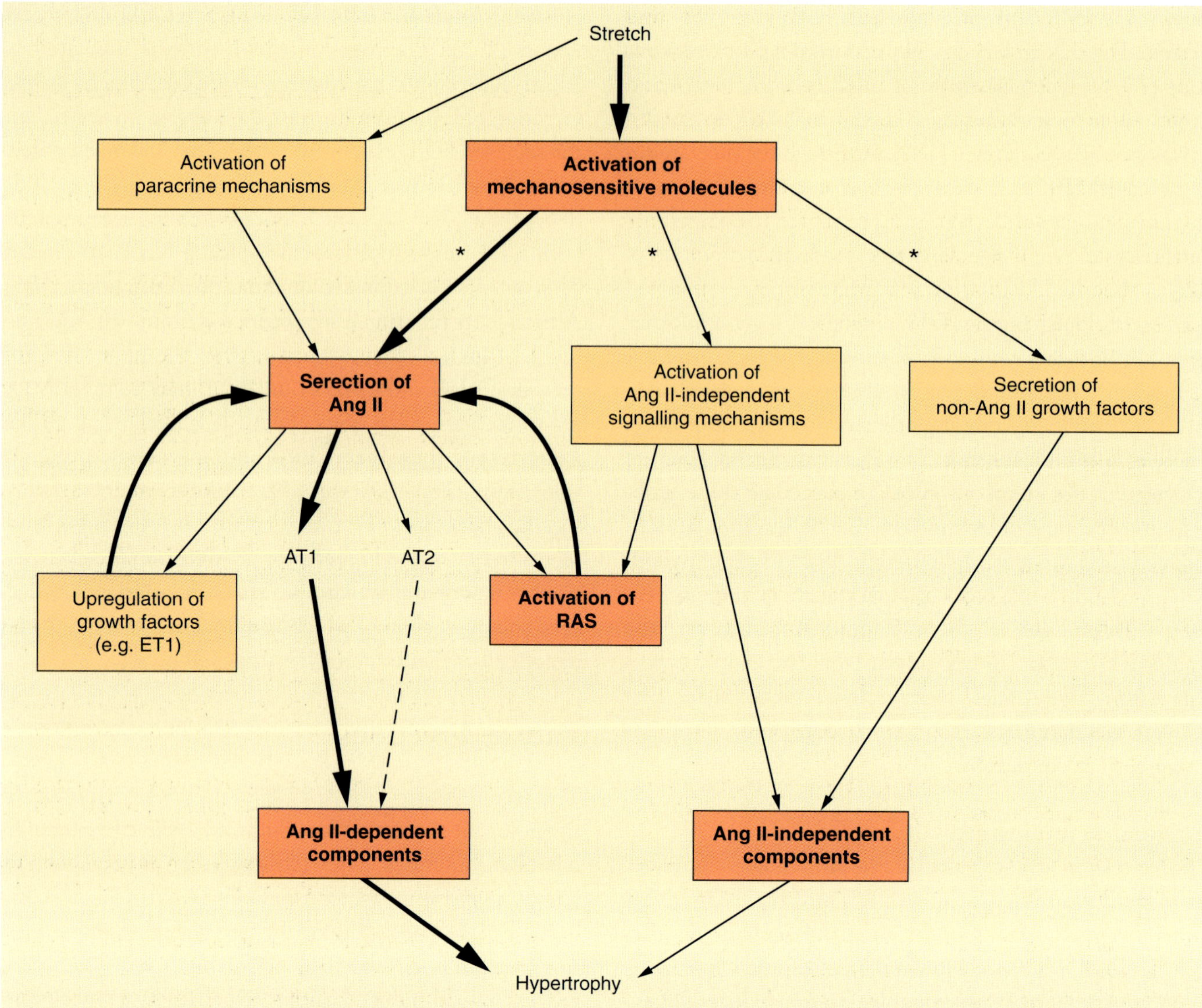


**Figure 9.2** *Current hypothesis of stretch-induced cardiac hypertrophy. Ang II: angiotensin II; RAS: renin angiotensin system; AT1: angiotensin II type I receptor; AT2: angiotensin II type II receptor. Thick lines indicate predominant signalling mechanisms in stretch-induced hypertrophy in cultured neonatal rat cardiac myocytes. Dashed line may be inhibitory. *Contribution of these three components may be affected by experimental conditions, including animal species, ages, types of mechanical stresses, etc.)*

hypertrophy, especially in humans. After growth factors activated by the defined mechanical stress have been identified, the cell signalling mechanism and the phenotype of hypertrophy must be characterized in detail. Although studies have focused on the qualitative aspects of cardiac hypertrophy thus far, they have not characterized its quantitative aspects or the long-term effects of each hypertrophic response. Careful comparison of the cardiac phenotype among different types of cardiac hypertrophy will clarify the feature of each hypertrophic stimulus and provide clues as to how a specific phenotype of cardiac hypertrophy can be modified. Although the signalling mechanism activated by growth factors was not discussed in this review, identification of the role of each signalling molecule in the development of the specific hypertrophic phenotype is also important. Targeted alteration of the activity of the signalling molecule is perhaps another way to modify an undesired phenotype of cardiac hypertrophy. Such alteration would change the natural history of cardiac hypertrophy and prevent the development of congestive heart failure. Finally, it is also important to identify the cell signal that causes or prevents cardiac dysfunction and cardiac myocyte death in response to growth factor stimulation. For example, AngII causes both hypertrophy and apoptosis of cardiac myocytes, but it is unknown whether these apparently opposite phenomena are sequential (hypertrophy leading to apoptosis) or independent events. It is important to identify the signalling mechanism responsible for these events. Further studies using *in vitro* culture systems with efficient gene expression as well as *in vivo* transgenic animals with conditional gene regulation will be required to address these issues.

## References


1. Ingber DE, Dike L, Hansen *et al.* Cellular tensegrity: exploring how mechanical changes in the cytoskeleton regulate cell growth, migration, and tissue pattern during morphogenesis. *Int Rev Cytol* 1994; 150: 173–224.
2. Vandenburgh HH. Mechanical forces and their second messengers in stimulating cell growth *in vitro*. *Am J Physiol* 1992; 262: R350–5.
3. Sadoshima J, Izumo S. The cellular and molecular response of myocytes to mechanical stress. *Annu Rev Physiol* 1997; 59: 551–71.
4. Morgan HE, Baker KM. Cardiac hypertrophy. *Circulation* 1991; 83: 13–25.
5. Vandenburgh HH, Kaufman S. *In vitro* model for stretch-induced hypertrophy of skeletal muscle. *Science* 1979; 203: 265–8.
6. Komuro I, Kaida T, Shibazaki Y *et al.* Stretching cardiac myocytes stimulates protooncogene expression. *J Biol Chem* 1990; 265: 3595–8.
7. Mann DL, Kent RL, Cooper G IV. Load regulation of the properties of adult feline cardiocytes: growth induction by cellular deformation. *Circ Res* 1989; 64: 1079–90.
8. Sadoshima J, Jahn L, Takahashi T, Kulik TJ, Izumo S. Molecular characterization of the stretch-induced adaptation of cultured cardiac cells: an *in vitro* model of load-induced cardiac hypertrophy. *J Biol Chem* 1992; 267: 10 551–60.
9. Izumo S, Nadal-Ginard B, Mahdavi V. Protooncogene induction and reprogramming of cardiac gene expression produced by pressure overload. *Proc Natl Acad Sci USA* 1988; 85: 339–43.
10. Sadoshima J, Izumo S. Mechanical stretch rapidly activates multiple signal transduction pathways in cardiac myocytes: potential involvement of an autorine/paracrine mechanism. *EMBO J* 1993; 12: 1681–92.
11. Yamazaki T, Tobe K, Hoh E *et al.* Mechanical loading activates mitogen-activated protein kinase and S6 peptide kinase in cultured rat cardiac myocytes. *J Biol Chem* 1993; 268: 12 069–76.
12. Baker KM, Booz GW, Dostal DE. Cardiac actions of angiotensin II: role of an intracardiac renin–angiotensin system. *Annu Rev Physiol* 1992; 54: 227–41.
13. Sadoshima J, Xu Y, Slayter HS, Izumo S. Autocrine release of angiotensin II mediates stretch-induced hypertrophy of cardiac myocytes *in vitro*. *Cell* 1993; 75: 977–84.
14. Chien KR, Zhu H, Knowlton KU *et al.* Transcriptional regulation during cardiac growth and development. *Annu Rev Physiol* 1993; 55: 77–95.
15. Komuro I, Yazaki Y. Control of cardiac gene expression by mechanical stress. *Annu Rev Physiol* 1993; 55: 55–75.
16. MacLellan WR, Schneider MD. Success in failure: modeling cardiac decompensation in transgenic mice (Editorial; Comment). *Circulation* 1998; 97: 1433–5.
17. Huxley AF, Simmons RM. Proposed mechanism of force generation in striated muscle. *Nature* 1971; 233: 533–8.
18. Sheetz MP, Dai J. Modulation of membrane dynamics and cell motility by membrane tension. *Trends Cell Biol* 1996; 6: 85–9.
19. Gudi SR, Lee AA, Clark CB, Frangos JA. Equibiaxial strain and strain rate stimulate early activation of G proteins in cardiac fibroblasts. *Am J Physiol* 1998; 274: C1424–8.
20. Hilal-Dandan R, Brunton LL. Transmembrane mechanochemical coupling in cardiac myocytes: novel activation of Gi by hyposmotic swelling. *Am J Physiol* 1995; 269: H798–804.
21. Vandenburgh HH, Shansky J, Solerssi R, Chromiak J. Mechanical stimulation of skeletal muscle increases prostaglandin F2 alpha production, cyclooxygenase activity, and cell growth by a pertussis toxin sensitive mechanism. *J Cell Physiol* 1995; 163: 285–94.
22. Gudi S, Nolan JP, Frangos JA. Modulation of GTPase activity of G proteins by fluid shear stress and phospholipid composition. *Proc Natl Acad Sci USA* 1998; 95: 2515–9.
23. Parsons JT. Integrin-mediated signalling: regulation by tyrosine kinases and small GTP-binding proteins. *Curr Opin Cell Biol* 1996; 8: 146–52.
24. Simpson DG, Terracio L, Terracio M *et al.* Modulation of cardiac myocyte phenotype *in vitro* by the composition and orientation of the extracellular matrix. *J Cell Physiol* 1994; 161: 89–105.
25. Baldwin HS, Buck CA. Integrins and other cell adhesion molecules in cardiac development. *Trends Cardiovasc Med* 1994; 4: 178–87.
26. Schwartz MA, Schaller MD, Ginsberg MH. Integrins: emerging paradigms of signal transduction. *Annu Rev Cell Dev Biol* 1995; 11: 549–99.
27. Wang N, Butler JP, Ingber DE. Mechanotransduction across the cell surface and through the cytoskeleton. *Science* 1993; 260: 1124–7.
28. Chen CS, Mrksich M, Huang S *et al.* Geometric control of cell life and death. *Science* 1997; 276: 1425–8.
29. Zhong C, Chrzanowska-Wodnicka M, Brown J *et al.* Rho-mediated contractility exposes a cryptic site in fibronectin and induces fibronectin matrix assembly. *J Cell Biol* 1998; 141: 539–51.
30. Pardo JV, Silicano JD, Craig SW. A vinculin-containing cortical lattice in skeletal muscle: transverse lattice element (costameres) mark sites of attachment between myofibrils and sarcolemma. *Proc Natl Acad Sci USA* 1983; 80: 1008–12.
31. Danowski BA, Imanaka-Yoshida K, Sanger JM, Sanger JW. Costameres are sites of force transmission to the substratum in adult rat cardiomyocytes. *J Cell Biol* 1992; 118: 1411–20.
32. Sadoshima J, Izumo S. Roles of integrins in cell swelling-induced tyrosine phosphorylation in cardiac myocytes (Abstract). *Circulation* 1994; 90: I-305.
33. MacKenna DA, Dolfi F, Vuori K, Ruoslahti E. Extracellular signal-regulated kinase and c-Jun $NH_2$-terminal kinase activation by mechanical stretch is integrin-dependent and matrix-specific in rat cardiac fibroblasts. *J Clin Invest* 1998; 101: 301–10.
34. Sharp WW, Simpson DG, Borg TK *et al.* Mechanical forces regulate focal adhesion and costamere assembly in cardiac myocytes. *Am J Physiol* 1997; 273: H546–56.
35. Ross RS, Pham C, Shai SY *et al.* Beta 1 integrins participate in the hypertrophic response of rat ventricular myocytes. *Circ Res* 1998; 82: 1160–72.

36. Sadoshima J, Takahashi T, Jahn L, Izumo S. Roles of mechanosensitive ion channels, cytoskeleton, and contractile activity in stretch-induced immediate-early gene expression and hypertrophy of cardiac myocytes. *Proc Natl Acad Sci USA* 1992; 89: 9905–9.
37. Lerman BB, Burkhoff D, Yue DT *et al.* Mechanoelectrical feedback: independent role of preload and contractility in modulation of canine ventricular excitability. *J Clin Invest* 1985; 76: 1843–50.
38. Ruknudin A, Sachs F, Bustamante JO. Stretch-activated ion channels in tissue-cultured chick heart. *Am J Physiol* 1993; 264: H960–72.
39. Sigurdson W, Ruknudin A, Sachs F. Calcium imaging of mechanically induced fluxes in tissue-cultured chick heart: role of stretch-activated ion channels. *Am J Physiol* 1992; 262: H1110–15.
40. Van Wagoner DR. Mechanosensitive gating of atrial ATP-sensitive potassium channels. *Circ Res* 1993; 72: 973–83.
41. Sasaki N, Mitsuiye T, Noma A. Effects of mechanical stretch on membrane currents of single ventricular myocytes of guinea-pig heart. *Jpn J Physiol* 1992; 42: 957–70.
42. Hagiwara N, Masuda H, Shoda M, Irisawa H. Stretch-activated anion currents of rabbit cardiac myocytes. *J Physiol* 1992; 456: 285–302.
43. Matsuda N, Hagiwara N, Shoda M *et al.* Enhancement of the L-tpe $Ca^{2+}$ current by mechanical stimulation in single rabbit cardiac myocytes. *Circ Res* 1996; 78: 650–9.
44. Sasaki N, Mitsuiye T, Wang Z, Noma A. Increase of the delayed rectifier $K^+$ and $Na(^+)$-$K^+$ pump currents by hypotonic solutions in guinea pig cardiac myocytes. *Circ Res* 1994; 75: 887–95.
45. Cingolani HE, Alvarez BV, Ennis IL, Camilion de Hurtado MC. Stretch-induced alkalinization of feline papillary muscle: an autocrine–paracrine system. *Circ Res* 1998; 83: 775–80.
46. Tung L, Zou S. Influence of stretch on excitation threshold of single frog ventricular cells. *Exp Physiol* 1995; 80: 221–35.
47. Clemo HF, Stambler BS, Baumgarten CM. Persistent activation of a swelling-activated cation current in ventricular myocytes from dogs with tachycardia-induced congestive heart failure. *Circ Res* 1998; 83: 147–57.
48. Hamill OP, McBride D Jr. The cloning of a mechano-gated membrane ion channel. *Trends Neurosci* 1994; 17: 439–43.
49. Sokabe M, Sachs F. Towards molecular mechanism of activation in mechanosensitive ion channels. In: *Advances in comp. env. physiology*. Volume 10. Berlin: Springer, 1992, 55–77.
50. Lansman JB, Hallam TJ, Rink TJ. Single stretch-activated ion channels in vascular endothelial cells as mechanotransducers? *Nature* 1987; 325: 811–13.
51. Awayda MS, Ismailov II, Berdiev BK, Benos DJ. A cloned renal epithelial $Na^+$ channel protein displays stretch activation in planar lipid bilayers. *Am J Physiol* 1995; 268: C1450–9.
52. Ordway RW, Petrou S, Kirber MT *et al.* Stretch activation of a toad smooth muscle $K^+$ channel may be mediated by fatty acids. *J Physiol* 1995; 484: 331–7.
53. Kernan M, Zuker C. Genetic approaches to mechanosensory transduction. *Curr Opin Neurobiol* 1995; 5: 443–8.
54. Sadoshima J, Qiu Z, Morgan JP, Izumo S. Tyrosine kinase activation is an immediate and essential step in hypotonic cell swelling-induced ERK activation and c-*fos* gene expression in cardiac myocytes. *EMBO J* 1996; 15: 5535–46.
55. Sadoshima J, Izumo S. Cell swelling rapidly activates src tyrosine kinase, a potential transducer of mechanical stress in cardiac myocytes. *Circulation* 1996; 94: I-409.
56. Kuppuswamy D, Kerr C, Narishige T *et al.* Association of tyrosine-phosphorylated c-Src with the cytoskeleton of hypertrophying myocardium. *J Biol Chem* 1997; 272: 4500–8.
57. Kijima K, Matsubara H, Murasawa S *et al.* Mechanical stretch induces enhanced expression of angiotensin II receptor subtypes in neonatal rat cardiac myocytes. *Circ Res* 1996; 79: 887–97.
58. Sorota S. Tyrosine protein kinase inhibitors prevent activation of cardiac swelling-induced chloride current. *Pflugers Arch Eur J Physiol* 1995; 431: 178–85.
59. Sawada Y, Suda M, Yokoyama H *et al.* Stretch-induced hypertrophic growth of cardiocytes and processing of brain-type natriuretic peptide are controlled by proprotein-processing endoprotease furin. *J Biol Chem* 1997; 272: 20 545–54.
60. Tyagi SC, Lewis K, Pikes D *et al.* Stretch-induced membrane type matrix metalloproteinase and tissue plasminogen activator in cardiac fibroblast cells. *J Cell Physiol* 1998; 176: 374–82.
61. Leri A, Claudio PP, Li Q *et al.* Stretch-mediated release of angiotensin II induces myocyte apoptosis by activating p53 that enhances the local renin–angiotensin system and decreases the Bcl-2-to-Bax protein ratio in the cell. *J Clin Invest* 1998; 101: 1326–42.
62. Samarel AM, Spragia LS, Maloney V *et al.* Contractile arrest accelerates myosin heavy chain degradation in neonatal rat heart cells. *Am J Physiol* 1992; 263: C642–52.
63. Knowlton KU, Rockman HA, Itani M *et al.* Divergent pathways mediate the induction of ANF transgenes in neonatal and hypertrophic ventricular myocardium. *J Clin Invest* 1995; 96: 1311–18.
64. Aoyagi T, Izumo S. Mapping of the pressure response element of the c-*fos* gene by direct DNA injection into beating hearts. *J Biol Chem* 1993; 268: 27 176–9.
65. Von Harsdorf R, Edwards JG, Shen Y-T *et al.* Identification of a *cis*-acting regulatory element conferring inducibility of the atrial natriuretic factor gene in acute pressure overload. *J Clin Invest* 1997; 100: 1294–304.
66. Hasegawa S, Sato S, Sato S *et al.* Mechanical stretching increases the number of cultured bone cells synthetizing DNA and alters their pattern of protein synthesis. *Calcif Tissue Int* 1985; 37: 431–6.
67. Herzig TC, Jobe SM, Aoki H *et al.* Angiotensin II $type_{1a}$ receptor gene expression in the heart: AP-1 and GATA-4 participate in the response to pressure overload. *Proc Natl Acad Sci USA* 1997; 94: 7543–8.
68. Vandenburgh HH, Shansky J, Karlisch P, Solerssi RL. Mechanical stimulation of skeletal muscle generates lipid-related second messengers by phospholipase activation. *J Cell Physiol* 1993; 155: 63–71.
69. Yamazaki T, Komuro I, Kudoh S *et al.* Mechanical stress activates protein kinase cascade of phosphorylation in neonatal rat cardiac myocytes. *J Clin Invest* 1995; 96: 438–46.
70. Rozengurt E. Neuropeptides as cellular growth factors: role of multiple signaling pathways. *Eur J Clin Invest* 1991; 21: 123–34.
71. Yamazaki T, Komuro I, Kudoh S *et al.* Angiotensin II partly mediates mechanical stress-induced cardiac hypertrophy. *Circ Res* 1995; 77: 258–65.
72. Li J, Hampton T, Morgan JP, Simons M. Stretch-induced VEGF expression in the heart. *J Clin Invest* 1997; 100: 18–24.
73. Wollert KC, Taga T, Saito M *et al.* Cardiotrophin-1 activates a distinct form of cardiac muscle cell hypertrophy. *J Biol Chem* 1996; 271: 9535–45.
74. Nyui N, Tanura K, Mizuno K *et al.* gp130 is involved in stretch-induced MAP kinase activation in cardiac myocytes. *Biochem Biophys Res Commun* 1998; 245: 928–32.

75. Pan J, Fukuda K, Kodama H *et al.* Role of angiotensin II in activation of the JAK/STAT pathway induced by acute pressure overload in the rat heart. *Circ Res* 1997; 81: 611–7.
76. Shioi T, Matsumori A, Kihara Y *et al.* Increased expression of interleukin-1 beta and monocyte chemotactic and activating factor/monocyte chemoattractant protein-1 in the hypertrophied and failing heart with pressure overload. *Circ Res* 1997; 81: 664–71.
77. Offermanns S, Zhao L-P, Gohla *et al.* Embryonic cardiomyocyte hypoplasia and craniofacial defects in Gαq/Gq11-mutant mice. *EMBO J* 1998; 17: 4304–12.
78. Akhter SA, Luttrell LM, Rockman HA *et al.* Targeting the receptor-Gq interface to inhibit *in vivo* pressure overload myocardial hypertrophy. *Science* 1998; 280: 574–7.
79. LaMorte VJ, Thorburn J, Absher D *et al.* Gq- and ras-dependent pathways mediate hypertrophy of neonatal rat ventricular myocytes following alpha 1-adrenergic stimulation. *J Biol Chem* 1994; 269: 13 490–6.
80. D'Angelo DD, Sakata Y, Lorenz JN *et al.* Transgenic Gαq overexpression induces cardiac contractile failure in mice. *Proc Natl Acad Sci USA* 1997; 94: 8121–6.
81. Sakata Y, Hoit BD, Liggett SB *et al.* Decompensation of pressure overload hypertrophy in Gαq-overexpressing mice. *Circulation* 1998; 97: 1488–96.
82. Hunter JJ, Tanaka N, Rockman HA *et al.* Ventricular expression of a MLC-2v-ras fusion gene induces cardiac hypertrophy and selective diastolic dysfunction in transgenic mice. *J Biol Chem* 1995; 270: 23 173–8.
83. Molkentin JD, Lu J-R, Antons CL *et al.* A calcineurin-dependent transcriptional pathway for cardiac hypertrophy. *Cell* 1998; 93: 215–28.
84. Wakasaki H, Koya D, Schoen FJ *et al.* Targeted overexpression of protein kinase C β2 isoform in myocardium causes cardiomyopathy. *Proc Natl Acad Sci USA* 1997; 94: 9320–5.
85. Sadoshima J. Versatility of the AT1 receptor. *Circ Res* 1998; 82: 1352–5.
86. Sadoshima J, Aoki H, Izumo S. Angiotensin II and serum differentially regulate expression of cyclin-dependent kinases and phosphorylation of pRb in neonatal cardiac myocytes. *Circ Res* 1997; 80: 228–41.
87. Baker KM, Chernin MI, Wixson SK, Aceto JF. Renin–angiotensin system involvement in pressure-overload cardiac hypertrophy in rats. *Am J Physiol* 1990; 259: H324–32.
88. Bruckschlegel G, Holmer SR, Jandeleit K *et al.* Blockade of the renin–angiotensin system in cardiac pressure-overload hypertrophy in rats. *Hypertension* 1995; 25: 250–9.
89. Kojima M, Shiojima I, Yamazaki T *et al.* Angiotensin II receptor antagonist TCV-116 induces regression of hypertensive left ventricular hypertrophy *in vivo* and inhibits the intracellular signaling pathway of stretch-mediated cardiomyocyte hypertrophy *in vitro*. *Circulation* 1994; 89: 2204–11.
90. Regan CP, Anderson PG, Bishop SP, Berecek KH. Pressure-independent effects of AT1-receptor antagonism on cardiovascular remodeling in aortic-banded rats. *Am J Physiol* 1997; 272: H2131–8.
91. Weinberg EO, Schoen FJ, George D *et al.* Angiotensin-converting enzyme inhibition prolongs survival and modifies the transition to heart failure in rats with pressure overload hypertrophy due to ascending aortic stenosis. *Circulation* 1994; 90: 1410–22.
92. Ruzicka M, Leenen FH. Relevance of blockade of cardiac and circulatory angiotensin-converting enzyme for the prevention of volume overload-induced cardiac hypertrophy. *Circulation* 1995; 91: 16–9.
93. Pfeffer JM, Fischer TA, Pfeffer MA. Angiotensin-converting enzyme inhibition and ventricular remodeling after myocardial infarction. *Annu Rev Physiol* 1995; 57: 805–26.
94. Schiefer B, Wirger A, Meybrunn M *et al.* Comparative effects of chronic angiotensin-converting enzyme inhibition and angiotensin II type I receptor blockade on cardiac remodeling after myocardial infarction in the rat. *Circulation* 1994; 89: 2273–82.
95. Pitt B, Segal R, Martinez FA *et al.* Randomised trial of losartan versus captopril in patient over 65 with heart failure. *Lancet* 1997; 349: 747–52.
96. Yamazaki T, Komuro I, Kudoh S *et al.* Endothelin-1 is involved in mechanical stress-induced cardiomyocyte hypertrophy. *J Biol Chem* 1996; 271: 3221–8.
97. Dostal DE, Baker KM. Angiotensin II stimulation of left ventricular hypertrophy in adult rat heart. Mediation by the AT1 receptor. *Am J Hypertens* 1992; 5: 276–80.
98. Schunkert H, Sadoshima J, Cornelius T *et al.* Angiotensin II-induced growth responses in isolated adult rat hearts. Evidence for load-independent induction of cardiac protein synthesis by angiotensin II. *Circ Res* 1995; 76: 489–97.
99. Kim S, Ohta K, Hamaguchi A *et al.* Angiotensin II induces cardiac phenotypic modulation and remodeling *in vivo* in rats. *Hypertension* 1995; 25: 1252–9.
100. Methot D, LaPointe MC, Touyz RM *et al.* Tissue targetting of angiotensin peptides. *J Biol Chem* 1997; 272: 12 994–9.
101. Hein L, Stevens M, Barsh G *et al.* Overexpression of angiotensin AT1 receptor transgene in the mouse myocardium produces a lethal phenotype associated with myocyte hyperplasia and heart block. *Proc Natl Acad Sci USA* 1997; 94: 6391–6.
102. Sadoshima J, Izumo S. Molecular characterization of angiotensin II-induced hypertrophy of cardiac myocytes and hyperplasia of cardiac fibroblasts. A critical role of the AT1 receptor subtype. *Circ Res* 1993; 73: 413–23.
103. Schorb W, Booz GW, Dostal DE *et al.* Angiotensin II is mitogenic in neonatal rat cardiac fibroblasts. *Circ Res* 1993; 72: 1245–54.
104. Malhotra R, Sadoshima J, Izumo S. Mechanical stretch upregulates expression of the local renin–angiotensin system genes in cardiac myocytes *in vitro* (Abstract). *Circulation* 1994; 90: I-195.
105. Sadoshima J, Izumo S. Rapamycin selectively inhibits angiotensin II-induced increase in protein synthesis in cardiac myocytes *in vitro*; a potential role of 70kDa S6 kinase. *Circ Res* 1995; 77: 1040–52.
106. Aoki H, Richmond M, Izumo S, Sadoshima J. The role of extracellular signal-regulated kinase pathway in angiotensin II-induced cardiac hypertrophy in cardiac myocytes *in vitro*. 1998; Submitted.
107. Aoki H, Izumo S, Sadoshima J. Angiotensin II activates RhoA in cardiac myocytes: a critical role of RhoA in angiotensin II-induced premyofibril formation. *Circ Res* 1998; 81: 666–76.
108. Baker KM, Aceto JF. Angiotensin II stimulation of protein synthesis and cell growth in chick heart cells. *Am J Physiol* 1990; 259: H610–18.
109. Burgess ML, Carver WE, Terracio L *et al.* Integrin-mediated collagen gel contraction by cardiac fibroblasts. Effects of angiotensin II. *Circ Res* 1994; 74: 291–8.
110. Liu Y, Leri A, Li B *et al.* Angiotensin II stimulation *in vitro* induces hypertrophy of normal and postinfarcted ventricular myocytes. *Circ Res* 1998; 82: 1145–59.

111. Kent RL, McDermott PJ. Passive load and angiotensin II evoke differential responses of gene expression and protein synthesis in cardiac myocytes. *Circ Res* 1996; 78: 829–38.
112. Pennica D, King KL, Shaw KJ *et al.* Expression cloning of cardiotrophin 1, a cytokine that induces cardiac myocyte hypertrophy. *Proc Natl Acad Sci USA* 1995; 92: 1142–6.
113. Asano K, Dutcher DL, Port JD *et al.* Selective downregulation of the angiotensin II AT1 receptor subtype in failing human ventricular myocardium. *Circulation* 1997; 95: 1193–200.
114. Matsubara H, Kanasaki M, Murasawa S *et al.* Differential gene expression and regulation of angiotensin II receptor subtypes in rat cardiac fibroblasts and cardiomyocytes in culture. *J Clin Invest* 1994; 93: 1592–601.
115. Villarreal FJ, Kim NN, Ungab GD *et al.* Identification of functional angiotensin II receptors on rat cardiac fibroblasts. *Circulation* 1993; 88: 2849–61.
116. Booz GW, Baker KM. Role of type 1 and type 2 angiotensin receptors in angiotensin II-induced cardiomyocyte hypertrophy. *Hypertension* 1996; 28: 635–40.
117. Hayashida W, Horiuchi M, Grandchamp J, Dzau VJ. Antagonistic actions of angiotensin type-1 and type-2 receptors on apoptosis in cultured neonatal rat ventricular myocytes. *Hypertension* 1996; 28: 535.
118. Tan LB, Jalil JE, Pick R *et al.* Cardiac myocyte necrosis induced by angiotensin II. *Circ Res* 1991; 69: 1185–95.
119. Cigola E, Kajstura J, Li B *et al.* Angiotensin II activates programmed myocyte cell death *in vitro*. *Exp Cell Res* 1997; 231: 363–71.
120. Kajstura J, Cigola E, Malhotra A *et al.* Angiotensin II induces apoptosis of adult ventricular myocytes *in vitro*. *J Mol Cell Cardiol* 1997; 29: 859–70.
121. Zechner D, Thuerauf DJ, Hanford DS *et al.* A role for the p38 mitogen-activated protein kinase pathway in myocardial cell growth, sarcomeric organization, and cardiac-specific gene expression. *J Cell Biol* 1997; 139: 115–27.
122. McDonough PM, Brown JH, Glembotski CC. Phenylephrine and endothelin differentially stimulate cardiac PI hydrolysis and ANF expression. *Am J Physiol* 1993; 264: H625–30.
123. Clerk A, Michael A, Sugden PH. Stimulation of the p38 mitogen-activated protein kinase pathway in neonatal rat ventricular myocytes by the G protein-coupled receptor agonists, endothelin-1 and phenylephrine: a role in cardiac myocyte hypertrophy? *J Cell Biol* 1998; 142: 523–35.
124. Dostal DE, Rothblum KN, Chernin MI *et al.* Intracardiac detection of angiotensinogen and renin: a localized renin–angiotensin system in neonatal rat heart. *Am J Physiol* 1992; 263: C838–50.
125. Dostal DE, Rothblum KN, Conrad KM *et al.* Detection of angiotensin I and II in cultured rat cardiac myocytes and fibroblasts. *Am J Physiol* 1992; 263: C851–63.
126. Inagami T. Intracellular renin: validation and function. In: JIS Robertson, MG Nicholls (eds) *The renin angiotensin system*. London: Gower Medical Publishing, 1993, 30.31–30.38.
127. Danser AH, van Kats JP, Admiraal PJ *et al.* Cardiac renin and angiotensins. Uptake from plasma versus *in situ* synthesis. *Hypertension* 1994; 24: 37–48.
128. van Kats JP, Danser AHJ, van Meegen JR *et al.* Angiotensin production by the heart: a quantitative study in pigs with the use of radiolabeled angiotensin infusions. *Circulation* 1998; 98: 73–81.
129. Dell'Italia LJ, Meng QC, Balcells E *et al.* Compartmentalization of angiotensin II generation in the dog heart: evidence for independent mechanisms in intravascular and interstitial spaces. *J Clin Invest* 1997; 100: 253–8.
130. Lin C, Baker KM, Thekkumkara TJ, Dostal DE. Sensitive bioassay for the detection and quantification of angiotensin II in tissue culture medium. *Biotechniques* 1995; 18: 1014–20.
131. Miyata S, Haneda T, Nakamura Y *et al.* The role of cardiac renin–angiotensin system in stretch-induced hypertrophy of cultured neonatal rat heart cells (Abstract). *Circulation* 1993; 88: I-614.
132. Liang F, Gardner DG. Autocrine/paracrine determinants of strain-activated brain natriuretic peptide gene expression in cultured cardiac myocytes. *J Biol Chem* 1998; 273: 14612–19.
133. Irons CE, Sei CA, Glembotski CC. Regulated secretion of atrial natriuretic factor from cultured ventricular myocytes. *Am J Physiol* 1993; 264: H282–5.
134. Macarthur H, Warner TD, Wood EG *et al.* Endothelin-1 release from endothelial cells in culture is elevated both acutely and chronically by short periods of mechanical stretch. *Biochem Biophys Res Commun* 1994; 200: 395–400.
135. Mangat H, de Bold AJ. Stretch-induced atrial natriuretic factor release utilizes a rapidly depleting pool of newly synthesized hormone. *Endocrinology* 1993; 133: 1398–403.
136. Persson K, Sando JJ, Tuttle JB, Steers WD. Protein kinase C in cyclic stretch-induced nerve growth factor production by urinary tract smooth muscle cells. *Am J Physiol* 1995; 269: C1018–24.
137. Wirtz HR, Dobbs LG. Calcium mobilization and exocytosis after one mechanical stretch of lung epithelial cells. *Science* 1990; 250: 1266–9.
138. Kaye D, Pimental D, Prasad S *et al.* Role of transiently altered sarcolemmal membrane permeability and basic fibroblast growth factor release in the hypertrophic response of adult rat ventricular myocytes to increased mechanical activity *in vitro*. *J Clin Invest* 1996; 97: 281–91.
139. Schunkert H, Dzau VJ, Tang SS *et al.* Increased rat cardiac angiotensin converting enzyme activity and mRNA expression in pressure overload left ventricular hypertrophy. Effects on coronary resistance, contractility, and relaxation. *J Clin Invest* 1990; 86: 1913–20.
140. Suzuki J, Matsubara H, Urakami M, Inada M. Rat angiotensin II (type 1A) receptor mRNA regulation and subtype expression in myocardial growth and hypertrophy. *Circ Res* 1993; 73: 439–47.
141. Zhang X, Dostal DE, Reiss K *et al.* Identification and activation of autocrine renin–angiotensin system in adult ventricular myocytes. *Am J Physiol* 1995; 269: H1791–802.
142. Meggs LG, Coupet J, Huang H *et al.* Regulation of angiotensin II receptors on ventricular myocytes after myocardial infarction in rats. *Circ Res* 1993; 72: 1149–62.
143. Nio Y, Matsubara H, Murasawa S *et al.* Regulation of gene transcription of angiotensin II receptor subtypes in myocardial infarction. *J Clin Invest* 1995; 95: 46–54.
144. Shyu KG, Chen JJ, Shih NL *et al.* Angiotensinogen gene expression is induced by cyclical mechanical stretch in cultured rat cardiomyocytes. *Biochem Biophys Res Commun* 1995; 211: 241–8.
145. Dell'italia LJ, Balcells E, Meng QC *et al.* Volume-overload cardiac hypertrophy is unaffected by ACE inhibitor treatment in dogs. *Am J Physiol* 1997; 273: H961–70.
146. Pierzchalski P, Reiss K, Cheng W *et al.* p53 Induces myocyte apoptosis via the activation of the renin-angiotensin system. *Exp Cell Res* 1997; 234: 57–65.
147. Fareh J, Touyz RM, Schiffrin G, Thibault G. Endothelin-1 and angiotensin II receptors in cells from rat hypertrophied heart: receptor regulation and intracellular $Ca^{2+}$ modulation. *Circ Res* 1996; 78: 302–11.

148. Harada M, Itoh H, Nakagawa O *et al.* Significance of ventricular myocytes and nonmyocytes interaction during cardiocyte hypertrophy: evidence for endothelin-1 as a paracrine hypertrophic factor from cardiac nonmyocytes. *Circulation* 1997; 96: 3737–44.
149. Lee YA, Liang CS, Lee MA, Lindpaintner K. Local stress, not systemic factors, regulate gene expression of the cardiac renin angiotensin system *in vivo*: a comprehensive study of all its components in the dog. *Proc Natl Acad Sci USA* 1996; 93: 11 035–40.
150. Lui Y-H, Yang X-P, Sharov VG *et al.* Effects of angiotensin-converting enzyme inhibitors and angiotensin II type 1 receptor antagonists in rats with heart failure. *J Clin Invest* 1997; 99: 1926–35.
151. Paul K, Ball NA, Dorn GWI, Walsh RA. Left ventricular stretch stimulates angiotensin II-mediated phosphatidylinositol hydrolysis and protein kinase C epsilon translocation in adult guinea pig hearts. *Circ Res* 1997; 81: 643–50.
152. Komuro I, Kudo S, Yamazaki T *et al.* Mechanical stretch activates the stress-activated protein kinases in cardiac myocytes. *FASEB J* 1995; 10: 631–6.
153. Weinberg EO, Lee MA, Weigner M *et al.* Angiotensin AT1 receptor inhibition. Effects on hypertrophic remodeling and ACE expression in rats with pressure-overload hypertrophy due to ascending aortic stenosis. *Circulation* 1997; 95: 1592–600.
154. Zierhut W, Zimmer HG, Gerdes AM. Influence of ramipril on right ventricular hypertrophy induced by pulmonary artery stenosis in rats. *J Cardiovasc Pharmacol* 1990; 16: 480–6.
155. Wiesner RJ, Ehmke H, Faulhaer J *et al.* Dissociation of left ventricular hypertrophy, β-myosin heavy chain gene expression, and myosin isoform sitch in rats after ascending aortic stenosis. *Circulation* 1997; 95: 1253–9.
156. Leskinen H, Vuolteenaho O, Ruskoaho H. Combined inhibition of endothelin and angiotensin II receptors blocks volume load-induced cardiac hormone release. *Circ Res* 1997; 80: 114–23.
157. Harada K, Komuro I, Shiojima I *et al.* Pressure overload induces cardiac hypertrophy in angiotensin II type 1A receptor knock out mice. *Circulation* 1998; 97: 1952–9.
158. Oliverio MI, Best CF, Kim HS *et al.* Angiotensin II responses in AT1A receptor-deficient mice: a role for AT1B receptors in blood pressure regulation. *Am J Physiol* 1997; 272: F515–20.
159. Sugaya T, Nishimatsu S, Tanimoto K *et al.* Angiotensin II type 1a receptor-deficient mice with hypotension and hyperreninemia. *J Biol Chem* 1995; 270: 18 719–22.
160. Nyui N, Tamura K, Mizuno K *et al.* Stretch-induced MAP kinase activation in cardiomyocytes of angiotensinogen-deficient mice. *Biochem Biophys Res Commun* 1997; 235: 36–41.
161. Delafontaine P, Lou H. Angiotensin II regulates insulin-like growth factor I gene expression in vascular smooth muscle cells. *J Biol Chem* 1993; 268: 16 866–70.
162. Itoh H, Mukoyama M, Pratt RE *et al.* Multiple autocrine growth factors modulate vascular smooth muscle cell growth response to angiotensin II. *J Clin Invest* 1993; 91: 2268–74.
163. Ito H, Hirata Y, Adachi S *et al.* Endothelin-1 is an autocrine/paracrine factor in the mechanism of angiotensin II-induced hypertrophy in cultured rat cardiomyocytes. *J Clin Invest* 1993; 92: 398–403.
164. Lee AA, Dillmann WH, McCulloch AD, Villarreal FJ. Angiotensin II stimulates the autocrine production of transforming growth factor-beta 1 in adult rat cardiac fibroblasts. *J Mol Cell Cardiol* 1995; 27: 2347–57.
165. Rajagopalan S, Laursen JB, Borthayre A *et al.* Role for endothelin-1 in angiotensin II-mediated hypertension. *Hypertension* 1997; 30: 29–34.
166. Ruiz-Opazo N, Hirayama K, Akimoto K, Herrera VL. Molecular characterization of a dual endothelin-1/angiotensin II receptor. *Mol Med* 1998; 4: 96–108.

# Molecular basis of cardiac hypertrophy

10

I. KOMURO AND Y. YAZAKI

## Introduction

Cardiac hypertrophy is a very important issue for cardiologists not only because it shows diastolic dysfunction and often leads to congestive heart failure but also because it is an independent risk factor for many cardiac diseases such as ischaemic heart disease and arrhythmia, and often results in sudden death [1]. Haemodynamic overload is a major cause of cardiac hypertrophy. Although the mechanisms by which haemodynamic overload induces cardiomyocyte hypertrophy have long been a subject of great interest for cardiologists, the lack of a good *in vitro* study system has hampered the understanding of the biochemical mechanisms. However, an *in vitro* system introduced in 1989, by which mechanical stress is imposed on cultured neonatal cardiocytes, has made it possible to examine the signal transduction of mechanical stress-induced cardiac hypertrophy [2]. Passive stretch of cardiac myocytes cultured on silicone membranes activates the protein kinase cascades of phosphorylation, and induces the expression of specific genes as well as increasing protein synthesis [2–4]. During this process, the secretion and production of vasoactive peptides such as angiotensin II (AngII) and endothelin-1 (ET-1) are increased and these peptides play critical roles in the induction of these hypertrophic responses [5–7]. Although these *in vitro* studies are useful for identifying the molecules that are involved in the development of cardiac hypertrophy, it is even more important to test whether the molecule really plays an important role in the development of cardiac hypertrophy *in vivo*. The study of genetics in mice has helped to elucidate the role of a molecule *in vivo*. Recently, the importance of $Ca^{2+}$/calcineurin for the development of cardiac hypertrophy has been proposed [8]. Transgenic mice overexpressing active calcineurin showed marked cardiac hypertrophy. Cardiac hypertrophy is an old issue but several novel findings have been accumulating.

## Mechanical stress induces cardiac hypertrophy

There has been controversy over whether a primary stimulus for cardiac hypertrophy is a mechanical stress itself or an increase in neurohumoral factors. Many studies have shown that the sympathetic nervous system is activated during the process of cardiac hypertrophy induced by haemodynamic overload (for review, see ref. 9). Various factors such as catecholamines, vasoactive peptides, growth factors, hormones, and cytokines have been reported to induce cardiac hypertrophy [10–17]. Almost all of these studies, however, only demonstrate that cardiomyocyte hypertrophy can be induced by infusion of these substances *in vivo* or by addition of these substances on cultured cardiac myocytes *in vitro*. There is not much evidence indicating that these substances are actually involved in the development of haemodynamic overload-induced cardiac hypertrophy. The evidence presented below suggests that humoral factors in the circulating blood may have a marginal effect on the development of cardiac hypertrophy in response to haemodynamic overload and that mechanical stress induces cardiac hypertrophy by increasing the local production of humoral factors. First, cardiac hypertrophy can be induced by a haemodynamic overload even after adrenoceptor blockade or sympathectomy [18]. Secondly, increased cardiac load stimulates protein synthesis in isolated hearts [19]. Thirdly, it has been shown that stretching cultured cardiomyocytes with no involvement of neural or humoral factors induces protein synthesis and specific gene expression [2–4].

How is mechanical stress perceived by a cardiomyocyte as a stimulus? With the use of a Langendorf preparation, it has been shown that the stretch of the ventricular wall as a consequence of increased aortic pressure is the mechanical parameter most closely related to an increase in protein synthesis [19]. This observation has been confirmed by the experiments on cardiocytes cultured in serum-free media. When cardiocytes cultured on deformable silicone membranes were stretched, an increase in protein synthesis was observed [2]. Stretching cardiocytes also induced expression of specific genes, such as immediate-early response genes (IEG) and foetal type genes [3, 4] (for review see refs. 20 and 21). These observations suggest that the stretching caused by mechanical stress (haemodynamic overload) induces cardiomyocyte hypertrophy.

## Mechanical stress activates a protein kinase cascade of phosphorylation

Cardiac hypertrophy is accomplished by an increase in protein synthesis and is usually accompanied by the assembly of sarcomeres and the expression of IEG and foetal genes. Among these hypertrophic responses, c-*fos* gene induction is the most rapid and prominent. Therefore, induction of the c-*fos* gene was first used to determine the molecular mechanism by which stretch induces cardiomyocyte hypertrophy [3, 4]. The serum response factor binding element (SRE) of the c-fos gene promoter was found to be an important requirement for response to mechanical stress, and protein kinase C (PKC) may be involved in stretch-induced *c-fos* gene expression. Experiments using *c-fos* gene promoter constructs containing fine mutations confirmed this conclusion [22]. Stretching cultured cardiac myocytes induces the activation of phospholipase C (PLC), which leads to the activation of PKC [4]. Stretch also activates phospholipases D and $A_2$ in cardiac myocytes [22]. Since these phospholipases directly bind and catalyse plasma membrane, it is possible that mechanical stretch of the plasma membrane directly activates these phospholipases. The molecular mechanism by which mechanical stress is converted into biochemical signals is described later in the chapter.

### Mitogen-activated protein kinases family

Several intracellular signals are transduced into a nucleus through a protein kinase cascade of phosphorylation [23]. Once a mechanical stimulus has been converted into biochemical signals involving phosphorylation events, how do these signals regulate protein synthesis and gene expression in cardiac myocytes? A growing body of evidence has suggested that a family of mitogen-activated protein kinases (MAPK) plays a critical role in cell proliferation, differentiation, and death [23–25]. Several members of the MAPK family have been isolated, three of which have been well characterized: extracellular signal-regulated kinases (ERKs), c-June N-terminal kinase/stress-activated protein kinase (JNK/SAPK, and p38MAPK).

#### *Extracellular signal-regulated kinases*

ERKs are activated by a variety of growth factors, hormones, cytokine, and phorbol esters, and play critical roles in cell proliferation and the differentiation of many cell types including cardiac myocytes [24, 25]. ERKs are important for the induction of hypertrophic responses including specific gene expression and an increase in protein synthesis [26]. Although the activation of ERKs is not sufficient or indispensable for the development of cardiomyocyte hypertrophy [27], antisense experiments showed that activated ERKs are critical for the induction of specific gene expression and sarcomere formation as well as an increase in protein synthesis [28]. Stretch of cultured cardiac myocytes by 20% for 10 min activated ERKs [22, 29]. Stretch also activated its upstream kinases such as Raf-1 kinase and MAPK kinase (MEK) (Fig. 10.1) [30]. Activation of PKC is known to increase the activity of Raf-1 kinase and ERKs in various cell types [31]. When PKC was depleted by preincubating myocytes with phorbol ester or its activity blocked by PKC inhibitors, stretch-induced ERK activity was decreased by more than 80%, suggesting that the stretch-induced increase in ERK activity occurs mainly through a PKC-dependent pathway. Although Ras exists upstream of ERKs in many cell types and stretch activates Ras [22], inhibition of Ras had no effect on stretch-induced ERK activation [32]. Although it is not clear why activated Ras does not lead to activation of ERKs, stretch-induced ERK activation is dependent on PKC but not on Ras. Stretch also activated p90 S6 kinase as a downstream kinase of ERKs [22, 29]. Although the signalling pathway remains to be determined, p70 S6 kinase was also activated by stretch. Stretch-induced activation of all of these kinases (PKC, Raf-1, MEK, ERKs, p90, and p70 S6) was partly suppressed by antagonists for AngII and ET-1 receptors, suggesting the involvement of vasoactive peptides in stretch-induced activation of protein kinases.

#### *C-Jun N-terminal kinase/stress-activated protein kinase*

JNK was first reported to be activated in response to cellular stresses such as osmotic stress, ultraviolet irradiation, oxidative stress, and heat shock [33]. JNK is activated not by

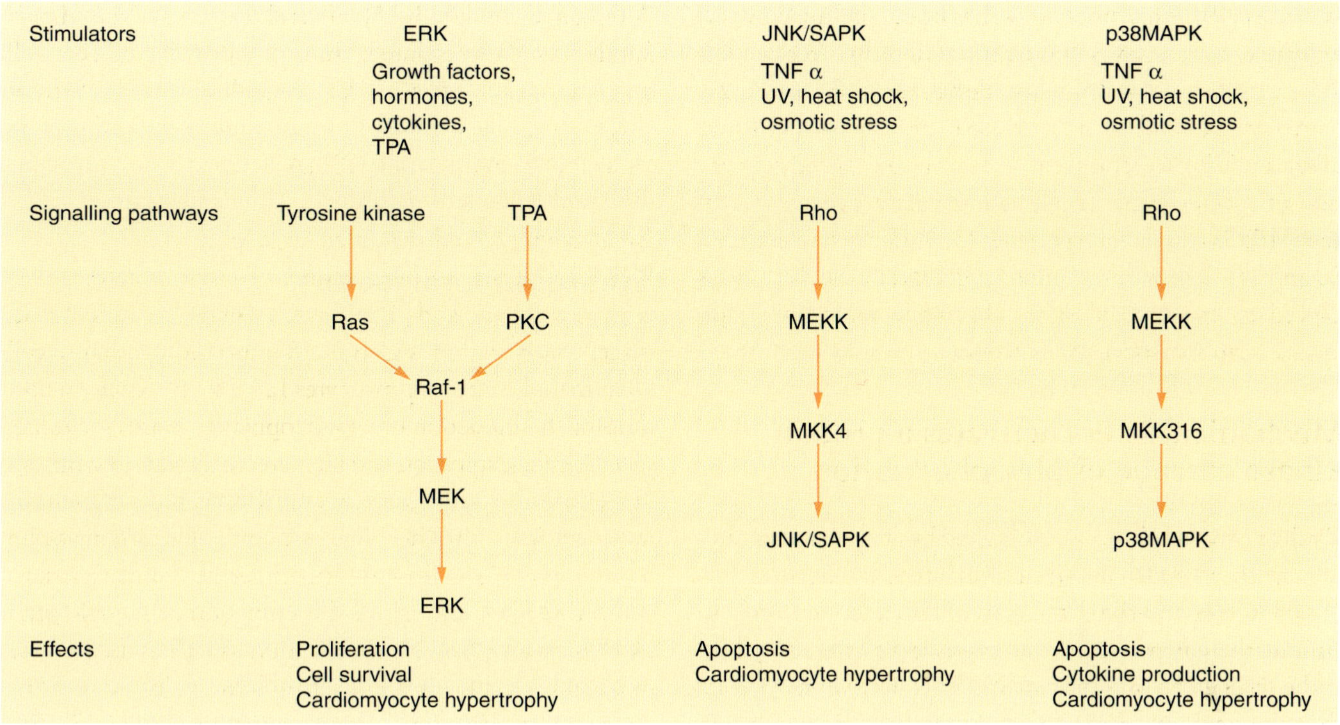


**Figure 10.1** *MAPK family.*

authentic growth factors such as epidermal growth factor (EGF) and basic fibroblast growth factor (FGF) but by proinflammatory cytokines including tumour necrosis factor-α (TNF-α). Since there are some similarities between osmotic stress and stretch, one study examined whether mechanical stretch activates JNK in cardiac myocytes. Stretch by 20% for 10 min strongly activates JNK in cultured cardiac myocytes [34]. Unlike ERKs, stretch-induced JNK activation is not inhibited by Ang II receptor antagonists. Although vasoactive peptides such as Ang II and ET-1 could activate JNK in cultured cardiac myocytes [35], the degree of activation by stretch was several-fold stronger than that by Ang II. These results suggest that mechanical stress itself may activate JNK. JNK is activated by a dual protein kinase, JNK kinase (JNKK/SEK/MKK4 or 7). MEKK1 is one of the JNK kinase kinases and is also activated by stretch in cardiac myocytes [30]. Recently, Ask 1 has been reported to be a JNK kinase kinase [36]. Stretch activates Ask 1 and inhibition of Ask1 attenuates stretch-induced JNK activation (komuro, unpublished observation). Elucidation of the molecular mechanism by which stretch activates JNK may pave the way to understanding how mechanical stress is converted into biochemical signals.

JNK has been reported to be involved in gene regulation by phosphorylating transcription factors such as c-Jun and ATF-2 [33]. Recently, JNK was reported to be involved in cardiomyocyte hypertrophy [37]. Wang *et al.* [37] reported that specific activation of the JNK pathway in cardiac myocytes induced characteristic features of hypertrophy, including an increase in cell size, elevated expression of atrial natriuretic peptide (ANP), and induction of sarcomere organization, and that coactivation of both JNK and p38MAPK in cardiomyocytes led to an induction of cytopathic responses and suppression of hypertrophic responses. In contrast. Nemoto *et al.* [38] reported that expression of constitutive active p38MAPK stimulated the expression of ANP and that activation of p38MAPK was required for ANP expression induced by the hypertrophic agonists. Activation of JNK led to inhibition of the ANP expression induced by MEKK1 and the hypertrophic agonists. It remains unknown why contradictory results were obtained; however, the effects of JNK and p38MAPK may be dependent on the way in which or the degree to which they are activated or inhibited. Both papers demonstrated that activation of either JNK to p38MAPK promotes cardiac hypertrophy and that the two kinases have opposing effects on the development of hypertrophy. Since both JNK and p38MAPK are usually activated by many stimuli, it remains to be determined how they are involved in the development of cardiac hypertrophy. Like ERKs, the precise role of JNK in the development of cardiac hypertrophy remains elusive.

### *p38MAPK*

p38MAPK is usually activated by stimuli similar to those for JNK: cellular stress such as osmotic stress, ultraviolet irradiation, oxidative stress, and heat shock, and anticancer agents [39]. p38MAPK has been reported to play an important role in the induction of apoptosis and the production of cytokines as well as in gene regulation [39]. Cytokines including interleukin-1β (IL-1β), IL-6, and TNF-α attracted great attention in the cardiovascular field because they may cause cardiac dysfunction [40]. It has been reported that p38MAPK is activated by hypertrophic agonists such as ET-1, phenylephrine, and the leukaemia inhibitory factor (LIF) [41]. As mentioned above, p38MAPK may have opposing effects against JNK on cardiomyocyte hypertrophy, but its precise role in cardiac hypertrophy remains controversial. Recently, Wang *et al.* [42] have reported interesting results with p38MAPK. There are four different isoforms of p38MAPK [43]. Activation of p38MAPKα elicits apoptosis in cardiac myocytes, whereas overexpression of p38MAPKβ induced characteristic hypertrophic responses. It remains to be determined how two similar isoforms elicit completely different effects on cardiac myocytes. Precise mapping of the region of p38MAPKα and β responsible for apoptosis and hypertrophy, respectively, may provide a clue.

### p70 S6 protein kinase

There are many pathways by which stretch induces cardiomyocyte hypertrophy (described later). Among them, the phosphorylation of S6 protein in 40S ribosome is well correlated to the efficiency of protein synthesis and p70 S6 protein kinase ($p70^{S6K}$) is reported to phosphorylate S6 protein *in vivo* [44]. Stretch by 20% for 15 min activated $p70^{S6K}$ in cardiac myocytes and inhibition of $p70^{S6K}$ by a specific inhibitor rapamycin strongly suppressed the stretch-induced increase in protein synthesis without affecting the activity of ERKs and expression of *c-fos* [45]. These results suggest that $p70^{S6K}$ is critically involved in stretch-induced cardiomyocyte hypertrophy and that the signalling pathway to $p70^{S6K}$ activation is different from that of ERKs and c-fos. Phosphoinositide-3 kinase (PI3-K) activates $p70^{S6K}$ in many cell types and, indeed, a PI3-K specific inhibitor, wortmannin, abolished stretch-induced activation of $p70^{S6K}$. However, activation of authentic PI3-K could not be detected after stretch (unpublished observation), suggesting that atypical PI3-K including PI3-Kγ may be activated by stretch, or $p70^{S6K}$ may be activated through a PI3-K-independent pathway in cardiac myocytes.

## Neurohumoral factors

The protein kinase cascade of phosphorylation activated by mechanical stress on cardiac myocytes is very similar to that evoked by the addition of growth factors and cytokines on many cell types. It is possible that cardiac myocytes and non-cardiomyocytes such as fibroblasts, endothelial cells, and smooth muscle cells secrete some hypertrophy-promoting factors following stretch and that they induce cardiac hypertrophy by an autocrine or a paracrine mechanism. Mechanical stress on myocardial cells has been reported to increase the synthesis of some growth-promoting factors [46]. Many growth factors, including acidic and basic FGF, transforming growth factor-β (TGF-β), and insulin-like growth factor I and II, have been reported to exist in the heart, and some of them can induce cardiac hypertrophy and specific gene expression in cultured cardiomyocytes (for review see ref. 14).

### Angiotensin II

A growing body of evidence has indicated that the local renin–angiotensin system plays a critical role in the development of cardiac hypertrophy (for review see ref. 47). All components of the renin–angiotensin system, such as angiotensinogen, renin, and angiotensin converting enzyme (ACE), have been identified at both the messenger ribonucleic acid (mRNA) and protein levels in the heart. Ang II stimulates protein synthesis in cultured cardiomyocytes [11]. Increases in angiotensinogen and ACE mRNA have been reported in the hypertrophied left ventricle of rats [48]. Subpressor doses of ACE inhibitors can prevent or cause regression of cardiac hypertrophy with no change in systemic systolic blood pressure [49]. An increase in left ventricular mass produced by abdominal aortic constriction, without significant increase in plasma renin activity, was completely prevented with an ACE inhibitor without any change in afterload [50]. These results strongly suggest that the local renin–angiotensin system but not the circulating one may play a critical role in pressure overload-induced cardiac hypertrophy.

AngII induces activation of ERKs and expression of the c-*fos* gene as well as increasing protein synthesis in neonatal rat cardiocytes through the activity of the AngII type 1 receptor (AT1) [51]. Activation of ERKs and upregulation of c-*fos* gene expression by AngII are blocked by PKC inhibitors, and AngII increases production of inositol phosphates and activates PKC [51, 52]. These signals elicited by AngII in cardiac myocytes are very similar to those evoked by mechanical stress, as mentioned above. The involvement of AngII in the stretch-induced hypertrophic response was examined using AT1-specific inhibitors. AT1 antagonists partially but significantly suppressed all stretch-induced hypertrophic responses, such as an increase in amino acid incorporation, the induction of c-*fos* gene expression, and the activation of ERKs [5, 6]. AngII is stored in secretory granules in neonatal ventricular myocytes and mechanical stretch causes its release from cultured cardiocytes (Fig. 10.2) [5]. Although it remains to be determined how stretch induces this release these results suggest that AngII is responsible at least in part for the hypertrophic responses evoked by mechanical stress on cardiac myocytes.

Several studies have demonstrated that when the AngII/AT1 signals are inhibited, mechanical stress-induced hypertrophic responses are abolished *in vivo* [50] and *in vitro* [5]. A series of studies tested whether AngII/AT1 signals are indispensable for mechanical stress-induced cardiac hypertrophy using AT1a knockout mice (KO mice) [53–55]. Reverse-transcriptase polymerase chain reaction analysis revealed that although the AT2 gene was expressed at almost the same levels in the heart of both types of mice, AT1 mRNA levels were detected in the hearts of wild-type (WT) mice but not in the hearts of KO mice. Acute pressure overload produced by constricting the transverse aorta induced expression of IEG and activation of ERKs in the heart of KO mice as well as WT mice [53]. Both basal and activated levels of all of these responses were significantly higher in KO mice than WT mice. Chronic pressure overload for 40 days produced by constriction of the abdominal aorta markedly increased the heart weight to body weight ratio and induced foetal gene expression in both mice to almost the same degree [54]. These results suggest that cardiac hypertrophy could be

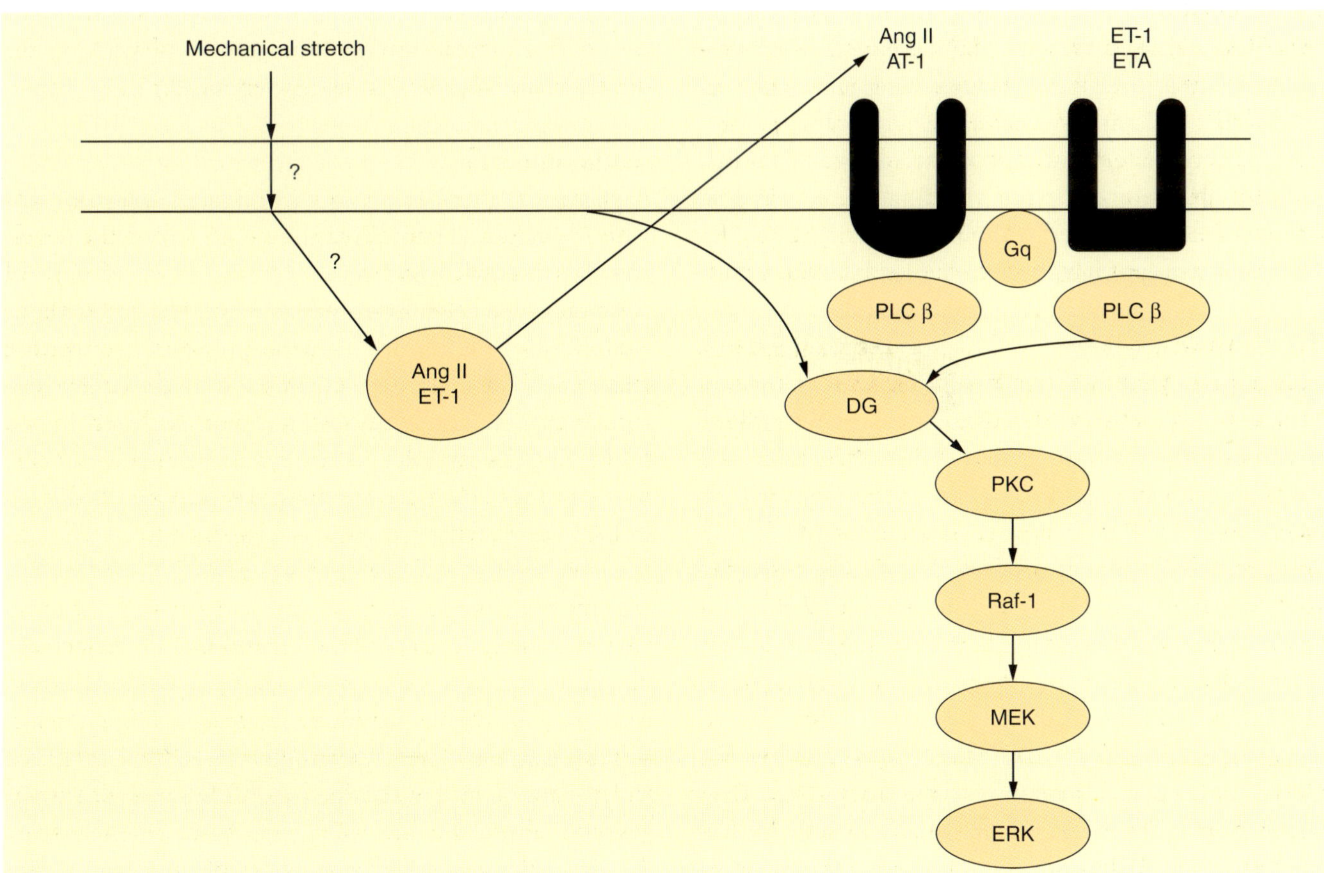


**Figure 10.2** *Mechanical stretch-induced signal transduction leading to cardiomyocyte hypertrophy*

induced by pressure overload *in vivo* without AT1a signalling.

The molecular mechanism by which mechanical stress induces hypertrophic responses without AngII/AT1 signalling was examined using cultured cardiac myocytes prepared from AT1a KO mice [55]. When cardiac myocytes were stretched by 20% for 10 min, ERKs were strongly activated in KO cardiomyocytes as well as WT myocytes. Both basal and stimulated levels of ERKs were higher in cardiomyocytes of KO mice than of WT mice. An AT1 antagonist attenuated stretch-induced ERK activation in WT myocytes but not in KO myocytes. Downregulation of PKC inhibited stretch-induced ERK activation in WT cardiocytes, while a tyrosine kinase inhibitor, genistein, suppressed the ERK activation in KO cardiac myocytes. Tyrphostins (AG1478 and B42), inhibitors for EGF receptor kinase, also significantly attenuated stretch-induced activation of ERKs. Stretch for 8 min significantly enhanced phosphorylation of the EGF receptor [55]. These results suggest that mechanical stretch could evoke hypertrophic responses in cardiac myocytes which lack AT1 signalling partly through tyrosine kinase activation. The clinical implication of this study is that since multiple factors mediate mechanical stress-induced cardiac hypertrophy, it is pivotal to suppress mechanical stress itself but there are no single mediator preventing the development of cardiac hypertrophy.

The intracellular signalling pathways evoked by AngII are different among cell types. AngII markedly activates ERKs in cardiac myocytes. Although AngII activates Fyn, a Src family tyrosine kinase and Ras [56], inhibition of these molecules has no effect on AngII-induced ERK activation. Instead, down-regulation of PKC or a PKC inhibitor, calphostin C, abolishes AngII-induced ERK activation [57]. AngII also activates Raf-1 kinase and MEK, and the activation of these kinases is also suppressed by inhibition of PKC. Since PKC has been reported to activate directly Raf-1 kinase, AngII may activate ERKs through PKC, Raf-1, and MEK. Signalling pathways from AT1 to ERKs are divergent among cell types. In smooth-muscle cells, pertussis toxin had no effects but PLC, $Ca^{2+}$, and Src family are critical for AngII-induced activation of ERKs. AngII activates ERKs, possibly through Gq-PLCγ- $Ca^{2+}$-$Ca^{2+}$-dependent tyrosine kinase Pyk2 and Src-Shc-Grb2-Sos-Ras ERKs [57]. Cardiac fibroblasts produce and secrete extracellular matrix proteins such as collagen and fibronectin in response to AngII, which induces fibrosis of the heart. In cardiac fibroblasts, AngII activates ERKs through pertussis toxin-sensitive G protein, possibly G1 protein. The βγ-subunit of G1 activates Src and then ERKs through Shc-Grb2-Sos-Ras [58]. It remains to be determined why signalling pathways are so divergent among cell types.

## Endothelin-1

ET-1 has been reported to be a strong inducer of cardiac hypertrophy [12]. The stretch-induced activation of ERKs is also suppressed by type A ET-1 (ETA) receptor antagonists [7], suggesting that ET-1 is also involved in mechanical stress-induced hypertrophic responses (Fig. 10.2). Since ET-1-induced activation of ERKs is also inhibited by downregulation of PKC, ET-1 activates ERKs, possibly through the same pathway as AngII. Recently, it was reported that AngII does not have direct potent hypertrophy-promoting effects on cardiac myocytes but may evoke hypertrophic responses in cardiac myocytes by inducing ET-1 secretion from cardiac fibroblasts [59]. Cross-talk among different cell types and among many molecules may be important not only for maintaining a highly differentiated phenotype but also for inducing cardiac hypertrophy. The beneficial effects of ET-1 receptor antagonists on myocardial infarction highlighted the importance of ET-1 in cardiovascular remodelling [60]. Recently, the importance of Gq protein in the development of pressure overload-induced cardiac hypertrophy was demonstrated using transgenic mice [61]. Class-specific inhibition of Gq-mediated signalling was produced in the heart of transgenic mice by targeted expression of a carboxyl-terminal peptide of the α-subunit of Gq. When pressure overload was surgically produced, the transgenic mice developed significantly less ventricular hypertrophy than control mice. Although the prevention of cardiac hypertrophy was not complete in the transgenic mice, this study suggests that Gq-coupled receptors such as AT1 and ETA, and seven other transmembrane receptors are important in the development of pressure overload-induced cardiac hypertrophy.

## Catecholamines

Catecholamines such as noradrenaline and phenylephrine are active in promoting hypertrophy [10]. Extensive pharmacological experiments have shown that noradrenaline induces cardiomyocyte hypertrophy through the α but not the β-receptor [10]. Since the α-adrenoceptor couples Gq protein, noradrenaline might induce cardiomyocyte hypertrophy through PKC activation, like AngII and ET-1. It has been observed that noradrenaline activates ERKs through the PKC-Raf-1 pathway [62]. The β-receptor agonist isoproterenol slightly but significantly activates ERKs. The β-adrenoceptor couples Gs protein and activates adenylate cyclase, resulting in an increase in cyclic adenosine monophosphate (cAMP) levels. In many types of cells, cAMP inhibits ERK activation by a variety of growth factors [63]. In cardiac myocytes, however, cAMP does not inhibit the activation of ERKs but rather activates them. Isoproterenol-induced ERK activation was blocked by a cAMP inhibitor RpcAMP, and a Gi inhibitor, pertussis toxin, suggesting that both β-receptor/Gs–cAMP–PKA and Gi are necessary for activation of ERKs by isoproterenol. Recently, Lefkowitz's group [64] reported that PKA phosphorylates the β-receptor, resulting in a change in affinity between the β-receptor and G proteins. Gi couples the phosphorylated β-receptor instead of Gs. Taken together, isoproterenol may activate ERKs in cardiac myocytes through Gs–cAMP–PKA first and then by phosphorylating β-receptor-Gi-βγ-Src-Ras ERKs. Overexpression of the β-receptor, which has a mutation in the phosphorylation site by PKA, inhibited isoproterenol-induced ERK activation in cultured cardiomyocytes. Inhibition of βγ and Src by overexpression of βARK minigene and Csk, respectively, also abolished isoproterenol-induced activation of ERKs (unpublished observations).

### Cytokines

Many cytokines have been isolated and studies revealed that they play important roles not only in inflammation but also in a wide variety of cell functions such as proliferation, differentiation, and death [65]. This is true in the case of cardiac myocytes. A novel cytokine was isolated from a cardiomyocyte differentiation system of embryonic stem cells as a factor which promotes cardiomyocyte hypertrophy [16]. This cytokine had potent hypertrophy-promoting activity and was named cardiotrophin-1 (CT-1). CT-1 is structurally similar to interleukin-6 (IL-6), ciliary neurotrophic factor (CNTF), and leukaemia inhibitory factor (LIF). All of these cytokine members use gp130 as a common receptor and elicit intracellular signals through it. LIF and CNTF as well as CT-1 can induce cardiomyocyte hypertrophy. Ligand binding activates a non-receptor type tyrosine kinase JAK family, followed by two signalling pathways, such as the STAT and Ras/ERK pathways (Fig. 10.3) [65]. The molecular mechanism by which CT-1 induces cardiomyocyte hypertrophy remains to be determined. KO and transgenic mouse technologies clearly demonstrated the important roles of the cytokines during embryonic cardiac development and in cardiac hypertrophy after birth, respectively. gp130-null mice have severe defects in cardiomyocyte proliferation during the embryonic stage and are embryonically [66]. Since expression of cardiac-specific genes and sarcomere formation are observed and the compact layer is thinner in KO mice, gp130 null mice have a defect of cardiomyocyte proliferation but not of differentiation. Recently, a similar phenotype was reported in K-ras KO mice [67]. It is noteworthy that Ha-ras or N-ras null mice had no apparent phenotype and that only K-ras null mice had severe defects in cardiac development. Since Ras is activated by gp130 stimulation, activation of K-ras through gp130 may be pivotal for the proliferation of cardiomyocytes during the mid-embryonic stage.

Double transgenic mice that overexpress IL-6 and soluble IL-6 receptor show marked cardiac hypertrophy [17]. Since there are few IL-6 receptors in cardiac myocytes, the transgenic mice that expressed only IL-6 did not show any cardiac hypertrophy. However, when both IL-6 and soluble IL-6 receptor were overexpressed in the same mice, gp130 was stimulated in the heart and cardiac hypertrophy was induced. These results suggest that stimulation of gp130 induces proliferation of cardiomyocytes during the foetal period and cardiomyocyte hypertrophy after birth.

Another role of gp130 activation was reported recently [68]. LIF and CT-1 protect cardiomyocytes from apoptosis. Two signalling pathways may be involved in preventing apoptosis of cardiac myocytes. One is the PI3-K pathway [69]: PI3-K activates a downstream kinase, Akt/PKB, which phosphorylates and inactivates a proapoptotic molecule, Bad [70]. Another is the ERK pathway. Inhibition of MEK blocks the antiapoptotic effects of CT-1 [68].

## Mechanisms by which mechanical stress is converted into biochemical signals

### Stretch-sensitive ion channels and exchangers

Many cells respond to a variety of environmental stimuli by activating ion channels in the plasma membrane. Mechanosensitive ion channels have been observed with single-channel recordings in more than 30 cell types of prokaryotes, plants, fungi, and all animals so far examined (for review see ref. 71). The activation of stretch-sensitive channels has been proposed as the transduction mechanism between load and protein synthesis in cardiac hypertrophy [72]. The stretch-sensitive channels allow the passage of

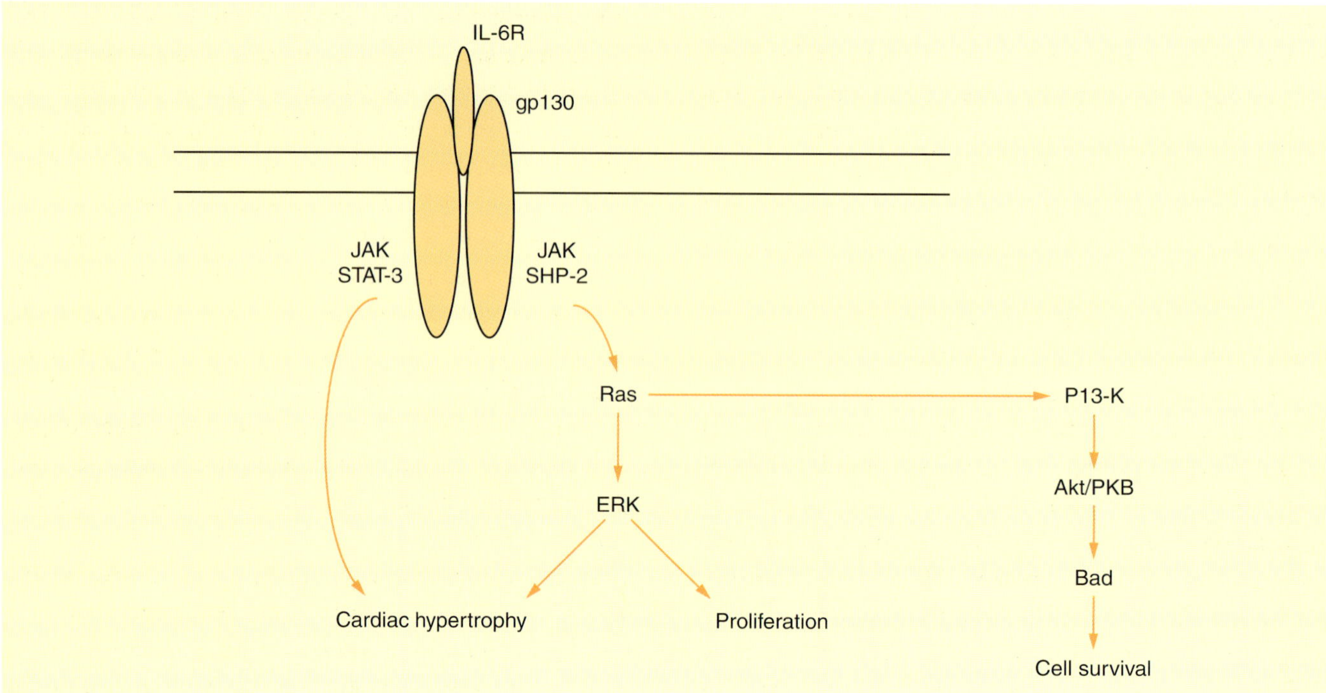


**Figure 10.3** *Signal transduction pathway through gp130.*

the major monovalent physiological cations, $Na^+$ and $K^+$, and the divalent cation, $Ca^{2+}$. With the use of a $Ca^{2+}$-binding fluorescent dye (fluo3) and the patch-clamp technique, mechanically induced $Ca^{2+}$ influx through stretch channels was shown to lead to waves of calcium-induced calcium release [73]. Therefore, stretch-sensitive ion channels may be the initial responder for mechanical stress. Experiments using inhibitors of stretch-sensitive ion channels, however, failed to confirm this hypothesis. Gadolinium and streptomycin (inhibitors of stretch-sensitive cation channels), glibenclamide (ATP-sensitive $K^+$ channels), and CsCl (hyperpolarization-activated inward channels) did not inhibit activation of ERKs by stretching [74]. Although preincubation with $Ca^{2+}$ channel blockers or short exposure to ethylenediaminetetra-acetate (EDTA) did not change the induction of c-*fos* mRNA after stretching [75], preincubation with ethyleneglycotetra-acetate (EGTA) attenuated stretch-induced activation of ERKs. This result suggests that $Ca^{2+}$ influx from the extracellular space may be involved in stretch-induced activation of ERKs. Since the importance of $Ca^{2+}$ in the development of cardiac hypertrophy was highlighted recently (see next section), the role of stretch-sensitive ion channels should be investigated more extensively.

Highly selective inhibitors of the $Na^+/H^+$ exchanger significantly attenuated the activation of ERKs by stretch [74]. Although the actual activity of the $Na^+/H^+$ exchanger was not determined, it may be activated by mechanical stress and function to convert mechanical stress into biochemical signals. Alkalization is necessary for proliferation in many cell types and may be also involved in stretch-induced activation of hypertrophic responses in cardiomyocytes.

## Extracellular matrix and the cytoskeleton

Data indicate that the mechanical stress is transduced into the cell from the sites at which cells attach to the extracellular matrix (ECM) (for review see ref. 76). Transmembrane ECM receptors, such as the integrin family, are good candidates for mechanoreceptors. A large extracellular domain of integrin receptor complex binds various ECM proteins, while a short cytoplasmic domain has been shown to interact with the cytoskeleton in the cell (for review see ref. 77). Since cytoskeleton proteins can potentially regulate plasma membrane proteins such as enzymes, ion channels, and antiporters, mechanical stress could modulate these membrane-associated proteins and stimulate second messenger systems through the cytoskeleton. Integrins can transmit signals not only by organizing the cytoskeleton but also by altering biochemical properties such as the extent of tyrosine phosphorylation of a complex of proteins including pp125$^{fak}$ [76]. Stretch of cultured mesangial cells enhances the phosphorylation of pp125$^{fak}$ [78].

The Rho small G protein family, consisting of Rho, Rac, and Cdc42, is important for the function of integrins by regulating the actin cytoskeleton [79]. When the functions of the Rho family were inhibited by C3 exoenzyme or by overexpression of Rho GDP dissociation inhibitor and dominant negative mutants, stretch-induced activation of ERKs and expression of IEG were strongly suppressed [32]. It has been reported that C3 exoenzyme inhibits MEKK- and phenylephrine-induced ANP expression but not actin organization, indicating that Rho regulates ANP gene expression but not sarcomere assembly [80]. Sah *et al.* [81] also reported that Rho is involved in phenylephrine- and G$\alpha$q-induced ANP expression but not in Ras-induced ANP expression. Activated RhoA and Ras produced synergistic effects on ANP gene expression, suggesting that Rho functions in a pathway separate from but complementary to Ras. Treatment of myocytes with AngII caused the formation of non-striated actin fibre (premyofibrils), which was abolished by C3 treatment [82]. Expression of constitutively active RhoA caused the formation of premyofibrils. These results suggest that RhoA is involved in premyofibril formation but not in mature myofibril formation.

## $Ca^{2+}$/calcineurin theory for cardiac hypertrophy

Using transgenic mouse technology, Molkentin *et al.* [8] clearly demonstrated that calcineurin plays a critical role in the development of cardiac hypertrophy. There have been several reports suggesting that a cardiac-enriched transcription factor, GATA4, plays a pivotal role in the induction of several genes by hypertrophy-promoting agents [83, 84]. These authors screened GATA4-associated proteins using a yeast two-hybrid system and isolated a transcription factor of a member of nuclear factor of activated T-cells (NF-AT). The NF-AT families, which have been well characterized in T-lymphocytes, are activated by an increase in intracellular $Ca^{2+}$ levels. When T-cells are activated, intracellular $Ca^{2+}$ levels are increased and $Ca^{2+}$/calmodulin activates a phosphatase calcineurin. Calcineurin then dephosphorylates NE-AT, which exists in the cytoplasm in a phosphorylated state. Dephosphorylated NF-AT moves into the nucleus and transactivates many genes with other transcription factors such as AP-1 [85].

In cardiac myocytes, NF-AT3 was shown to associate with GATA4 and both transcription factors activated cardiac specific genes in concert. Cotransfection of NF-AT3 and GATA4 synergistically activated the brain natriuretic peptide (BNP) promoter. When calcineurin was inhibited by a calcineurin-specific inhibitor, cyclosporin A, AngII-induced cardiomyocyte hypertrophy was suppressed. Both transgenic mice overexpressing constitutively activated calcineurin and NF-AT3 showed marked cardiac hypertrophy. All of these results strongly indicate that calcineurin/NF-AT3 is critically involved in the development of cardiac hypertrophy (Fig. 10.4).

This study is interesting because the totally novel theory is clearly demonstrated by transgenic mouse strategy as well as by the *in vitro* culture system. At the same time, however, this study proposed many new questions regarding the role of $Ca^{2+}$ in the development of cardiac hypertrophy. The importance of calcineurin was clearly shown, but there is no clear evidence indicating that hypertrophy-promoting agents increase intracellular $Ca^{2+}$ levels. Although it may depend on the species and the stages, developmental it remains controversial whether AngII or other inositol trisphosphate ($IP_3$)-elevating agents increase $Ca^{2+}$ levels. In cardiac myocytes, unlike many types of cells including smooth muscle cells, $IP_3$ does not release $Ca^{2+}$ from the sarcoplasmic reticulum. In mice, cardiac myocytes are beating and intracellular $Ca^{2+}$ levels change more than 500 times/min. First, in this situation, how is calcineurin activated? Prolonged elevation of $Ca^{2+}$ levels is necessary for activation of calcineurin. Secondly, how does the activation of NF-AT3 lead to an increase in total protein synthesis? NF-AT3 is a transcription factor, so some genes including the BNP gene could be upregulated, but it is difficult to explain an increase in total protein synthesis by the single transcription factor. Thirdly, what is the relationship between protein kinases and NF-AT? Since cyclosporin A and FK506 have no effect on AngII-induced ERK activation, protein kinases and NF-AT may be independently involved in the development of cardiac hypertrophy. There may be multiple pathways which lead to cardiac hypertrophy. Fourthly, haemodynamic overload is the most important cause of cardiac hypertrophy, as mentioned before. Does mechanical stress also increase intracellular $Ca^{2+}$ levels and activate calcineurin/NF-AT3? Fifthly,

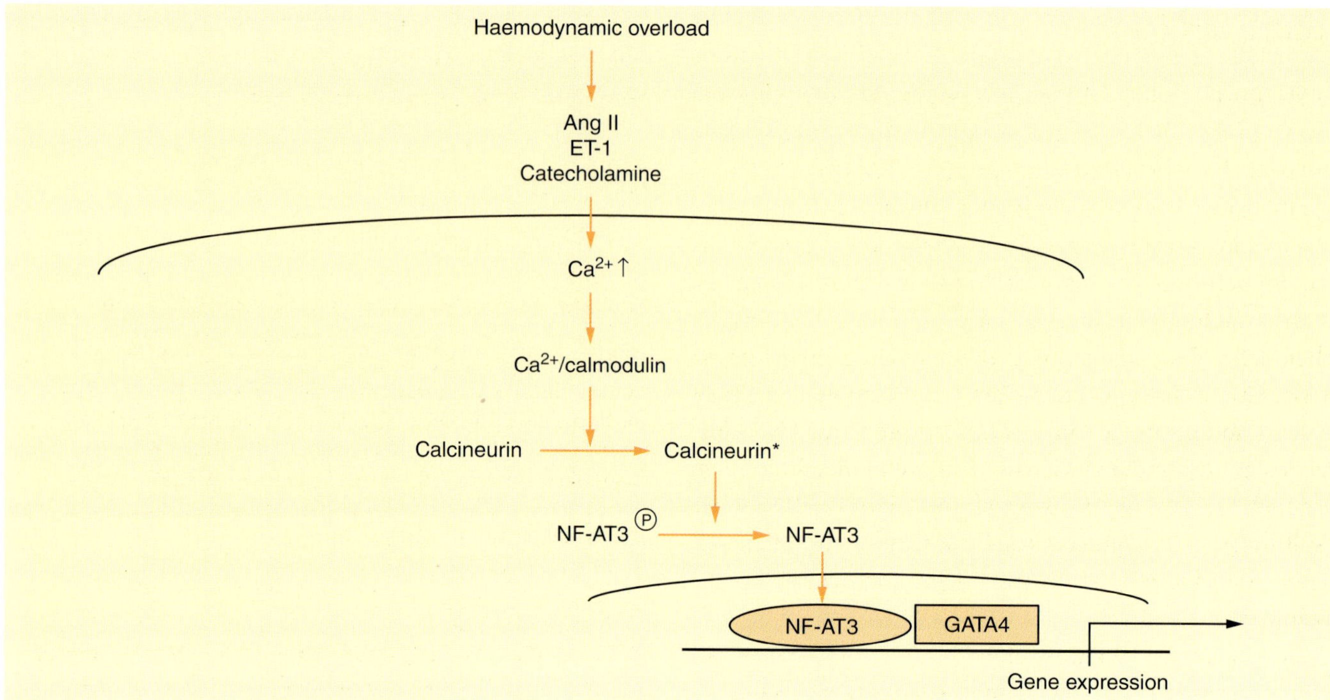


**Figure 10.4** *$Ca^{2+}$/Calcineurin theory for cardiac hypertrophy.*

transgenic mice that overexpress constitutively activated calcineurin show marked cardiac hypertrophy first and at later stages, and some of them show dilated cardiomyopathy. Cardiac hypertrophy can be treated with cyclosporin A. Can cyclosporin A prevent the progress from cardiac hypertrophy to dilated cardiomyopathy? Many interesting and important questions remain to be answered.

## Mechanism of an increase in protein synthesis

In cardiac hypertrophy, the rate of protein degradation is not changed but that of synthesis increases. There are several mechanisms by which protein synthesis is enhanced. As described in the first two sections of this chapter, expression of foetal genes is specifically enhanced at the transcriptional level during cardiac hypertrophy. Phosphorylation of S6 protein in the 40S ribosome may be one of the mechanisms for increasing global protein synthesis at the translational level.

### Ribosomal DNA transcription

The increased capacity for protein synthesis that is a constant feature in all forms of cardiac hypertrophy is largely mediated by accelerated ribosome biogenesis. Hypertrophy-promoting agonists such as noradrenaline, ET-1, and contraction, all increase the rate of DNA transcription. The cellular content of ribosomal DNA (rDNA) transcription factor UBF is increased in adrenergic- and contraction-induced models of cardiac hypertrophy [86], while ET-1 and phorbol ester phosphorylate increase the activity of UBF [87]. Overexpression of UBF increased rDNA transcription in cultured cardiac myocytes [88]. These observations suggest that enhancement of rDNA transcription by UBF plays a role in the development of cardiac hypertrophy; however, the role of UBF in this process remains to be determined.

### Translational initiation

Eucariotic initiation factor 4E (eIF-4E) is rate limiting for translational initiation. Electorically stimulated contraction of cultured cardiomyocytes and acute pressure overload in the *in vivo* heart increased phosphorylation of eIF-4E [89]. Inhibition of actin–myosin cross-bridge cycling and development of active tension inhibited the phosphorylation of eIF-4E *in vitro*. It remains to be determined how eIF-4E is phosphorylated during the process of cardiac hypertrophy.

## Future directions

As shown in Figure 10.1, mechanical stress can evoke a variety of signals in cardiac myocytes. Once mechanical stress has been received and converted into biochemical signals, the signal transduction pathway leading to an increase in protein synthesis is similar to the pathway that is activated by various humoral factors such as growth factors, hormones, and cytokines in many other cells. Recently, yeast genes encoding members of MAP kinase have been isolated by complementation of yeast mutations as an essential protein for restoring the osmotic gradient across the cell membrane in response to increased external osmolarity [90]. This result suggests that mechanical stress-induced intracellular signal transduction pathways are highly conserved in evolution.

Although many biochemical events that occur in cardiac myocytes subsequent to mechanical stretch have been clarified, a main intriguing question remains unanswered: how is mechanical stress converted into biochemical signals? In other words, what is the mechanoreceptor or the transducer for mechanical stress in cardiac myocytes? It is conceivable that by stretching the plasma membrane, mechanical stress directly changes conformations of the functional proteins in the membrane such as enzymes and G proteins, or directly activates enzymes such as phospholipases by physically placing the enzymes close to their phospholipid substances in the plasma membrane. As mentioned above, the integrin–cytoskeleton complex seems to be an alternative candidate structure for a mechanoreceptor and a transducer. Integrin–cytoskeleton proteins not only play a 'passive' role, such as maintaining the cell structure, but may also play 'active' roles in the regulation of cellular functions, such as protein phosphorylation and activation of an antiporter. Integrin $\alpha_5\beta_1$ was shown to activate the $Na^+H^+$ antiporter by binding to fibronectin, suggesting that integrin can behave similarly to a growth factor receptor in activating signalling pathways [91]. The cytoskeleton has been also shown to play an important role in secretion. Mechanical stress may stimulate the secretion of some cytokines, which generate multiple intracellular signals as a secondary event. Further studies are necessary to identify specific signalling molecules, including mechanoreceptors and mechanotransducers, and characterization of these molecules may pave the way to understanding the definite mechanism of mechanical stress-induced cardiac hypertrophy and finally clarifying the mechanisms by which adaptive cardiac hypertrophy deteriorates into congestive heart failure.

## References


1. Levy D, Garrison RJ, Savage DD *et al. N Engl J Med* 1990; 322: 1561–6.
2. Mann DL, Kent RL, Cooper G. *Circ Res* 1989; 64: 1079–90.
3. Komuro I, Kaida T, Shibasaki Y *et al. J Biol Chem* 1990; 265: 3595–8.
4. Komuro I, Katoh Y, Kaida T *et al. J Biol Chem* 1991; 266: 1265–8.
5. Sadoshima J, Xu Y, Slayter HS, Izumo S. *Cell* 1993; 95: 977–84.
6. Yamazaki T, Komuro I, Kudoh S *et al. Circ Res* 1995; 77: 258–65.
7. Yamazaki T, Komuro I, Kudoh S *et al. J Biol Chem* 1996; 271: 3221–8.
8. Molkentin JD, Lu J-R, Antos CL *et al. Cell* 1998; 93: 215–28.
9. Zak R. In: R Zak (ed.) *Growth of the heart in health and disease*. New York: Raven Press, 1984, 165–85.
10. Simpson P. *Circ Res* 1985; 56: 884–94.
11. Baker KM, Aceto JF. *Am J Physiol* 1990; 259: H610–18.
12. Ito H, Hirata Y, Adachi S *et al. J Clin Invest* 1993; 92: 398–403.
13. Parker TG, Schneider MD. *Annu Rev Physiol* 1991; 53: 179–200.
14. Ito H, Hiroe M, Hirata Y *et al. Circulation* 1993; 87: 1715–21.
15. Tanaka N, Ryoke T, Hongo M *et al. Am J Physiol* 1998; 275: H393–9.
16. Pennica D, King KL, Shaw KJ *et al. Proc Natl Acad Sci USA* 1995; 92: 1142–6.
17. Hirota H, Yoshida K, Kishimoto T, Taga T. *Proc Natl Acad Sci USA* 1995; 92: 4862–6.
18. Cooper G, Kent RL, Uboh CE *et al. J Clin Invest* 1985; 75: 1403–14.
19. Kira Y, Kochel PJ, Gordon EE; Morgan HE. *Am J Physiol* 1984; 246: C247–58.
20. Komuro I, Yazaki Y. *Annu Rev Physiol* 1993; 55: 55–75.
21. Sadoshima J, Izumo S. *Annu Rev Physiol* 1997; 59: 551–71.
22. Sadoshima J, Izumo S. *EMBO J* 1993; 12: 1681–92.
23. Cantley LC, Auger KR, Carpenter C *et al. Cell* 1991; 64: 281–302.
24. Blenis J. *Cancer Cells* 1991; 3: 445–9.
25. Nishida E, Gotoh Y. *Trends Biochem Sci* 1993; 18: 128–31.
26. Thorburn J, Frost JA, Thorburn J. *J Cell Biol* 1994; 126: 1565–72.
27. Post GR, Goldstein D, Thuerauf DJ *et al. J Biol Chem* 1996; 271: 8452–7.
28. Glennon PE, Kaddoura S, Sale EM *et al. Circ Res* 1996; 78: 954–61.
29. Yamazaki T, Tobe K, Hoh E *et al. J Biol Chem* 1993; 268: 12 069–76.
30. Yamazaki T, Komuro I, Shiojima I *et al. J Clin Invest* 1995; 96: 438–46.
31. Kyriakis JM, App H, Zhang X *et al. Nature* 1992; 358: 417–21.
32. Aikawa R, Komuro I, Yamazaki T *et al. Circ Res* (in press).
33. Ip YT, Davis RJ. *Curr Opin Cell Biol* 1998; 10: 205–19.
34. Komuro I, Kudoh S, Yamazaki T *et al. FASEB J* 1996; 10: 631–6.
35. Kudoh S, Komuro I, Mizuno T *et al. Circ Res* 1997; 80: 139–46.
36. Ichijo H, Nishida E, Irie K *et al. Science* 1997; 275: 90–4.
37. Wang Y, Su B, Sah VP *et al. J Biol Chem* 1998; 273: 5423–6.
38. Nemoto S, Sheng Z, Lin A. *Mol Cell Biol* 1998; 18: 3518–26.
39. New L, Han J. *Trends Cardiovasc Med* 1998; 8: 220–8.
40. Bozkurt B, Kribbs SB, Clubb FJ *et al. Circulation* 1998; 97: 1382–91.
41. Clerk A, Fuller SJ, Michael A, Sugden PH. *J Biol Chem* 1998; 273: 7228–34.
42. Wang Y, Huang S, Sah VP *et al. J Biol Chem* 1998; 273: 2161–8.
43. Jiang Y, Chen C, Li Z *et al. J Biol Chem* 1996; 271: 17 920–6.
44. Erikson RL. *J Biol Chem* 1990; 266: 6007–10.

45. Sadoshima J, Izumo S. *Circ Res* 1995; 77: 1040–52.
46. Hammond GL, Wieben E, Market CL. *Proc Natl Acad Sci USA* 1979; 76: 2455–9.
47. Baker KM, Booz GW, Dostal DE. *Annu Rev Physiol* 1992; 54: 227–41.
48. Schnkert H, Dzau VJ, Tang SS *et al*. *J Clin Invest* 1990; 86: 1913–20.
49. Linz W, Schoelkens BA, Ganten D. *Clin Exp Hypertens* 1989; 11: 1325–50.
50. Baker KM, Cherin MI, Wixon SK, Aceto JF. *Am J Physiol* 1990; 259: H324–32.
51. Sadoshima J, Izumo S. *Circ Res* 1993; 73: 413–23.
52. Katoh Y, Komuro I, Shibasaki Y *et al*. (Abstract). *Circulation* 1989; 80: II–450.
53. Harada K, Komuro I, Kudoh S *et al*. *Circulation* 1998; 97: 1952–9.
54. Harada K, Komuro I, Kudoh S *et al*. *Circ Res* 1998; 82: 779–85.
55. Kudoh S, Komuro I, Hiroi Y *et al*. *J Biol Chem* 1998; 273: 24 037–43.
56. Sadoshima J, Izumo S. *EMBO J* 1996; 15: 775–87.
57. Zou Y, Komuro I, Yamazaki T *et al*. *Circ Res* 1998; 82: 337–45.
58. Zou Y, Komuro I, Yamazaki T *et al*. *J Biol Chem* 1996; 271: 33 592–7.
59. Harada M, Itoh H, Nakagawa O *et al*. *Circulation* 1997; 96: 3737–44.
60. Sakai S, Miyauchi T, Kobayashi M *et al*. *Nature* 1996; 384: 353–5.
61. Akhter SA, Luttrell LM, Rockman HA *et al*. *Science* 1998; 280: 574–7.
62. Yamazaki T, Komuro I, Kudoh S *et al*. *Circulation* 1997; 95: 1260–8.
63. Wu J, Dent P, Jelinek T *et al*. *Science* 1993; 262: 1065–9.
64. Daaka Y, Luttrell LM, Lefkowitz RJ. *Nature* 1997; 390: 88–91.
65. Taga T, Kishimoto T. *Annu Rev Immunol* 1997; 15: 797–819.
66. Yoshida K, Taga T, Saito M *et al*. *Proc Natl Acad Sci USA* 1996; 93: 407–11.
67. Koera K, Nakamura K, Nakao K *et al*. *Oncogene* 1997; 15: 1151–9.
68. Sheng Z, Knowlton K, Chen J *et al*. *J Biol Chem* 1997; 272: 5783–91.
69. Oh H, Fujio Y, Kunisada K *et al*. *J Biol Chem* 1998; 273: 9703–10.
70. Datta SR, Dudek H, Tao X *et al*. *Cell* 1997; 91: 231–41.
71. Morris CE. *J Membrane Biol* 1990; 113: 93–107.
72. Bustamante JO, Ruknudin A, Sachs F. *J Cardiovasc Pharmacol* 1991; 17: S110–17.
73. Sigurdson W, Ruknudin A, Sachs F. *Am J Physiol* 1992; 262: H1110–15.
74. Yamazaki T, Komuro I, Kudoh S *et al*. *Circ Res* 1998; 82: 430–7.
75. Komuro I, Katoh Y, Hoh E *et al*. *Jpn Circ J* 1991; 55: 1149–57.
76. Juliano RL, Haskill S. *J Cell Biol* 1993; 120: 577–85.
77. Hynes RO. *Cell* 1992; 69: 11–25.
78. Hamasaki K, Mimura T, Furuya H *et al*. *Biochem Biophys Res Commun* 1995; 212: 544–9.
79. Mackay DJ, Hall A. *J Biol Chem* 1998; 273: 20 685–8.
80. Thorburn J, Xu S, Thorburn A. *EMBO J* 1997; 16: 1888–900.
81. Sah VP, Hoshijima M, Chien KR, Brown JH. *J Biol Chem* 1996; 271: 31 185–90.
82. Aoki H, Izumo S, Sadoshima J. *Circ Res* 1998; 82: 666–76.
83. Herzig TC, Jobe SM, Aoki H *et al*. *Proc Natl Acad Sci USA* 1997; 94: 7543–8.
84. Hasegawa K, Lee SJ, Jobe SM *et al*. *Circulation* 1997; 96: 3943–53.
85. Rao A, Luo C, Hogan PG. *Annu Rev Immunol* 1997; 15: 707–47.
86. Hannan RD, Luyken J, Rothblum LI. *J Biol Chem* 1995; 270: 8290–7.
87. Luyken J, Hannan R, Cheung J, Rothblum L. *Circ Res* 1996; 78: 354–61.
88. Hannan RD, Stefanovsky V, Taylor L *et al*. *Proc Natl Acad Sci USA* 1996; 93: 8750–5.
89. Wada H, Ivester CT, Carabello BA *et al*. *J Biol Chem* 1996; 271: 8359–64.
90. Brewster JL, de Valoir T, Dwyer ND *et al*. *Science* 1993; 259: 1760–3.
91. Schwartz MA, Lechene C, Ingber DE. *Proc Natl Acad Sci USA* 1991; 88: 7849–53.

# Endothelin in myocardial remodelling and failure 11

W. S. COLUCCI

## Introduction

Endothelin (ET) is a potent vasoconstrictor peptide, first identified in vascular endothelial cells by Masaki and colleagues in 1988 [1]. Since then it has been appreciated that ET exerts potent effects on the biochemistry and biology of essentially all cell types in the cardiovascular system, and thereby influences many aspects of normal cardiovascular system development, physiology, and structure. More recently it has become apparent that ET is an important mediator of cardiovascular system remodelling in response to environmental stresses. This suggests that ET could play a central role in the pathophysiology of cardiovascular disease. This chapter focuses on the role of ET in pathological myocardial remodelling.

## Endothelin physiology

### Synthesis

ET is a 21 amino acid peptide which is synthesized as a larger peptide, termed prepro-ET. Prepro-ET is cleaved by one or more endothelin-converting enzymes (ECEs) first to form a 38–39 amino acid peptide, pro-ET, and again to form the final 21 amino acid molecule. ETs are rapidly cleared from the circulation by the lung, live, and kidney [2].

Multiple ECEs have been cloned and characterized [3, 4]. The various ECEs have different preferences for big ET-1, big ET-2, and big ET-3 as substrates. The ECEs are membrane-bound proteases, structurally related to neutral endopeptidase 24.11 and Kell blood group protein, with a single transmembrane spanning domain, conserved zinc-binding motifs, N-glycosylation sites, a short N-terminal tail, and a large extracytoplasmic portion that contains the catalytic domain. These distinct ECE-1 isoforms, ECE-1a, ECE-1b, and ECE-1c, have been identified in humans, and appear to be differentially localized within the cell, with ECE-1a and ECE-1c located at the cell surface, and ECE-1b associated with the trans-Golgi network [5]. ECE-1a is expressed in endothelial cells in all organs, and in epithelial cells in the airway, gastroentestinal tract, and urinary tract. ET-1 inhibits the expression of ECE-1 mRNA via stimulation of $ET_B$ receptors, thereby exerting feedback regulation of levels of ET [6]. ECE-2 is present in human umbilical cord endothelial cells, and bovine adrenal cortex and endothelial cells. The ECEs are potential targets for the pharmacological interruption of the ET system [7].

### Isoforms

Three isoforms of ET, termed ET-1, ET-2, and ET-3, have been identified. ET-1 predominates in the human vasculature and, on a weight basis, is the most potent vasoconstrictor yet identified. ET-2 is not found in human plasma but is expressed in the kidney, brain, adrenal gland, and intestine, and like ET-1, has vasoconstrictor properties. The primary source of ET-3 is not known, and unlike ET-1 and ET-2, it has minimal vasoconstrictor properties.

### Receptors

Two major subtypes of ET receptors have been identified, $ET_A$ and $ET_B$ [8]. At the pharmacological level, the subtypes differ with regard to selectivity for ET-1-2 and -3. The $ET_A$ receptor binds the ETs in the order ET-1 $\geq$ ET-2 $\gg$ ET-3, with about a 100-fold greater affinity for ET-1 than ET-3. The $ET_B$ receptor shows no binding selectivity for the ETs (i.e. ET-1 = ET-2 = ET-3). $ET_A$ receptors predominate on vascular smooth-muscle cells and cardiac myocytes, but are not found on endothelial cells. $ET_B$ receptors are found on vascular smooth-muscle cells, endothelial cells and, to a lesser extent, cardiac myocytes. Both subtypes are found on cardiac fibroblasts [9].

The ET receptor subtypes are encoded by distinct genes which have been isolated, sequenced, and related to human homologues [8]. The $ET_A$ and $ET_B$ receptors have about 63% homology at the amino acid level, and both belong to the G protein-coupled heptahelical superfamily. In contrast to most members of this family, they have a long N-terminal extracellular portion which may be involved in peptide binding. The third cytoplasmic loop and the C-terminal tail have multiple serine/threonine residues which may be substrates for the protein kinases involved in the regulation of receptor function.

Both subtypes couple to multiple signalling pathways, including activation of phospholipase C via a G protein, activation of L-type calcium channels, and stimulation of mitogen-activated protein kinase [10]. In endothelial cells, $ET_B$ receptors are coupled to the endothelial isoform of nitric oxide synthase. NOS-3, so that stimulation of this receptor causes endothelium-dependent vasodilatation [11]. Other $ET_B$ receptors located on vascular smooth-muscle cells, which may or may not be distinguishable pharmacologically [12, 13], are coupled to contraction, and appear not to stimulate NOS-3. A third receptor subtype, termed $ET_C$, has been identified in *Xenopus laevis* dermal malanophores, but has yet to be found in mammals [14].

## Endothelin receptor antagonists

A large number of non-peptide molecules that specifically block ET receptors has been developed [15]. The availability of these antagonists has contributed greatly to an understanding of the actions of ET-1. Some of these agents are non-selective (e.g. bosentan), whereas others are selective for the $ET_A$ (e.g. BQ-123) or $ET_B$ (e.g. BQ-788) receptor. The use of these antagonists *in vitro* and in animals has helped to define the relative roles of the ET receptor subtypes in normal physiology and development. Furthermore, their use in animal models has helped to clarify the role of ET-1 in myocardial remodelling and failure, and has led to the investigational use of some of the antagonists as therapy in patients with heart failure.

## Cardiovascular actions of endothelin

### Development effects

Mice homozygous for a ET-1 gene null mutation die of respiratory failure soon after birth. These mice have extensive morphological abnormalities of the pharyngeal arch-derived craniofacial tissues and organs, including cardiovascular malformations of the heart and great vessels. The latter include anomalies of the aortic arch and aorticopulmonary septation defects in the cardiac outflow tract [16, 17]. These mice have phenotypic similarities to some human disorders that involve defects in neural crest-derived tissues, including DiGeorge syndrome and conotruncal-anomoly face syndrome [18]. In contrast, ET-3 knockout mice die at 3–4 weeks of age of toxic megacolon, and have a spotted coat owing to a regional lack of melanocytes. These mice exhibit a phenotype similar to Hirschsprung's disease in humans or its genetic rat model.

The phenotype seen in ET-1 knockout mice is mimicked by mice with knockout of the $ET_A$ receptor, or by treatment of embryonic animals with an $ET_A$-selective antagonist (e.g. BQ-123) or antibodies to $ET_A$ receptors. Conversely, mice with $ET_B$ receptor knockout have a phenotype similar to that of ET-3 knockout mice. These findings indicate that ET-1 and ET-3 are involved in normal embryonic development, and that the developmental effects of ET-1 and ET-3 are mediated by the $ET_A$ and $ET_B$ receptors, respectively.

### Vascular tone

ET is the most potent vasoconstrictor yet identified on a weight basis. The stimulation of $ET_A$ receptors on vascular smooth-muscle cells causes constriction. In contrast, the stimulation of $ET_B$ receptors on endothelial cells causes vasodilation owing to the release of endothelium-dependent relaxing factor (EDRF), the active moiety of which is nitric oxide (NO) (Fig. 11.1). Although the constrictor effect generally predominates, there appears to be substantial variability depending on the vascular bed. Furthermore, in some vessels it appears that $ET_B$ receptors located on vascular smooth-muscle cells mediate constriction. It is not clear whether these receptors differ from $ET_B$ receptors on endothelial cells, couple to different signalling pathways, or both [12, 13].

Although ET-1 is a potent vasoconstrictor, mice heterozygous for a null mutation of ET-1 have a reduced tissue expression of ET-1 which is associated with a modest increase in systemic blood pressure [16]. This surprising result may reflect the counter-regulatory actions of $ET_A$ and $ET_B$ receptors or the secondary involvement of other regulatory mechanisms such as the sympathetic nervous system.

### Myocardial contraction

In the myocardium, $ET_A$ receptors predominate on myocytes, whereas both $ET_A$ and $ET_B$ subtypes are

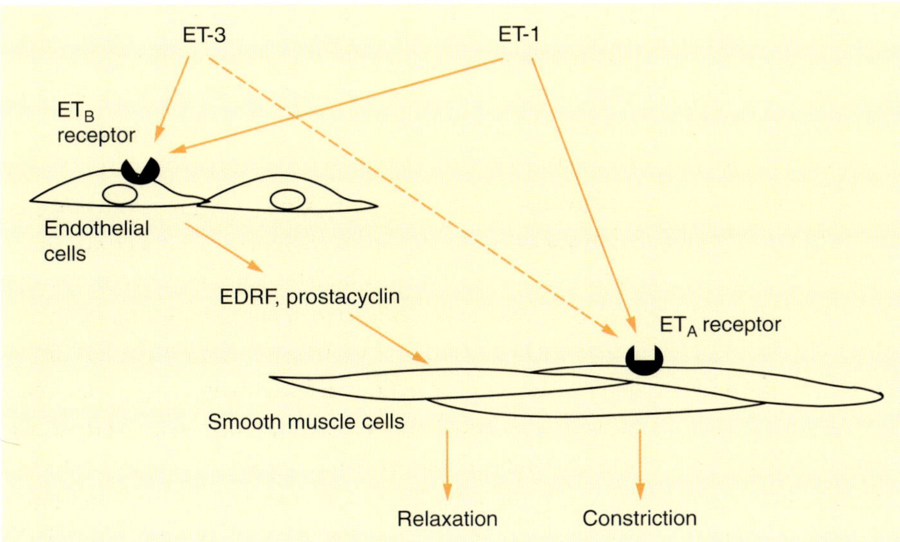


**Figure 11.1** *Roles of the $ET_A$ and $ET_B$ receptor subtypes in mediating vascular smooth-muscle response to endothelin ET. ET-1, the major endothelin in the vasculature, acts directly on $ET_A$ receptors on vascular smooth-muscle cells to cause contraction. In endothelial cells, ET-1 acts via $ET_B$ receptors to cause the release of endothelium-dependent relaxing factor (EDRF) and thereby attenuating the magnitude of the contractile response. (From ref. 8 with permission.)*

expressed on fibroblasts. In myocytes, ET can stimulate contractility, at least in part through an increase in the myofilament sensitivity to calcium [19, 20]. At picomolar concentrations, ET-1 increases both the extent and velocity of shortening in cardiac myocytes isolated from adult rat hearts [21]. This effect is attenuated by pertussis toxin, suggesting the involvement of a G protein. In contrast to contraction, the stimulation of phophoinositide turnover by ET is not sensitive to pertussis toxin, suggesting that these actions are mediated either by distinct receptors or by a common receptor that couples to different signalling pathways with differential sensitivity to pertussis toxin.

## Myocyte growth and phenotype

ET stimulates cell growth in several cell types, including cardiac myocytes and fibroblasts. In cardiac myocytes *in vitro*, ET causes cellular hypertrophy as manifested by an increase in cell size [22, 23]. This effect is associated with increased assembly of sarcomeres, activation of inositol phospholipid hydrolysis, expression of atrial natriuretic peptide (ANP), induction of several immediate-response genes (e.g. c-*fos*, *egr*-1), and expression of myosin light chain-2. Recently, in adult cardiac myocytes exposure to ET-1 for 24 h caused a marked decrease in the expression of several genes that are important for the regulation of calcium homoeostasis, including decreased expression of sarcoplasmic reticulum ATPase (SERCA2) and the calcium release channel (CRC), and increased expression of the sodium–calcium exchanger [24]. Thus, ET-1 causes myocyte hypertrophy associated with a shift to a foetal contractile phenotype.

ET-1 may mediate the hypertrophic effects of other stimuli in cardiac myocytes *in vitro*. Ito *et al.* [25] found that angiotensin stimulated the expression of ET-1 in neonatal rat cardiac myocytes and caused hypertrophy. The hypertrophic effect of angiotensin was blocked by both an $ET_A$-selective antagonist (BQ123) and antisense mRNA directed against the coding region of prepro-ET.

Likewise, Yamazaki *et al.* [26] found that ET expression in neonatal rat cardiac myocytes was increased by a mechanical stretch which was sustained for 24 h, resulting in an approximately three-fold increase in the concentration of ET-1 in the culture media. They further found that addition of the $ET_A$-selective antagonist BQ123 attenuated the stretch-induced increase in protein synthesis and activation of growth pathways, including Raf-1 kinase and mitogen-activated protein kinase. In contrast, the $ET_B$-selective blocker BQ788 had no effect on any of these stretch-induced effects. These observations suggest that ET could play an autocrine or a paracrine role in mediating the growth responses to angiotensin and mechanical stretch via the $ET_A$ receptor.

## Fibroblast and collagen regulation

In cardiac fibroblasts ET stimulates DNA replication, cell proliferation, and protein synthesis. In addition, ET acting on fibroblasts regulates both the synthesis and degradation of extracellular matrix collagen. Guarda *et al.* [9] found that

**Table 11.1** Effects of endothelin (ET) receptor subtypes on fibrillar collagen turnover in cardiac fibroblasts

| Receptor subtype | $ET_A$ | $ET_B$ |
|---|---|---|
| Synthesis | No effect | Increased |
| Degradation | Increased | No effect |
| Net fibrillar collagen | Decreased | Increased |

(Adapted from ref. 9.)

both ET-1 and ET-3 stimulated the synthesis of type I and II collagen in adult rat cardiac fibroblasts (Table 11.1). These effects were mediated by the $ET_B$ receptor since they were not blocked by an $ET_A$-selective antagonist. Conversely, they found that only ET-1 stimulated collagenase activity, and that this action was mediated by the $ET_A$ receptor since it was inhibited by an $ET_A$-selective antagonist. Taken together, these findings suggest that stimulation of the fibroblast $ET_B$ receptor would favour collagen accumulation, whereas stimulation of the $ET_A$ receptor would favour a decrease in fibrillar collagen. Given the role of fibrillar collagen in determining myocardial structure, strength, and other physical properties, its net increase or decrease could have important effects on myocardial stiffness or chamber dilation, respectively.

## Myocardial expression of endothelin-1

ET-1 can be synthesized by several cell types present in the myocardium, including endothelial cells, cardiac myocytes [27], and fibroblasts [28]. Several stimuli that are associated with myocardial remodelling or heart failure increase the expression of ET-1 and its mRNA *in vitro*. As noted above, both angiotensin and mechanical stretch induce the expression of ET in cardiac myocytes, and the hypertrophic response to each is attenuated by an $ET_A$-selective antagonist. Other demonstrated stimuli for ET-1 in a variety of cell types include hypoxia, catecholamines, arginine vasopressin, transforming growth factor-1β, thrombin, ischaemia, and interleukin-1β.

ET-1 is expressed in the myocardium and is increased in pathological circumstances [29–31]. In rats, the myocardial levels of ET-1 mRNA are increased with pressure overload induced hypertrophy caused by aortic constriction [32] or after myocardial infarction [33]. In a rabbit model of ischaemia–reperfusion, there were increased levels of myocardial ET-1 mRNA in the ischaemic zone (compared with the non-ischaemic zone), and administration of the non-selective ET receptor antagonist PD-145065 reduced infarct size, suggesting a role in ischaemic damage [34]. In addition, ET-1 can stimulate the synthesis and release of ET-1.

Although ET-1 is present in the plasma, it is likely that its physiological and pathological actions are mediated at the cellular level by much higher local concentrations. The evidence that ET production can be stimulated in the myocardium and that ET can regulate many features of cardiac myocyte and fibroblast biology has led to the thesis that ET, acting in an autocrine or a paracrine manner, may play a role in myocardial remodelling (Fig. 11.2).

## Myocardial remodelling

Myocardial remodelling is the process by which progressive changes occur in the structure and function of the myocardium in response to physiological or pathological stimuli [35]. Myocardial remodelling is a feature of normal tissue development and may be a useful adaptation to increased demands (e.g. with athletic training) in the adult. However, when this process occurs in response to pathological stimuli (e.g. abnormal wall stresses or noradrenaline release), the remodelling that ensues may be maladaptive in the long term and often results in further myocardial dysfunction.

Myocardial remodelling consists of an array of molecular and cellular events that determine the structure, function, and phenotype of the myocardium. At the cellular level, there may be hypertrophy and apoptosis of cardiac myocytes, re-expression of a foetal phenotype, and alterations in the quantity and composition of the extracellular matrix. Numerous factors have been identified that can mimic some or all of the features of myocardial remodelling. Best characterized among these are mechanical stress, angiotensin, and nor adrenaline.

Interest in the potential role of ET-1 in myocardial remodelling has been spurred by the demonstration that ET-1 can mimic many features of myocardial remodelling and, as discussed below, the observation that ET-1 expression is increased in animal models and humans with heart failure. As reviewed elsewhere [36], it appears likely that additional factors produced primarily within the myocardium may be involved in myocardial remodelling, including inflammatory cytokines, peptide growth factors, nitric oxide, and reactive oxygen species.

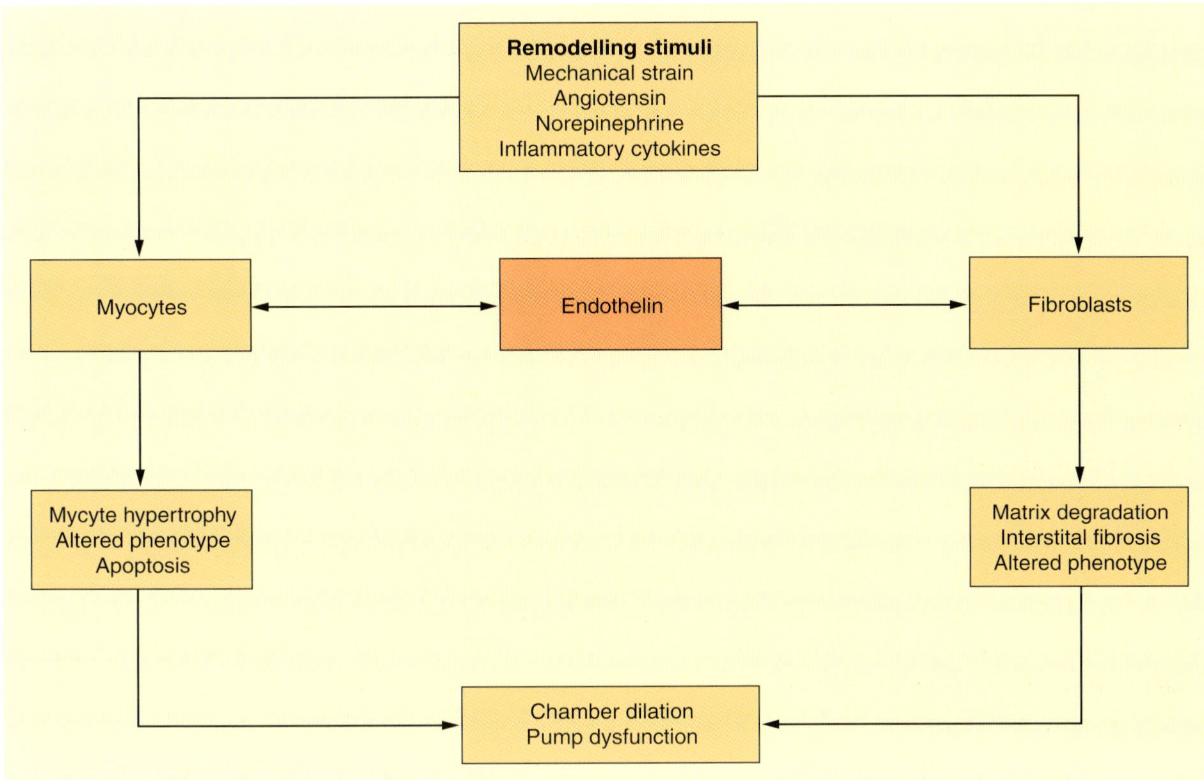


**Figure 11.2** *Schematic depicting the possible central role of endothelin in mediating the effects of stimuli such as mechanical stress and angiotensin on myocardial remodelling.*

## Increased plasma endothelin levels in heart failure

The levels of plasma ET are increased in a variety of pathological cardiovascular conditions including hypertension, angina, cardiogenic shock, myocardial infarction, Raynaud's phenomenon, cerebral vasospasm, and atherosclerosis. Elevated plasma ET-1 levels in patients with heart failure have been observed by several groups [37–41]. In general, the resting ET-1 levels are two to three times higher than in control subjects without heart failure, and the degree of elevation is related to the severity of symptoms [42]. ET-1 levels in patients with congestive heart failure correlate inversely with left ventricular (LV) ejection fraction and cardiac index, and positively with New York Heart Association functional class and LV end-diastolic volume [42]. In some studies, the level of plasma ET-1 correlates best with the degree of pulmonary hypertension, as reflected by the pulmonary artery pressure or pulmonary vascular resistance (Fig. 11.3) [37]. Although most studies have found that plasma ET-1 does not increase with exercise in patients with heart failure [38, 43], one study found that ET-1 levels increased during isometric handgrip exercise [40].

Plasma ET-1 levels may predict clinical outcome. Plasma ET-1 levels correlate inversely with exercise capacity, leading to the suggestion that ET-1 is an important determinant of exercise dysfunction in heart failure [44]. An elevated plasma ET-1 level following myocardial infarction predicts a reduced 1 year survival rate [45]. In patients with moderate to severe heart failure, Pacher *et al.* [46] found that plasma levels of big ET-1 predicted mortality better than haemodynamic variables such as ejection fraction or level of ANP. Furthermore, plasma ET-1 levels may indicate the clinical response to drug therapy. Krum *et al.* [47] found that the change in ET-1 level was a sensitive independent marker of the clinical response to the β-blocker carvedilol.

The mechanism for increased plasma ET-1 in heart failure appears to be increased production, possibly from the pulmonary vasculature, rather than decreased clearance [48]. Circulating ET-1 reflects spillover from production sites and, therefore, local concentrations at the tissue and cellular levels are almost certainly much higher.

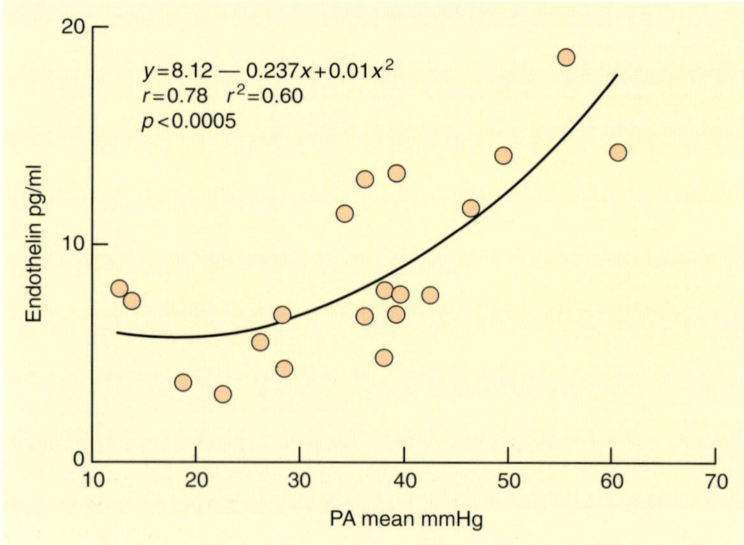


**Figure 11.3** *Relationship between plasma endothelin levels and mean pulmonary artery pressure in patients with congestive heart failure. A highly significant relationship was found between pulmonary artery pressure and plasma endothelin across a wide range of pulmonary artery pressures. The fit was best when a polynomial equation was used. (Adapted from ref. 37 with permission.)*

## Animal models of myocardial hypertrophy and failure

In the rat aortic banding model of pressure overload, Ito *et al.* [31] found that that there was a transient increase in the level of prepro-ET-1 mRNA in the left ventricle at day 1, which returned to baseline at day 4. In the same model, they showed that infusion of the $ET_A$-selective blocker BQ123 prevented ventricular hypertrophy and expression of the foetal markers ANP and α-skeletal actin at 1 week after banding, but that the effect was lost at 2 weeks. These observations suggested that myocardial ET-1 might be involved in the early growth response to pressure overload.

In another rat model of myocardial remodelling due to a continuous 7 day infusion of noradrenaline, Kaddoura *et al.* [49] found that there was likewise a transient increase in expression of ET-1 mRNA in the ventricular myocardium. As with pressure overload, the expression of ET-1 mRNA was highest on day 1 and had returned to baseline by day 5 despite continued noradrenaline infusion. In this model they found that treatment with bosentan prevented ventricular hypertrophy for 7 days, and attenuated the induction of β-myosin heavy chain and skeletal α-actin mRNA, but did not prevent the increase in ANP mRNA.

Both ET-1 and $ET_A$ receptors are increased in the surviving myocardium of rats after myocardial infarction [50]. In this model, Teerlink *et al.* [51] showed that plasma ET-1 increased from 1 to 16 weeks after infarction, and that ET-3 increased transiently in 1 week. Big ET-1 was not increased, suggesting that there may be increased conversion to ET-1. The oral administration of the non-selective blocker bosentan from weeks 2 to 8 caused a decrease in arterial pressure which was additive to that of the converting enzyme inhibitor cilazapril.

Several studies have determined the effect of ET receptor blockade on remodelling and survival in this model. Sakai *et al.* [52] showed that the administration of the $ET_A$ receptor-selective antagonist BQ123 improved survival at 12 weeks after coronary artery ligation from 43% to 85% (Fig. 11.4). Mulder *et al.* [53] examined two doses of the non-selective antagonist bosentan which was added to the chow for up to 9 months after infarction. The lower dose (30 mg/kg per day) had little effect, but the higher dose (100 mg/kg per day) reduced the extent of LV dilatation and improved contractility in the surviving myocardium (Fig. 11.5). These structural and functional changes, which were apparent by 2 months of therapy, were associated with improved survival. Likewise, Fraccarollo *et al.* [54] demonstrated that the early (3 h postinfarction) administration of bosentan at a high dose (100 mg/kg) resulted in improved haemodynamics and prevented LV dilatation 8 weeks postinfarction.

Recently, the effects of oral administration of the $ET_A$-selective antagonist TBC11254 were examined in rats after myocardial infarction [55]. Over a period of 6 weeks, there was no effect on LV weight or end-diastolic pressure measured when the rats were killed. At 6 weeks, LV volume and isovolumic function were determined in isolated blood-perfused hearts by the Langendorf method. In placebo-

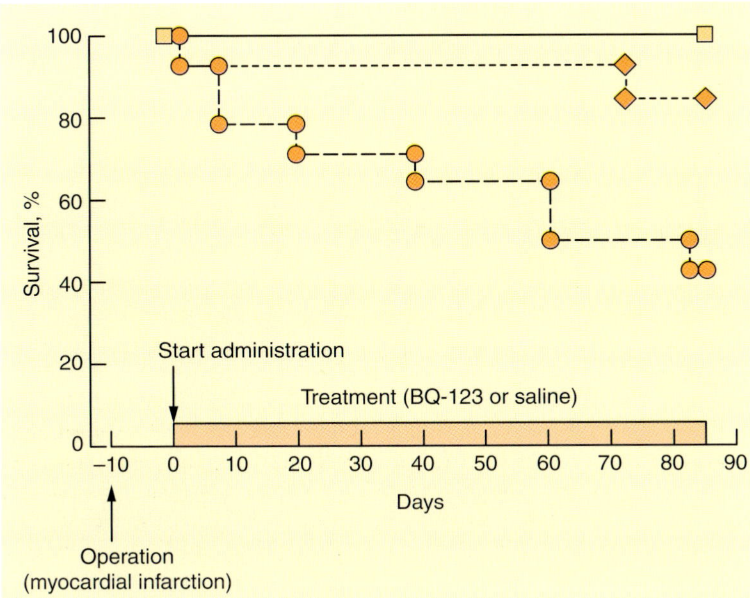


**Figure 11.4** *Effect of the $ET_A$ selective receptor antagonist BQ123 on the survival of rats after myocardial infarction. Addition of BQ123 to the drinking water beginning 10 days after coronary artery ligation (●) resulted in a significant improvement in survival over animals treated with saline (◆). ■ = Sham-operated animals treated with saline. (From ref. 52 with permission.)*

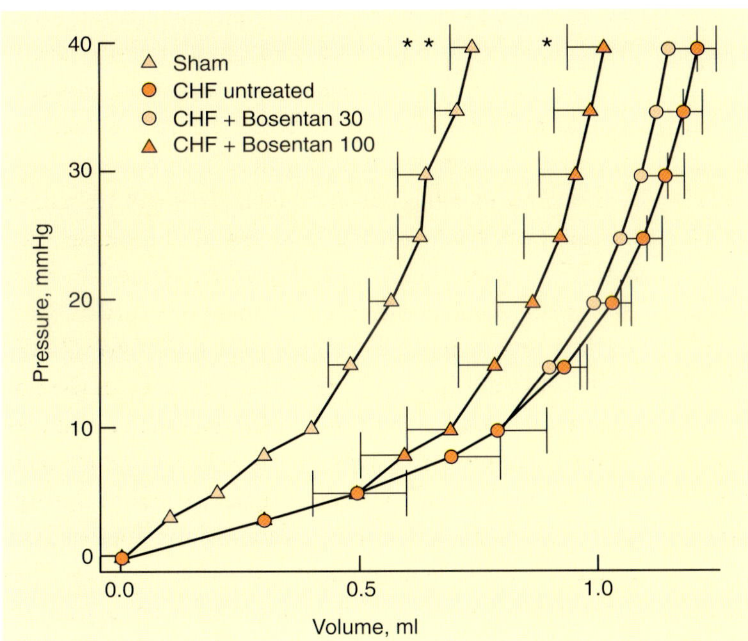


**Figure 11.5** *Effect of treatment with the non-selective endothelin-1 receptor antagonist bosentan on left ventricular (LV) pressure–volume relationships in rats with chronic myocardial infarction. Two months after myocardial infarction, the LV pressure–volume relationship was shifted rightwards (●) compared with sham-operated animals (▲). Treatment with bosentan 100 mg/kg per day resulted in a significant attenuation of the rightward shift, although a lower dose (30 mg/kg per day) had no effect. (Adapted from ref. 53 with permission).*

treated rats, there was a marked rightward shift in the LV pressure–volume relationship, indicating chamber dilation, and a depression in the LV developed pressure–volume relationship, indicating reduced pumping capacity. In hearts from rats treated with TBC11254 there was attenuation of both chamber dilatation and decrease in pump function.

Spinale *et al.* [56] studied rabbits with pacing-induced heart failure. They found that plasma ET-1 increased with pacing-induced failure, in association with an increase in LV end-diastolic diameter and a decrease in LV shortening fraction. Treatment with the $ET_A$-selective antagonist PD-156707 improved LV pump function (increased shortening fraction and decreased LV diameter) and reduced LV peak wall stress. In this study, heart failure was associated with a decrease in the shortening velocity of isolated myocytes. In animals treated with the $ET_A$ receptor blocker, myocyte shortening velocity improved, leading to the suggestion that ET blockade caused an improvement at the cellular level. Shimoyama *et al.* [57] examined the acute haemodynamic effect of bosentan in dogs with chronic heart failure after embolic infarction. At 60 min, bosentan had no effect on heart rate or mean arterial pressure, but caused decreases in LV end-diastolic pressure and systemic vascular resistance, and increases in cardiac output, LV fractional shortening, and $+dP/dt$.

## Endothelin-1 antagonists in patients with heart failure

The observed increase in ET-1 levels in patients with heart failure and the results of *in vitro* and animal studies have led to the suggestion that interruption of the ET system with an ET-1 receptor antagonist or ECE inhibitor would exert beneficial effects in patients with chronic heart failure [58–60]. In an important proof of principle experiment, Love *et al.* [61] administered the ECE inhibitor phosphoramidon or the $ET_A$-selective antagonist BQ123 via selective infusion into the brachial artery of patients with chronic heart failure while measuring forearm blood flow by venous occlusion plethysmography. Phosphoramidon and BQ123 increased forearm blood flow by 52 ± 10% and 31 ± 6%, respectively [61]. This result suggested that ET contributes to increased systemic vascular tone in patients with heart failure, and that the effect is mediated, at least in part, by the $ET_A$ receptor.

Kiowski *et al.* [62] reported the first systemic administration of an $ET_A$ blocker in patients with heart failure (Fig. 11.6). They gave the non-selective antagonist bosentan by intravenous infusion (100 mg followed after 60 min by 200 mg) to 24 patients with chronic heart failure. Bosentan caused modest decreases in mean arterial pressure (−8%), mean pulmonary artery pressure (−14%), right atrial pressure (−18%), systemic vascular resistance (−17%), and pulmonary wedge pressure (−9%). Heart rate was unchanged and cardiac index increased by 14%. The most pronounced effect of bosentan was a 33% decrease in the pulmonary vascular resistance.

Sutsch *et al.* [63] examined the acute and subacute (14 days) effects of bosentan administered orally (0.5 g twice daily) to patients with chronic heart failure. The subjects were receiving standard triple therapy consisting of diuretics, digitalis, and angiotensin-converting enzyme inhibitors. The acute haemodynamic effects of oral bosentan were similar to those observed with intravenous administration of the drug. With continuous oral administration for 14 days, the drug was well tolerated, and the haemodynamic effect of the drug was sustained or possibly augmented compared with the early haemodynamic effects at 24 h. Plasma ET-1 levels increased with both acute and 14 day bosentan treatment, whereas noradrenaline, renin, and angiotensin were unchanged.

Although to date most of the clinical data relate to bosentan, several other receptor blockers have entered clinical trials [64, 65]. The acute haemodynamic effects of intravenous administration of two doses of the $ET_A$-selective blocker TBC11254 have recently been examined in patients with chronic stable heart failure [66]. In 24 patients studied, both low (1.5 mg/kg) and high (3 mg/kg) doses caused significant decreases in mean pulmonary artery pressure and pulmonary vascular resistance, but had no effect on systemic vascular resistance, pulmonary capillary wedge pressure, cardiac index, or heart are. Since the non-selective antagonist bosentan decreased both systemic and pulmonary resistance, this early finding raises the possibility that $ET_A$ receptors predominate in the pulmonary vasculature.

An important question is whether ET receptor selectivity is of clinical value. Because of their differential effects on vascular contraction and relaxation, it might be anticipated that $ET_A$-selective blockade would result in more effective vasodilatation than $ET_B$-selective blockade. However, based on the limited data available this may not prove to be true, at least in the short term. It is also possible that the benefits of long-term treatment with an ET blocker have little or nothing to do with the drug's acute haemodynamic actions, but rather are a function of the ability of the drug to prevent myocardial remodelling. The relative contributions of the $ET_A$ and $ET_B$ subtypes to myocardial remodelling and failure are not known. However, two *in vitro* observations suggest that $ET_A$-selective blockade may be preferable: (1) the $ET_A$ subtype predominates on myocytes; and (2) although both $ET_A$ and $ET_B$ subtypes are present on cardiac fibroblasts, the $ET_A$ subtype causes degradation of fibrillar collagen, whereas the $ET_B$ subtype increases collagen synthesis. The former effect may be important in preventing LV dilatation, whereas the latter could play a role in acute wound healing and chronic fibrosis. Although these observations provide some theoretical insight, ultimately, the clinical effects of specific ET receptor blockers or ECE antagonists can only be determined from trials in humans.

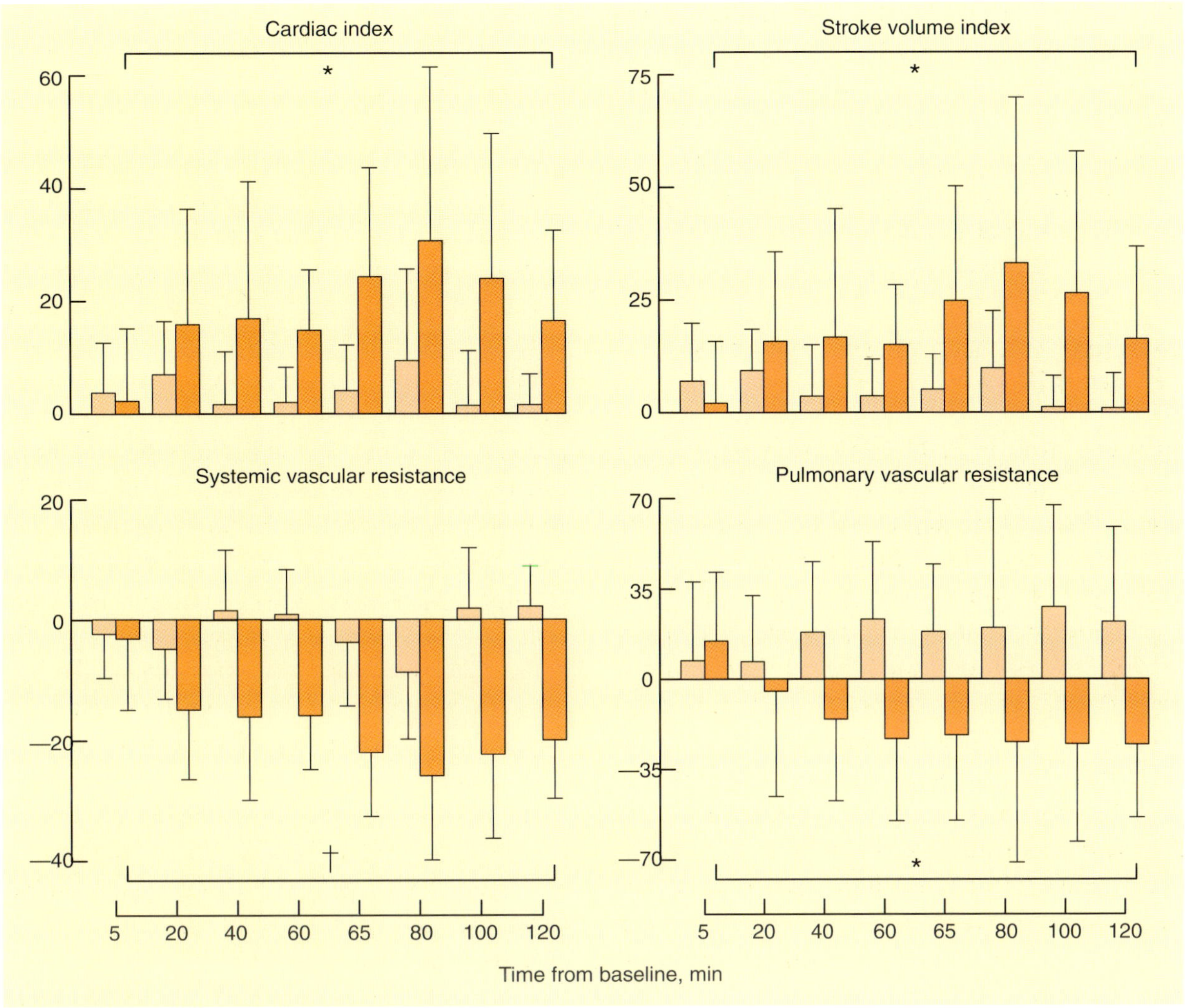


**Figure 11.6** *Short-term haemodynamic effects of bosentan in patients with chronic heart failure. An intravenous bolus of bosantan (100 mg) given at time 0 and again at 60 min increased cardiac index and stroke volume, and decreased systemic and pulmonary vascular resistance. Heart rate was unchanged, and there were decreases in right atrial, pulmonary artery, pulmonary capillary wedge, and systemic arterial pressure (not shown). (Adapted from ref. 62 with permission).*

## References


1. Yanagisawa M, Kurihara H, Kimura S *et al.* A novel potent vasoconstrictor peptide produced by vascular endothelial cells. *Nature* 1988; 332: 411–15.
2. Fukuroda T, Fujikawa T, Ozaki S *et al.* Clearance of circulating endothelin-1 by ETB receptors in rats. *Biochem Biophys Res Commun.* 1994; 199: 1461–5.
3. Xu D, Emoto N, Giaid A *et al.* ECE-1: a membrane bound metalloprotease that catalyzes the proteolytic activation of big endothelin-1. *Cell* 1994; 78: 473–85.
4. Vane J, Botting R, Vanhoutte PM. Up-to date on endothelins. *J Cardiovasc Pharmacol* 1995; 26 (Suppl 3): xi–xii.
5. Schweizer A, Valdenaire O, Nelbock P *et al.* Human endothelin-converting enzyme (ECE-1): three isoforms with distinct subcellular localizations. *Biochem J* 1997; 328: 871–7.
6. Naomi S, Iwaoka T, Disashi T *et al.* Endothelin-1 inhibits endothelin-converting enzyme-1 expression in cultured rat pulmonary endothelial cells. *Circulation* 1998; 97: 234–6.
7. Takahashi T, Kanda T, Inoue M *et al.* Endothelin converting enzyme inhibitor protects development of right ventricular overload and medial thickening of pulmonary arteries in rats with monocrotaline-induced pulmonary hypertension. *Life Sci* 1998; 63: PL137–43.
8. Sakurai T, Yanagisawa M, Masaki T. Molecular characterization of endothelin receptors. *Trends Pharmacol Sci* 1992; 13: 103–8.
9. Guarda E, Katwa LC, Myers PR *et al.* Effects of endothelins on collagen turnover in cardiac fibroblasts. *Cardiovasc Res* 1993; 27: 2130–4.
10. Wang Y, Rose PM, Webb ML, Dunn MJ. Endothelins stimulate mitogen-activated protein kinase cascade through either $ET_A$ or $ET_B$. *Am J Physiol* 1994; 267: C1130–5.

11. Gellai M, De Wolf R, Fletcher T, Nambi P. Contribution of endogenous endothelin-1 to the maintenance of vascular tone: role of nitric oxide. *Pharmacology* 1997; 55: 299–308.
12. Warner TD, Allcock GH, Mickley EJ *et al.* Comparative studies with the endothelin receptor antagonists BQ-123 and PD 142893 indicate at least three endothelin receptors. *J Cardiovasc Pharmacol* 19xx; 22 (Suppl 8): S117–20.
13. Nambi P, Pullen M, Kincaid J *et al.* Identification and characterization of a novel endothelin receptor that binds both ETA- and ETB-selective ligands. *Mol Pharmacol* 1997; 52: 582–9.
14. Karne S, Jayawickreme CK, Lerner MR. Cloning and characterization of an endothelin-3 specific receptor (ETC receptor) from *Xenopus laevis* dermal melanophores. *J Biol Chem* 1993; 268: 19 126–33.
15. Webb ML, Meek TD. Inhibitors of endothelin. *Med Res Rev* 1997; 17: 17–67.
16. Kurihara Y, Kurihara H, Suzuki H *et al.* Elevated blood pressure and craniofacial abnormalities in mice deficient in endothelin-1. *Nature* 1994; 368: 703–10.
17. Kurihara Y, Kurihara H, Oda H *et al.* Aortic arch malformations and ventricular septal defect in mice deficient in endothelin-1. *J Clin Invest* 1995; 96: 293–330.
18. Chien KR. Close encounters with ET-1. *J Clin Invest* 1995; 96: 1–3.
19. Kelly RA, Eid H, Kramer BK *et al.* Endothelin enhances the contractile responsiveness of adult rat ventricular myocytes to calcium by a pertussis toxin-sensitive pathway. *J Clin Invest* 1990; 86: 1164–71.
20. Endoh M, Fujita S, Yang HT *et al.* Endothelin: receptor subtypes, signal transduction, regulation of $CA^{2+}$ transients and contractility in rabbit ventricular myocardium. *Life Sci* 19xx; 62: 1485–9.
21. Jones LG, Rozich JD, Tsutsui H, Cooper GIV. Endothelin stimulates multiple responses in isolated adult ventricular cardiac myocytes. *Am J Physiol* 1992; 263: H1447–54.
22. Ito H, Hirata Y, Hiroe M *et al.* Endothelin-1 induces hypertrophy with enhanced expression of muscle-specific genes in cultured rat cardiomyocytes. *Circ Res* 1991; 69: 209–15.
23. Shubeita HE, McDonough PM, Harris AN *et al.* Endothelin induction of inostol phospholipid hydrolysis, sarcomere assembly, and cardiac gene expression in ventricular myocytes. *J Biol Chem* 1990; 265: 20 555–62.
24. Satoh N, Suter TM, Liao R, Colucci WS, α-Adrenergic stimulation and endothelin-1 upregulate expressionof Na/Ca exchanger mRNA and increase sensitivity to $[Na]_i$ in adult rat ventricular myocytes. *Circulation* 1997; 96 (Suppl I): I–629.
25. Ito H, Hirata Y, Adachi S *et al.* Endothelin-1 is an autocrine/paracrine factor in the mechanism of angiotensin II-induced hypertrophy in cultured rat cardiomyocytes. *J Clin Invest* 1993; 92: 398–403.
26. Yamazaki, Komuro I, Kudoh S *et al.* Endothelin-1 is involved in mechanical stress-induced cardiomyocyte hypertrophy. *J Biol Chem* 1996; 271: 3221–8.
27. Thomas PB, Liu EC, Webb ML *et al.* Exogenous effects and endogenous production of endothelin in cardiac myocytes: potential significance in heart failure. *Am J Physiol* 1996; 271: H2629–37.
28. Fujisaki H, Ito H, Hirata Y *et al.* Natriuretic peptides inhibit angiotensin II-induced proliferation of rat cardiac fibroblasts by blocking endothelin-1 gene expression. *J Clin Invest* 1995; 96: 1059–65.
29. Nunez DJ, Brown MJ, Davenport AP *et al.* Endothelin-1 mRNA is widely expressed in porcine and human tissues. *J Clin Invest* 1990; 85: 1537–41.
30. Plumpton C, Ashby MJ, Kuc RE *et al.* Expression of endothelin peptides and mRNA in the human heart. *Clin Sci* 1996; 90: 37–46.
31. Ito H, Hiroe M, Hirata Y *et al.* Endothelin ETA receptor antagonist blocks cardiac hypertrophy provoked by hemodynamic overload. *Circulation* 1994; 89: 2198–203.
32. Arai M, Yoguchi A, Iso T *et al.* Endothelin-1 and its binding sites are upregulated in pressure overload cardiac hypertorphy. *Am J Physiol* 1995; 268: H2084–91.
33. Tonnessen T, Christensen G, Oie E *et al.* Increased cardiac expression of endothelin-1 mRNA in ischemic heart failure in rats. *Cardiovasc Res* 1997; 33: 601–10.
34. Vitola JV, Forman MB, Holsinger JP *et al.* Role of endothelin in a rabbit model of acute myocardial infarction: effects of receptor antagonists. *J Cardiovasc Pharmacol* 1996; 28: 774–83.
35. Cohn JN, Structural basis for heart failure. Ventricular remodeling and its pharmacological inhibition. *Circulation* 1995; 91: 2504–7.
36. Colucci WS. Molecular and cellular mechanisms of myocardial failure. *Am J Cardiol* 1997; 80: 15–25L.
37. Cody RJ, Haas GJ, Binkley PF *et al.* Plasma endothelin correlates with the extent of pulmonary hypertension in patients with congestive heart failure. *Circulation* 1992; 85: 504–9.
38. McMurray JJ, Ray SG, Abdullah I *et al.* Plasma endothelin in chronic heart failure. *Circulation* 1992; 85: 1374–9.
39. Good JM, Nihoyannopoulos P, Ghatei MA *et al.* Elevated plasma endothelin concentrations in heart failure, an effect of angiotensin II? *Eur Heart J* 1994; 15: 1634–40.
40. Mangieri E, Tanzilli G, Barilla F *et al.* Isometric handgrip exercise increases endothelin-1 plasma levels in patients with chronic congestive heart failure. *Am J Cardiol* 1997; 79: 1261–3.
41. Lerman A, Kubo SH, Tschumperlin LK, Burnett JC Jr. Plasma endothelin concentrations in humans with end-stage heart failure and after heart transplantation. *J Am Coll Cardiol* 1992; 20: 849–53.
42. Wei CM, Lerman A, Rodeheffer RJ *et al.* Endothelin in human congestive heart failure. *Circulation* 1994; 89: 1580–6.
43. de Groote P, Millaire A, Racadot A *et al.* Plasma levels of endothelin-1 at rest and after exercise in patients with moderate congestive heart failure. *Int J Cardiol* 1995; 51: 267–72.
44. Krum H, Goldsmith R, Wilshire-Clement M *et al.* Role of endothelin in the exercise intolerance of chronic heart failure. *Am J Cardiol* 1995; 75: 1282–3.
45. Omland T, Lie RT, Aakvaag A *et al.* Plasma endothelin determination as a prognostic indicator of 1-year mortality after acute myocardial infarction. *Circulation* 1994; 89: 1573–9.
46. Pacher R, Stanek B, Hulsmann M *et al.* Prognostic impact of big endothelin-1 plasma concentrations compared with invasive hemodynamic evaluation in severe heart failure. *J Am Coll Cardiol* 1996; 27: 633–41.
47. Krum H, Gu A, Wilshire CM *et al.* Changes in plasma endothelin-1 levels reflect clinical response to beta-blockade in chronic heart failure. *Am Heart J* 1996; 131: 337–41.
48. Margulies KB, Hildebrand FL Jr, Lerman A *et al.* Increased endothelin in experimental heart failure. *Circulation* 1990; 82: 2226–30.
49. Kaddoura S, Firth JD, Boheler KR *et al.* Endothelin-1 is involved in norepinephrine-induced ventricular hypertrophy *in vivo*. Acute effects of bosentan and orally active mixed endothelin $ET_A$ and $ET_B$ receptor antagonists. *Circulation* 1996; 92: 2068–79.
50. Sakai S, Miyauchi T, Sakurai T *et al.* Endogenous endothelin-1 participates in the maintenance of cardiac function in rats with congestive heart failure: marked increase in endothelin-1 production in the failing heart. *Circulation* 1996; 93: 1214–22.

51. Teerlink JR, Loffler B-M, Hess P *et al.* Role of endothelin in the maintenance of blood pressure in conscious rats with chronic heart failure. Acute effects of the endothelin receptor antagonist Ro 47-0203 (bosentan). *Circulation* 1994; 90: 2510–8.
52. Sakai S, Miyauchi T, Kobayashi M *et al.* Inhibition of myocardial endothelin pathway improves long-term survival in heart failure. *Nature* 1996; 384: 353–5.
53. Mulder P. Richard V, Derumeaux G *et al.* Role of endogenous endothelin in chronic heart failure: effect of long-term treatment with an endothelin antagonist on survival, hemodynamics, and cardiac remodeling. *Circulation* 1997; 96: 1976–82.
54. Fraccarollo D, Hu K, Galuppo P *et al.* Chronic endothelin receptor blockade attenuates progressive ventricular dilation and improves cardiac function in rats with myocardial infarction. *Circulation* 1997; 96: 3963–73.
55. Podesser BK, Siwik DA, Eberli FR *et al.* $ET_A$-receptor blockage matrix metalloprotein ase activation late post myocardial infarction in the rat. *Am J Physiol* (*Heart Circ Physiol*) 2001; 280: H984–91.
56. Spinale FG, Walker JD, Mukherjee R *et al.* Concomitant endothelin receptor subtype-A blockade during the progression of pacing-induced congestive heart failure in rabbits. Beneficial effects on left ventricular and myocyte function. *Circulation* 1997; 95: 1918–29.
57. Shimoyama H, Sabbah HN, Borzak S *et al.* Short-term hemodynamic effects of endothelin receptor blockade in dogs with chronic heart failure. *Circulation* 1996; 94: 779–84.
58. Colucci WS. Myocardial endothelin. Does it play a role in myocardial failure? *Circulation* 1996; 93: 1069–72.
59. Cohn JN. Is there a role for endothelin in the natural history of heart failure? *Circulation* 1996; 94: 604–6.
60. Yazaki Y, Yamazaki T. Reversing congestive heart failure with endothelin receptor antagonists. *Circulation* 1997; 95: 1752–4.
61. Love MP, Haynes WG, Gray GA *et al.* Vasodilator effects of endothelin-converting enzyme inhibition and endothelin ETA receptor blockade in chronic heart failure patients treated with ACE inhibitors. *Circulation* 1996; 94: 2131–7.
62. Kiowski W, Sutsch G, Hunziker P *et al.* Evidence for endothelin-1-mediated vasoconstriction in severe chronic heart failure. *Lancet* 1995; 346: 732–6.
63. Sutsch G, Bertel O, Kiowski W. Acute and short-term effects of thenonpeptide endothelin-1 receptor antagonist bosentan in humans. *Cardiovasc Drugs Ther* 1997; 10: 717–25.
64. Webb DJ, Strachan FE. Clinical experience with endothelin antagonists. *Am J Hypertens* 1998; 11: 71–9S.
65. Noll G, Wenzel RR, Lüscher TF. Endothelin and endothelin antagonists: potential role in cardiovascular and renal disease. *Mol Cell Biochem* 1996; 157: 259–67.
66. Givertz MM, Colucci WS, LeJemtel TH *et al.* Acute endothelin A receptor causes selective pulmonary vasodilation in patients with chronic heart failure. *Circulation* 2000; 101: 2922–7.

# Mitochondrial abnormalities in cardiomyopathy 12

E. ARBUSTINI, P. MORBINI, B. DAL BELLO AND J. NARULA

## Introduction

The steady state in living cells is maintained by biochemical processes that produce and consume energy [1], and the majority of the energy is produced by oxidative phosphorylation in mitochondria [2–4]. Mitochondria are intracellular organelles found in all mammalian cells [5]. Their number in each cell and their morphology vary, depending on the function and activity of the cell [6]. Cells with high metabolic activity, such as hepatocytes, contain thousands of mitochondria [7]. An increase in metabolic activity or demand, such as during hyperactivity in skeletal muscle [8], or during cardiac myocyte hypertrophy [9, 10], induces an increase in the total number of mitochondria in cells.

## Mitochondrial structure and function

### Origin of mitochondria

Mitochondria represent external micro-organisms that were incorporated within the cell and developed a symbiotic relationship with multicellular organisms, some time early in evolution [11]. The timing of this event is difficult to establish and probably corresponds to the ecological change from an erstwhile reducing atmosphere to the present oxidizing environment, approximately a billion years ago. Facing the change from an environment rich in hydrogen, ammonia, and methane, to one rich in oxygen, nitrogen, and carbon dioxide, organisms survived the lethal effects of oxygen and free radicals by the intracellular incorporation of bacteria that were capable of adjusting to rapid changes in the environment. These incorporated prokaryotes captured and utilized oxygen in benign oxidation–reduction metabolic reactions. The endosymbiotic mechanisms led to progressive reciprocal adaptation; more than 99% of the original bacterial genome was lost because the nutritional supply was provided by the host organism. Of the original 4000 prokaryotic genes, only 37 were retained by the incorporated prokaryotes and are present in the modern mitochondria. The symbiotic bacteria lost their autonomy and became increasingly dependent on the host cell genome, which encoded factors controlling mitochondrial DNA (mtDNA) replication, transcription, and translation [12]. To prevent translation of messenger RNAs escaping from the mitochondrion into the host cell cytoplasm, the original prokaryotic genetic code mutated, degenerating from the nuclear genetic code (Table 12.1). The few genes that remained in the modern mitochondrion are uniquely necessary for local aerobic respiration and oxidative phosphorylation. During the symbiotic evolution, the eukaryotes have become almost entirely dependent on mitochondrial aerobic reactions for viability.

All human mtDNAs derive from a single phylogenetic tree; today, mtDNAs from people from single continents cluster together. African mtDNAs are the oldest and most divergent, followed by Asian and then European mtDNAs [13, 14]. Comparison of the human mtDNA tree in Africa and chimpanzee mtDNA suggests an estimated coalescence time of 149 000 years before present (YBP; 95% confidence interval 81 000–231 000) [14], whereas the European coalescence time is between 40 000 and 50 000 YBP [15].

### Morphology of mitochondria

The basic structure of mitochondria was established by electron microscopy [16]. The mitochondrion consists of

**Table 12.1** Mitochondrial genetic code

| Codon | Mitochondrial code of mammals | 'Universal' code |
|---|---|---|
| UGA | Tryptophan | STOP |
| AUA | Methionine | Isoleucine |
| AGA | STOP | Arginine |
| AGG | STOP | Arginine |

two membranes: an outer membrane derived from the phagocytic phase of the host organism, and an inner membrane of bacterial origin infolded to form mitochondrial cristae. The space between the two membranes is called the intermembrane space and the space enclosed by the inner membrane is referred to as matrix. Inner and outer membranes differ in composition and function. The lipid content of the outer membrane is nearly 50% by weight, whereas the inner membrane is richer in proteins and contains less than 30% lipid. Cardiolipin predominates in the inner membrane and phosphatidyl inositol is abundant in the outer membrane [17]. The inner mitochondrial membrane is the site of cellular respiratory chain and energy-transduction processes because the respiratory enzymes responsible for oxygen uptake are attached to this membrane [2]. Mitochondrial ribosomes are smaller than those found in the cytoplasm [13].

The permeability characteristics of outer and inner mitochondrial membranes are significantly different: the outer is very permeable whereas the inner is not [17, 18]. Inner membrane is, in fact, the major permeability barrier within the cell, even to relatively small molecules. Lipid insoluble non-electrolytes higher than 100 molecular weight (mol. wt), as well as charged ions such as $Na^+$, $K^+$ and $Cl^-$, do not pass through the inner membrane [18]. The outer membrane of isolated mitochondria is permeable to most ions, substrates, and various molecules of up to 10 000 mol. wt. It contains a protein called porin, which makes it largely permeable to molecules less than 1500 mol. wt. [19].

## Mitochondrial function

Mitochondria are the major site of energy production within the cell [1]. Most of the cellular adenosine triphosphate (ATP) is synthesized by the oxidative phosphorylation that takes place across the inner membrane [2, 18]. A pivotal role in oxidative phosphorylation is played by the electron transport chain. In this process, electrons flow through a chain of protein carriers bound to the inner mitochondrial membrane and are finally delivered to molecular oxygen. In normal conditions, the electron flow from energetic substrates to molecular oxygen is coupled with the active transport of protons across the inner mitochondrial membrane into the intermembrane space. This results in a higher concentration of protons in the intermembrane space than in the matrix. The subsequent transmembranous flow of protons, down the concentration gradient back to mitochondrial matrix, provides energy for the synthesis of ATP (Fig. 12.1). The normal respiratory state of mitochondria is defined as tightly coupled when the concentration of oxygen consumed is proportional to the amount of adenosine diphosphate (ADP) phosphorylated into ATP [1] with active production of energy. In tightly coupled mitochondria, the substrate oxidation rate directly depends on the presence of ADP and on the efficiency of the ATP/ADP exchange across the inner mitochondrial membrane [20]. In loosely coupled mitochondria, oxidation is maintained even in the absence of ADP and energy is dispersed as heat [20].

The energy substrates for the respiratory chain, such as the reduced form of nicotinamide adenine dinucleotide (NADH) and succinate, are provided by the citric acid cycle enzymes and pyruvate dehydrogenase, which are located in the mitochondrial matrix [21]. The mitochondrial respiratory chain works in serially ordered complexes, each containing electron carrier molecules and oxidative enzymes. The major electron carriers are ubiquinone (coenzyme Q, a hydrophobic, two-electron carrier), which moves in the lipid phase of the inner membrane, and cytochromes which contain an iron atom bound to haeme group [22, 23]. The presence of one of three different haeme groups characterizes three classes of cytochromes

**Table 12.2** Mitochondrial oxidative complexes

| | Name | Number of peptides | Number of mtDNA coded peptides |
|---|---|---|---|
| Complex I | NADH dehydrogenase | 44 | 7 |
| Complex II | Succinate dehydrogenase | 7 | 0 |
| Complex III | Dihydroubiquinone–cytochrome *c* oxidoreductase | 11 | 1 |
| Complex IV | Cytochrome *c* oxidase | 13 | 3 |
| Complex V | ATP synthase | > 20 | 2 |

NADH = reduced form of micotinamide adenine dinucleotide; mtDNA = mitochondrial DNA.

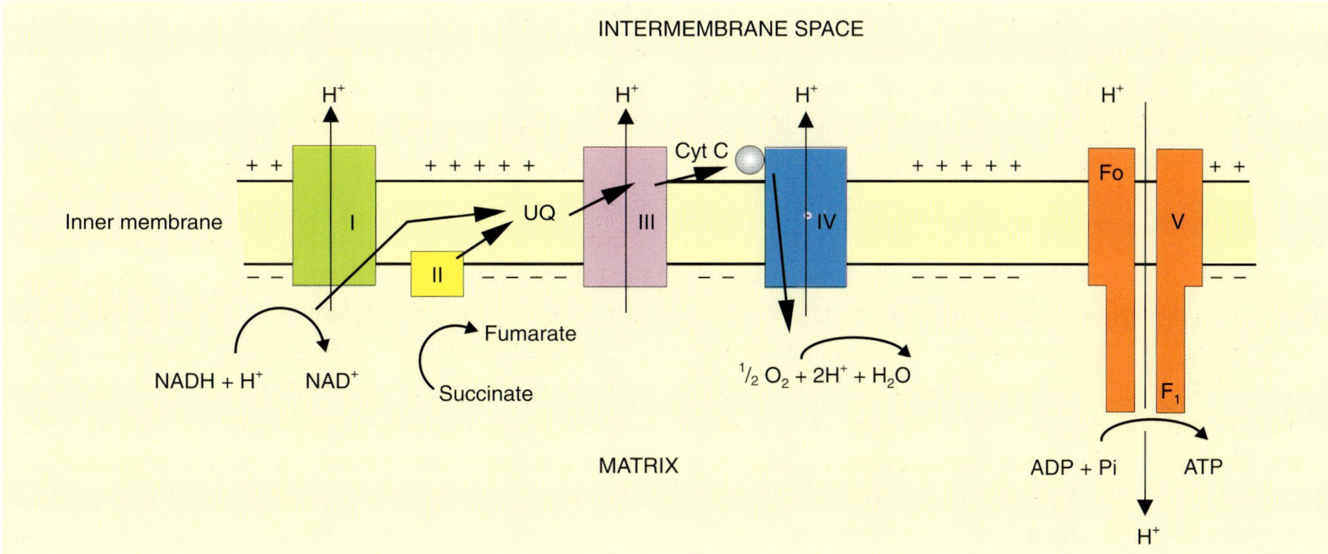


**Figure 12.1** *Simplified overview of electron from and ATP synthesis in the inner mitochondrial membrane. I, II, III, IV, and V: complexes I, II, III, IV, and V; NADH: nicotinamide adenine dinucleotide; UQ: ubiquinone; Cyt C: Cytochrome C; ADP: adenosine diphosphate; ATP: adenosine triphosphate. See text for complete explanation.*

(*a*, *b*, and *c*) [23]. The oxidative complexes (Table 12.2) comprise five distinct subgroups [3], all associated to the inner mitochonial membrane.

- Complex I, NADH dehydrogenase, catalyses electron transfer from NADH to ubiquinone [24]. It is composed of 44 subunits embedded in the inner mitochondrial membrane. Seven subunits are encoded by mtDNA (NDI–VII), and the remainder by nuclear genome. The electron flow through complex I from NADH to ubiquinone is accompanied by proton flow from the matrix to the intermembrane space.
- Complex II, succinate dehydrogenase (SDH) is the only membrane-bound enzyme of the citric acid cycle [25]. It is composed of at least seven proteins, all encoded by nuclear DNA, and also contains one flavin adenin dinucleotide (FAD). Electrons are transferred from succinate to FAD and then to ubiquinone.
- Complex III, dihydroubiquinone–cytochrome *c* oxidoreductase, contains 11 peptides, including two different cytochromes *b* and one cytochrome *c* [26]. The apoprotein of cytochrome *b* is encoded by mtDNA, while the other proteins of complex III are of nuclear origin. Complex III carries the electrons from ubiquinone to cytochrome *c*, and releases protons to the intermembrane space.
- Complex IV or cytochrome *c* oxidase (COX), is a transmembrane enzyme complex located in the inner mitochondrial membrane. It contains 13 peptides, three of which are encoded by mtDNA (CX I–III), and two cytochrome *a* [27]. Electrons are transferred from cytochrome *c* to molecular oxygen, with the production of water and the passage of protons from the matrix to the intermembrane space.
- ATP synthase (also called complex) is another large protein complex embedded in the inner mitochondrial membrane [28]. The protein has a headpiece, which is water soluble and extends into the matrix. The headpiece is composed of five peptides, all of which are encoded by nuclear genes, and catalyses the synthesis of ATP. The membrane sector of ATP synthase is composed of a basepiece and a stalk. The latter is highly hydrophobic and is comprised of a large number of peptides, two of which are coded by mtDNA. The synthase also contains an ATPase inhibitor moiety, which is encoded by nuclear DNA.

The proton gradient, created across the inner membrane along the electron transfer chain, drives the synthesis of ATP from ADP and $P_i$ during passive flow of protons into the matrix through pores formed by the inner membrane sector of the ATP synthase. Mitochondria synthesize about three ATPs per pair of electrons passed to oxygen when NADH is the electron donor. When succinate is the electron donor, two ATPs are produced [2]. Matrix ATP, produced by ATP synthase, is transferred across the inner mitochondrial membrane to the cellular cytosol by a specific carrier, adenine nucleotide translocator [29]. This transmembrane homodimer of 30 000 mol. wt, which is encoded by a nuclear gene, exchanges mitochondrial matrix ATP for cytosolic ADP. The energy produced in the mitochondrion is thus transferred to the whole cell [30, 31].

## Mitochondrial genome

### *Structure*

The human mitochondrial genome is a circular, 16.569 bp, double-stranded DNA which was completely sequenced by Sanger and co-workers in 1981 [32]. Mitochondrial DNA comprises 37 genes, including 22 transfer RNA (tRNA), two ribosomal RNA (12 S and 16 S rRNA), and 13 polypeptide coding genes [33, 34]. All genes are densely packed since there are no introns, and only tiny gaps exist between successive genes (Fig. 12.2).

The base composition of mtDNA is highly asymmetric. The heavy (H) mtDNA strand has a higher guanine and adenine (purine) content, whereas the light (L) strand is rich in cytosine and thymine (pyrimidine) [32]. The two strands can be resolved on a caesium chloride gradient, and show different buoyancy. Of the 37 mitochondrial genes, 28 are located in the H strand [32]. The H strand is transcribed in a clockwise direction as a single RNA molecule which starts from the heavy strand promoter (HT), while the L strand is transcribed anticlockwise from the light strand promoter (LT) [35, 36].

### *Replication*

Analogous to prokaryotes, there is only one origin of replication (O) in mtDNA, which has been divided into two parts: one for the H and another for the L strand [35]. OH is located in the (only) region of the mtDNA genome that contains no genes. This control region is called the D loop or displacement loop. Here, a locally synthesized fragment of RNA, quiescent until replication starts at the end of the D loop, displaces a large segment of the H strand. When replication starts, the mtDNA polymerase gamma, encoded by nuclear genes and imported from the cytosol, synthesizes daughter H strand DNA beginning at the 1 o'clock position and progresses clockwise around the circular genome molecule [37]. This process exposes the origin for the light chain. When polymerase passes OL at the 9 o'clock position, DNA synthesis on the template L strand starts and progresses in the opposite direction. When synthesis is completed on both H and L strands, the linked rings are divided to generate two

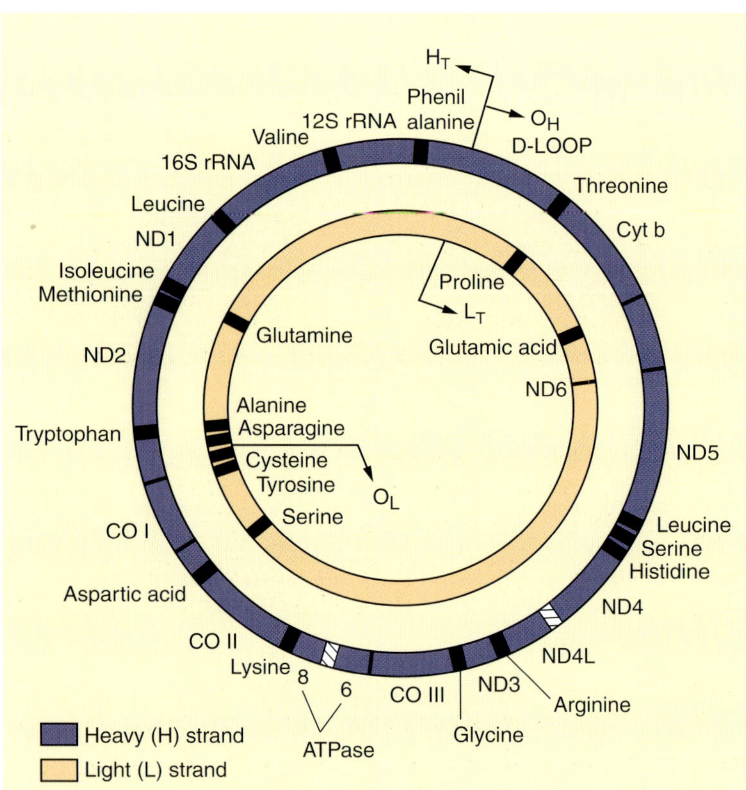


**Figure 12.2** *The human mitochondrial DNA map. Black bars represent regions coding for mitochondrial transfer RNAs.*

daughter duplex DNA molecules [37]. Overall, mtDNA replication takes about 2 h.

*Transcription*

Transcription of mtDNA differs from that of nuclear DNA genes because there is only one promoter region, which is located in the D loop. The HT and LT initiate transcription of the respective strands and progress to generate large polycistronic products [38]. The punctuated localization of tRNA genes among rRNA and mRNA allows separation of the single gene products. Endogenous nucleases cleave rRNA at both the 5′ and 3′ ends, thus releasing both mature tRNA and flanking rRNA and mRNA [39]. After transcription, tRNA receives a 3′ CCA triplet, and polyA binds to mRNA [39]. Given that the 2 rRNA transcribed with the 13 mRNA in each process cannot accommodate the translation requirements of the 13 mRNA, shorter transcripts of the region including HT, 12S rRNA, and 16S rRNA are synthesized 25-fold more quickly than the full-length transcript [40, 41]. Immediately downstream of the end of the 16S rRNA, a terminator protein binds a DNA region within the tRNA $Leu^{uur}$. This protein stops RNA polymerase progression and blocks transcription. If this block does not occur, polymerases continue to synthesize a full-length transcript [42, 43]. This parallel transcription yields a sufficient number of rRNA to make up the mitochondrial ribosomes for translation of the 13 mRNA.

*Translation*

Translation of the 13 mRNA takes place on mitochondrial ribosomes, which contain ribosomal proteins encoded by nuclear genes and the two ribosomal RNA (12S and 16S) of mitochondrial origin [41].

## Interaction between nuclear and mitochondrial genome

Mitochondrial structure and function are the result of the integration of nuclear and mitochondrial DNA-encoded proteins [44]. Structural proteins, transport factors, enzymes, and regulatory peptides of both nuclear and mitochondrial origin are precisely integrated in a unique intergenomic collaborative programme [45]. The number of nuclear DNA encoded proteins largely outnumbers mtDNA encoded proteins. Therefore, the probability of a mitochondrial disorder caused by a nuclear defect is much higher than that caused by a mitochondrial DNA defect [45]. At present, however, knowledge in the field of mitochondrial disorders is dominated by phenotypes associated with mitochondrial DNA defects [12]. The reasons are two-fold. First, mtDNA is a small molecule and its sequence, structure, and function are completely known. As a result, the related genetic defects can be more easily identified. In contrast, nuclear genes encoding mitochondrial structural, enzymatic, regulatory, and transport elements are still largely unknown. Secondly, a series of peculiar characteristics of mtDNA strongly influences the proportion of mitochondrial defects.

*Nucleosomes and other proteins*

- Nuclear DNA is bound by the nuclear membrane and thus more is protected from mutagenic effects, while mtDNA is naked in the matrix and exposed to damage induced by free radicals generated during oxidative phosphorylation processes [46].
- The mtDNA mutation rate is ten to 15 times higher than that of nuclear DNA.
- mtDNA lacks DNA repair systems, which operate efficiently in nuclear DNA [47].
- mtDNA genes are densely packed, so that mutations are likely to affect either coding genes or ribosomal or transfer RNA genes [34]. Conversely, in nuclear DNA, most mutations occur in non-coding regions.
- mtDNA defects accumulate within mitochondria, and corresponding phenotypes only appear after the amount of mutant has reached a threshold value [48]. In most cases, mutations are lethal only for very large amounts of mutated DNA so that they do not interfere with reproductive activity [49].
- The amount of mutant DNA varies from tissue to tissue and from cell to cell [49, 50]. Consequently, it is almost impossible to quantify the risk of a mtDNA defect-associated disease unless the amount of a given mutant in target tissues is known.

Therefore, although the number of nuclear genes encoding mitochondrial proteins is much higher than that of mtDNA-coded peptides, the peculiar characteristics of mitochondrial DNA make the expected proportion of nuclear DNA/mtDNA defects causing mitochondrial diseases unpredictable.

## Mitochondrial proteins encoded by nuclear DNA

As discussed above, nuclear DNA encodes a larger number of mitochondrial proteins than those encoded by the mitochondrial genome itself. Some important nuclear genome-encoded proteins are summarized below.

*Translocases*

Metabolites are carried across the mitochondrial membrane by specific translocases, which are encoded by nuclear DNA [45]. Recently, attention has focused on the adenine nucleotide translocator (ANT), which is responsible for the ATP/ADP exchange [30, 31]. There are three isoforms of the ANT protein (ANT1-3) in humans, which demonstrate tissue-specific expression [51]. ANT1 is predominantly expressed in cardiac and skeletal muscle, and has been designated the heart-muscle specific isoform. The ATP/ADP translocator is the most abundant mitochondrial protein [30]. It forms a gated pore through which ATP is moved from the matrix to the cytoplasm (29). However, in heart mitochondria, the transport of ATP/ADP seems to be, at least partially, mediated by ANT2. ANT1 gene maps on 4q35 [31]. Among other mitochondrial–membrane carrier proteins, defects in carnitine–acylcarnitine translocase have been recently related to disorders of mitochondrial fatty and oxidation [52]. The protein, which is coded by a gene mapping on 3p21.31, transfers fatty acylcarnitines across the inner mitochondrial membrane in exchange for free carnitine [52].

*Protein transport factors*

Most mitochondrial proteins encoded by nuclear DNA are synthesized in the cytoplasm and imported into the mitochondria, where they are delivered to their proper subcompartments, such as the inner and outer membrane systems, intermembrane space, or matrix [53, 54]. Importation is based both on generally needed transport factors, such as chaperonins, and on mitochondrial specific factors. The latter are basic peptides attached to the N-terminus of most imported proteins and capable of guiding proteins to the mitochondrion [45]. Genetic errors affecting nuclear genes encoding general proteins lead to severe multisystem disorders, and are likely to be lethal early in life. The myocardium is one of the affected tissues [55, 56]. In contrast, errors affecting nuclear genes encoding specific mitochondial carrier factors are likely to cause a single enzyme defect [53].

*Respiratory chain enzyme subunits*

Most defects of the various nuclear DNA coded subunits of the respiratory chain cause multiorgan diseases which are often fatal early after birth [45]. The heart may be involved, and may determine the final outcome of the disease, even when it is not the primarily affected target organ.

*Regulators of iron metabolism*

Frataxin, the mutation of which is responsible for a common form of hereditary neurodegenerative disorder, Friedreich's ataxia, has recently been identified in the inner membrane and cristae, of the mitochondria, where it is believed to regulate iron efflux [57, 58]. The pathology and target tissues in Friedreich's ataxia are consistent with mitochondrial diseases that affect tissues with high metabolic activity, such as central nervous system, heart, and pancreas. In yeast strains, deletion of the frataxin homologue causes excess iron to accumulate and damage mitochondria. [58]. Frataxin deficiency results in an alteration of mitochondrial iron homoeostasis, loss of iron catalytic activity on free radicals, and oxidative damage. In particular, reduced activity of iron-sulphur (Fe-S) cluster-containing subunits of mitochondrial respiratory complexes I, II, and III, as well as of aconitase, has been shown in cardiac tissue in patients with Friedreich's ataxia [59]. Since Fe-S proteins are extremely sensitive to free radicals, the iron overload should be responsible for the reduction in mitochondrial respiratory activity in target tissues.

## Identification of abnormalities of mitochondrial morphology, function, and mitochondrial DNA

Although morphological, histochemical, immunohistochemical, biochemical, and molecular analysis of myocardial samples can be performed, two major factors limit wider application of such studies. First, the cardiac disorders wherein investigation for mitochondrial function is necessary are predominantly represented by idiopathic cardiomyopathies, and the myocardial samples for diagnosis can only be obtained by endomyocardial biopsy (EMB). An invasive procedure such as EMB has inherent risks and complications [60]. Secondly, even when successfully performed, the biopsy only allows sampling of a limited number of small-sized myocardial samples, on which all mitochondrial investigations such as conventional histopathology, electron microscopy, histoenzymatic reactions, protein extraction for Western blotting studies, DNA and RNA extraction for molecular studies [multiple polymerase chain reaction (PCR) screening techniques such as denaturing gradient gel electrophoresis (DGGE) or single-strand conformational polymorphism (SSCP)] and DNA sequencing need to be undertaken. Although each technique increases the yield of information, given the small size and number of samples it becomes necessary to select the most appropriate and informative investigations. The selection of tests can be guided by clinical, histochemical, biochemical, and ultrastructural observations [9, 61, 62].

## Ultrastructural mitochondrial changes in the myocardium

Mitochondria undergo morphological modifications in almost all cardiac disorders [9, 10, 63]. Most ultrastructural changes in cardiomyopathic hearts are non-specific and may be found in normal hearts as well. These alterations can be grouped as follows.

### *Alterations in number of mitochondria*

The most common mitochondrial abnormality is proliferation of mitochondria. In cardiac myocytes, proliferating mitochondria are characteristically localized in paranuclear/perinuclear areas, and among myofibrils [10]; less frequently they accumulate under the sarcolemma. In myocardial cells, proliferating mitochondria do not arrange in ordinate arrays or lines. This pattern is in contrast to skeletal muscle fibres, where proliferating mitochondria characteristically accumulate under sarcolemma and distribute radially along myofibrils. The ordinate arrangement in skeletal muscle induces the typical ragged red fibre pattern on

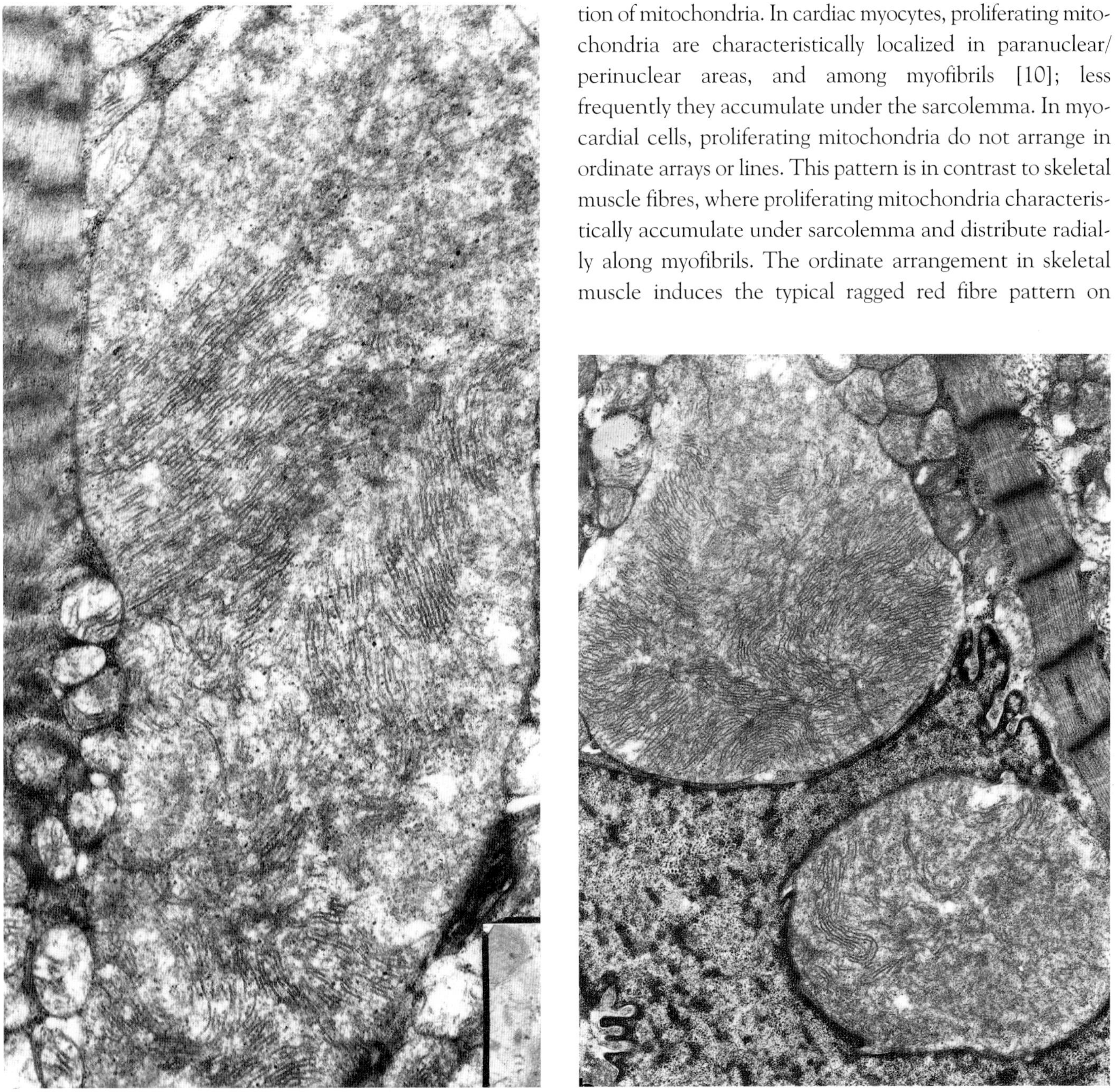

**Figure 12.3** *Electron micrographs showing giant mitochondria in cardiac myocytes with abnormal cristae. Compare large organelles with smaller mitochondria and sarcomere units (uranyl acetate, lead citrate).*

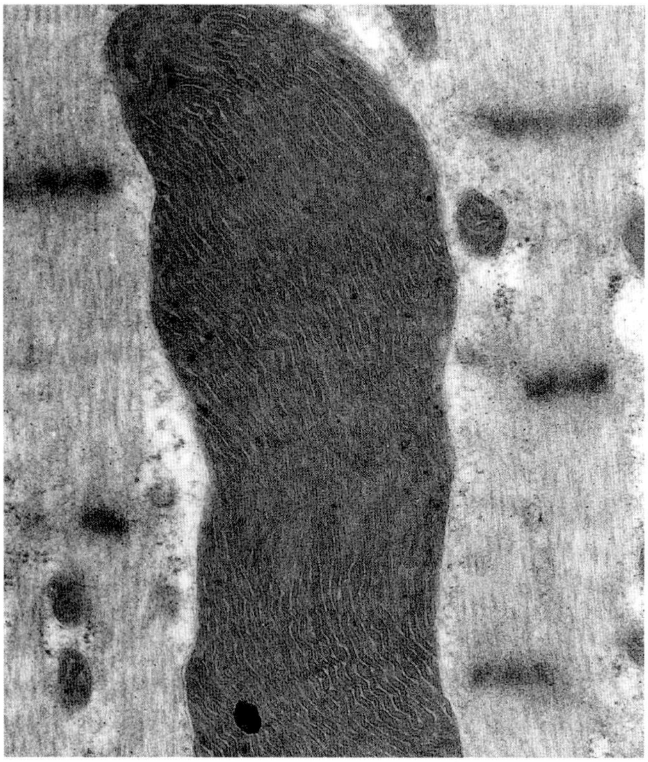

Figure 12.3 *(Continued)*

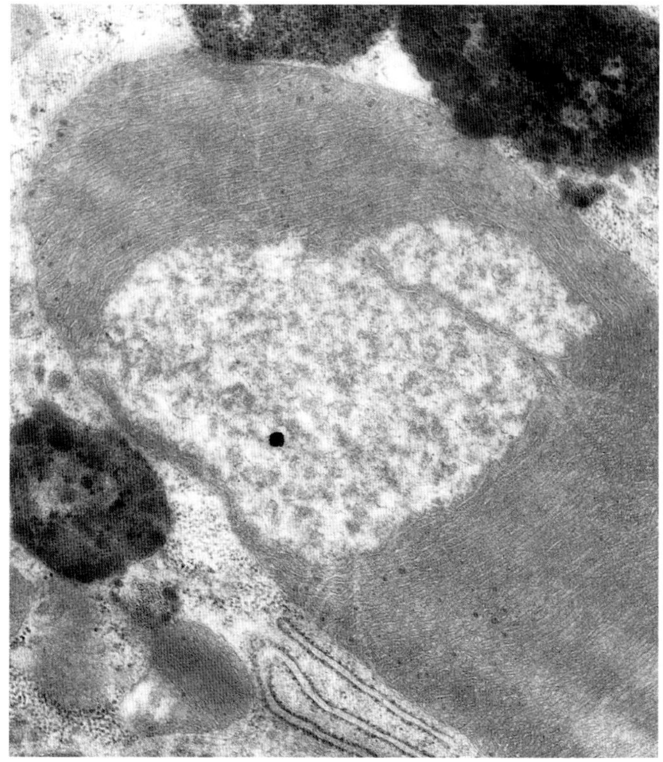

modified Gomori stain, and is characteristic of mitochondrial myopathy such as myoclonic epilepsy with ragged red fibres (MERRF) [64]. It is conceivable that in unabatedly contracting cardiac myocytes with centrally located nuclei, proliferating mitochondria are forced to localize in any available space. Conversely, in the skeletal muscle, proliferating mitochondria first accumulate in the most permissive subsarcolemmal space and then move to the centre via intermyofibrillar spaces.

Multiple major mtDNA large rearrangements, such as deletions, which are associated with the loss of several mitochondrial genes, molecules and organelles, represent a strong proliferation trigger in ischaemic cardiomyopathy [65, 66]. Deletions are favoured by free radical generation during the oxidative phosphorylation process in mitochondria of the ischaemic tissue [67]. In cardiac hypertrophy, the energy demand of hypertrophic myocytes is higher than in normotrophic cells and mitochondrial proliferation represents an adaptive response [9, 68].

Less frequently than proliferation, the amount of mitochondria appears reduced. This may occur in hypotrophic myocytes or in the cells wherein myofibrillar lysis leaves an empty sarcolemmal sheath with a residual reticular structure and organelles.

***Ultrastructural changes in size of mitochondria***

Increased size, up to giant organelles (10 $\mu$m or more), may be seen in myocyte hypertrophy (Fig. 12.3) [63]. Giant organelles could derive from fusion of multiple single organelles (Fig. 12.4), incomplete/abnormal division (too fast replication?), and abnormal growth.

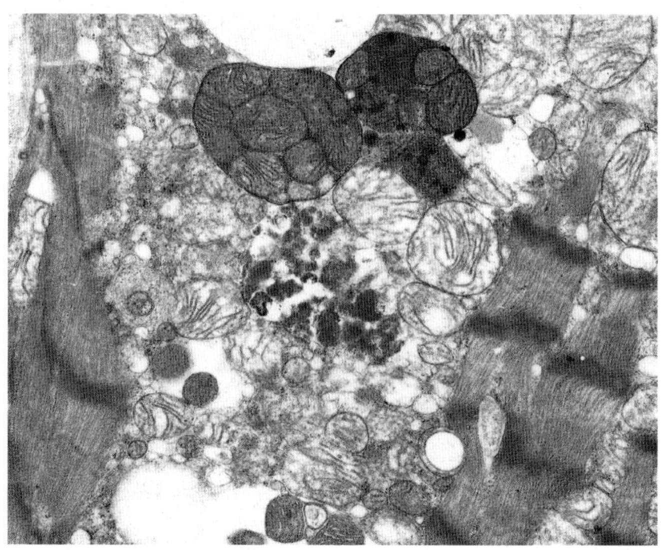

**Figure 12.4** *Electron micrograph showing damaged mitochondria with a fusion pattern (uranyl acetate, lead citrate).*

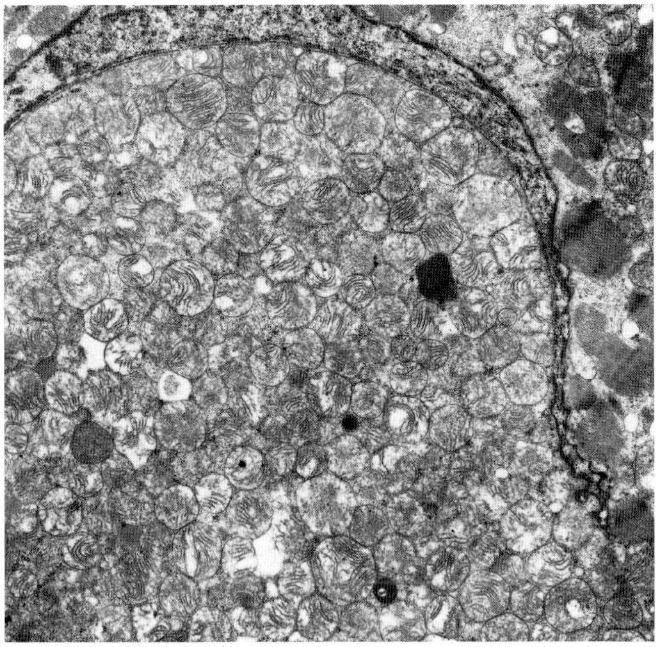

**Figure 12.5** *Electron micrograph showing a high number of mitochondria with an irregular size and shape, clear matrix and cristolysis (uranyl acetate, lead citrate).*

***Alteration in both number and size of mitochondria***

A large number of both large and small organelles in the heart is generically termed mitochondriosis (Fig. 12.5) [9].

***Changes in mitochondrial shape and appearance***

The bacterium-like shape of mitochondria may be lost in myocardial diseases and they may appear thinner than normal or rounded [9, 62]. In hypertrophic myocytes, mitochondria are often densely packed, and their morphology is influenced by the reciprocal proximity that induces the assumption of secondary 'polygonal' shapes.

In some myocardial diseases, the cristae may appear whorled, tubular, angulated, or concentrically arranged (Fig. 12.6). In addition, intramitochondrial inclusions of

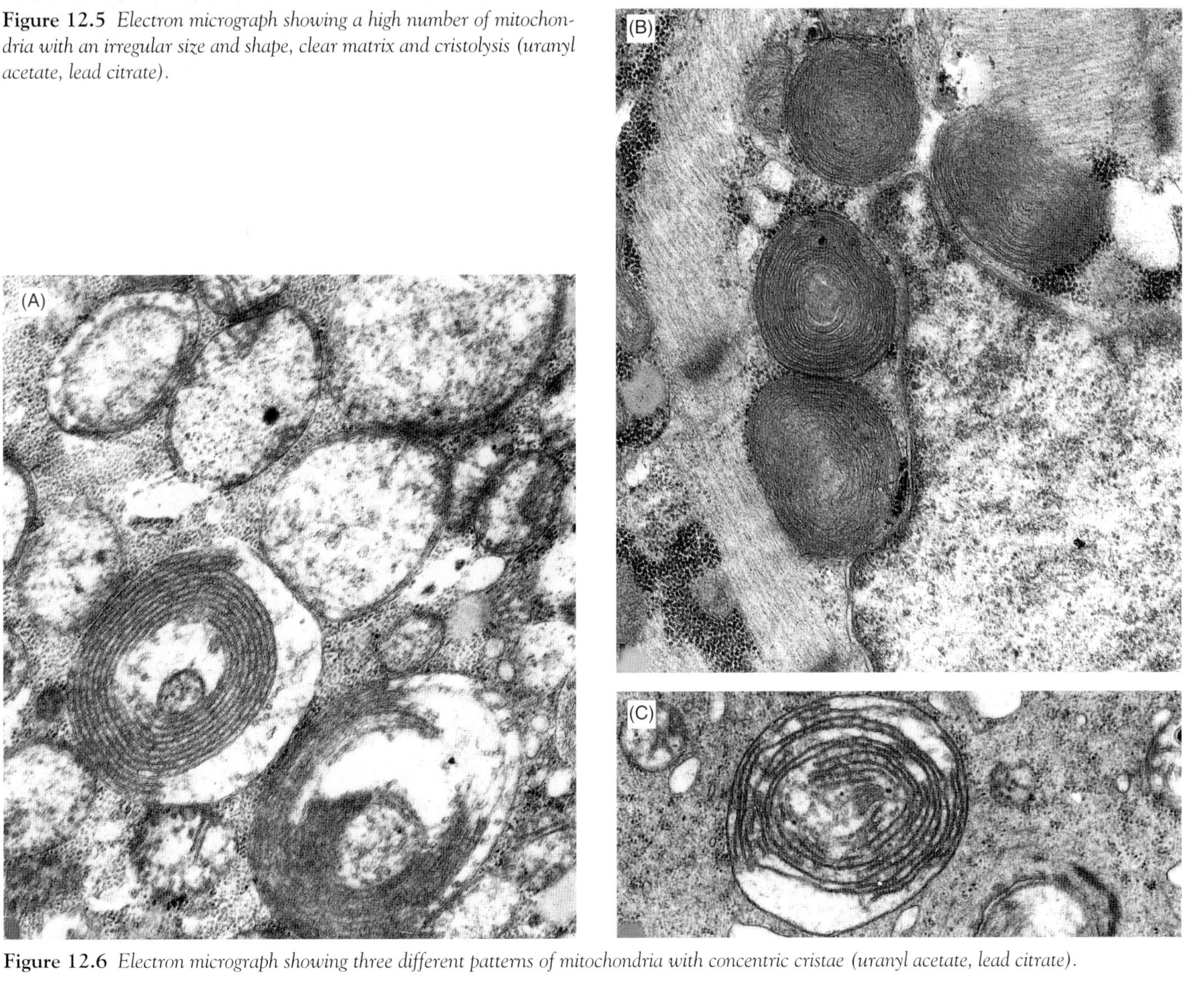


**Figure 12.6** *Electron micrograph showing three different patterns of mitochondria with concentric cristae (uranyl acetate, lead citrate).*

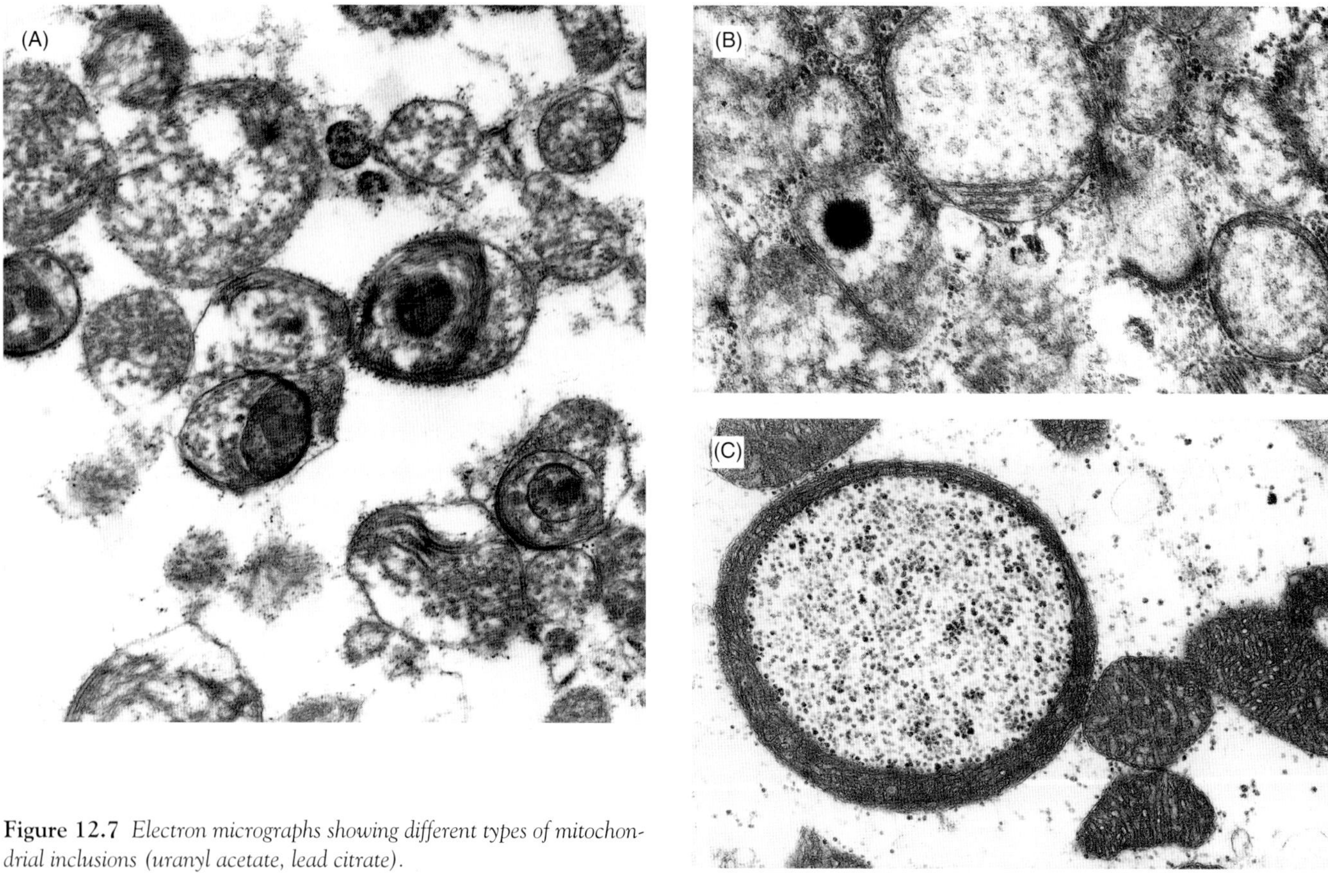


**Figure 12.7** *Electron micrographs showing different types of mitochondrial inclusions (uranyl acetate, lead citrate).*

crystalline or osmiophylic bodies, lipid material, or glycogen may be observed. In cardiac myocytes, crystalline inclusions are less frequent than in skeletal muscle and, when present, they look different from skeletal muscle cell inclusions (Fig. 12.7). Furthermore, matrix density may be abnormally reduced or increased in cardiomyopathy mitochondria. The combination of quantitative changes such as increase in number and size of mitochondria, and qualitative modifications including concentric cristae and mitochondrial inclusions provide a useful morphological guide for molecular analysis of mtDNA [62]. Although this pattern is not obligatorily specific for mtDNA-related cardiomyopathies, it allows triage of EMB samples to different types of investigation. In fact, the small number and size of biopsy samples obtained from patients affected by cardiomyopathies limit the variety of diagnostic procedures that can be performed for pathological and molecular studies. With the ultrastructural screening approach, pathological mtDNA mutations have been reported in more than 20% of patients whose cardiac mitochondria show the above abnormalities [62].

## Ultrastructural immunocytochemical changes

This technique provides *in situ* information about the enzyme subunits and substrates. Specific antibodies reactive against each protein subunit of the respiratory chain allow assessment of the protein expression and location in the mitochondria, as well as quantitation and comparison of expression of the target protein in different mitochondria and cells. For instance, cytochrome *c* expression has been shown to be preferentially concentrated in the mitochondria of normal hearts, whereas in hearts with cardiomyopathy cytochrome *c* is released from the mitochondria into the sarcoplasm [69]. However, ultrastructural immunocytochemistry cannot provide information on the effective functional status of normally expressed enzymes.

## Histochemical mitochondrial alterations

Histoenzymatic techniques investigate the mitochondrial enzyme activity and distribution in the muscle cells. The application of these studies is somewhat limited as snap-frozen tissue samples are mandatory, in order to preserve enzyme integrity. For histoenzymatic reactions the tissue sections are incubated with the specific enzyme substrate coupled with a chromogen. The oxidation of the substrate is associated with the chromogen reduction, which precipitates in a coloured, insoluble form. Although a large number of enzymes has been investigated, NADH dehydrogenase, succinate dehydrogenase, and cytochrome *c* oxidase are those most useful for mitochondrial study [69, 70]. Cardiomyocytes stain homogeneously and intensely with histoenzymatic reactions similar to smooth muscle cells but unlike skeletal myocytes which show different intensity of staining in type 1 and type 2 cells. However, in small EMB samples with artefactual contraction bands, the histoenzymatic stains may appear abnormally distributed, and only very severe enzyme deficiency can be suspected in small biopsy samples. In larger myocardial samples, histoenzymatic stains may clearly demonstrate abnormalities in the distribution and magnitude of the reaction (Fig. 12.8).

The modified Gomori trichrome histochemical stain has been routinely used to identify subsarcolemmal deposits of mitochondria in skeletal mitochondrial myopathy. The Gomori reaction, however, cannot be applied to myocardial samples, since proliferating mitochondria in cardiac myocytes do not preferentially accumulate in subsarcolemmal spaces.

### Biochemical and spectrophotometric assays of mitochondrial enzyme activity

Enzymatic activity of mitochondrial complexes I–IV can be quantified in tissue homogenates by spectrophotometric assays [71–73]. The change in the optical density of the preparation reflects the rate of reduction of a specific electron acceptor by the oxidative enzyme, in the presence of the appropriate enzyme substrate. Spectrophotometric assays, histoenzymatic reactions, and immunoelectron microscopy are complementary in quantifying the overall activity of the mitochondrial enzymes, assessing the cell distribution of enzyme defects and identifying the absence of specific enzyme subunits [62].

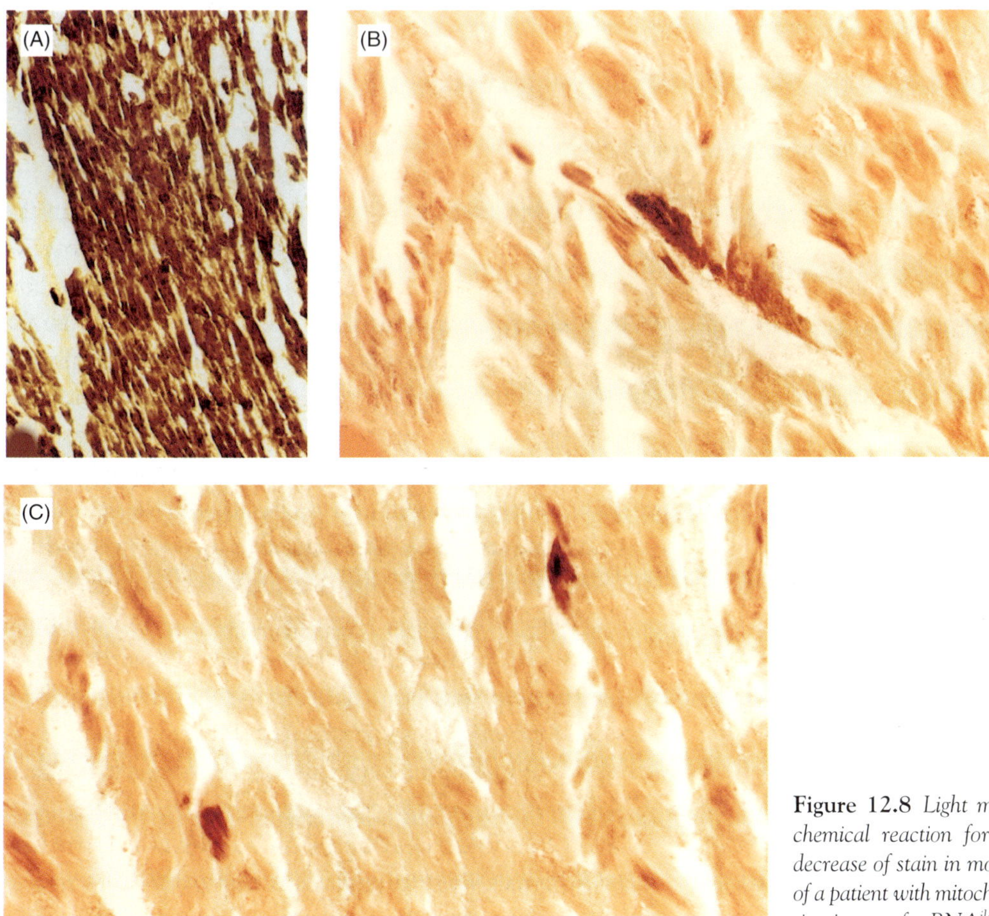


**Figure 12.8** *Light micrographs showing: (a) normal histochemical reaction for cytochrome* c *oxidase; (b, c) severe decrease of stain in most cardiac myocytes in the myocardium of a patient with mitochondrial DNA heteroplasmic point mutation in transfer* $RNA^{ile}$ *(COX histoenzymatic reaction).*

## Mitochondria in cardiomyopathy

### Classification of mitochondrial defects in cardiomyopathy

Mitochondrial defects in cardiomyopathic hearts can be grouped as follows.

#### *Disorders that primarily or dominantly affect hearts*

Patients diagnosed with cardiomyopathy causally linked to mtDNA defect may be clinically undistinguishable from patients in whom the disease is caused by viral infections or nuclear gene defects [72, 74–83]. When skeletal muscle involvement in such patients is subclinical or absent and other mitochondrial DNA defect-related phenotypes are not apparent in both probands and relatives, clinicians do not have any useful markers to attribute the disease to the mitochondrial defects. In these cases, biochemical analysis of EMB as well as molecular analyses of mtDNA and of nuclear genes governing mitochondrial structure and function may help in the diagnosis. Most of these disorders include adult-onset cardiomyopathies that are not associated with lactic acidosis, diabetes mellitus, or mental retardation [62, 83].

#### *Disorders affecting heart and other organ/tissue function*

Cardiac involvement in patients with encephalomyopathies constitutes the major determinant of the poor outcome [84–88]. Such defects often occur in children and result in major metabolic and neurological deficits. Cardiologists are often consulted for the management of conduction disturbances or congestive heart failure [84]. In mitochondrial disorders such as Kearns–Sayre syndrome (KSS), the cardiac involvement is often mild, affects atrioventricular conduction, and may be managed by pacemaker implantation [84]. In patients with myoclonic epilepsy lactic acidosis and stroke (MELAS), the systolic dysfunction of the heart can be severe and may necessitate transplantation as the treatment option [84].

#### *Secondary mitochondrial abnormalities in cardiovascular diseases*

Mitochondrial alterations may be observed in myocyte hypertrophy of variable origin or in ischaemic heart disease [65, 89–91]. Although such mitochondrial defects are likely to be widely prevalent, little is known about their morphological functional or genomic characterization with the exception of large mtDNA deletions causing loss of several genes [65, 90, 91].

### Classification of genomic defects in mitochondrial cardiomyopathy

Genome defects causing cardiomyopathic disorders can be classified as mtDNA and nuclear DNA defects [45].

#### *Mitochondrial DNA defects*

Since the first description of mtDNA defects in Leber's hereditary optic neuropathy (LHON)[92], several mutations have been found to be associated with cardiomyopathies [62, 74–83, 93]. Most of them affect mitochondrial tRNA genes. Pathologic mutations are not found in healthy controls and are heteroplasmic, with a large amount of mutated DNA in the heart than in other tissues. Phenotypes segregate with progressively increasing percentages of mutated DNA in the heart, where the threshold value (for clinical presentation) is in most cases higher than 80%. Functional defects corresponding to an increasing proportion of mutant DNA are not well elucidated. The defects affecting tRNAs limit or impair the correct amino acid placement in the polypeptide chains. As far as the number of mutated molecules increases, the likelihood of loss of integer peptide formation becomes higher. In most cardiomyopathies with tRNA pathological mutations, the mitochondrial activity of cytochrome *c* oxidase is commonly affected, followed by activity of NADH dehydrogenase [62]. In contrast, a missense mutation in a coding gene only affects the corresponding protein. Given the negligible replication of myocytes [94], the amount of mutant increases with time, thus influencing the age of phenotype manifestation.

A major limitation in the understanding of the pathogenetic role of mtDNA mutations in cardiomyopathies is the large number of polymorphisms affecting mtDNA which are not associated with any phenotype, especially when the polymorphisms are heteroplasmic [93]. Polymorphic changes could be associated with other pathological mutations, either nuclear or mitochondrial, particularly in cardiomyopathies, wherein a pathological defect has been documented in nuclear and mitochondrial genes [70], in two nuclear genes [95], and in two different exons of the same gene [96]. In patients presenting with familial forms of hypertrophic cardiomyopathy, pathological mtDNA mutations were found to combine with nuclear DNA mutations in the β-myosin heavy chain gene [70]. The mtDNA mutation was associated with a severe reduction in cytochrome *c* oxidase activity in most cardiac myocytes. In one family, an inheritance that was potentially both maternal and autosomal dominant demonstrated an association of nuclear DNA mutation with the disease and an associated contribution of the mtDNA defect. In another family in which both mother and son underwent heart transplantation the inheritance was clearly autosomal dominant as the young daughter of the male proband was affected. This family highlights the role of nuclear mutation and suggests that mitochondrial mutation may be a modifier factor of the phenotype. In other words, the molecular basis of cardiomyopathies, even those that originally appeared as single gene defects are likely more complex than previously suspected.

#### *Nuclear gene defects*

Mitochondrial disorders secondary to nuclear gene mutations are more numerous than those secondary to mitochondrial gene mutations because the number of mitochondrial peptides encoded by nuclear genes exceeds that of mitochondrial genes. Although most of the nuclear genes encoding mitochondrial peptides are still unknown, recent studies have started to elucidate these defects. The role of the adenosine nucleotide translocator (ANT) in mitochondrial metabolism and pathology has recently been reported [97], and a mouse model defective for the ANT1 gene ($ANT1^{PGKneo}$ mice) developed exercise intolerance, myopathy with ragged red fibres, and hypertrophic cardiomyopathy with the eventual development of congestive heart failure [98]. Biochemical and ultrastructural studies in such transgenic mice have demonstrated a four-fold reduction in cytochrome *c* oxidase activity, and proliferation of giant mitochondria. Failure of ATP/ADP transport across the mitochondrial membrane results in a global reduction in electron transport activity with upstream accumulation of substrates such as NADH. The excess of NADH leads to the reduction of pyruvate to lactate and the accumulation of other Krebs cycle intermediates. The consequent increase in free radical production results in mitochondrial damage, while the development of giant mitochondria and proliferation represents a compensatory response to the energy production defect. Mutations in the carnitine–acylcarnitine translocase gene [52] are associated with a disease in newborns characterized by coma, hypoketosis, muscle weakness, and cardiomyopathy [52, 99, 100]. In these infants, the cardiac involvement is secondary to the cardiotoxic effect of long-chain acycarnitine. Isolated defects of complex I [101] and III [102] subunits, unrelated to mtDNA mutations, have been described in fatal multiorgan diseases with severe cardiac involvement. Finally, mutations of frataxin in patients with Friedreich's ataxia are frequently associated with heart involvement. Electrocardiography and echocardiography show concentric ventricular or asymmetric septal hypertrophy [103]. Myocyte hypertrophy and iron overload are observed by EMB in these patients [104].

In most cardiomyopathies it is not possible to exclude nuclear DNA mutations unless extensive screening of all disease-related genes is completed, especially since many disease genes are still unknown. Although linkage analysis provides useful help, most of the families are not large enough for satisfactory, linkage study. Therefore, to make order in such a complex field, only screening studies on large population samples help to subgroup these diseases according to their molecular defects [59].

## Approach to the diagnosis of mitochondrial cardiomyopathies

#### *Clinical studies*

While both dilated and hypertrophic cardiomyopathies may be associated with mitochondrial defects, there is no evidence of association of mtDNA defects in pure restrictive phenotypes. Medical history, evaluation of the skeletal muscle, biochemical data such as lactic acidosis and creatine phosphokinase levels may provide helpful information during clinical assessment. However, in a recent study done in a large number of patients with dilated cardiomyopathy, pathological mtDNA defects were found in young adults who had presented with exclusive cardiac involvement [62]. Other phenotypic markers, known to be associated with mtDNA defects, such as palpebral ptosis, hearing loss, and clinically overt signs of encephalopathy, were not found in any of these patients.

#### *Familial and maternal inheritance studies*

A major contribution to the clinical suspicion of a mtDNA defect-related cardiomyopathy would derive from family studies. If the disorder is familial (two or more members with proven disease), and the inheritance pattern is clearly maternal and non-X-linked, then the investigation should be directed to mtDNA analysis. However, maternal inheritance often simulates autosomal dominant inheritance, especially in smaller families. Transmission from males to offspring is the only scenario in which maternal inheritance can be excluded. When the number of family members suitable for pedigree analysis is low, the family tree is not very helpful. The effort necessary to convince all family members to be analysed, is very demanding and their evaluation becomes expensive. Therefore, the authors prefer population screening wherein EMB demonstrating ultrastructural abnormalities of mitochondria is included for genetic analyses. Patients with mtDNA defect-related cardiomyopathy often present as sporadic phenotype, although the maternal relatives carry the same pathological mutations but without clinical manifestations of cardiomyopathy. The key role played by heteroplasmy in phenotype as well as the ethical limitation to invasive studies in healthy subjects limit the predictive value of molecular findings.

#### *Endomyocardial biopsy*

Conventional histopathological examination of EMB usually does not provide any diagnostic clue in dilated cardiomyopathy since most histopathological changes are shared by several disorders with different aetiologies. EMB may only be useful when investigation includes ultrastructural, histochemical, biochemical, and immunochemical studies.

#### *Mitochondrial DNA analysis*

Evaluation of mtDNA is easy and quick. Screening techniques, such as DGGE and SSCP, are helpful to identify point mutations [105–107]. Although DGGE has a very high sensitivity, much higher than that of SSCP, it is time consuming and the requirements of additional primers with the GC clamp add to procedural cost. Furthermore, the high number of mtDNA polymorphisms [93] complicates the screening. Overall, the cost and time for sequences that have to be performed in each case, combined with those of the screening techniques, approach those of direct sequencing without a screening phase. The microchip-based new technology is promising [108], but can only be used for the detection of pathological mutations which have been well characterized for the given disorder. Therefore, a presently used strategy is to sequence the entire mtDNA in all patients in whom either histochemistry, ultrastructural study, or familial inheritance pattern indicates the possibility of a mitochondrion-related disorder [62]. Pathological significance is assigned to a given point mutation when conventional rules are respected, including heteroplasmy, absence in normal subjects, presence in a conserved region, higher amount of mutant DNA in affected than in non-affected tissues, and an associated corresponding biochemical defect. Many mtDNA-related disorders are associated with more than one mutation contributing to a phenotype such as in LHON [109] or predisposition to Alzheimer's disease [110], and therefore sequencing of entire mtDNA should constitute a preferred strategy of investigation.

After the mtDNA analysis, the significance of large mitochondrial genome rearrangements needs to be critically evaluated. mtDNA deletions, in particular, may simply constitute an age-related change [65]. The key role is played by the amount of deleted mtDNA and, therefore, by the threshold value that exclusively explains a phenotype, such as in KSS. Deletions are very common in cardiomyopathies, as well as in many other long-lasting myocardial diseases. A parallel investigation was performed with PCR and Southern blot in patients with dilated cardiomyopathy, valvular and ischaemic heart disease, and normal donor hearts, and compared them with the disorders associated with mtDNA deletions such as KSS. This study aimed at concretizing the investigational strategy and optimizing methods in the laboratory (unpublished data). Whereas deletions were found in cardiomyopathy and in some normal hearts by PCR, the parallel use of Southern blot technique allowed identification of deletions only in KSS. Therefore, a pathogenetic role for PCR-detected deletions in cardiomyopathy should not be accepted unless quantitative studies are done and the threshold values of observed deletions are established.

### Genetic counselling

Genetic counselling for nuclear gene defects in mitochondrial cardiomyopathy relies on the established rules that govern mendelian disorders barring the penetrance-related alterations which are common to all mendelian diseases. However, counselling becomes extremely difficult when a pathological mutation has been identified in mtDNA and has proved to segregate with the phenotype since the information about the risk of development of disease in clinically healthy but mutated relatives is poor, owing to heteroplasmic presentation. In particular, it is impossible to calculate the risk for cardiac involvement. Although the mtDNA is always of maternal origin [49], as a result of the mitotic segregation, the likelihood of transmission of a pathological mutation from mother to offspring in a sufficient amount to cause a clinical phenotype cannot be estimated. It is difficult to predict the severity of clinical phenotype since the same degree of mutation (especially when measured in DNA from peripheral blood) may result in very mild diseases, allowing a good quality of life, or in an extremely severe and lethal phenotype.

## References


1. Rolfe DF, Brown GC. Cellular energy utilization and molecular origin of standard metabolic rate in mammals. *Physiol Rev* 1997; 77: 731–58.
2. Klingenberg M. The respiratory chain. In: Singet TP (ed.) *Biological oxidations*. New York: Wiley, 1968, 3–54.
3. Hatefi Y. The mitochondrial electron transport and oxidative phosphorylation system. *Annu Rev Biochem* 1985; 54: 1015–69.
4. Wikstrom M, Saraste M. The mitochondrial respiratory chain. In: L Ernster (ed.) *New comprehensive biochemistry*. Volume 6. Amsterdam: Elsevier, 1984, 49–94.
5. Tzagoloff A. *Mitochondria*. New York: Plenum, 1982.
6. Lehninger AL. *The mitochondrion. Molecular basis of structure and function*. New York: WA Benjamin, 1965.
7. Lestienne P. Mitochondrial DNA mutations in human diseases. A review. *Biochemie* 1992: 74: 123–30.
8. Hood DA, Balaban A, Connor MK *et al*. Mitochondrial biogenesis in striated muscle. *Can J Appl Physiol* 1994; 19: 12–48.
9. Ferrans VJ, Butany JW. Ultrastructural pathology of the heart. In: BF Trump, RT Jones (eds) *Diagnostic electron microscopy*. New York: John Wiley and Sons, 1983, 319–473.
10. Barth E, Stammler G, Speiser B, Schaper J. Ultrastructural quantitation of mitochondria and myofilaments in cardiac muscle from 10 different animal species including man. *J Mol Cell Cardiol* 1992; 24: 669–81.
11. Margulis L. *Origin of eukaryotic cells*. New Haven: Yale University Press, 1970.
12. Di Mauro S, Wallace DC. *Mitochondrial DNA in human pathology*. New York: Raven Press, 1993.
13. Jorde LB, Bamshad M, Rogers AR. Using mitochondrial and nuclear DNA markers to reconstruct human evolution. *Bioessays* 1998; 20: 126–36.
14. Vigilant L, Stoneking M, Harpending H *et al*. African populations and evolution of human mitochondrial DNA. *Science* 1991; 253: 1503–7.
15. Calafell F, Underhill P, Tolun A *et al*. From Asia to Europe: mitochondrial DNA sequence variability in Bulgarians and Turks. *Ann Hum Genet* 1996; 60: 35–49.
16. Munn EA. *The structure of the mitochondria*. London: Academic Press, 1974.
17. Ernster L, Kuylenstierna B. *Outer membrane of mitochondria and chloroplasts*. New York: van Nostrand-Reinhold, 1970, 172–212.
18. Mitchell P. Coupling of phosphorylation to electron and hydrogen transfer by a chemioosmotic type of mechanism. *Nature* 1961; 191: 144–8.
19. Benz R. Permeation of hydrophilic solutes through mitochondrial outer membranes: review on mitochondrial porins. *Biochem Biophys Acta* 1994; 1197: 167–96.
20. Van Dam K. Uncoupling and loose coupling. In: Busch HFM, Jennekens FGI, Scholte HR (eds) *Mitochondria and muscular diseases*. Beetsterzwaag: Mefar 1981: 65–9.
21. Robinson JB Jr, Srere PA. Organization of Krebs tricarboxylic acid cycle enzyme mitochondria. *J Biol Chem* 1985; 260: 1800–5.
22. Brown GG, Beattie DS. Role of coenzyme Q in the mitochondrial respiratory chain. Reconstitution of activity in coenzyme Q deficient mutants of yeasts. *Biochemistry* 1977; 16: 4449–54.
23. Singer TP, Ramsey RR, Peach C. The flavoproteins of the respiratory chain. In: CP Lee, G Dallner, G Schatz (eds) *Mitochondria and microsomes*. Reading, M: Addison-Wesley, 1981, 155–90.
24. Weiss H, Friedrich T, Hofhaus G, Preis D. The respiratory chain NADH dehydrogenase (complex I) of mitochondria. *Eur J Biochem* 1991; 197: 563–76.
25. Ohnishi T. Structure of the succinate ubiquinone oxidoreductase (complex II). In: CP Lee (ed.) *Current topics in bioenergetics*. Volume 16. New York: Academic Press, 1987, 37–65.
26. Nelson BD. The composition, structure, topology and function of complex III (ubiquinone–cytochrome *c* reductase). In: CP Lee, G Dallner, G Schatz (eds) *Mitochondria and microsomes*. Reading, MA: Addison-Wesley, 1981, 217–47.
27. Malmstrom BG. Cytochrome *c* oxidase. Structure and catalytic activity. *Biochim Biophys Acta* 1979; 549: 281–303.
28. Penefsky HS, Cross RL. Structure and mechanism of $F_0F_1$-type ATP synthases and ATPases. *Adv Enzymol* 1991; 64: 173–214.
29. Klingenberg M. Structure–function of the ADP/ATP carrier. *Biochem Soc Trans* 1992; 20: 547–50.
30. Li K, Warner CK, Hodge JA *et al*. A human muscle adenine nucleotide translocator gene has four exons, is located on chromosome 4, and is differentially expressed. *J Biol Chem* 1989; 264: 13 998–4004.
31. Haraguchi Y, Chung AB, Torroni A *et al*. Genetic mapping of human heart–skeletal muscle adenine nucleotide translocator and its relationship to the facioscapulohumeral muscular dystrophy locus. *Genomics* 1993; 16: 479–85.
32. Anderson S, Bankier AT, Barrell BG *et al*. Sequence and organization of the human mitochondrial genome. *Nature* 1981; 290: 457–65.
33. Wallace DC. Report of the Committee on human mitochondrial DNA. *Cytogenet Cell Genet* 1989; 51: 612–21.
34. Clayton DA. Structure and function of the mitochondrial genome. *J Inherited Metab Dis* 1992; 15: 439–47.
35. Clayton DA. Replication of animal mitochondrial DNA. *Cell* 1982; 28: 693–705.
36. Chang DD, Clayton DA. Precise identification of individual promoters for transcription of each strand of human mitochondrial DNA. *Cell* 1984; 36: 635–43.
37. Poulton J. Duplications of mitochondrial DNA: implications for pathogenesis. *J Inherited Metab Dis* 1992; 15: 487–98.
38. Clayton DA. Transcription of the mammalian mitochondrial genome. *Annu Rev Biochem* 1984; 53: 573–94.
39. Oyala D, Montoya J, Attardi G. tRNA punctuation model of RNA processing in human mitochondria. *Nature* 1981; 290: 470–4.
40. Attardi G, Chomyn A, King MP *et al*. Regulation of mitochondrial gene expression in mammalian cells. *Biochem Soc Trans* 1989; 18: 509–13.
41. Gelfand R, Attardi G. Synthesis and turnover of mitochondrial nucleic acid in HeLa cells: the mature ribosomal and messenger ribonucleic acid species are metabolically unstable. *Mol Cell Biol* 1981; 1: 497–511.
42. Christianson TW, Clayton DA. *In vitro* transcription of human mitochondrial DNA: accurate termination requires a region of DNA sequence that can function bidirectionally. *Proc Natl Acad Sci USA* 1986; 83: 6277–81.

43. Kruse B, Narasimhan N, Attardi G. Termination of transcription in human mitochondria: identification and purification of a DNA binding factor that promotes termination. *Cell* 1989; 58: 391–7.
44. Zeviani M, Antozzi C. Nuclear DNA contribution to the synthesis of the respiratory chain enzymes. *Mol Hum Reprod* 1997; 3: 133–48.
45. DiMauro S, Hirano M. Mitochondria and heart disease. *Curr Opin Cardiol* 1998; 13: 190–7.
46. Richter C, Park JW, Ames BN. Normal oxidative damage to mitochondrial and nuclear DNA synthesis in mouse L-cells. *J Biol Chem* 1976; 251: 2938–44.
47. Clayton DA, Doda JN, Friedberg EC. The absence of a pyrimidine dimer repair mechanism in mammalian mitochondria. *Proc Natl Acad Sci USA* 1974; 71: 2777–81.
48. Wallace DC. Mitochondrial diseases: genotype versus phenotype. *Trends Genet* 1993; 9: 128–33.
49. Zeviani M, Tiranti V, Piantadosi C. Mitochondrial disorders. *Medicine* 1998; 77: 59–72.
50. Giles RE, Blanc H, Cann RM. Maternal inheritance of human mitochondrial DNA. *Proc Natl Acad Sci USA* 1980; 83: 9611–15.
51. Stepien G, Torrona A, Chung AB *et al.* Differential expression of adenine nucleotide translocator isoforms in mammalian tissues and during muscle cell differentiation. *J Biol Chem* 1992; 267: 14592–7.
52. Huizing M, Iacobazzi V, Ijlst P *et al.* Cloning of the human carnitine-acylcarnitine carrier cDNA and identification of the molecular defects in a patient. *Am J Hum Genet* 1997; 61: 1239–45.
53. Fenton WA. Mitochondrial protein transport — a system in search of mutations. *AM J Hum Genet* 1995; 57: 235–8.
54. DiMauro S, Tanji K. Mitochondrial disorders. *Jpn J Human Genet* 1997; 42: 473–87.
55. Agsteribbe E, Huckriede A, Veenhuis M *et al.* A fatal, systemic mitochondrial disease with decreased mitochondrial enzyme activities, abnormal ultrastructure of the mitochondria and deficiency of heat shock protein 60. *Biochem Biophys Res Commun* 1993; 193: 46–154.
56. Briones P, Villaseca MA, Ribes A *et al.* A new case of multiple mitochondrial enzyme deficiencies with decreased amount of heat shok protein 60. *J Inherit Metab Dis* 1997; 20: 569–77.
57. Campuzano V, Montermini L, Lutz Y *et al.* Frataxin is reduced in Friedreich ataxia patients and is associated with mitochondrial membranes. *Hum Mol Genet* 1997; 6: 1771–80.
58. Radisky DC, Babcock MC, Kaplan J. The yeast frataxin homologue mediates mitochondrial iron efflux. Evidence for a mitochondrial iron cycle. *J Biol Chem* 1999; 274: 4497–9.
59. Rotig A, de Lonlay P, Chretien D *et al.* Aconitase and mitochondrial iron-sulphur protein deficiency in Friedreich ataxia. *Nat Genet* 1997; 17: 215–17.
60. Sakakibira S, Konno S. Endomyocardial biopsy. *Jpn Heart J* 1962; 3: 537–40.
61. Arbustini E, Burke AP, Diegoli M *et al.* Ultrastructural findings in dilated cardiomyopathy: are they clinically relevant? *Am J Pathol* 1999 (submitted).
62. Arbustini E, Diegoli M, Fasani R *et al.* Mitochondrial DNA mutations and mitochondrial abnormalities in dilated cardiomyopathy. *Am J Pathol* 1998; 153: 1501–10.
63. Challice LE, Viragh S. *Ultrastructure of the mammalian heart.* New York: Academic Press, 1973.
64. Schoffner JM, Lott MT, Lezza AMS *et al.* Myoclonic epilepsy and ragged red fiber disease (MERRF) is associated with a mitochondrial tRNALys mutation. *Cell* 1990; 61: 931–7.
65. Hattori K, Tanaka M, Sugiyama S *et al.* Age-dependent increase in deleted mitochondrial DNA in the human heart: possible contributory factor to 'presbycardia' *Am Heart J* 1991; 121: 1735–42.
66. Takeda N, Tanamura A, Iwai T *et al.* Mitochondrial DNA deletion in human myocardium. *Mol Cell Biochem* 1993; 199: 105–8.
67. Herman D. Free radical theory of aging: consequences of mitochondrial aging. *Age* 1983; 6: 86–94.
68. Zak R, Rabinowitz M, Rajamanickam C *et al.* Mitochondrial proliferation in cardiac hypertrophy. *Basic Res Cardiol* 1980; 75: 171–8.
69. Cumming WJK, Fulthorpe J, Hudgson P, Mahon M. *Muscle pathology.* London: Mosby-Wolfe, 1994.
70. Arbustini E, Fasani R, Morbini P *et al.* Coexistence of mitochondrial DNA and β-myosin heavy chain mutations in hypertrophic cardiomyopathy with late congestive heart failure. *Heart* 1998; 80: 548–58.
71. Sottocasa GL, Kuylenstierna B, Ernster L, Bergstrand A. An electron transfer system associated with the outer membrane of the mitochondria. *J Cell Biol* 1967; 32: 415–38.
72. King TE, Howard RL. Preparation and properties of soluble NADH dehydrogenase from cardiac muscle. *Methods Enzymol* 1967; 10: 332–5.
73. King TE, Howard RL. Preparation of succinate dehydrogenase and reconstitution of succinate oxidase. *Methods Enzymol* 1967; 10: 322–31.
74. Silvestri G, Bertini E, Servidei S *et al.* Maternally inherited cardiomyopathy: a new phenotype associated with the A to G at nt 3243 of mitochondrial DNA (MELAS mutation). *Muscle Nerve* 1997; 20: 221–5.
75. Casali C, Santorelli FM, D'Amati G *et al.* A novel mtDNA mutation in maternally inherited cardiomyopathy. *Biochem Biophys Res Commun* 1995; 213: 588–93.
76. Merante F, Tein I, Benson L, Robinson BH. Maternally inherited hypertrophic cardiomyopathy due to a novel T-to-C transition at nucleotide 9997 in the mitochondrial tRNAGlycine gene. *Am J Hum Genet* 1994; 55: 437–46.
77. Merante F, Myint T, Tein I *et al.* An additional mitochondrial tRNAIle point mutation (A-to-G at nucleotide 4295) causing hypertrophic cardiomyopathy. *Hum Mutat* 1996; 8: 216–22.
78. Obayashi T, Hattori K, Sugiyama S *et al.* Point mutations in mitochondrial DNA in patients with hypertrophic cardiomyopathy. *Am Heart J* 1992; 124: 1263–9.
79. Taniike M, Fukushima H, Yanagihara I *et al.* Mitochondrial tRNAIle mutation in fatal cardiomyopathy. *Biochem Biophys Res Commun* 1992; 186: 47–53.
80. Ito T, Hattori K, Obayashi T *et al.* Mitochondrial DNA mutations in cardiomyopathy. *Jpn Circ J* 1992; 56: 1045–53.
81. Silvestri G, Santorelli FM, Shanske SB *et al.* A new mitochondrial DNA mutation in the tRNALeu(UUR) gene associated with maternally inherited cardiomyopathy. *Hum Mut* 1994; 3: 37–43.
82. Vilarinho L, Santorelli FM, Rosas MJ *et al.* The mitochondrial A3243G mutation presenting as severe cardiomyopathy. *J Med Genet* 1997; 34: 607–9.
83. Li YY, Maisch B, Rose ML, Hengstenberg C. Point mutations in mitochondrial DNA of patients with dilated cardiomyopathy. *J Mol Cell Cardiol* 1997; 29: 2699–709.
84. Anan R, Nakagawa M, Miyata M *et al.* Cardiac involvement in mitochondrial diseases: a study of 17 patients with mitochondrial DNA defects. *Circulation* 1995; 91: 955–61.
85. Santorelli FM, Mak S, Vazquez-Aceredo M *et al.* A novel mitochondrial DNA point mutation associated with mitochondrial

encephalocardiomyopathy. *Biochem Biophys Res Commun* 1995; 216: 835–40.

86. Zeviani M, Gellera C, Antozzi C. Maternally inherited myopathy and cardiomyopathy: association with mutation in mitochondrial DNA tRNALeu(UUR). *Lancet* 1991; 338: 143–7.
87. Pastores GM, Santorelli FM, Shanske S *et al.* Leigh syndrome and hypertrophic cardiomyopathy in an infant with a mitochondrial DNA point mutation (T8993). *Am J Med Genet* 1994; 50: 265–71.
88. Manfredi G, Schon EA, Moraes CT *et al.* A new mutation associated with MELAS is located in a mitochondrial DNA polypeptide-coding gene. *Neuromusc Disord* 1995; 5: 391–8.
89. Wallace DC. Mitochondrial DNA mutations and bioenergetic defects in aging and degenerative diseases. In: RN Rosenberg, SB Prusiner, S DiMauro, RL Barchi (eds) *The molecular and genetic basis of neurological disease* 2nd edn. Boston: Butterworth-Heinemann, 1997, 237–69.
90. Ozawa T. Genetic and functional changes in mitochondria associated with ageing. *Physiol Rev* 1997; 77: 425–64.
91. Ozawa T, Tanaka M, Sugiyama S *et al.* Multiple mitochondrial DNA deletions exist in cardiomyocytes of patients with hypertrophic or dilated cardiomyopathy. *Biochem Biophys Res Commun* 1990; 170: 830–6.
92. Wallace DC, Singh G, Lott MT *et al.* Mitochondrial DNA mutation associated with Leber's hereditary optic neuropathy. *Science* 1988; 242: 1427–30.
93. Kogelnik AM, Lott MT, Brown MD *et al.* MITOMAP: a human mitochondrial genome database 1998 — update. *Nucl Acids Res* 1998; 26: 112–15.
94. Arbustini E, Diegoli M, Grasso M *et al.* Expression of proliferating cell markers in normal and diseased human hearts. *Am J Cardiol* 1993; 72: 608–14.
95. Isnard R, Richard P, Dubourg O *et al.* Identification of a double heterozygosity for a mutation in the β-myosin heavy chain gene and in the cardiac binding protein C gene in familial hypertrophic cardiomyopathy: phenotype–genotype relationship. *Eur Heart J* 1998; 19: 607.
96. Havndrup O, Bundgaard H, Andersen PS *et al.* Double missense mutation in codon 390 in the cardiac β-myosin heavy chain gene, a probable cause of hypertrophic cardiomyopathy. *Eur Heart J* 1998; 19: 606.
97. Bakker HD, Scholte HR, Van den Bogert C *et al.* Deficiency of the adenine nucleotide translocator in muscle of a patient with myopathy and lactic acidosis: a new mitochondrial defect. *Pediatr Res* 1993; 33: 412–17.
98. Graham BH, Waymire KG, Cottrell B *et al.* A mouse model for mitochondrial myopathy and cardiomyopathy resulting from a deficiency in the heart/muscle isoform of the adenine nucleotide translocator. *Nat Genet* 1997; 16: 226–34.
99. Stanley CA, Hale DE, Berry GT *et al.* A deficiency of carnitine–acylcarnitine translocase in the inner mitochondrial membrane. *J Med* 1992; 327: 19–23.
100. Di Donato S. Disorders associated with defects of beta-oxidation. In: RN Rosenberg, SB Prusiner, S DiMauro, RL Barchi (eds) *The molecular and genetic basis of neurological disease.* 2nd edn. Boston: Butterworth-Heinemann, 1997, 939–56.
101. Pitkanen S, Merante F, McLeod DR *et al.* Familial cardiomyopathy with cataracts and lactic acidosis: a defect in complex 1 (NADH dehydrogenase) of the mitochondria respiratory chain. *J Pediatr Res* 1996; 39: 513–21.
102. Mourmans J, Wendel U, Bentlage HACM *et al.* Clinical heterogeneity in respiratory chain complex III deficiency in childhood. *J Neurol Sci* 1997; 149: 111–17.
103. Morvan D, Komaijda M, Doan LD *et al.* cardiomyopathy in Friedreich ataxia: a Doppler–echocardiographic study. *Eur Heart J* 1992; 13: 1393–8.
104. Lamarche JB, Cote M, Lemieux B. The cardiomyopathy of Friedreich's ataxia morphological observations in 3 cases. *Can J Neurol Sci* 1980; 7: 389–96.
105. Myers RM, Maniatis T, Lerman LS. Detection and localization of single base change by denaturing gradient gel electrophoresis. *Methods Enzymol* 1987; 155: 501–527.
106. Hayashi K. PCR-SSCP: a method for detection of mutations. *Genet Anal Tech Appl* 1992; 9: 73–9.
107. Iolascon A, Parrella T, Perrotta S *et al.* Fortina P: Rapid detection of medium chain acyl-CoA dehydrogenase gene mutations by non-radioactive, single strand conformation polymorphism minigels. *J Med Genet* 1994; 31: 551–4.
108. Cheng J, Waters LC, Fortina P *et al.* Degenerae oligonucleotide primed-polymerase chain reaction and capillary electrophoretic analysis of human DNA on microchip-based devices. *Anal Biochem* 1998; 257: 101–6.
109. Brown MD, Voljavec AS, Lott MT *et al.* Mitochondrial DNA complex I and III mutations associated with Leber's hereditary optic neuropathy. *Genetics* 1992; 130: 163–73.
110. Gearing M, Salvo R, Watts RL *et al.* Mitochondrial DNA variations observed in Alzheimer disease and Parkinson disease patients. *Genomics* 1993, 17: 171–84.

# Altered receptor-mediated signalling in cardiomyopathy 

M. BÖHM, G. NICKENIG, P. SCHNABEL AND O. ZOLK

## Introduction

This chapter summarizes alterations in relevant cardiac receptors as well as their signal transduction in cardiac failure. The overview is restricted to G protein-coupled receptors and signal transduction mechanisms. It focuses on the adrenergic receptors and peptide hormone receptors involved in hypertrophy and remodelling, namely angiotensin II–AT1 receptors as well as endothelin receptors.

## Physiological regulation of signal transduction cascades

### The β-adrenergic signalling pathway

In the mammmalian heart, signalling through β-adrenergic receptors and the subsequent activation of the G protein–adenylyl cyclase signal transduction cascade are essential for the regulation of inotropy, chronotropy, dromotropy, lusitropy, and growth. The following chapter reviews the components generally involved in β-adrenergic signalling and in alterations in expression or function in heart failure.

### β-Adrenergic receptors

β-Adrenergic receptors belong to the large family of G protein-coupled receptors. This family includes several hundred members characterized by a typical structure with an extracellular N-terminus, seven transmembrane domains, and an intracellular C-terminus [1]. While the putative ligand-binding domain is formed by the amino-terminus and certain portions of the transmembrane domains, the intracellular loops, particularly the third one, seem to be involved in the interaction with signal-transducing G proteins. The C-terminal portion of the receptors contains phosphorylation sites which serve as targets for protein kinase A (PKA), protein kinase C (PKC), and β-adrenergic receptor kinases (β-ARK). Three types of β-adrenergic receptors, designated $\beta_1$-, $\beta_2$-, and $\beta_3$-adrenoceptors, have been cloned from mammalian tissues [1, 2]. In the heart, the $\beta_1$-adrenoceptor subtype is predominant, but functional coupling has also been demonstrated for the $\beta_2$ subtype. Several authors identified a third cardiac β-adrenergic receptor population; it is controversial however, whether these receptors are identical to the $\beta_3$-adrenoceptor present in adipose tissue, as suggested by Gauthier *et al.* [3]. These authors suggest that $\beta_3$-adrenoceptors are expressed in the human heart and, in contrast to $\beta_1$- and $\beta_2$-adrenergic receptors, mediate negative inotropic effects like Gi-coupled receptors. Other investigators [4–6] also postulate the presence of a third β-adrenergic receptor population in the mammalian heart, but report it to be distinct from the $\beta_3$-adrenergic receptors cloned from adipose tissue. Cardiac β-adrenergic receptors are primarily activated by noradrenaline locally released from sympathetic nerve endings rather than circulating adrenaline. Noradrenaline exerts the highest affinity for the $\beta_1$-adrenoceptor subtype, suggesting the predominant physiological importance of this particular subtype.

β-adrenergic receptor signalling can be desensitized at the receptor level, i.e. receptor expression or function can be reduced in response to prolonged or repeated receptor stimulation. Receptor expression is regulated within several hours; a reduction in receptor messenger ribonucleic acid (mRNA) and protein levels, i.e., receptor downregulation, is caused by a decrease in receptor synthesis or an increase in receptor degradation or sequestration into an intracellular compartment, a process which seems to be reversible [7]. In addition, the numbers of $\beta_2$-adrenergic receptors can be decreased by mRNA destabilization in response to agonist exposure [8]. Destabilization of $\beta_2$-adrenergic receptor mRNA is associated with induction of proteins binding to AU-rich areas in the 3' untranslated region of receptor mRNA [9, 10]. For the cardiac $\beta_1$-adrenergic receptor, regulation of mRNA stability has not yet been shown. However, $\beta_1$-adrenoceptor downregulation has been suggested to be due to decreased transcriptional activity [11]. Since these data have been obtained from different cellular systems, it is not possible to draw definitive conclusions concerning the mechanisms of β-adrenergic receptor downregulation in the mammalian heart.

In contrast to receptor downregulation (changes in β-adrenoceptor expression) a loss of receptor function as a result of uncoupling from the signal-transducing G protein, Gs, may occur within a few seconds. This rapid process can be induced by receptor phosphorylation in the C-terminal domain by protein kinases A and C, and β-ARK. Protein kinases A and C are activated by the second messenger molecules cyclic adenosine monophosphate (cAMP) and diacyl glycerol, respectively. These second messengers are generated in response to activation of G protein-coupled receptors: the β- and α-adrenergic receptors, respectively. Receptor phosphorylation by protein kinases A and C blocks the interaction of the receptor with the stimulatory G protein, Gs [12]. A highly specific, homologous desensitization mechanism for β-adrenergic receptors is supplied by βARK, a serine/threonine kinase belonging to the family of G protein-coupled receptor kinases (GRKs) (for review see ref. 13). There are two isoforms, designated βARK-1 and βARK-2 (corresponding to GRK-2 and GRK-3 in the GRK terminology), both of which are expressed in the mammalian heart [14]. βARK phosphorylates agonist-liganded receptors, which then become a substrate for β-arrestin, a cytosolic protein which binds to the receptor and leads to uncoupling from G Gs. βARK is a cytosolic protein and requires translocation to the plasma membrane prior to enzymatic activity. There is evidence that this membrane association is accomplished by interaction with G protein βγ subunits [15] and takes place in the C-terminal region of the βARK polypeptide [16], stimulating βARK activity [17]. There are two isoforms of β-arrestin, β-arrestin-1 and β-arrestin-2, both of which are expressed in the mammalian heart. The predominant cardiac isoform is β-arrestin-1 [14].

## Signal-transducing G proteins

Heterotrimeric G proteins coupe the signals of many hormones, neurotransmitters, growth factors, and primary sensory stimuli from seven transmembrane-spanning receptors to intracellular effector moieties (for review see ref. 18). Effectors are enzymes such as adenylyl cyclase, phospholipase C (PLC), or cyclic guanosine monophosphate (cGMP) phosphodiesterase, or ion channels such as potassium and calcium channels. Heterotrimeric G proteins are composed of three distinct polypeptide chains designated α (39 000–52 000 mol. wt), β (35 000–36 000 mol. wt), and γ (7000–8000 mol. wt) subunits. There is considerable diversity among the different subunits [19, 20]. To date, the complementary deoxyribonucleic acid (cDNA) of 16 α-, five β-, and ten γ-subunits has been cloned. The α-subunits are, according to their overall sequence homology, divided into four groups designated αs, αi, αq, and α12, each containing several members.

All known G proteins are activated and inactivated in a similar manner: an activated receptor interacts with the heterotrimeric G protein. This interaction triggers the replacement of guanosine diphosphate (GDP), which is bound to the α-subunit in the inactive state, by guanosine triphosphate (GTP). Subsequently, the heterotrimer dissociates into a free, GTP-liganded α-subunit and the βγ-dimer. Both α-subunits and βγ-dimers can interact with effectors such as phospholipase C and adenylyl cyclase. The activation cycle is terminated by the intrinsic GTPase activity of the α-subunit which cleaves the α-subunit-bound GTP into GDP and inorganic phosphate (Pi). The GDP-

**Table 13.1** $\alpha_1$-Adrenergic signal transduction in different models of cardiac hypertrophy and failure

| Condition | $\alpha_1$-Adrenoceptor density | Positive inotropic effect |
|---|---|---|
| SHR rats | ↓ | ↑↓ |
| TG(mREN2)27 rats | ↑ | ↓ |
| Cardiomyopathic Syrian hamsters | = | ↑ |
| Human heart failure | ↑= | ↓= |

SHR = spontaneously hypertensive rats; TG(mREN2)27 = rats with somatic overexpression of the mouse renin gene *ren*$^{2d}$. Alterations are given in comparison with the respective controls. For details and references see text.

bound α-subunit reassociates with the βγ-dimer to form the heterotrimer present in the inactive state (for review see ref. 18).

Adenylyl cyclase is dually regulated by αs and αi proteins. αs stimulates adenylyl cyclase and activates calcium channels. It is also the substrate for covalent modification by the cholera toxin. The toxin cleaves nicotinamide-adenine dinucleotide (NAD) into nicotinamide and adenosine diphosphate (ADP) ribose, and links the ADP-ribose moiety covalently to an arginine residue of the αs polypeptide chain. This results in inhibition of the GTPase activity and constitutive activation of αs. The human αs gene has been mapped to chromosome 20 [21] and is composed of 13 exons and 12 introns. There are four splice variants generated by alternate use of exon 3 and two different 3' splice sites of intron 3 which are functionally indistinguishable.

The family of adenylyl cyclase-inhibiting αi proteins is comprised of three members: $\alpha i_1$, $\alpha i_2$, and $\alpha i_3$. Each αi-subunit is the product of a distinct gene (for review see ref. 22). The amino acid composition of these three genes is approximately 85%. The three human αi genes are composed of eight coding exons and seven introns, and have an identical exon–intron organization. *In vitro*, all three αi-subunits inhibit adenylyl cyclase, but they are also able to interact with other effector systems such as potassium channels (for review see ref. 18). αi proteins are substrates to ADP-ribosylation by pertussis toxin, which covalently links ADP-ribose to a cysteine residue close to the C-terminus common to $\alpha i_1$, $\alpha i_2$, and $\alpha i_3$. In contrast to αs, which is constitutively activated, αi proteins are uncoupled from the receptor by this modification. The αi-subunit predominantly expressed in the mammalian heart is $\alpha i_2$, although $\alpha i_3$ is also present [23, 24]. The significance of this molecular diversity within one tissue is not yet clear, and it is not known whether there is specificity concerning the interaction with certain cardiac receptors or adenylyl cyclase isozymes.

βγ-Subunits are important players in G protein-mediated signalling (for review see ref. 25). The dimer remains tightly associated during the entire activation cycle of the G protein. β-Subunits are predicted to form coiled-coil structures in their N-terminal region, which are stabilized α-helices important for protein–protein interactions, especially with the γ-subunit. The γ-subunits, which share a lower sequence homology than the β-subunits, are subject to a cascade of post-translational modifications [26]. First, a cysteine residue four amino acids upstream from the C-terminus is isoprenylated. Secondly, the C-terminal three residues are cleaved by proteolysis. Thirdly, carboxymethylation of the isoprenylated cysteine residue occurs. These steps are important for the function of the βγ-subunits. In rat heart, the expression of $\beta_1$, $\beta_2$, $\gamma_3$, $\gamma_5$, and $\gamma_7$ has been demonstrated [27]. However, it is not clear which combinations are formed *in vivo* and whether there is specificity of certain βγ-combinations for certain receptors, α-subunits, or effectors. Evidence for a high degree of specificity of βγ interactions has been presented by Kleuss *et al.* [28–30]. An increasing number of effectors such as adenylyl cyclase, PLC, βARK, phosphoinositide-3-kinase, and many others (for review see ref. 20) has been shown to be regulated by βγ-subunits in either a stimulatory or an inhibitory manner. In the mammalian heart, it has not yet been systematically investigated which βγ-dimers are formed. A review of the regulation of adenylyl cyclase by G protein α- and βγ-subunits follows.

## Adenylyl cyclases

Adenylyl cyclase converts ATP into cAMP, an intracellular second messenger molecule involved in the regulation of important cell functions such as metabolism and growth. Many of the actions of cAMP are mediated by cAMP-dependent protein kinases. In the heart, an increase in intracelluar cAMP by adenylyl cyclase leads to activation of cAMP-dependent PKA, which phosphorylates L-type calcium channels, resulting in increased trans-sarcolemmal calcium influx, increased sarcoplasmic reticulum calcium ATPase activity and, consequently, increased contractility. Adenylyl cyclase activity is modulated in a stimulatory or an inhibitory manner by hormones and neurotransmitters, which exert their action through seven transmembrane spanning receptors and Gs or Gi proteins, respectively.

Mammalian adenylyl cyclases are membrane-bound proteins with a short amino-terminal region (N), a hydrophobic domain (M1) predicted to cross the plasma membrane six times, a cytoplasmic domain (C1), a second hydrophobic domain with six transmembrane stretches (M2), and a C-terminal cytoplasmic domain (C2) (for review see ref. 31). The cytoplasmic domains are highly conserved among the mammalian isozymes and between adenylyl and guanylyl cyclases, and are required for catalytic activity.

Six distinct adenylyl cyclase isozymes, designated AC I to AC VI, have been cloned from mammalian tissues (for review see ref. 31). All are stimulated by αs. In addition, AC II and IV are sensitive to stimulation by G protein βγ-subunits [32, 33]. In contrast, AC I is inhibited by βγ-subunits, and AC III, V, and VI are unaffected by βγ-subunits. The dimers of β- and γ-subunits that regulate adenylyl cyclase are not yet identified. In contrast to PLC activation, activation of adenylyl cyclase by βγ-subunits is only observed in the presence of activated αs. Thus, AC II and AC IV are molecular machines that integrate coincident signals [34]. The mammalian heart contains the adenylyl cyclase isozymes AC IV [35], AC V, and AC VI [31]. Thus, βγ-subunit-sensitive as well as -insensitive isozymes are present. The question of whether myocardial adenylyl cyclase activity is stimulated or inhibited by free βγ-subunits has not yet been addressed. In general αs-αi-, and βγ-subunits are involved in the regulation of adenylyl cyclase. The exact molecular interactions taking place in mammalian myocardium remain to be identified.

## Phospholipase C

Phosphoinositide-specific PLC generates two second messengers, inositol-(1,4,5)-trisphosphate (Ins $P_3$) and diacylglycerol (DAG). Nine PLC isozymes are known, four of which ($PLC\beta_{1-4}$) are regulated by G proteins [36]. Within the group of PLCβ isozymes, $PLC\beta_4$ is the most distantly related member. It is expressed solely in the retina and regulated by αq-, but not by βγ-subunits. $PLC\beta_{1-3}$, in contrast, are regulated by the α-subunits of the Gq family as well as by free βγ-subunits (for review see ref. 36). $PLC\beta_1$ is expressed mainly in the brain, $PLC\beta_2$ in haematopoietic tissue, and $PLC\beta_3$ is the most ubiquitously expressed PLCβ isozyme known. While activated αs is required for adenylyl cyclase stimulation by βγ-subunits, PLCβ is stimulated by βγ-subunits independently from α-subunits.

In the heart, PLC is involved in the mediation of positive inotropic effects [37] by PLC-coupled receptors. However, the significance of this signal transduction pathway for contractile force is controversial. In contrast, the relevance of the PLC pathway in myocardial hypertrophy is well established (see below). In the rat heart, the predominant PLCβ isozyme seems to be $PLC\beta_3$ [27]. However, Jhon *et al.* [38] detected only marginal amounts of $PLC_3$ in the rat heart. No $PLC\beta_3$ was found in the human heart. In contrast, PLCβ1 was detected by polymerase chain reaction (PCR) amplification [39]. The PLC activity present in human myocardial tissue is regulated by G protein α- and βγ-subunits [39]. This corresponds to the pharmacological profile of $PLC\beta_1$. It is also possible that $PLC\beta_1$ is amplified from the nerve cells present in myocardial tissue and that the predominant PLC isozyme of the cardiomyocyte remains to be identified.

The complexity of the pathways of signal transduction in the heart and in other tissues increases with the possibilities of cross-talk between different receptor/G protein effector systems. Activation of any G protein coupled receptor results in a release of free βγ-subunits, which could theoretically stimulate an effector distinct from the one stimulated by the α-subunit released. Such a setting has been accomplished *in vitro* [40]. Another method of cross-talk exists for adenylyl cylase and PLC (for review see ref. 41). DAG, one of the second messengers generated by PLC, stimulates PKC (for review see ref. 42). Adenylyl cyclase isozymes AC II and AC VII are activated by PKC, indicating that receptor-mediated stimulation of PLC can also lead to adenylyl cyclase stimulation [41]. The other second messenger formed by PLC, $InsP_3$, leads to a release of calcium ions from intracellular stores (for review see ref. 43). Again, there are certain adenylyl cyclase isozymes which are sensitive to calcium: AC I, AC III, and AC VIII are stimulated, while AC V and AC VI are inhibited by calcium ions.

## Endothelin receptors

Endothelin (ET) receptors are distributed throughout a variety of tissues including the heart and the vasculature [44, 45]. At least two major subtypes, $ET_A$ and $ET_B$, are defined by the rank order of affinity for ET-1, ET-2, ET-3, and sarafotoxin. $ET_A$ receptors are characterized by high and equal affinity for ET-1 and ET-2, approximately 100-fold lower affinity for ET-3, and 1000-fold lower affinity for sarafotoxin [46]. In contrast, the $ET_B$-receptor subtype displays high and similar affinity for all ET-related peptides [47]. Paralleling this functional classification, two classes of cDNA clones encoding ET receptors have been isolated from mammalian tissues [46, 48–50]. The structures of the mature ET receptors have been deduced from the nucleotide sequences of the cDNAs. The receptors are homologous to other heptahelical receptors of the rhodopsin superfamily. They are characterized by seven regions of 20–27 hydrophobic amino acid residues predicted to form transmembrane helices. Various alternative splicing variants for the human $ET_A$ [51] and $ET_B$ [52, 53] receptor have been described. The $ET_B$ splice variant $ET_B1$ is characterized by an increase in the length of the second cytoplasmic domain by ten amino acids. This alteration, however, does not result in significant differences in functional properties between $ET_B$ and $ET_B1$ [52]. In contrast, another splice variant with a modification of the C-terminal region is incapable of stimulating a functional response even though this $ET_B$ receptor splice variant displays the same binding properties as the wild-type [53]. These examples underline the diversity of ET receptors. However, the physiological role of ET receptor splice variants and their possible participation in pathophysiological processes remain to be clarified.

The tissue distribution of the two main ET receptor subtypes has been extensively investigated. There is consensus that the $ET_A$ receptor subtype predominates in most compartments of the mammalian heart. In the human heart, *in situ* binding experiments demonstrate a ratio of $ET_A$/total ET receptors of about 70% in atrial and ventricular myocardium [54], about 50% in the atrioventricular conducting system, about 85% in the media of epicardial coronary artery, and about 100% in the media of intramyocardial resistance vessels [55].

The direct cardiac actions of the ETs include positive inotropic and chronotropic effects as well as prolongation of the action potential duration and vasoconstriction of coronary arteries. Ishikawa *et al.* [56] were the first to demonstrate positive inotropic effects of ET-1 (delayed onset and a prolonged duration of action) in isolated guinea-pig atria. ET-1 has subsequently been demonstrated to increase contractility in isolated perfused hearts [57, 58], isolated human and rat atria [59], human and rabbit papillary muscle [44, 60], and isolated adult human, rat, and rabbit ventricular myocytes [44, 61]. In isolated rat ventricular myocytes, ET-1 at concentrations less that 1 nmole/l, caused a maximum inotropic response without a detectable increase in intracellular $[Ca^{2+}]_i$ [61], suggesting that ET-1 sensitizes the myofilaments to $Ca^{2+}$. Amiloride, an inhibitor of sarcolemmal $Na^+/H^+$ exchange, prevented the intracellular alkalinization response to ET-1 and attenuated the inotropic effect [62]. At higher concentrations, ET-1 triggers the mobilization of intracellular $Ca^{2+}$ and stimulates the transmembrane $Ca^{2+}$ current in isolated rat and rabbit myocytes [61]. Cardiac ET receptors couple via a pertussis-insensitive G protein, presumably Gq/11 [63], to the PLC/$IP_3$/DAG system as the major intracellular signalling pathway [64]. In rat cardiac myocytes and human right atrium, ET receptors couple to inhibit adenylyl cyclase activity via a pertussis toxin-sensitive G protein [65–68]. These findings suggest that multiple G proteins may be involved in ET-1-induced cardiac signal transduction. In human atrial tissue, $ET_A$ receptors stimulate PLC via Gq/11 and inhibit adenylyl cyclase via Gi, whereas in ventricular myocardium they only couple to Gq/11 [69]. Moreover, ET-1-induced IP formation in right atrial and left ventricular myocardial slices is nearly completely suppressed by the $ET_A$ receptor antagonist BQ-123, suggesting that the $ET_B$ receptor in the human myocardium is not coupled to the PLC/$IP_3$/DAG pathway [69]. From *in vitro* studies on human astrocytoma and endothelial cells [70, 71] and from *in vivo* animal studies [72, 73], there is emerging evidence that a major function of the $ET_B$ receptor is to clear ET by rapid internalization.

ET also has potent effects on cell growth (Fig. 13.1). The growth-promoting effects on cardiomyocytes are associated with stimulation of cardiac protein synthesis [74] and the induction of muscle-specific genes, such as ventricular myosin light chain-2 and cardiac $\alpha$-actin. Immediate-early genes (c-*fos*, c-*jun*, and *egr*-1) that encode transcription factors are rapidly and transiently expressed. Furthermore, genes that are normally expressed in the foetal ventricle, $\beta$-myosin heavy chain, and skeletal muscle $\alpha$-actin, are re-expressed [75–77]. Locally generated and secreted ET-1 may play an important role as an autocrine/paracrine factor in angiotensin II- and noradrenaline-induced hypertrophy [78, 79].

Besides the inotropic effects of ETs, positive chronotropic [80] and arrythmogenic effects [81] have been demonstrated in various species. In the guinea-pig atria, the positive chronotropic effects of ETs are negatively modulated mainly through the $ET_A$ receptor subtype [82]. $ET_A$ and $ET_B$ receptors, like other G protein-coupled receptors, are subject to agonist-induced downregulation [83, 84]. Receptor desensitization by GRK-mediated phosphorylation of serine and threonine residues plays an important role in the rapid homologous desensitization of the $ET_A$ and $ET_B$ receptors [85]. An alternative mechanism of ET receptor regulation is the ET-1-induced endocytosis of cell surface $ET_A$ receptors. Findings from stably $ET_A$ receptor-transfected CHO cells indicate that ET-1 bound to the receptor remains intact for up to 2 h after endocytosis [86]. From this observation it has been hypothesized that internalized ET-1 bound to $ET_A$ receptors continues to activate a signal-transducing G protein, thus accounting for the prolonged physiological effects observed after a single administration of ET-1 [86].

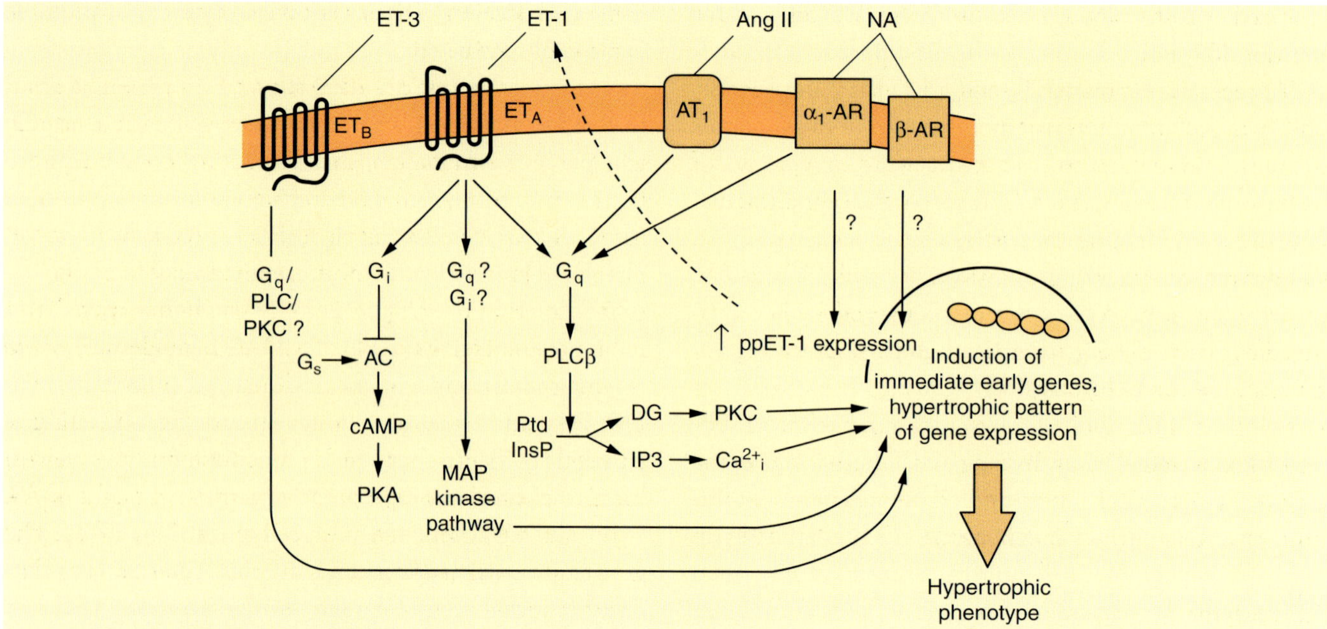


**Figure 13.1** *Signalling pathways leading to cardiomyocyte hypertrophy. Mitogenesis is dependent on both pertussis toxin-sensitive and -insensitive pathways. The first one corresponds to the phospholipase C/PKC pathway. ET-1 binding to the $ET_A$ receptor activates heterotrimeric G proteins of the Gq and Gi classes. The Gq α-subunit stimulates phospholipase C (PLCβ) to hydrolyse the membrane phosphoinotisol-4,5-bisphosphate (Ptdlns) to diacylglycerol (DAG) and inositol 1,4,5-trisphosphate ($IP_3$). DG-dependent protein kinase C (PKC) activation and $Ca^{2+}$ mobilization lead to induction of immediate-early genes, a hypertrophic pattern of gene expression, and a hypertrophic phenotype. The second pathway could be identified in the activation of MAP kinase via Gq. In addition, Gi may couple to growth responses in cardiac myocytes independent of inhibition of adenylyl cyclase (AC) (which generates the second messenger cAMP which, in turn, activates PKC) possibly though activation of Ras and subsequent activation of MAP kinases. Beside $ET_A$ receptors, selective stimulation of $ET_B$ receptors increases protein synthesis, indicating a role of the $ET_B$-receptor in the production of cardiac hypertrophy. Angiotensin II, norepinephrine, ET-3, and ET-1 generate prepro-ET-1 (ppET-1)-specific transcripts and stimulate secretion of ET-1. This may explain, in part, the synergism in mitogenic activities of these neurohormones.*

## Angiotensin II receptors

The biological effects of angiotensin (AT) II are mediated by the AT and AT receptors. Both receptors have recently been cloned and are thought to play a pivotal role in the pathogenesis of cardiovascular disease.

### *AT1 receptor*

The AT1 receptor is a G protein coupled receptor consisting of 359 amino acids that form the typical seven transmembrane loops [87–89]. The genomic organization among species. In rats, there are two AT1 receptors, AT1a and AT1b, which differ in their expression pattern but share common functions. Humans do not express an AT1b receptor. The rat AT1a receptor gene consists of four exons covering more than 80 kb. The third exon contains the complete coding region. Similarly, the human AT1 receptor is composed of four exons spread over 60 kb genomic DNA. The AT1 receptor is expressed in most tissues; nevertheless, most receptors are found in the vascular media, liver, kidney, adrenal, gland, brain, and heart [89–91].

Stimulation of AT1 receptors causes activation of multiple signalling pathways. First, stimulation of PLC causes hydrolysis of phosphatidylinositol in DAG and inositol triphosphates. The latter are decisively involved in the release of cytocolic calcium. DAG activates PKC. Secondly, AT1 receptor activation stimulates phospholipase D, leading to the release of choline and phosphatidic acid which then form DAG. Thirdly, the adenylate cyclase system may be activated or inhibited (via Gi proteins) resulting in an increase or decrease of intracellular cAMP. Fourthly, via AT1 receptors, angiotensin II activates NADH and NADPH oxidases, which are involved in the release of reactive oxygen species. Fifthly, angiotensin II phosphorylates intracellular kinases such as Jak2 and Tyk2, which phosphorylate STAT 1 and 2. Furthermore, angiotensin II activates the mitogen-activated protein (MAP) kinase pathway [89–94]. These intracellular pathways lead to the biological effects of AT1 receptor activation, namely, vasoconstriction, cellular growth, release of catecholamines, vasopression and aldosterone release, enhanced thirst, blood pressure increase, and water retention [89–91].

AT1 receptor expression is regulated via internalization and downregulation. Internalization occurs within minutes of agonist stimulation and is caused by internalization of receptor–ligand complexes in lysosomal compartments. Some of these complexes are lysed, while some are recycled as intact receptor molecules towards the cell surface. The downregulation of AT1 receptors is caused by the prolonged exposure of cells to various agonists. Down regulation can be homologous (angiotensin II induced) or heterologous (induced by growth factors, insulin, or low-density lipoprotein.The underlying mechanism involves the down regulation of AT1 receptor mRNA via transcriptional and post-transcriptional mechanisms [89–91, 95–105].

#### *AT2 receptor*

The AT2 receptor, cloned in 1993 [106, 107], also belongs to the family of G protein-coupled receptors, although it shares only a 34% homology with the AT1 receptor. The AT2 receptor is expressed in the adrenal, gland uterus, and brain, in the pathological setting of vascular balloon injury, cardiac hypertrophy and failure, as well as after skin injury. A functional coupling to signalling pathways typical for AT1 receptor activation (e.g. calcium) could not be shown, but the AT2 receptor may be coupled to tyrosine phosphatases and MAP kinase phosphatases. Based on recent observations, the AT2 receptor is involved in the control of cell growth. So far it has been shown that AT2 receptor activation may inhibit growth as well as apoptosis in various tissues [108–113].

## Pathophysiology of signal transduction in heart disease

### Sympathetic activation in heart failure

Heart failure is characterized by inadequate cardiac output due to impaired performance of cardiac muscle. The heart is unable to supply oxygen and substrates to the periphery. In the early stages of heart failure, several neuroendocrine mechanisms are activated to increase blood pressure and maintain blood flow to vital organs [114]. These compensatory mechanisms include activation of the renin–angiotensin–aldosterone system [115] increased release of vasopressin [116], and activation of the sympathetic nervous system [117]. Although these mechanisms are relevant in acute shock, they potentially worsen the outcome and accelerate the progression of heart failure when chronically activated.

Several investigations have shown that general activation of the sympathetic nervous system occurs in heart failure [117]. Consistently, noradrenalone concentrations increase at rest [118] and during exercise [119]. As a result of this pre-existing elevation of resting noradrenaline the relative increase during exercise has been reported to be attenuated [119]. When patients with heart failure are divided into groups with high, moderate, or low plasma concentrations of noradrenaline, a close correlation between noradrenaline levels and the worsening of survival has been observed [118]. These findings suggest but do not prove that sympathetic activation might not be a harmless bystander in the pathophysiology of chronic heart failure but rather is a relevant contributor to cardiac deterioration.

#### *Presynaptic alteration*

Swedberg *et al.* [120] reported an increased release of noradrenaline from the myocardium, indicating that activation of myocardial sympathetic nerve terminals contributes to the elevation of noradrenaline plasma concentrations. In addition, there is evidence that diminished noradrenaline uptake and release also contribute to these alterations [121, 122]. Rundqvist *et al.* [123] showed that extraction of noradrenaline is impaired but that spillover is enhanced (Fig. 13.2). In addition, direct measurements of noradrenaline uptake I carrier sites have been reported to be reduced by about 40% [121] (Fig. 13.3). These observations suggest that local and systemic release of noradrenaline not only chronically stimulate the failing heart, but may also be involved in the postsynaptic alteration of cardiomyocytes in heart failure.

### Alteration of β-adrenergic signal transduction in heart failure

#### *β-Adrenoceptors*

Downregulation of β-adrenoceptors is well established in the failing human heart. Bristow *et al.* [124] described a decline in their number in this situation. Later, these findings were confirmed by many investigators (for review, see ref. 125). The downregulation of β-adrenoceptors is dependent on the severity of the heart failure but not on its underlying cause (Fig. 13.4). As shown in Figure 13.4, 75–80% of β-adrenergic receptors are downregulated in hearts of patients with terminal heart failure due to dilated

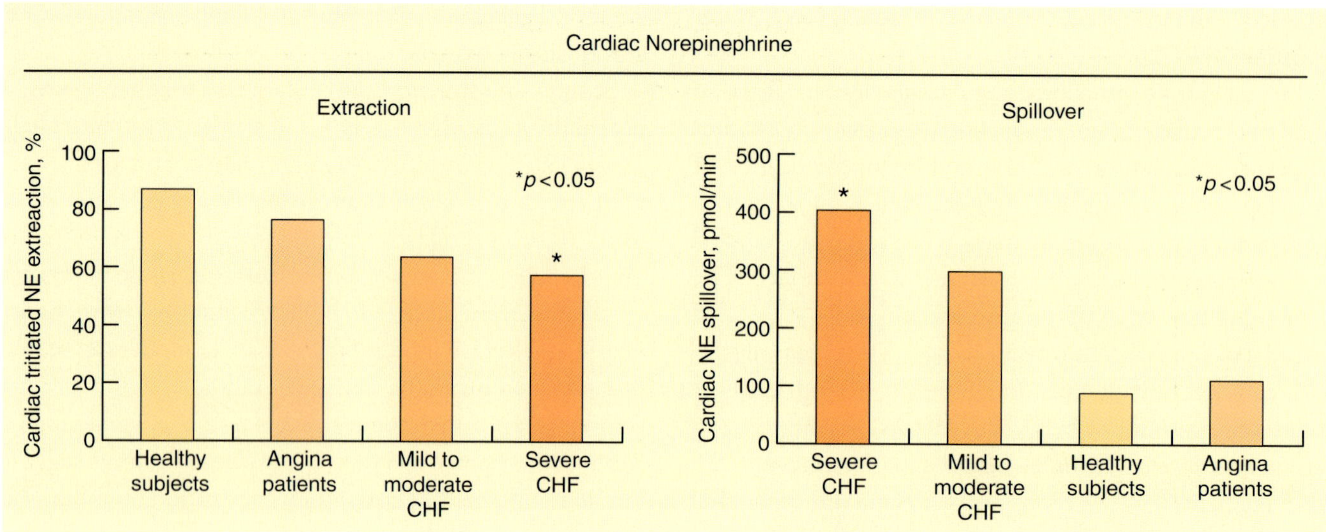


**Figure 13.2** *Myocardial extraction* (left) *and spillover* (right) *of noradrenaline from patients with cardiac diseases and in healthy subjects as controls. (Modified from ref. 123.)*

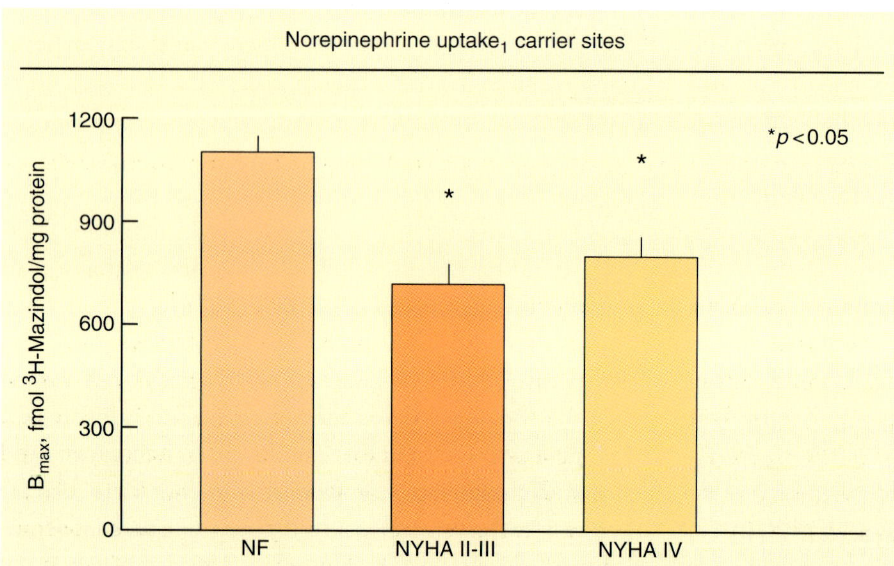


**Figure 13.3** *Norepinephrine uptake$_1$ carrier sites in left ventricular myocardium from patients with moderate (NYHA II–III) or severe (NYHA IV) heart failure and in non-failing hearts (NF). (Modified from ref. 121.)*

cardiomyopathy. However, in patients in moderate heart failure, the decline in receptor number is about 50%, indicating that in compensated heart failure β-adrenergic desensitization also occurs. The downregulation of β-adrenoceptors is due to a reduction in the number of β1-adrenoceptors, whereas the number of $\beta_2$-adrenoceptors remains unchanged [125]. Downregulation occurs because of either an increase in β-adrenoceptor breakdown or a reduction in the *de novo* synthesis of β-adrenoceptors. Evidence in favour of the latter suggestion has recently been provided by studies on steady-state levels of β-adrenoceptor mRNA. With quantitative polymerase chain reaction [126] and nuclease protection assays [127], a reduction in steady-state mRNA levels of $\beta_1$-adrenoceptors but not $\beta_2$-adrenoceptors has been observed. These findings suggest that a reduction in receptor protein synthesis due to reduced mRNA synthesis or enhanced mRNA degradation could play a role in the decline in myocardial β-adrenoceptors. The effect of cAMP on PKA activity is unchanged in failing and non-failing myocardium [128, 129]. The consequence of the reduction in β-adrenoceptors is reduced formation of cAMP and an impaired posi-

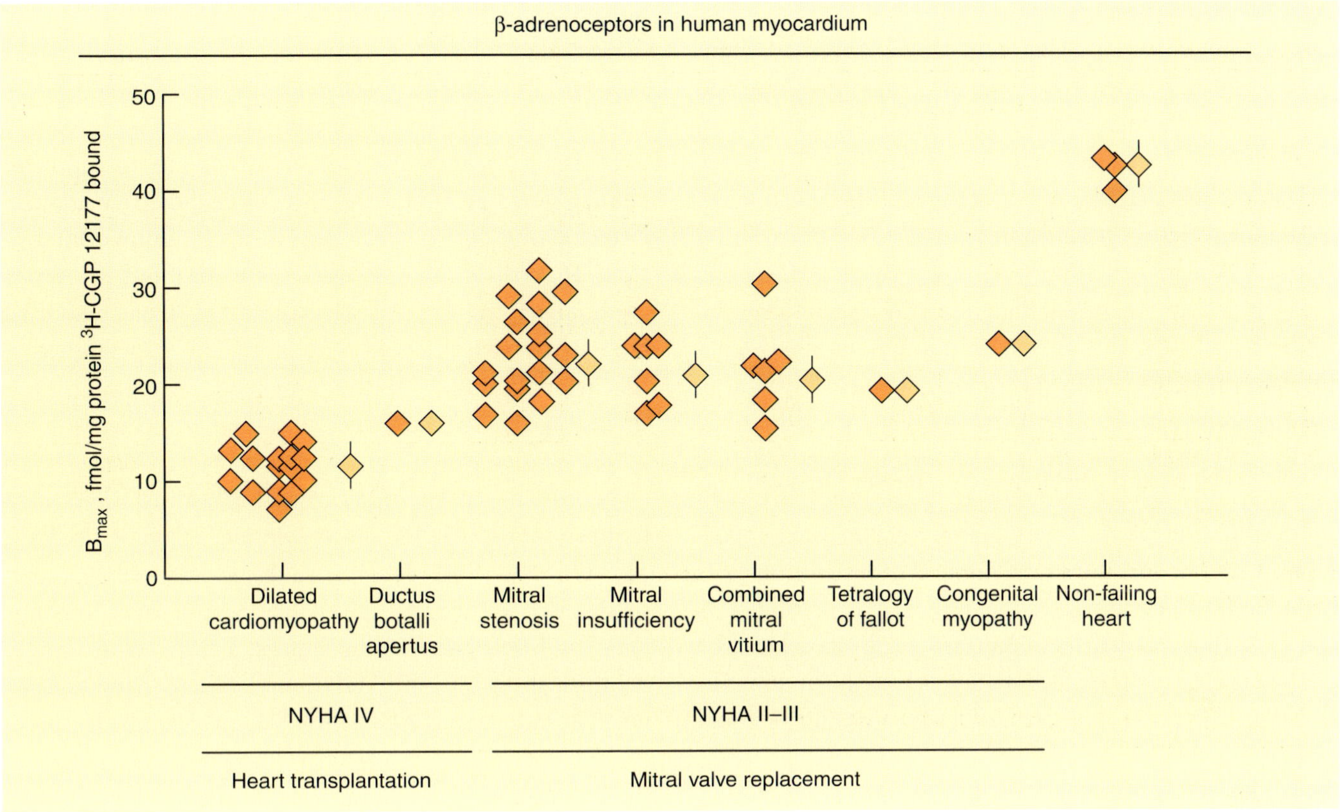


**Figure 13.4** *Density of β-adrenergic receptors in left ventricular myocardium (papillary muscle specimen) from patients with various cardiac diseases.*

tive inotropic effect following activation with β-agonists. Recently, $\beta_3$-adrenoceptors have been identified in the human heart [3]. $\beta_3$-Adrenoceptors are different from $\beta_1$- and $\beta_2$-adrenoceptors and share only 40–50% of their amino acid sequence [130, 131]. They lack the phosphorylation sites for the β-ARKs and cAMP-dependent protein kinase [131, 132]. It has recently been shown that in the presence of the $\beta_1$- and $\beta_2$-antagonist nadolol, isoprenaline produced negative inotropic effects. The negative inotropic effect was antagonized by the non-selective β-adrenoceptor antagonist bupranolol and was sensitive to pertussis toxin [3]. Thus, there is evidence that in the human heart, $\beta_3$-adrenoceptors are coupled to inhibitory G protein α-subunits, thereby producing negative inotropic effects. In heart failure. $\beta_1$-adrenoceptors are downregulated and $\beta_2$-receptors are apparently uncoupled [125, 129]. The $\beta_3$-adrenoceptor might depress the force of contraction during catecholamine stimulation. Further studies, in particular on the functional role and the regulation of $\beta_3$-adrenoceptors, are necessary to elucidate their role in the pathophysiology of heart failure.

### *β-Adrenergic receptors in circulatory shock*

The desensitization of β-adrenergic receptors has been shown to be accompanied by reduced positive inotropic effects of β-adrenoceptor agonists [125, 129]. Therefore, treatment of endstage heart failure in the decompensated state with β-adrenoceptor agonists is questionable. Nevertheless, the agents can acutely produce marked haemodynamic effects [133]. However, after application of dobutamine in patients with heart failure a complete tolerance towards the β-adrenoceptor agonist has been described [133]. One potential mechanism of this phenomenon is depicted in Figure 13.5. Four patients awaiting cardiac transplantation were treated with catecholamines to maintain cardiac output. β-Adrenoceptors were analysed following transplantation. In patients on catecholamine treatment, there was a 40% decline in the number of β-adrenergic receptors compared with patients with heart failure without catecholamine treatment. The reduction in receptors amounted to 80% compared with that of the non-failing myocardium and was at the lower margin for detecting β-adrenergic receptors by radioligand binding experiments.

***Signal-transducing G proteins***

Gs is the heterotrimeric G protein which couples β-adrenergic receptors to adenylyl cyclase. αs can be visualized and quantified by cholera toxin-induced [$^{32}$P]ADP-ribosylation using [$^{32}$P]NAD as a substrate, with subsequent separation on sodium dodecyl sulfate–polyacrylamide gel and autoradiography. Cholera toxin-induced [$^{32}$P]ADP-ribosylation of αs is similar in human failing and non-failing hearts [134]. However, the signals obtained by this technology are rather weak. The authors' group partially purified ADP-ribosylation factor (ARF), a cofactor of cholera toxin, from bovine brain cytosol to enhance cholera toxin-induced [$^{32}$-P]ADP-ribosylation of αs in human left ventricular membranes [135]. This method revealed that [$^{32}$P]ADP-ribosylation signals in heart failure remain unchanged. However, even this improved method of visualizing αs is hampered by data suggesting that only a small portion of αs present in myocardial membranes is ADP-ribosylated by cholera toxin [136]. αs mRNA levels have been reported to be similar [137] or increased [138] in failing human hearts. The bioactivity of αs was investigated by solubilization from myocardial membranes and reconstitution with S49 cyc$^-$ membranes. The cyc$^-$ mutant of S49 mouse lymphoma cells is genetically deficient in αs. This method revealed unchanged αs activity during heart failure as judged by unchanged isoprenaline- and Gpp(NH)p-stimulated adenylyl cyclase activity in the reconstituted lipid vesicles [134]. Taken together, the results obtained by different techniques and different authors strongly suggest unchanged amounts and bioactivity of αs in human heart failure. However, in human heart failure due to Chagas cardiomyopathy [139], as well as in several animal models, such as aortic banding in dogs [140, 141] and hereditary cardiomyopathy in Syrian hamsters [142], decreased αs bioactivity was observed, indicating the dependence of the regulation of the β-adrenergic/G protein/adenylyl cyclase system on the species and the pathogenesis of the failure.

αi proteins can be visualized and quantified by pertussis toxin-induced [$^{32}$P]ADP-ribosylation. Several authors [23, 134, 143, 144] observed a substantial increase in pertussis toxin-induced [$^{32}$P]ADP-ribosylation of αi in failing compared with non-failing human hearts. However, αi quantification by [$^{32}$P]ADP-ribosylation is hampered by possible endogenous ADP-ribosylation [145] or other kinds of covalent modification such as phosphorylation [146] at the C-terminus. In addition, several factors such as βγ-subunits enhance ADP-ribosylation and differences in these factors can influence the results. Quantification of αi by Western blot analysis using polyclonal rabbit antisera [147]

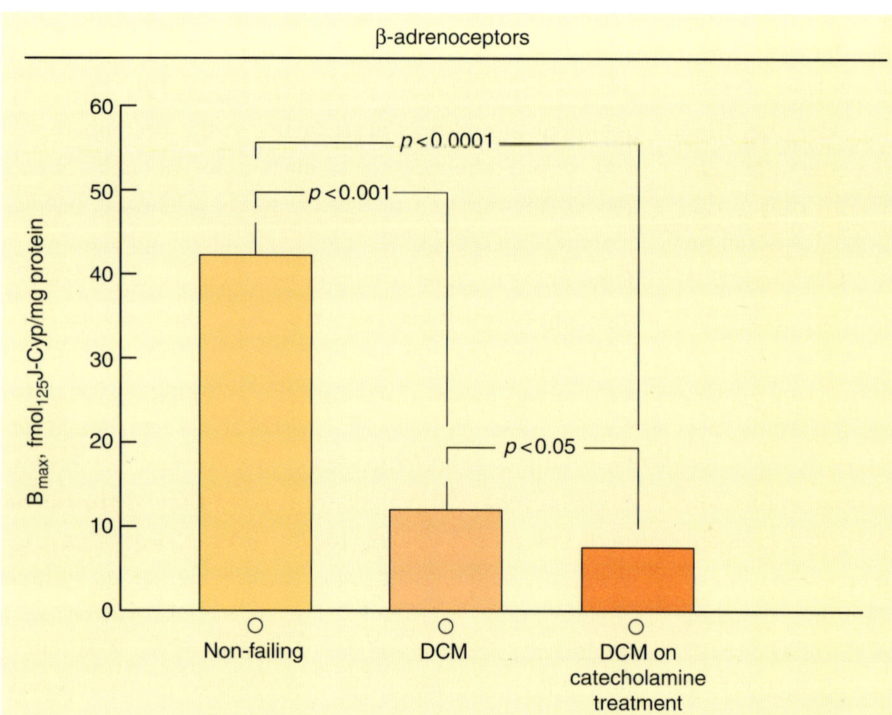


**Figure 13.5** *β-Adrenergic receptors in left ventricular myocardium from patients with severe heart failure due to dilated cardiomyopathy (DCM) and in non-failing hearts. Receptor densities in patients with or without catecholamine treatment prior to transplantation were compared.*

that recognizes all αi subtypes has been done by several groups with discrepant results. Böhm *et al.* [23] found increased immunoreactivity in left ventricles from patients with dilated cardiomyopathy and unchanged amounts of αi in ischaemic cardiomyopathy, (Fig. 13.6). Feldman *et al.* [149] observed unchanged amounts of αi in dilated cardiomyopathy. The reason for this discrepancy is not clear. The results of Böhm *et al.* [150], revealing a marked increase in immunoreactive αi proteins were confirmed by a radioimmunoassay with purified retinal transducin as standard and the $^{125}$I-labelled C-terminal decapeptide of transducin-α as tracer. A differentiation between the different αi subtypes ($\alpha i_2$ and $\alpha i_3$ are expressed in the heart) was not possible with the antibodies applied. At the level of mRNA, a subtype-specific increase in $\alpha i_2$ has been demonstrated, while $\alpha i_3$ mRNA is similar in failing and non-failing human hearts [151]. At this point there is again a discrepancy with a very useful animal model, namely isoprenaline-treated rats. In the hearts of these animals, an increase in both $\alpha i_2$ and $\alpha i_3$ mRNA is observed [137]. The increase in $\alpha i_2$ mRNA was paralleled by an increased transcriptional rate of the $\alpha i_2$ gene, as assessed by nuclear run-on assays performed with nuclear extracts from isoprenaline-treated rat cardiomyocytes [152] (Fig. 13.7). Thus, increased transcriptional activity contributes to the upregulation of $\alpha i_2$ in this system. The upregulation of αi is not observed in S49 cyc$^-$ or kin$^-$ cells lacking or PKA, respectively, indicating that an intact Gs–adenylyl cyclase–PKA signalling cascade is required for this process in rat cardiomyocytes. In the human heart, no data are yet available on this issue.

Although β-adrenergic receptors do not transduce their signals via Gi proteins, Gi influences the balance between stimulatory and inhibitory effects on adenylyl cyclase and thus might contribute to decreased adenylyl cyclase and inotropic response to β-adrenergic agonists. This hypothesis is supported by the finding that adenylyl cyclase activity in the failing human left ventricle [134] is restored when the membranes are pretreated with pertussis toxin, which uncouples Gi from inhibitory receptors. In pertussis toxin-treated isolated human cardiomyocytes from patients with heart failure, an isoprenaline-stimulated contractile force was restored to the level of cardiomyocytes from non-failing hearts [153]. It appears likely that the upregulation of

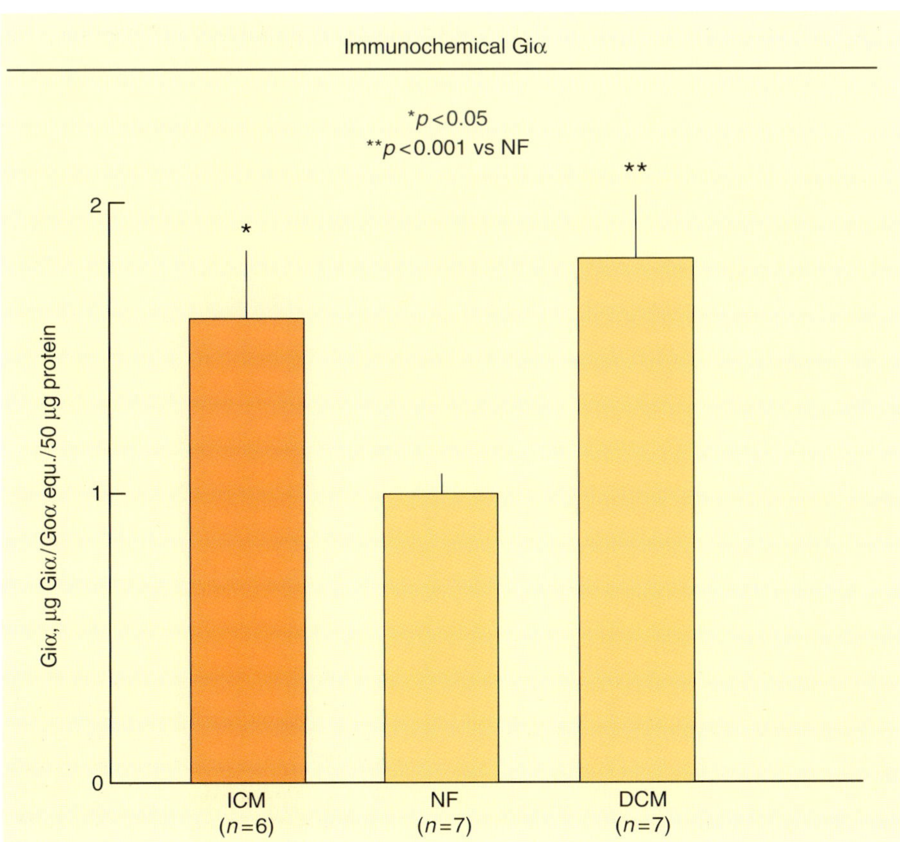


**Figure 13.6** *Representative Western blot* (left) *and immunochemical quantification* (right) *of inhibitory G-protein α-subunits* (Giα) *in left ventricular myocardium from patients with ischaemic* (ICM) *or dilated* (DCM) *cardiomyopathy and nonfailing myocardium. (Modified from ref. 148.)*

$\alpha i_2$ contributes to the decreased inotropic response to β-adrenergic agonists and is of pathophysiological relevance in heart failure.

### *G proteins in shock*

Recently, the concentration of myocardial Giα proteins during terminal catecholamine-refractory shock was evaluated. Postmortem samples were controlled for the stability of Giα proteins. Immunochemical detection as well as [$^{32}$P]ADP-ribosylation with pertussis toxin revealed an increase in Giα proteins in patients in shock compared with those who died of carcinoma and in whom clinical and morphological evidence of heart disease was lacking. Patients treated with high doses of catecholamines for septic or cardiogenic shock who died in catecholamine refractory shock had a four-fold higher level of myocardial Giα (Fig. 13.8). The increase in Giα was similar in patients with septic multiorgan failure, who also died in catecholamine refractory shock [154, 155]. In addition to chronic heart failure in humans, other conditions, such as catecholamine refractory septic or cardiogenic shock, which increase myocardial Giα concentrations may contribute to catecholamine refractoriness and contractile failure. The mechanism of Giα upregulation appears to be an increase in the gene transcription rate of $Gi\alpha_2$ genes, whereas a destabilization of mRNA contributes to the reduction in β-adrenergic receptors (Fig. 13.9).

### *Adenylyl cyclases*

As mentioned above, adenylyl cyclase types IV, V, and VI are the isozymes present in the mammalian heart. Surprisingly, not many studies have dealt with the qualitative or quantitative changes of adenylyl cyclase isozyme expression patterns in heart failure. In human heart failure due to dilated or ischaemic cardiomyopathy, the mRNA of type V adenylyl cyclase, the predominant cardiac isozyme, is increased [156]. The mechanism of this increase has not yet been addressed. The observation suggests that adenylyl cyclase might not be impaired in heart failure, consistent with the previous observation [23] that maximal adenylyl cyclase activity as assessed by stimulation with forskolin is not compromised in human heart failure. However, Holmer *et al.* [156] only investigated adenylyl cyclase type V and not types IV and VI. In contrast, in pacing-induced heart failure in dogs, AV V and VI mRNA levels are decreased [157]. The data obtained in human myocardial tissue are not convincing enough to draw final conclusions on possible changes in adenylyl cyclase isoform expression.

### *α-Adrenoceptors*

Catecholamines such as noradrenaline activate not only cardiac β-, but also $\alpha_1$-adrenoceptors. Three different $\alpha_1$-adrenoceptor subtype, $\alpha_{1A}$, $\alpha_{1B}$, and $\alpha_{1D}$, have been cloned. Pharmacological studies using subtype-selective

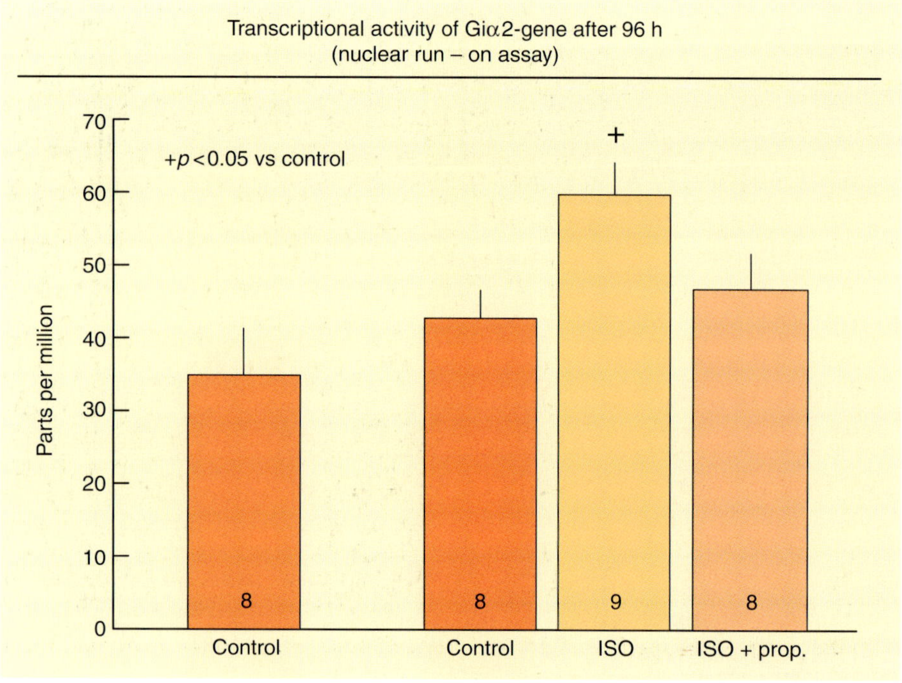


**Figure 13.7** *Transcriptional activity of the $Gi\alpha_2$ gene in rat hearts following treatment of the annimals with isoprenaline or isoprenaline plus propanolol. (Modified from ref. 152.)*

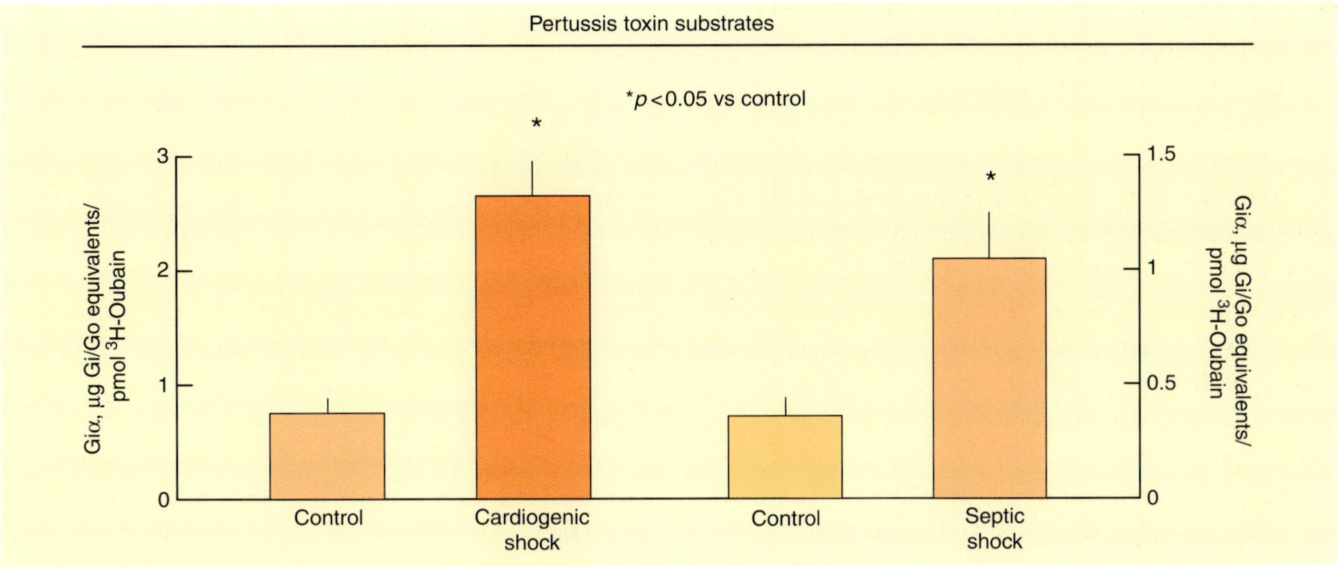


**Figure 13.8** *Immunochemical Giα proteins in left ventricular myocardium of patients who died in catecholamine-refractory cardiogenic* (left) *or septic* (right) *shock. Controls are myocardial samples from patients, who died of cancer and had no evidence for cardiac disease. (Modified from ref. 155.)*

antagonists suggest that in addition to the above three 'classic' $\alpha_1$-adrenoceptor subtypes, an additional putative $\alpha_{1L}$ adrenoceptor is expressed in rat heart [158]. The physiological significance of this diversity is not yet understood. $\alpha_1$-Adrenoceptors are, like β-adrenoceptors, G protein-coupled receptors. Agonist binding leads to increased formation of intracellular inositol phosphate by PLCβ isozymes through the mediation of Gq proteins. $\alpha_1$-Adrenoceptor stimulation induces a positive inotropic effect (for review see ref. 37).

In hypertensive transgenic rats that overexpress the mouse renin gene TG(mREN2)27, indicating massive cardiac hypertrophy but no heart failure, circulating catecholamine levels are increased [150]. $\alpha_1$-Adrenoceptor density is increased, but the pathway is desensitized at the level of PLC [135]. In contrast, in another rat model of cardiac hypertrophy spontaneously hypertensive rats (SHR), $\alpha_1$-adrenoceptor density is decreased [159], while the reports on $\alpha_1$-adrenoceptor-stimulated PLC activity are contradictory: Ivorra *et al.* [159] reported a decrease and Kawaguchi *et al.* [160] an increase in the PLC response to noradrenaline.

In the heart failure model of cardiomyopathic Syrian hamsters, the positive inotropic response to $\alpha_1$-adrenoceptor agonists is increased [161], while $\alpha_1$-adrenoceptor density is unchanged [162]. In human heart failure,

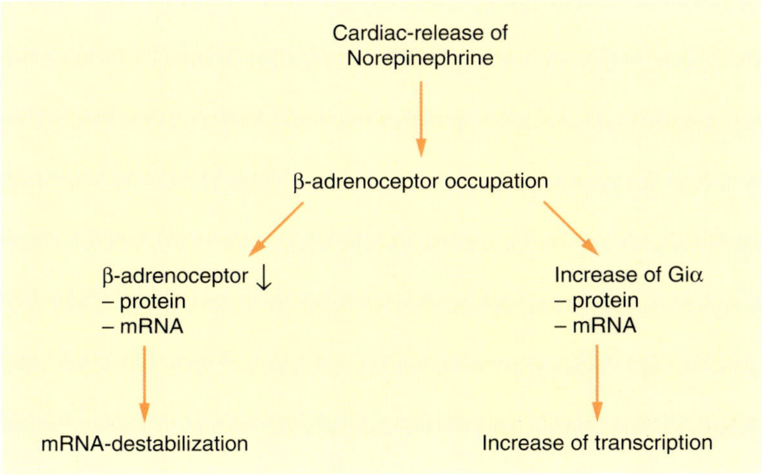


**Figure 13.9** *Mechanisms of β-adrenergic signal transduction defects in heart failure.*

Steinfath *et al.* [163] observed a reduced inotropic response to $\alpha_1$-adrenoceptor agonists despite an increased receptor density. Other studies performed in human hearts reported an unchanged responsiveness to $\alpha_1$-adrenoceptor agonists [164, 165] accompanied by unchanged receptor densities. The levels of αq/11 proteins and maximal PLC activity are unchanged in failing compared with non-failing human myocardium (Schnabel and Böhm, unpublished data). In heart failure, the $\alpha_1$-adrenergic signal transduction pathway is of particular relevance because it may be a reserve mechanism to maintain inotropy in a state in which the β-adrenergic system is desensitized. The results of the studies cited above show that the regulation of the $\alpha_1$-adrenergic pathway is not simply dependent on the level of circulating noradrenaline, but also on whether there is hypertrophy or failure and its pathogenesis, or other factors yet to be determined. There are considerable differences among species regarding $\alpha_1$-adrenoceptor density, the degree of α1-adrenoceptor-mediated PLC activation, and the degree of positive inotropic effects. However, the physiological significance of the $\alpha_1$-adrenoceptor–G protein–PLC signalling system for the mediation of hypertrophic effects may be even greater than for the regulation of contractility in heart failure.

## Phospholipase C-coupled receptor system in heart disease

### *Phospholipase* C

A second G protein-coupled pathway that is important in the pathophysiology of hypertrophy is the PLC pathway. Many stimuli that induce myocardial hypertrophy, such as noradrenaline [166, 167], angiotensin II [168, 169], and endothelin [77], use this enzyme as an intracellular effector. All of these agonists activate receptors which couple to PLC via Gq. The $\alpha_1$-adrenergic receptor pathway seems to be of particular interest, as the sympathetic nervous system is activated in hypertrophy [170]. The hypertrophic response of isolated neonatal rat cardiomyocytes to α-adrenergic receptor stimulation has been shown to be dependent on the presence of αq [171]. Thus, it is tempting to speculate that alterations in the Gq–PLC system might be involved in the pathogenesis of mycardial hypertrophy. Animal studies addressing this issue are sparse. In cardiomyocytes prepared from SHR, noradrenaline-induced inositol phosphate formation is increased compared with control cells [160]. However, the level of the signal transduction cascade at which activation takes place has not yet been determined.

The hypothesis that the PLC pathway is activated in hypertrophy, which can be understood as an adaptation to increased workload, is confirmed by the finding that not only receptor agonists, but also mechanical stretch activates PLC (for review see ref. 172). This has been shown in perfused rat hearts [173] and in cultured rat cardiomyocytes [174]. Thus, PLC may be the trigger that translates mechanical into biochemical signals. This issue has not yet been investigated in humans and the αq and PLC isoforms involved have not yet been identified.

### *Endothelin receptors*

Many studies have shown that endothelin levels are increased in patients with heart failure, irrespective of aetiology. As with noradrenaline, plasma levels of ET-1 and big ET-1, the inactive precursor peptide of ET-1, are of prognostic significance [175–178]. Elevated circulating irET-1 levels were also reported in experimental animal models of heart failure [179, 180]. Furthermore, elevated ET-1 tissue concentrations in the ventricular myocardium are well documented in animals and humans with congestive heart failure [181, 182]. Thus, the ET receptors are chronically exposed to high concentrations of ET-1 and, therefore, they may be downregulated or desensitized during congestive heart failure. However, total ET receptor density is found to be unchanged or even upregulated in the failing human left ventricle [69, 182] and in failing rat myocardium after coronary artery ligation [183–185] (Table 13.2). In human heart failure, a change in ventricular ET receptor expression in favour of the $ET_A$ receptor has been observed [182, 190]. In a rabbit model of congestive heart failure induced by combined aortic valvular stenosis and insufficiency, the density of the $ET_A$ and $ET_B$ receptors was decreased in the right and left ventricles [187].

Findings about the regulation of ET receptor expression in animals with compensated cardiac hypertrophy are inconsistent. In SHR [188] and aortocaval shunt rats [195], ET receptor density did not differ between samples from hypertrophied ventricles and controls. Another study demonstrated a selective increase in $ET_A$ receptor mRNA expression in all chambers, whereas [$^{125}$I]ET-1 binding was not changed in the aortocaval shunt model, suggesting rapid turnover of ET receptors balanced by increased transcription [189]. Ventricular ET-1 levels were markedly increased and the density of ET-1 binding sites was decreased in rats with constriction of the suprarenal aorta [186]. One factor may explain in part the diversity of results obtained from the different animal models. Chronic pressure overload may lead to quite different pathophysiological alterations in the ET system than chronic volume overload, although both mechanisms lead to cardiac hypertrophy. This suggestion is supported by the observation that cardiac ET gene expression is increased only in rats with aortic banding and not in rats with aortic valve regurgitation [196]. Although alterations in ET receptor regulation in heart failure and cardiac hypertrophy have been described, the pathophysiological significance *in vivo* remains to be investigated.

### *Angiotensin II receptors*

The AT1 receptor that mediates most of the biological effects of the renin–angiotensin system is thought to be decisively involved in the pathogenesis of heart failure [90, 97]. There is ample evidence that inhibition of AT1 receptor activation is of substantial benefit for patients suffering from heart failure. Angiotensin-converting enzyme (ACE) inhibitors and probably also AT1 receptor antagonists decrease mortality rates in patients with heart failure based on either cardiomyopathy or coronary heart disease [197–201]. Despite these convincing data, the mechanisms underlying this pivotal role of AT1 receptor activation in the setting of heart failure ar still poorly understood. The AT1 receptor is, besides other localizations, expressed in the heart as well as the vasculature [90, 97, 202]. Since AT1 receptor activation causes vasoconstriction and increased afterload [90, 97, 197–202] inhibition of its activation goes along with decreased afterload, which is preferable in heart failure. In addition to these general circulatory effects, the AT1 receptor is involved in various cardiac events such as hypertrophy, fibrosis, and remodelling following myocardial infarction [202]. Several animal models have been used to elucidate the role of AT1 receptor activation and AT1 receptor regulation in cardiac

**Table 13.2** Expression of endothelin (ET) receptor protein and messenger RNA in humans and animal models with cardiac hypertrophy and heart failure

| | Total ET receptor binding sites | $ET_A$ receptor binding sites | $ET_B$ receptor binding sites | $ET_A$ receptor mRNA | $ET_B$ receptor mRNA |
|---|---|---|---|---|---|
| Animal models | | | | | |
| Rat, constriction of suprarenal aorta | ↑ [186] | | | ↓ ventricle [191]<br>↔ atrium [191] | ↓ ventricle [191]<br>↔ atrium [191] |
| Rabbit, combined aortic valvular insufficiency and stenosis | ↑ [187] | | | | |
| Spontaneous hypertensive rat | ↔ [188] | | | ↓ [192] | ↓ [192] |
| Rat, aortocaval shunt | ↔ [189] | | | ↑ [189] | |
| Rat, coronary artery ligation | ↔ [184]<br>↑ [183, 185] | | | ↑ [193] | ↑ [193] |
| Dahl salt-sensitive rat | | | | ↔ [192] | ↔ [192] |
| Humans | | | | | |
| Hypertrophic cardiomyopathy | | | | ↔[194] | |
| Heart failure | ↔ [69, 182]<br>↑ [190] | ↑ [182, 190]<br>↔ [69] | ↓ [182]<br>↔ [69, 190] | ↔ [182] | ↓ [182] |

disease (summarized in Table 13.3). Whereas the AT1 receptor is downregulated in the hearts of renin-transgenic animals as well as in the models of aortic banding and arteriovenous shunting, it is upregulated in the myocardium of SHR and rats with renovascular hypertensive disease. The state of activation of other components of the renin–angiotensin system (e.g. ACE) may influence cardiac AT1 receptor regulation by negative or positive feedback regulation. Rats with, for example, a clipped renal artery, as well as renin-transgenic rats, display a stimulated local or circulating renin–angiotensin system but show either upregulation or downregulation of cardiac AT1 receptor expression, suggesting renin–angiotensin-independent regulation of AT1 receptor expression. Possibly, in these experiments, AT1 receptor expression was assessed at different times with regard to the individual and time-dependent development of cardiac hypertrophy and heart failure. Cardiac AT1 receptor expression may not always be comparable between animal models. Additional experiments at various time-points are needed to clarify this hypothesis.

Heart failure in humans is associated with cardiac AT1 receptor downregulation, which is possibly independent of the aetiology of heart failure [218, 219]. There are two putative explanations for this observation: AT1 receptor downregulation may be secondary to neurohumoral changes such as activation of renin–angiotensin, or the transition to heart failure is based on AT1 receptor downregulation (together with calcium-handling proteins, contractile protein, and β-adrenergic receptors). In other words, intracellular molecular changes such as AT1 receptor downregulation initiate the development of heart failure due to the reduced growth-stimulating effect of AT1 receptor activation.

Although clinical intervention studies with patients in heart failure clearly demonstrate the marked beneficial effect on mortality, morbidity, and hospitalization of ACE inhibition, further animal studies using modern genetic approaches such as inducible gene disruption in combination with AT1 receptor antagonism or ACE inhibition treatment are required to elucidate the significance of AT1 receptor activation and regulation, as well as the role of kinins in the diseased heart. The development of cardiac hypertrophy and its relation to the expression of the components of the renin–angiotensin system (renin, ACE, AT1 receptor) awaits further study.

## Perspectives

During the past few years, alterations in cardiac receptors as well as their signal transduction mechanisms have been identified. The characterization of these alterations have led to a better understanding not only of the dysregulation of the force of contraction but also of the initiation of cardiac remodelling, namely, the mechanisms of cardiac hypertrophy. The major task of the future will be the development of strategies and drugs that enable the physician to interact selectively with various steps in the cardiac receptor-coupled signal transduction mechanisms in order to prevent heart failure or to reverse contractile dysfunction in later stages.

## Acknowledgement

This experimental work was supported by the Deutsche Forschungsgemeinschaft.

**Table 13.3** Expression of myocardial angiotensin-converting enzyme (ACE), angiotensin (AT)1 and AT2 receptors and plasma renin concentrations in experimental animal models of cardiac hypertrophy and heart failure

| Model | Plasma renin | Cardiac ACE | Cardiac AT1 receptor | Cardiac AT2 receptor |
|---|---|---|---|---|
| TG(mREN2)27 rats | ↑/= | ↑ | ↓ | |
| SHR rats | | | ↑ | |
| Renal hypertension | ↑ | ↑ | ↑ | |
| Volume overload | ↑ | ↑ | ↓ | ↑ |
| Aortic-banded model | | ↑ | ↓ | ↑/= |
| Pacing-induced heart failure | ↑ | ↓ | ↓ | ↓ |
| Myocardial infarction | | ↑ | ↑ | |

Data from ref. 101–103, 111, 195, 203–217.
TG(mREN2)27 = rats with somatic overexpression of the mouse renin gene $ren^{2d}$; SHR = spontaneously hypertensive rats.

## References


1. Gudermann T, Nürnberg B, Schultz G. Receptors and G proteins as primary components of transmembrane signal transduction. Part 1. G-protein-coupled receptors: structure and function. *J Mol Med* 1995; 73: 51–63.
2. Dohlman HG, Thorner J, Caron MG, Lefkowitz RJ. Model systems for the study of seven-transmembrane-segment receptors. *Annu Rev Biochem* 1991; 60: 653–88.
3. Gauthier C, Tavernier G, Charpentier F *et al.* Functional β3-adrenoceptor in the human heart. *J Clin Invest* 1996; 98: 556–62.
4. Krief S, Lönnqvist F, Raimbault S *et al.* Tissue distribution of β3-adrenergic receptor mRNA in man. *J Clin Invest* 1993; 91: 344–9.
5. Evans BA, Papaioannou M, Bonazzi VR *et al.* Expression of β-adrenoceptor mRNA in rat tissues. *Br J Pharmacol* 1996; 117: 210–16.
6. Kaumann AJ, Molenaar P. Differences between the third cardiac β-adrenoceptor and the colonic β3-adrenoceptor in the rat. *Br J Pharmacol* 1996; 118: 2085–98.
7. Pippig S, Andexinger S, Lohse MJ. Sequestration and recycling of β2-adrenergic receptors permit receptor resensitization. *Mol Pharmacol* 1995; 47: 666–76.
8. Hadcock JR, Wang H, Malbon CC. Agonist-induced destabilization of β-adrenergic receptor mRNA attenuation of glucocorticoid-induced up-regulation of β-adrenergic receptors. *J Biol Chem* 1989; 264: 19 928–33.
9. Port JD, Huang LJ, Malbon CC. β-Adrenergic agonists that down-regulate receptor mRNA up-regulate a Mr 35,000 protein(s) that selectively binds to β-adrenergic receptor mRNAs. *J Biol Chem* 1992; 267: 24 103–8.
10. Tholanikunnel BG, Granneman JG, Malbon CC. The Mr 35,000 β-adrenergic receptor mRNA-binding protein binds transcripts of G-protein-linked receptors which undergo agonist-induced destabilization. *J Biol Chem* 1995; 270: 12 787–93.
11. Hosoda K, Feussner GK, Rydelek-Fitzgerald L *et al.* Agonist and cyclic AMP-mediated regulation of β1-adrenergic receptor mRNA and gene transcription in rat C6 glioma cells. *J Neurochem* 1994; 63: 1635–45.
12. Bouvier M, Leeb-Lundberg LMF, Benovic JL *et al.* Regulation of adrenergic receptor function by phosphorylation. II. Effects of agonist occupancy on phosphorylation of α1- and β2-adrenergic receptors by protein kinase C and the cyclic AMP-dependent protein kinase. *J Biol Chem* 1997; 262: 3106–13.
13. Lefkowitz RJ. G protein-coupled receptor kinases. *Cell* 1993; 74: 409–12.
14. Ungerer M, Parruti G, Böhm M *et al.* Expression of β-arrestins and β-adrenergic receptor kinases in the failing human heart. *Circ Res* 1994; 74: 206–13.
15. Pitcher JA, Inglese J, Higgins JB *et al.* Role of βγ subunits of G proteins in targeting the β-adrenergic receptor kinase to membrane-bound receptors. *Science* 1992; 257: 1264–7.
16. Koch WJ, Inglese J, Stone WC, Lefkowitz RJ. The binding site for the βγ subunits of heterotrimeric G proteins on the β-adrenergic receptor kinase. *J Biol Chem* 1993; 268: 8256–60.
17. Inglese J, Koch WJ, Caron MG, Lefkowitz RJ. Isoprenylation in regulation of signal transduction by G-protein-coupled receptor kinases. *Nature* 1992; 359: 147–50.
18. Birnbaumer L, Abramowitz J, Brown AM. Receptor-effector coupling by G proteins. *Biochim Biophys Acta* 1990; 1031: 163–224.
19. Simon MI, Strathmann MP, Gautam N. Diversity of G proteins in signal transduction. *Science* 1991; 252: 802–8.
20. Nürnberg B, Gudermann T, Schultz G. Receptors and G proteins as primary components of transmembrane signal transduction. Part 2. G proteins: structure and function. *J Mol Med* 1995; 73: 123–32.
21. Levine MA, Modi WS, O'Brien SJ. Mapping of the gene encoding the α subunit of the stimulatory G protein of adenylyl cyclase (GNAS1) to 20q13.2-q13.3 in human by *in situ* hybridization. *Genomics* 1991; 11: 478–9.
22. Kaziro Y, Itoh H, Kozasa T *et al.* Structure and function of signal-transducing GTP-binding proteins. *Annu Rev Biochem* 1991; 60: 349–400.
23. Böhm M, Gierschik P, Jakobs KH *et al.* Increase of Giα in human hearts with dilated but not ischemic cardiomyopathy. *Circulation* 1990; 82: 1249–65.
24. Eschenhagen T. G proteins in the heart. *Cell Biol Int* 1993; 17: 723–49.
25. Clapham DE, Neer EJ. New roles for G-protein βγ-dimers in transmembrane signalling. *Nature* 1993; 365: 403–6.
26. Wedegaertner PB, Wilson PT, Bourne HR. Lipid modifications of trimeric G proteins. *J Biol Chem* 1995; 270: 503–6.
27. Hansen CA, Schroering AG, Robishaw JD. Subunit expression of signal transducing G proteins in cardiac tissue: Implications for phospholipase C-β regulation. *J Mol Cell Cardiol* 1995; 27: 471–84.
28. Kleuss C, Hescheler J, Ewel C *et al.* Assignment of G-protein subtypes to specific receptors inducing inhibition of calcium currents. *Nature* 1991; 353: 43–8.
29. Kleuss C, Scherübl H, Hescheler J *et al.* Different β-subunits determine G-protein interaction with transmembrane receptors. *Nature* 1993; 358: 424–6.
30. Kleuss C, Scherübl H, Hescheler J *et al.* Selectivity in signal transduction determined by γ subunits of heterotrimeric G proteins. *Science* 1993; 259: 832–4.
31. Tang WJ, Gilman AG. Adenylyl cyclases. *Cell* 1992; 70: 869–72.
32. Tang WJ, Gilman AG. Type-specific regulation of adenylyl cyclase by G protein βγ subunits. *Science* 1991; 254: 1500–3.
33. Taussig R, Quarmby LM, Gilman AG. Regulation of purified type I and type II adenylylcyclases by G protein βγ subunits. *J Biol Chem* 1993; 268: 9–12.
34. Bourne HR, Nicoll RA. Molecular machines integrate coincident synaptic signals. *Cell/Neuron* 1993; 72/12: 65–75.
35. Gao B, Gilman AG. Cloning and expression of a widely distributed (type IV) adenylyl cyclase. *Proc Natl Acad Sci USA* 1991; 88: 10 178–82.
36. Rhee SG, Choi KD. Regulation of inositol phospholipid-specific phospholipase C isozymes. *J Biol Chem* 1992; 267: 12 393–6.
37. Terzic A, Puceat M, Vassort G, Vogel SM. Cardiac $\alpha_1$-adrenoceptors: an overview. *Pharmacol Rev* 1993; 45: 147–75.
38. Jhon DY, Lee HH, Park D *et al.* Cloning, sequencing, purification, and Gq-dependent activation of phospholipase C-β3. *J Biol Chem* 1993; 268: 6654–61.
39. Schnabel P, Böhm M. Mutations of signal-transducing G proteins in human disease. *J Mol Med* 1995; 73: 221–8.
40. Katz A, Wu D, Simon MI. Subunits βγ of heterotrimeric G protein activate α2 isoform of phospholipase C. *Nature* 1992; 360: 686–9.
41. Cooper DMF, Mons N, Karpen JW. Adenylyl cyclases and the interaction between calcium and cAMP signalling. *Nature* 1995; 374: 421–4.

42. Nishizuka Y. Intracellular signalling by hydrolysis of phospholipids and activation of protein kinase C. *Science* 1992; 258: 607–14.
43. Berridge MJ. Inositol triphosphate and calcium signalling. *Nature* 1993; 361: 315–25.
44. Moody CJ, Dashwood MR, Sykes RM *et al.* Functional and autoradiographic evidence for endothelin 1 receptors on human and rat cardiac myocytes. Comparison with single smooth muscle cells. *Circ Res* 1990; 67: 764–9.
45. Rubanyi GM, Polokoff MA. Endothelins: molecular biology, biochemistry, pharmacology, physiology, and pathophysiology. *Pharmacol Rev* 1994; 46: 325–415.
46. Arai H, Hori S, Aramori I *et al.* Cloning and expression of a cDNA encoding an endothelin receptor. *Nature* 1990; 348: 730–2.
47. Sakin *et al.* 1990.
48. Hosoda K, Nakao K, Hiroshi A *et al.* Cloning and expression of human endothelin-1 receptor cDNA. *FEBS Lett* 1991; 287: 23–6.
49. Saito Y, Mizuno T, Itakura M *et al.* Primary structure of bovine endothelin $ET_B$ receptor and identification of signal peptidase and metal proteinase cleavage sites. *J Biol Chem* 1991; 266: 23 433–7.
50. Sakamoto A, Yanagisawa M, Sakurai T *et al.* Cloning and functional expression of human cDNA for the $ET_B$ endothelin receptor. *Biochem Biophys Res Commun* 1991; 178: 656–63.
51. Hokimoto S, Yasue H, Fujimoto K *et al.* Expression of angiotensin-converting enzyme in remaining viable myocytes of human ventricles after myocardial infarction. *Circulation* 1996; 94: 1513–18.
52. Shyamala V, Moulthrop TH, Stratton-Thomas J, Tekamp Olson P. Two distinct human endothelin B receptors generated by alternative splicing from a single gene. *Cell Mol Biol Res* 1994; 40: 285–96.
53. Elshourbagy NA, Adamou JE, Gagnon AW *et al.* Molecular characterization of a novel human endothelin receptor splice variant. *J Biol Chem* 1996; 271: 25 300–7.
54. Molenaar P, O'Reilly G, Sharkey A *et al.* Characterization and localization of endothelin receptor subtypes in the human atrioventricular conducting system and myocardium. *Circ Res* 1993; 72: 526–38.
55. Davenport AP, Kuc RE, Maguire JJ, Harland SP. ETA receptors predominate in the human vasculature and mediate constriction. *J Cardiovasc Pharmacol* 1995; 26 (Suppl 3): S265–7.
56. Ishikawa T, Yanagisawa M, Kimura S *et al.* Positive inotropic action of novel vasoconstrictor peptide endothelin on guinea pig atria. *Am J Physiol* 1988; 255: H970–3.
57. Baydoun AR, Peers SH, Cirino G, Woodward B. Effects of endothelin-1 on the rat isolated heart. *J Cardiovasc Pharmacol* 1989; 13 (Suppl 5): S193–6.
58. Firth JD, Roberts AF, Raine AE. Effect of endothelin on the function of the isolated perfused working rat heart. *Clin Sci (Colch)* 1990; 79: 221–6.
59. Davenport AP, Nunez DJ, Hall JA *et al.* Autoradiographical localization of binding sites for porcine $[^{125}I]$endothelin-1 in humans, pigs, and rats: functional relevance in humans. *J Cardiovasc Pharmacol* 1989; 13 (Suppl 5): S166–70.
60. Watanabe T, Kusumoto K, Kitayoshi T, Shimamoto N. Positive inotropic and vasoconstrictive effects of endothelin-1 in *in vivo* and *in vitro* experiments: characteristics and the role of L-type calcium channels. *J Cardiovasc Pharmacol* 1989; 13 (Suppl 5): S108–11.
61. Kelly RA, Eid H, Kramer BK *et al.* Endothelin enhances the contractile responsiveness of adult rat ventricular myocytes to calcium by a pertussis toxin-sensitive pathway. *J Clin Invest* 1990; 86: 1164–71.
62. Krämer BK, Smith TW, Kelly RA. Endothelin and increased contractility in adult rat ventricular myocytes. Role of intracellular alkalosis induced by activation of the protein kinase C-dependent $Na(^+)$-$H^+$ exchanger. *Circ Res* 1991; 68: 269–79.
63. Takigawa M, Sakurai T, Kasuya Y *et al.* Molecular identification of guanine-nucleotide-binding regulatory proteins which couple to endothelin receptors. *Eur J Biochem* 1995; 228: 102–8.
64. Sugden PH, Bogoyevitch MA. Endothelin-1-dependent signaling pathways in the myocardium. *Trends Cardiovasc Med* 1998; 6: 87–94.
65. Hilal-Dandan R, Merck DT, Lujan JP, Brunton LL. Coupling of the type A endothelin receptor to multiple responses in adult rat cardiac myocytes. *Mol Pharmacol* 1994; 45: 1183–90.
66. Hilal-Dandan R, Urasawa K, Brunton LL. Endothelin inhibits adenylate cyclase and stimulates phosphoinositide hydrolysis in adult cardiac myocytes. *J Biol Chem* 1992; 267: 10 620–4.
67. Vogelsang M, Broede-Sitz A, Schafer E *et al.* Endothelin $ET_A$-receptors couple to inositol phosphate formation and inhibition of adenylate cyclase in human right atrium. *J Cardiovasc Pharmacol* 1994; 23: 344–7.
68. Jones LG, Rozich JD, Tsutsui H, Cooper G. Endothelin stimulates multiple responses in isolated adult ventricular cardiac myocytes. *Am J Physiol* 1992; 263: H1447–54.
69. Pönicke K, Vogelsang M, Heinroth M *et al.* Endothelin receptors in the failing and nonfailing human heart. *Circulation* 1998; 97: 744–51.
70. Wu-Wong JR, Chiou WJ, Magnuson SR, Opgenorth TJ. Endothelin receptor in human astrocytoma U373MG cells: binding, dissociation, receptor internalization. *J Pharmacol Exp Ther* 1995; 274: 499–507.
71. Ozaki S, Ohwaki K, Ihara M *et al.* $ET_B$-mediated regulation of extracellular levels of endothelin-1 in cultured human endothelial cells. *Biochem Biophys Res Commun* 1995; 209: 483–9.
72. Fukuroda T, Fujikawa T, Ozaki S *et al.* Clearance of circulating endothelin-1 by $ET_B$ receptors in rats. *Biochem Biophys Res Commun* 1994; 199: 1461–5.
73. Dupuis J, Goresky CA, Fournier A. Pulmonary clearance of circulating endothelin-1 in dogs *in vivo*: exclusive role of $ET_B$ receptors. *J Appl Physiol* 1996; 81: 1510–15.
74. Sugden PH, Fuller SJ, Mynett JR *et al.* Stimulation of adult rat ventricular myocyte protein synthesis and phosphoinositide hydrolysis by the endothelins. *Biochim Biophys Acta* 1993; 1175: 327–32.
75. Suzuki T, Hoshi H, Mitsui Y. Endothelin stimulates hypertrophy and contractility of neonatal rat cardiac myocytes in a serum-free medium. *FEBS Lett* 1990; 268: 149–51.
76. Ito H, Hirata Y, Hiroe M *et al.* Endothelin-1 induces hypertrophy with enhanced expression of muscle-specific genes in cultured neonatal rat cardiomyocytes. *Circ Res* 1991; 69: 209–15.
77. Shubeita HE, McDonough PM, Harris AN *et al.* Endothelin induction of inositol phospholipid hydrolysis, sarcomere assembly, and cardiac gene expression in ventricular myocytes. A paracrine mechanism for myocardial cell hypertrophy. *J Biol Chem* 1990; 265: 20 555–62.

78. Ito H, Hirata Y, Adachi S *et al.* Endothelin-1 is an autocrine/paracrine factor in the mechanism of angiotensin II-induced hypertrophy in cultured rat cardiomyocytes. *J Clin Invest* 1993; 92: 398–403.
79. Kaddoura S, Firth JD, Boheler KR *et al.* Endothelin-1 is involved in norepinephrine-induced ventricular hypertrophy *in vivo*. Acute effects of bosentan, an orally active, mixed endothelin $ET_A$ and $ET_B$ receptor antagonist. *Circulation* 1996; 93: 2068–79.
80. Ishikawa T, Yanagisawa M, Kimura S *et al.* Positive chronotropic efffects of endothelin, a novel endothelium-derived vasoconstrictor peptide. *Pflugers Arch* 1988; 413: 108–10.
81. Toth M, Solti F, Merkely B *et al.* Ventricular tachycardias induced by intracoronary administration of endothelin-1 in dogs. *J Cardiovasc Pharmacol* 1995; 26 (Suppl 3): S153–5.
82. Ono K, Eto K, Sakamoto A *et al.* Negative chronotropic effect of endothelin 1 mediated through $ET_A$ receptors in guinea pig atria. *Circ Res* 1995; 76: 284–92.
83. Clozel M, Löffler BM, Breu V *et al.* Downregulation of endothelin receptors by autocrine production of endothelin-1. *Am J Physiol* 1993; 265: C188–92.
84. Hirata Y, Yoshimi H, Takaichi S *et al.* Binding and receptor down-regulation of a novel vasoconstrictor endothelin in cultured rat vascular smooth muscle cells. *FEBS Lett* 1988; 239: 13–17.
85. Freedman NJ, Ament AS, Oppermann M *et al.* Phosphorylation and desensitization of human endothelin A and B receptors. Evidence for G protein-coupled receptor kinase specificity. *J Biol Chem* 1997; 272: 17 734–43.
86. Chun M, Lin HY, Henis YI, Lodish HF. Endothelin-induced endocytosis of cell surface ETA receptors. Endothelin remains intact and bound to the $ET_A$ receptor. *J Biol Chem* 1995; 270: 10 855–60.
87. Carini DJ, Johnson AL, Mccall DE *et al.* Nonpeptide angiotensin II receptor antagonists. II. Pharmacology of S-8308. *Eur J Pharmacol* 1988; 157: 13–21.
88. Murphy TJ, Alexander RW, Griendling KK *et al.* Isolation of a cDNA encoding the vascular type-1 angiotensin II receptor. *Nature (Lond)* 1991; 351: 233–6.
89. Campanile CPJK, Crane MJ, Peach MJ, Garrison JC. The hepatic angiotensin II receptor, I. Characterization of the membrane-binding site and correlation with physiological responses in hepatocytes. *J Biol Chem* 1982; 257: 4951–8.
90. Peach MJ. Renin-angiotens in system: biochemistry and mechanism of action. *Physiol Rev* 1977; 57: 313–70.
91. Dzau VJH, Sasamura, Hein L. Heterogeneity of angiotensin synthetic pathways and receptor subtypes: physiological and pharmacological implications. *J Hypertens* 1993; 11 (Suppl 3): 13–18.
92. Duff JL, Marrero MM, Paxton WG *et al.* Angiotensin II signal transduction and the mitogen-activated protein kinase pathway. *Cardiovasc Res* 1995; 30: 511–17.
93. Marrero MB, Schieffer B, Paxton WG *et al.* The role of tyrosine phosphorylation in angiotensin II-mediated intracellular signalling. *Cardiovasc Res* 1995; 30: 530–6.
94. Murphy TJK, Takeuchi, Alexander RW. Molecular cloning of AT1 angiotensin receptors. *Am Hypertens* 1992; 5: 236–42.
95. Aguilera G, Catt K. Regulation of vascular angiotens in II receptors during altered sodium intake. *Circ Res* 1981; 49: 751–8.
96. Belluci A, Wilkes BM. Mechanism of sodium modulation of glomerular angiotens in receptors in the rat. *Circ Res* 1989; 49: 751–8.
97. Caponi AM, Aguilera G, Fakunding JL, Catt KJ. Angiotens in II: receptors and mechanisms of action. In: RL Soffer (ed.) *Biochemical regulation of blood pressure*. New York: John Wiley & Sons, 1981, 205–62.
98. Griendling KK, Minieri CA, Ollerenshaw JD, Alexander RW. Angiotensin II stimulates NADH and NADPH oxidase activity in cultured smooth muscle cells. *Circ Res* 1994; 74: 1141–8.
99. Griendling KK, Lassegue B, Murphy TJ, Alexander RW. Angiotensin II receptor pharmacology. *Adv Pharmacol* 1994; 28: 269–306.
100. Lassegue B, Alexander RW, Nickenig G *et al.* Angiotensin II down regulates the vascular smooth muscle AT1 receptor by transcriptional and posttranscriptional mechanisms: evidence for homologous and heterologous regulation. *Mol Pharmacol* 1995; 48: 601–9.
101. Nickenig G, Murphy TJ. Enhanced AT1 receptor mRNA degradation and induction of polyribosomal mRNA binding proteins by angiotensin II in vascular smooth muscle cells. *Mol Pharmacol* 1996; 50: 743–51.
102. Nickenig G, Murphy TJ. Down-regulation by growth factors of vascular smooth muscle angiotens in receptor gene expression. *Mol Pharmacol* 1994; 46: 653–9.
103. Nickenig G, Laufs U, Schnabel P *et al.* Down-regulation of aortic and cardiac AT1 receptor gene expression in TG (mREN2)27 rats. *Br J Pharmacol* 1997; 121: 134–40.
104. Nickenig G, Sachinidis A, Michaelsen F *et al.* Up-regulation of vascular angiotensin II receptor gene expression by low density lipoprotein in vascular smooth muscle cells. *Circulation* 1997; 95: 473–8.
105. Nickenig G, Jung O, Strehlow K *et al.* Hypercholesterolemia is associated with enhanced angiotensin AT1 receptor expression. *Am J Physiol* 1997; 272: H2701–7.
106. Sasaki K, Yamano Y, Bardhan S *et al.* Cloning and expression of a complementary DNA encoding a bovine adrenal angiotensin II type-1 receptor. *Nature (Lond)* 1991; 351: 230–2.
107. Mukoyama M, Nakajima M, Horiuchi M *et al.* Expression cloning of type 2 angiotensin II receptor of a unique class of seven membrane receptors. *J Biol Chem* 1992; 268: 24 539–42.
108. Ichiki T, Kambayashi Y, Inagami T. Transcription of the rat angiotensin II type 2 receptor gene. *Biochem Biophys Res Commun* 1996; 22: 566–71.
109. Nakajima M, Hutchinson HG, Fujinaga M *et al.* The angiotensin II type 2 (AT2) receptor anatgonizes the growth effects of the AT1 receptor: gain-of-function study using gene transfer. *Proc Natl Acad Sci USA* 1995; 92: 10 663–7.
110. Warnholtz A, Nickenig G, Schulz E *et al.* Increased NADH-oxidase-mediated superoxide production in the early stages of atherosclerosis. *Circulation* 1999; 99: 2027–2033.
111. Nio Y, Matsubara H, Murasawa S *et al.* Regulation of gene transcription of angiotensin II receptor subtypes in myocardial infarction. *J Clin Invest* 1995; 95: 46–54.
112. Stoll M, Steckelings UM, Paul M *et al.* The angiotensin AT2 receptor mediates inhibition of cell proliferation in coronary endothelial cells. *J Clin Invest* 1995; 95: 651–7.
113. Yamada T, Horiuchi M, Dzau VJ. Angiotensin II type 2 receptor mediates programmed cell death. *Proc Natl Acad Sci USA* 1996; 93: 150–60.
114. Packer M. Neurohormonal interactions and adaptations in congestive heart failure. *Circulation* 1988; 77: 721–30.

115. Dzau V, Colucci W, Hollenberg N, Williams G. Relation of renin–angiotensin–aldosterone system to clinical state in concestive heart failure. *Circulation* 1981; 63: 645–56.
116. Bayliss J, Norell M, Capena-Anson R *et al.* Untreated heart failure. Clinical and neuroendocrine effects of introducing diurestics. *Br Heart J* 1987; 57: 17–21.
117. Cohn JN. The sympathetic nervous system in heart failure. *J Cardiovasc Pharmacol* 1989; 14 (Suppl 5): 57–61.
118. Cohn JN, Levine TB, Olivari MT *et al.* Plasma norepinephrine as a guide to prognosis in patients with chronic congestive heart failure. *N Engl J Med* 1984; 311: 819–23.
119. Francis GS, Goldsmith SR, Ziesche SM, Cohn JN. Response of plasma norepinephrine and epinephrine to dynamic exercise in patients with congestive heart failure. *Am J Cardiol* 1982; 49: 1152–9.
120. Swedberg K, Viquerat C, Rouleau JL *et al.* Comparison of myocardial catecholamine balance in chronic congestive heart failure and in angina pectoris without failure. *Am J Cardiol* 1984; 54: 783–9.
121. Böhm M, La Rosée K, Schwinger RHG, Erdmann E. Evidence for reduction of norepinephrine uptake sites in the failing human heart. *J Am Coll Cardiol* 1995; 25: 146–53.
122. Rose CP, Burgess JH, Cousineau D. Tracer norepinephrine kinetics in coronary circulation of patients with heart failure secondary to chronic pressure and volume overload. *J Clin Invest* 1985; 76: 1740–7.
123. Rundqvist B, Elam M, Bergmann-Sverrisdottir Y *et al.* Increased cardiac adrenergic drive precedes generalized sympathetic activation in human heart failure. *Circulation* 1997; 95: 169–75.
124. Bristow MR, Ginsburg R, Minobe W *et al.* Decreased catecholamine sensitivity and β-adrenergic receptor density in failing human hearts. *N Engl J Med* 1982; 307: 205–11.
125. Brodde OE. $\beta_1$- and $\beta_2$-adrenoceptors in the human heart: properties, function, and alterations in chronic heart failure. *Pharmacol Rev* 1991; 43: 203–42.
126. Ungerer M, Böhm M, Elce JS *et al.* Altered expression of β-adrenergic receptor kinase and $\beta_1$-adrenergic receptors in the failing human heart. *Circulation* 1993; 87: 454–63.
127. Bristow MR, Minobe WA, Raynolds MV *et al.* Reduced $\beta_1$-receptor messenger RNA abundance in the failing human heart. *J Clin Invest* 1993; 92: 2737–45.
128. Böhm M, Reiger B, Schwinger RHG, Erdmann E. cAMP-concentrations, cAMP-dependent protein kinase activity and phospholamban in nonfailing and failing myocardium. *Cardiovasc Res* 1994; 28: 1713–19.
129. Böhm M. Alterations of β-adrenoceptor–G-protein-regulated adenylyl cyclase in heart failure. *Mol Cell Biochem* 1995; 147: 147–60.
130. Granneman JG, Lahners KN, Chaudhry A. Characterization of the human $\beta_3$-adrenoceptor receptor gene. *Mol Pharmacol* 1993; 44: 264–70.
131. Strosberg AD. Structure, function, and regulation of adrenoceptor receptors. *Protein Sci* 1993; 2: 1198–209.
132. Manara L, Bianchetti A. The phenylethanoaminotetralines: new selective agonists for atypical $\beta_3$-adrenoceptors. *Trends Pharmacol Sci* 1990; 11: 229–30.
133. Unverferth DV, Blanford M, Kates RE, Leier CV. Tolerance to dobutamine after a 72-hour continuous infusion. *Am J Med* 1980; 69: 262–6.
134. Feldman AM, Cates AE, Veazey WB *et al.* Increase in the 40,000 mol wt perussis toxin substrate (G-protein) in the failing human heart. 1988.
135. Schnabel P, Nohr T, Nickenig G *et al.* α-Adrenergic signal transduction in renin transgenic rats. *Hypertension* 30: 1356–61.
136. Insel PA, Ransnäs LA. G-proteins and cardiovascular disease. *Circulation* 1988; 78: 1511–13.
137. Eschenhagen T, Mende U, Nose M *et al.* Long term β-adrenoceptor-mediated upregulation of Giα- and Goα-mRNA levels and pertussis toxin sensitive G-proteins in rat heart. *Mol Pharmacol* 1992; 42: 773–83.
138. Feldman AM, Cates AE, Bristow MR, Van Dop C. Altered expression of the α-subunits of G-proteins in failing human hearts. *J Mol Cell Cardiol* 1989; 21: 359–65.
139. Morris SA, Tanowitz H, Wittner M, Bilezilian JP. Pathophysiological insights into the cardiomyopathy of Chagas' disease. *Circulation* 1990; 82: 1900–9.
140. Vatner DE, Vatner SF, Fujii AM, Homcy CJ. Loss of high affinity cardiac beta-adrenergic receptors in dogs with heart failure. *J Clin Invest* 1985; 76: 2259–64.
141. Longabaugh JP, Vatner DE, Vatner SF, Homcy CJ. Decreased stimulatory guanosine triphosphate binding protein in dogs with pressure overload left ventricular failure. *J Clin Invest* 1988; 81: 420–4.
142. Kessler PD, Cates AE, Van Dop C, Feldman AM. Decreased bioactivity of the guanine nucleotide-binding protein that stimulates adenylate cyclase in hearts from Cardiomyopathic Syrian hamsters. *J Clin Invest* 1989; 84: 244–52.
143. Neumann J, Scholz H, Döring V *et al.* Increase in myocardial Gi-proteins in heart failure. *Lancet* 1988; ii: 936–7.
144. Hershberger RE, Feldman AM, Bristow MR. A1-adenosine receptor inhibition of adenylate cyclase in failing and nonfailing human myocardium. *Circulation* 1991; 83: 1343–51.
145. Tanuma S, Kawashima K, Endo H. Eukaryotic mono (ADP) ribosyltransferase that ADP-ribosylates GTP-binding regulatory Giα protein. *J Biol Chem* 1988; 263: 5485–9.
146. Watanabe Y, Imaizumi T, Misaki N *et al.* Effects of phosphorylation of inhibitory GTP-binding protein by cyclic AMP-dependent protein kinase on its ADP-ribosylation by pertussis toxin, islet activating protein. *FEBS Lett* 1988; 236: 372–4.
147. Goldsmith P, Gierschik P, Milligan G *et al.* Antibodies directed against synthetic peptides distinguish between GTP-binding proteins in neutrophils and brain. *J Biol Chem* 1987; 262: 14 683–8.
148. Flesch M, Schwinger RHG, Schnabel P *et al.* Sarcoplasmatic reticulum $Ca^{2+}$ATPase and phospholamban mRNA and protein levels in end-stage heart failure due to ischemic or dilated cardiomyopathy. *J Mol Med* 1996; 74: 321–32.
149. Feldman AM, Jackson DG, Bristow MR *et al.* Immunodetectable levels of the inhibitory guanine nucleotide-binding regulatory proteins in failing human heart. *J Mol Cell Cardiol* 1991; 23: 439–52.
150. Böhm M, Moll M, Schmid B *et al.* α-Adrenergic neuroeffector mechanisms in cardiac hypertrophy of renin transgenic rats. *Hypertension* 1994; 24: 653–62.
151. Eschenhagen T, Mende U, Nose M *et al.* Increased messenger RNA level of the inhibitory G-protein α-subunit Giα-2 in human end-stage heart failure. *Circ Res* 1992; 70: 688–96.
152. Müller FU, Boheler KR, Eschenhagen T *et al.* Isoprenaline stimulates gene transcription of the inhibitory G-protein α-subunit Giα2 in rat heart. *Circ Res* 1993; 72: 696–700.

153. Brown LA, Harding SE. The effect of pertussis toxin on β-adrenoceptor responses in isolated cardiac myocytes from noradrenaline-treated guinea pigs and patients with heart failure. *Br J Pharmacol* 1992; 106: 115–22.
154. Böhm M, Kirchmayr R, Erdmann E. Myocardial Giα-protein levels in patients with hypertensive cardiac hypertrophy, ischemic heart disease and cardiogenic shock. *Cardiovasc Res* 1995; 30: 611–18.
155. Böhm M, Kirchmayr R, Gierschik P, Erdmann E. Increase of myocardial inhibitory G-proteins in catecholamine-refractory septic shock or in septic multiorgan failure. *Am J Med* 1995; 98: 183–6.
156. Holmer SR, Eschenhagen T, Nose M, Riegger GAJ. Expression of adenylyl cyclase and G-protein beta subunit in end-stage human heart failure. *J Cardiac Failure* 1996; 2: 279–83.
157. Ishikawa Y, Sorota S, Kiuchi K *et al.* Downregulation of adenylylcyclase types V and VI mRNA levels in pacing-induced heart failure in dogs. *J Clin Invest* 1994; 93: 2224–9.
158. Noguchi H, Muraoka R, Kigoshi S, Muramatsu I. Pharmacological characterization of α1-adrenoceptor subtypes in rat heart: a binding study. *Br J Pharmacol* 1995; 114: 1026–30.
159. Ivorra D, Gascon S, Vila E, Badia A. α-Adrenoceptor subtypes and inositol phosphates production in heart ventricles of spontaneously hypertensive rats. *J Cardiovasc Pharmacol* 1993; 21: 931–6.
160. Kawaguchi H, Sano H, Iizuka K *et al.* Phosphatidylinositol metabolism in hypertrophic rat heart. *Circ Res* 1993; 72: 966–72.
161. Böhm M, Mende U, Schmitz W, Scholz H. Increased sensitivity to α-adrenoceptor stimulation but intact muscarinergic and purinergic isoprenaline-antagonistic effect in prehypertensive cardiac hypertrophy of spontaneously hypertensive rats. *Naunyn-Schmiedeberg's Arch Pharmacol* 1986; 333: 284–9.
162. Kagiya T, Hori M, Iwakura K *et al.* Role of increased α1-adrenergic activity in cardiomyopathic syrian hamster. *Am J Physiol* 1991; 260: H80–8.
163. Steinfath M, Danielsen W, von der Leyen H *et al.* Reduced $\alpha_1$- and $\alpha_2$-adrenoceptor-mediated positive inotropic effects in human end-stage heart failure. *Br J Pharmacol*, 1992; 105: 463–9.
164. Bristow MR, Minobe W, Rasmussen R *et al.* $\alpha_1$-Adrenergic receptors in nonfailing and failing human heart. *J Pharmacol Exp Ther* 1988; 247: 1039–45.
165. Böhm M *et al.* 1988
166. Simpson PC. Norepinephrine-stimulated hypertrophy of cultured rat myocardial cells is an alpha 1 adrenergic response. *J Clin Invest* 1983; 72: 732–8.
167. Knowlton KU, Michel MC, Itani M *et al.* The α1A-adrenergic receptor subtype mediates biochemical, molecular, and morphologic features of cultured myocardial cell hypertrophy. *J Biol Chem* 1993; 268: 15 374–80.
168. Sadoshima JI, Izumo S. Molecular characterization of the angiotensin II-induced hypertrophy of cardiac myocytes and hyperplasia of cardiac fibroblasts. Critical role of the AT1 receptor subtype. *Circ Res* 1993; 73: 413–23.
169. Sadoshima JI, Izumo S. Signal transduction pathways of angiotensin II-induced c-fos gene expression in cardiac myocytes *in vivo*. Roles of phospholipid-derived second messengers. *Circ Res* 1993; 73: 424–38.
170. Goldstein DS, Kopin. The autonomic nervous system and catecholamines in normal blood pressure control and in hypertension. In: JH Laragh, BM Brenner (eds) *Hypertension pathophysiology: diagnosis and management*. New York: Raven Press, 1990, 711–47.
171. LaMorte VJ, Thorburn J, Absher D *et al.* Gq- and ras-dependent pathways mediate hypertrophy of neonatal rat ventricular myocytes following α1-adrenergic stimulation. *J Biol Chem* 1994; 2690: 811.
172. Yamazaki T, Komuro I, Yazaki Y. Molecular mechanism of cardiac cellular hypertrophy by mechanical stress. *J Mol Cell Cardiol* 1995; 27: 133–40.
173. von Harsdorf R, Lang RE, Fullerton M, Woodcock EA. Myocardial stretch stimulates phosphatidylinositol turnover. *Circ Res* 1989; 65: 494–501.
174. Sadoshima J, Izumo S. Mechanical stretch rapidly activates multiple signal transduction pathways in cardiac myocytes: potential involvement of an autocrine/paracrine mechanism. *EMBO J* 1993; 12: 1681–92.
175. McMurray JJ, Ray SG, Abdullah I *et al.* Plasma endothelin in chronic heart failure. *Circulation* 1992; 85: 1374–9.
176. Rodeheffer RJ, Lerman A, Heublein DM, Burnett JCJ. Increased plasma concentrations of endothelin in congestive heart failure in humans. *Mayo Clin Proc* 1992; 67: 719–24.
177. Hiroe M, Hirata Y, Fujita N *et al.* Plasma endothelin-1 levels in idiopathic dilated cardiomyopathy. *Am J Cardiol* 1991; 68: 1114–15.
178. Nakamura M, Arakawa N, Yoshida H *et al.* Increased plasma endothelin concentrations in patients with acute heart failure after myocardial infarction. *Jpn Circ J* 1993; 57: 371–8.
179. Cavero PG, Miller WL, Heublein DM *et al.* Endothelin in experimental congestive heart failure in the anesthetized dog. *Am J Physiol* 1990; 259: F312–17.
180. Margulies KB, Hildebrand FLJ, Lerman *et al.* Increased endothelin in experimental heart failure. *Circulation* 1990; 82: 2226–30.
181. Wei CM, Lerman A, Rodeheffer RJ *et al.* Endothelin in human congestive heart failure. *Circulation* 1994; 89: 1580–6.
182. Zolk O, Quattek J, Schrader T *et al.* Expression of endothelin receptors, endothelin-1 and endothelin converting enzyme in chronic human heart failure (Abstract). *Hospitalis* 1998; 68: 25S.
183. Fraccarollo D, Hu K, Galuppo P *et al.* Chronic endothelin receptor blockade attenuates progressive ventricular dilation and improves cardiac function in rats with myocardial infarction: possible involvement of myocardial endothelin system in ventricular remodeling. *Circulation* 1997; 96: 3963–73.
184. Kohzuki M, Kanazawa M, Yoshida *et al.* Cardiac angiotensin converting enzyme and endothelin receptor in rats with chronic myocardial infarction. *Jpn Circ J* 1996; 60: 972–80.
185. Miyauchi T, Sakai S, Ihara M *et al.* Increased endothelin-1 binding sites in the cardiac membranes in rats with chronic heart failure. *J Cardiovasc Pharmacol* 1995; 26 (Suppl 3): S448–51.
186. Arai M, Yoguchi A, Iso T *et al.* Endothelin-1 and its binding sites are upregulated in pressure overload cardiac hypertrophy. *Am J Physiol* 1995; 268: H2084–91.
187. Löffler BM, Roux S, Kalina B *et al.* Influence of congestive heart failure on endothelin levels and receptors in rabbits. *J Mol Cell Cardiol* 1993; 25: 407–16.
188. Thibault G, Arguin C, Garcia R. Cardiac endothelin-1 content and receptor subtype in spontaneously hypertensive rats. *J Mol Cell Cardiol* 1995; 27: 2327–36.
189. Brown LA, Nunez DJ, Brookes CI, Wilkins MR. Selective increase in endothelin-1 and endothelin A receptor subtype in the hypertrophied myocardium of the aorto-venacaval fistula rat. *Cardiovasc Res* 1995; 29: 768–74.

190. Pieske B, Beyermann B, Duis J *et al.* Endothelin-1 increases contractility in human dilated cardiomyopathy via an upregulated $ET_A$-receptor subtype (Abstract). *Circulation* 1996; 94 (Suppl 1): 1–406.
191. Sirvio ML, Uhlenius N, Stewen P, Metsarinne K, Fyhrquiest F. The effect of aortic coaractaion on expression of endothelin-1 and endothelin-receptors in the heart and lungs. *Blood Press* 1995; 4: 320–3.
192. Hayzer DJ, Cicila G, Cockerham C, Griendling KK, Delafontaine P, Ng SC, Runge MS. Endothelin A and B receptors are down-regulated in the heart of hypertensive rats. Am J Med Sci 1994; 307: 222–7.
193. Picard P, Smith PJ, Monge JC, Rouleau JL, Nguyen QT, Calderone A, Stewart DJ. Coordinated upregulation of the cardiac endothelin system in a rat model of cardiac failure. *J Cardiovasc Pharmacol* 1998; 31(Suppl. 1): 294–7.
194. Hasegawa K, Fujiwara H, Koshiji M *et al.* Endothelin-1 and its receptor in hypertrophic cardiomyopathy. *Hypertension* 1996; 27: 259–64.
195. Fareh J, Touyz RM, Schiffrin EL, Thibault G. Endothelin-1 and angiotensin II receptors in cells from rat hypertrophied heart. Receptor regulation and intracellular $Ca^{2+}$ modulation. *Circ Res* 1996; 78: 302–11.
196. Sakai S, Yorikane R, Miyauchi T *et al.* Altered production of endothelin-1 in the hypertrophied rat heart. *J Cardiovasc Pharmacol* 1995; 26 (Suppl 3): S452–5.
197. CONSENSUS Trial Study Group. Effects of enalapril on mortality in severe congestive heart failure: results of the Cooperative North Scandinavian Enalapril Survival Study (CONSENSUS). *N Engl J Med* 1987; 316: 1429–35.
198. Acute Infarction Ramipril Efficacy (AIRE) Study Investigators. Effect of ramipril on mortality and morbidity of survivors of acute myocardial infarction with clinical evidence of heart failure. *Lancet* 1993; 342: 812–28.
199. Hall AS, Murray GD, Ball SG, on behalf of the AIREX Study Investigators. Follow-up study of patients randomly allocated ramipril or placebo for heart failure after acute myocardial infarction: AIRE Extension (AIREX) study. *Lancet* 1997; 349: 1493–7.
200. SOLVD Investigator. Effect of enalapril on survival in patients with reduced leftventricular ejection fraction and congestive heart failure. *N Engl J Med* 1991; 325: 293–302.
201. Pitt B, Segal R, Martinez FA *et al.* Randomised trial of losartan versus captopril in patients over 65 with heart failure (Evaluation of Losartan in the Elderly Study, ELITE). *Lancet* 1997; 349: 747–52.
202. Timmermans PBMWM, Wong PC, Chiu AT *et al.* Angiotensin II receptors and angiotensin II receptor antagonists. *Pharmacol Rev* 1993; 45: 205–51.
203. Mullins JJ, Peters J, Ganten D. Fulminant hypertension in transgenic rats harbouring the mouse Ren-2 gene. *Nature* 1990; 3: 541–4.
204. Böhm M, Gierschik P, Knorr A *et al.* Role of altered G-protein expression in the regulation of spontaneously hypertensive cardiomyopathy. *J Hypertens* 1992; 10: 1115–28.
205. Suzuki J, Matsabura H, Urakami M, Inada M. Rat angiotensin II (type 1A) receptor mRNA regulation and subtype expression in myocardial growth and hypertrophy. *Circ Res* 1993; 73: 439–47.
206. Poole TD, Holder MS, Gipson D. Cardiac angiotensin II receptor populations during aortocaval fistulae, AII and β-adrenergic receptor blockade. *Biochem Biophys Res Commun* 1994; 203: 1865–74.
207. Mohabir R, Young SD, Strosberg AM. Role of angiotensin in pressure overload-induced hypertrophy in rats: effects of angiotensin-converting enzyme inhibitors, an AT1 receptor antagonist, and surgical reversal. *J Cardiovasc Pharmacol* 1994; 23: 291–9.
208. Regan CP, Anderson PG, Bishop SP, Berecek KH. Pressure-independent effects of AT1 receptor antagonism on cardiovascular remodeling in aortic-banded rats. *Am J Physiol* 1997; 272 (*Heart Circ Physiol*): H2131–8.
209. Weinberg EO, Lee MA, Weigner M *et al.* Angiotensin AT1 receptor inhibition. Effects on hypertrophic remodeling and ACE expression in rats with pressure-overload hypertrophy due to ascending aortic stenosis. *Circulation* 1997; 95: 1592–600.
210. Lopez JJ, Lorell BH, Ingelfinger JR *et al.* Distribution and function of cardiac angiotensin AT1- and AT2-receptor subtypes in hypertrophied rat hearts. *Am J Physiol* 1994; 267: H844–50.
211. Cheng CP, Suzuki M, Ohte N *et al.* Altered ventricular and myocyte response to angiotensin II in pacing-induced heart failure. *Circ Res* 1996; 78: 880–92.
212. Pfeffer MA, Braunwald E. Ventricular remodeling after myocardial infarction. Experimental observations and clinical implications. *Circulation* 1990; 81: 1161–72.
213. Rademaker MT, Fitzpatrick MA, Charles CJ *et al.* Central angiotensin II AT1 receptor antagonism in normal and heart-failed sheep. *Am J Physiol* 1995; 269: H425–32.
214. Spinale FG, Gasparo M, Whitebread S *et al.* Modulation of the renin angiotensin pathway through enzyme inhibition and specific receptor blockade in pacing-induced heart failure. *Circulation* 1997; 96: 2385–96.
215. Sladek T, Sladkova J, Kolar F *et al.* The effect of AT1 receptor antagonist on chronic cardiac response to coronary artery ligation in rats. *Cardiovasc Res* 1996; 31: 568–76.
216. Schieffer B, Wirger A, Meybrunn M *et al.* Comparative effects of chronic angiotensin-converting enzyme inhibition and angiotensin II type I receptor blockade on cardic remodelling after myocardial infarction in the rat. *Circulation* 1994; 89: 2273–82.
217. Liu YH, Yang XP, Sharov VG *et al.* Effects of angiotensin II Type 1 receptor antagonists in rats with heart failure. *J Clin Invest* 1997; 99: 1926–35.
218. Asano K, Dutcher DL, Port D *et al.* Selective downregulation of the angiotensin II AT1 receptor subtype 1 in failing human ventricular myocardium. *Circulation* 1997; 95: 1193–200.
219. Regitz-Zagrosek V, Friedel N, Heymann A *et al.* Regulation, chamber localization, and subtype distribution of angiotensin II receptors in human hearts. *Circulation* 1995; 91: 1461–71.

# Role of altered ion-channel expression in sudden death in heart failure

14

M. NÄBAUER, S. KÄÄB AND E. MARBAN

## Introduction

Electrical instability is a characteristic feature of the failing heart. Despite advances in the treatment of heart failure in recent years, annual mortality exceeds 10%, and 35–50% of those deaths are sudden, presumably due to ventricular tachyarrhythmias [1–3]. The mechanisms of the increased electrical instability of failing myocardium are not known. While in ischaemic heart disease, fibrosis and myocardial scarring may provide a substrate for re-entrant ventricular tachycardia, other mechanisms appear to be responsible for the propensity of failing myocardium to potentially fatal arrhythmias, such as abnormal intracellular and transmembrane $Ca^{2+}$ handling [4–7], stretch-induced changes due to altered ventricular loading conditions [8–10], and changes in myocyte electrical properties [8, 11–13].

A substantial amount of evidence indicates a crucial role for the altered expression of sarcolemmal ion channels in the electrically unstable failing myocardium, causing abnormalities in repolarization. Prolongation of the cardiac action potential is the most consistent finding in a wide variety of experimental models of cardiac hypertrophy and failure, and in terminal heart failure in humans. Recent data indicate that downregulation of potassium currents, particularly of the transient outward current, is a prominent feature, and contributes significantly to the increased lability of repolarization and electrical instability of the failing myocardium [13–17]. Clinically, these abnormalities may manifest as a spatial or temporal dispersion of repolarization, as observed in patients with heart failure and increased risk of sudden cardiac death [18–20]. Identification of the mechanisms involved in altered ion-channel expression and associated repolarization abnormalities might provide options to interfere with these potentially detrimental adaptive changes, and for the development of new strategies to prevent sudden cardiac death in heart failure.

## Ion channels controlling the cardiac action potential

Voltage-gated ion channels open in response to a change in membrane potential, permitting the transmembrane passage of specific ions according to inherent voltage- and time-dependent properties. Even though many more ion currents have been described in myocardial cells, most features of the cardiac action potential can be adequately reproduced by including the fast sodium current ($I_{Na}$) and the calcium current ($I_{Ca,L}$) as inward currents, the Na/Ca-exchange current, and four outward potassium currents ($I_{to1}$, $I_{Kr}$, $I_{Ks}$, $I_{K1}$) with different densities and kinetic properties (Fig. 14.1) [21–24]. Depolarization of the cardiac action potential is a robust 'all-or-none' process carried initially by a large $I_{Na}$ and continued by $I_{Ca,L}$. Repolarization is controlled by outward potassium currents, with $I_{to1}$ determining the voltage level of the early plateau, and $I_{Kr}$ and $I_{Ks}$ controlling terminal repolarization. In addition to potassium channels, chloride channels and currents generated by ion pumps and Na/Ca exchange influence the repolarization process. No significant differences in the macroscopic characteristics of the two major inward currents have been found in different species. In contrast, a large diversity of repolarizing outward potassium currents has been observed, with expression of different channels and densities in different species and myocardial regions (Figs. 14.2, 14.7) [21, 25–29]. Thus, depending on the species studied, different ion channels underlie the normal action potential and potentially contribute to the phenotypic prolongation of the action potential in cardiac hypertrophy or failure.

It is important to note that the plateau of the cardiac action potential is a phase of very low conductance [13, 30] where even small current changes can critically influence the balance between inward and outward currents, and markedly alter the time-course of repolarization. The late

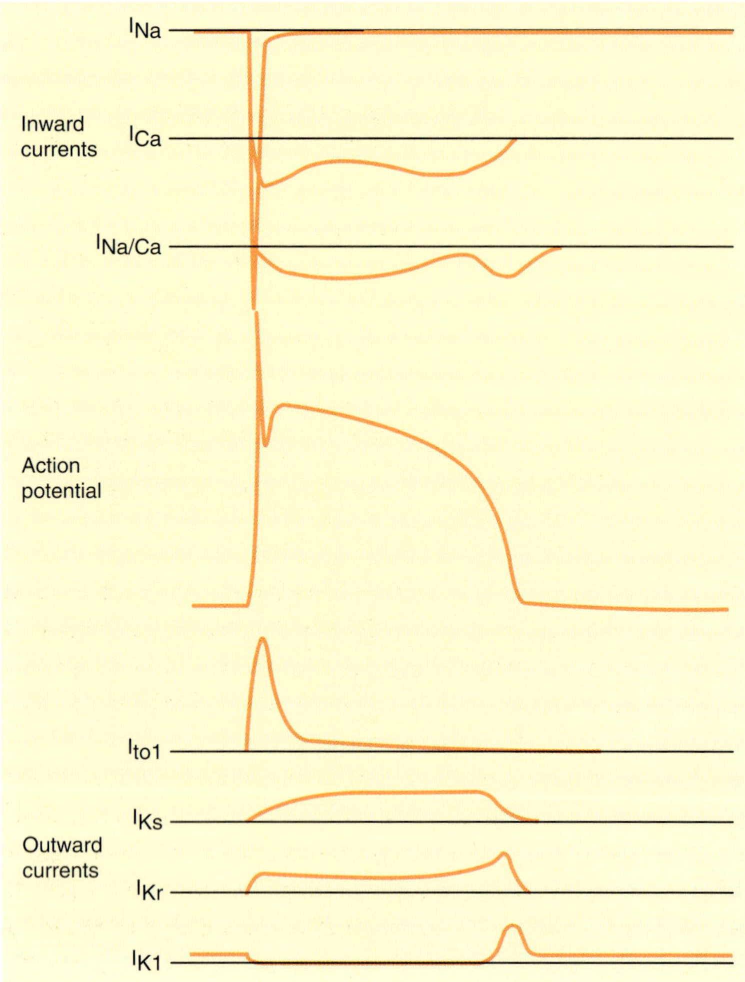


**Figure 14.1** *Ventricular action potential and time-dependent contribution of major inward currents ($I_{Na}$, $I_{Ca,L}$), Na/Ca-exchange current, and outward currents ($I_{to1}$, $I_{Ks}$, $I_{Kr}$, $I_{K1}$). Tracings are graphical representations of the time dependence of the contribution of various currents to the depolarization and repolarization process. The relative size of the currents is not correctly represented; downward deflections indicate the contribution of an inward current. The initial depolarization is induced by rapid activation of $I_{Na}$, followed by activation of the L-type Ca current. While $I_{to1}$ causes early repolarization of the action potential plateau leading to a notch in the action potential shape, activation of the delayed rectifier currents $I_{Kr}$ and $I_{Ks}$, together with a decrease in $I_{Ca,L}$, control final repolarization. The late phase of the final repolarization is further accomplished by current contributed by $I_{K1}$.*

repolarization phase is therefore a labile condition which is highly sensitive to alterations in the ionic environment (e.g. hypokalaemia), block of potassium channels by drugs, and alterations in ion-channel function or density by disease processes. Delay of the repolarization process may initiate arrhythmias by causing abnormal impulse generation due to early after depolarizations and triggered activity or, when spatial or temporal inhomogeneity of repolarization ensues, to abnormal impulse conduction which promotes reentrant arrhythmias. Alterations in various genes involved in myocardial repolarization (HERG, KvLQT1, minK, SCN5A) have recently been shown to underlie the propensity to ventricular tachyarrhythmias and sudden cardiac death in patients with the congenital form of the long-QT syndrome (Table 14.1) [13]. Similarly, disease processes or neurohumoral adaptations may lead to acquired alterations in channel density or function and cause abnormalities in repolarization, providing a substrate for arrhythmias.

Prolongation of the corrected QT (QTc) interval of the electrocardiogram, the clinical representation of action potential duration, has long been recognized to occur in cardiomyopathies [32]. More recent data consistently support this prolongation of the QTc interval in patients with hypertrophy or congestive heart failure [20, 33, 34]. Even though prolongation of action potential duration, if homogeneous, is not necessarily deleterious, the risk of generating arrhythmias can predominate when there is spatial or temporal inhomogeneity of repolarization.

Disease-induced abnormalities of repolarization in myopathic hearts are capable of disturbing the physiological electrical heterogeneity of the ventricular myocardium which underlies the normal transmural repolarization sequence in the myocardial wall. This heterogeneity involves at least the transient outward potassium current ($I_{to1}$) [28, 29, 35]. In addition, $I_{Ks}$ may be smaller in the central myocardium, possibly accompanied by a more

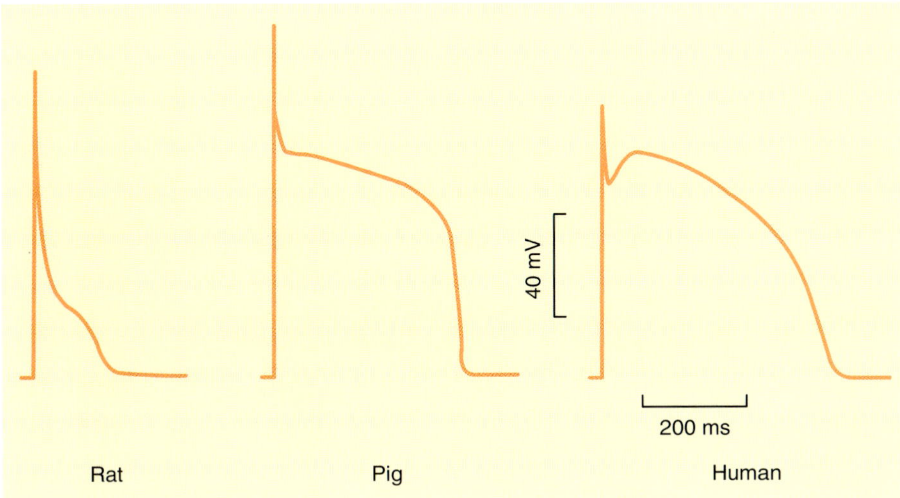


**Figure 14.2** *Species difference in configuration of the ventricular action potential in a rat ventricular myocyte, and a pig and human ventricular myocyte isolated from the epicardium. Rat ventricular myocardium, unlike most other species, does not exhibit an action potential plateau in the positive voltage range. Despite the similarity of human and pig ventricular action potentials, the underlying potassium currents are different in both species, with the transient outward current being absent in pig ventricle. Recordings are from isolated ventricular cells made at 35°C using the patch-clamp technique.*

prominent non-inactivating component of $I_{Na}$ [36]. Even if ion-channel expression were altered identically in all regions, the physiological heterogeneous distribution of ion channels across the wall would cause electrical properties to change differently in different regions. This is most evident in $I_{to1}$, which is large in central and subepicardial layers, but small in subendocardial layers (Fig. 14.7). In the subendocardium, it may even be encoded by a different gene with possibly different regulation [26, 28]. A differential regulation of $I_{to1}$ in subepicardial and subendocardial myocytes has recently been reported in the hypertrophied rat ventricle [37, 38]. Furthermore, regional cellular electrical properties may be affected differentially by hypertrophy [28, 37, 38] or by localized disease processes such as ischaemia, inhomogeneous mechanical load in ventricular remodelling, or variability of sympathetic innervation [39].

The action potential in hypertrophy begins to diverge from control soon after the maximum overshoot, which suggests that the currents responsible for the prolongation are operative very early in the plateau (Fig. 14.3) [15, 40, 41]. The major currents active during that time include $I_{Ca,L}$ and $I_{to1}$, even though other currents ($I_{Na}$, $I_{to2}$, $I_{Kr}$, $I_{Na/Ca}$, $I_{Ca,T}$) may also be involved. In principle, any increase

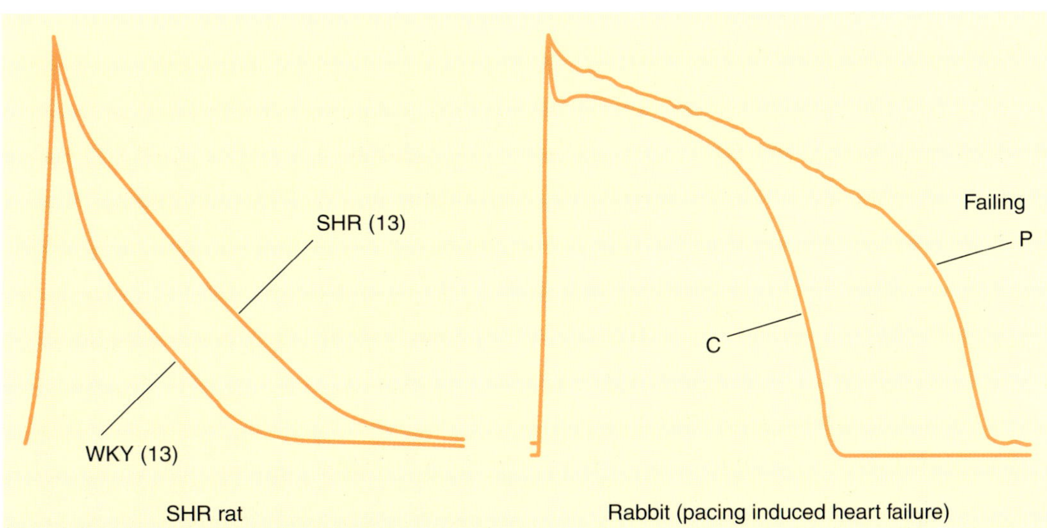


**Figure 14.3** *Early deviation of action potential configuration in rat hypertrophy, indicating that currents active during the early plateau are altered in ventricular hypertrophy and failure. Data are from rats with spontaneous hypertension [41]* (left) *and rabbits with pacing-induced heart failure [15].*

**Table 14.1** Ion currents affected in long-QT syndrome causing ventricular arrhythmias and sudden cardiac death

| | Chromosome | Gene | Current |
|---|---|---|---|
| LQT-1 | 11p15.5 | KvLQT1 | $I_{Ks}$ |
| LQT-2 | 7q35–36 | HERG | $I_{Kr}$ |
| LQT-3 | 3q21–24 | SCN5A | $I_{Na}$ |
| LQT-4 | 4q25–27 | ? | ? |
| LQT-5 | 21q22 | minK | $I_{Ks}$ |

**Table 14.2** Gene families expressing transient outward potassium currents

| Gene family | Gene | Type of current expressed |
|---|---|---|
| Shaker | Kv1.4 | Transient outward |
| Shab | Kv2 | Transient outward |
| Shaw | Kv3 | Transient outward |
| Shal | Kv4.2 | Transient outward |
| | Kv4.3 | Transient outward |

At least Kv1.4, Kv4.2, and Kv4.3 have been shown to be expressed in ventricular myocytes. Expression of Shab and Shaw-type potassium channels in ventricular myocardium has not yet been reported.

in inward or decrease in outward currents during the plateau phase of the action potential is capable of causing a prolongation of the cardiac action potential, while a simultaneous decrease in inward and outward currents generates a more labile plateau at lower conductance levels without necessarily affecting action potential duration.

The recent linkage of arrhythmias and sudden cardiac death in patients with congenital long-QT syndrome to potassium-channel gene defects (LQT-1, -2, -4, -5) (Table 14.1) [31, 32] demonstrated the arrhythmogenic potential of altered repolarization due to decreased outward potassium currents. The long-QT syndrome also shares polymorphic ventricular tachycardia (VT) as the characteristic arrhythmia (called torsade de pointes in long-QT syndrome), often triggered by short-long-short sequences [43, 44]. The crucial role of a reduction in potassium conductance for the

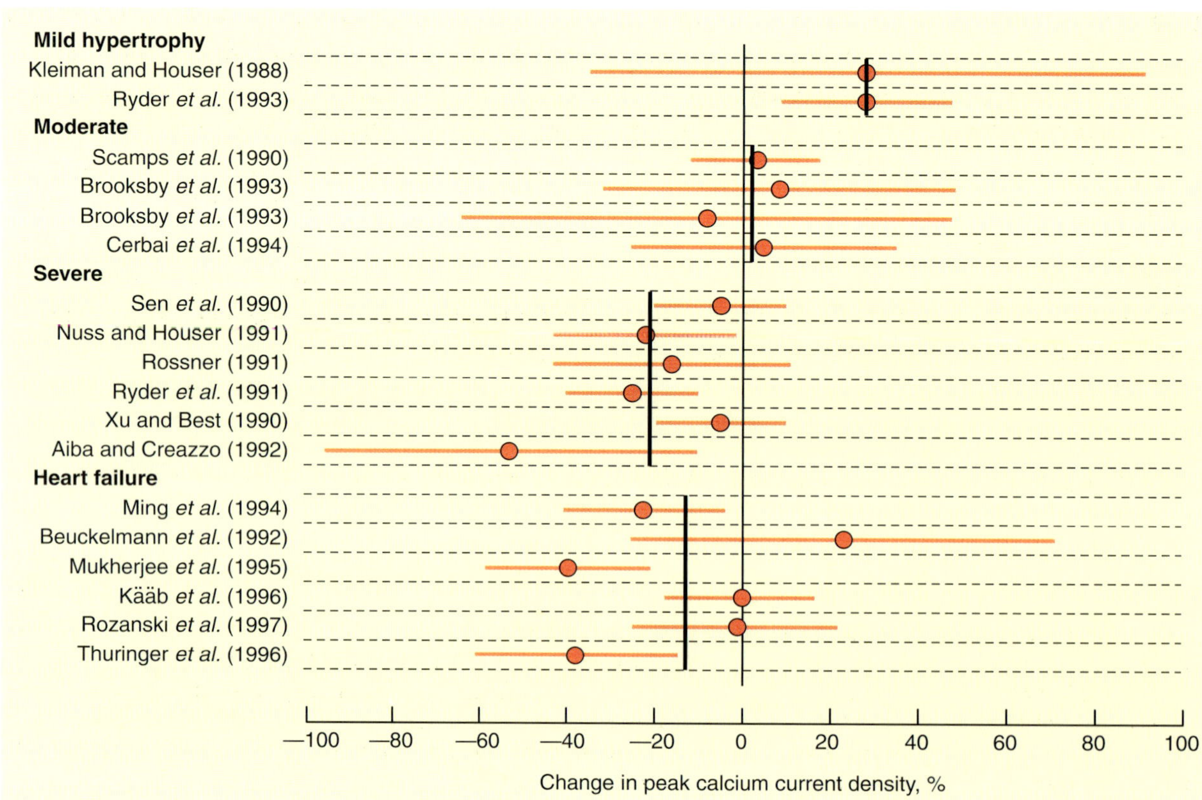


Figure 14.4

occurrence of polymorphic VT has been strengthened by numerical simulations which indicate that small decreases in potassium conductance can lead to destabilization of a spiral re-entry process, causing increased occurrence of polymorphic VT and ventricular fibrillation [45].

Two recent developments have set the stage for identification of the cellular changes underlying alterations in ion-channel expression in cardiomyopathies. The patch clamp technique and its application to isolated cardiac myocytes has enabled selective characterization of the various ion currents, demonstrating that the electrical abnormalities in cardiomyopathy are due to cellular alterations in ion-channel expression; simultaneously, progress in molecular biology allowed identification of the genes encoding cardiac sodium, calcium, and potassium channels [46–48], and heterologous expression of the channels with correlation of expressed ion-channel properties to native myocardial channels.

## Altered ion-channel expression in cardiomyopathies

Usually, some degree of hypertrophy is present during the development of heart failure, often due to pressure or volume overload. Moreover, the presence of compensatory hypertrophy in non-infarcted myocardium during ischaemic heart failure and in myocytes from hearts with dilated cardiomyopathy suggests similarities and overlap between electrophysiological changes in cardiac hypertrophy and failure [6, 8].

Conventional microelectrode studies first demonstrated alterations in repolarization in myopathic hearts. An increase in the action potential duration and voltage level of the early plateau was observed in cat hearts failing because of right ventricular pressure overload [49]. In the same model, prolongation of action potential duration was already evident during hypertrophy [50]. Similarly, action potential duration was prolonged in rat hearts with renovascular hypertension [51–53] and in chronically infarcted rat hearts with myocyte hypertrophy [54]. Prolongation of the action potential is the most consistent electrophysiological finding in myocardium and myocytes from myopathic hearts (Table 14.3). However, some reports indicated no change or even shortening of the action potential duration in hypertrophied myocardium [49, 60], suggesting that species differences or degree of hypertrophy may be of importance. Specifically, shortening of the action potential duration is usually observed in cardiomyopathy due to chronic doxorubicin application [40, 61, 62].

In the failing human ventricular myocardium, prolongation of the action potential has been reported in isolated cardiac preparations [4] as well as in isolated myocytes [5, 16]. Importantly, the prolongation of action potential duration in isolated myocytes was conserved under conditions in which intracellular $Ca^{2+}$ transients would have been suppressed, indicating that the changes in electrical properties exist independently of altered intracellular $Ca^{2+}$ handling in heart failure. Nevertheless, when considering studies in human tissue, it must be kept in mind that end-stage heart failure is a highly variable clinical entity with respect to aetiology, duration, clinical course, age of the patient, treatment, and the clinical condition at the time of transplantation, all of which may influence ion-channel expression.

**Table 14.3** Prolongation of action potential duration (APD) in experimental models of heart failure and terminal heart failure in humans

| Reference | Species | Model details | APD |
|---|---|---|---|
| Ryder *et al.* (1991) [55] | Guinea-pig | Thoracic aortic banding | =/↑ |
| Beuckelmann *et al.* (1992) [5] | Human | Terminal heart failure transplant ($[Ca]_i$-transient present) | ↑ |
| Beuckelmann *et al.* (1993) [16] | Human | Terminal heart failure transplant ($[Ca]_i$ buffered) | ↑ |
| Vermeulen *et al.* (1994) [56] | Rabbit | Pressure and volume overload | ↑ |
| Koumi *et al.* (1995) [57] | Human | Dilated CMP vs ischaemic CMP or valvular disease | ↑ |
| Kääb *et al.* (1996) [58] | Dog | Pacing-induced failure | ↑ |
| Thuringer *et al.* (1996) [59] | Hamster | Hereditary CMP | ↑ |
| Rozanski *et al.* (1997) [15] | Rabbit | Pacing-induced failure | ↑ |

CMP = cardiomyopathy.

## Inward currents

### *Sodium current*

Owing to the large size of the fast inward sodium current ($I_{Na}$), measurement of the whole-cell current under physiological conditions is prohibited and most studies rely on upstroke velocity of the action potential as an indirect parameter of sodium current density. Usually, no significant changes in maximum upstroke velocity are detected in hypertrophic myocardium, even though changes in both directions have been reported [24, 40, 63]. In failing myocardium, the peak current density of $I_{Na}$ was unchanged in pacing-induced heart failure in dog [58] and cardiomyopathic human ventricular myocardium [64], but altered sodium channels have also been suspected [65]. The kinetic properties of $I_{Na}$ have not yet been studied in detail, even though an increase in the inward sodium window current would clearly affect repolarization (similarly to the defect in congenital long QT-3 syndrome). Taken together, the available data do not indicate changes in $I_{Na}$ density relevant to repolarization in myopathic hearts.

### *Calcium current*

Because of its important role in cardiac excitation–contraction coupling, the L-type calcium current ($I_{Ca,L}$) has been studied more thoroughly than other currents in myocytes from hypertrophied and failing hearts. An increase in peak $I_{Ca,L}$ density or a slowing of its voltage- and calcium-dependent inactivation could be responsible for a prolongation of the cardiac action potential in cardiomyopathic hearts. A variety of models has been studied, including hypertrophied feline right ventricle [66], renal or spontaneous hypertension in rats [67, 68], congenital cardiomyopathy in hamsters [69, 70], aortic constriction in guinea-pigs [71, 72], and cardiomyopathic hearts in humans [73, 74]. Data from various models on peak $I_{Ca,L}$ are compiled in Figure 14.5. Even though changes in of $I_{Ca,L}$ are critical for repolarization, no studies adequately address potential alterations in the inactivation process in myopathic cells. Most studies report no difference in fast and slow time constants during inactivation of $I_{Ca,L}$, while some studies find one or both time constants to be prolonged in hypertrophy [40, 75]. Data in guinea-pigs with pressure overload indicate that a shift in activation and inactivation parameters could cause an increase in the L-type calcium window current, despite a decrease in unstimulated peak $I_{Ca,L}$, which might offset the decrease in $I_{Ca,L}$ with respect to the late repolarizing phase of the action potential [55]. Others report no change in the steady-state

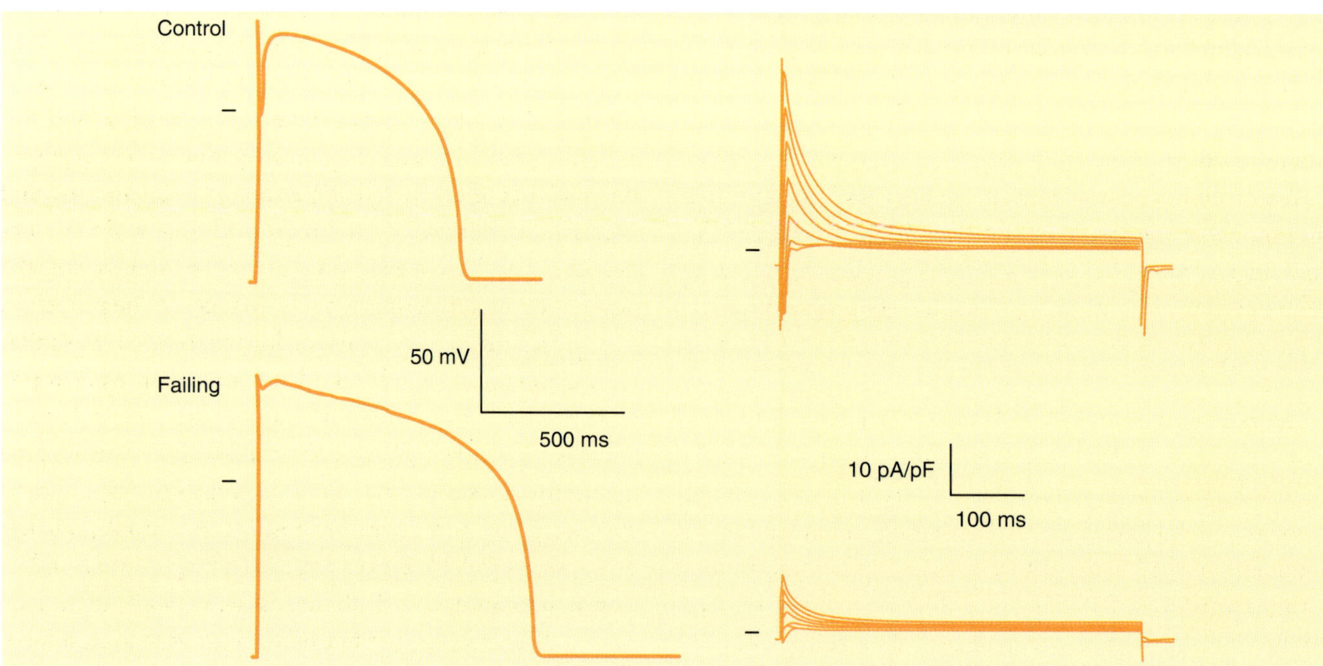


**Figure 14.5** *Prolongation of action potential duration in dogs with pacing-induced heart failure. The figure shows action potentials (left) recorded in myocytes isolated from central regions of the non-failing (upper panel) and failing (lower panel) canine left ventricular myocardium. The density of $I_{to1}$ is illustrated, indicating a marked decrease in $I_{to1}$ in isolated myocytes from failing hearts, corresponding to the smaller notch during early repolarization of the action potential. Short bars indicate zero voltage and current level. (Adapted from ref. 58.)*

inactivation variable, and activation was unchanged or slightly shifted to more positive potentials, suggesting that the calcium window current was not increased in hypertrophy [40]. Clarification of the influence of a late L-type calcium current on repolarization is hampered by the complex interaction of $Ca^{2+}$-channel inactivation with $Ca^{2+}$ release from the sarcoplasmic reticulum and the intracellular $Ca^{2+}$ level, both of which appear to be altered in heart failure [5, 76, 77].

Available data indicate that in most models studied, the prolongation of the action potential cannot be adequately explained by alterations in $I_{Ca,L}$. When unstimulated peak $Ca^{2+}$ is used to assess changes in $I_{Ca,L}$ density in myopathic hearts, an increase in L-type $Ca^{2+}$ current suitable to explain prolonged action potentials in severe hypertrophy or heart failure is not observed. Rather, even though $I_{Ca,L}$ may be slightly increased in mild hypertrophy, it appears unchanged in moderate degrees of hypertrophy, and reduced in severe hypertrophy or in heart failure (Fig. 14.5; see also ref. 40). In addition, as a result of desensitization of the β-receptor/adenylate-cyclase system, peak $I_{Ca,L}$ in response to β-adrenoceptor stimulation is consistently found to be reduced in myopathic cells [78, 79].

Nevertheless, some data indicate that $Ca^{2+}$-channel composition is altered in cardiomyopathy. In hypertrophic rat heart and myocardium from terminally failing human hearts, alternatively spliced isoforms of the pore-forming α-subunit have been observed [80–82], while in hypertrophied infarcted rat heart, re-expression of foetal $Ca^{2+}$-channel isoforms were reported [83]. β-Subunit expression was significantly decreased in the denervated transplanted human heart, while α-subunit levels appeared to be unchanged [84]. Therefore, changes at a functional level may occur. At present, the significance of these findings for macroscopic current density or properties of $I_{Ca,L}$ is not known.

Apart from the L-type $Ca^{2+}$ current, a T-type $Ca^{2+}$ current has been reported to be present in adult ventricular myocardium of some species [85, 86]. In myocytes isolated from adult feline left ventricles with longstanding pressure overload-induced hypertrophy [87] and in hereditary cardiomyopathy in the Syrian hamster [88], expression of T-type $Ca^{2+}$ current has been observed, which might also increase the early plateau voltage. However, no evidence for a contribution of T-type $Ca^{2+}$ current to transmembrane $Ca^{2+}$ influx was found in myocytes isolated from failing human ventricular myocardium [78], indicating that expression of $I_{Ca,T}$ may not be important in the failing human ventricle.

## Outward potassium currents

### *Transient outward current*

*Hypertrophy.* The $Ca^{2+}$-independent transient outward potassium current, $I_{to1}$, is a large current present in the ventricular myocardium of most species (notable exceptions being the guinea-pig and pig) [89]. Despite the kinetic similarity of the macroscopic current in various species, the genetic basis of this current appears to differ among species (Table 14.2). While the kinetics of rapid inactivation of $I_{to1}$ (time constant of decay ~8 ms at physiological temperatures in human myocardium [28]) make it unlikely that this current contributes directly to the final phase of repolarization, $I_{to1}$ is nevertheless very important during early repolarization at the initial level of the plateau, affecting the activation of all other plateau currents and, by this means, the duration of the action potential [58]. In species expressing a significant $I_{to1}$ (rat, ferret, hamster, rabbit, dog, cat, and humans), a decrease in this current may contribute to early deviation of the action potential configuration and prolongation of the action potential.

Various models of pressure overload hypertrophy have been used to delineate the role of $I_{to1}$ in the prolongation of the duration of the action potential. In hypertrophied myocardium from spontaneously hypertensive rats, prolongation of the action potential duration was reported in tissue [90] and in single isolated myocytes [41], which correlated to the decrease in $I_{to1}$. Prolongation of action potential and decrease in $I_{to1}$ depended on the degree and duration of hypertrophy and increased from a 37% reduction at 3 months to a 48% reduction at 18 months after the development of hypertension. No changes in the properties of $I_{to1}$, late outward current, or $I_{K1}$ were noted. A similar reduction was observed when left ventricular hypertrophy was induced by abdominal aortic ligation, where a decrease in $I_{to1}$ by 35% was observed without any change in current properties [91], or was accompanied by a shift of current activation to more positive potentials, further decreasing available current at a specific potential [37].

When pharmacological means were used to induce cardiac hypertrophy in rats treated with growth hormone, a decrease in $I_{to1}$ by 37.7% was found [92]. In rats treated with deoxycorticosterone acetate (DOCA) salt, $I_{to1}$ density was reduced depending on the severity of hypertrophy, by 53% in moderately hypertrophic and 94% in severely hypertrophic hearts, with no changes in sustained outward currents or $Ca^{2+}$-handling systems [93, 94]. Catecholamine-stimulated cardiac hypertrophy in rats also resulted in a 50% reduction in $I_{to1}$ with no change in voltage dependence or kinetic properties [95].

Similar reductions in $I_{to1}$ during hypertrophy were observed in other species. In ferrets with pulmonary artery banding, $I_{to1}$ decreased by approximately 35% [96], activation and inactivation parameters were not altered, and recovery from inactivation was found to be slowed, further reducing the available current at physiological frequencies [96]. $I_{Ca}$ was unchanged in this model [97].

Notable exceptions to this almost uniform reduction in $I_{to1}$ in cardiac hypertrophy were reported [98], while $I_{Ca,L}$ and outward currents were unchanged in spontaneously hypertensive rats despite prolongation of the action potential duration. In a one-clip/two-kidney model of renovascular hypertension, action potential duration was prolonged, but the transient component of the outward current was increased by approximately 35% [99]. Action potential prolongation was suggested to be due to increased $I_{Ca,L}$ in this model [67, 99]. This indicates that the same phenotype of a prolonged action potential in hypertrophy may be due to diverse changes in ionic channels. An increase in $I_{to1}$ was observed in myocytes from hypertrophied feline right ventricles after pulmonary artery banding [100], without changes in channel kinetics. The reason for an unchanged or increased $I_{to1}$ in cardiac hypertrophy is unknown, but may be related to the different species and models used, or the degree and time-course of development of the hypertrophy.

*Heart failure.* Evidence for the downregulation of cardiac potassium currents in heart failure has been derived from studies of a hereditary cardiomyopathy of the Syrian hamster [101], rabbit and dog models of pacing-induced heart failure [14, 15, 58], and terminally failing human myocardium at the time of cardiac transplantation [16, 102]. Common to these conditions is a prolongation of action potential duration, similar to that found in most models of pressure overload cardiac hypertrophy.

In hereditary cardiomyopathy of the Syrian hamster, several electrophysiological alterations have been reported, including a decrease in $I_{Ca,L}$ by 37% [59], an increase in $I_{Ca,L}$ and the Na/Ca-exchange current [88, 103], and alterations in sarcoplasmic reticulum calcium handling [69]. Prolongation of action potential duration has been observed in multicellular preparations [59, 104] and isolated myocytes, indicating that the intrinsic properties of the cells were altered. Deviation of the configuration of the action potential in failing myocardium and myocytes from control traces was evident immediately after the upstroke and in the voltage range above 0 mV, where the Na/Ca-exchange current is unlikely to play a major role. Analysis of $I_{to1}$ revealed a dramatic decrease of 70.6% which was considered to be responsible for the prolongation of the action potential duration [59].

Two models of heart failure induced by rapid ventricular pacing have recently been implemented and analysed, both displaying a significant prolongation of action potential duration together with a dramatic decrease in $I_{to1}$ [15, 58]. In the dog model, heart failure was induced by rapid ventricular pacing at a frequency of 240 beats/min for 3–4 weeks, when animals develop clinical signs of cardiac failure [58]. These hearts were considered to be in terminal failure when analysed and showed an increased left ventricular end-diastolic pressure, depressed $dP/dt_{max}$, and delayed relaxation time. The QT interval, the surface manifestation of action potential duration, and the monophasic action potential duration were increased in failing hearts, as was dispersion of repolarization determined by recordings of the monophasic action potential. Importantly, these animals showed a propensity to die from sudden cardiac death [14]. When measured in single isolated cells, action potential prolongation was preserved (and possibly accentuated) when intracellular calcium transients were reduced or eliminated, showing that these alterations exist independently of intracellular $Ca^{2+}$-handling processes. Analysis of inward currents revealed $I_{Na}$ and unstimulated peak $I_{Ca,L}$ to be unchanged, suggesting that these currents were not responsible for the prolonged duration of the action potential. A substantial reduction in $I_{to1}$ density by 65.5% was found in myocytes from failing hearts without differences in kinetics or voltage dependence (Fig. 14.6). Using single channel conductance measurements and non-stationary fluctuation analysis, the reduction in $I_{to1}$ density could be attributed to a reduction in the number of functional channels. The observed changes in the action potential of failing myocytes could be reproduced by blocking $I_{to1}$ with 4-aminopyridine in myocytes from non-failing hearts, and reversed by introducing an $I_{to1}$-like repolarizing current pulse during the early plateau of the action potential in cells from failing myocardium (Fig. 14.7) [58]. This indicates

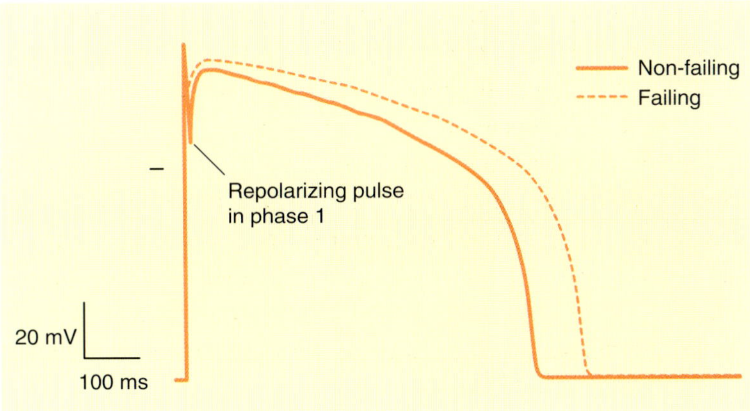


**Figure 14.6** *Relevance of $I_{to1}$ current density for late repolarization: application of a repolarizing current pulse immediately after the upstroke caused the action potential to shorten in a myocyte from the failing dog ventricle. [58]. Owing to the rapid inactivation of $I_{to1}$, this effect on action potential duration is expected to be mediated by the influence of $I_{to1}$ on the activation of other ion currents during the early plateau. (Adapted from ref. 58.)*

that $I_{to1}$, despite its transient nature, can influence the overall shape and duration of the ventricular action potential.

In rabbits with pacing-induced heart failure, similar changes in $I_{to1}$ were reported [15]. After 2–3 weeks of rapid ventricular pacing, animals were considered to be in an early stage of heart failure. Analysis of ion currents found $I_{Ca,L}$ and $I_{K1}$ to be unchanged, while $I_{to1}$ was reduced by 65%. The reduction in $I_{to1}$ was considered to account at least partly for the changes in action potential duration observed in this model.

In human ventricular myocytes isolated from failing and non-failing myocardium obtained at the time of transplantation, $I_{to1}$ was found to be markedly decreased, by 37%, in central myocardial layers from failing hearts. Evaluation of regional differences of $I_{to1}$ also demonstrated a decrease of 26% in epicardial myocytes from failing hearts but no difference in the subendocardial layer [28] (Fig. 14.3). In subendocardial layers of the human left ventricle, $I_{to1}$ exhibits different electrophysiological properties (a more negative steady-state inactivation parameter and an approximately 70-fold slower recovery from inactivation [28]), suggesting that a different channel is carrying the transient outward current in the subendocardium. Other studies, however, reported a decrease in $I_{to1}$ of 47% in the subendocardium but not in the subepicardium of the human left ventricle [102].

If generalizations can be made from these observations, $I_{to1}$ is significantly reduced in hypertrophied and failing

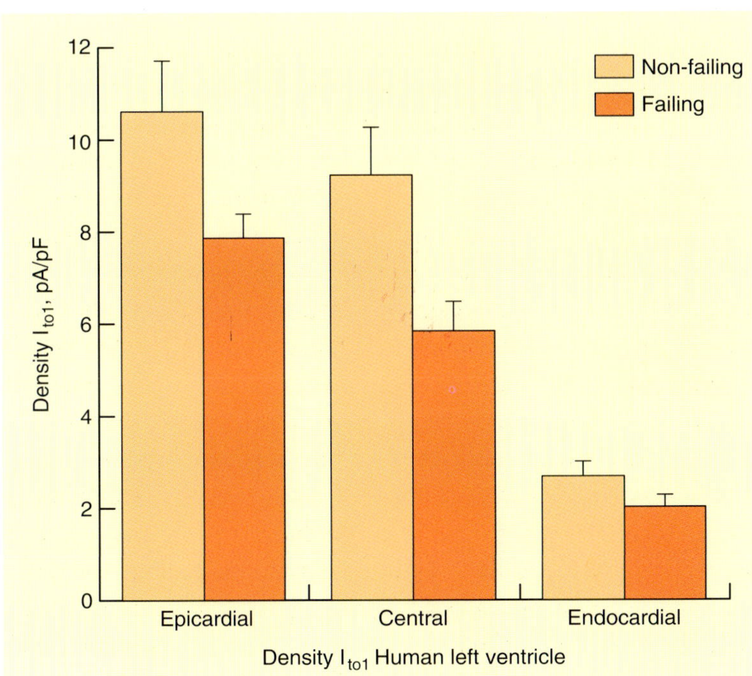


**Figure 14.7** *Current density of $I_{to1}$ in myocytes isolated from subepicardial, central and subendocardial layers of non-failing and failing (black) human left ventricle. There was a significant reduction in current density of $I_{to1}$ in the subepicardial and central layers. On the endocardial side, no significant difference in transient outward current density was observed, and the transmural gradient in $I_{to1}$ was altered compared with the myocardial wall of the non-failing myocardium. (Compiled from refs. 16 and 28.)*

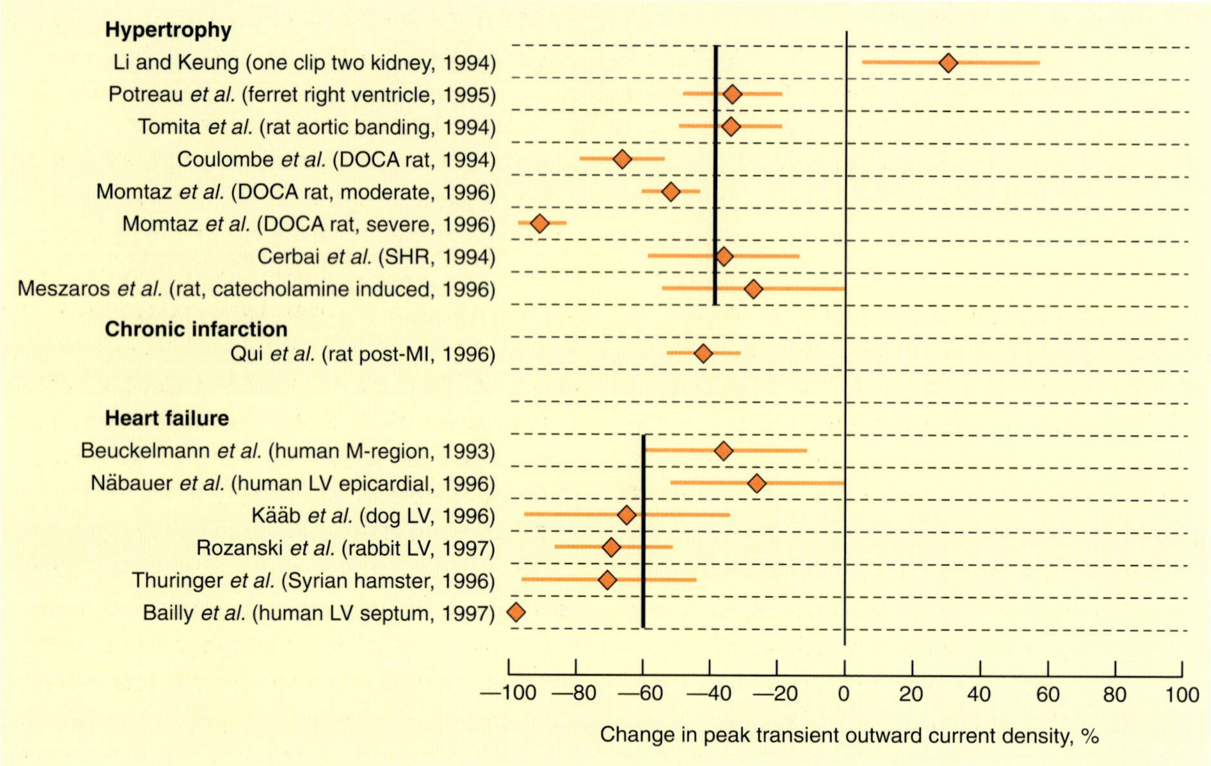


**Figure 14.8** *Reduction in $I_{to1}$ in myocytes from hypertrophic or failing hearts. Bars denote 95% confidence intervals. Bars not crossing the zero line indicate significant differences between groups; thick vertical bars indicate group means.*

myocardium, and the reduction appears to be related to the degree of hypertrophy, with a greater reduction in more severe stages and in heart failure. The average reduction in $I_{to1}$ in myocytes from hypertrophic myocardium was 40.0 ± 12.4%, and 61.5 ± 10.5% (mean ± SD) in myocytes from failing myocardium (Fig. 14.8).

### *Inward rectifier current*

Only a few observations on changes in the inward rectifier current, $I_{K1}$, are available in myopathic hearts. In mildly hypertrophied feline right ventricular myocytes after pulmonary artery banding, the magnitude of $I_{K1}$ was found to be increased [105]. In contrast, in rats with spontaneous hypertension [41] and guinea-pigs with mild hypertrophy due to abdominal aortic constriction [71], no changes in $I_{K1}$ density were observed. In myocytes isolated from failing human hearts, a small reduction in $I_{K1}$ was observed compared with cells from non-failing hearts; however, the difference was significant only at voltages negative to the potassium reversal potential, a voltage range that does not contribute to final repolarization [16]. Similarly, in dogs with heart failure due to rapid ventricular pacing, $I_{K1}$ was found to be reduced slightly, but significantly, mostly at voltages more negative than –90 mV [58]. In the voltage range relevant to repolarization (positive to the potassium reversal potential), a significant difference from control was observed only at –60 mV, indicating that a reduced $I_{K1}$ may be involved in slowing the terminal repolarization in heart failure. In a rabbit model of pacing-induced heart failure, $I_{K1}$ current density was not different in myocytes isolated from failing and non-failing myocardium [15].

Koumi *et al.* [57, 106] studied alterations in whole-cell current density and single-channel properties in isolated myocytes from human hearts with a variety of diseases. $I_{K1}$ density was lower in cells from hearts with dilated cardiomyopathy than in those with ischaemic cardiomyopathy [57]. Another study from the same group, however, could not verify significant differences in basal $I_{K1}$ density [106].

The available data do not support the generalization that $I_{K1}$ is significantly altered in myopathic hearts. However, a tendency towards a lower current density in heart failure has been observed in several studies.

### *Delayed rectifier potassium currents*

Data on altered expression of delayed rectifier-type currents ($I_K$) in cardiac hypertrophy are limited, and there is no study available discriminating the two components of this current, $I_{Ks}$ and $I_{Kr}$, as described recently [21]. This is of special importance as the relative contribution of the two channels to repolarization may vary in different species, with $I_{Kr}$ appearing to be more prominent in cat [107] and rabbit [108] than guinea-pig [21]. In addition, the various component genes are located on different chromosomes and expression would be expected to be selectively regulated. Both types of delayed rectifier current can be detected in human ventricular myocytes and are of functional importance, as evident in the long-QT syndromes 1 and 2.

In isolated myocytes from cats with right ventricular hypertrophy due to pulmonary artery banding, $I_K$ was found to be reduced in hypertrophied cells, which was accompanied by slower activation, more rapid deactivation, and steeper rectification properties [105, 109]. Together with an increase in $I_{Ca,L}$, this was considered to be responsible for the prolongation of the action potential duration. In feline left ventricular hypertrophy due to abdominal aortic constriction, the density of $I_K$ was also found to be reduced, by approximately 31% (Fig. 14.4) [110], with delayed activation and faster deactivation kinetics. The decreased delayed rectifier current was considered to be involved in the prolongation of the action potential duration and a propensity to early after-depolarization during reperfusions in hypertrophied cells [111].

Data in guinea-pigs with mild hypertrophy due to abdominal aortic constriction indicated no changes in the density of $I_K$ [71], and the prolongation of the action potential duration was attributed to an increased $I_{Ca,L}$ and Na/Ca-exchange current. Similarly, in hearts from spontaneously hypertensive rats, Brooksby *et al.* found no evidence for altered delayed rectifier currents measured at the end of a 500 ms depolarizing pulse [98].

Presently, no definitive data on the regulation of any of the delayed rectifier channels at a molecular level are available, but some preliminary data suggest a reduction in mRNA levels of HERG (the gene encoding the pore-forming unit of $I_{Kr}$) in failing compared with non-failing human hearts [112, 113]. Nevertheless, given the generally poor correlation between steady-state mRNA levels and the final product, further studies at the functional and protein levels are required.

## Mechanisms of altered ion-channel expression in cardiomyopathy

Knowledge of the signalling pathways involved in cardiac adaptation processes, specifically the regulation of ion-channel expression in cardiac hypertrophy and failure, is of considerable interest since it may provide targets for therapeutic intervention aimed at blocking or correcting potentially detrimental changes. Even though involvement of several mechanisms has been demonstrated, present understanding is limited. Adaptive changes may be initiated by pathways intrinsic to the myocytes, such as mechanical stress or electrical activity, or occur in response to paracrine or neurohumoral signals [114, 115].

While short-term adjustment of cardiac output is achieved by heart rate, preload (Frank–Starling mechanism), and β-adrenergic stimulation, chronic cardiac overload in myocardial hypertrophy has been recognized to alter cardiac gene expression, with changes at a cellular and molecular level. Alterations in gene expression similar to those in hypertrophy are often observed in heart failure, not all of which are beneficial [114–116]. Even though altered gene expression in biological adaptation is considered to be compensatory, some of these changes may turn out to be maladaptive and detrimental [114]. Cardiac failure indicates the limits of the process of compensation and adaptation.

One of the main cellular features of the adaptation process in cardiomyopathy is the slowing of the kinetics of contraction, presumably driven by improved contractile economy [117–119]. A second important feature of heart failure is a depressed sarcoplasmic reticulum Ca-ATPase function, and increased transsarcolemmal $Ca^{2+}$ cycling appears to be required for compensation [5, 103, 117, 120, 121]. Both a prolonged time-course of the mechanical cycle and an increased transsarcolemmal $Ca^{2+}$ transport are facilitated by action potential prolongation, so that delayed repolarization by potassium channel downregulation is a useful adaptive change in cardiac hypertrophy and failure.

Adaptive changes may be effected by several signalling systems known to be activated in cardiac hypertrophy and failure, such as cAMP- [122] and protein kinase C-dependent pathways [123, 124] or elevation of intracellular calcium [123], all of which have been demonstrated to regulate ion-channel expression in myocardial cells. With respect to the calcium channel, β-adrenergic transmembrane signalling increased DHP receptor mRNA and a number of functional calcium channels, while α-adrenergic signalling had a reciprocal effect [125]. Contact with sympathetic neurons also increased expression of $I_{Ca,L}$ [126], while activation of protein kinase C was found to reduce calcium and potassium channel ($I_{to1}$) gene expression [127]. However, despite the induction of altered calcium channel expression in isolated cell systems, changes in macroscopic peak $I_{Ca,L}$ in hypertrophic or failing myocardium were, on average, found to be small or absent (Fig. 14.5). This contrasts with the marked changes in potassium-channel currents, specifically the downregulation of the transient outward current by 40–70% in myopathic hearts.

Potassium-channel expression has been shown to be affected by chronic membrane depolarization, which causes a significantly reduced density of the transient outward current ($I_{to1}$) without affecting channel kinetics and voltage dependence; in contrast, $I_{Kr}$ and $I_{Ks}$ were enhanced by depolarization [128]. Another study found Kv1.5 mRNA (the gene encoding $I_{Kur}$, a delayed rectifier type current) expression to be enhanced by chronic membrane depolarization in atrial myocytes [122]. However, in spontaneously beating neonatal rat myocytes, membrane depolarization with potassium chloride, or stimulation with a calcium-channel activator or phorbol ester, resulted in a substantial increase in Kv1.4 mRNA (encoding a transient outward current), while Kv1.5 mRNA was depressed [123].

Outward potassium-channel density has been shown to be strongly affected by the state of the thyroid gland. Earlier studies described marked decreases and increases in $I_{to1}$ in hypothyroid and hyperthyroid animals, respectively [129, 130]. Recent preliminary data indicate that other potassium currents are similarly affected by thyroid hormone: a pronounced decrease in KvLQT1 mRNA expression and a corresponding decrease in $I_{Ks}$ were observed in hypothyroid guinea-pigs [131]. Whether these findings are relevant to myopathic hearts is presently unknown. The renin–angiotensin system, which is known to play a key role in cardiac adaptation, also appears to be involved in the regulation of potassium-channel properties, specifically $I_{to1}$ [132, 133].

Resolving the pathways of regulation of the transient outward current is complicated by the fact that more than one gene appears to encode currents with similar macroscopic appearance. At least three potassium-channel genes encoding transient outward currents (Kv1.4, Kv4.2, and Kv4.3) have been shown to be present in ventricular myocardium (Table 14.2) [26, 27, 134, 135]. While some species appear to express one of the channels preferentially, others may express two or more channels with different regional distribution [26, 28]. Therefore, regulation of the transient outward current may differ depending on the channel expressed in the species and the myocardial region studied. Present data indicate that mRNA transcripts encoding $I_{to1}$ in the rat (presumably Kv4.2 [134]) are reduced in parallel with the current density of $I_{to1}$ in hypertrophied myocytes of the chronically infarcted rat heart [54]. In the central layers of failing human left ventricular myocardium, Kv4.3 mRNA (the putative gene encoding $I_{to1}$ in epicardial and central layers of human left ventricle [28, 135]) was reduced by a similar extent as $I_{to1}$, indicating that functional expression of $I_{to1}$ is at least in part transcriptionally regulated (Fig. 14.9) [113]. However, before the incorporation of functional channel protein into the membrane, other steps may also be altered. In addition to the channel protein, β-subunits may be altered, significantly affecting the properties of the ion channel [136–138].

Potassium-channel density could be altered by metabolic factors independent of gene expression, as may be the case in the reduction of $I_{to1}$ density by metabolic alterations in rats with diabetes mellitus, which has been found to be reversed by pyruvate, an activator of pyruvate dehydrogenase [139]. Moreover, different mechanisms may be involved in the short-term and long-term regulation of potassium-channel density, as suggested in electrical remodelling in atrial fibrillation, where a calcium-dependent mechanism has been implicated to be responsible for changes occurring within the first few hours [140, 141], while in the long run, altered gene expression of atrial ion channels has been reported [142].

Myocardial potassium channels appear to be actively regulated by several signalling systems involved in the regulation of cardiac growth and hypertrophy, and metabolic state. Regulation of potassium-current expression may therefore be a mechanism of biological adaptation that alters electrical excitability in the myocardium, as proposed for other excitable cells [122, 143].

## Functional implications of altered ion-channel expression in cardiomyopathy

Adaptive changes to cardiac hypertrophy or failure, originating as a compensatory response, have been shown not

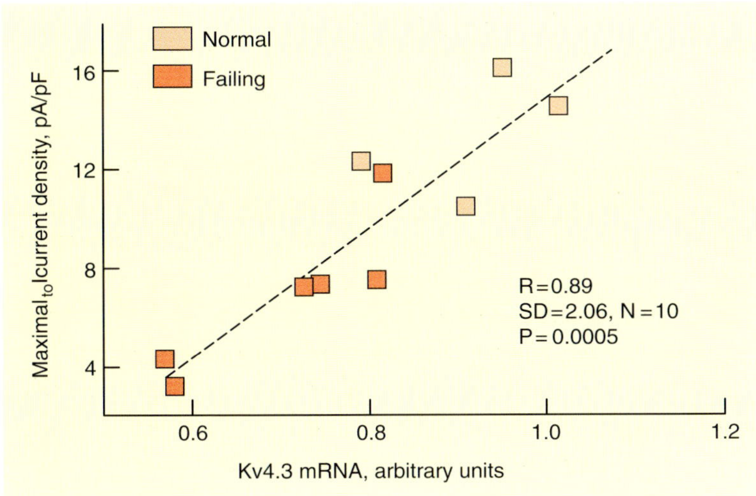


**Figure 14.9** *Expression of Kv4.3 mRNA in normal (non-failing) and failing human left ventricle. mRNA levels of Kv4.3 (using ribonuclease protection assays, upper panel) and* $I_{to1}$ *(using the patch-clamp technique) measured from the same hearts were found to be reduced to a similar degree. The close correlation suggests that in central myocardium of the human heart,* $I_{to1}$ *is at least in part transcriptionally regulated. hH1 marks the labelling of the human ventricular sodium channel mRNA.*

to be beneficial from all perspectives [114, 144], and there is increasing evidence that this may also be true for alterations in ion-current expression. Heart failure results in a high risk of cardiac death, which can be reduced by interfering with the mechanisms involved in the adaptation processes [115]. Even though deterioration of heart failure may be responsible for a significant number of deaths, many patients die of ventricular tachyarrhythmias, notably polymorphic ventricular tachycardia [13, 145]. Depressed left ventricular function is the strongest predictor of arrhythmic death, independent of the aetiology of heart failure [114, 146–148], indicating that common mechanisms may be involved in the electrical instability of the failing heart. However, even at the stage of hypertrophy when haemodynamics are not compromised, the risk of sudden cardiac death is increased significantly [149]. Interestingly, as shown above, cardiac hypertrophy is also characterized by prolonged action potential duration and thus increased instability of the repolarization process, as shown, for example, by the facilitated provocation of early after-depolarizations [150].

While no major changes in inward currents can be delineated in cardiac hypertrophy and failure, potassium currents, specifically $I_{to1}$, appear to be downregulated. Animal studies have provided a close correlation between delayed repolarization, reduction in potassium currents, and increased propensity to ventricular arrhythmias in cardiac hypertrophy and failure. Earlier studies have shown that hypertrophied rat hearts had a longer action potential duration and higher incidence of early after-depolarizations and triggered activity when tetraethylammonium ($TEA^+$) was used to destabilize the repolarization process by partial block of potassium channels [11, 53]. In feline left ventricular hypertrophy, enhanced sensitivity to metabolic inhibition was attributed to decreased delayed rectifier currents [110]. Similarly, reperfusion-induced early afterdepolarizations and arrhythmias could be related to decreased outward potassium currents [111]. A postinfarct model of myocyte hypertrophy in rat demonstrated increased susceptibility to ventricular tachycardia, increased dispersion of repolarization, triggered activity from early and delayed after depolarizations, and re-entrant excitation which were shown to be accompanied by decreases in $I_{to1}$ and a slowly decaying transient outward current, $I_{to\text{-}s}$ [54]. In the hypertrophied canine ventricle, prolongation of action potential duration was found to facilitate early afterdepolarizations which triggered ventricular tachyarrhythmias [150]. These correlations suggest that reduction in potassium currents may contribute to the propensity to ventricular arrhythmias in cardiac hypertrophy.

For failing myocardium, substantial evidence connecting potassium-channel downregulation to abnormalities of repolarization, arrhythmias, and sudden cardiac death has recently been provided in dogs with pacing-induced cardiac failure [14, 58, 151]. A dramatic 65% decrease in $I_{to1}$ was found to be accompanied by an increased effective refractory period, monophasic action potential duration, and dispersion of repolarization, and a high incidence of ventricular arrhythmias and sudden cardiac death. In addition, sensitivity to caesium chloride (CsCl), which challenges repolarization by reducing potassium currents, was greatly enhanced, leading to excessive prolongation and dispersion of monophasic action potential, and generation of early

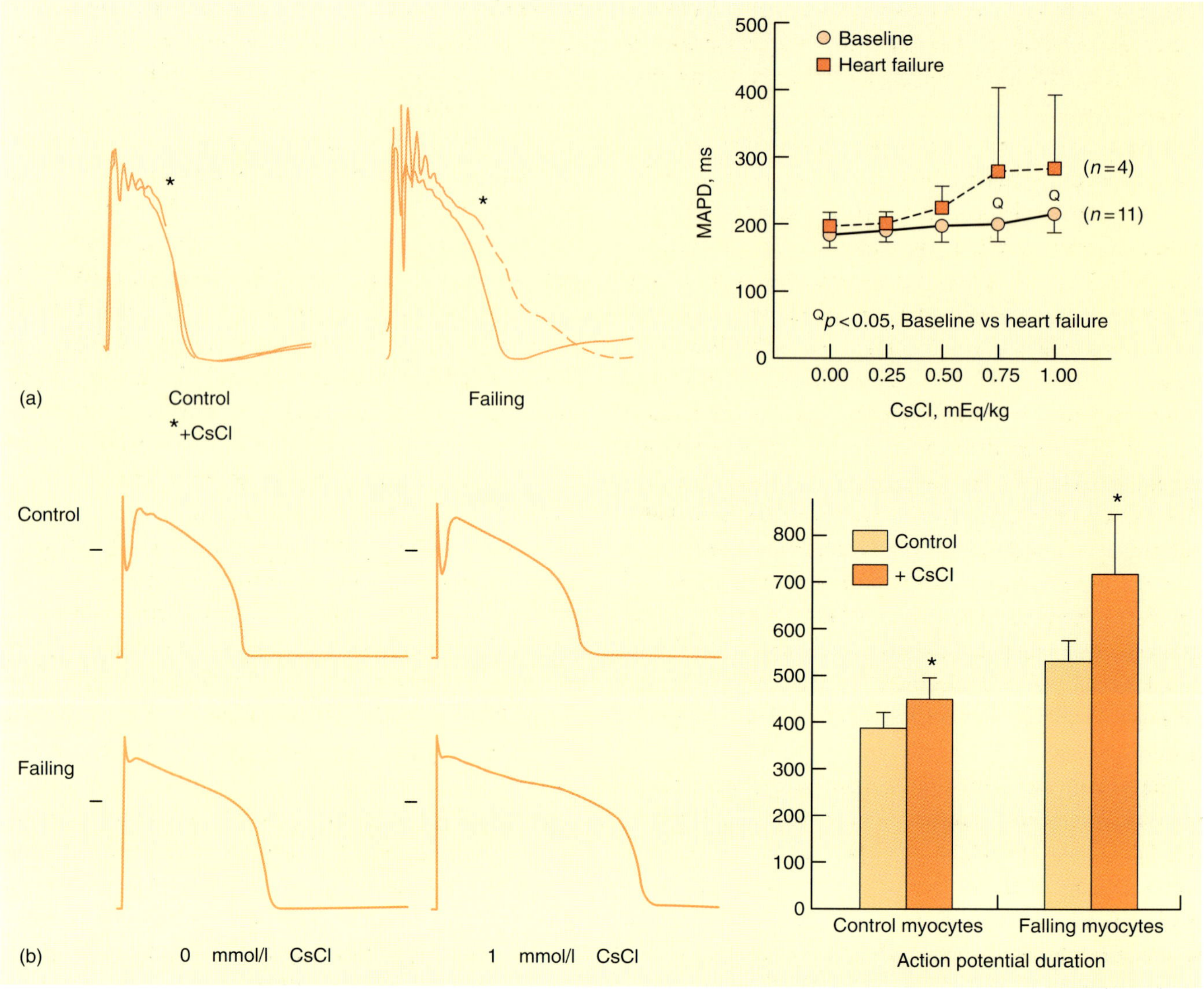


**Figure 14.10** *Excessive prolongation of action potential duration in dogs with pacing-induced heart failure, measured as monophasic action potentials (MAP; A) and in isolated myocytes (action potential duration; B). In intact myocardium as well as isolated myocytes, provocation or repolarization abnormalities with CsCl (1 mmol/l) caused excessive prolongation in failing tissue or cells. (Adapted from ref. 14.)*

after-depolarizations in failing myocardium (Fig. 14.10). This correlated to a similar propensity to excessive action potential prolongation and early after-depolarizations in response to CsCl at the level of the single myocyte, demonstrating that this repolarization abnormality was due to a cellular alteration in ion-channel expression [14]. Thus, potassium-channel downregulation appears to enhance sensitivity to measures disturbing repolarization, such as ischaemia, sympathetic activation, low extracellular potassium, or drugs with class III antiarrhythmic activity.

However, more subtle changes possibly important in the genesis of arrhythmias may also arise from altered ion-current expression in cardiomyopathy, such as abnormal rate adaptation of the QT interval as recently reported in hypertensive patients [34]. Clinical correlates to an increased spatial and temporal lability of repolarization are currently under investigation. While spatial inhomogeneity may be difficult to resolve in a 12-lead surface electrocardiogram (ECG), increased temporal variability of the repolarization process may be accessible from the surface ECG and possibly allow risk stratification of patients with cardiomyopathy [152].

Present evidence on potassium-channel downregulation in heart failure clearly indicates the involvement of $I_{to1}$.

With respect to $I_{K1}$, alterations reported [16, 58] did not extend to the voltage range positive to the potassium reversal potential, which is relevant to the final repolarization process. Thus, data on $I_{K1}$ remain conflicting, even though most studies find only small or no changes. Further studies will be required to clarify potential alterations in $I_{K1}$ in heart failure. Preliminary reports also suggest a reduction in mRNA levels of HERG in failing human myocardium [112, 113]; if these findings translate into reduced functional expression of $I_{Kr}$, a more widespread reduction in potassium currents may be occurring in failing human hearts.

Even though potassium channel downregulation is a prominent feature in cardiomyopathy, this does not exclude the contribution of other ion currents (such as increased sodium window current, L-type calcium current [55], or Na/Ca-exchange current [103]. However, any decrease in outward current will shift the repolarization process towards later repolarization and greater lability for any given inward currents. Even if a simultaneous reduction in inward currents counteracts action potential prolongation, membrane impedance at the action potential plateau would still be increased, producing an increased lability of the repolarizing process.

The recent discovery of a causative role of decreased or altered repolarizing potassium currents in congenital long-QT syndrome (LQT-1, LQT-2, LQT-4) provides a strong argument for linking potassium-channel downregulation and action potential prolongation to enhanced lability of repolarization and sudden cardiac death. Genetic alterations in $I_{Ks}$ (KvLQT 1) and $I_{Kr}$ (HERG) are probably responsible for the majority of long-QT syndromes [31], which are characterized by repolarization abnormalities with prolongation and increased lability of the action potential duration as manifested by an increased dispersion of repolarization and sudden cardiac death. Even more importantly, QT prolongation and dispersion appear to be reversible by interventions increasing $I_{Kr}$ (such as elevation of extracellular potassium concentration) [153], demonstrating a crucial role of reduced potassium currents in the instability of the repolarization process in heart failure.

To some degree, action potential prolongation in cardiac hypertrophy and failure may be viewed as a form of acquired long-QT syndrome, sharing the characteristics of action potential prolongation with increased lability and dispersion, reduction in outward potassium currents (or possibly increased inward currents such as $I_{Na}$ in LQT-3), and propensity to early after-depolarizations, polymorphic ventricular tachycardia or torsade de pointes, and sudden cardiac death. As in long-QT syndrome, heart failure shows a greater sensitivity to further prolongation of the action potential duration in hypokalaemia [14] or following exposure to antiarrhythmic agents such as sotalol, which has been shown to exert greater proarrhythmic effects in failing hearts and to cause excess mortality [19]. Further validation of the critical role of reduced potassium currents in electrical instability in heart failure might be obtained by demonstrating that repolarization can be stabilized by increasing outward potassium currents, as has been demonstrated for genetic LQT-2 [153]. Recent preliminary data suggest that this may indeed be true, as increasing $I_{Kr}$ (by elevation of $[K^+]_o$) was capable of reducing QT prolongation and dispersion in congestive heart failure in humans [33]. Downregulation of potassium currents and the associated electrical instability may also be counteracted by introducing suitable potassium-channel constructs into the myocardial cell using molecular genetic techniques [154, 155]. Owing to the low membrane conductance of the cardiac action potential at plateau voltages, a low density of additional outward current would be capable of counteracting potassium-channel downregulation in cardiomyopathy.

The clinical efficacy of elevation of extracellular potassium in stabilizing ventricular arrhythmias in long-QT syndrome and congestive heart failure suggests that despite disappointing results with most current antiarrhythmic drugs, there may be a potential for new strategies, possibly by increasing potassium currents or specific current components. However, a much deeper level of understanding of the electrical activity in the myocardium under normal and pathological conditions, as well as the structure and function of the ion channels, will be an essential prerequisite.

## Future aspects

Most cardiac potassium channels exhibit a pronounced regional heterogeneity throughout the ventricular wall, from base to apex and between septum, left ventricle, and right ventricle [25, 28, 35, 156, 157]. Therefore, when studying current densities and properties or mRNA levels of ion channels, great care has to be taken to prevent any influence possibly arising from tissue sampling. Even in the rat heart, regional differences in action potential configuration and current densities have been clearly recognized [37]. As evident from the rapid changes in $I_{to1}$ density towards the deeper subendocardium [158], even a small local sampling error may cause significant differences in current density. In addition, more than one gene appears to encode transient outward-type channels in the ventricular myocardium, at least in some species including humans [26, 28] (Table 14.2). The channel (or channels) underlying the macroscopic current in the respective species and the myocardial region need to be characterized before ion-channel expression and current densities can be correlated.

As shown recently, the delayed rectifier current $I_K$ consists of two components which can be separated based on kinetic criteria and pharmacological sensitivity [21]. Considering that the two channels are encoded by different genes [31] and may be regulated independently, these channels need to be evaluated separately. However, at present no study has attempted to quantify separately the alterations in current density of $I_{Kr}$ and $I_{Ks}$ in hypertrophied or failing myocardium.

Finally, little is known about the mechanisms regulating the altered expression of potassium currents in cardiac hypertrophy and failure, such as mechanical stress, neurohumoral activation, or membrane potential. A deeper understanding might allow interference with these mechanisms and prevention of potentially detrimental processes.

Treatment of electrical instability and prevention of sudden cardiac death require a broad knowledge of the basic mechanisms underlying the electrical activity of the myocardium. Increasing the cellular and molecular understanding of the determinants of normal and abnormal cardiac electrogenesis will allow the development of new approaches for safe and effective treatment of cardiac arrhythmias in myopathic hearts.

## Acknowledgements

Supported by the Deutsche Forschungsgemeinschaft and by the National Institutes of Health (Specialized Center of Research P50 HL52307). The authors thank Drs Gordon Tomaselli and Dirk Beuckelmann for their help and collaboration.

## References

1. Cohn JN, Johnson G, Ziesche S *et al.* A comparison of enalapril with hydralazine isosorbide dinitrate in the treatment of chronic congestive heart failure. *N Engl J Med* 1991; 325: 303–10.
2. CONSENSUS Study Trial Group. Effect of enalapril on survival in patients with reduced left ventricular ejection fractions and congestive heart failure. The SOLVD investigators. *N Engl J Med* 1991; 325: 293–302.
3. CONSENSUS Study Trial Group. Effect of enalapril on mortality and the development of heart failure in asymptomatic patients with reduced left ventricular ejection fractions. The SOLVD investigators. *N Engl J Med* 1992; 327: 685–91.
4. Gwathmey JK, Copelas L, MacKinnon R *et al.* Abnormal intracellular calcium handling in myocardium from patients with end-stage heart failure. *Circ Res* 1987; 61: 70–6.
5. Beuckelmann DJ, Näbauer M, Erdmann E. Intracellular calcium handling in isolated ventricular myocytes from patients with terminal heart failure. *Circulation* 1992; 85: 1046–55.
6. Davies CH, Harding SE, Poole-Wilson PA. Cellular mechanisms of contractile dysfunction in human heart failure. *Eur Heart J* 1996; 17: 189–98.
7. Gomez AM, Valdivia HH, Cheng H *et al.* Defective excitation contraction coupling in experimental cardiac hypertrophy and heart failure. *Science* 1997; 276: 800–6.
8. Pye MP, Cobbe SM. Mechanisms of ventricular arrhythmias in cardiac failure and hypertrophy. *Cardiovasc Res* 1992; 26: 740–50.
9. Crozatier B. Stretch induced modifications of myocardial performance: from ventricular function to cellular and molecular mechanisms. *Cardiovasc Res* 1996; 32: 25–37.
10. Pye MP, Cobbe SM. Arrhythmogenesis in experimental models of heart failure: the role of increased load. *Cardiovasc Res* 1996; 32: 248–57.
11. Aronson RS. Afterpotentials and triggered activity in hypertrophied myocardium from rats with renal hypertension. *Circ Res* 1981; 48: 720–7.
12. Aronson RS, Ming Z. Cellular mechanisms of arrhythmias in hypertrophied and failing myocardium. *Circulation* 1993; 87: VII-76–83.
13. Tomaselli GF, Beuckelmann DJ, Calkins HG *et al.* Sudden cardiac death in heart failure. The role of abnormal repolarization. *Circulation* 1994; 90: 2534–9.
14. Pak PH, Nuss HB, Tunin RS *et al.* Repolarization abnormalities, arrhythmia and sudden death in canine tachycardia-induced cardiomyopathy. *J Am Coll Cardiol* 1997; 30: 576–84.
15. Rozanski GJ, Xu Z, Whitney RT *et al.* Electrophysiology of rabbit ventricular myocytes following sustained rapid ventricular pacing. *J Mol Cell Cardiol* 1997; 29: 721–32.
16. Beuckelmann DJ, Näbauer M, Erdmann E. Alterations of $K^+$-currents in isolated human ventricular myocytes from patients with terminal heart failure. *Circ Res* 1993; 73: 379–85.
17. Näbauer M, Kääb S. Potassium channel down-regulation in heart failure. *Cardiovasc Res* 1998; 37: 324–34.
18. Misier AR, Opthof T, van Hemel NM *et al.* Dispersion of 'refractoriness' in noninfarcted myocardium of patients with ventricular tachycardia or ventricular fibrillation after myocardial infarction. *Circulation* 1995; 91: 2566–72.
19. Waldo AL, Camm AJ, deRuyter H *et al.* Effect of D-sotalol on mortality in patients with left ventricular dysfunction after recent and remote myocardial infarction. The SWORD Investigators. Survival With Oral D-Sotalol. *Lancet* 1996; 348: 7–12.
20. Fu G-S, Meissner A, Simon R. Repolarization dispersion and sudden cardiac death in patients with impaired left ventricular function. *Eur Heart J* 1997; 18: 218–89.

21. Sanguinetti MC, Jurkiewicz NK. Two components of cardiac delayed rectifier $K^+$ current. Differential sensitivity to block by class III antiarrhythmic agents. *J Gen Physiol* 1990; 96: 195–215.
22. Woosley R, Zaza A. The Sicilian Gambit. A new approach to the classification of antiarrhythmic drugs based on their actions on arrhythmogenic mechanisms. *Circulation* 1991; 84: 1831–51.
23. Surawicz B. Role of potassium channels in cycle length dependent regulation of action potential duration in mammalian cardiac Purkinje and ventricular muscle fibres. *Cardiovasc Res* 1992; 26: 1021–9.
24. Boyden PA. Cellular electrophysiologic basis of cardiac arrhythmias. *Am J Cardiol* 1996; 78: 4–11.
25. Liu DW, Gintant GA, Antzelevitch C. Ionic bases for electrophysiological distinctions among epicardial, midmyocardial, and endocardial myocytes from the free wall of the canine left ventricle. *Circ Res* 1993; 72: 671–87.
26. Brahmajothi MV, Morales MJ, Liu S *et al.* *In situ* hybridization reveals extensive diversity of $K^+$ channel mRNA in isolated ferret cardiac myocytes. *Circ Res* 1996; 78: 1083–9.
27. Deal KK, England SK, Tamkin MM. Molecular physiology of cardiac potassium channels. *Physiol Rev* 1996; 76: 49–67.
28. Näbauer M, Beuckelmann DJ, Uberfuhr P, Steinbeck G. Regional differences in current density and rate-dependent properties of the transient outward current in subepicardial and subendocardial myocytes of human left ventricle. *Circulation* 1996; 93: 168–77.
29. Antzelevitch C, Sicouri S, Litovsky SH *et al.* Heterogeneity within the ventricular wall — electrophysiology and pharmacology of epicardial, endocardial, and M-cells. *Circ Res* 1991; 69: 1427–49.
30. Weidmann S. Effect of current flow on the membrane potential of cardiac muscle. *J Physiol (Lond)* 1951; 115: 227–36.
31. Roden DM, Lazzara R, Rosen M *et al.* Multiple mechanisms in the long-QT syndrome. Current knowledge, gaps, and future directions. The SADS Foundation Task Force on LQTS. *Circulation* 1996; 94: 1996–2012.
32. Surawicz B, Knoebel SB. Long QT: good, bad or indifferent? *J Am Coll Cardiol* 1984; 4: 398–413.
33. Choy AM, Lang CC, Chomsky DB *et al.* Normalization of acquired QT prolongation by IV potassium (Abstract). *Pace-Pac Clin Electrophys* 1997; 20: 1235.
34. Singh JP, Johnston J, Sleight P *et al.* Left ventricular hypertrophy in hypertensive patients is associated with abnormal rate adaptation of QT interval. *J Am Coll Cardiol* 1997; 29: 778–84.
35. Litovsky SH, Antzelevitch C. Transient outward current prominent in canine ventricular epicardium but not endocardium. *Circ Res* 1988; 62: 116–26.
36. Sicouri S, Antzelevitch C. Electrophysiologic characteristics of m cells in the canine left ventricular free wall. *J Cardiovasc Electrophysiol* 1995; 6: 591–603.
37. Benitah JP, Gomez AM, Bailly P *et al.* Heterogeneity of the early outward current in ventricular cells isolated from normal and hypertrophied rat hearts. *J Physiol (Lond)* 1993; 469: 111–38.
38. Bryant SM, Shipsey SJ, Hart G. Regional differences in electrical and mechanical properties of myocytes from guinea-pig hearts with mild left ventricular hypertrophy. *Cardiovasc Res* 1997; 35: 315–23.
39. Ungerer M, Hartmann F, Karoglan M *et al.* Regional *in vivo* and *in vitro* characterization of autonomic innervation in cardiomyopathic human heart. *Circulation* 1998; 97: 174–80.
40. Hart G. Cellular electrophysiology in cardiac hypertrophy and failure. *Cardiovasc Res* 1994; 28: 933–46.
41. Cerbai E, Barbieri M, Li Q, Mugelli A. Ionic basis of action potential prolongation of hypertrophied cardiac myocytes isolated from hypertensive rats of different ages. *Cardiovasc Res* 1994; 28: 1180–7.
42. Keating MT, Sanguinetti MC. Molecular genetic insights into cardiovascular disease. *Science* 1996; 272: 681–5.
43. Meyerfeldt U, Schirdewan A, Wiedemann M *et al.* Natural trigger mechanisms of ventricular fibrillation in patients with chronic heart failure (Abstract). *Eur Heart J* 1997; 18: 189.
44. Schaumann A, Neufert C, Poppinga A *et al.* Short–long–short sequences are an important trigger mechanism of spontaneous ventricular arrhythmias (Abstract). *Eur Heart J* 1997; 18: 191.
45. Starmer CF, Romashko DN, Reddy RS *et al.* Proarrhythmic response to potassium channel blockade. Numerical studies of polymorphic tachyarrhythmias. *Circulation* 1995; 92: 595–605.
46. Noda M, Ikeda T, Suzuki H *et al.* Expression of functional sodium channels from cloned cDNA. *Nature* 1986; 322: 826–8.
47. Tanabe T, Takeshima H, Mikami A *et al.* Primary structure of the receptor for calcium channel blockers from skeletal muscle. *Nature* 1987; 328: 313–18.
48. Miller C. 1990: Annus mirabilis of potassium channels. *Science* 1991; 252: 1092–6.
49. Gelband H, Bassett AL. Depressed transmembrane potentials during experimentally induced ventricular failure in cats. *Circ Res* 1973; 32: 625–34.
50. Tritthart H, Luedcke H, Bayer R *et al.* Right ventricular hypertrophy in the cat — an electrophysiological and anatomical study. *J Mol Cell Cardiol* 1975; 7: 163–74.
51. Aronson RS. Characteristics of action potential of hypertrophied myocardium from rats with renal hypertension. *Circ Res*1980; 47: 443–54.
52. Gülch RW. The effect of elevated chronic loading on the action potential of mammalian myocardium. *J Mol Cell Cardiol* 1980; 12: 415–20.
53. Keung EC, Aronson RS. Transmembrane action potentials and the electrocardiogram in rats with renal hypertension. *Cardiovasc Res* 1981; 15: 611–14.
54. Qin D, Zhang ZH, Caref EB *et al.* Cellular and ionic basis of arrhythmias in postinfarction remodeled ventricular myocardium. *Circ Res* 1996; 79: 461–73.
55. Ryder KO, Bryant SM, Winterton SJ *et al.* Electrical and mechanical characteristics of isolated ventricular myocytes from guinea-pigs with left ventricular hypertrophy and congestive heart failure (Abstract) *J Physiol (Lond)* 1991; 443: 181P.
56. Vermeulen JT, McGuire MA, Opthof T *et al.* Triggered activity and automaticity in ventricular trabeculae of failing human and rabbit hearts. *Cardiovasc Res* 1994; 28: 1547–1554.
57. Koumi S, Backer CL, Arentzen CE. Characterization of inwardly rectifying $K^+$ channel in human cardiac myocytes. Alterations in channel behavior in myocytes isolated from patients with idiopathic dilated cardiomyopathy. *Circulation* 1995; 92: 164–74.
58. Kääb S, Nuss HB, Chiamvimonvat N *et al.* Ionic mechanisms of action potential prolongation in ventricular myocytes from dogs with pacing-induced heart failure. *Circ Res* 1996; 78: 262–73.
59. Thuringer D, Coulombe A, Deroubaix E *et al.* Depressed transient outward current density in ventricular myocytes from cardiomyopathic Syrian hamsters of different ages. *J Mol Cell Cardiol* 1996; 28: 387–401.

60. Cameron JS, Gaide MS, Epstein K *et al.* Regional distribution of action potential abnormalities induced by subacute right ventricular pressure overload. *J Mol Cell Cardiol* 1984; 16: 321–30.
61. Doherty JD, Cobbe SM. Electrophysiological changes in animal model of chronic cardiac failure. *Cardiovascular Res* 1990; 24: 309–16.
62. Shenasa H, Calderone A, Vermeulen M *et al.* Chronic doxorubicin induced cardiomyopathy in rabbits: mechanical, intracellular action potential, and beta adrenergic characteristics of the failing myocardium. *Cardiovasc Res* 1990; 24: 591–604.
63. Boyden PA, Jeck CD. Ion channel function in disease. *Cardiovasc Res* 1995; 29: 312–18.
64. Sakakibara Y, Furukawa T, Singer DH *et al.* Sodium current in isolated human ventricular myocytes. *Am J Physiol* 1993; 265: H1301–9.
65. Maltsev VA, Sabbah HN, Goldstein S *et al.* Sarcolemma-related abnormalities of excitation–contraction coupling in cardomyocytes from dogs with heart failure (Abstract). *J Am Coll Cardiol* 1997; 29: 405A.
66. Kleiman RB, Houser SR. Calcium currents in normal and hypertrophied isolated feline ventricular myocytes. *Am J Physiol* 1988; 255: H1434–42.
67. Keung EC. Calcium current is increased in isolated adult myocytes from hypertrophied rat myocardium. *Circ Res* 1989; 64: 753–63.
68. Brooksby P, Levi AJ, Jones JV. Investigation of the mechanisms underlying the increased contraction of hypertrophied ventricular myocytes isolated from the spontaneously hypertensive rat. *Cardiovasc Res* 1993; 27: 1268–77.
69. Kruger C, Erdmann E, Näbauer M, Beuckelmann DJ. Intracellular calcium handling in isolated ventricular myocytes from cardiomyopathic hamsters (strain bio 14.6) with congestive heart failure. *Cell Calcium* 1994; 16: 500–8.
70. Harding SE, MacLeod KT, Davies CH *et al.* Abnormalities of the myocytes in ischaemic cardiomyopathy. *Eur Heart J* 1995; 16 (Suppl I): 74–81.
71. Ryder KO, Bryant SM, Hart G. Membrane current changes in left ventricular myocytes isolated from guinea pigs after abdominal aortic coarctation. *Cardiovasc Res* 1993; 27: 1278–87.
72. Ming Z, Nordin C, Siri F, Aronson RS. Reduced calcium current density in single myocytes isolated from hypertrophied failing guinea pig hearts. *J Mol Cell Cardiol* 1994; 26: 1133–43.
73. Beuckelmann DJ, Erdmann E. $Ca^{2+}$-currents and intracellular $Ca^{2+}$ transients in single ventricular myocytes isolated from terminally failing human myocardium. *Basic Res Cardiol* 1992; 87: 235–43.
74. Mewes T, Ravens U. L-type calcium currents of human myocytes from ventricle of non-failing and failing hearts and from atrium. *J Mol Cell Cardiol* 1994; 26: 1307–20.
75. Meszaros J, Coutinho JJ, Bryant SM *et al.* L-type calcium current in catecholamine-induced cardiac hypertrophy in the rat. *Exp Physiol* 1997; 82: 71–83.
76. Hasenfuss G, Mulieri LA, Leavitt BJ *et al.* Contractile protein function in failing and nonfailing human myocardium. *Basic Res Cardiol* 1992; 87: 107–16.
77. Morgan JP. Abnormal intracellular modulation of calcium as a major cause of cardiac contractile dysfunction. *N Engl J Med* 1992; 323: 625–32.
78. Beuckelmann DJ, Näbauer M, Erdmann E. Characteristics of calcium-current in isolated human ventricular myocytes from patients with terminal heart failure. *J Mol Cell Cardiol* 1991; 23: 929–37.
79. Spinale FG, Tempel GE, Mukherjee R *et al.* Cellular and molecular alterations in the beta adrenergic system with cardiomyopathy induced by tachycardia. *Cardiovasc Res* 1994; 28: 1243–50.
80. Yang Y, Toaldo GL, Bailey BA *et al.* Multiple alternative spliced isoforms of the alpha-1c subunit of the calcium channels in normal and diseased human and rat heart (Abstract). *Circulation* 1996; 94: I-223.
81. Yang Y, Hefner CA, Pollack PS *et al.* Failing human ventricular myocytes express the smooth muscle isoform of the L-type calcium channel alpha-1c subunit. *Circulation* 1997; 96: I-54.
82. Yang Y, Margulies KB, Pollack PS, Houser SR. N-terminal L-type calcium channel alpha-1c isoform switching in normal and failing human heart. *Circulation* 1997; 96: I-54.
83. Gidh-Jain M, Huang B, Jain P *et al.* Reemergence of the fetal pattern of I-type calcium channel gene expression in non infarcted myocardium during left ventricular remodeling. *Biochem Biophys Res Commun* 1995; 216: 892–7.
84. Hullin RA, Asmus F, Berger HJ, Boekstegers P. Differential expression of the subunits of the human cardiac L-type calcium channel in diastolic failure of the transplanted heart. *Circulation* 1997; 96: I-55.
85. Mitra R, Morad M. Two types of calcium channels in guinea pig ventricular myocytes. *Proc Natl Acad Sci USA* 1986; 83: 5340–4.
86. Nuss HB, Marban E. Electrophysiological properties of neonatal mouse cardiac myocytes in primary culture. *J Physiol (Lond)* 1994; 479: 265–79.
87. Nuss HB, Houser SR. T-type $Ca^{2+}$ current is expressed in hypertrophied adult feline left ventricular myocytes. *Circ Res* 1993; 73: 777–82.
88. Sen L, Smith TW. T-type $Ca^{2+}$ channels are abnormal in genetically determined cardiomyopathic hamster hearts. *Circ Res* 1994; 75: 149–55.
89. Näbauer M, Barth A, Kääb S. Repolarization in pig left ventricle: Absence of a relevant Ito1 and control by IKR and IKS. *Circulation* 1997; 96: I-500.
90. Barbieri M, Varani K, Cerbai E *et al.* Electrophysiological basis for the enhanced cardiac arrhythmogenic effect of isoprenaline in aged spontaneously hypertensive rats. *J Mol Cell Cardiol* 1994; 26: 849–60.
91. Tomita F, Bassett AL, Myerburg RJ, Kimura S. Diminished transient outward currents in rat hypertrophied ventricular myocytes. *Circ Res* 1994; 75: 296–303.
92. Xu XP, Best PM. Decreased transient outward $K^+$ current in ventricular myocytes from acromegalic rats. *Am J Physiol* 1991; 260: H935–42.
93. Coulombe A, Momtaz A, Richer P *et al.* Reduction of calcium-independent transient outward potassium current density in DOCA salt hypertrophied rat ventricular myocytes. *Pflugers Arch* 1994; 427: 47–55.
94. Momtaz A, Coulombe A, Richer P *et al.* Action potential and plateau ionic currents in moderately and severely DOCA-salt hypertrophied rat hearts. *J Mol Cell Cardiol* 1996; 28: 2511–22.
95. Meszaros J, Ryder KO, Hart G. Transient outward current in catecholamine-induced cardiac hypertrophy in the rat. *Am J Physiol* 1996; 271: H23670–7.
96. Potreau D, Gomez JP, Fares N. Depressed transient outward current in single hypertrophied cardiomyocytes isolated from the right ventricle of ferret heart. *Cardiovasc Res* 1995; 30: 440–8.
97. Bouron A, Potreau D, Raymond G. The L-type calcium current in single hypertrophied cardiomyocytes isolated from the right ventricle of ferret heart. *Cardiovasc Res* 1992; 26: 662–70.
98. Brooksby P, Levi AJ, Jones JV. The electrophysiological characteristics of hypertrophied ventricular myocytes from the spontaneously hypertensive rat. *J Hypertens* 1993; 11: 611–22.

99. Li Q, Keung EC. Effects of myocardial hypertrophy on transient outward current. *Am J Physiol* 1994; 266: H1738–45.
100. Ten Eick RE, Zhang K, Harvey RD, Bassett AL. Enhanced functional expression of transient outward current in hypertro-phied feline myocytes. *Cardiovasc Drugs Ther* 1993; 7 (Suppl 3): 611–19.
101. Hano O, Mitsuoka T, Matsumoto Y *et al.* Arrhythmogenic properties of the ventricular myocardium in cardiomyopathic Syrian hamster, B10 14.6 strain. *Cardiovasc Res* 1991; 25: 49–57.
102. Wettwer E, Amos GJ, Posival H, Ravens U. Transient outward current in human ventricular myocytes of subepicardial and subendocardial origin. *Circ Res* 1994; 75: 473–82.
103. Hatem SN, Sham JSK, Morad M. Enhanced $Na^+$–$Ca^{2+}$ exchange activity in cardiomyopathic Syrian hamster. *Circ Res* 1994; 74: 253–61.
104. Rossner KL, Sachs HG. Electrophysiological study of Syrian hamster hereditary cardiomyopathy. *Cardiovasc Res* 1978; 12: 436–43.
105. Kleiman RB, Houser SR. Outward currents in normal and hypertrophied feline ventricular myocytes. *Am J Physiol* 1989; 256: H1450–61.
106. Koumi S, Backer CL, Arentzen CE, Sato R. Beta-adrenergic modulation of the inwardly rectifying potassium channel in isolated human ventricular myocytes. Alteration in channel response to beta-adrenergic stimulation in failing human hearts. *J Clin Invest* 1995; 96: 2870–81.
107. Follmer CH, Colatsky TJ. Block of delayed rectifier potassium current, IK, by flecainide and E-4031 in cat ventricular myocytes. *Circulation* 1990; 82: 289–93.
108. Carmeliet E. Voltage-dependent and time-dependent block of the delayed $K^+$ current in cardiac myocytes by dofetilide. *J Pharmacol Exp Ther* 1992; 262: 809–17.
109. Kleiman RB, Houser SR. Outward currents in hypertrophied feline ventricular myocytes. *Prog Clin Biol Res* 1990; 334: 65–83.
110. Furukawa T, Myerburg RJ, Furukawa N *et al.* Metabolic inhibition of ICa,L and IK differs in feline left ventricular hypertrophy. *Am J Physiol* 1994; 266: H1121–31.
111. Furukawa T, Bassett AL, Furukawa N *et al.* The ionic mechanism of reperfusion-induced early after depolarizations in feline left ventricular hypertrophy. *J Clin Invest* 1993; 91: 1521–31.
112. Choy AM, Kupershmidt S, Lang CC *et al.* Regional expression of HERG and KVLQT1 in heart failure (Abstract). *Circulation* 1996; 94: I-164.
113. Kääb S, Duc J, Ashen D *et al.* Quantitative analysis of K channel mRNA expression in normal and failing human ventricle reveals the molecular identity of Ito1 (Abstract). *Circulation* 1996; 94: I-592.
114. Moalic JM, Charlemagne D, Mansier P *et al.* Cardiac hypertrophy and failure — a disease of adaptation. Modifications in membrane proteins provide a molecular basis for arrhythmogenicity. *Circulation* 1993; 87: IV21–6.
115. Eichhorn EJ, Bristow MR. Medical therapy can improve the biological properties of the chronically failing heart. A new era in the treatment of heart failure. *Circulation* 1996; 94: 2285–96.
116. Roden DM. Ionic mechanisms for prolongation of refractoriness and their proarrhythmic and antiarrhythmic correlates. *Am J Cardiol* 1996; 78: 12–16.
117. Hasenfuss G, Mulieri LA, Leavitt BJ *et al.* Alteration of contractile function and excitation–contraction coupling in dilated cardiomyopathy. *Circ Res* 1992; 70: 1225–32.
118. Alpert NR, Mulieri LA, Hasenfuss G, Holubarsch C. Optimization of myocardial function. *Basic Res Cardiol* 1993; 88: 29–41.
119. Hasenfuss G, Mulieri LA, Holubarsch C *et al.* Nyocardial adaptation to stress from the viewpoint of adaptation and development. *Basic Res Cardiol* 1993; 88: 91–102.
120. Mercadier J, Lompre A, Duc P *et al.* Altered sarcoplasmic reticulum $Ca^{2+}$-ATPase gene expression in the human ventricular during end-stage heart failure. *J Clin Invest* 1990; 85: 305–9.
121. Studer R, Reinecke H, Bilger J *et al.* Gene expression of the cardiac $Na^+$–$Ca^{2+}$ exchanger in end-stage human heart failure. *Circ Res* 1994; 75: 443–53.
122. Mori Y, Matsubara H, Folco E *et al.* The transcription of a mammalian voltage-gated potassium channel is regulated by cAMP in a cell-specific manner. *J Biol Chem* 1993; 268: 26 482–93.
123. Matsubara H, Suzuki J, Inada M. Shaker-related potassium channel, Kv1.4, mRNA regulation in cultured rat heart myocytes and differential expression of Kv1.4 and Kv1.5 genes in myocardial development and hypertrophy. *J Clin Invest* 1993; 92: 1659–66.
124. Zhang ZJ, Jurkiewicz NK, Folander K *et al.* $K^+$ currents expressed from the guinea pig cardiac IsK protein are enhanced by activators of protein kinase C. *Proc Natl Acad Sci USA* 1994; 91: 1766–70.
125. Maki T, Gruver EJ, Davidoff AJ *et al.* Regulation of calcium channel expression in neonatal myocytes by catecholamines. *J Clin Invest* 1996; 97: 656–63.
126. Ogawa S, Barnett JV, Sen L *et al.* Direct contact between sympathetic neurons and rat cardiac myocytes *in vitro* increases expression of functional calcium channels. *J Clin Invest* 1992; 89: 1085–93.
127. Gaughan JP, Hefner C, Houser SR. Alpha-adrenergic modulation produces hypertrophy and alters ion channel expression in neonatal rat ventricular myocytes (Abstract). *Circulation* 1995; 92: I-503.
128. Guo W, Kamiya K, Toyama J. Differential effects of chronic membrane depolarization on the $K^+$ channel activities in cultured rat ventricular cells. *Cardiovasc Res* 1997; 33: 139–46.
129. Shimoni Y, Banno H, Clark RB. Hyperthyroidism selectively modified a transient potassium current in rabbit ventricular and atrial myocytes. *J Physiol (Lond)* 1992; 457: 369–89.
130. Shimoni Y, Severson D, Giles W. Thyroid status and diabetes modulate regional differences in potassium currents in rat ventricle. *J Physiol (Lond)* 1995; 488: 673–88.
131. Bosch RF, Wible BA, Wang Z *et al.* Hypothyreose verringert die Expression des KvLQT1 Gens und von IKs im Meerschweinchenventrikel. *Z Kardiol* 1998; 87: I-126.
132. Schöll E, Markwardt F, Holtz J. Chronic modulation of the transient outward current in rat left ventricular myocytes by the renin–angiotensin-system? (Abstract). *Circulation* 1996; 94: I-714.
133. Yu H, Rosen MR, Danilo P *et al.* Angiotensin II alters Ito properties in cardiac ventricular myocytes. *Circulation* 1997; 96: I-295.
134. Dixon JE, McKinnon D. Quantitative analysis of potassium channel mRNA expression in atrial and ventricular muscle of rats. *Circ Res* 1994; 75: 252–60.
135. Dixon JE, Shi W, Wang HS *et al.* Role of the Kv4.3 $K^+$ channel in ventricular muscle. A molecular correlate for the transient outward current. *Circ Res* 1996; 79: 659–68.
136. England SK, Uebele VN, Kodali J *et al.* A Novel $K^+$ channel beta-subunit (hKv beta 1.3) is produced via alternative mRNA splicing. *J Biol Chem* 1995; 270: 28 531–4.
137. England SK, Uebele VN, Shear H *et al.* Characterization of a voltage-gated $K^+$ channel beta subunit expressed in human heart. *Proc Natl Acad Sci USA* 1995; 92: 6309–13.
138. Morales MJ, Castellino RC, Crews AL *et al.* A novel beta subunit increases rate of inactivation of specific voltage-gated potassium channel alpha subunits. *J Biol Chem* 1995; 270: 6272–7.

139. Xu Z, Patel KP, Rozanski GJ. Metabolic basis of decreased transient outward $K^+$ current in ventricular myocytes from diabetic rats. *Am J Physiol* 1996; 271: H2190–6.
140. Goette A, Honeycutt C, Langberg JJ. Electrical remodeling in atrial fibrillation. Time course and mechanisms. *Circulation* 1996; 94: 2968–74.
141. Tieleman RG, De Langen C, Van Gelder IC *et al.* Verapamil reduces tachycardia-induced electrical remodeling of the atria. *Circulation* 1997; 95: 1945–53.
142. Yue L, Feng J, Gaspo R *et al.* Ionic remodeling underlying action potential changes in a canine model of atrial fibrillation. *Circ Res* 1997; 81: 512–25.
143. Heinemann S, Rettig J, Scott V *et al.* The inactivation behaviour of voltage-gated K-channels may be determined by association of alpha- and beta-subunits. *J Physiol Paris* 1994; 88: 173–80.
144. Katz AM. Cardiomyopathy of overload. A major determinant of prognosis in congestive heart failure. *N Engl J Med* 1990; 322: 100–10.
145. Stevenson WG, Stevenson LW, Middlekauff HR, Saxon LA. Sudden death prevention in patients with advanced ventricular dysfunction. *Circulation* 1993; 88: 2953–61.
146. Kjekshus J. Arrhythmias and mortality in congestive heart failure. *Am J Cardiol* 1990; 65: 421–81.
147. Goldman S, Johnson G, Cohn JN *et al.* Mechanism of death in heart failure. The vasodilator-heart failure trials. The V-HeFT VA cooperative studies group. *Circulation* 1993; 87 (6 Suppl): VI24–31.
148. Kottkamp H, Budde T, Lamp B *et al.* Clinical significance and management of ventricular arrhythmias in heart failure. *Eur Heart J* 1994; 15 (Suppl D): 155–63.
149. Levy D, Garrison RJ, Savage DD *et al.* Prognostic implications of echocardiographically determined left ventricular mass in the Framingham Heart Study. *N Engl J Med* 1990; 322: 1561–6.
150. Ben David J, Zipes DP, Ayers GM, Pride HP. Canine left ventricular hypertrophy predisposes to ventricular tachycardia induction by phase 2 early after depolarizations after administration of BAY K 8644. *J Am Coll Cardiol* 1992; 20: 1576–84.
151. Li HG, Jones DL, Yee R, Klein GJ. Electrophysiologic substrate associated with pacing-induced heart failure in dogs: potential value of programmed stimulation in predicting sudden death. *J Am Coll Cardiol* 1992; 19: 444–9.
152. Berger RD, Kasper EK, Baughman KL *et al.* Beat-to-beat QT interval variability: novel evidence for repolarization lability in ischemic and nonischemic dilated cardiomyopathy. *Circulation* 1997; 96: 1557–65.
153. Compton SJ, Lux RL, Ramsey MR *et al.* Genetically defined therapy of inherited long-QT syndrome. Correction of abnormal repolarization by potassium. *Circulation* 1996; 94: 1018–22.
154. Lawrence JH, Johns DC, Chiamvimonvat N *et al.* Prospects for genetic manipulation of cardiac excitability. *Adv Exp Med Biol* 1995; 382: 41–8.
155. Nuss HB, Johns DC, Kääb S *et al.* Reversal of potassium channel deficiency in cells from failing hearts by adenoviral gene transfer: a prototype for gene therapy for disorders of cardiac excitability and contractility. *Gene Ther* 1996; 3: 900–12.
156. Liu DW, Antzelevitch C. Characteristics of the delayed rectifier current (IKr and IKs) in canine ventricular epicardial, midmyocardial, and endocardial myocytes. A weaker IKs contributes to the longer action potential of the M cell. *Circ Res* 1995; 76: 351–65.
157. Di Diego JM, Sun ZQ, Antzelevitch C. Ito and action potential notch are smaller in left vs. right canine ventricular epicardium. *Am J Physiol* 1996; 271: H548–61.
158. Sicouri S, Fish J, Antzelevitch C. Distribution of M cells in the canine ventricle. *J Cardiovasc Electrophysiol* 1994; 5: 824–37.

# Viral myocardial disease 15

H. ZHANG, D. CHIN, P. RICHARDSON AND L. ARCHARD

## Introduction

Viruses are important agents in the pathogenesis of heart muscle disease and are implicated in acute myocarditis and the subsequent development of chronic, dilated cardiomyopathy (DCM). Between 1 and 5% of the virus infected population have cardiovascular signs and symptoms [1]. Because of seasonal, geographical, epidemic, and institutional variations, the true incidence of viral heart muscle disease remains uncertain. The majority of patients with viral myocardial disease have no specific cardiac symptoms or signs; cardiac involvement is often subclinical and may manifest only as transient electrocardiographic (ECG) changes [2]. In symptomatic patients with suspected inflammatory heart muscle disease, the clinical presentation is variable, with about 30% giving a history of preceding 'viral illness', including upper respiratory or gastrointestinal symptoms, myalgia, or fever [1]. An important subset of patients has risk factors for, or a proven diagnosis, of human immunodeficiency virus (HIV) or hepatitis C virus (HCV) infection. Complaints reflecting myocardial involvement include pleuritic or exertional chest pains related to myopericarditis (37% in one cohort), fatigue or exertional dyspnoea (90%) due to cardiac failure, and palpitations due to arrhythmia. In a small proportion of patients the course of illness is fulminant, leading to sudden cardiac death [3, 4] although a less aggressive course is seen in most cases.

## Clinical presentation and management

Three major cardiac syndromes are recognized: (1) myopericarditis with predominant chest pain and ECG abnormalities, with or without pericardial effusion; (2) dilated heart failure with pulmonary or peripheral congestion, low cardiac output, or cardiogenic shock and (3) arrhythmia, with palpitations, loss of consciousness, or even sudden death. Physical examination occasionally reveals a pericardial friction rub and low-grade pyrexia; in more severe or chronic cases, clinical signs reflect cardiac decompensation. Congestion of the left heart may be evident with dyspnoea at rest, a summation gallop with added third and fourth heart sounds, inspiratory crepitations in the lungs, and the stony dullness of pleural effusion. Right heart failure may manifest as peripheral oedema, ascites, and hepatomegaly. The jugular venous pressure is also elevated; the a wave is absent in atrial fibrillation and the v wave is prominent in tricuspid regurgitation. Low cardiac output and neuroendocrine activation with poor peripheral perfusion and reduced systolic blood pressure are seen [2, 5]. Routine investigations in the acute phase may show a raised erythrocyte sedimentation rate, leucocytosis, and elevated cardiac enzymes. The ECG demonstrates ST and T wave abnormalities, atrial and ventricular arrhythmias, and conduction block [2]. Pulmonary congestion and cardiomegaly are present on the chest radiograph. Echocardiography is essential in determining the size and haemodynamic effects of any pericardial effusion, the severity of ventricular involvement (which may be regional) and the presence of valvular regurgitation or intracardiac thrombi [5].

The diagnosis of viral cardiomyopathy is based on evidence of recent infection and of myocardial inflammation. However, isolation of virus from stool or body fluids is generally unsuccessful [1] and the criterion of a four-fold rise in antibody titre from paired sera is rarely met. Endomyocardial biopsy can be performed in clinically stable patients and allows the histological diagnosis of myocarditis or DCM and the detection of viral nucleic acids by molecular techniques [1, 5]. This provides prognostic information [5] and can be performed following haemodynamic measurements and coronary angiography as part of assessment for cardiac transplantation. In selected patients, radionuclide scanning with gallium-67- or indium-111-labelled antimyosin antibody may be helpful in identifying myocardial inflammation or damage (6–10].

The treatment for viral heart muscle disease is supportive. Concurrent pericarditis may be treated with non-steroidal anti-inflammatory agents and occasionally with corticosteroids, while cardiac failure is treated with diuretics, digitalis, vasodilators, and angiotensin-converting enzyme inhibitors. Patients in cardiogenic shock may require inotropes, mechanical support, or cardiac transplantation. Tachyarrhythmias may be treated with digitalis and amiodarone, while pacemakers and implantable defibrillators may be required in survivors of cardiac arrest. Anticoagulation as prophylaxis against cardiogenic embolism should be considered with care, given the risk of haemorrhagic pericardial effusion [1, 11].

## Pathophysiology

The pathogenesis of viral myocarditis or DCM is not clear. The wide clinical spectrum of disease, ranging from asymptomatic ECG changes to fulminant heart failure, is dependent on the virulence or persistence of particular viruses, the host immune response to infection and the extent to which cardiac structures are affected. As the diagnosis of viral myocardial disease is often one of exclusion when coronary, valvular, or other causes are absent, the correlation of cardiomyopathy with infection is difficult and frequently not attempted as no definitive therapy is yet available.

Numerous viruses can infect the heart, although the enteroviruses in general and Coxsackie B viruses in particular are thought to be responsible for most viral myocardial diseases [12]. There is no doubt that viruses cause acute myocarditis both in humans and in animal models, as characterized by mononuclear cell infiltrates and myocyte necrosis. One series, documented by the histology of serial endomyocardial biopsies, suggests the progression of clinical myocarditis to DCM [13]. Mouse models of experimental enterovirus infection show that the primary immune response, when virus may be isolated from myocardium, is followed by the development of secondary cellular and humoral autoimmunity [1]. This autoimmunity may continue to cause cardiac damage independently of the effects of the viral infection and so the hypothesis that persistent inflammation leads to the development of DCM is plausible.

Immune system activation is seen in both myocarditis and DCM. Elevated levels of circulating cytokines [14] and their receptors [15] are found in both conditions. Soluble interleukin-2 receptor levels correlate with T-cell activation in the myocardium and are associated with more severe DCM [15]. Autoantibodies against cardiac antigens such as sarcolemma, myofibrils, actin, and myosin are produced following viral myocarditis [16–19]; antibodies to laminin [20], myosin heavy chain [2], myosin light chain-1, tropomyosin, actin [22], $\beta_1$- and $\beta_2$-adrenoceptors [23], muscarinic acetylcholine, and angiotensin II-AT1 receptors [24] are also found in DCM. This autoimmunity may be simply a consequence of cellular necrosis and the exposure of previously occult intracellular antigens, but molecular mimicry between cardiac and viral antigens has been proposed and antibodies against the myolemma [25] and adenine nucleotide translocator (ANT) [26] show some cross-reactivity with enteroviral proteins. Antiheart antibodies found in serum from patients with DCM can mediate complement-dependent cytolysis [22, 27]. Anti-ANT antibody interferes with myocyte energy metabolism [28–30], while the anti-$\beta_1$-adrenoceptor antibody has a positive inotropic effect [23, 31]. The extent of cardiac autoantibody production is reduced in experimental infection with attenuated strains of Coxsackie B virus [32].

Elevated nitric oxide production in response to virus infection may be important in the development of DCM. Excess nitric oxide exerts a negative inotropic effect which exacerbates heart failure [33] and contributes to cardiac dilatation. This hypothesis is supported by the increase in activity of inducible nitric oxide synthase (iNOS) in the myocardium of patients with myocarditis, DCM, or postpartum cardiomyopathy, but not in those with ischaemic or valvular heart disease [34, 35]. The inflammatory cytokine tumour necrosis factor (TNF) $\alpha$ stimulates nitric oxide production and colocalization with iNOS seen in the myocardium of patients with DCM [36, 37]. TNF-$\alpha$ is elevated in hearts explanted from patients with DCM, but not in non-failing donor hearts [38].

The relationship between viral myocarditis and DCM remains open to debate because of the consistent difficulty in culturing viral pathogens from the myocardium of DCM patients [39, 40]. But clinical studies provide circumstantial evidence of this pathophysiological link. High Coxsackie B virus titres are more frequent in patients with DCM than in controls [39, 41] and patients with serological evidence of Coxsackie virus infection may develop chronic impairment of cardiac function after several years [42, 43]. Endomyocardial biopsies from patients with suspected inflammatory heart muscle disease showed histological features ranging from acute myocarditis (7%) to healing myocarditis (29%) and the changes of DCM (64%), in a cohort of 153 patients [1]. In patients with biopsy-proven acute myocarditis, 14–21% subsequently developed DCM [26, 44].

Molecular techniques such as *in situ* hybridization or polymerase chain reaction (PCR) have been used to demonstrate, for example, enteroviral RNA in endomyocardial biopsies from patients with myocarditis or DCM [1, 45] and in explanted hearts following transplantation for DCM [46–50], while cytomegalovirus (CMV) sequences have been detected in tissue from patients with myopericarditis [1]. The presence of enteroviral RNA in DCM is as associated with increased myocardial fibrosis [45] and higher mortality [50, 51].

## Perimyocarditis known virus involvement

### Mumps virus

Severe, often fatal myocarditis was associated with mumps virus infection in 1980 [52, 53]. This viral myocarditis was suspected as an initial step in the pathogenesis of endocardial fibroelastosis (EFE), previously a common disease of children which often resulted in congestive heart failure and death [54]. While the incidence of EFE has declined dramatically during the 1980s and 1990s, myocardial samples analysed recently for association with virus infection showed that 21 of 29 cases (72%) were positive by reverse transcription (RT) PCR for mumps virus RNA sequences, compared with none of 65 control samples; interestingly, adenovirus DNA was detected in the remaining eight cases (28%). These data provide direct evidence of a viral (in particular, mumps) role in the aetiology of EFE [55] and support the view that since the introduction of mumps vaccine, the incidence of mumps virus-induced myocarditis has decreased and so a dramatic decline in the incidence of EFE has been seen. Similarly, future immunization programmes against adenoviruses (types to be determined) and Coxsackie B viruses (see below) may prevent much viral myocardial disease [56].

### Hepatitis C virus

HCV is a single-strand, positive RNA virus and the major cause of non-A, non-B hepatitis; it was recovered as a complementary DNA clone from virus genomic RNA in sera. Anti-HCV antibodies in sera and the PCR-based detection of HCV RNA in sera or in myocardial samples from patients with DCM have been reported from Japan [57], but a significant association between HCV infection and myocardial diseases was not seen in other geographical regions. Of 102 patients with established chronic HCV infection and 55 patients with DCM in north-western Greece, none of the patients with chronic HCV had evidence of DCM from history and laboratory findings and none of the patients with DCM had antibodies to HCV or was viraemic on testing for HCV RNA [58]. A low prevalence of HCV antibodies or virus RNA in patients with myocarditis or DCM was also observed in Germany [59]. Investigation of HCV involvement in myocardial disease is still at an early stage.

### Adenoviruses

Adenoviruses are a group of double-stranded, linear DNA viruses containing at least 47 human serotypes, based on serological neutralization. They cause mainly respiratory tract infections, conjunctivitis and infant diarrhoea, although some serotypes are more frequently associated with a particular disease than others, e.g. serotypes 8, 19, and 37 with epidemic keratoconjunctivitis [4].

There are early reports of adenovirus-associated myocarditis, particularly in children [60], although research in this area is recent. Among 26 of 38 (68%) myocardial samples from patients with acute myocarditis found positive for viral genomic sequences by PCR, 15 (22%) contained adenovirus DNA while eight (12%) contained enterovirus RNA; all 17 comparison samples from patients with congenital heart disease or hypertrophic cardiomyopathy and associated blood samples were negative [61]. As few as ten copies of adenovirus genomic DNA can be detected by PCR in formalin-fixed, paraffin-embedded tissue; archival tissue examined by PCR permitted a retrospective diagnosis of adenoviral myocarditis in two paediatric patients [62]. Of 29 myocardial samples from patients with autopsy-proven EFE investigated similarly, 21 (72%) were positive for mumps viral RNA (see above) but adenovirus DNA was detected in eight, supporting an aetiological role in EFE and the hypothesis that EFE is a sequela of viral myocarditis [55]. Recent identification of a receptor common for adenovirus and Coxsackie B virus may explain why these two unrelated agents both cause myocardial disease [63].

### Human cytomegalovirus

Like other human herpesviruses, CMV persists in various tissues following primary infection, due to a mechanism of latency fundamental to its replication. Latent CMV is widespread in the population. Virus reactivation is seen frequently in immunosuppression, whether iatrogenic (e.g. following transplantation), associated with infection (e.g. HIV) or with malignancy. CMV infection is associated with atherosclerosis [64] and there are sporadic reports implicating CMV as a cause of myocardial disease. A 60-year-old woman developed CMV myocarditis following a respiratory infection [65], CMV was isolated from the explanted heart of a patient who developed DCM following cardiac transplantation [66] and CMV-induced myocarditis has been seen in previously healthy persons [67]. Again, recent evidence of an association with myocardial diseases was obtained by *in situ* hybridization and PCR. Endomyocardial biopsies from 27 patients with a histological diagnosis of active myocarditis, 35 with healing myocarditis, 41 with healed myocarditis, 25 with ongoing myocarditis, and 52 with dilated cardiomyopathy were compared with tissue from 25 healthy heart donors [68]. CMV DNA was detected in the myocardium in 5–14% of patients with different stages of myocarditis and in 22% of patients with DCM. Virus DNA was localized to all cell types, including cardiac myocytes, in the patient group but was restricted to interstitial cells only in the two positive samples of 25 in the comparison group. Investigation of paraffin-embedded endomyocardial biopsy specimens from a different ethnic group of patients with myocardial diseases gave similar results [69].

### Herpes simplex virus

Like human CMV, herpes simplex virus (HSV) is occasionally detected in patients with myocardial disease. In a survey of the frequency of different viruses implicated in myocarditis, PCR was used to investigate myocardial tissue from patients with suspected acute viral myocarditis and from a comparison group with congenital heart disease or hypertrophic cardiomyopathy. Viral sequences were detected in 26 of 38 (68%) myocarditic samples and were mostly adenovirus or enterovirus, but were HSV in two instances and CMV in one; all myocardial and associated blood samples from the comparison group were negative [61].

### Human immunodeficiency virus

While HIV primarily infects $CD4^+$ T-helper cells, it is clear that many tissues can be damaged directly or indirectly by the virus and that heart muscle disease is emerging as a significant cause of morbidity in patients with acquired immunodeficiency syndrome (AIDS) consequent on HIV infection [70, 71]. All parts of the heart can be affected and while the true prevalence of myocarditis in HIV infection is not yet clear, it was found postmortem in 37 of 71 (52%) AIDS patients [72]. Some of these cases were not recognized until postmortem examination and there was no evidence of secondary infection, suggesting that HIV was the primary agent of myocyte damage [72, 73]. HIV-induced damage to cardiac myocytes may also occur indirectly through autoimmune mechanisms as high levels of circulating cardiac autoantibodies are found in HIV patients with myocardial disease [3]. This is accompanied by induction of class I major histocompatiability complex (MHC) antigens within the myocardium. Other mechanisms of myocarditis in HIV infection are various opportunistic infections consequent on immunosuppression [74] including *Toxoplasma* [75], CMV [76], *Cryptococcus neoformans* [77, 78], *Histoplasma capsulatum* [79], and *Aspergillus fumigatus* [80].

Myocardial disease other than myocarditis has been seen in HIV infection, particularly in late-stage disease [81], and is referred to as HIV heart muscle disease. Heart failure was described in three HIV-positive patients [82]. Postmortem examination of two showed global dilatation of the cardiac chambers; there was no evidence of coronary artery disease or myocarditis. Several *in vivo* or retrospective postmortem studies have confirmed the existence of HIV heart muscle disease [75, 83, 84], and the presence of cardiac dysfunction in late-stage HIV infection is a particularly poor prognostic factor [85].

### Enteroviruses

Enteroviruses are a group of more than 65 serotypes within the family picornavirus. They are small, non-enveloped viruses with a single-stranded, positive (messenger function) RNA genome of about 7.4 kilobases (kb). The route of infection is mainly faecal–oral (although it can be respiratory), usually resulting in trivial or subclinical enteric disease involving limited virus replication in lymphoid tissue in the gut. In a proportion of cases, there is spread via the lymphatics, a transient viraemia, and an episode of febrile illness. In a proportion of those, particular enteroviruses may then replicate cytolytically in tissues for which they have a tropism, including heart, pancreas, or elements of the central nervous system, leading to significant disease. The frequency of infection with these ubiquitous pathogens means that these uncommon disease progressions are a major public-health problem [86]. Some serotypes, particularly the Coxsackie viruses, are myotropic and members of the Coxsackie B group are strongly associated with human heart muscle disease. The prototype Coxsackie virus B3, strain Nancy, was isolated in 1949 in Connecticut [87].

That enteroviruses are the most common human agents of viral myocarditis and cardiomyopathy was shown by early virological and retrospective serological studies [12, 39, 88, 89]. More recent investigations using molecular biological techniques such as slot-blot hybridization [46, 47], *in situ* hybridization [90–92], reverse transcription PCR, or nested PCR [93–95] confirm these observations and the association of enterovirus infection with myocardial disease has been extensively reviewed [96]. The presence of enteroviral RNA in the myocardium is a significant independent factor in predicting poor prognosis in DCM [50].

Many studies have focused on the detection of any of a range of enterovirus serotypes implicated in various cases by using group-specific hybridization probes or PCR primers, usually targeting conserved regions of the enteroviral genome such as 5′- or 3′-non-translated regions or the viral RNA polymerase gene. To characterize the enteroviruses involved in myocardial disease, the high sensitivity of reverse transcription-nested PCR (RT-NPCR) has been coupled to direct nucleotide sequencing of the PCR products. In a prospective investigation of 35 consecutive endomyocardial biopsies nine of 21 (42.9%) patients with a histologically confirmed diagnosis of DCM were positive for enterovirus by RT-NPCR compared with only one of 14 (7.1%) patients with other myocardial pathologies (odds ratio 9.75). The nucleotide sequence of the PCR products differed, indicating no cross-contamination. However, a computerized comparison showed that each had the greatest homology with the 5′-non-translated region of Coxsackie B virus, but contained up to 11% sequence variations compared with prototype Coxsackie B3 strain [93]. Repetitive direct sequencing of the uncloned PCR products from a mouse model of Coxsackie virus B3-induced myocarditis or from other prototype enteroviruses demonstrates that this generates accurate consensus DNA sequence data and that random errors introduced into individual amplicons by reverse transcription and enzymatic amplification are not seen [97]. In a recent interlaboratory trial, five of eight experimental samples were made positive for enteroviral RNA and supplied blinded. Each positive sample was detected by RT-NPCR, with no false positives. Direct sequencing of the PCR products correctly identified the Coxsackie virus B3 variant employed [98] with no sequence errors, the results matching the sample provider's data (B. Maisch, personal communication). Although RT-PCR of RNA extracted from fixed-embedded tissue is more difficult than from frozen tissue, one such study found enterovirus sequences in five of six myocardial samples with histological evidence of myocarditis but in none of eight control samples; again, direct nucleotide sequencing identified these as being most closely related to group B Coxsackie viruses [99]. These data suggest that the enteroviruses most often associated with human heart muscle disease are natural variants of Coxsackie virus B3, although frequently the sequence determined was from the 5′-non-translated region rather than the capsid protein coding region which ultimately defines serotype. These data support the link between enteroviral infection and dilated heart muscle disease and suggest that Coxsackie B serotypes are particularly cardiovirulent. This approach has also been useful in genetic typing of other clinical isolates of enteroviruses [100].

While the association with infection is clear, the pathogenesis of enterovirus-induced myocardial disease remains contentious. Enteroviruses generally replicate cytolytically and some myocardial damage results directly from virus replication in myocytes and other cardiac cells. This invokes a cellular immune response *in vivo* with the induction of inflammatory cytokines, nitric oxide synthase, and a mononuclear cell infiltration; T-cell-mediated cytolysis produces the characteristic histopathology of acute focal myocarditis. However, immunopathology following virus infection also has a role in myocardial damage and disease progression; as noted previously, patients with myocarditis or DCM have autoantibodies directed against various cardiac antigens [101, 102]. Experimental studies show increases in antimyosin heavy chain, antiactin, and antitropomyosin antiheart antibodies in mice infected with cardiovirulent CVB3. These were not seen in mock-infected mice and were significantly less in mice receiving an attenuated virus derived directly from the cardiovirulent wild-type [32, 56]. The relative importance of immunopathological factors differs in genetically different mice; experimental enteroviral myocarditis in Balb/c or DBA/2 mice is progressed by cellular or humoral mechanisms, respectively [103, 104], while animals with severe combined immunodeficiency (SCID) have fulminant disease. These results suggest that attenuation of cardiovirulence may involve failure to induce immunopathogenic mechanisms, possibly through reduced levels of virus replication. Comparative nucleotide sequence analysis of cardiovirulent Coxsackie B3, an attenuated mutant derived from it, and a subsequent revertant to virulence has identified several changes related to attenuation [105]. The relative effect of these is not yet known, although analogously with attenuation of neurovirulence in poliovirus, a change within the 5′-non-translated region seems important.

Increased activity of inducible nitric oxide synthase (iNOS) produces excess nitric oxide (NO), which plays a role in inflammatory myocardial disease [34, 35]. Increased expression of iNOS is associated with increased severity of myocarditis and contractile depression [106]. This is confirmed in mouse models of CVB3-induced myocarditis where iNOS increased by day 4 and peaked on day 8 after infection; iNOS messenger RNA in heart was detected by RT-PCR on day 4 and remained elevated for 1 month [107, 108]. Attenuated mutants of CVB3 induce less NOS. However, the cytotoxic effector molecule, NO, also inhibits enterovirus replication. CVB3-infected mice fed NOS inhibitors had increased titres of virus and higher mortality [109]. Coxsackie virus B3 replicates to higher titres and myocarditis is more severe in homozygous iNOS knockout (NOS2 −/−) mice. These results demonstrate that NO is required at an appropriate level in the host response to Coxsackie virus infection.

Inflammation is not a feature of DCM yet enterovirus RNA can be detected in the myocardium from some cases presumed a postinflammatory sequela of a previous viral myocarditis [45, 46, 91, 93, 94] and is a predictor of poor prognosis [50]. Evidence of persisting enterovirus is seen even in some cases of end-stage disease requiring cardiac transplantation [47]. The mechanism by which a cytolytic virus which normally replicates productively is able to persist in myocardium without attracting an inflammatory response is not known. The emergence of replication-defective mutants in which sequence changes alter the specificity of the viral RNA-dependent RNA polymerase or a cleavage site for the major viral protease has been proposed.

## Outlook

Antiviral agents are available and used empirically in patients with CMV, herpes, and HIV infections, and potentially may prevent the development of DCM following viral myocarditis. Despite the initial inflammatory response to virus infection of the myocardium and the known immunopathogenic factors in the progression to DCM, there is no clear benefit from immunomodulatory treatments. An extensive randomized trial of immunosuppression in myocarditis found no improvement in myocardial function or survival and its use remains controversial [110]. The use of interferon-α or thymic hormones [111] or the immunoadsorption of immunoglobulins [112, 113] shows some promise in small studies. As enteroviruses, predominantly Coxsackie B3, seem to be the most common agents of human heart muscle disease, a more directed approach is justified. Given that stable, attenuated strains that induce CVB3-specific neutralizing antibodies and protect mice against subsequent challenge with cardiovirulent wild-type virus exist [56], should another component be added to the sugar lump in the poliovirus immunization programme?

## References

1. Richardson PJ, Why HJF, Maisch B. Myocarditis, myopericarditis and DCM. In: D Julian, J Camm, K Fox *et al.* (eds) *Diseases of the heart*. WB Saunders, London, 1996, 489.
2. Peters NS, Poole-Wilson PA. Myocarditis — continuing clinical and pathologic confusion. *Am Heart* 1991; 121: 942.
3. Herskowitz A, Ansari AA. Myocarditis. In: WH Abelmann, E Braunwald (eds) *Cardiomyopathies, myocarditis and pericardial disease. Atlas of heart diseases*. Volume 2. Philadelphia, PA: Current Medicine, 1995.
4. Sharp IR, Wadell G, Adenovirus. In: AJ Zuckerman, JE Banatvala, JR Pattison (eds) *Principles and practice of clinical virology*. 3rd edition. New York: John Wiley & Sons, 1994.
5. Richardson P, Chin D. Dilated cardiomyopathy. In: S Dalla Volta (ed.) *Cardiology*. London: McGraw-Hill, 1999, 581.
6. Marti V, Coll P, Ballester M *et al.* Enterovirus persistence and myocardial damage detected by $^{111}$In-monoclonal antimyosin antibodies in patients with dilated cardiomyopathy. *Eur Heart J* 1996; 17: 545–9.
7. Matsumori A, Yamada T, Sasayama S. Antimyosin antibody imaging in clinical myocarditis and cardiomyopathy: principle and application. *Int J Cardiol* 1996; 54: 183.
8. O'Connell JB, Robinson JA, Henkin RE, Gunnar RM. Immunosuppressive therapy in patients with congestive cardiomyopathy and myocardial uptake of gallium-67. *Circulation* 1981; 64: 780.
9. Rezkella S, Khoer RA, Khaw BA *et al.* Detection of experimental myocarditis by monoclonal antimyosin antibody FAB fragments. *Am Heart J* 1989; 117: 391.
10. Yasuda TS, Palacios IF, Dec W *et al.* Indium-111 monoclonal antimyosin antibody imaging in the diagnosis of acute myocarditis. *Circulation* 1987; 76: 306.
11. Wynne J, Braunwald E. The cardiomyopathies and myocarditides. In: E Braunwald (ed.) *Heart disease — a textbook of cardiovascular medicine*. 5th edition. Philadelphia, PA: WB Saunders, 1997, 1404.

12. Woodruff JF. Viral myocarditis: a review. *Am J Pathol* 1980; 101: 427.
13. Quigley PJ, Richardson PJ, Meany BT *et al.* Long-term follow-up of acute myocarditis. Correlation of ventricular function and outcome. *Eur Heart J* 1987; 8 (Suppl J): 39.
14. Matsumori A, Yamada T, Suzuki H *et al.* Increased circulating cytokines in patients with myocarditis and cardiomyopathy. *Br Heart J* 1994; 72: 561.
15. Limas CJ, Goldenberg IF, Limas C. Soluble interleukin-2 receptor levels in patients with DCM. Correlation with disease severity and cardiac autoantibodies. *Circulation* 1995; 91: 631.
16. Maisch B, Trostel-Soeder R, Stechermesser E *et al.* Diagnostic relevance of humoral and cell-mediated immune reactions in patients with acute viral myocarditis. *Clin Exp Immunol* 1982; 48: 533.
17. Maisch B. Surface antigens of adult heart cells and their use in diagnosis. *Basic Res Cardiol* 1985; 80 (Suppl 1): 47.
18. Maisch B, Bueschel G, Izumi T *et al.* Four years of experience in endomyocardial biopsy. An immunohistologic approach. *Heart Vessels* 1985; (Suppl 1): 59.
19. Wittner B, Maisch B, Kochsiek K. Quantification of antimyosin antibodies in experimental myocarditis by a new solid-phase fluorometric assay. *J Immunol Methods* 1983; 64: 239.
20. Wolff PG, Kuhl U, Schultheiss HP. Laminin distribution and autoantibodies to laminin in DCM and myocarditis. *Am Heart J* 1989; 117: 1303.
21. Caforio ALP, Grazzini M, Mann JM *et al.* Identification of alpha- and beta-cardiac myosin heavy chain isoforms as major autoantigens in DCM. *Circulation* 1992; 85: 1734.
22. Latif N, Baker CS, Dunn MJ *et al.* Frequency and specificity of anti-heart antibodies in patients with DCM detected using SDS–PAGE and Western blotting. *J Am Coll Cardiol* 1993; 22: 1378.
23. Chiale PA, Rosenbaum MB, Elizari MV *et al.* High prevalence of antibodies against beta-1 and beta-2 adrenoceptors in patients with primary electrical cardiac abnormalities. *J Am Coll Cardiol* 1995; 26: 864.
24. Matsui S, Fu ML. Distribution of serum autoantibodies against G-protein coupled cardiovascular receptors in Japanese patients with cardiomyopathy. *Blood Press* 1996; Suppl 3: 328.
25. Maisch B, Bauer E, Cirsi M, Kochsiek K. Cytolytic cross-reactive antibodies directed against the cardiac membrane and viral proteins in Coxsackie B3 and B4 myocarditis — characterisation and pathogenetic relevance. *Circulation* 1993; 87 (Suppl): IV49.
26. Schwimbeck PL, Schultheiss HP, Strauer BE. Identification of a main autoimmunogenic epitope of the adenine nucleotide translocator which cross-reacts with coxsackie B3 virus. use in the diagnosis of myocarditis and DCM. *Circulation* 1989; 80 (Suppl II): II642.
27. Latif N, Smith J, Dunn MJ *et al.* Complement-mediated cytotoxic activity of anti-heart antibodies present in the sera of patients with DCM. *Autoimmunity* 1994; 119: 99.
28. Schultheiss HP. The significance of autoantibodies against the ADP/ATP carrier for the pathogenesis of myocarditis and DCM: clinical and experimental data. *Springer Semin Immunopathol* 1989; 11: 15.
29. Schulze K, Becker BF, Schultheiss HP. Antibodies to the ADP/ATP carrier, an autoantigen in myocarditis and DCM, penetrate into myocardial cells and disturb energy metabolism *in vivo*. *Circ Res* 1989; 64: 179.
30. Schulze K, Becker BF, Strauer B, Schultheiss HP. Antibodies to ADP/ATP carrier — an autoantigen in myocarditis and DCM — impair cardiac function. *Circulation* 1990; 81: 959.
31. Magnusson Y, Wallukat G, Waagstein F *et al.* Autoimmunity in idiopathic DCM. Characterization of antibodies against the beta-1 adrenoceptor with positive chronotropic effect. *Circulation* 1994; 89: 2760.
32. Latif N, Zhang HY, Archard LC *et al.* Characterisation of anti-heart antibodies in mice after infection with Coxsackie B3 virus. *Clin Immunol* (in press).
33. de Belder A, Moncada S. Cardiomyopathy: a role for nitric oxide? *Int J Cardiol* 1995; 50: 263.
34. de Belder A, Radomski MW, Why HJ *et al.* Nitric oxide synthase activities in human myocardium. *Lancet* 1993; 341: 84.
35. de Belder A, Radomski MW, Why HJ *et al.* Myocardial calcium-independent nitric oxide synthase activity is present in DCM, myocarditis and postpartum cardiomyopathy but not in ischaemic or valvar heart disease. *Br Heart J* 1995; 74: 426.
36. Habib FM, Springall DR, Davies GJ *et al.* Tumour necrosis factor and inducible nitric oxide synthase in DCM. *Lancet* 1996; 347: 1151–5.
37. Satoh M, Nakamura M, Tamura G *et al.* Inducible nitric oxide synthase and tumour necrosis factor-alpha in myocardium in human DCM. *J Am Coll Cardiol* 1997; 29: 716.
38. Torre-Amione G, Kapadia S, Lee J *et al.* Tumour necrosis factor-alpha and tumour necrosis factor receptors in the failing human heart. *Circulation* 1996; 93: 704.
39. Cambridge G, MacArthur CGC, Waterston AP *et al.* Antibodies to Coxsackie B viruses in congestive cardiomyopathy. *Br Heart J* 1979; 41: 692.
40. Morgan-Capner P, Richardson PJ, McSorley C *et al.* Virus investigations in heart muscle disease. In HD Bolte (ed.) *Viral heart disease*. Berlin: Springer, 1984, 99.
41. Kawai C. Idiopathic cardiomyopathy. A study on the infectious immune theory as a cause of the disease. *Jpn Circ J* 1971; 35: 765.
42. Levi GF, Proto C, Quadri A, Ratti S. Coxsackie virus heart disease and cardiomyopathy. *Am Heart J* 1977; 93: 419.
43. Levi GF, Scalvini S, Volterrani M *et al.* Coxsackie virus heart disease. 15 years later. *Eur Heart J* 1988; 9 (Suppl J): 1303.
44. Hiramitsu S, Morimoto S, Uemura A *et al.* Long-term outcome of 28 patients with viral or idiopathic myocarditis. In: M Sekiguchi, PJ Richardson (eds) *Prognosis and treatment of cardiomyopathies and myocarditis*. Tokyo: University of Tokyo Press, 1994, 201.
45. Satoh M, Tamura G, Segawa I *et al.* Enteroviral RNA in DCM. *Eur Heart J* 1994; 15: 934.
46. Bowles NE, Richardson PJ, Olsen EJ, Archard LC. Detection of Coxsackie B virus specific sequences in myocardial biopsies from cases of myocarditis and dilated cardiomyopathy. *Lancet* 1986; i: 1120–2.
47. Bowles NE, Rose ML, Taylor P *et al.* End-stage DCM: persistence of enterovirus RNA in myocardium at cardiac transplantation and lack of immune response. *Circulation* 1989; 80: 1128.
48. Hilton DA, Variend S, Pringle JH. Demonstration of Coxsackie virus RNA in formalin-fixed tissue sections from childhood myocarditis cases by *in situ* hybridization and the polymerase chain reaction. *J Pathol* 1993; 170: 45–51.
49. Kandolf R, Canu A, Klinger K *et al.* Molecular studies in enteroviral heart diseases. In: MA Brinton, FX Henry (eds) *New aspects of positive-strand RNA viruses*. Washington, DC: American Society for Microbiology, 1990, 340.

50. Why HJF, Meany BT, Richardson PJ *et al.* Clinical and prognostic significance of detection of enteroviral RNA in the myocardium of patients with myocarditis or DCM. *Circulation* 1994; 89: 2582.
51. Sekiguchi M, Shin-ichi N, Hiroe M, Richardson PJ. Prognosis of patients with acute viral myocarditis in whom endomyocardial biopsies and/or autopsies were performed. an ISFC survey. In: M Sekiguchi, PJ Richardson (eds) *Prognosis and treatment of cardiomyopathies and myocarditis*. Tokyo: University of Tokyo Press, 1994, 189.
52. Arita M, Ueno Y, Masuyama Y. Complete heart block in mumps myocarditis. *Br Heart J* 1981; 46: 342–4.
53. Brown NJ, Richmond SJ. Fatal mumps myocarditis in an 8-month-old child. *BMJ* 1980; 281: 356–7.
54. St Geme JW Jr, Peralta J, Farias E *et al.* Experimental gestational mumps virus infection and endocardial fibroelastosis. *Pediatrics* 1971; 48: 821–6.
55. Ni J, Bowles NE, Kim YH *et al.* Viral infection of the myocardium in endocardial fibroelastosis. Molecular evidence for the role of mumps virus as an etiologic agent. *Circulation* 1997; 95: 133–9.
56. Zhang H, Morgan-Capner P, Pandolfino YA *et al.* Coxsackievirus B3-induced myocarditis: characterisation of stable attenuated variants which protect against infection with the wild-type strain. *Am J Pathol* 1997; 150: 2197–208.
57. Matsumori A, Matoba Y, Sasayama S. Dilated cardiomyopathy associated with hepatitis C virus infection. *Circulation* 1995; 92: 2519–25.
58. Dalekos GN, Achenbach K, Christodoulou D *et al.* Idiopathic dilated cardiomyopathy: lack of association with hepatitis C virus infection. *Heart* 1998; 80: 270–5.
59. Grumbach IM, Heermann K, Figulla HR. Low prevalence of hepatitis C virus antibodies and RNA in patients with myocarditis and dilated cardiomyopathy. *Cardiology* 1998; 90: 75–8.
60. Henson D, Mufson MA. Myocarditis and pneumonitis with type 21 adenovirus infection. Association with fatal myocarditis and pneumonitis. *Am J Dis Child* 1971; 121: 334–6.
61. Martin AB, Webber S, Fricker FJ *et al.* Acute myocarditis. Rapid diagnosis by PCR in children. *Circulation* 1994; 90: 330–9.
62. Lozinski GM, Davis GG, Krous HF *et al.* Adenovirus myocarditis: retrospective diagnosis by gene amplification from formalin-fixed, paraffin-embedded tissues. *Hum Pathol* 1994; 25: 831–4.
63. Bergelson JM, Cunningham JA, Droguett G *et al.* Isolation of a common receptor for Coxsackie B viruses and adenoviruses 2 and 5. *Science* 1997; 275: 1320–3.
64. Adam E, Melnick JL, DeBakey ME. Cytomegalovirus infection and atherosclerosis. *Cent Eur J Public Health* 1997; 5: 99–106.
65. Wilson RSE, Morris TII, Rees JR. Cytomegalovirus myocarditis. *Br Heart J* 1972; 34: 865–8.
66. Gowna TA, Capehart JE, Pilcher JW, Alivizatos PA. Cytomegalovirus myocarditis as a cause of cardiac dysfunction in a heart transplant recipient. *Transplantation* 1989; 47: 197–8.
67. Waris E, Raesaenen O, Kreus KE, Kreus R. Fatal cytomegalovirus disease in a previously healthy adult. *Scand J Infect Dis* 1972; 4: 61–7.
68. Schonian U, Crombach M, Maser S, Maisch B. Cytomegalovirus-associated heart muscle disease. *Eur Heart J* 1995; 16 Suppl O: 46–9.
69. Li W, Crombach M, Schonian U *et al.* Detection of cytomegalovirus genome by in situ hybridization in paraffin embedded endomyocardial biopsy specimens of viral myocarditis. *Chin Med J (Engl)* 1994; 107: 888–91.
70. Acierno LJ. Cardiac complications in acquired immunodeficiency syndrome (AIDS): a review. *J Am Coll Cardiol* 1989; 13: 1144–54.
71. Herskowitz A, Willoughby SB, Vlahov D *et al.* Dilated heart muscle disease associated with HIV infection. *Eur Heart J* 1995; 16 (Suppl O): 50–5.
72. Anderson DW, Virmani R, Reilly JM *et al.* Prevalent myocarditis at necropsy in the acquired immunodeficiency syndrome. *J Am Coll Cardiol* 1988; 11: 792–9.
73. Baroldi G, Corallo S, Moroni M *et al.* Focal lymphocytic myocarditis in acquired immunodeficiency syndrome (AIDS): a correlative morphologic and clinical study in 26 consecutive fatal cases. *Am Coll Cardiol* 1988; 12: 463–9.
74. Lewes D, Rainfall DJ, Lane WE. Symptomless myocarditis and myalgia in viral and mycoplasma pneumoniae infections. *Br Heart J* 1974; 36: 924.
75. Adair OV, Randive N, Krasnow N. Isolated toxoplasma myocarditis in acquired immunodeficiency syndrome. *Am Heart J* 1989; 118: 856–7.
76. Drew WL. Other virus infections in AIDS. I. Cytomegalovirus. *Immunol Ser* 1989; 44: 507–34.
77. Cammarosano C, Lewis W. Cardiac lesions in acquired immune deficiency syndrome (AIDS). *J Am Coll Cardiol* 1985; 5: 7036.
78. Lafont A, Wolff M, Marche C *et al.* Overwhelming myocarditis due to *Cryptococcus neoformans* in an AIDS patient. *Lancet* 1987; ii: 1145–6.
79. Altieri PI, Climent C, Lazala G *et al.* Opportunistic invasion of the heart in Hispanic patients with acquired immunodeficiency syndrome. *Am J Trop Med Hyg* 1994; 51: 56–9.
80. Cox JN, di Dio F, Pizzolato GP *et al.* *Aspergillus* endocarditis and myocarditis in a patient with the acquired immunodeficiency syndrome (AIDS). A review of the literature. *Virchows Arch A Pathol Anat Histopathol* 1990; 417: 255–9.
81. Levy WS, Simon GL, Rios JC, Ross AM. Prevalence of cardiac abnormalities in human immunodeficiency virus infection. *Am J Cardiol* 1989; 63: 86–9.
82. Cohen IS, Anderson DW, Virmani R *et al.* Congestive cardiomyopathy in association with the acquired immunodeficiency syndrome. *N Engl J Med* 1986; 315: 628–30.
83. Blanchard DG, Hagenhoff C, Chow LC *et al.* Reversibility of cardiac abnormalities in human immunodeficiency virus (HIV)-infected individuals: a serial echocardiographic study. *J Am Coll Cardiol* 1991; 17: 1270–6.
84. Corallo S, Mutinelli MR, Moroni M *et al.* Echocardiography detects myocardial damage in AIDS: prospective study in 102 patients. *Eur Heart J* 1988; 9: 887–92.
85. Himelman RB, Chung WS, Chernoff DN *et al.* Cardiac manifestations of human immunodeficiency virus infection: a two-dimensional echocardiographic study. *Am Coll Cardiol* 1989; 13: 1030–6.
86. Melnick JL. Enteroviruses: polioviruses, coxsackieviruses, echoviruses, and newer enteroviruses. In: BN Field *et al.* (eds) *Virology*. 3rd edition. New York: Lippincott-Raven, 1996; 655–712.
87. Melnick JL, Ledinko N. Immunological reactions of the coxsackie viruses I. The neutralisation test: technic and application. *J Exp Med* 1950; 92: 463–82.

88. El-Hagrassy MMO, Banatvala JE, Coltart DJ. Coxsackie B virus IgM responses in patients with cardiac and other diseases. *Lancet* 1980; ii: 1160–2.
89. Grist NR, Bell EJ. A six year study of coxsackie B virus infections in heart disease. *J Hygiene* 1984; 73: 165–72.
90. Easton AJ, Eglin RP. The detection of coxsackievirus RNA in cardiac tissue by *in situ* hybridisation. *J Gen Virol* 1988; 69: 285–91.
91. Kandolf R. The impact of recombinant DNA technology on the study of enteroviral heart disease. In: M Bendinelli, H Friedman (eds) *Coxsackieviruses: a general update*. New York: Plenum Press, 1988, 293–318.
92. Tracy S, Chapman NM, McManus BM *et al.* A molecular and serologic evaluation of enteroviral envolvement in human myocarditis. *JM Cell Cardiol* 1990; 22: 403–14.
93. Archard LC, Khan MA, Soteriou BA *et al.* Characterisation of Coxsackie B virus RNA in myocardium from patients with dilated cardiomyopathy by nucleotide sequencing of reverse-transcription-nested polymerase chain reaction products. *Hum Pathol* 1998; 29: 578–84.
94. Jin O, Sole MJ, Butany JW *et al.* Detection of enterovirus RNA in myocardial biopsies from patients with myocarditis and cardiomyopathy using gene amplification by polymerase chain reaction. *Circulation* 1990; 82: 8–16.
95. Weiss LM, Movahed LA, Billingham ME, Leary ML. Detection of coxsackievirus B3 RNA in myocardial tissues by the polymerase chain reaction. *Am J Pathol* 1991; 138: 497–503.
96. Baboonian C, Davies MJ, Booth JC, McKenna WJ. Coxsackie B viruses and human heart disease. In: S Tracy, NM Chapman, BWJ Mahy (eds) *The Coxsackie B viruses*. Berlin: Springer, 1997, 31–32.
97. Zhang H, Soteriou B, Knowlson S *et al.* Characterisation of genomic RNA of Coxsackievirus B3 in murine myocarditis: reliability of direct sequencing of reverse transcription-nested polymerase chain reaction products. *J Virol Meth* 1997; 69: 7–17.
98. Knowlton KU, Jeon ES, Berkley N *et al.* A mutation in the puff region of VP2 attenuates the myocarditic phenotype of an infectious cDNA of the Woodruff variant of coxsackievirus B3. *J Virol* 1996; 70: 7811–18.
99. Nicholson F, Ajetunmobi JF, Li M *et al.* Molecular detection and serotypic analysis of enterovirus RNA in archival specimens from patients with acute myocarditis. *British Heart J* 1995; 74: 522–7.
100. Arola A, Santti J, Ruuskanen O *et al.* Identification of enteroviruses in clinical specimens by competitive PCR fellowed by genetic typing using sequence analysis. *J Clin Microbiol* 1996; 34: 313–18.
101. Maisch B, Berg PA, Kochsiek K. Clinical significance of immunopathological findings in patients with post-pericardiotomy syndrome. I. Relevance of antibody pattern. *Clin Exp Immunol* 1979; 38: 189–97.
102. Maisch B, Deeg P, Liebau G, Kochsiek K. Diagnostic relevance of humoral and cytotoxic immune reactions in primary and secondary dilated cardiomyopathy. *Am J Cardiol* 1983; 52: 1072–8.
103. Huber SA, Lodge PA Coxsackievirus B-3 myocarditis. Identification of different pathogenic mechanisms in DAB/2 and Balb/c mice. *Am J Pathol* 1984; 122: 284–91.
104. Liao L, Sindhwani R, Rojkind M *et al.* Antibody-mediated autoimmune myocarditis depends on genetically determined target organ sensitivity. *J Exp Med* 1995; 181: 1123–31.
105. Cameron-Wilson CL, Pandolfino YA, Zhang HY *et al.* Nucleotide sequence of an attenuated mutant of Coxsackievirus B3 compared with the cardiovirulent wildtype: assessment of candidate mutations by analysis of a revertant to cardiovirulence. *Clin Diagn Virol* 1998; 9: 99–105.
106. Freeman GL, Colston JT, Zabalgoitia M, Chandrasekar B. Contractile depression and expression of proinflammatory cytokines and iNOS in viral myocarditis. *Am J Physiol* 1998; 274: H249–58.
107. Mikami S, Kawashima S, Kanazawa K *et al.* Expression of nitric oxide synthase in a murine model of viral myocarditis induced by coxsackievirus B3. *Biochem Biophys Res Commun* 1996; 220: 983–9.
108. Zhang H, Bevan A, Inniss H *et al.* Differential expression of inducible nitric oxide synthase in murine myocardium infected with wildtype or attenuated Coxsackievirus B3. *Biochem Soc Trans* 1997; 25: 415S.
109. Lowenstein CJ, Hill SL, Lafond-Walker A *et al.* Nitric oxide inhibits viral replication in murine myocarditis. *Clin Invest* 1996; 97: 1837–43.
110. Mason JW, O'Connell JB, Herskowitz A *et al.* A clinical trial of immunosuppressive therapy for myocarditis. *N Engl J Med* 1995; 333: 269.
111. Miric M, Vasiljevic J, Bojic M *et al.* Long-term follow-up of patients with dilated heart muscle disease treated with human leucocytic interferon alpha or thymic hormones. Initial results. *Heart* 1996; 75: 596.
112. Doerffel WV, Felix SB, Wallukat G *et al.* Short-term haemodynamic effects of immunoadsorption in DCM. *Circulation* 1997; 95: 1994.
113. Wallukat G, Reinke P, Doerffel WV *et al.* Removal of autoantibodies in DCM by immunoadsorption. *Int J Cardiol* 1996; 54: 191.

# Autoimmune basis of myocardial disease 16

M. FU AND F. WAAGSTEIN

## Introduction

The heart is susceptible to immune-mediated injury during or after an immune response to endogenous or exogenous cardiac antigens. Such immune-mediated myocyte injury may be either reversible, with manifestations of a transient depression of ventricular function and/or electrical instability, or irreversible, leading ultimately to myocyte necrosis. The mechanisms of immune-mediated injury are mainly classified into humoral or cellular immunity. Humoral immunity requires recognition of epitope(s) by antibody molecules expressed by B-lymphocytes. It depends on circulating antibodies to initiate injury, mainly through the activation of complements via the classical pathway, involving binding of the C1 component by an antigen–antibody complex on the surface of the target cell. A cascade of reactions is initiated that results in the formation of the membrane attack complex, which is arranged into a plasma membrane pore. Cellular immunity may be another mechanism underlying cardiac dysfunction. Normally, cellular immunity is initiated when antigen-specific T-lymphocytes recognize an immunogenic epitope. This initial recognition and subsequent activation are effected by helper T-cells, and require the presence of histocompatible antigen-presenting cells (APCs). The presentation of myocardial antigens to T-lymphocytes by APCs can result in the clonal expansion and differentiation of cytotoxic T-cells, stimulated by the release of immune cytokines. The consequent myocyte necrosis results in fibrosis [1, 2].

In dilated cardiomyopathy and myocarditis, abnormalities in cell-mediated immunity have been demonstrated clinically by the findings of altered lymphocyte function, altered relative proportions of lymphocyte subsets, an activated immune cytokine system, inappropriate expression of the major histocompatibility complex on cardiac tissue, and expression of adhesion molecules on cardiac myocytes [3–12]. The relative contribution of cellular and humoral immune disturbances to the pathogenesis of myocyte injury in various heart diseases has not been determined.

Accumulated evidence has demonstrated a variety of circulating autoantibodies in the sera of patients with idiopathic dilated cardiomyopathy (DCM). The list includes autoantibodies directed against myosin [8, 13–16], the mitochondrial adenine nucleotide translocator and M7 [17–20], the branched-chain $\alpha$-ketoacid dehydrogenase dihydrolipoyl transacylase (BCKD-E2) [21], laminin [22], $\beta$-adrenoceptors [23–28], and $M_2$-muscarinic receptors [27–29]. According to the locations of major cardiac autoantigens, autoantibodies can be roughly divided into three subtypes: (1) directed against cell-surface proteins which have a reasonable chance of causing damage to the cell, e.g. antiadrenergic or muscarinic receptor autoantibodies; (2) directed against intracellular proteins which are not pathogenic unless the cell membrane is already leaky; it is unclear how these autoantibodies escape lysosomal degradation under this circumstance; and (3) directed against intracellular proteins cross-reacting with another surface molecule through molecular mimicry, e.g. antimyosin autoantibodies. Myosin may cross-react with anti-$M_2$-muscarinic receptor autoantibodies: at concentrations of 0.1 μg/ml, 1 μg/ml, and 10 μg/ml, myosin is able to inhibit the muscarinic stimulatory effect of anti-$M_2$-muscarinic receptor autoantibodies in neonatal rat myocytes from DCM, in terms of the negative chronotropic activity, by 8%, 26%, and 64%, respectively (to be published). According to the distribution spectrum in DCM, the autoantibodies can be classified as those mainly detectable in DCM and those detectable in DCM and other diseases. For example, antiadenine nucleotide translocator autoantibodies, antilaminin autoantibodies, and antiheart autoantibodies exist in both DCM and myocarditis, whereas autoantibodies against $\beta$-adrenergic receptors and cardiac $M_2$-muscarinic acetylcholine receptors are mainly confined to DCM.

## Distribution spectrum of antireceptor autoantibodies

Since Venter *et al.* [31] in 1980 reported autoantibodes against $\beta_2$-adrenoceptors in patients with allergic rhinitis and asthma, a great amount of evidence has been published describing autoantibodies against $\beta_1$-adrenoceptors in patients with DCM. In 1987, Wallukat and Wollenberger [24] found that the immunoglobulin G (IgG) fraction in patients with DCM displayed a positive chronotropic effect on cultured neonatal rat myocytes. By using ligand binding of DCM sera on rat cardiac membranes, Limas *et al.* [32] in 1989 demonstrated autoantibodies against β-adrenergic receptors in 40% of patients with DCM. Magnusson *et al.* [26] in 1990 used synthetic peptides corresponding to the second extracellular loops of human $\beta_1$- and $\beta_2$-adrenergic receptors as coated antigens in an enzyme-linked immunoabsorbent assay (ELISA) and found autoantibodies against $\beta_1$-adrenergic receptor peptide in 31% of patients with DCM but no autoantibodies against $\beta_2$-adrenergic receptor peptide.

An Ig component with the capacity for interacting with cardiac muscarinic receptors was discovered in mice with Chagas' myocarditis by Sterin-Borda *et al.* [33] in 1991, indicating that muscarinic receptor autoimmunity may be involved in the pathogenesis of this disease. However, limited information is available about the possible involvement of muscarinic receptor autoimmunity in DCM. Since autoantibodies against β-adrenoceptors have been repeatedly demonstrated in patients with DCM and both muscarinic receptors and β-adrenoceptors are equally predominant cardiac receptors for myocardial functional and metabolic regulation, it is assumed that autoantibodies against muscarinic receptors in DCM also exist.

Muscarinic receptors, as a member of the G protein-coupled receptor superfamily, have structural, biochemical, and immunological bases which allow them to act as an autoimmune target. Hydropathicity analysis of muscarinic receptors indicates that they contain seven hydrophobic and potential transmembrane domains, similar to those adopted for rhodopsin and β-adrenoceptors, with an extracellular amino-terminus and intracellular carboxy-terminus. Different subtypes of muscarinic receptors share a high degree of homology (65%) in these membrane-spanning segments and short-connecting loops. Based on the putative structure of the human $M_2$ muscarinic receptors, a sequence was predicted, V-R-T-V-E-D-G-E-C-Y-I-Q-F-F-S-N-Ȧ-A-V-T-F-G-T-A-I, corresponding to the second extracellular loop of human $M_2$-muscarinic receptor, which might be involved in the autoimmune recognition of this receptor. In previous studies, it was demonstrated that the sera from patients with DCM recognized the $M_2$-muscarinic receptor peptide (36–37%) and $\beta_1$-adrenoceptor peptide (31%) [27–29].

More studies were performed to ensure the fine specificity of these antireceptor autoantibodies in patients with the same disease, i.e. DCM, but from different geographical origins such as Sweden and Japan, were studied to see whether they have a similar frequency of occurrence of antireceptor autoantibodies in their sera. The results demonstrated that anti-$M_2$-muscarinic receptors and $\beta_1$-adrenoceptor autoantibodies have an almost identical spectrum of frequencies of occurrence in patients with DCM from different geographical origins [27–29]. In addition, patients with other cardiovascular diseases, such as essential or secondary malignant hypertension and hypertrophic cardiomyopathy and myocarditis, were used to study the disease specificity. Both anti-$\beta_1$-adrenoceptor autoantibodies and anti-$M_2$-muscarinic receptor autoantibodies are mainly present in patients with DCM but not in those with hypertension and hypertrophic cardiomyopathy [27] and myocarditis. Studies were also performed to determine whether anticardiovascular receptor autoantibodies in DCM patients could be extended to other cardiovascular receptors that are also coupled to the G protein, as $\alpha_1$-adrenoceptors and angiotensin II receptor subtype 1 (AT1) receptors belong to the superfamily of G protein-coupled receptors. These receptors are important to cardiovascular function. By examining autoantibodies against these G protein-coupled cardiovascular receptors, such as $\alpha_1$-adrenoceptors, $\beta_1$-adrenoceptors, and AT1 receptors, as well as $M_2$-muscarinic receptors, in a well-defined group of patients with DCM, it was found that autoantibodies against $\alpha_1$-adrenoceptors and AT1 receptors were present only in 14% and 4% of cases, respectively, whereas autoantibodies against either $M_2$-muscarinic receptors or $\beta_1$-adrenoceptors were detected in over 30% of cases [28]. In contrast, in secondary malignant hypertension due mainly to renovascular diseases, autoantibodies against $\alpha_1$-adrenoceptors and AT1 receptors were demonstrated in 64% and 44% of cases, respectively [34, 35], which were

**Table 16.1** Representative findings of main autoantibodies against cardiac autoantigens in dilated cardiomyopathy

| Autoantibodies to | Frequency of occurrence (%) |
|---|---|
| Heart (mainly myosin heavy chain) | 20–35 |
| Adenine nucleotide translocator | 95 |
| Laminin | 78 |
| $\beta_1$-adrenoceptor | 30–32 |
| $M_2$-muscarinic receptor | 36–38 |

**Table 16.2** Representative pathophysiological studies of antireceptor autoantibodies

| Parameters | Anti-$\beta_1$ antibody | Anti-$M_2$ antibody |
|---|---|---|
| *In vitro*[a] | | |
| Receptor binding sites | Decrease | Decrease |
| Recognition of blotted membrane | Yes | Yes |
| Localization of receptor | Yes | Yes |
| Chronotropic effect | Positive | Negative |
| Resistance to desensitization | Yes | Yes |
| *In vivo*[b] | | |
| Maximal rate of rise of ventricular pressure | Not done | Decrease |
| cAMP accumulation in guinea-pig ventricles | Not done | Decrease |
| Induction of cardiomyopathic changes: | | |
| 6 month immunization | Not done | Pathological changes |
| 1 year immunization | Pathological changes Heart dysfunction | Pathological changes |

[a]Autoantibodies from patients with dilated cardiomyopathy.
[b]Rabbit antibodies.

shown in a later study to be confined to the malignant phase rather than the renovascular disease [30]. These investigations suggest that the prevalence of antimuscarinic receptor and $\beta_1$-adrenoceptor autoantibodies is largely specific to DCM (Table 16.1), although these studies need to be extended to other ethnic populations and other cardiovascular diseases. A correlation study was performed between the degree of autoimmune response as expressed by the optical density of autoantibodies in ELISA and the clinical characteristics of DCM. No correlation was found in the optical density of sera positive for $\beta_1$-adrenoceptors or $M_2$-muscarinic receptors and the clinical characteristics as expressed by the ejection fraction (%) of the patient group studied. However, this study should be extended to include multiple clinical parameters, therapeutic effectiveness, and prognosis. Since there are at least two different types of antireceptor autoantibody in patients with DCM, the question is raised as to whether these two antibodies belong to two distinct antibody populations that react exclusively with their own target receptors or whether they belong to one antibody population that possesses a property enabling it to cross-react with both target receptors. The results of one study showed ambiguously that the former is the case [27]. However, what the above data mean in the context of the development of DCM remains unresolved.

## Possible pathophysiological importance of autoantibodies

A given autoantibody may be present in DCM for three different reasons: (1) for involvement in the pathogenesis of DCM, i.e. to have pathogenic importance; (2) for prognostic value; or (3) both. To clarify this issue, studies are needed on the *in vitro* functional activity of autoantibodies, as assessed by an antigen-mediated cellular and intracellular system. In addition, the *in vivo* functional activity can be verified in an animal model to determine whether the autoantibody can interfere with heart function acutely and whether the autoantigen as a function of time can induce DCM-like disease. The autoantibodies against G protein-coupled cardiac receptors may play an important role in the pathogenesis of DCM and have prognostic value. Although this remains speculative, it is becoming more convincing. Below are three lines of evidence that add weight to this hypothesis (Table 16.2).

### *In vitro* studies

Wallukat and Wollenberger [24] used cultured, beating neonatal rat heart cells as a sensitive adrenergic effector system to demonstrate that the IgG fractions from patients with DCM were able to increase the beating rate of the myocytes and that autoantibodies were able to recognize epitopes on the first and second extracellular loops of the $\beta_1$-adrenoceptors [36]. Limas *et al.* [32] found that positive sera from patients with DCM were able to immunoprecipitate the β-adrenergic receptors from solubilized cardiac membranes and to inhibit isopreterenol-stimulated adenylyl cyclase activity. Using affinity-purified anti-$\beta_1$-adrenergic receptor autoantibodies from patients with DCM, Magnusson *et al.* [26, 37, 38] demonstrated that these purified autoantibodies not only decrease the binding sites without a change in antagonist affinity on C6 rat glioma cell membranes (C6 cells express 80% of $\beta_1$-adrenergic receptors and 20% of $\beta_2$-adrenergic receptors) but also recognize the target receptors by both immunoblot and immunocytochemistry. Krause *et al.* [39] showed that autoantibodies against $\beta_1$-adrenergic receptors from patients with DCM increase the activity of cAMP-dependent protein kinase (PKA). Fu *et al.* [27, 29] demonstrated a specific localization of muscarinic receptors in human myocardium from patients with DCM using anti-$M_2$-muscarinic receptor autoantibodies, suggesting that autoantibodies can interact with their target receptors in failing heart tissue. The localization of $M_2$-muscarinic receptors in human myocardium is specific, since it can be blocked by preincubation of autoantibodies with the peptide and staining did not occur when using control human IgG or conjugate alone. Further studies showed that autoantibodies were capable of decreasing [$^3$H]quinuclidinyl benzylate (QNB) binding sites on rat ventricular membranes, suggesting that autoantibodies can also interfere with the ligand binding function [27, 29].

The functional effects of both anti-$\beta_1$-adrenergic receptor autoantibodies and anti-$M_2$-muscarinic receptor autoantibodies were assessed by examining their chronotropic effects on rat neonatal cardiomyocytes. Their ability to change the cell beating frequency of the myocytes, which is generally accepted as one of the most important functional parameters for both adrenergic and muscarinic acetylcholine activity at the cellular level, was assessed. It was shown that anti-$\beta_1$-adrenergic receptor and anti-$M_2$-muscarinic receptor autoantibodies from DCM patients display positive (increasing frequency of cell beats) [37] and negative (decreasing frequency of cells beats) chronotropic effect, respectively [30]. Moreover, such chronotropic effects were sustained over a period of more than 5 h, even after the autoantibodies had been washed away. This property of autoantibodies differs from that of the classical β-adrenergic receptor agonist isoprenaline and the muscarinic receptor agonist carbachol, which can induce desensitization after a short duration. For example, anti-$M_2$-muscarinic receptor autoantibodies were able to decrease the cell beating frequency in a dose-dependent manner (50–500 nM); the frequency was sustained for more than 5 h and was persistent even after washing and subsequent incubation for a few hours in fresh culture medium without autoantibodies. This negative chronotropic effect was, however, completely and rapidly reversed by the addition of the muscarinic receptor antagonist atropine (1 μM), suggesting that the chronotropic effect induced by the autoantibodies was specific to the muscarinic receptor. In contrast, the negative chronotropic action by the muscarinic receptor agonist carbachol (100 μM) was subject to relatively rapid desensitization, since the negative chronotropic effect waned after 1 h.

These results indicate that antiheart muscarinic receptor autoantibodies have stimulatory muscarinic receptor activity *in vitro*, which differs from that of normal muscarinic agonists by its non-desensitization [40]. As this property of non-desensitization or resistance to desensitization is shared by anti-$\beta_1$-adrenergic receptors autoantibodies and anti-$M_2$ muscarinic receptor autoantibodies, it seems that this is a common feature of antireceptor autoantibodies. However, the detailed mechanism remains unknown. Anti-$\beta_1$-adrenergic receptor autoantibodies had only a marginal effect on cAMP accumulation, suggesting that they may act in a different way to isoprenaline [37]. There may be other mechanisms involved in anti-$M_2$-muscarinic receptor autoantibodies. The autoantibodies were not able to induce internalization of muscarinic receptors. The radiolabelled hydrophilic ligand *N*-methylscopolamine (NMS) was used to study the internalization of the muscarinic receptors. After preincubating cultured cardiomyocytes for 3 h with carbachol (1000 μM), the number of NMS binding sites ($4.2 \pm 0.7 \times 10^{-12}$ M) decreased by 57% compared with the control (in the absence of carbachol, $9.9 \pm 1.7 \times 10^{-12}$ M). However, no such decrease in NMS binding sites was found in autoantibody-treated cardiomyocytes ($11.9 \pm 2.2 \times 10^{-12}$ M), suggesting that carbachol can induce a decrease in plasma membrane-localized muscarinic receptors whereas autoantibodies have no such effect. The association constants in both groups remained unchanged [40]. The fact that anti-$M_2$-muscarinic receptor autoantibodies from DCM patients were unable to induce internalization may explain, at least partly, to their non-desensitizing property. This resistance may be the result of cross-linking of receptors by the bivalent autoantibodies inhibiting the internalization of the receptors in the same manner as reported for bivalent lectins.

Antireceptor autoantibodies from DCM patients are not the only examples of *in vitro* functional activities. Autoantibodies against the ADP/ATP translocator of the mitochondrial membrane have also been shown to impair energy metabolism in an animal model [18].

### Acute *in vivo* studies

*In vivo* studies have been regarded as a further step in elucidating the role of autoantibodies in the development of DCM. This has been done mostly in animal models, not in humans, for ethical reasons. Wang *et al.* [41] demonstrated that rabbit antimuscarinic receptor antibodies can exert acute negative chronotropic and inotropic effects in rats, as does the muscarinic receptor agonist carbachol. Autoantibodies against the ADP/ATP translocator were also shown to disturb energy metabolism *in vivo* [42].

### Chronic *in vivo* studies: induction of cardiomyopathy-like changes in animal models

Muscarinic stimulatory antibodies can be induced in rabbits after immunization with a synthetic peptide corresponding to the second extracellular loop of the $M_2$-acetylcholine receptor, one of the targets for autoantibodies in patients with DCM [27, 29]. By studying these animals, the development of the antibodies and the possible effects on the heart of their interaction with the target receptors can be shown. A continuing monthly boosting of the rabbit immune system for 6 months increased the IgG fraction of the antiserum. These results confirm that the immunizing peptide contains at least one T-cell epitope, responsible for the switch to IgG of the immune response as well as for the induction of memory cells, increasing the immune response over time. The histopathological findings of a 6 month immunization schedule showed a bioenergetic degradation of the myocardial cells (mitochondrial alterations) that could lead to sarcolemmal damage [43]. Similar observations have been made on heart biopsy specimens from patients with DCM [44]. In contrast to myosin-induced myocarditis [45], which is a cellular immunological disease, the structural and functional changes induced by immunization with the $M_2$ acetylcholine peptide occur with only a minor infiltration of inflammatory cells. Moreover, the ultrastructural changes also occur in regions in which there is no such infiltration, indicating that these changes are mediated by the pharmacological properties of anti-$M_2$-muscarinic receptor antibodies.

In order to observe the maximal change by immunization with receptor peptide and to mimic the situations in DCM in which both anti-$\beta_1$-adrenoceptor antibody and anti-$M_2$ muscarinic receptor antibody are present, the experimental set-up prolonged the immunization duration from 6 months to 1 year with both receptor peptides in rabbits. It was shown that both groups of rabbits immunized with either $\beta_1$-adrenoceptor peptide or $M_2$-muscarinic receptor peptide displayed significantly enlarged ventricles and thinner walls, compared with the control group. However, in contrast to the $\beta_1$ group, which showed enlarged cavities in both left and right ventricles, the $M_2$ group was mainly affected in the right ventricles. Moreover, morphological examination of the rabbit hearts from both groups demonstrated mainly degenerative changes such as focal myofibrillar lysis, loss of myofilament, mitochondrial swelling and condensation, sarcoplasmic vacuolation, and deposition of dense granules in the sarcoplasma and the myofibrils [46]. These results suggest that immunization by peptides, corresponding to the target sequences for antireceptor autoantibodies in DCM, induces morphological changes in the heart similar to those found in the human disease. These finding are especially interesting as they add weight to the hypothesis that anti-$\beta_1$-adrenoceptor autoantibodies and/or anti-$M_2$-muscarinic receptor autoantibodies play a pathophysiological role in the development of DCM. The limitation of this study was that it did not include a group of rabbits immunized with both receptor peptides since around 50% of patients with DCM who had autoantibodies against the $\beta_1$-adrenoceptor also had autoantibodies against the $M_2$-muscarinic receptor [27–29]. A further study investigated whether the rabbits immunized with both receptor peptides showed similar or distinct cardiomyopathic changes after 1 year compared with rabbits immunized with either $\beta_1$-adrenoceptor peptide or $M_2$-muscarinic receptor peptide alone [46]. As before, the cardiomyopathic changes were identified by examining the anatomical, histochemical, and ultrastructural alterations. At the anatomical level, the wall thickness of the interventricular septum was 3.99 ± 0.97 mm, which was significantly thicker than previously reported in the control group (2.75 ± 0.57 mm), $\beta_1$ group (2.44 ± 0.64 mm), and $M_2$ group (2.96 ± 0.26 mm) [46]. The wall thickness in the left ventricle was 3.87 ± 0.82 mm, which was not significantly thicker than previously reported in the control group (3.16 ± 0.49 mm), $\beta_1$ group (2.53 ± 0.64 mm), and $M_2$ group (2.95 ± 0.41 mm). The total ventricular wall area was 207.4 ± 27.8 $mm^2$, which was significantly larger that that of the previously reported control group (158.6 ± 12.8 $mm^2$), $\beta_1$ group (158.4 ± 23.5 $mm^2$), and $M_2$ group (160.5 ± 15.1 $mm^2$) [46]. At the light-microscopic level, the hearts displayed myocardial cell hypertrophy, particularly in the left ventricular wall and interventricular septum. The inflammatory reaction was mild, although scattered mononuclear cells such as lymphocytes and macrophages were present in the wall of both ventricles. There was no evidence of active necrosis of myocardial cells. In one rabbit, interstitial fibrosis with myocardial degeneration and mononuclear cell infiltration was found in the right ventricular wall. Sudden death occurred in two rabbits; there was extensive infiltration of inflammatory cells together with myocardial degeneration and necrosis involving the right ventricular wall. The inflammatory cells were mainly lymphocytes and macrophages. Rare polymorphonuclear leucocytes were present. Patchy interstitial fibrosis was also found in both ventricular walls. As shown previously [46], the ultrastructural changes of the hearts of rabbits immunized with either $\beta_1$-receptor peptide or $M_2$-muscarinic receptor peptide have been degenerative, characterized by focal myofibrillar lysis, loss of normal myofilament banding patterns with hypercontraction bands, mitochondrial swelling and condensation, sarcoplasmic vacuolation, and deposition of dense granules in both the sarcoplasma and myofibrils. In the present study, however, the morphological findings in the hearts immunized with both $\beta_1$-receptor peptide and the $M_2$-muscarinic receptor peptide were mainly hypertrophic changes rather than degenerative changes of myocardial cells. The major ultrastructural change in the myocytes was a marked increase in the number of mitochondria. Degenerative changes in myocardial cells were milder in the group immunized with both the $\beta_1$- and $M_2$-receptor peptides than those in the group immunized with $\beta_1$- or $M_2$-receptor peptide alone.

The difference in the morphological changes between the group immunized with both receptor peptides and the group immunized with a single receptor peptide [47] correlate with antireceptor autoantibodies since the levels of both anti-$\beta_1$-adrenoceptor autoantibodies and anti-$M_2$-muscarinic receptor autoantibodies were high throughout the experimental period but not in the preimmune sera or the control sera. There was a significantly positive correlation ($p$ = 0.0494) between the titres of anti $\beta_1$-adrenoceptor and anti-$M_2$-muscarinic receptor autoantibodies in the rabbits after 12 months of immunization. Moreover, the anti-$M_2$-acetylcholine receptor antibodies decreased significantly from 7 to 12 months at the same time that their cross-reactivity with the $\beta_1$-adrenoceptor increased. Cross-reactive autoanitibodies are a feature of Chagas' disease, an autoimmune cardiomyopathy caused by the parasite *Trypanosoma cruzi* [48].

Ligand binding studies of myocardial β-adrenoceptors and muscarinic receptors showed downregulation of β-adrenoceptors without changes in muscarinic receptors. The density of β-adrenoceptors was 55.6 ± 13.8 fmol//mg, significantly lower than that of either the control group (104.3 ± 48.0 fmol/mg) or the $\beta_1$-receptor group (132.8 ± 38.7 fmol/mg) [46], whereas the density of muscarinic receptors was 37.5 ± 11.3 fmol/mg and was identical to that of the control group, the $\beta_1$ group, and the $M_2$ group [46]. A high inverse correlation ($p$ = 0.0056) was found between this downregulation and the anti-$M_2$-acetylcholine receptor antibodies, whereas no correlation was found between the anti-$\beta_1$-adrenoceptor antibodies and receptor downregulation. The downregulation of myocardial β-adrenoceptors from rabbits immunized with both $\beta_1$-receptor peptide and $M_2$-receptor peptide cannot due to fibrosis, since (1) interstitial fibrosis has been found only in the right but not the left ventricle and only in one rabbit; and (2) a similar extent of fibrosis has been shown previously in the $\beta_1$-adrenoceptor peptide-immunized group without affecting the myocardial $\beta_1$-receptor receptor density [46]. The monospecific anti-$M_2$-acetylcholine receptor autoantibodies could at least partially compensate for this downregulation, as suggested by the inverse correlation between the anti-$M_2$-acetylcholine autoantibody titres and $\beta_1$-adrenoceptor downregulation. This phenomenon could be explained by the agonist-like activity of the anti-$M_2$-acetylcholine antibodies [27], which can inhibit the stimulatory activity of anti-$\beta_1$-adrenoceptor autoantibodies [37]. Since the anti-$M_2$-acetylcholine receptor response decreases as function of time, the pathogenic role of the anti-$\beta_1$-adrenoceptor autoantibodies predominates.

Heart function has also been determined in rabbits immunized with anti-$\beta_1$-adrenoceptors for 1 year. Zhao *et al.* demonstrated heart dysfunction in the form of a decrease in $dP/dt$ max in both left and right ventricles in immunized rabbits (to be published).

## Possible prognostic value of autoantibodies

As stated above, the specific distribution of autoantibodies in patients with DCM may have prognostic value, with or without being involved in the pathogenesis of the disease. The evaluation of the prognostic value is limited since previous studies have focused on correlating clinical severity and antibody titre. This is partly due to the incomplete clinical parameters chosen during retroactive study, and partly because it is not possible to determine the exact amount of autoantibody for all patients studied. In a recent study of patients from the Metoprolol in Dilated Cardiomyopathy (MDC) trial, chronic metoprolol treatment was not effective in improving cardiac function in patients who had anti-$\beta_1$-adrenergic receptor autoantibodies compared with similar autoantibody-positive patients in the placebo group [38]. The reason for the inefficiency of metoprolol in this case may be that autoantibodies can have β-adrenergic antagonist-like effects and prevent sympathetic overstimulation, similar to metoprolol, with improvement in cardiac function. It may also be that the presence of autoantibodies is a marker of patients with a better prognosis, but with limited pathophysiological importance. Nevertheless, it seems that autoantibodies are beneficial, but do not participate in the pathogenesis of DCM. Autoimmunity-related mechanisms are more complicated than anticipated. There are many kinds of autoantibody, with different properties, different targets, different actions, and different mechanisms. An antibody against the second extracellular loop of the receptor can have agonist-like activity, whereas another antibody against the first extracellular loop of the same receptor may have antagonist-like activity. It all depends on how these different antibodies against the same target protein or against different target proteins reach an equilibrium in the body. A typical example for DCM can be the delicate balance between the stimulatory antimuscarinic receptor autoantibodies and the stimulatory anti-β-adrenergic receptor autoantibodies. This multiple autoimmunity makes any findings difficult to interpret.

## Clinical implication of the presence of circulating autoantibodies in patients with dilated cardiomyopathy

The way in which autoantibodies work in patients with DCM and functional activity has clinical implications since the autoimmune mechanism plays an important role in the pathogenesis of DCM. Although there are distinctive clinical clues and experimental approaches, as discussed above, supporting DCM as an 'autoimmune disease', the available evidence does not entirely meet the criteria of an autoimmune disease as suggested by Rose and Bona [49]. A clear-cut definition of DCM as an autoimmune disease needs additional evidence. DCM can be transferred from patients to severely combined immunodeficiency (SCID) mice. These mice lack functional T- and B-lymphocytes in the peripheral blood owing to a genetic defect and are suitable for transfer experiments, to receive allogenic or xenogenic transplants, as in transferring lupus erythematodes, primary biliary cirrhosis, and Grave's disease. Schwimmbeck *et al.* [50] successfully transferred peripheral blood leucocytes of patients with chronic myocarditis into SCID mice, which developed human cellular infiltrates of the myocardium and an impairment in left ventricular function within 60 days, indicating that sensitized T-cells play an important role in the pathogenesis of myocarditis. The agonistic activities of anti-$\beta_1$- and $M_2$-receptor autoantibodies may also have therapeutic importance. There are three different subgroups of DCM patients: those with only anti-$\beta_1$-adrenoceptor autoantibodies; those with only anti-$M_2$-muscarinic receptor autoantibodies; and those with both types of autoantibody. For the group containing only one type of antireceptor autoantibody, the therapy theoretically, should be aimed at blocking the active autoantibodies of pathogenic importance by either modulating the immune system or direct blockading of antibody activity. A recent study has shown that a specific $\beta_1$-adrenergic receptor blocker, bisoprolol (3 mg/day), was able to protect the myocardium of the rabbits immunized with $\beta_1$-adrenergic receptor peptide from immune-mediated injury after 1 year [51]. However, for the group with both types of autoantibody, the situation is more complicated and a delicate balance between autoantibodies is needed. Since the two antibodies have different affinities, avidities, and biochemical, biophysical, and immunological properties, such a balance is difficult. The concentration of autoantibodies needed to affect the $\beta_1$-adrenoceptor pharmacologically is ten times lower than that needed to affect the $M_2$-muscarinic receptor [27, 29]. It is hard to judge the overall effect on cardiac function of the simultaneous presence of both anti-$\beta_1$- and anti-$M_2$-receptor autoantibodies. Moreover, in patients with DCM, the sympathetic nervous system is markedly activated and myocardial $\beta_1$-adrenoceptor density is downregulated, while vagal control of the heart is impaired, but $M_2$-receptor density is not decreased and the effects of the $M_2$-receptor agonist carbachol are not attenuated [52–55]. More studies are needed to determine how such antireceptor autoantibodies could interfere with the delicate balance between the sympathetic and vagal stimulation of cardiac function and thus contribute to the overall symptomatology of DCM. This remains a prerequisite for effective and specific immune therapy [56].

Recently, the effect of immunoadsorption give on 5 consecutive days to nine patients with severe DCM (who were on stable drug therapy including angiotensin-converting enzyme inhibitors, digitalis, diuretics, and β-blockers) was studied. Immunoadsorption resulted in a decrease in anti-$\beta_1$-adrenergic receptor antibodies and an improvement in cardiac function, suggesting that immunoadsorption may be an additional therapeutic possibility for haemodynamic stabilization of patients with severe DCM [57, 58].

## Unanswered questions and future directions

During the 1990s, the role of autoimmune mechanism in the pathogenesis of DCM has been greatly elucidated. Today we can say that DCM is very likely an autoimmune disease. Further studies in which DCM is transferred from humans to SCID mice are needed to confirm this. The authors' ongoing study using this technique will hopefully provide an answer. The following knowledge is required before a specific immune therapy regimen can be developed. (1) How much is known about the targets of autoimmune response and the mechanisms that trigger and regulate such response? How are they balanced? (2) How is the autoantigen presented and recognized by the immune system? (3) Does autoimmune response damage myocytes by the direct effect of autoantibody to the antigen-expressing myocytes, by the release of cytokines produced by infiltrating T-lymphocytes, or both? (4) As the pathophysiology of DCM is heterogeneous, how important is the autoimmune mechanism in relation to other mechanism? Since there are so many unanswered questions, it is clear that there is a great deal yet to be understood before the specific role of the autoimmune mechanism in DCM can be fully elucidated and a specific immune therapy introduced.

Although many efforts have been made to understand the relationship between autoimmunity and DCM, there is still a large gap between hypothesis and reality. Future studies should focus on: (1) the properties of autoantibodies by both *in vitro* and *in vivo* means; (2) the molecular and cellular mechanisms for the actions of autoantibodies; (3) the mechanisms that modulate autoantibody action; and (4) techniques to reproduce DCM using pathogenic putative autoantigens. It is hoped that a breakthrough in the understanding of the relationship between the autoimmune mechanism and DCM will take place in the near future. This will certainly add a new therapeutic potential to the management of DCM.

## References


1. Barry WH. Mechanisms of immune-mediated myocyte injury. *Circulation* 1994; 89: 2421–32.
2. Rose NR, Herskowitz A, Neumann D, Neu N. Autoimmune myocarditis: a paradigm of post-infection autoimmune disease. *Immunol Today* 1988; 9: 117–20.
3. Fowles RE, Bieber CP, Stinson EB. Defective *in vitro* suppressor cell function in idiopathic congestive cardiomyopathy. *Circulation* 1979; 59: 483–91.
4. Eckstein R, Mempel W, Bolte HD. Reduced suppressor cell activity in congestive cardiomyopathy and in myocarditis. *Circulation* 1982; 65: 1224–9.
5. Anderson JL, Carlquist JF, Hammond EH. Deficient natural killer cell activity in patients with idiopathic dilated cardiomyopathy. *Lancet* 1982; ii: 1124–7.
6. Sanderson JE, Koech D, Iha D, Ojiambo H. T-lymphocyte subsets in idiopathic dilated cardiomyopathy. *Am J Cardiol* 1985; 55: 755–8.
7. Rönnblom LE, Forsberg H, Evrin PE. Increased level of HLA-DR-expressing T lymphocytes in peripheral blood from patients with idiopathic dilated cardiomyopathy. *Cardiology* 1991; 78: 161–7.
8. Caforio ALP, Stewart JT, Bonifacio E *et al.* Inappropriate major histocompatibility complex expression on cardiac tissue in dilated cardiomyopathy. Relative for autoimmunity? *J Autoimmun* 1990; 3: 187–200.
9. Koike S. Immunological disorders in patients with dilated cadiomyopathy. With special reference to the production of interleukin-2 receptors in the patients' peripheral blood lymphocytes. *Jpn Heart J* 1989; 30: 799–807.
10. Limas CJ, Goldenberg IF, Limas C. Soluble interleukin-2 receptor levels in patients with dilated cardiomyopathy. *Circulation* 1995; 91: 631–43.
11. Seko Y, Yamazaki T, Shinkai Y *et al.* Cellular and molecular bases for the immunopathology of the myocardial damage involved in acute viral myocarditis with special reference to dilated cardiomyopathy. *Jpn Circ J* 1992; 56: 1062–72.
12. Toyozaki T, Saito T, Takano H *et al.* Expression of intercellular adhesion molecule-1 on cardiac myocytes for myocarditis before and during immuno-suppressive therapy. *Am J Cardiol* 1993; 72: 441–4.
13. Das SK, Cassidy JT, Petty RE. Antibodies against heart muscle and nuclear constitutents in cardiomyopathy. *Am Heart J* 1972; 83: 159–66.
14. Latif N, Baker CS, Dunn MJ *et al.* Frequency and specificity of anti-heart antibodies in patients with dilated cardiomyopathy detected

using SDS-PAGE and western blotting. *J Am Coll Cardiol* 1993; 22: 1378–84.

15. Neumann DA, Burek CL, Baughman KL *et al.* Circulating heart-reactive antibodies in patients with myocarditis or cardiomyopathy. *J Am Coll Cardiol* 1990; 16: 839–46.
16. Caforio ALP, Grazzini M, Mann JM *et al.* Identification of alpha and β myosin heavy chain isoforms as major autoantigens in dilated cardiomyopathy. *Circulation* 1992; 85: 1734–42.
17. Schultheiss HP, Schwimmbeck P, Bolte HD, Klingenberg M. The antigenic characteristics and the significance of the adenine nucleotide translocator as a major autoantigen to antimitochondrial antobodies in dilated cardiomyopathy. *Adv Myocardial* 1985; 6: 311–27.
18. Schulze K, Becker BF, Schauer R, Schultheiss HP. Antibodies to ADP-ATP carrier-an autoantigen in myocarditis and dilated cardiomyopathy-impaired cardiac function. *Circulation* 1990; 81: 959–69.
19. Ansari AA, Herskowitz A, Danner DJ. Identification of mitochondrial proteins that serve as targets for autoimmunity in human dilated cardiomyopathy. *Circulation* 1988; 78 (Suppl): 457.
20. Klein R, Maisch B, Kochsiek K, Berg PA. Demonstration of organ-specific antibodies against heart mitochondria (anti-M7) in sera from patients with some forms of heart diseases. *Clin Exp Immunol* 1984; 58: 283–92.
21. Ansari AA, Neckemann N, Villinger F *et al.* Epitope mapping of the branched chain alpha-ketoacid dehydrogenase dihydrolipoyl transacylase (BCKD-E2) protein that reacts with serA from patients with idiopathic dilated cardiomyopathy. *J Immunol* 1994; 153: 4754–65.
22. Wolff PG, Kuhl U, Schultheiss HP. Laminin distribution and autoantibodies to laminin in dilated cardiomyopathy and myocarditis. *Am Heart J* 1989; 117: 1303–9.
23. Sterin-Borda LA, Cremaschi G, Pascual J *et al.* Alloimmune IgG binds and modulates cardiac β-adrenergic receptors. *Clin Exp Immunol* 1984; 58: 223–8.
24. Wallukat G, Wollenberger A. Effects of the serum gammal globulin fraction of patients with allergic asthma and dilated cardiomyopathy on chronotropic beta-adrenoceptor function in cultured neonatal rat heart myocytes. *Biomed Biochim Acta* 1987; 46: 634–9.
25. Limas CJ, Limas C, Kubo SH, Olivari MT. Anti-β receptor antibodies in human dilated cardiomyopathy and correlation with HLA-DR antigens. *Am J Cardiol* 1990; 65: 483–7.
26. Magnusson Y, Marullo S, Hoyer S *et al.* Mapping of a functional autoimmune epitope on the $\beta_1$-adrenergic receptor in patients with idiopathic dilated cardiomyopathy. *J Clin Invest* 1990; 86: 1658–63.
27. Fu LXM, Hoebeke J, Matsui S *et al.* Autoantibodies against cardiac G-protein-coupled receptors define different populations with cardiomyopathies but not with hypertension. *Clin Immunol Immunopathol* 1994; 72: 15–20.
28. Matsui S, Fu LXM, Shimizu M *et al.* Dilated cardiomyopathy defines serum autoantibodies against G-protein coupled cardiovascular receptors. *Autoimmunity* 1995; 21: 85–8.
29. Fu LX, Magnusson Y, Bergh C *et al.* Locatlization of functional autoimmune epitope on the muscarinic acetylcholine receptor-2 in patients with idiopathic dilated cardiomyopathy. *J Clin Invest* 1993; 91: 1964–8.
30. Fu LXM, Herlitz H, Schulze W *et al.* Autoantibodies against the angiotensin receptor (AT1) in patients with hypertension. *J Hypertens* 2000; 18(7): 945–53.
31. Venter JC, Fraser CM, Harrison LC. Autoantibodies to $\beta_2$ adrenergic receptors: a possible cause of adrenergic hyporesponsiveness in allergic rhinitis and asthma. *Science* 1980; 207: 1361.
32. Limas CJ, Goldenberg IF, Limas C. Autoantibodies against β-adrenoreceptors in human dilated cardiomyopathy. *Circ Res* 1989; 97–103.
33. Sterin-Borda L, Gorelik G, Borda ES. Chagasic IgG binding with cardiac muscarinic cholinergic receptors modifies cholinergic-mediated cellular transmembrane signals. *Clin Immunol Immunopathol* 1991; 61: 387–91.
34. Fu LXM, Herlitz H, Wallukat G *et al.* Functional autoimmune epitope on $\alpha_1$-adrenergic receptors in patients with malignant hypertension. *Lancet* 1994; 344: 1660–3.
35. Fu LXM, Herlitz H, Schulze W *et al.* Autoantibodies against an extracellular domain on human angiotensin II receptor subtype 1 in patients with malignant hypertension (Abstract). *Circulation* 1995; (Suppl): 1337.
36. Wallukat G, Wollenberger A, Morwinski R, Pitschner H-F. Anti-β1-adrenoceptor autoantibodies with chronotropic activity from the serum of patients with dilated cardiomyopathy: mapping of epitopes in the first and second extracellular loops. *J Mol Cell Cardiol* 1995; 27: 397–406.
37. Magnusson Y, Wallukat G, Waagstein F *et al.* Autoimmunity in idiopathic dilated cardiomyopathy: characterization of antibodies against the $\beta_1$-adrenoceptor with positive chronotropic effect. *Circulation* 1994; 89: 2760–7.
38. Magnusson Y, Hoebeke J, Waagstein F, Hjalmarson Å and the MDC Trial Group. Predictive role of the beta 1-autoantibodies in patients with idiopathic dilated cardiomyopathy treated with metoprolol (Abstract). *Circulation* 1994; 90: I-543.
39. Krause EG, Bartel S, Beyerdorfer I, Wallukat G. Activation of cyclic AMP-dependent protein kinase in cardiomyocytes by anti-beta 1-adrenoceptor autoantibodies from patients with idiopathic dilated cardiomyopathy. *Blood Press* 1996; 3 (Suppl): 37–40.
40. Wallukat G, Fu HM, Matsui S *et al.* Autoantibodies against M2 muscarinic receptors in patients with cardiomyopathy display non-desensitized agonist-like effects. *Life Sci* 1999; 64: 465–9.
41. Wang WZ, Zhao R, Wu BW *et al.* Effects of anti-pepptide antibodies against human M2 muscarinic receptors on cardiac function in rats *in vivo*. *Blood Press* 1996; 3: 25–7.
42. Schulze K, Becker BF, Schultheiss HP. Antibodies to the ADP — ATP carrier — an autoantigen in myocarditis and dilated cardiomyopathy–penetrate into myocardial cells and disturb energy metabolism *in vivo*. *Circ Res* 1989; 64: 179–92.
43. Fu LXM, Schulze W, Wallukat G *et al.* A synthetic peptide corresponding to the second extracellular loop of the human $M_2$ muscarinic receptor induces pharmacological and morphological changes in cardiomyocytes by active immunization during 6 months in rabbits. *Clin Immunol Immunopathol* 1996; 78: 203–207.
44. McKinneyy B. *Pathology of the cardiomyopathy*. Bath: Butterworth, 1974, 29–47.
45. Neu N, Rose NR, Beisel KW *et al.* Cardial myosin induces myocarditis in genetically predisposed mice. *J Immunol* 1987; 139: 3630–6.
46. Matsui S, Fu LX, Katsuda S *et al.* Peptides derived from cardiovascular G-protein coupled receptors induce morphological cardiomyopathic changes in immunized rabbits. *J Mol Cell Cardiol* 1997; 29: 641–55.
47. Matsui S, Fu LXM, Hayase M *et al.* Active immunization of combined beta 1 adrenoceptor and M2 muscarinic receptor peptides

induces cardiac hypertrophy in rabbits. *J Cardiac Failure* 1999; 5(3): 246–54.
48. Elies R, Fu LXM, Eftekhari P *et al.* Immunocytochemical and functional characterization of an agonist-like monoclonal antibodies against the M2 acetylcholine receptors. *Eur J Biochem* 1998; 251: 659–66.
49. Rose NR, Bona C. Defining criteria for autoimmune diseases. *Immunol Today* 1993; 14: 426–30.
50. Schwimmbeck PL, Badorff C, Rohn G *et al.* The role of sensitized T-cells in myocarditis and dilated cardiomyopathy. *Int J Cardiol* 1996; 54: 117–25.
51. Matsui S, Fu LXM, Katsuda S *et al.* Beneficial effect of beta-blockade on dilated cardiomyopathy induced by autoimmune mechanism against beta 1-adrenoceptor (Abstract). *J Mol Cell Cardiol* 1998 (Suppl): 98.
52. Matsui S, Persson M, Katsuda S *et al.* Protective effect of bisoprolol on beta 1 adrenoceptor peptide induce autoimmune myocardial damage in rabbits. *Herz* 2000; 25(3): 267–70.
53. Francis GS, Benedict C, Johnstone DE *et al.* for the SOLVD Investigators. Comparisons of neuroendocrine activation in patients with and without congestive heart failure. A substudy of the Studies of Left Ventricular Dysfunction (SOLVD). *Circulation* 1990; 82: 1724–9.
54. Porter TR, Eckberg DL, Fritsch JM *et al.* Autonomic pathophysiology in heart failure patients: sympathetic–cholinergic interrelations. *J Clin Invest* 1990; 85: 1362–71.
55. Fu LXM, Waagstein F, Hjalmarson Å. An overview of β-adrenoceptor signal transduction system: desensitization in heart failure and effect of β-blockade. *Int J Cardiol* 1991; 30: 261–8.
56. Fu LXM, Liang QM, Waagstein F *et al.* Increase in functional activity rather than in amount of Gi in failing human heart with dilated cardiomyopathy. *Cardiovasc Res* 1992; 26: 950–5.
57. Fu LXM. Anti-M2 muscarinic receptor autoantibodies and idiopathic dilated cardiomyopathy. *Int J Cardiol* 1996; 54: 127–35.
58. Dorffel WV, Felix SB, Wallukat G *et al.* Short-term hemodynamic effects of immunoadsorption in dilated cardiomyopathy. *Circulation* 1997; 95: 1994–7.
59. Wallukat G, Reinke P, Dorffel WV *et al.* Removal of autoantibodies in dilated cardiomyopathy by immunoadsorption. *Int J Cardiol* 1996; 54: 191–5.

# Myocardial inflammation and myocellular damage 17

M. RITTER AND W. H. BARRY

## Introduction

Myocardial inflammation occurs in cardiac transplant rejection, myocarditis, and in some cases of idiopathic dilated cardiomyopathy. The inflammation can be associated with abnormal cardiac systolic and diastolic function and may be caused by a highly differentiated immunological reaction against the myocardium or the vascular tissue. Myocytes are the central functioning unit within the myocardium and their involvement in the inflammatory process is the main focus of this discussion. The immunological reaction consists of both cellular and humoral components. Cellular and humoral factors may damage myocytes either by direct interaction or indirectly by altering structures such as vascular endothelial cells or interstitial tissue, leading to, for example, ischaemia and fibrosis. The degree of damage can range from slight impairment of function to necrosis or apoptosis of individual myocytes, and subsequent loss of contractile mass. The effects of the cellular components of the immune reaction are primarily considered here.

## Cellular components of myocardial inflammatory infiltrates

The nature of the cellular infiltrate that occurs in immune-mediated cardiac inflammation has been investigated in a number of animal models, and the findings are summarized in Table 17.1. Lymphocytes and macrophages predominate in infiltrates, although other cell types, including neutrophils, are also present. Considerable effort has been directed towards defining the characteristics of the inflammatory infiltrate in various types of clinical myocarditis, and in human heart transplant rejection. Based on the working formulation of the International Society of Heart Transplantation for the Standardization of Nomenclature in the Diagnosis of Heart Rejection [8] and the Dallas Criteria for myocarditis [9], grading systems for the severity of inflammatory infiltrates seen in cardiac biopsies have been established.

In acute cardiac rejection the infiltrates range from large lymphocytes in grade 1a (mild acute rejection) to

**Table 17.1** Infiltrating cells in myocardial inflammation

| Authors [ref.] | | Lymphocytes (%) | Macrophages (%) | Neutrophils (%) | Animal model |
|---|---|---|---|---|---|
| Tilney *et al.* | [1] | 75 | 15–25 | 5 | Rat heterotopic heart transplantation |
| Barry | [2] | 44 | 36 | 20 | Mouse heterotopic heart transplantation |
| Cramer *et al.* | [3] | 37[a] | 63 | | Rat heterotopic heart transplantation |
| Ruderman *et al.* | [4] | <5 | >90 | | Murine Lyme carditis |
| Kelleher *et al.* | [5] | ~10 | ~90 | | Murine Lyme carditis |
| Saeki *et al.* | [6] | | 70 | | Rat myosin-induced myocarditis |
| Smith *et al.* | [7] | ~30 | ~30 | ~30 | Murine myosin-induced myocarditis |

[a]16% of total infiltrate is due to natural killer cell infiltration.

'aggressive' lymphocytes, eosinophils, and neutrophils in grade 4 (severe acute rejection). T-lymphocytes are present in every infiltrate in rejecting hearts and appear to be absolutely required [10]. Infiltrates due to rejection of an acute allograft need to be distinguished from those of perioperative ischaemic myocardial injury [11]. Thought to be secondary to coagulative myocyte necrosis, these infiltrates are primarily composed of polymorphonuclear leucocytes (PMNs) and histiocytes, including plasma cells and occasional lymphocytes.

The idiopathic or primary form of myocarditis is usually characterized by exclusively lymphocytic inflammatory infiltrates with occasional PMNs, especially in the early course. According to the Dallas criteria, myocarditis is defined by an inflammatory infiltrate that is adjacent to degenerating or necrotic myocytes. Inflammatory processes secondary to a known cause may differ substantially and can be used for differential diagnosis. For example, the infiltrate in Lyme carditis is composed primarily of macrophages and a small number of T-cells [4, 5], whereas in viral myocarditis natural killer (NK) cells and T-cells are predominant [12]. The infiltrate in giant cell myocarditis, a rapidly fatal myocarditis, contains macrophagic giant cells, cytotoxic lymphocytes, and eosinophils [13].

Recent evidence supports the hypothesis that idiopathic dilated cardiomyopathy (DCM) might be a sequela of a myocarditis. In a recent study up to 38% of biopsies showed increased infiltrating lymphocytes [14], indicating borderline or ongoing myocarditis. Recent advances, including improved immunohistochemical methods, may provide means to subclassify infiltrating cells further. It appears that different types of cardiac infiltrate can lead to myocardial damage, suggesting that a variety of cell types can cause myocyte injury during immunologically stimulated reactions. The possible cell types and mechanisms involved in this process are considered next.

## Interaction of lymphocytes and cardiac myocytes

Several types of lymphocyte are involved in cellular immune reactions. NK lymphocytes recognize viral antigens and immunoglobulin-$\gamma$ (IgG) molecules on the surface of target cells, resulting in NK cell degranulation. Helper T-lymphocytes (HTLs, $CD4^+$), via their T-cell receptor (TCR)–CD3 complex, recognize endocytosed peptides that are bound to major histocompatibility complex (MHC) class II molecules on antigen-presenting cells (APCs). Cytotoxic T-lymphocytes (CTLs $CD8^+$) recognize endogenously synthesized peptide antigens associated with MHC class I molecules on the target cell. Binding of the HTL and CTL CD3 complex to MHC antigens is supported by accessory molecules. Although interaction of the TCR with the MHC complex is responsible for the specificity of the immune response, non-antigen-specific accessory molecules are required to activate T-cells fully [15, 16].

Activation of T-cells involves an increase in phospholipase C activity, and a rise in intracellular calcium concentration ($[Ca^{2+}]_i$) due to both an inositol 1, 4, 5-triphosphate ($IP_3$)-induced $Ca^{2+}$ release from intracellular stores and an increase in $Ca^{2+}$ influx via an intracellular $Ca^{2+}$ store-dependent pathway [17]. In HTL, $Ca^{2+}$ activates the $Ca^{2+}$ calmodulin-dependent phosphatase, calcineurin, which dephosphorylates nuclear factors of activated T-cells (NF-ATs) [18]. These dephosphorylated NF-ATs then gain access to the nucleus, where they activate immune regulatory genes, thus initiating cytokine production. The commonly used immunosuppressant drugs cyclosporin A and FK 506 inhibit the effect of calcineurin on NF-ATs [19].

The degree of MHC expression is of particular clinical importance in modulating lymphocyte–myocyte interaction. Herskowitz *et al.* [20] reported up to a ten-fold increase in MHC class I and II expression within microvascular endothelium and myocytes in patients with active myocarditis. Biopsy specimens from human hearts before transplantation showed basically no expression of MHC class I (except at intercalated discs) or class II on the surface of the myocytes [21]. However, after transplantation, although no increase in class II antigens on the myocytes was seen, strong expression of class I could be detected. Expression of MHC classes I and II on interstitial cells increased post-transplant. The MHC increase was noted in some cases even before an infiltrate was seen, indicating the importance of cytokines in regulating MHC expression.

Experiments with MHC class I or II knockout mice further underline the importance of these molecules in the rejection process. A significant prolongation of heart allograft survival time was observed in donors deficient in either class I or II antigens [22]. The extent of the MHC compatibility also significantly influences the heart allograft survival time in humans. In a multicentre trial with more than 8000 heart-transplant patients, that the Opelz *et al.*

[23] showed 3-year survival rate when there were zero and one MHC mismatches was 93%, compared with 71% when there were three to six mismatches.

Accessory molecules strengthen cell adhesion and transduce biochemical signals for costimulation. For the cardiac inflammatory process, the adhesion of infiltrating cells to endothelium and myocytes is of special interest. Members of the integrin family on the lymphocyte surface [leucocyte function-associated antigen (LFA-1), very late antigens 4–6 (VLA-4 to VLA-6) and their ligands on the target cell surface, intercellular adhesion molecules 1–3 (ICAM-1 to ICAM-3), vascular cell adhesion molecule (VCAM-1), as well as matrix molecules] are responsible for cell adhesion [24]. At least two other accessory molecules [CD28 and CD40L (former gp39, now called CD154)] on the surface of T-cells are known to serve costimulatory purposes [16]. CD28 binds to B7-1 (CD80) and B7-2 (CD86) mainly on APCs and endothelial cells [25], while CD40L conjugates with CD40 expressed on a variety of cells such as B-cells, macrophages, endothelial cells, and dendritic cells [24].

Cardiac myocytes constitutively express ICAM-1 (CD54) and LFA-3 (CD58), but not LFA-1 (CD11), and their expression can be increased by cytokines such as interleukin-1 (IL-1)-$\alpha$ and IL-1$\beta$, interferon-$\gamma$ (IFN-$\gamma$), and tumour necrosis factor-$\alpha$ (TNF-$\alpha$) [26, 27]. In a recent study Wang *et al.* [28] demonstrated that ICAM-1 expression is related to cardiac performance. In a syngenic heterotopic mouse cardiac transplant model, which included 2 h of cold ischaemia, ICAM-1-positive grafts had a reduced left ventricular compliance and an increased neutrophil infiltration compared with ICAM-1-negative grafts.

Most of the cytotoxic effects of lymphocytes are mediated by activated $CD8^+$ CTL or NK cells, although under certain circumstances $CD4^+$ cells may also be cytotoxic [2, 24, 29]. This discussion focuses on the effects of $CD4^+$ and $CD8^+$ lymphocytes.

## Helper T-lymphocytes ($CD4^+$)

There are two subgroups of HTL, evolving from the same precursor cell called $Th_0$, which can be distinguished by the cytokine types that they secrete (Fig. 17.1). $Th_1$ HTLs produce IL-2, IFN-$\gamma$, and lymphotoxin, which promote CTL development, delayed-type hypersensitivity (DTH) responses, and IgG2a antibody isotope switching, which facilitates antibody-dependent cellular cytotoxicity (ADCC). Th2 HTLs produce IL-4, IL-5, IL-6, IL-9, IL-10, and IL-13, thereby promoting humoral, allergic, and mucosal responses [30–32]. As will be discussed below, CTLs and macrophages, stimulated by $Th_1$ HTLs, are known to induce myocellular dysfunction and damage, both directly and, in the case of macrophages, indirectly, by the cytokines that they produce. The $Th_2$-mediated contribution is still under investigation. IL-4, initially secreted by mast cells [33] and NK1. 1 $CD4^+$ T-cells [34], is believed to be required for the development of $Th_2$ CTLs [32, 35], which could be cytotoxic. However, IL-4 decreases IL-2 receptor expression [36] and antagonizes IFN-$\gamma$-mediated effects [32], thus inhibiting $Th_1$ development. Furthermore, IL-10 produced by $Th_2$ inhibits IL-12 production [35], possibly providing another way of downregulating $Th_1$ responses.

Some experimental work helped to profile the different cytokines involved in myocardial inflammation. Cytokine profiles were analysed in murine cardiac allografts in which tolerance is induced by treating the recipient with either anti-CD4 monoclonal antibodies (mAbs) [37] alone or in combination with donor-specific blood transfusion and cyclosporine A [38]. IL-4 and IL-10 were increased while IFN-$\gamma$ and IL-2 were reduced compared with rejecting controls. As discussed later, blocking ICAM-1 and LFA-1 leads to long-term survival of cardiac allografts [39]. Analysis of cytokine profiles in these experiments shows that predominance of $Th_2$ over $Th_1$ is essential for the induction of tolerance. Mouse models of neonatal tolerance revealed similar results. Neonatal mice primed with allogenic splenocytes tolerated skin grafts from the same donor while rejecting third-party grafts [40]. Lymph-node cells draining the tolerated grafts showed a IL-4 to IFN-$\gamma$ ratio 100 times higher than that in rejecting grafts. These results seem to favour the hypothesis that $Th_2$ THLs are responsible for graft tolerance.

However, considerable evidence exists that questions the importance of $Th_2$ HTLs for tolerance. VanBuskirk *et al.* [41] transfused severe combined immunodeficiency (SCID) mice after allogenic heart transplantation with $Th_1$- or $Th_2$-like graft-reactive cells, generated by *in vitro* stimulation of splenocytes with donor strain alloantigens using IL-4 or IL-4 mAbs, respectively. As expected, $Th_1$-like cells led to acute allograft rejection; however, $Th_2$-like cells had the same effect. In both cases the transfused cells were found in the allograft and histological analyses showed sim-

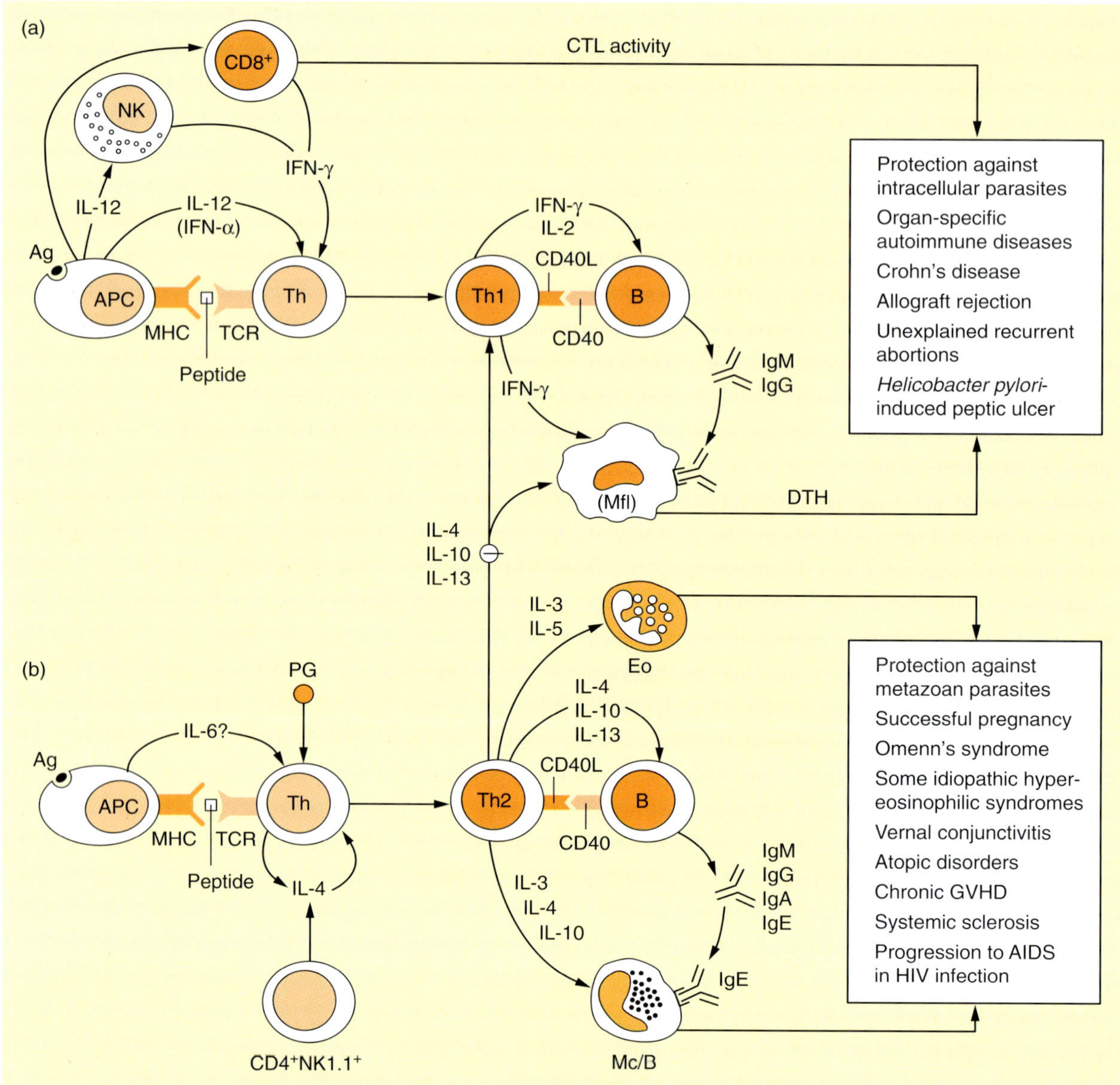


**Figure 17.1** *Functions of $Th_1$ and $Th_2$ helper T-lymphocytes. (a) Early production of interleukin-12 (IL-12) and interferons by cells of the innate immune system promotes the development of $Th_1$ cells, which induces the activation of macrophages (Mφs) which can elicit a delayed-type hypersensitivity (DTH) reaction. $Th_1$ responses, together with frequently associated cytotoxic T-lymphocyte (CTL) activity, are responsible for acute allograft rejection, but may result in organ-specific autoimmune disease and other immunopathological disorders. (b) Autonomous IL-4 production by the naive Th cell, possibly stimulated by antigen-presenting cell (APC)-derived IL-6, or early production of IL-4 provided by the $CD4^+NK1.1^+$ subset, promotes the development of $Th_2$ cells, which stimulate high antibody production (including IgE), eosinophil and mast cell activity, and inhibit (indicated by the minus sign) $Th_1$ cells and macrophages. $Th_2$ responses hamper the rejection of the foetal 'allograft', but can be responsible for the development of atopy and other immunopathological disorders. Ag=antigen; B=B-cell; Eo= eosinophil; GVHD= graft-versus-host disease; IFN-γ= interferon-γ; Mc/B = mast cell/basophil; MHC = major histocompatibility complex; NK = natural killer; PG= progesterone; T= T-cell; TCR = T-cell receptor; $Th_1$ = T-helper-1. (From ref. 30 with permission.)*

ilar rejection processes. Rejecting cardiac allografts accumulate large numbers of $CD8^+$ CTLs, indicating a $Th_1$-like immune reaction. Chan *et al.* [42] depleted recipients of $CD8^+$ cells; despite depletion, rejection still occurred, showing a cellular infiltrate rich in eosinophils and large mononuclear cells. Compared with non-depleted controls, grafts showed increased $Th_2$ cytokine gene expression. The authors suggest that $CD8^+$ CTLs inhibit intragraft production of $Th_2$-like cytokines, thus promoting $Th_1$ dominance, while $CD8^+$ depletion allows $Th_2$ production, which has different but still deleterious effects on the graft.

As mentioned above, blocking IL-12 gives a $Th_2$-like cytokine response. In a murine cardiac allograft model, Piccotti *et al.* [43] showed that IL-12 antagonism induces intragraft $Th_2$-like cytokine expression; however, the rejection was exacerbated. In this model, IL-12 antagonism did not completely abrogate $Th_1$-like cytokines, as IFN-$\gamma$-producing cells could still be found. Conversely, it has been shown recently that IL-12 can trigger a $Th_1$-like response in experimental autoimmune myocarditis [44]. Myosin-specific T-lymphocytes cultured with cardiac myosin peptide in the presence of IL-12 were more potent in inducing experimental autoimmune myocarditis after being transferred in a naive rat than those cultured in the presence of IL-2. Using a different approach to block a $Th_1$-like immune response, Qian *et al.* [45] administered IL-10 in a murine heart-transplant model. Instead of protecting the graft, rejection was enhanced. IL-10 increased both the circulating complement-dependent cytotoxic antibody titre and cytotoxic T-lymphocyte activity.

The above evidence shows that $Th_2$ cell-mediated immune reactions can be both protective and deleterious. Further studies will be needed to clarify their roles and the mechanisms involved during rejection and other types of myocardial inflammation.

## Mechanisms and importance of cytotoxic T-lymphocyte-mediated myocyte injury

After conjugation to the target cell, the CTLs have two known ways to deliver a 'lethal hit': a granule exocytosis-dependent (perforin/granzyme-mediated) and a granule exocytosis-independent (Fas ligand-mediated) pathway [24]. In the former, perforin monomers are exocytosed to reassemble as a polymer in a calcium-dependent manner in the target cell membrane. This polymer forms an unselective ion channel, also allowing water to enter the cell and thus osmotically leading to cell swelling and, eventually, cell lysis. Granzyme B, a serine protease, is exocytosed from CTLs together with perforin and can cross the target cell membrane in a perforin-independent, energy-dependent mechanism [46]. Perforin is required for granzyme B to enter the nucleus, where it mediates apoptosis through an interleukin-1-converting enzyme (ICE)-dependent pathway, similar to that of Fas/Fas ligand. The exact mechanism of apoptosis is beyond the scope of this chapter (for review see refs. 24 and 47).

The Fas/Fas-ligand pathway seems to be even more complex as it can induce apoptosis on the one hand and immunotolerance on the other. Usually, the Fas ligand on CTLs induces apoptosis in Fas-bearing target cells. Tissues constitutively expressing high levels of Fas ligand, such as the cornea and testis, however, enjoy a state of immune privilege. They seem to cause apoptosis in infiltrating cells when binding, for example, to the Fas antigen of the CTL, thus leading to immunotolerance [48].

There is some uncertainty as to the significance of these pathways in myocyte injury. It has been demonstrated in human cardiac transplant biopsies that the expression of granzyme A and perforin correlates with rejection [49]. Chen *et al.* [50] showed that in murine cardiac allografts in which tolerance was induced by donor-specific transfusion and anti-CD4 treatment, the expression of granzyme and perforin is decreased compared with rejecting grafts. However, in a murine cardiac transplant model, perforin-deficient recipients rejected fully MHC-mismatched allografts in the same period (6 days) as did perforin-positive recipients [51]. As a possible explanation Fas-dependent killing might come into play. However, in the same study, Fas-negative donor hearts transplanted into perforin-negative recipients were almost equally rejected within 7 days. Secreted factors or yet unknown cell contact-dependent cytotoxic mechanisms may contribute to this phenomenon. This same group showed the importance of perforin-mediated rejection in a model using only one MHC class I mismatch. Grafts in perforin-deficient mice survived about three times longer than in control mice (31 vs 87 days). Under these special conditions, MHC class II restricted HTLs are not activated initially, perhaps resulting in a lack of the lymphokines usually secreted by these HTLs. Together with a low class I antigenicity, this might reduce the intensity of other cellular injury mechanisms such as DTH, making perforin more important for the rejection process.

Results from the present authors' laboratory also indicate the importance of CTL degranulation-dependent myocyte target cell injury [52]. Allosensitized CTLs were able to decrease the amplitude of myocyte motion, and action potential and decrease calcium transients in cultures of donor-type foetal ventricular myocytes; the diastolic membrane potential was also decreased. These effects were abolished by pretreating the cells with 4,4′-diisothiocyano-2,2′disulfonic acid stilbene (DIDS), an inhibitor of lymphocyte degranulation. This work is consistent with results from Binah *et al.* [53], who demonstrated that granules from CTLs could induce similar electrophysiological changes (shortening of action potential duration, reduction of resting potential, and reduction in action potential amplitude followed by a progressive contracture and elevation in cytosolic calcium associated with cell lysis) in isolated adult ventricular myocytes.

Evidence for the existence of Fas-mediated myocyte damage comes from a recent study by Felzen *et al.* [54], who showed the presence of Fas on freshly isolated murine ventricular myocytes. Alloreactive CTLs from peritoneal exudates, derived from perforin gene knockout mice and coincubated with donor-specific myocytes, caused decreased myocyte resting membrane potential, decreased action potential amplitude, prolonged action potential duration at 80% repolarization, diastolic $[Ca^{2+}]_i$ increase, delayed after-depolarizations, and arrhythmogenic activity. All these effects could be reproduced by an anti-Fas mAb, Jo2. Their data also suggest that $IP_3$ is a second messenger in the Fas pathway. Blocking $IP_3$ with heparin prevented the myocyte dysfunction induced by the Fas receptor, while the above results could be reproduced by applying $IP_3$ via a patch pipette directly into the myocyte.

Although these *in vitro* studies suggest a potential role for the Fas/Fas-ligand pathway in immune-mediated myocyte injury, the results of Seino *et al.* [55] indicate that the *in vivo* situation is more complex. Transplanting murine hearts into Fas- or Fas-ligand-deficient recipients led to prolonged survival, while Fas-deficient grafts transplanted into regular recipients were rejected in the same period as controls. To explain why Fas-deficient recipients had a prolonged survival, the authors postulate that either Fas might be needed as a T-cell costimulator or Fas ligand produced by alloreactive T-cells might interact with Fas on the recipient-derived macrophages in the allograft to initiate the additional cytokine release possibly required for a competent immune response. These results are consistent with findings from Schulz *et al.* [51], who also showed that Fas-negative grafts are rejected even in perforin-deficient mice.

While it is well established that CTLs can produce myocyte injury *in vitro* [52, 56, 57], the significance of CTL-mediated injury *in vivo* is less certain. When heart infiltrating cells (HICs) isolated from cardiac allografts were used as effector cells, a small portion of myocyte cytotoxicity caused by HICs could be prevented by CTL depletion [57]. A recent report [58] showed that *in vivo* depletion of CTLs improved the function of the rejecting murine heart early (at 5 days post-transplant) in the rejection process (Fig. 17.2). However, Chan *et al.* [42] and Menon *et al.* [58] found that *in vivo* depletion of $CD8^+$ cells in the recipient animal, which virtually eliminated CTLs from the infiltrating cell population, did not cause prolonged survival of the allograft. It is clear that $CD8^+$ cells can cause myocyte injury but their contribution to myocyte necrosis during advanced heart transplant rejection *in vivo* appears to be relatively minor.

## Effects or macrophages

Macrophages are present in considerable numbers in myocardial inflammatory lesions, and may contribute to myocyte dysfunction and injury (Table 17.1). Initial studies by Christmas and MacPherson [59, 60] demonstrated that macrophages infiltrating a rejecting transplanted rat heart inhibited spontaneous contractions of cultured neonatal rat ventricular myocytes but did not cause cell lysis. Pinsky *et al.* [61] have shown that J774 macrophages activated by exposure to IFN-$\gamma$ and lipopolysaccharides (LPS) cause lysis of isolated adult rat cardiac myocytes, which was; inhibited by the addition of the competitive nitric oxide (NO) synthesis inhibitor L-*N*-monomethyl-arginine (L-NMMA) to the culture medium.

These findings are consistent with the report by Higuchi *et al.* [62] that TNF-$\alpha$ production and L-arginine-dependent mechanisms act synergistically as a major cytolytic mechanism of isolated macrophages when assessed against L929 and P815 target cells. Hibbs *et al.* [63] showed that L-arginine-dependent NO production by activated macrophages can inhibit mitochondrial respiration in some target cells. Isolated activated primary murine macrophages can induce lysis of cultured adult mouse ventricular myocytes [64], although this effect of macrophages could not be consistently diminished by nitric oxide synthase (NOS) inhibition. Other potential mechanisms by which macrophages could produce cytotoxicity include the generation of hydrogen peroxide [65], cytolytic proteases [66], and reactive nitrogen intermediates [67].

Effects on myocyte function can be caused by macrophages. The work of Christmas and MacPherson [59, 60] has been mentioned. In addition, Balligand *et al.* [68] demonstrated that impaired contractile responses of iso-

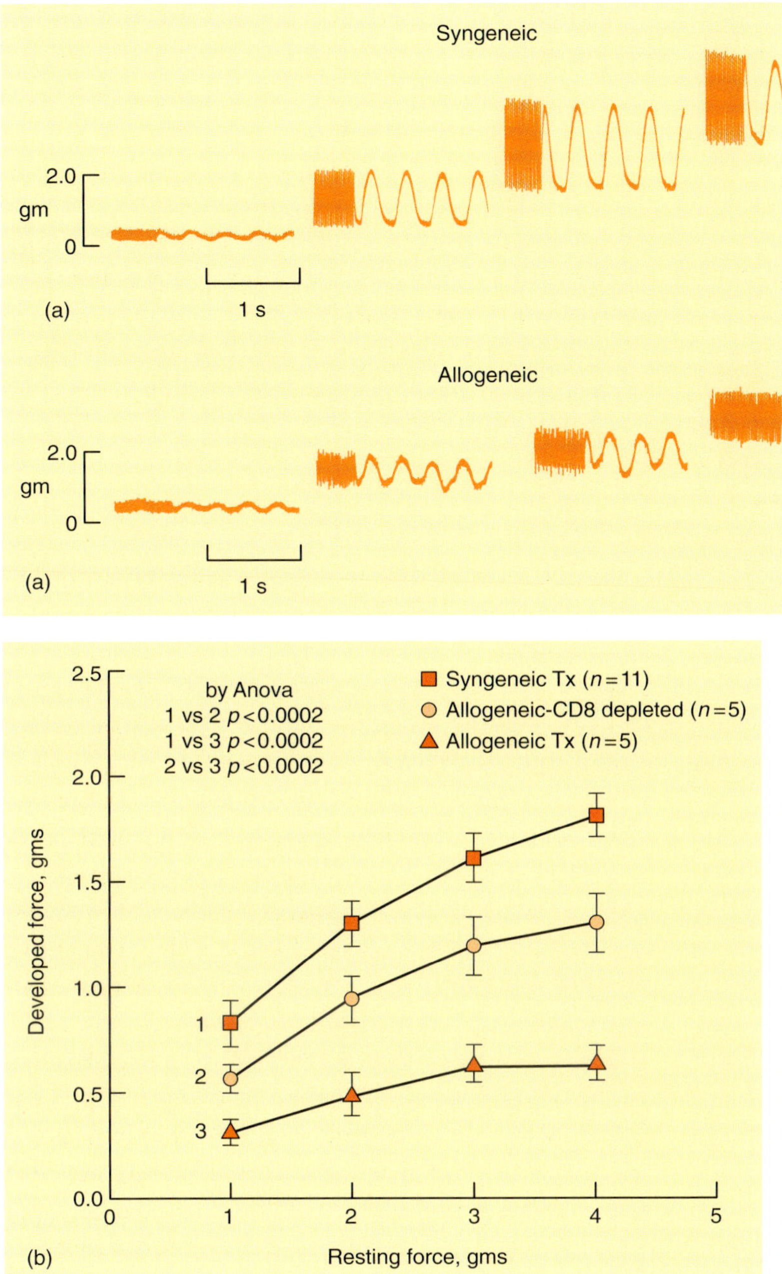


**Figure 17.2** *(A) Example of force measurements contractions made with a strain gauge attached by a suture to an intra-abdominal heterotopic heart transplant* in vivo *at varying degrees of diastolic stretch (resting force changed with a micromanipulator to which the strain gauge was attached). A syngeneic transplanted heart* (upper trace) *and an allogeneic rejecting heart* (lower trace) *are shown 5 days after transplant, at fast and slow recorder speed. A decrease in developed force is apparent in the rejecting heart. There was no significant difference in the spontaneous beating rates (approx. 200 min) between the two transplanted hearts. (B) Average developed force as a function of diastolic stretch (force) for syngeneic, allogeneic and allogeneic transplants in which CD8⁺ CTLs were depleted by injectioin of monoclonal antibody, at day 5. There was a significant decrease in developed force associated with the rejection process and this was partially but incompletely reversed by depletion of CTL. (From ref. 58 with permission.)*

lated rat ventricular myocytes to catecholamine stimulation can be induced by exposure to a medium conditioned by activated macrophages. This effect on catecholamine responsiveness was blocked by the presence of L-NMMA in the preincubation medium. They concluded that the cytokines produced by activated macrophages induced NO synthesis in ventricular myocytes, and that this was responsible for the inhibition of the inotropic response to catecholamines, possibly mediated by activation of soluble intracellular guanylate cyclase. The mechanisms by which cytokines increase NO, and by which NO alters myocyte function by cyclic guanosine monophosphate (cGMP)- and non-cGMP-dependent mechanisms, have been well summarized by [69] and are discussed in more detail below.

Not all negative inotropic effects of macrophage-derived cytokines are due to enhanced production of NO. Yokoyama *et al.* [70] found that TNF-α caused a direct negative inotropic effect in feline myocardium, intact ventricle, and isolated cardiac myocytes. In cat myocytes, this negative inotropic effect was associated with a decrease in the calcium transient, had no effect no the calcium current, and was not inhibited by NOS blockers. Thus, it seems likely that macrophages may cause some myocyte injury and dysfunction via the cytokines that they produce. The effects on myocytes of cytokines produced by inflammatory cells are considered next.

## Cytokine effects on myocytes

Cytokines have important immunoregulatory effects, for example, by directing immune responses into a $Th_1$- or $Th_2$-mediated pathway, possibly influencing tolerance versus rejection in transplantation. It is also well established that certain cytokines have direct effects on the myocardium. The clinical importance of cytokines is supported by several studies that have shown elevated circulating cytokine levels in patients with different cardiac illnesses: congestive heart failure due to coronary artery disease or hypertension, myocarditis, cardiomyopathy, and heart-transplant recipients [71–76]. Testa *et al.* [71] demonstrated a correlation between cyokine levels (TNF-α, IL-1β, and IL-6), and New York Heart Association (NYHA) functional class.

Experimental work has supported the validity of these observations. Kumar *et al.* [77] examined the effect of human serum from patients with septic shock on neonatal rat cardiac myocytes. They found that TNF-α and IL-1β were responsible for significant concentration-dependent depression of maximum extent and peak velocity of neonatal rat myocyte shortening *in vitro*. Removing TNF-α and IL-1β (but not either alone) from the serum by immunoabsorption eliminated the myocardial depressant activity. While each cytokine alone was effective in depressing myocyte function, they acted synergistically at concentrations well within the serum range documented in human septic shock. In this study, IL-2, IL-4, Il-6, IL-8, IL-10, and IFN-γ in a wide range of concentrations had no effect on myocytes. Many other studies using different models, including intact animals [78], isolated hearts [79], isolated papillary muscles [80], and cardiomyocytes [79], have shown that TNF-α and IL-1β depress cardiac function. A summary of the cytokines that decrease myocardial contractility is given in Table 17.2.

TNF-α has two different time-courses of action: an immediate effect within 30 min [79–81] and a delayed effect after 24–72 h [90]. The delayed effect seems to be mediated by an NO-dependent pathway. However, Oral *et al.* [81] found that sphingosine mediates the immediate effect of TNF-α. They were able to show in isolated adult feline myocytes that treatment with TNF-α led to a rapid increase in free sphingosine, possibly mediated by cytokine-induced activation of neutral sphingomyelinase. Sphingosine applied to isolated myocytes mimicked the immediate effect of TNF-α and sphingosine production blocked with oleoylethanolamine completely abrogated the TNF-α effect. Neither precursors nor metabolites of sphingosine were able to reproduce its effects. McDonough *et al.* [82] used whole-cell patch clamping of adult and neonatal rat ventricular myocytes to demonstrate that sphingosine directly inhibits L-type calcium current in a does-dependent fashion. Furthermore, caffeine-induced calcium transients were reduced, indicating impaired sarcoplasmic reticulum function. Thus, the amount of entering 'trigger calcium' is reduced by sphingosine, while the

**Table 17.2** Cytokines that decrease myocardial contractility

| Cytokine | Mediated by | Produced by | Refs. | Inotropic effect | |
|---|---|---|---|---|---|
| | | | | ⇓ basal function | ⇓ β-adrenergic response |
| TNF-α | Sphingosine, NO | Macrophages, myocytes, endothelial cells | [81–85] [86] | | — |
| IFN-γ | NO | Activated T-cells | [87][a] | — | |
| IL-1 | NO | Activated macrophases, endothelial cells | [85, 86] | — | — |
| IL-2 | NO | Activated T-cells | [88] | — | |
| IL-6 | NO | Macrophages, monocytes, T-cells, endothelial cells | [89] | — | |

[a]Interferon-γ (IFN-γ) in combination with lipopolysaccharide.
TNF-α = tumour necrosis-factor-α; IL = interleukin; NO = nitric oxide.

threshold of the ryanodine receptor for calcium-induced calcium release is increased, explaining the decrease in the $[Ca^{2+}]_i$ transient and the negative inotropic effect induced by TNF-α.

TNF-α can cause severe myocardial dysfunction. Bryant *et al.* [83] recently developed a transgenic mouse model in which TNF-α was overexpressed in myocytes driven by the promoter of the α-myosine heavy chain. They found a severe panmyocarditis with an intiltrate rich in macrophages and small T-cells, which clinically progressed into heart failure and premature mortality. Although the direct action of TNF-α on cardiac myocytes may not account entirely for the effects noted, myocyte TNF-α production can at least trigger an immunological response, and possibly produce significant direct negative inotropic effects.

## Nitric oxide-mediated cytokine effects

NO is generated by a family of enzymes called nitric oxide synthases (NOS) during the conversion of L-arginine to L-citruline in the presence of $O_2$ and NADPH [69]. While the isoenzyme NOS-1 seems only to play a minor role within the myocardium [91–93], the calcium-independent, cytokine-inducible NOS-2 and the calcium-dependent, constitutive NOS-3 [93–96] are more important. NOS-2 mRNA and activity in myocytes are increased by LPS, IL-1β, TNF-α, IFN-γ, and IL-6 [84, 96–98]. The most important cell types within the heart producing NO via the NOS-2 pathway are believed to be myocytes, endothelial cells and, in inflammation, infiltrating inflammatory cells, especially macrophages [96, 99]. NOS-3 has also been identified in myocytes and cardiac microvascular endothelium cells [93–96, 100].

NO can have significant effects on myocardial function [69]. Schulz *et al.* [85] showed that perfusing isolated whole hearts with a cytokine combination of IL-1β and TNF-α led to decreased contractile function with a time-course consistent with NOS-2 induction. Furthermore, it has been shown that the effects of NOS-2 induction are not limited to depressing function. Pinsky *et al.* [61] showed that exposure of adult rat ventricular myocytes to the combination of recombinant IL-1β, TNF-α, and IFN-γ resulted in significant myocyte injury and death. NOS inhibitors or prevention of myocyte NOS-2 induction by transforming growth factor-β (TGF-β) prevented the deleterious effects of the cytokines on myocyte survival.

Several reports have confirmed NOS-2 induction in inflammatory cells, microvasculature, and cardiac myocytes in allogenic transplants but not in syngenic controls [101, 102]. A reasonable hypothesis is that increased NO production is responsible for impaired contraction and graft loss during cardiac transplant rejection. Consistent with this idea, blocking NOS-2 with aminoguanidine was shown to improve graft survival, and increase tension development in right ventricular papillary muscles and shortening in isolated myocytes obtained from allografted but not isografted hearts [101, 103, 104]. Similar results were shown in studies by Menon *et al.* (Fig. 17.3) [58]. In a heterotopic abdominal cardiac mouse transplant model, continuous subcutaneous L-NMMA was administered by an osmotic pump to block NOS. In allogenic hearts treated with L-NMMA the developed force was significantly improved compared with non-treated hearts, although still slightly depressed compared with syngenic hearts treated with L-NMMA. Inhibition of NOS only slightly prolonged average graft survival from 10 to 11 days. These findings suggest that NO is an important mediator of contractile dysfunction during rejection, but that other factors are important in influencing graft survival.

Besides a possibly deleterious effect, NO may have some important function in regulating immune response [105]. Cytokines characterized as mediators of innate or natural immunity such as TNF-α, IL-1β, or IL-6 are all related to NOS-2 induction. $NO_x$ generated by NOS-2 has been shown to suppress viral replicating or reactivation and to promote bacterial killing [106, 107]. Thus, NOS-2 knockout mice were susceptible to lethal infection with facultative intracellular and opportunistic pathogens at rates much higher than the wild-type mice [108, 109].

## Effects of neutrophils on myocytes

As shown in Table 17.1, neutrophils comprise a significant component of the inflammatory response. Neutrophils can also cause direct injury of cardiac myocytes, an effect that may be modulated by cytokines. Youker *et al.* [27] showed that exposure of adult canine cardiac myocytes to cytokines such as IL-1 and TNF-α produces surface expression of ICAM-1 on the myocyte. Subsequent exposure to activated neutrophils allows a neutrophil–myocyte adhesion mediated by the CD18–ICAM-1 interaction.

Entman *et al.* [110] further demonstrated that shortly after neutrophil adherence to an individual myocyte,

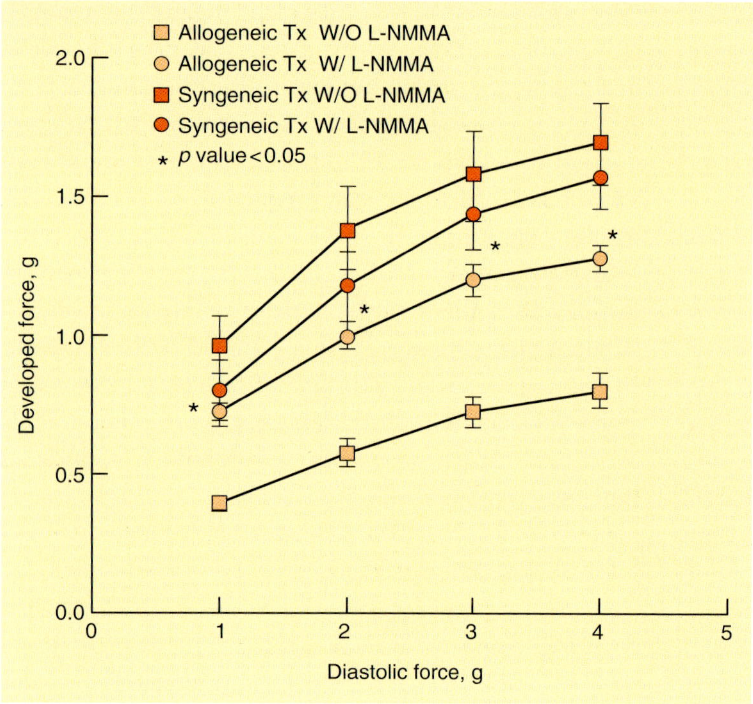


**Figure 17.3** *Effect of inhibition of nitric oxide synthase (NOS) by subcutaneous infusion of* L*-N-monomethyl-arginine (*L*-NMMA) on contractile function measured* in vivo *on day 5 after transplantation. Inhibition of NOS produced a significant improvement in contractile function in rejecting allogeneic hearts, although function remained slightly depressed relative to syngeneic hearts, and to syngeneic hearts in animals treated with* L*-NMMA alone. (From ref. 58 with permission.)*

myocyte contracture is induced, which is associated with intracellular oxidation as monitored by the fluorescent probe dichlorofluorescein. The fluorescence and myocyte injury can be inhibited by the intracellular hydroxyl radical scavenger dimethylthiourea. The conclusion was that neutrophil–myocyte interaction dependent on expression of the Mac-1 (CD11B/CD18) complex on the neutrophil and ICAM-1 on the myocyte results in activation of neutrophil respiratory burst, in turn resulting in compartmentalized, iron-dependent, myocyte oxidative injury. Semb *et al.* [111] showed that activated leucocytes cause structural changes in the heart through the combined action of oxygen free radicals and arachidonic acid metabolites. Isolated rat hearts were perfused with PMNs activated with phorbol 12-myristate 13-acetate. Coperfusion with scavengers (superoxide dismutase + catalase + thiourea) or in combination with ibuprofen, a cyclooxygenase inhibitor; diethylcarbamazine, a lipoxygenase inhibitor; or BW755C, a dual inhibitor of cyclooxygenase and lipoxygenase, and an oxygen free radical scavenger ameliorated the effect of activated leucocytes on mitochondria and the capillary walls. It was recently also demonstrated that $\alpha_4$-integrin is important for the myocyte–neutrophil adhesion process once the neutrophils have migrated into the tissue [112]. Upregulated by chemokines such as CINC-gro or fMLP, $\alpha_4$ expression is increased and binds to fibronectin, a myocyte matrix protein, thus potentially bringing neutrophils into close contact with myocytes.

In a rat heart-transplant model, Oubenaissa *et al.* [113] suggested the involvement of LFA-1 (CD11a) in neutrophil-mediated early reperfusion injury. Applying anti-LFA-1 mAB to the recipient in a single dose 35 min before reperfusing the allograft resulted in significantly improved recovery of contractility compared with controls pretreated with saline. The improved haemodynamic parameters went hand in hand with a reduction in myocardial accumulation of neutrophils in the anti-LFA-1 mAB-treated group.

As mentioned previously, neutrophils can be found in inflammatory lesions associated with cardiac rejection or with myocarditis. It is possible therefore, that a component of myocyte injury induced in inflammatory infiltrates of the myocardium is due to the neutrophil–myocyte interaction. However, a murine transplant study by Schowengerdt *et al.* [114] demonstrated that in mice homozygous for a gene-targeted mutation of ICAM-1, cardiac allograft survival did not differ significantly from controls when ICAM-1-deficient mutants were used either as donor or as recipient. Histological examination of the rejection of both normal and ICAM-1-deficient cardiac allografts revealed similar patterns of infiltration of mononuclear and granulocytic leucocytes, and myocyte necrosis. While this might suggest that neutrophils are not important contributors to myocyte injury during rejection, the interpretation of this result is complicated by the fact that there are, as previously discussed, multiple pathways causing myocyte injury during cardiac transplant rejection. In many instances, elimination of one pathway may be insufficient to have a dramatic effect on the intensity of the rejection injury, possibly owing to upregulation of other alternative pathways.

## Possible new approaches to treatment

Conventional immunosuppressants such as cyclosporin A, prednisone, immuran, and OKT-3 have markedly improved results in cardiac transplantation, but chronic rejection remains a major problem. This is particularly true with respect to graft arteriopathy resulting from immune-mediated vascular injury. However, some promising new approaches are being studied in animal models that may eventually prove useful clinically.

With respect to transplant rejection, the molecular identification of the various adhesion molecules involved in the interaction of lymphocytes with various target cells and with lymphocyte activation has permitted the development of monoclonal antibodies and other agents that significantly alter the immune response. For example, blocking ICAM-1 and LFA-1 with monoclonal antibodies (mABs) induced immunotolerance and long-term survival greater (> 100 days) in mice with cardiac transplants [115, 116], compared with blocking either of them alone. Although mABs were only administered for 7 days post-transplant, long-term survival still occurred.

The function and effect of VCAM-1 seem to be similar to those seen with ICAM-1. Expressed mainly on the surface of endothelial cells, VCAM-1 can be upregulated by inflammatory cytokines [117] and blocking it leads to long-term cardiac allograft survival in the heterotopic murine transplant model. Orosz *et al.* [118] showed that anti-VCAM-1 treatment for 20 days led to graft survival of at least 60 days. They observed only a mild T-cell infiltrate with few macrophages and could not detect any mRNA of IL-2, IL-4, and IFN-$\gamma$ by polymerase chain reaction.

CTLA4-Ig, an immunoglobulin fusion protein that binds to CD80 and CD86, in combination with anti-CD40L mAB, caused long-term cardiac allograft survival [119]. Grafts were remarkably free from lymphocytic infiltrates, and the parenchyma and blood vessels were virtually indistinguishable from those found in normal hearts. Treatment with CTLA4-Ig or anti-CD40L resulted in a more extensive lymphocytic infiltrate, with interstitial fibrosis and signs of coronary vasculopathy characteristic of chronic rejection, although the overall survival was prolonged compared with non-treated animals with transplants. Others have demonstrated that blocking only the CD-28/B7 pathway with CTLA4-Ig was sufficient to induce long-term survival in mice with allogenic heart transplants [120, 121]. Other evidence exists to show that CTLA4-Ig can only induce tolerance in conjunction with donor antigens [122].

Hancock *et al.* [25] reported a 70% long-term survival rate in mice with allografts by using anti-CD40L mAB alone. By combining this treatment with donor-specific lymphocyte transfusion (DST), indefinite survival was achieved, but the exact mechanism of DST action remains unclear. DST alone had no major effect on survival. However, indirect effects of anti-CD40L mAB via altered expression of other costimulatory molecules such as CD80 and/or CD86 remain a possibility. Although CD80 induction was almost completely abolished by anti-CD40L mAB plus DST, CD86 expression was not affected, ruling out a significant impact on the CD86-mediated pathway. Additional experiments using anti-CD80 mAB in combination with DST could not reproduce the long-term survival seen with anti-CD40L mAB plus DST, making it unlikely that impaired induction of CD80 was responsible for the anti-CD40L effect, and arguing for a direct costimulatory effect of the CD40L pathway in T-cell activation in this model. Further development of this type of approach may result in a reduced incidence of chronic rejection in clinical heart transplantation.

Mason *et al.* [123] and Parrillo *et al.* [124] showed that conventional immunosuppression does not improve clinical outcome in humans with myocarditis. However, a better characterization of inflammatory cell infiltrates by means of specific immunohistochemical techniques may allow identification of patients in whom immunosuppression will be of benefit [125]. As the molecular events involved in the initiation and maintenance of the immune response are better defined, the ability to diagnose and treat immune-mediated cardiac dysfunction will increase substantially.

## References

1. Tilney NL, Strom TB, Macpherson SG *et al.* Surface properties and functional characteristics of infiltrating cells harvested from acutely rejecting cardiac allografts in inbred rats. *Transplantation* 1975; 22: 1385–8.

2. Barry WH. Mechanisms of immune-mediated myocyte injury. *Circulation* 1994; 89: 2421–32.
3. Cramer DV, Wu GD, Chapman FA *et al.* Lymphocytic subsets and histopathologic changes associated with the development of heart transplant arteriosclerosis. *J Heart Lung Transplant* 1992; 11(3Pt1): 458–66.
4. Ruderman E, Kerr J, Telford S *et al.* Early murine lyme carditis has a macrophage predominace and is independent of major histocompatibility complex class II-Cd4$^+$ T cell interactions. *J Infect Dis* 1995; 171: 362–70.
5. Kelleher M, Telford S, Criscione L *et al.* Cytokines in murine lyme carditis: Th1 cytokine expression follows expression of proinflammatory cytokines in a susceptible mouse strain. *J Infect Dis* 1998; 177: 242–6.
6. Saeki M, Kodama M, Hanawa H *et al.* Morphological analysis of infiltrates in experimental autoimmune myocarditis. *Cardiomyopathy update 5. Prognosis and treatment of cardiomyopathies and myocarditis*. University of Tokyo Press: 1994; 241–3.
7. Smith SC, Allen PM. Neutralization of endogenous tumor necrosis factor ameliorates the severity of myosin-induced myocarditis. *Circ Res* 1992; 70: 856–63.
8. Billingham ME, Cary N, Hammond ME *et al.* A working formulation for the standardization of nomenclature in the diagnosis of heart and lung rejection: heart rejection study group. *Heart Transplant* 1990; 9: 587–93.
9. Aretz HT, Billingham ME, Edwards WD. Myocarditis: a histopathologic definition and classification. *Am J Cardiovasc Pathol* 1987; 1: 3–14.
10. Krensky A, Weiss A, Crabtree G *et al.* T-lymphocyte–antigen interactions in transplant rejection. *N Engl J Med* 1990; 322: 510–17.
11. Fyfe B, Loh E, Gayle L *et al.* Heart transplantation — associated perioperative ischemic myocardial injury. *Circulation* 1996; 93: 1133–40.
12. Seko Y, Takahashi N, Yagita H *et al.* Expression of cytokine mRNAs in murine hearts with acute myocarditis caused by coxsackievirus B3. *J Pathol* 1997; 183: 105–8.
13. Litovsky S, Burke A, Virmani R. Giant cell myocarditis an entity distinct from sarcoidosis characterized by multiphasic myocyte destruction by cytotoxic T cells and histiocytic giant cells. *Mod Pathol* 1996; 9: 1126–34.
14. Kuehl U, Noutsias M, Schultheiss H. Immunohistochemistry in dilated cardiomyopathy. *Eur Heart J* 1995; 16 (Suppl): 100–6.
15. Janeway CH, Bottomly K. Signals and signs for lymphocyte responses. *Cell* 1994; 76: 275–85.
16. Sayegh M, Turka L. The role of T-cell costimulatory activation pathways in transplant rejection. *N Engl J Med* 1998; 338: 1813–21.
17. Clapham DE. Calcium signaling. *Cell* 1995; 80: 259–68.
18. Jalin J, McCaffrey PG, Miner Z *et al.* The T-cell transcription factor $NFAT_p$ is a substrate for calcineurin and interacts with FOS and JUN. *Nature* 1993; 365: 352–5.
19. Alberola-Ila J, Takaki S, Kerner JD, Perlmutter RM. Differential signaling by lymphocyte antigen receptors. *Annu Rev Immunol* 1997; 15: 125–54.
20. Herskowitz A, Ansari A, Neumann D *et al.* Induction of major histocompatibility complex antigens within the myocardium of patients with active myocarditis: a nonhistologic marker of myocarditis. *J Am Coll Cardiol* 1990; 15: 624–32.
21. Rose M, Coles M, Griffin R *et al.* Expression of class I and class II MHC antigens in normal and transplanted human heart. *Transplantation* 1986; 41: 776–80.
22. Qian S, Fu F, Li Y *et al.* Impact of donor MHC class I or class II antigen deficiency on first- and second-set rejection of mouse heart or liver allografts. *Immunology* 1996; 88: 124–9.
23. Opelz G, Wujciak TH, for the Collaborative Transplant Study. The influence of HLA compatibility on graft survival after heart transplantation. *N Engl J Med* 1994; 330: 816–19.
24. Abbas A, Lichtman A, Pober J. Cellular and molecular immunology. *Saunders text and review series*, Philadelphia, PA: WB Saunders, 1997.
25. Hancock W, Sayegh M, Zheng X, Turka L. Costimulatory function and expression of CD40 ligand, CD80, and CD86 in vascularized murine cardiac allograft rejection. *Immunology* 1996; 93: 13 967–72.
26. Ansari A, Sudstrom J, Runnels H, Herskowitz A. The absence of constitutive and induced expression of critical cell-adhesion molecules on human cardiac myocytes. *Transplantation* 1994; 57: 942–9.
27. Youker K, Smith C, Anderson D *et al.* Neutrophil adherence to isolated adult cardiac myocytes: induction by cardiac lymph collected during ischemia and reperfusion. *J Clin Invest* 1992; 89: 602–9.
28. Wang C, Naka Y, Liao H, Pinsky C. Cardiac graft intercellular adhesion molecule-1 (ICAM-1) and interleukin-1 expression mediate primary isograft failure and induction of ICAM-1 in organs remote from the site of transplantation. *Circ Res* 1998; 82: 762–72.
29. Barry WH. Effects of cellular elements of the immune response on myocyte function and survival. *Heart Failure Rev* 1996; 1: 183–91.
30. Romagnani S. The Th1/Th2 paradigm. *Immunol Today* 1997; 18: 263–6.
31. Piccotti J, Chan S, VanBuskirk A *et al.* Are Th2 helper T lymphocytes beneficial, deleterious, or irrelevent in promoting allograft survival? *Transplantation* 1997; 63: 619–24.
32. Mosmann T, Sad S. The expanding universes of T-cell subsets: Th1, Th2 and more. *Immunol Today* 1996; 178: 138–46.
33. Ben-Sasson S, Gros G, Conrad D *et al.* Cross-linking Fc receptors stimulate splenic non-B, non-T cells to secrete interleukin 4 and other lymphokines. *Proc Natl Acad Sci USA* 1990; 87: 1421–5.
34. Yoshimoto T, Paul W. CD4 pos, NK1.1pos T cells promptly produce interleukin 4 in respone to *in vivo* challenge with anti-CD3. *J Exp Med* 1994; 179: 1285–95.
35. Trinchieri G. Interleukin-12: a proinflammatory cytokine with immunoregulatory functions that bridge innate resistance and antigen-specific adaptive immunity. *Annu Rev Immunol* 1995; 13: 251–76.
36. Martinez O, Gibbons R, Garovoy M, Aronson F. IL-4 inhibits IL-2 receptor expression and IL-2 dependent proliferation of human T cells. *J Immunol* 1990; 144: 2211–17.
37. Mottram P, Han W, Purcell L *et al.* Increased expression of IL-4 and IL-10 and decreased expression of IL-2 and interferon-gamma in long-surviving mouse heart allografts after brief CD4-mAB therapy. *Transplantation* 1995; 59: 559–65.
38. Takeuchi T, Lowry R, Konieczny B. Heart allografts in murine systems. *Transplantation* 1992; 53: 1281–94.
39. Isobe M, Suzuki J, Yamazake S *et al.* Regulation by differential development of Th1 and Th2 cells in peripheral tolerance to cardiac allograft induced by blocking ICAM-1/LFA-1 adhesion. *Circulation* 1997; 96: 2247–53.
40. Chen N, Field E. Enhanced type 2 and diminished type 1 cytokines in neonatal tolerance. *Transplantation* 1995; 59: 933–41.

41. VanBuskirk A, Wakely M, Oroz CH. Transfusion of polarized $Th_2$-like cell populations into SCID mouse cardiac allograft recipients results in acute allograft rejection. *Transplantation* 1996; 62: 229–38.
42. Chan SH, DeBruyne L, Goodman R *et al. In vivo* depletion of $CD8^+$ T cells results in Th2 cytokine production and alternate mechanisms of allograft rejection. *Transplantation* 1995; 59: 1155–61.
43. Piccotti J, Chan SH, Goodman R *et al.* IL-12 antagonism induces T helper 2 responses, yet exacerbates cardiac allograft rejection. *J Immunol* 1996; 157: 1951–7.
44. Okura Y, Takeda K, Honda S *et al.* Recombinant murine interleukin-12 facilitates induction of cardiac myosin-specific type 1 helper T cells in rats. *Circ Res* 1998; 82: 1035–42.
45. Qian S, Li W, Li Y *et al.* Systemic administration of cellular interleukin-10 can exacerbate cardic allograft rejection in mice. *Transplantation* 1996; 62: 1709–14.
46. Shi L, Mai S, Israels S, Greenberg A. Granzyme B (GraB) autonomously crosses the cell membrane and perforin initiates apoptosis and GraB nuclear localization. *J Exp Med* 1997; 185: 855–66.
47. Kaegi D, Ledermann B, Buerki K *et al.* Molecular mechanisms of lymphocyte-mediated cytotoxicity and their role in immunological protection and pathogenesis *in vivo. Annu Rev Immunol* 1996; 14: 207–32.
48. Kabelitz D. Apoptosis, graft rejection, and transplantation tolerance. *Transplantation* 1998; 65: 869–75.
49. Griffiths G, Namikawa R, Mueller C *et al.* Granzyme A and perforin as markers for rejection in cardiac transplantion. *Eur J Immunol* 1991; 21: 687–93.
50. Chen R, Bushell A, Fuggle S, Morris P. Expression of granzyme A and perforin in mouse heart transplants immunosuppressed with donor-specific transfusion and anti-CD4 monoclonal AB. *Transplantation* 1996; 61: 625–9.
51. Schulz M, Schuurman H, Zinkernagel R, Ledermann B. Acute rejection of vascular heart allografts by perforin-deficient mice. *Eur J Immunol* 1995; 25: 474–80.
52. Ensley R, Ives M, Zhao L *et al.* Effects of alloimmune injury on contraction and relaxation in cultured myocytes and intact cardiac allografts. *J Am Coll Cardiol* 1994; 24: 769–78.
53. Binah O, Marom S, Rubinstein I *et al.* Immunological rejection of heart transplant: How lytic granules from cytotoxic T lymphocytes damage guinea pig ventricular myocytes. *Eur J Physiol* 1992; 420: 172–9.
54. Felzen B, Shilkrut M, Less H, Binah O. FAS (CD95/Apo-1)-mediated damage to ventricular myocytes induced by cytotoxic T lymphocytes from perforin-deficient mice. *Circ Res* 1998; 82: 438–50.
55. Seino K, Kayagaki N, Bashuda H, Yagita H. Contribution of FAS ligand to cardiac allograft rejection. *Int Immunol* 1996; 8: 1347–54.
56. Woodley W, McMillan M, Shelby J, Barry WH. Myocyte injury and contraction abnormalities produced by cytotoxic T lymphocytes. *Circulation* 1991; 83: 1410–18.
57. Wagoner L, Zhao L, Bishop D *et al.* Lysis of adult ventricular myocytes by cells infiltrating rejecting murine cardiac allografts. *Circulation* 1996; 93: 111–19.
58. Menon SG, Zhao L, Xu S *et al.* Relative importance of cytotoxic T lymphocytes (CTL) and nitric oxide (NO) dependent cytotoxicity in contractile dysfunction associated with rejecting mouse cardiac allografts. *Transplantation* 1998; 66(4): 413–19.
59. Christmas SE, MacPherson GG. The role of mononuclear phagocytes in cardiac allograft rejection in the rat, II: characterization of nomonuclear phagocytes extracted from rat cardiac allografts. *Cell Immunol* 1982; 69: 271–80.
60. Christmas SE, MacPherson GG. The role of mononuclear phagocytes in cardiac allograft rejection in the rat, III: the effect of cells extracted from rat cardiac allografts upon beating heart cell cultures. *Cell Immunol* 1982; 69: 281–90.
61. Pinksy DJ, Cai B, Yang X *et al.* The lethal effects of cytokine-induced nitric oxide on cardiac myocytes are blocked by nitric oxide synthase antagonism or transforming growth factor β. *J Clin Invest* 1995; 95: 677–85.
62. Higuchi M, Higashi N, Taki H, Osawa T. Cytolytic mechanisms of activated macrophages: tumor necrosis factor and L-arginine-dependent mechanisms act synergistically as the major cytolytic mechanisms of activated macrophages. *J Immunol* 1990; 144: 1425–31.
63. Hibbs JB Jr, Vavrin Z, Taintor RR. L-arginine is required for expression of the activated effector mechanism causing selective metabolic inhibition in target cells. *J Immunol* 1987; 138: 550–65.
64. Barry WH, Zhao L. The role of heart infiltrating cells in myocyte injury. In: Schultheiss HP, Schwimmbeck P (eds) *The role of immune mechanisms in cardiovascular disease.* Berlin: Springer, 1996.
65. Babiar BM. The respiratory burst of macrophages. *J Clin Invest* 1984; 73: 599–601.
66. Adams DO, Kao K-J, Farb R, Pizzo SV. Effector mechanisms of cytolytically activated macrophages. II. Secretion of a cytolytic factor by activated macrophages and its relationship to secreted neutral proteases. *J Immunol* 1980; 124: 293–300.
67. Ding AH, Nathan CF, Stuehr DJ. Release of reactive nitrogen intermediates and reactive oxygen intermediates from mouse peritoneal macrophages: comparison of activating cytokines and evidence for independent production. *J Immunol* 1988; 141: 2407–12.
68. Balligand JL, Ungureanu D, Kelly RA *et al.* Abnormal contractile function due to induction of nitric oxide synthesis in rat cardiac myocytes follows exposure to activated macrophage-conditioned medium. *J Clin Invest* 1993; 91.
69. Kelly R, Balligand J, Smith T. Nitric oxide and cardiac function. *Circ Res* 1996; 79: 363–80.
70. Yokoyama T, Vaca L, Rossen RD *et al.* Cellular basis for the negative inotropic effects of tumor necrosis factor-α in the adult mammalian heart. *J Clin Invest* 1993; 92: 2303–12.
71. Testa M, Yeh M, Lee P *et al.* Circulating levels of cytokines and their endogenous modulators in patients with mild to severe congestive heart failure due to coronary artery disease or hypertension. *J Am Coll Cardiol* 1996; 28: 964–71.
72. Matsumori A, Yamada T, Suzuki H *et al.* Increased circulating cytokines in patients with myocarditis and cardiomyopathy. *Br Heart J* 1994; 72: 561–6.
73. Habib F, Springall D, Davies G *et al.* Tumor necrosis factor and inducible nitric oxide synthase in dilated cardiomyopathy. *Lancet* 1996; 347: 1151–5.
74. Grant S, Lamb W, Brooks M *et al.* Serum cytokines in human heart transplant recipients. *Transplantation* 1996; 62: 480–91.
75. Torre-Amione G, Kapadia S, Lee J *et al.* Tumor necrosis factor-alpha and tumor necrosis factor receptors in the failing human heart. *Circulation* 1996; 93: 704–11.
76. Kapadia S, Oral H, Lee J *et al.* Hemodynamic regulation of tumor necrosis factor-alpha gene and protein expression in adult feline myocardium, *Circ Res* 1997; 81: 187–95.

77. Kumar A, Thota V, Dee L *et al.* Tumor necrosis factor alpha and interleukin 1beta are responsible for *in vitro* myocardial cell depression induced by human septic shock serum. *J Exp Med* 1996; 183: 949–58.
78. Murray D, Freeman G. Tumor necrosis factor alpha induces a biphasic effect on myocardial contractility in conscious dogs. *Circ Res* 1996; 78: 154–60.
79. Yokoyama T, Vaca L, Rossen R *et al.* Cellular basis for the negative inotropic effects of tumor necrosis factor alpha in the adult mammalian heart. *J Clin Invest* 1993; 92: 2303–12.
80. Finkel M, Oddis C, Jacob T *et al.* Negative inotropic effects of cytokines on the heart mediated by nitric oxide. *Science* 1992; 257: 387–9.
81. Oral H, Dorn W II, Mann D. Sphingosine mediates the immediate negative inotropic effects of tumor necrosis factor alpha in the adult mammalian cardiac myocyte. *J Biol Chem* 1997; 272: 4836–42.
82. McDonough P, Yasui K, Betto R *et al.* Control of cardiac calcium levels — inhibitory actions of sphingosine on calcium transients and L-type calcium channel conductance. *Circ Res* 1994; 75: 981–9.
83. Bryant D, Becker L, Richardson J *et al.* Cardiac failure in transgenic mice with myocardial expression of tumor necrosis factor alpha. *Circulation* 1998; 97: 1375–81.
84. Ungureanu-Longrois D, Balligand J, Simmons W *et al.* Induction of nitric oxide synthase activity by cytokines in ventricular myocytes is necessary but not sufficient to decrease contractile responsiveness to beta-adrenergic agonists. *Circ Res* 1995; 77: 494–502.
85. Schulz R, Panas D, Catena R *et al.* The role of nitric oxide in cardiac depression induced by interleukin-1beta and TNF alpha. *Br J Pharmacol* 1995; 114: 27–34.
86. Gulick R, Chung M, Pieper S *et al.* Interleukin 1β and tumor necrosis factor inhibit cardiac myocyte beta adrenergic responsiveness. *Proc Natl Acad Sci USA* 1989; 86: 6753–7.
87. Sun X, Delbrigde L, Dusting G. Cardiodepressant effects of interferon-gamma and endotoxin reversed by inhibition of NO synthase 2 in rat myocardium. *J Mol Cell Cardiol* 1998; 30: 989–97.
88. McGowan FX, Takeuchi K, del Nido PJ *et al.* Myocardial effects of interleukin 2. *Transpl Proc* 1994; 26: 209–10.
89. Kinugawa K, Takahashi T, Kohmoto O *et al.* Nitric oxide-mediated effects of interleukin-6 on $[Ca^{2+}]_i$ and cell contraction in cultured chick ventricular myocytes. *Circ Res* 1994; 75: 285–95.
90. Chung M, Gulick T, Rotondo R *et al.* Mechanism of cytokine inhibition of beta-adrenergic agonist stimulation of cyclic AMP in rat cardiac myocytes. *Circ Res* 1990; 67: 753–63.
91. Kobzik L, Reid M, Bredt D, Stamler J. Nitric oxide in skeletal muscle. *Nature* 1994; 372: 546–8.
92. Schwarz P, Kiem R, Dun N, Foerstermann U. Endogenous and exogenous nitric oxide inhibits norepinephrine release from rat heart sympathetic nerves. *Circ Res* 1995; 77: 841–8.
93. Balligand J, Kobzik L, Han X *et al.* Nitric oxide-dependent parasympathetic signaling is due to activation of constitutive endothelial (type III) nitric oxide synthase in cardiac myocytes. *J Biol Chem* 1995; 270: 14 582–6.
94. Schulz R, Nava E, Moncada S. Induction and potential biological relevance of a calcium-independent nitric oxide synthase in the myocardium. *Br J Pharmacol* 1992; 105: 575–80.
95. Han X, Kobzik L, Balligand J *et al.* Nitric oxide synthase (NOS3)-mediated cholinergic modulation of calcium current in adult rabbit atrioventricular nodal cells. *Circ Res* 1996; 78: 998–1008.
96. Balligand J, Ungureannu-Longrois D, Simmons W *et al.* Cytokine-inducible nitric oxide synthase (iNOS) expression in cardiac myocytes. *J Biol Chem* 1994; 269: 27 580–8.
97. Balligand J, Ungureanu D, Kelly R *et al.* Abnormal contractile function due to induction of nitric oxide synthesis in rat cardiac myocytes follows exposure to activated macrophage-conditioned medium. *J Clin Invest* 1993; 91: 2314–19.
98. Brady A, Poole-Wilson P, Haring S, Warren J. Nitric oxide production within cardiac myocytes reduces their contractility in endotoxemia. *Am J Physiol* 1992; 263: H1963–6.
99. Balligand J, Ungureanu-Longrois D, Simmons W *et al.* Induction of No synthase in rat cardiac microvascular endothelial cells by IL-1beta and IFN-gamma. *Am J Physiol* 1995; 268: H1293–303.
100. Schulz R, Smith J, Lewis M, Moncada S. Nitric oxide synthase in cultured endocardial cells of pig. *Br J Pharmacol* 1992; 104: 21–4.
101. Worral N, Douglas W, Misko T *et al.* Modulation of *in vivo* alloreactivity by inhibion of inducible nitric oxide synthase. *J Exp Med* 1995; 181: 63–70.
102. Yang X, Chowdhury N, Cai B *et al.* Induction of myocardial nitric oxide synthase by cardiac allograft rejection. *J Clin Invest* 1994; 94: 714–21.
103. Ziolo M, Dollinger S, Wahler G. Myocytes isolated from rejecting transplanted rat hearts exhibit reduced basal shortening which is reversible by aminoguanidine. *J Mol Cell Cardiol* 1998; 30: 1009–17.
104. Worrall N, Pyo R, Botney M *et al.* Inflammatory cell-derived NO modulates cardiac allograft contractile and electrophysiological function. *Am J Physiol* 1997; 273: H28–37.
105. Nathan C. Natural resistance and nitric oxide. *Cell* 1995; 82: 873–6.
106. Karupiah G, Harris N. Inhibition of viral replication by nitric oxide and its reversal by ferrous sulfate and tricarboxylic acids cycle metabolites. *J Exp Med* 1995; 181: 2171–9.
107. Mannick J, Asano K, Izumi K *et al.* Nitric oxide produced by human B lymphocytes inhibits apoptosis and Epstein–Barr virus reactivation. *Cell* 1995; 79: 1137–46.
108. Wei X, Charles I, Smith A *et al.* Altered immune responses in mice lacking inducible nitric oxide synthase. *Nature* 1995; 375: 408–11.
109. MacMicking J, Nathan C, Hom G *et al.* Altered responses to bacterial infection and endotoxic shock in mice lacking inducible nitric oxide synthase. *Cell* 1995; 81: 641–50.
110. Entman M, Youker K, Shoji T *et al.* Neutrophil induced oxidative injury of cardiac myocytes. *J Clin Invest* 1992; 90: 1335–45.
111. Semb A, Ytrehus K, Vaage J, Myklebust R. Cardiac injury by activated leukocytes: effect of cyclooxygenase and lipoxygenase inhibition evaluated by electron microscopical morphometry. *J Mol Cell Cardiol* 1996; 28: 311–20.
112. Reinhardt P, Ward C, Giles W, Kubes P. Emigrated rat neutrophils adhere to cardiac myocytes via alpha4 integrin. *Circ Res* 1997; 81: 196–201.
113. Oubenaissa A, Mouas C, Bourgeois F *et al.* Evidence for an involvement of the neutrophil integrin lymphocyte function-associated antigen-1 in early failure of heart transplants. *Circulation* 1996; 94(Suppl I): II254–9.
114. Schowengerdt K, Zhu J, Stepkowski ST, Ballantyne CH. Cardiac allograft survival in mice deficient in intercellular adhesion molecule-1. *Circulation* 1995; 92: 82–7.

115. Isobe M, Yagita H, Okumura K, Ihara A. Specific acceptance of cardiac allograft after treatment with antibodies to ICAM-1 and LFA-1. *Science* 1992; 255(5048): 1125–7.
116. Xu X, Honjo K, Deore-Carter D, Bucy R. Immunosuppression by inhibition of cellular adhesion mediated by leukocyte function-associated antigen-1/intercelllular adhesion molecule-1 in murine cardiac transplantation. *Transplantation* 1997; 63: 867–85.
117. Masinovsky B, Urdal D, Gallatin W. IL-4 acts synergistically with IL-1 beta to promote lymphocyte adhesion to microvascular endothelium by induction of vascular cell adhesion molecue-1. *J Immunol* 1990; 145: 2886–93.
118. Orosz CH, Ohye R, Pelletier R *et al.* Treatment with anti-vascular cell adhesion molecule 1 monoclonal antibody induces long-term murine cardiac allograft acceptance. *Transplantation* 1993; 56: 453–60.
119. Larsen CP, Elwood ET, Alexander DZ *et al.* Long-term acceptance of skin and cardiac allografts after blocking CD40 and CD28 pathways. *Nature* 1996; 381: 434–8.
120. Lakkis F, Konieczny B, Baddoura F *et al.* Blocking the CD28-B7 T cell costimulation pathway induces longterm cardiac allograft acceptance in the absence of IL-4. *J Immunol* 1997; 158: 2443–8.
121. Turka L, Linsley P, Lin H *et al.* T cell activation by the CD28 ligand B7 is required for cardiac allograft rejection *in vivo*. *Proc Natl Acad Sci USA* 1992; 89: 11 102–5.
122. Sayegh M, Zheng X, Magee C *et al.* Donor antigen is necessary for the prevention of chronic rejection in CTLA4Ig-treated murine cardiac allograft recipients. *Transplantation* 1997; 64: 1646–50.
123. Mason JW, O'Connell JB, Herskowitz A *et al.* A clinical trial of immunosuppressive therapy for myocarditis. *N Engl J Med* 1995; 333: 269–75.
124. Parillo JE, Cunnion RE, Epstein SE *et al.* A prospective, randomized controlled trial of prednisone for dilated cardiomyopathy. *N Engl J Med* 1989; 321: 1061–8.
125. Maisch B, Hufnagel G, Schonian U, Hengstenberg C. The European study of epidemiology and treatment of cardiac inflammatory disease (ESETCID). *Eur Heart J* 1995; 16 (Suppl): 173–5.

# Apoptosis in congestive heart failure 18

R. R. BALIGA, Y. CHANDRASHEKHAR AND J. NARULA

## Introduction

Congestive heart failure affects about 1% of adults in the USA [1], including 1.5 million people younger than 65 years of age, and is a contributing factor in over 250 000 deaths annually. It is diagnosed in 400 000 Americans each year and is the primary diagnosis for over 900 000 hospitalizations annually. Congestive heart failure is the single most frequent cause of hospitalization for people age 65 years and older [2]. The direct health-care costs (drugs, nursing home care, and professional services) have been estimated as approximately US$17.8 billion each year. These numbers will likely increase as the US population ages. In 1990, the age-adjusted death rate from congestive heart failure was 106.4 per 100 000 [3], more than that from acquired immunodeficiency syndrome and breast cancer combined [4, 5]. The median survival after the diagnosis of heart failure is 1.7 years in men and 3.2 years in women, with a 5 year survival rate of less than 50% [6]. The process of left ventricular remodelling has been shown to be an important predictor of morbidity and mortality in patients with heart failure. Therefore, identifying the cascade of molecular and cellular events that contributes to left ventricular modelling is likely to provide novel targets for preventing disease progression in heart failure [7].

Advances in the understanding of the pathophysiology of heart failure have been accompanied by an impressive expansion in the modalities available for treatment [8]. In the first half of the twentieth century heart failure was viewed as an 'oedematous state' and treatment involved using diuretics to ameliorate symptoms. Subsequently, it was viewed as a 'haemodynamic disorder' and therapies focused on the improvement of haemodynamic function. Although short-term haemodynamic stabilization remains an important goal in the in-hospital management of heart failure [9, 10], it is now well recognized that haemodynamic improvement is only one aspect of successful long-term therapy. The recognition that heart failure is a 'neurohormonal disorder' resulted in the use of angiotensin-converting enzyme (ACE) inhibitors and β-blockers. Evidence from several large, controlled trials has shown that therapy of heart failure with converting enzyme inhibitors and β-blockers not only alleviates symptoms and improves functional capacity, but also reduces mortality. These agents are now being used to prevent adverse ventricular remodelling and diminish the symptoms of heart failure. The success of these agents has validated the importance of neurohormonal factors in influencing clinical events. Recently, there has been a paradigm shift in our understanding of the pathophysiology of heart failure and it is now widely recognized that apoptosis or programmed cell death plays a major role in the progressive decline in left ventricular function and ventricular remodelling [11]. Understanding the role of apoptosis in cardiac failure should aid in the development of novel antiapoptotic therapies to prevent progressive congestive cardiac failure.

## Apoptosis or programmed cell death

Historically, pathologists have viewed cell death using light and electron microscopy, and have described the morphological characteristics of necrosis. In 1910, von Recklinghausen proposed the term 'oncosis' (Greek: *Óncosis*, swelling) precisely to mean cell death with sweiling. As early as 1885 another morphological form of cell death was recognized by Walther Flemming, who called it 'chromatolysis'. He noticed that the epithelial lining of regressing ovarian follicles was littered with cells wherein the nuclei were breaking up. A few months later the same observation was made by Franz Nissen in lactating mammary glands. By 1914 enough data were available for a German anatomist, Ludwig Graper, to publish a paper entitled (in translation)

'A new point of view regarding the elimination of cells'. In 1967, Frans Wackers [12] used the term 'bionecrosis' to describe changes in human mammary glands. He noticed that dead and dying cells existed among living cells without provoking a cellular reaction. He also commented that although the cells were dead it was still possible to recognize them as cells. These milestone papers made no significant impact until 'chromatolysis' and 'bionecrosis' resurfaced in 1971 when Kerr described what he called at first 'shrinkage necrosis' and a year later, 'apoptosis' (Greek: *apo-tosis*, falling off, as in the petals of a flower or the leaves of a tree) [13]. Apoptosis leads to necrosis with karyorhexis and cell shrinkage, and stands in contrast to oncosis which leads to necrosis with karyolysis and cell swelling.

Wyllie *et al.* [14] subsequently demonstrated discrete internucleosomal DNA fragmentation in apoptosis and thereby added a specific biochemical marker to the distinctive morphological changes of apoptosis. DNA fragmentation, which is the hallmark of apoptosis, can be identified in homogenized tissue extracts by agarose gel DNA electrophoresis, in which the fragmental DNA imparts a laddering pattern to the gel. DNA fragmentation in the nuclei of individual cells can be recognized by histochemical techniques, often referred to as TUNEL or ISEL techniques. In addition, transmission electron microscopic examination of tissues of interest allows ultrastructural characterization of nucleus, cytoplasmic, and sarcolemmal alterations of apoptotic myocytes.

The first suggestion that apoptosis may play a role in ventricular remodelling and cardiac failure in patients with end-stage heart failure [11] provided impetus for further research into the role of apoptosis in a variety of cardiovascular disorders [15–18]. Until these recent reports it was generally believed that apoptosis did not occur in terminally differentiated adult cardiac cells [19]. Subsequent evidence from several human studies, animal models, and *in vitro* systems further suggests that apoptosis does occur in the myocardium in response to a variety of insults, including myocardial infarction [20, 21], reperfusion injury [22], heart failure [23], mechanical stretch [24], and pressure overload [25]. Improvement in the apoptotic regulatory paradigm by the implantation of a left ventricular assist device has been demonstrated by Packer and other investigators [26, 27]. The premise that the cardiac myocyte is a terminally differentiated cell has been recently challenged [28]. Several factors known or suspected to be present in the failing myocardium (e.g. angiotensin, catecholamines, cytokines, reactive oxygen species, mechanical stress, and natriuretic peptides) have been shown to cause apoptosis of cardiac myocytes. Many of these factors also cause hypertrophy of the cardiac myocytes and thus there appears to be some unknown paradigm shift that causes 'growth factors' to become 'death factors' [29].

## Apoptosis in animal models of heart failure

Apoptosis has been described in two dog models of heart failure [23, 30]. Sharov *et al.* [30], using a model of chronic heart failure caused by multiple sequential microembolizations of the coronary arteries, documented apoptosis by immunohistochemical staining for nuclear DNA breaks using the TUNEL method and characterized the ultrastructural features of apoptosis using transmission electron microscopy. Electron microscopy identified apoptosis in left ventricular tissue from every dog with heart failure but in none of the tissue specimens obtained from normal dogs. They confirmed that the apoptotic cells were myocytes and not interstitial cells by using a monoclonal mouse ventricular heavy chain muscle antimyosin antibody. In the early stages of apoptosis there was evidence of compaction of nuclear chromatin into sharply circumscribed, uniformly dense masses abutting the nuclear envelope of cardiac myocytes. In these myocytes, the inner organelles were intact and the sarcolemma was preserved but with blebbing. In advanced stages of apoptosis, the sarcolemma was still intact but the inner organelles were highly disorganized. Only remnants of myofibrils and Z-band material allowed recognition that these apoptotic bodies had indeed originated from cardiac myocytes. Sharov and coworkers [30] further demonstrated that the majority of apoptotic myocytes in dogs with heart failure was preferentially located in ventricular regions bordering old infarcts and these were often encircled by large amounts of collagen. The apoptosis was not associated with an inflammatory response. In contrast, in normal dogs, TUNEL-positive cells (if any) did not stain for antimyosin antibody, suggesting that apoptosis of cardiac myocytes was rare in the normal myocardium. In a subsequent study, the apoptosis of cardiac myocytes was quantified using histomorphometry [31]: the severity of the apoptosis was the number of myocytes that labelled for nuclear DNA strand breaks per 1000 cardiomyocytes. They found $4.0 \pm 0.5$ nuclear DNA fragmentation events in left ventricular regions bordering old infarcts compared with 0.5 ± 0.3 in left ventricular regions remote from the infarct. These findings suggest that apoptosis in the peri-infarct zone may lead to chronic centrifugal progression of myocardial damage towards the development of ventricular remodelling and heart failure.

Liu *et al.* [23] described apoptosis of myocytes in a canine model of heart failure induced by rapid ventricular pacing. They documented and quantified apoptosis using DNA laddering, TUNEL staining, and immunochemical Fas labelling of myocytes. DNA laddering was observed in the myocardium of dogs with heart failure but not in sham-operated control animals. Using the TUNEL method, they demonstrated that 3700 myocyte nuclei per million were undergoing apoptosis. Analogous to Sharov *et al.* [30] they also found that apoptotic myocytes were in areas with significant replacement fibrosis. Fas immunostaining was positive in over 11 000 myocytes per million in the failing hearts but absent in the sham-operated animals. These data not only confirm the occurrence of apoptosis in this canine model but also suggest that the death receptor pathways may contribute to the development of heart failure. Further confirmatory studies using soluble Fas or Fas ligand, and myocyte expression of Fas L are required.

Apoptosis has also been documented in two murine models of heart failure secondary to either large acute myocardial infarction (Fischer 344 rat) or progressive hypertension [the spontaneously hypertensive rat (SHR)]. Kajstura *et al.* [32] documented both myocyte necrosis and apoptosis in Fischer 344 rats of varying ages. Apoptosis was demonstrated by the TUNEL method and DNA laddering, and necrosis by staining with antimyosin antibodies for necrosis. There were 80 myocytes per million in rats with heart failure compared with only ten myocytes per million in those without heart failure. Cell necrosis occurred earlier than apoptosis in this model, which suggested that cell necrosis may trigger apoptosis in viable myocardial regions that border the fibrous scar in these hearts [18, 23, 30, 33] and in failing human hearts. More recently, the same group of investigators demonstrated in the same animal model that an increase in diastolic calcium occurred which activated DNAse I to trigger apoptosis. The DNAse activation was independent of the expression of p53, Bax, and Bcl-2 in cardiac myocytes [34].

In 1994, Bing [35] proposed the hypothesis that the gradual loss of cardiac myocytes through apoptosis may be responsible, in part, for the transition from cardiac hypertrophy to heart failure. Li *et al.* [36] examined this hypothesis in the SHR, which initially develop cardiac hypertrophy and finally heart failure between 18 and 24 months. They employed the TUNEL method to demonstrate apoptosis in failing and non-failing SHR hearts, as well as in age-matched Wistar–Kyoto (WKY) rat hearts, and used double staining for α-sarcomeric actin to identify cardiomyocytes. In failing SHR hearts, approximately 40 cells per 100 000 harboured apoptotic nuclei compared with approximately eight cells per 100 000 nuclei in the non-failing SHR hearts with cardiac hypertrophy. In age-matched control WKY rats, the incidence of apoptotic nuclei of myocyte origin was approximately two cells per 100 000 nuclei. In the same study, Li *et al.* [36] found that WAF-1 mRNA, a gene known to promote apoptosis, was higher in failing than in non-failing SHRs. However, there was no difference in the Bcl-2 protein expression, an inhibitor of apoptosis, in all three rat groups. Baliga *et al.* [37] found that the expression of $\beta_1$-integrin mRNA was increased in SHRs compared with age-matched WKY controls and the density of $\beta_1$-integrin was higher in failing SHR, hearts than in non-failing hearts [37]. *Anoikis* is the term used for apoptosis due to loss of integrin-mediated anchorage of the cell to the extracellular matrix [38]. It is well recognized that integrins regulate Bcl-2 expression levels [38]. The increase in the expression of $\beta_1$-integrins is likely to be a compensatory mechanism to increased apoptosis; however, the role of integrins in cardiac remodelling needs further investigation [39].

Plasma membrane changes occur in apoptosis. In early apoptosis, there is a conformational change in the plasma membrane of the cell, resulting in predominance of the phosphatidylserine (PS) groups on the outer face of the plasma membrane secondary to loss of membrane enzymes that flip PS to the inner side of the membrane [40]. Strauss and co-workers [41] have shown that neo-expression of PS can be identified using a fluorescein-labelled ligand termed annexin-V, making it a promising technique for detecting apoptosis *in vivo*, the 'aposcan'.

## Apoptosis in human heart failure

In 1996, Narula *et al.* [11] examined seven human explanted failing hearts for apoptosis. Four of their patients had idiopathic dilated cardiomyopathy (IDC), whereas the remaining three had ischaemic cardiomyopathy (ICM). All patients with IDC and one patient with ICM had evidence of nuclear DNA fragmentation. Subsequently, Olivetti *et al.* [16] provided more precise estimates of apoptosis in cardiomyopathic hearts. They reported that in eight normal donor hearts, apoptotic nuclei were rare and seen on average in only ten nuclei per million. In contrast, in 15 failing hearts there were up to 6549 nuclei per million with a minimum of 673 nuclei. No differences were observed in the number of apoptotic nuclei in patients with IDC (2366 nuclei per million, $n = 5$) or ICM (2436 nuclei per million, $n = 9$). Sharov *et al.* [18] demonstrated that there was a higher incidence of apoptosis in cardiac myocyte of ICM than in those of IDC (0.31 vs 0.10 apoptotic myocytes per 1000). There was nearly a three-fold higher incidence of apoptosis in regions bordering old infarcts compared with myocardial regions remote from any infarcts (0.50 vs 0.06 apoptotic myocytes per 1000).

## Triggers of apoptosis of heart failure

During ventricular remodelling the mediators of hypertrophy (growth factors) cause apoptosis as well (death factors). Cell-specific pathways resulting in cell growth and cell death are mediated by various triggers including increased sympathetic activity, mechanical factors, the renin–angiotensin system (RAS), endothelin, reactive oxygen species, nitric oxide, paracrine growth factors, cytokines, and cell cycle inhibitors. The identification of these factors has led to the development of novel therapeutic strategies which are now being tested clinically.

### Mechanical factors

Haemodynamic overload and the resulting increase in wall stress are common stimuli for ventricular remodelling. Mechanical stretch results not only in increased myocyte length and hypertrophy [42], but also in apoptosis [24]. Apoptosis has been demonstrated in pressure overload-induced myocardial hypertrophy in the rat [25] and greater mechanical stretch has been shown to induce both hypertrophy and apoptosis in neonatal cardiac myocytes [43]. The latter investigators found that MnTMPyp, a cell-permeable superoxide dismutase mimetic, reduced apoptosis in response to stretch, suggesting a central role for reactive oxygen species in mediating apoptosis. Leri *et al.* [44] reported that the stretch-mediated release of angiotensin II is coupled with the activation of p53, which may be responsible for the prolonged upregulation of the local renin–angiotensin system and the increased susceptibility of myocytes to apoptosis. Endothelin is another peptide that is released on mechanical stretch [45] but further studies are required to determine its role in myocardial apoptosis.

### Sympathoadrenergic activity

It is well recognized that the activity of the sympathetic nervous system is increased in patients with heart failure [46–48]. The evidence of sympathetic activation is based on increased plasma noradrenaline, an increased aorta/coronary sinus norepinephrine gradient [49], radiotracer studies of norepinephrine turnover [50], and increased sympathetic traffic to skeletal muscle [51]. It appears that the availability of noradrenaline to the cardiac myocyte is due to both increased sympathetic activity and decreased noradrenaline clearance. For several years it was believed that exposure to high levels of catecholamines is lethal to cardiac myocytes. Mann *et al.* [52] proposed that exposure to noradrenaline exerted a direct toxic effect on cardiac myocytes in cell culture that was mediated by increases in both cyclic adenosine monophosphate (cAMP) and calcium influx [52]. Matsui *et al.* [53] showed that noradrenaline induced apoptosis in neonatal rat ventricular myocytes and that blockade of both α- and β-adrenergic receptors was required for prevention of apoptosis. Colucci and co-workers [54] observed myocyte death by apoptosis in adult rat ventricular myocytes exposed in culture to noradrenaline for 24 h; this was inhibited by the β-adrenergic antagonist propranolol but not by the α-adrenergic antagonist prazosin [54]. β-adrenergic stimulation using isoproterenol also leads to apoptosis [55]. Use of β-blockers such as carvedilol protects hypoxia/reoxygenation-induced apoptosis in cardiac myocytes [56, 57]. Apoptosis in cardiac myocytes is also induced by forskolin and inhibited by the protein kinase inhibitor H-89 or calcium channel blockers such as diltiazem and nifedipine, implicating the role of the adrenergic pathway [54]. The same investigators demonstrated that Gi protein protects adult rat ventricular myocytes from β-adrenergic receptor-stimulated apoptosis [58]. These observations are supported by the development of dilated cardiomyopathy in transgenic mice overexpressing the Gs protein α-subunit [59], which is associated with an increased rate of myocyte apoptosis [60, 61]. Cardiac myocytes cultured from these mice also develop apoptosis when exposed to isoproterenol [62]. New evidence suggests that the activation of $\beta_1$-adrenergic receptors results in apoptosis of cardiac myocytes [63]; this is supported by the fact that transgenic mice that overexpress the $\beta_2$-adrenergic receptors do not develop dilated cardiomyopathy [64].

Neuropeptide Y (NPY) is a 36-amino acid peptide that is widely distributed in the hearts of mammals [65–67] and is known to modify catecholamine signalling in the cardiovascular system [68–71]. NPY is present in postganglionic sympathetic neurons, being colocalized and coreleased with catecholamines. Circulating levels of NPY are elevated in patients with congestive heart failure [72–77], whereas depletion of NPY has been reported in explanted human myocardial tissue [78]. NPY, in a paracrine manner, improves survival in adult rat ventricular cardiomyocytes [68] and its depletion in heart failure is likely to contribute to apoptosis.

## Vasoactive humoral factors

### *Renin–angiotensin system*

Angiotensin II modulates myocardial performance [79] and inhibition of ACE improves survival in patients with heart failure [80] and delays the development of heart failure in those with asymptomatic left ventricular dysfunction [81]. ACE is predominantly found in tissues, with only 1–10% in the peripheral circulation [82, 83]. The tissue RAS is often activated during compensated heart failure, although the circulating RAS is relatively normal [84]. In animals with heart failure the activity of the tissue and circulating RAS systems is regulated differently [85]. Increased expression of angiotensinogen [86] and ACE [79, 87] occurs in experimental animal models of heart failure. It has been suggested that the direct autocrine effect of angiotensin on cardiac angiotensin receptors plays a central role in modifying structure and function of the myocardium in patients with heart failure by differential alteration of cell growth and gene expression in cardiac myocytes and fibroblasts. Anversa *et al.* [88] showed that angiotensin II induces apoptosis of adult rat ventricular myocytes in culture, an effect that appears to be linked to the activation of the angiotensin I receptor [89, 90]. They also observed the translocation of the major protein kinase C (PKC) isoforms, but whether PKC-$\varepsilon$ and -$\delta$ singularly or in concert are involved in the initiation of apoptosis remains unclear. However, the elevation of intracellular calcium via a PKC-dependent mechanism was responsible for the activation of double-strand cleavage of the DNA. They also demonstrated that the angiotensin I receptor blocker losartan completely abrogated angiotensin II-induced apoptosis. Dzau and co-workers showed that angiotensin II receptors also mediate apoptosis [91–93]. Li *et al.* [36] observed that in failing SHR hearts there was a 4.5-fold increase in apoptosis compared with control animals and the administration of captopril reduced the magnitude of apoptosis. Sabbah and co-workers [94] also demonstrated attenuation of cardiomyocyte apoptosis by ACE inhibition in a canine model of heart failure. One study has suggested similar effects of ACE antagonism in patients with left ventricular failure [27].

### *Endothelin*

Several studies have demonstrated elevated plasma endothelin (ET) in patients with heart failure [95–99] and animal models [100–108]. Plasma endothelin was increased in patients with mild heart failure [New York Heart Association (NYHA) functional class I–II], and further elevated in severe heart failure (NYHA III–IV). This increase in plasma endothelin did not appear to be related to the cause of the heart failure (ischaemic versus cardiomyopathic) or to reduced renal clearance of the peptide. The myocardium expresses both $ET_A$ and $ET_B$ receptors and the evidence suggests that myocardial endothelin is induced in response to pressure or volume overload [109, 110]. Endothelin has positive inotropic effects [111, 112], stimulates foetal gene expression [113], and has recently emerged as a novel and potent inhibitor of apoptosis [114–116]. However, its role in cardiomyocyte apoptosis needs to be characterized.

### *Natriuretic peptides and arginine vasopressin*

Early heart failure is characterized by elevated plasma atrial natriuretic peptide (ANP) [117, 118]. In the SOLVD study, the level of ANP was increased in asymptomatic patients and further elevated in symptomatic patients with heart failure. Although normally ANPs are present at low levels in the ventricular myocardium, in patients with heart failure the ventricular production (generated by wall tension) contributes to circulating serum levels. A recent study showed that ANP induces apoptosis in neonatal rat cardiac myocytes [119] through the cyclic guanosine monophosphate (cGMP) pathway. In addition, ANP decreased the level of expression of Mcl-1, a homologue of Bcl-2, thereby reducing the rescue efforts of the Bcl-2 pathway [119].

## Cytokines and lymphokines

Cytokines are secreted by cells in response to a variety of different stimuli including environmental stress. Tumour necrosis factor-α (TNF-α) is an example of a cytokine that was originally considered to be produced by cells of the immune system. It has recently been demonstrated that the failing heart is capable of producing TNF-α [120–123]. TNF-α exerts its effects by binding to two specific receptors, TNFR1 and TNFR2, both of which have been described recently in non-failing and failing human hearts [122, 124]. Activation of TNFR1 produces negative inotropic effects in isolated cardiac myocytes [124], and leads to apoptosis in cultured rat cardiac myocytes [125]. Since the original report by Levine *et al.* [126] there have been at least 11 publications confirming the finding that circulating levels of TNF-α are elevated in patients with advanced chronic heart failure [122, 127–136]. The elaboration of TNF-α leads to left ventricular dysfunction, pulmonary oedema, and left ventricular remodelling in humans, all of which are seen in patients with advanced heart failure [137–139]. The SOLVD investigators reported a significant increase in circulating levels of TNF-α in patients with heart failure compared with age-matched controls free of cardiovascular disease or comorbid conditions. The peripheral TNF-α concentration increased in direct relation to symptomatic NYHA functional class: there was an eight-fold increase in TNF-α levels in patients with functional NYHA class III and IV heart failure. Bozkurt *et al.* [140] showed that pathological concentrations of TNF-α result in left ventricular systolic dysfunction and remodelling in rats, while Kubota *et al.* [141] showed that overexpression of TNF-α leads to dilated cardiomyopathy and induces the expression of multiple members of the apoptosis pathways in transgenic mice. More recently it has been shown that TNF-α stimulation of neonatal ventricular myocytes results in a 2.1-fold increase in nuclear factor-κβ (NFκβ) gene transcription and nuclear binding [142], suggesting that this is an important mechanism of apoptosis in these cells. One study showed that a combination of macrophage-derived cytokines, interleukin-1β (IL-1β), TNF-α, and interferon-γ caused a time-dependent apoptosis of cardiomyocytes that was preceded by a 50-fold induction of inducible nitric oxide synthase (iNOS) mRNA and a release of large amounts of nitric oxide (NO) metabolites [143]. The apoptosis was completely blocked by an NOS inhibitor and attenuated by antioxidants (*N*-acetylcyteine and DTT and the caspase inhibitor ZVAD-fmk. These investigators concluded that cytokine toxicity to neonatal cardiac myocytes results from the induction of NO and the subsequent activation of apoptosis, at least in part through the generation of oxygen free radicals. The rate and extent of this apoptosis were modulated by alterations in the cellular balance of Bak and Bcl-xL, which respond differentially to cytokine-induced and exogenous NO, and by the availability of oxidant species [143]. Future efforts will need to address the role of other cytokines, such as IL-1β and IL-6, which are also elevated in the failing myocardium and are known to play a role in cardiomyocyte apoptosis.

## Intracellular couplers of triggers and executors of apoptosis

### Reactive oxygen radicals

Several studies have demonstrated that reactive oxygen radicals are produced in patients with heart failure [144–148] and in animal models of heart failure [149–151]. Plasma malondialdehyde-like activity (MDA), a marker of lipid peroxidation, is elevated in patients with congestive cardiac failure [144, 145] and correlates directly with the duration and severity of symptoms and inversely with exercise capacity and ejection fraction [146, 147]. Another index of oxidative stress, 8-iso-$PGF_{2\alpha}$ is increased in the pericardial fluid of patients with congestive heart failure in direct relationship with the severity of functional class and echocardiographic indices of ventricular dilatation [148]. Several reports have indicated that reactive oxygen species (ROS) result in apoptosis and scavengers of ROS inhibit the death of myocytes induced by diverse stimuli. Although short-term deleterious effects of free radicals have been noted during hypoxia and reperfusion injury of the myocardium, much less is known about the effects from prolonged exposure to relatively low levels of oxidative stress in the myocardium. Mechanical stress and inflammatory cytokines such as TNF-α can increase oxidative stress in the tissue.

Oxygen free radicals can induce the expression of immediate-early genes associated with myocyte growth and apoptosis. Oxidative stress has also been shown to stimulate fibroblast proliferation and to activate *ras* signalling. Oxidative stress (decreased ratio of reduced to oxidized glutathione, increased lipid peroxidation) appears to be increased in the myocardium during the transition from compensated hypertrophy to heart failure. The potential importance of this apparent increase in oxidative stress has been confirmed by the prevention of the development of congestive cardiac failure by an endogenous antioxidant, vitamin E [152]. Several enzymes, including glutathione peroxidase and superoxide dismutase, prevent oxidative and free radical damage to cells. Selenium is an important component of these enzymes and deficiency of selenium can result in a selenium-responsive cardiomyopathy, such as in patients on total parenteral nutrition or in those with selenium deficiency, e.g. Keshan disease in China.

These observations suggest that increased oxidative stress and the consequent apoptosis contribute to myocardial remodelling and failure. In one study, oxidative stress caused the relocation of the lysosomal enzyme cathepsin D to the cytosol, resulting in apoptosis of neonatal rat cardiomyocytes [153]. Other mechanisms of oxidative stress-induced apoptosis need to be explored further. Although there is no doubt that reactive oxygen radicals are involved in some way in apoptosis, the question of cause and effect remains unanswered: 'Are they the molecules that cause the cells to die? Or are they a consequence of cells dying?'

## Nitric oxide

Excessive production of NO in the heart, and specifically in the myocytes, is one of the mechanisms proposed for myocardial dysfunction in heart failure [154, 155]. The ubiquitous distribution of NOS isoforms as well as prominent upregulation in heart failure [156] implicate NO as an important regulator of cell viability. NO is produced by the myocardium at low levels by two constitutive NOS (eNOS and nNOS) and in much greater levels by iNOS. NO at high concentrations has negative inotropic effects [157, 158] and has recently emerged as a potent inducer of apoptosis [159–161]. In contrast, low levels of NO inhibit apoptosis in cardiac myocytes [24] and other cell types, including human B-lymphocytes [162], splenocytes, eosinophils, ovarian follicles, and endothelial cells.

*In vivo* gene transfection of human eNOS in cardiomyocytes results in apoptosis [159] and a recent study suggested that increased eNOS expression in the failing human ventricular myocardium was also associated with apoptosis of cardiac myocytes [160]. Because NO is readily diffusible it can affect many molecular targets including molecular oxygen. NO reacts with free radical superoxide to form the highly reactive peroxynitrate. Peroxynitrate leads to direct damage of DNA and consequently triggers the p53- and Bax-related cascade of apoptosis. The formation of peroxynitrate is determined by the ratio of NO to superoxide, and the cellular susceptibility to peroxynitrate is dependent in large part on the levels of antioxidants (e.g. thiols).

Several mechanisms have been proposed for the antiapoptotic effects of NO [163], including induction of cytoprotective stress proteins, cGMP-dependent inhibition of apoptosis signal transduction, suppression of caspase activity, and inhibition of cytochrome *c* release. Inhibition of caspase activity by S-nitrosylation is the best characterized mechanism for the inhibition of apoptosis by NO and is likely to be effective in cells that can efficiently carry out S-nitrosylation. High rates of NO production overwhelm cellular protective mechanisms and shift the balance towards apoptosis. The presence of superoxide may also divert NO to a toxic activity by leading to the formation of peroxynitrate. Whether NO is cytotoxic or protective for cardiac myocytes is probably determined by local myocardial concentrations of NO and the generation of free oxygen [143, 161].

## Growth factors

Several peptide growth factors have important effects on the myocardium and vasculature, and are involved in heart failure. Peptide growth factors induce growth, prevent apoptosis, and induce foetal gene expression in cardiac myocytes, cardiac microvascular endothelial cells, and fibroblasts. The growth factors can be expressed by myocardial ischaemia or haemodynamic overload and may play a central role in the ventricular remodelling that occurs in heart failure [164, 165]. Numerous distinct growth factors have been identified in the myocardium, including endothelin-1, angiotensin-II, insulin-like growth factor-1 (IGF-1) [166], transforming growth factor-β (TGF-β), cardiotrophin-1 (CT-1) [167], leukaemia inhibitory factor [168], and neuregulins [169]. Overexpression of IGF-1 promotes myocardial salvage and apoptosis in murine myocardial infact models. IGF-1 therapy inhibits apoptosis and improves cardiac function in a canine model of dilated cardiomyopathy [166]. Higher expression of IGF-1 in women may partly explain the lower incidence of apoptosis in end-stage cardiac failure in females [170]. Sheng *et al.* [167] have demonstrated that CT-1, a novel growth factor, reduces apoptosis in neonatal rat ventricular myocytes. The antiapoptotic action of CT-1 has been shown to require the activation of Ras/Raf/MEK mitogen-activated protein kinase (MAPK) pathway, since inhibition of p42/p44 MAPK with the MEK inhibitor PD98059 prevented CT-1s antiapoptotic activity. Another mechanism by which CT-1 treated cardiac myocytes are protected from ischaemic apoptosis is by increasing the synthesis of heat shock proteins [171]. Kelly *et al.* [165] showed that neuregulins (a family of locally acting peptide autocoids known to be important in the development of the central and peripheral nervous system) promoted survival and inhibited apoptosis in neonatal and adult rat ventricular myocytes [169, 172]. Neuregulins also activate MAPK pathways in myocytes [173, 174]. However, the activation of this MAPK pathway alone cannot be sufficient for the antiapoptotic effects of these ligands since several other growth factors, including angiotensin II [175], IL-1β, and interferon-γ, also activate this signal transduction cascade, which promotes apoptosis in both adult [90] and neonatal rat ventricular myocytes. Similarly to CT-1, fibroblast growth factor plays a role in promoting myocyte survival through suppression of apoptosis [176, 177]. Several other growth factors exert variable effects on cardiac myocytes: while phenylephrine and leukaemia inhibitory factor completely prevented apoptosis induced by hypoxia and starvation in neonatal rat ventricular myocytes, endothelin-1 had only a partial protective effect and angiotensin-II had no antiapoptotic effect [168]. Leukaemia inhibitory factor also protects cardiomyocytes from apoptosis induced by oxidative stress via the activation of the JAK/STAT and MAPK cascade [178]. Further studies are required to determine how these peptide growth factors differentially affect cardiomyocyte survival and apoptosis. Regardless of the eventual outcome, growth factors lead to expression of transcription factors, induce myocyte hypertrophy, and prepare the cell for entry into the cell cycle.

## Cell-cycle regulators

Recently, Williams [179] suggested that manipulation of the cell cycle in the cardiac myocyte is a potential therapeutic strategy for the management of heart failure. In the absence of mitogenic stimuli, or under the influence of dominantly acting signals that suppress cell growth, the cell cycle stops, a condition characterized as phase $G_0$. Upon mitogenic stimulation, the mammalian cell cycle is driven by sequential activation of specific cyclin/cyclin-dependent kinase pairs. DNA replication (S phase) and mitosis (M phase) are separated by periods characterized by unreplicated ($G_1$) or replicated ($G_2$) DNA. The restriction point (R) is the checkpoint in $G_1$ after which the decision to replicate DNA no longer requires the continued presence of mitogenic growth stimuli. Adult cardiomyocytes are resistant to mitogens (postmitotic) and appear to be locked permanently in $G_0$. A complex combination of molecular mechanisms serves to maintain the postmitotic state of adult cardiac myocytes. Agents that force the terminally differentiated cell, such as the cardiac myocyte, to re-enter the cell cycle are all potent inducers of apoptosis. The coordination of events that occur during a cell cycle is dependent on a series of cyclin-dependent kinases (Cdks), that when activated consist of the combination of a kinase and a cyclin. The combination of Cdk4 with cyclin E or A is essential for DNA replication, whereas the combination of Cdk2 with cyclin A or B is important for the progression from $G_2$ (the second phase of the growth cycle) to mitosis. Entry into $G_1$, the first phase of the cell cycle, is associated with increased expression of a number of genes encoding enzymes involved in DNA and nucleotide synthesis, and DNA binding proteins which, in turn, induce the expression of regulatory proteins such as polymerase-α, histone H3, and proliferating cell nuclear antigen (PCNA). Progression through $G_1$ also requires inactivation of several tumour suppressor genes including *p53*, *p21*, *p16*, *p15*, *p27* (discussed below), and the retinoblastoma gene, *Rb*, that inhibit the kinase activity of the cyclin/Cdk complexes. *p53* and *p21* are also required to sustain G2 arrest after DNA damage [180]. Survivin is a new inhibitor of apoptosis that is expressed in the $G_2$/M phase of the cell cycle in a cycle-regulated manner [181]. At the beginning of mitosis, survivin associates with microtubules of the mitotic spindle. Disruption of survivin–microtubule interactions results in the loss of survivin's antiapoptosis function and increased caspase-3 activity, a mechanism involved in cell death [182]. Overexpression of survivin may overcome this apoptotic checkpoint and may be a potential therapeutic strategy to prevent and ameliorate apoptosis in dilated cardiomyopathy. It has been shown that myocytes react to heart failure by activating cyclins and Edks which are coupled with cell regeneration and the recovery of muscle mass [183]. One study showed that there is a reversion to the foetal pattern of Cdk inhibitor expression in acute and end-stage heart failure [184].

It has been suggested that overexpression of Cdk inhibitors, e.g. *p21* and *p16*, may protect myocytes from apoptosis, whereas others have disputed this suggestion [185]. Cdk inhibitors act as the traffic police of cell division. There are three potential ways in which these proteins might stop and start cellular proliferation: (1) as a restriction-point regulator that controls entry into both differentiation and division; (2) as a checkpoint system that stops division in response to genetic damage; and (3) as a holding function that keeps cells in a non-proliferative state [186]. A recent study showed that adenoviral delivery of *E2F-1* to postmitotic ventricular myocytes results in cell cycle re-entry and a *p53*-independent apoptosis [187]. These results suggest that re-entry of the postmitotic ventricular myocytes results in apoptosis. Another study also showed that induction of DNA synthesis by E1A oncoprotein results in apoptosis [188]. It is possible that in response to remodelling factors the cell cycle occurs in an asymmetric fashion in the cardiac myocyte. This asymmetric cell response, albeit mediated by the same signal transduction pathways, causes hypertrophy of most of the ventricular myocytes and apoptosis of a minority of its neighbouring myocytes to make room for the hypertrophied cell. Asymmetric cell responses have been identified in several cell systems [189] but the determinants that control the fate of the individual myocyte remain to be characterized. Replenishing the myocardium with a sufficient number of new cardiac myocytes by manipulating the cell cycle may be a potential therapeutic strategy for the management of heart failure [179].

## Intracellular calcium excess

Excessive entry of calcium into myocytes may be the underlying mechanism of cardiac damage following ischaemia [190]. Numerous experimental studies have suggested that a sustained elevation of calcium, e.g. by exposure of cells to ionophores, causes cell death, and that alterations in calcium signalling pathways (e.g. alterations in calcium currents) or prevention of free calcium elevation can prevent cell death [191]. The duration and extent of calcium influx may determine whether cells survive, die by apoptosis, or undergo necrotic lysis. Accordingly, continuous but moderate increases in calcium, such as those produced by a sustained low influx, may cause apoptosis, whereas an exceedingly high influx rate would cause rapid cell necrosis. Unlike excessive sodium, which damages cells by direct osmotic effects, increased calcium probably does not elicit apoptosis by itself. Rather, it activates enzymes in signalling pathways, some of which depend on the continuous presence of elevated calcium or require calcium signal as a trigger. A modest increase in calcium promotes cell survival and does so through calmodulin kinase kinase activation of the protein kinase B pathway, which in turn phosphorylates apoptotic proteins such as Bad [192]. The nature of these processes and their contribution to calcium-induced apoptosis have only been partially elucidated.

The possible targets for calcium elevations include signal transduction intermediates, calcium-activated proteases, calcium-activated endonucleases, calcium-dependent transglutaminase, and exposure of cell surface phosphatidylserine. Activation of calcium-dependent protein kinases and/or phosphatases leads to alterations in gene transcription and is one way in which calcium may regulate apoptosis. Most support comes from the hypothesis that cyclosporin A, an inhibitor of the calcium–calmodulin-dependent protein serine/threonine phosphatase, calcineurin, can block calcium-dependent apoptosis [193–195]. Transgenic mice that express activated forms of calcineurin develop dilated cardiomyopathy and heart failure, which can be prevented by the administration of cyclosporin [196, 197]. It is likely that in this model of cardiomyopathy, calcium excess is responsible for apoptosis. If this prediction comes to pass, calcineurin-blocking drugs may be part of the treatment of early stage heart failure.

High intracellular calcium can also activate various hydrolytic enzymes that have been implicated as effectors of calcium-elicited apoptosis, including proteases, endonucleases, and lipases (discussed below). Recent work indicates that the movement of PS from the inner to the outer surface of the plasma membrane, a process that functions in the removal of apoptotic cells and bodies by both professional phagocytic cells (macrophages) and neighbouring cells in tissues, is another component of apoptosis [40, 41] that appears to be regulated by alterations in cytosolic calcium. The mechanism of calcium-mediated PS exposure is not yet clear but closely parallels the formation of cytoskeleton-free lipid microvesicles and other phenomena such as calpain activation and the formation of phosphatidylinositol (4,5)-bisphosphate [Ins (4,5)] $P_2$–calcium complexes. However, neither direct calcium effects, calpain-mediated protein degradation, Ins(4,5)$P_2$ accumulation, nor inhibition of the flipase can singularly explain the membrane rearrangements. Furthermore, an increase in diastolic calcium in the cardiac myocyte may activate DNAse I, triggering apoptosis independently from the expression of *p53*, *Bax* and *Bcl-2* in the cells [34]. Another group found that blocking extracellular calcium influx with nifedipine, an L-type calcium channel blocker, protected the cardiac myocyte from apoptosis induced by hypoxia [191].

Depletion of the calcium stored of the sarcoplasmic reticulum may serve as a signal for apoptosis. DNAse I and the extranuclear scaffold protease are localized to the endoplasmic reticulum and it is possible that the loss of calcium leads to the release of these factors into the perinuclear region or into the nuclear matrix. It is known that depletion of the sarcoplasmic reticulum calcium pool results in the release of a small biomolecule that participates in a retrograde signal for plasma membrane calcium influx, and may promote apoptosis. To rest this hypothesis, Chen *et al.* [191] examined the efficacy of dantrolene, a drug that decreases the release of calcium from the sarcoplasmic reticulum. Dantiolene inhibited cell death and morphological changes as efficiently as nifedipine, suggesting that calcium influx/release is required for executing myocyte apoptosis. They also found that specific inhibition of PKC exerted a prominent dose-dependent protective effect. Inhibition of calcium/calmodulin-dependent protein kinases was also protective, although less effective than the inhibitor of PKC. In contrast, specific inhibition of protein kinase A had no appreciable effect even at higher concentrations.

Depletion of mitochondrial calcium stores may also participate in the signal for apoptosis. Inhibition of mitochondrial calcium uptake blocks or inhibits apoptosis in various cell systems. Further efforts are required to determine the relationship between this event and the activation of proteases and nucleases of the effector pathway.

## Modulators of the apoptotic process in heart failure

The mechanism by which growth factors become death factors will only become apparent once the molecular regulators of apoptosis are understood. Until recently attention has focused on the *p53* tumor suppressor gene, which exists in a kind of yin–yang balance with the Bcl-2 family of proteins (including Bax, Bcl-x, Bad, and Bak) in preventing apoptosis. The cast of characters has expanded to include several more antiapoptotic and proapoptotic proteins such as the MAPK family and molecular chaperones. Most of these proteins come in two forms, the inactive and the active. Each receives and sends messages via a maze of signal transduction pathways. Extracellular signals through the TNF receptor or a related receptor (Fas), or intracellular signals related to *p53* detection of irreparable DNA damage lead to the activation of a series of cellular proteases. Activated proteases cleave specific proteins at asparagine residues and activate the cell death pathway.

### *p53* tumour suppressor genes

*p53* gene expression either arrests stable growth or leads to programmed cell death. The *p53* gene is like a security guard, deployed when cellular DNA is damaged, to prevent the cell from becoming neoplastic. It either inhibits cell growth until the damage is repaired or leads the cell to apoptosis. *p53* deficient homozygous mice are normal at birth but become increasingly susceptible to tumours [198]. Mutations of *p53* have been observed in approximately 50% of patients with tumours, underscoring its importance as a tumour suppressor gene. Several mechanisms by which the *p53* gene may initiate apoptosis have been postulated. In human colorectal cancers, growth arrest is dependent on p53-mediated transcriptional induction of protein $p21^{WAF1/CIP1}$. Alternatively, *p53* may lead to apoptosis through a stepwise process. *p53* transcriptionally activates a specific subset of genes referred to as *p53*-induced genes (PIGs), including oxidoreductases, long before biochemical or morphological evidence of cell death becomes apparent. The proteins encoded by these genes collectively increase the formation of reactive oxygen species, which damage mitochondria, and the resulting leakage of calcium and respiratory chain proteins activates the caspases that are ubiquitously activated during the apoptotic process.

The apoptotic effect of *p53* in heart failure has resulted in it being viewed as the 'terminator'. Apoptosis-associated proteins, C-myc and p53, are expressed in cardiomyocytes isolated from dogs with chronic heart failure [30, 33]. This has been confirmed in dogs with pacing-induced heart failure [199]. Pierzchalski *et al.* [89] and Leri *et al.* [44] have suggested that p53-induced apoptosis of cardiac myocytes occurs by the activation of the renin–angiotensin system. Another induction mechanism may be the activation of apoptotic genes such as *bax*; however, a study in mice showed that myocyte apoptosis during acute myocardial infarction localized to hypoxic regions occurred independently of the *p53* gene [200] and this was confirmed recently [201]. In addition, El-Deiry *et al.* [202] have shown that p53 elevates the cellular concentration of a death receptor, DR5, that binds to a cytotoxic factor, TNF-related apoptosis-inducing ligand (TRAIL), which suggests a contributory role of the TRAIL system or its decoy receptor for enhanced apoptosis in failing human hearts [203]. Although DR5 is regulated by p53, it is unclear whether this regulation is direct. A region of the DR5 gene resembles the p53 binding site and strengthens the notion that p53 can directly activate the transcription of DR5. DR5 may be a novel target for antiheart failure therapy. Drugs or hormones that stimulate or inhibit DR5 may allow effective control of p53-induced apoptosis.

*p53* was thought to have no close relatives, but now researchers have discovered a long-lost cousin in the *p73* gene, which bears a strong resemblance to *p53* [204]. *p73* shares the growth-inhibiting and apoptosis-promoting effects of *p53*, although it is unknown what triggers it and exactly what its cellular role is. *p73* is located on a region near the tip of chromosome 1 that is often deleted in cancers such as neuroblastoma. Proteins made by *p73* are somewhat larger than p53. One section of p73 closely binds to the core-binding region of p53. Of the 177 amino acids in this region, 112 are identical. Additional similarities are observed in two other sections: one is needed for its gene regulatory effects and another where it apparently binds to itself. Whether both *p53* and *p73* are progeny of a gene duplicated in some ancient cellular event needs to be explored. In addition, *p73* latches on to stretches of DNA to which *p53* normally attaches itself when instructing a cell to self-destruct. Despite these similarities, there are several differences between p53 and p73. Unlike p53 protein, p73 does not seem to be produced in response to DNA damage, i.e. it is not a cell security guard. In addition, *p53* genes require two hits for inactivation: a partial or complete deletion of one of the two gene copies and another lesser change which cripples the second copy, whereas in *p73*, the only copy of the gene is already inactive in normal cells, owing to a mysterious process called 'imprinting' (during embryonic development, imprinting alters certain genes so that the copy inherited from the mother or the father is specifically shut down). The role of the *p73* gene in apoptosis and cell-cycle control of terminally differentiated cardiac myocytes remains to be explored.

By using the degenerate polymerase chain reaction (PCR) approach, various other tumour suppressor proteins have been identified. p40 and p51, both encoded by an additional *p53* family member [205, 206], are the products of alternatively spliced mRNAS encoded by a single gene located on chromosome 3q. Preliminary data suggest that *p51*, like *p53* and *p73*, can activate transcription and induce apoptosis [205]. The primary sequences of *p51* and *p73* resemble each other more closely than either resembles *p53*. *p51* exists in the heart as two major splicing variants of the latter gene, *p51A* and *p51B* (a human homologue of murine *Ket*). The function of *p73* and *p51* remains to be elucidated, as do their potential roles in cardiac failure. *p63* is yet another *p53* homologue which has remarkably divergent abilities to induce apoptosis [207]. Similarly, a novel alternative splice form of *p53* in rat cardiac myocytes has recently been reported but its significance remains to be determined [208].

## Molecular chaperones

Diverse physiological and pathological stresses, such as those seen in heart failure and myocardial ischaemia, result in protein damage and affect protein structure and function [209, 210]. Molecular chaperones are one of the many endogenous pathways that are engaged in restoring cellular homoeostasis. Several recent studies have implicated molecular chaperones in cell survival pathways, particularly during cell differentiation and damage due to oxidative stress. Molecular chaperones, such as heat shock protein (Hsp)70 and αB-crystallin, are proteins that facilitate folding, assembly, and dissembly of other proteins but are not part of the finished product [211]. Molecular chaperones, in particular, heat shock proteins, are rapidly expressed through mechanisms of transcriptional activation and preferential translation in response to ischaemic–reperfusion injury and oxidative stress [212]. Splicing alterations and stabilization of mRNA are adaptive mechanisms used to translate efficiently stress proteins, which can reach 15–25% of total intracellular protein within minutes after physiological stress. At the same time, several cytosolic chaperones translocate to the nucleus where inhibition of DNA chromatin assembly exposes a nuclease-sensitive conformation, a pathognomonic feature of ischaemia-induced apoptosis [213]. Cessation of the noxious stimulus is followed by rapid and efficient degradation of Hsp mRNA. In addition, TNF-α-treated cardiac myocytes induce transient gene expression of cytoprotective molecules such as Hsp27 and Hsp70 [214]. Hsp70 expression inhibits apoptosis through a mechanism involving cell-cycle control. It has been suggested that the Hsp70 chaperone inhibits apoptosis by preventing activation of stress kinases [215]. Overexpression of Hsp25/27, like the antiapoptotic protein Bcl-2, results in an increase in the levels of antioxidant glutathione and resistance to Fas/Apo-1-mediated apoptosïs. Antisense-mediated reduction of Hsp25/27 inhibits apoptosis through reduction of glutathione levels and prolongation of the cell cycle. In embryonic stem cells, withdrawal from the cell cycle results in upregulation of Hsp25/27 mRNA, which is accompanied by an increase in oligomerization of the Hsp25/27 protein. These studies suggest that during differentiation and proliferation of myocardial cells, the Hsp25/27 chaperone and others can reduce oxidative stress and prevent apoptosis through a redox-dependent mechanism [216]. The aging rodent myocardium is associated with increased apoptosis [32, 88] and a decrease in the expression of Hsp genes and the DNA-binding activity of HSF-1 [217]. A recent study demonstrated differential expression of heat shock proteins in normal and failing human hearts. Hsp27 was increased almost two-fold in dilated cardiomyopathy compared with normal hearts and was significantly greater than in ischaemic hearts [218]. Hsp60 was doubled in both dilated cardiomyopathy and ischaemic hearts, whereas Hsp72, Hsp70, and Hsp90 were not significantly changed. The mechanism of heat shock proteins in cardiomyocyte apoptosis needs to be characterized. The current availability of transgenic mouse models should clarify the role of heat shock gene expression in apoptosis of the ventricular myocardium.

## The *bcl-2* family of genes

*Bcl-2* is a member of a multigene family of proteins with a homologous structure, some of which, such as *Bcl-2* itself, A-1, *Mcl-1*, and *Bcl-xl*, inhibit apoptosis [219, 220] and others, such as *Bax*, *Bcl-x-s*, *bad*, *bid*, and *bak*, promote apoptosis. Stretch-induced apoptosis in myocardial cells has been shown to be associated with a decrease in the *Bcl-2*/*Bax* ratio [44, 221] and when the Bcl-2 protein is transfected into ventricular myocytes, *p53*-induced apoptosis is blunted [222], confirming that Bcl-2 plays a protective role in cardiac myocytes. Adenoviral-mediated gene transfer of *Bcl-2* prevents apoptosis of neonatal rat ventricular myocytes induced by TNF-α [142]. In the myocardium of spontaneously hypertensive rats with heart failure, expression of Bcl-2 was unchanged compared with non-failing controls, and facilitated apoptosis in the former group [36]. Infarcted myocardium from human autopsies reveals an increase in Bcl-2 protein, whereas the Bax protein is overexpressed at later stages of the infarct [223]. In contrast, apoptosis in end-stage heart failure was associated with near doubling of the expression of Bcl-2 in the myocardium without changes in expression of Bax [16].

It remains unknown precisely know how Bcl-2/caspase-like proteins work. If they prevent apoptosis by blocking cytochrome c release, would they need to bind to caspase proteins, and what is the role for Bcl-2 in other locations, such as on the endoplasmic reticulum and nuclear membrane? If Bcl-2-like proteins function by binding to and inhibiting caspases, why would they need to prevent cytochrome *c* release? It may be that Bcl-2 proteins perform both functions. Another possibility is that Bcl-2 may retain cytochrome *c* in the mitochondria indirectly. If cytochrome *c* were only one of a number of factors that can activate caspase, induction of apoptosis by these alternative pathways may lead to a secondary loss of mitochondrial function, release of cytochrome *c*, and amplification of the apoptotic cascade. In such a scenario, Bcl-2-like proteins would only act as caspase inhibitors, indirectly preventing cytochrome *c* release by inhibiting the initial premitochondrial activation of caspase. It has been suggested that Bcl-2 suppresses apoptosis by activating transcription factor NF-κβ [224]. Bax and Bax-like proteins may mediate caspase-independent death via channel-forming activity, which could promote mitochondrial permeability or puncture the mitochondrial outer membrane [225]. However, because the evidence for caspase-independent apoptosis relies largely on overexpression and chemical inhibitors, its pathophysiological significance remains disputed [225].

## Mitogen-activated protein kinase family

Using adenoviral vectors, Chien and co-workers [226] characterized the role of the p38 MAPK pathway in cardiac hypertrophy, apoptosis, and failure. They found that transfection of cardiac myocytes with adenoviral vectors expressing upstream inducers for p38 kinases activated mutants of MAPK kinase 3b(E)(MKK3bE) and MAPK kinase 6b(E) to elicit characteristic hypertrophic responses, including an increase in cell size, enhanced sarcomeric organization, and elevated atrial natriuretic factor expression. The hypertrophic response was suppressed by the p38β-dominant negative mutant. Overexpression of the activated MKK3bE in cardiomyocytes led to an increase in apoptosis. The MKK3bE-induced cell death was increased by co-transfection of wild-type p38α, and was suppressed by the dominant negative p38α mutant. Cardiac selective p38 MAPK inhibitors may be potential therapeutic agents to ameliorate apoptosis in cardiac failure. A recent study suggested that activation of p38 MAPK protects cardiac cells from apoptosis [227]; however, the investigators did not characterize the isoform of p38 kinase, unlike the previous study [226].

## Executors of apoptosis in heart failure

Narula and co-workers [228] showed that caspases are required for the execution of apoptosis in heart failure. Caspases refer to a family of proteases that are central mediators of apoptosis. They are synthesized and stored in the cells as zymogens and are activated in response to diverse apoptotic triggers. Caspase activation is one of the final steps required for the execution phase of apoptosis. The cellular targets for these proteases include other inactive caspase zymogens, cytoskeletal proteins, nuclease precursors, and nuclear envelope proteins. Caspases are activated broadly by two major pathways: the first is triggered by cytokines and involves death receptor assembly, and the other is initiated by diverse stress stimuli including ischaemia, calcium excess, and reactive oxygen radicals, and is mediated by release of cytochrome *c* from mitochondria. Both cascades interact at various levels. A recent study has demonstrated that cytokine-induced activation of caspase-8 cleaves the proapoptotic protein, Bid, which overwhelms the protection provided to cytochrome *c* by antiapoptotic proteins such as Bcl-2. In addition to caspases, various other proteases may lead to intracellular digestion of the cell.

### Death receptor-related pathway

The Fas–Fas ligand (FasL) system is the representative system of apoptosis-signalling receptor molecules. Fas (CD95) is a cell-surface protein consisting of 319 amino acids with a single membrane domain, belonging to the nerve growth factor receptor or TNF receptor family [229–233]. Fas ligand (FasL), a type II membrane protein belonging to the TNF family, induces apoptotic cell death when bound to the Fas antigen [234]. Fas–Fas interaction leads to the aggregation of the death domain of Fas. [Fas-associating protein with death domain (FADD)], which physically links with caspase-8 and triggers apoptosis [235, 236]. Others have shown that triggering of Fas/Apo-1 induces activation of c-Jun N-terminal kinases (JNK) [237]. Activation of this characteristic set of kinases precedes nuclear DNA fragmentation and is dependent on the activity of ICE-like proteases [237]. Molecular cloning and nucleotide sequence analysis have revealed a human Fas mRNA variant that encodes a soluble Fas (sFas) molecule that lacks the membrane domain because of a deletion of an exon encoding this region [238]. The membrane-bound FasL is converted to a soluble form of FasL (sFasL) by a metalloproteinase [239, 240]. Human sFas-L, a 26 000 mol.wt glycoprotein, consists of the extracellular region of the FasL. In mice, FasL is predominantly expressed in activated T-cells, whereas Fas is expressed in various tissues including the thymus, heart, liver, and ovary but not in the brain or spleen [241, 242]. The binding of FasL, sFasL, or agonistic anti-Fas antibodies to Fas induces apoptosis [234, 241, 242]. Extrinsic sFas blocks apoptosis in cells by inhibiting the binding of the Fas-L or sFasL to Fas on the cell membrane [238, 240]. Fas mRNA is induced by hypoxia in cultured neonatal rat myocytes [243]. In patients with chronic congestive heart failure, plasma sFasL does not increase, while plasma sFas levels increase relative to the severity of the functional class [244]. sFas levels were significantly higher even in patients in functional NYHA class II than in normal subjects and those in functional class I, and were highest in functional class IV patients. Plasma sFas levels were significantly higher in patients with elevated pulmonary artery wedge pressure and a decreased cardiac index than in those with values in the normal range. In patients in functional class IV, there was no significant difference in plasma sFas levels between the survivors and non-survivors during a 6-month follow-up. However, plasma levels of sFas tended to decrease in nine clinically improved patients but were similar in patients with no change in functional class [244]. Others have demonstrated that serum levels of sFasL are significantly higher in myocarditis [245, 246]. The disparate results may be explained by the pathogenesis of these cardiac diseases. In myocarditis, activated T-lymphocytes stimulated by viruses or other antigens may produce sFasL, leading to myocardial injury, followed by cell death and cardiac failure. Using reverse transcription (RT) PCR, Schumann *et al.* [247] found mRNA for Fas and five isoforms in the non-failing left ventricles, whereas Fas and only one isoform (FasExo6Del) were detectable in the failing left ventricle. Standard calibrated, competitive RT-PCR revealed no significant increase in Fas mRNA in failing compared with non-failing ventricles. However, the mRNA for FasExo6Del, expressed nearly on the same level as Fas in non-failing ventricles, was decreased about three-fold in the failing ventricle. They proposed that this altered expression of the Fas system renders the myocardium more susceptible to Fas-mediated apoptosis in end-stage heart failure. A recent study suggested that Fas-mediated damage to ventricular myocytes, at least in part, is mediated by inositol 1,4,5-triphosphate [248].

In addition to the well-characterized death receptors, Fas (CD95 or Apo-1) and TNFR-1 (also called p55 or CD120a), other death receptors such as avian CAR1, death receptor DR-3 (also called Apo-3, WSL-1, TRAMP, or LARD), DR-4, DR-5 (also called Apo-2, TRAIL-Rs, TRICK 2, or KILLER), and DR-6 have been implicated in apoptosis. The ligands that activate these receptors are structurally related to the TNF gene superfamily. Dixit and co-workers [249] recently found abundant DR-6 transcript in the heart. DR-6 interacts with TRADD, which has previously been shown to associate with TNFR-1. Furthermore, ectopic expression of DR-6 in mammalian cells induces apoptosis and activation of NF-κβ and JNK [249]. Although these death receptors remain to be characterized on cardiac myocytes, the idea of targeting specific receptors to inhibit apoptosis in heart failure is attractive, because death receptors have direct access to the caspase machinery.

## Cytochrome c release and caspase activation in heart failure

Narula *et al.* [11] found that in human explanted hearts cytochrome *c* release and caspase activation occurred during apoptosis. This work has been supported by other investigations in ventricular myocytes [250–253] and in rats with acute myocardial infarction [254], based on the ability of pharmacological inhibitors such as ZVAD-fmk partially to inhibit apoptosis. ACE inhibitors prevent apoptosis by inhibiting proteases, and caspases constitute attractive potential targets in this respect. Peptidyl caspase inhibitors have been found to be effective in animal models of myocardial ischaemia–reperfusion injury. Elegant work on cysteine protease inhibition has provided a starting point, leading to the identification of several classes of potent reversible and irreversible caspase inhibitors [255]. Studies with these compounds will no doubt provide answers to many questions regarding the therapeutic potential of caspase inhibition. Although the relative importance of apoptotic and non-apoptotic cell death in myocardial ischaemia is not known, the use of the caspase inhibitor zVAD-fmk leads to a reduction in acute functional parameters after myocardial infarct. However, these changes were recorded within 24 h of infarction, and it is unclear whether the effects of zVAD-fmk persist for longer periods [256]. The recent identification of ARC, an inhibitor of apoptosis expressed in skeletal muscle and heart that selectively interacts with caspases, may provide an exciting therapeutic strategy in the treatment of heart failure [257]. The role of caspase inhibitors in preventing or ameliorating heart failure needs to be investigated.

## Calcium-related and- unrelated proteases and proteinases

Calpains are a family of calcium-dependent cysteine proteases that absolutely require calcium for catalytic activity. There are two major isoforms: calpain μ and calpain *m*, which require micromolar and millimolar levels of calcium, respectively. Upon autoproteolytic activation, the proteases can selectively cleave a subset of cellular proteins, including membrane receptors, G proteins, cytoskeletal proteins, protein kinases, and transcription factors, particularly fodrin. The involvement of calpain seems to be independent of the caspase family, but may be related to p53. A recent study found that the execution phase of cardiomyocyte apoptosis is marked by increased calpain expression and cell death [191]. A slight increase in calpain mRNA levels occurs at the onset of the execution phase and this increase becomes prominent during the execution phase, resulting in a greater than five-fold increase in the steady-state levels of calpain transcripts. They also found that calpeptin, a specific and cell-permeable calpain inhibitor, prevented cardiomyocyte apoptosis induced by chemical hypoxia. These studies suggest that calpains may be centrally involved in the regulation of cardiomyocyte apoptosis. These conclusions are supported by other studies demonstrating that calpain activation is associated with hypoxic injury both in cultured myocytes and in the ischaemic heart [258–260].

To understand better calpain-induced apoptosis, the effects of proteasome and lyzozomal proteases must be eliminated. The largest area of uncertainty is perhaps the nature of the protein substrates which become cleaved in various phases of the cell cycle, only some of which are known. Calpain has a role in the destruction of cyclin D1, however, the majority of the substrates is degraded by the ubiquitin–proteasome route. Field and Clark [261] hypothesized the role of inappropriate ubiquitin conjugation in heart failure. In many cell types, including cardiac myocytes, the proteasome, a multicatalytic complex of proteases, is responsible for the degradation of essentially all of the intracellular protein within the dying cell [142]. Using immunofluorescence, the mammalian ubiquitin-conjugating enzyme has been localized to Z-bands and intercalated discs in rat cardiac myocytes [262]. Treatment of cardiac myocytes with TNF-$\alpha$ results in a four-fold increase in ubiquitin mRNA [214]. Recent studies demonstrate that proteasomes are required for apoptosis induced by a wide variety of signals in cultured cell lines, suggesting that proteasomes take part in the common portion of the cell-death pathway. How the proteasome functions is not understood, but in some cell types, a proteasome is required for the activation of caspase-3. In neonatal ventricular myocytes, the proteasome inhibitor lactacystin prevents Bcl-2-mediated loss of I$\kappa$B. Lactacystin, which covalently modifies the active site of proteasome, is an inhibitor of apoptosis; however, since it acts on several cell types it may not be a rational therapeutic agent in heart failure. Although other molecules may also be involved, a recent study suggests that stabilization and accumulation of p53 play a key role in the apoptosis induced by proteasome inhibitors [142, 263].

## Conclusions

Although there is sufficient evidence to suggest that apoptosis is associated with end-stage heart failure, the relative roles of apoptosis, necrosis, and hypertrophy of the cardiac myocyte in the pathogenesis of heart failure remain to be defined. The mechanisms of apoptosis and its accurate quantification, including the rate and duration of the apoptotic therapy is to be developed. The work ahead necessary to develop and refine clinically useful antiapoptotic therapy is daunting. There are many unanswered questions: What will be the most practical method for delivering this therapy to the cardiac myocyte? Will antiapoptotic agents act selectively on affected myocytes to provide clinical efficacy? Will antiapoptotic agents be effective or will they be limited by dose heterogeneity? If the antiapoptotic is proven to have long-lasting efficacy, should it be used for all patients with myocardial infarction or confined only to patients with left ventricular dysfunction? Will antiapoptotic therapy be so effective that it replaces ACE inhibitors and $\beta$-adrenergic antagonists, or will it always be used as an adjunct? These questions lay the foundation for the next decade of investigation.

## Acknowledgement

The authors thank Ralph A. Kelly, MD, for reading the manuscript and for his useful comments.

## References

1. Schocken DD, Arrieta MI, Leaverton PE, Ross EA. Prevalence and mortality rate of congestive heart failure in the United States. *J Am Coll Cardiol* 1992; 20: 301–6.
2. American Heart Association. 1999 Heart and Stroke Statistical Update, Dallas, Texas. American Heart Association, 1998.
3. MMWR. Mortality from congestive heart failure — United States, 1980–1990. *MMWR Morb Mortal Wkly Rep* 1994; 53: 77–81.
4. MMWR. Breast cancer incidence and mortality — United States, 1992. *MMWR Morb Mortal Wkly Rep* 1996; 45: 833–7.
5. MMWR. Update: trends in AIDS, incidence, deaths and prevalence — United States, 1996. *MMWR Morb Mortal Wkly Rep* 1997; 46: 165–73.
6. Ho KKL, Pinsky JL, Kannel WB, Levy D. The epidemiology of heart failure: the Framingham Study. *J Am Coll Cardiol* 1993; Suppl A: 6–13A.
7. Lenfant C. Fixing the failing heart. *Circulation* 1997; 95: 771–2.
8. Packer M. Evolution of the neurohormonal hypothesis to explain the progression of chronic heart failure. *Eur Heart J* 1995; 16 Suppl F:4–6.
9. Konstam MA, Dracup K, Baker DW *et al. Heart failure evaluation and care of patients with left-ventricular systolic dysfunction.* Rockville, MD: Agency for Health Care Policy and Research Publication 94–0612, June 1994.
10. Stevenson LW, Massie BM, Francis GS. Optimizing therapy for complex or refractory heart failure: an advanced algorithm from the Advanced Heart Failure Group. *Am Heart J* 1998; 135: S293–309.
11. Narula J, Haider N, Virmani R *et al.* Programmed myocyte death in end-stage heart failure. *N Engl J Med* 1996; 335: 1182–9.
12. Wackers FJ, Vogt-Hoerner G. Presence of focal bionecrosis in the epithelium of the acini in the human mammary gland. *Ann Anat Pathol* 1967; 12: 21–34.
13. Kerr JFR, Wyllie AH, Currie AR. Apoptosis: a basic biologic phenomenon with wide-ranging implications in tissue kinetics. *Br J Cancer* 1972; 26: 239–57.
14. Wyllie AH, Morris RG, Smith AL, Dunlap D. Chromatin cleavage in apoptosis: association with condensed chromatin morphology and dependent on macromolecular synthesis. *J Pathol* 1984; 142: 67–77.
15. Mallat Z *et al.* Evidence of apoptosis in arrhythmogenic right ventricular dysplasia. *N Engl J Med* 1996; 335: 1190–6.
16. Olivetti G, Abbi Quaini F *et al.* Apoptosis in failing human heart. *N Engl J Med* 1997; 336: 1131–41.
17. Saraste A *et al.* Apoptosis in the heart. *N Engl J Med* 1997; 336: 1025–6.
18. Sharov VG, Goussev A, Higgins RSD *et al.* Higher incidence of cardiocyte apoptosis in failing explanted hearts of patients with ischemic versus idiopathic dilated cardiomyopathy (Abstract). *Circulation* 1997; 96: I-17.
19. Colucci WS. Apoptosis in the heart. *N Engl J Med* 1996; 335: 1224–6.

20. Kajsutra J, Cheng W, Reiss K *et al.* Apoptotic and necrotic myocyte cell deaths are independently contributing variables of infarct size in rats. *Lad Invest* 1996; 74: 86–107.
21. Saraste A, Pulkki K, Kallajoki M *et al.* Apoptosis in human myocardial infarction. *Circulation* 1997; 95: 320–3.
22. Gottlieb RA, Buresldon KO, Kloner RA *et al.* Reperfusion injury induces apoptosis in rabbit cardiac myocytes. *J Clin Invest* 1994; 74: 86–107.
23. Liu Y, Cigola E, Cheng W *et al.* Myocyte nuclear mitotic division and programmed myocyte death characterize the cardiac myopathy induced by rapid ventricular pacing in dogs. *Lab Invest* 1995; 73: 771–87.
24. Cheng W, Li B, Kajustura J *et al.* Stretch-induced programmed myocyte cell death. *J Clin Invest* 1995; 96: 2247–59.
25. Teiger E, Dam T-V, Richard L *et al.* Apoptosis in pressure overload-induced heart hypertrophy in the rat. *J Clin Invest* 1996; 97: 2891–7.
26. Spanier T, Wang J, Oz M *et al.* Improvement in the apoptotic regulatory paradigm with left ventricular device (LVAD) implantation. *Circulation* 1998; Suppl 1: I-719.
27. Bartling B, Milting H, Schumann H *et al.* Improved myocardial expression of anti-apoptotic genes under support by ventricular assist devices in terminal heart failure. *Circulation* 1998; Suppl 1: I-200.
28. Kajstura J *et al.* Myocyte proliferation in end-stage cardiac failure in humans. *Proc Natl Acad Sci USA* 1998; 95: 8801–5.
29. Adams JW *et al.* Enhanced Gα-q signaling; a common pathway mediates cardiac hypertrophy and apoptotic heart failure. *Proc Natl Acad Sci USA* 1990; 95: 10 140–5.
30. Sharov VG, Sabbah HN, Shimoyama H *et al.* Evidence of cardiomyocyte apoptosis in myocardium of dogs with chronic heart failure. *Am J Pathol* 1996; 148: 141–9.
31. Sabbah HN, Sharov VG, Goussev A *et al.* Evidence of ongoing loss of cardiomyocytes in dogs with progressive left ventricular dysfunction and heart failure. *Circulation* 1997; 96: I-754.
32. Kajstura J, Cheng W, Sarangrajan R *et al.* Necrotic and apoptotic myocyte cell death in the aging heart of Fischer 344 rats. *Am J Physiol* 1996; 271: H1215–28.
33. Sharov VG, Sabbah HN, Goussev A *et al.* Apoptosis associated proteins c-myc and p53 are expressed in cardiomyocytes isolated from dogs with chronic heart failure. *Circulation* 1996; 94: I–171.
34. Nitahara JA, Cheng W, Liu Y *et al.* Intracellular calcium, DNase activity and myocyte apoptosis in aging Fischer 344 rats. *J Mol Cell Cardiol* 1998; 30: 519–35.
35. Bing OH, Hague NL, Perreault CL *et al.* Thyroid hormone effects on intracellular calcium and inotropic responses of rat ventricular myocardium. *Am J Physiol* 1994; 267(3 Pt 2): H1112–21.
36. Li Z, Bing OHL, Long X *et al.* Increased cardiomyocyte apoptosis during transition to heart failure in the spontaneously hypertensive rat. *Am J Physiol* 1997; 272: H2313–19.
37. Baliga RR, Brooks WW, Bing OH, Singh K. Beta-1 integrins in cardiac hypertrophy and failure. *Circulation* 1998; Suppl 1: I–648.
38. Frisch SM, Ruoshlahti E. Integrins and anoikis. *Curr Opin Cell Biol* 1997; 9: 701–6.
39. Hsueh WA, Law RE, Do YS. Integrins, adhesion and cardiac remodeling. *Hypertension* 1998; 31: 176–80.
40. Maulik N, Kagan VE, Tyurin VA, Das DK. Redistribution of phosphatidylethanolamine and phosphatidylserine precedes reperfusion-induced apoptosis. *Am J Physiol* 1998; 274: H242–8.
41. Blankenberg FG *et al.* *In vivo* detection and imaging of phosphatidylserine expression during programmed cell death. *Proc Natl Acad Sci USA* 1998; 95: 6349–54.
42. Sadoshima J-I, Xu Y, Slayter HS, Izumo S. Autocrine release of angiotensin II mediates stretch-induced hypertrophy of cardiac myocytes *in vitro*. *Cell* 1993; 75: 977–84.
43. Pimental DR, Amin JK, Baliga RR *et al.* Reactive oxygen species mediate hypertrophy and apoptosis in cyclically-stretched cardiac myocytes. *Circulation* 1998; Suppl 1: I-743.
44. Leri A, Claudio PP, Li Q *et al.* Stretch-mediated release of angiotensin II induced myocyte apoptosis by activating p53 that enhances the local renin-angiotensin system and decreases the Bcl-2 to bax protein ratio in the cell. *J Clin Invest* 1998; 101: 1326–42.
45. Yamazaki T, Komouro I, Kudoh S *et al.* Endothelin is involved in mechanical stress-induced cardiomyocyte hypertrophy. *J Biol Chem* 1996; 271: 3221–7.
46. Chidsey CA, Braunwald E. Sympathetic activity and neurotransmitter depletion in congestive heart failure. *Pharmacol Rev* 1966; 18: 685–700.
47. Thomas JA, Marks BH. Plasma norepinephrine in congestive heart failure. *Am J Cardiol* 1978; 41: 233–43.
48. Levine TB, Francis GS, Goldsmith SR *et al.* Activity of the sympathetic nervous system and renin angiotension system assessed by plasma hormone levels and their relation to hemodynamic abnormalities in congestive heart failure. *Am J Cardiol* 1982; 49: 1659–66.
49. Swedberg K, Viquerat C, Rouleau JL *et al.* Comparison of myocardial catecholamine balance in congestive heart failure and angina pectoris without heart failure. *J Clin Pharmacol* 1984; 54: 783–6.
50. Hasking GJ, Esier MD, Jennings GL *et al.* Norepinephrine spillover to plasma in patients with congestive heart failure. Evidence of increased overall and cardiorenal sympathetic nervous activity. *Circulation* 1986; 73: 615–21.
51. Leimbach JR, Wallin BG, Victor RG *et al.* Direct evidence from intraneural recordings for increased central sympathetic outflow in patients with heart failure. *Circulation* 1986; 73: 913–19.
52. Mann DL, Kent RL, Parsons B, Cooper G IV. Adrenergic effects on the biology of the adult mammalian cardiocyte. *Circulation* 1992; 85: 790–804.
53. Matsui T, Hajjar R, Kang JX *et al.* Norepinephrine directly induces apoptosis in neonatal rat myocytes. *J Am Coll Cardiol* 1997; 29: 230A.
54. Communal C, Singh K, Pimentel DR, Colucci WS. Norepinephrine stimulates apoptosis in adult rat ventricular myocytes by activation of the β-adrenergic pathway. *Circulation* 1998; 98: 1329–34.
55. Shizukuda Y, Buttrick PM, Geenen DL *et al.* Beta-adrenergic stimulation causes cardiocyte apoptosis: influence of tachycardia and hypertrophy. *Am J Physiol* 1998; 275: H961–8.
56. Sigel AV, Romanic AM, Hart TK *et al.* Hypoxia and reoxygenation related injuries in cardiac myocytes are enhanced by programmed cell death. Differential protective effects of beta-adrenergic receptor blockers. *Circulation* 1998; Suppl 1: I-742.
57. Yue TL, Ma XL, Wang X *et al.* Possible involvement of stress-activated protein kinase signaling pathway and Fas receptor expression in prevention of ischemia/reperfusion-induced cardiomyocyte apoptosis by carvedilol. *Circ Res* 1998; 82: 166–74.
58. Communal C, Singh K, Colucci WS. Gi protein protects adult rat ventricular myocytes from β-adrenergic receptor-stimulated apoptosis *in vitro*. *Circulation* 1998; Suppl 1: I-742.
59. Iwase M, Uechi M, Vatner DE *et al.* Cardiomyopathy induced by cardiac Gsα overexpression. *Am J Physiol* 1997; 41: H585–9.

60. Geng YJ, Ishikawa Y, Vatner DE *et al.* Over-expression of Gs-$\alpha$ accelerates programmed cell death (apoptosis) of cardiomyocytes in transgenic mice. *Circulation* 1996; 94 (Suppl 1): 1640.
61. Geng Y-J, Ishikawa Y, Vatner DE *et al.* Apoptosis of cardiac myocytes in Gs$\alpha$ transgenic mice. *Circ Res* 1999; 84: 34–42.
62. Geng YJ, Homcy CJ, Kim SJ *et al.* Persistent stimulation of $\beta$-adrenergic signaling triggers degeneration and apoptosis of cardiac myocytes. *Circulation* 1997; 96 (Suppl I): I-116.
63. Remmers U, Fink C *et al.* Intrinsic receptor activity of $\beta$1-adrenoceptors overexpressed in rat ventricular cardiac myocytes. *Circulation* 1998; Suppl 1: I-123.
64. Milano CA, Allen LF, Rockman HA *et al.* Enhanced myocardial function in transgenic mice overexpressing the $\beta$2-adrenergic receptor. *Science* 1994; 264: 582–6.
65. Gu J, Polak JM, Adrian TE *et al.* Neuropeptide tyrosine (NPY) — a major cardiac neuropeptide. *Lancet* 1983; i: 1008–10.
66. Gu J, Polak JM, Allen JM *et al.* High concentrations of a novel peptide, neuropeptide Y, in the innervation of mouse and rat heart. *J Histochem Cytochem* 1984; 32: 467–72.
67. Gulbenkian S, Costa Andrade N, Wharton J *et al.* Immunocytochemical localization of neuropeptide Y and its C-terminal flanking peptide in the human heart. *Ann NY Acac Sci* 1990; 611: 429–31.
68. Millar BC, Schluter KD, Zhou XJ *et al.* Neuropeptide Y stimulates hypertrophy of adult ventricular cardiomyocytes. *Am J Physiol* 1994; 266: C1271–7.
69. Selbie LA, Darby K, Schmitz PC *et al.* Synergistic interaction of Y1-neuropeptide Y and $\alpha_{1b}$-adrenergic receptors in the regulation of phospholipase C, protein kinase C, and arachidonic acid production. *J Biol Chem* 1995; 270: 11 789–96.
70. Baliga RR, Simmons WW, Kelly RA. Neuropeptide Y stimulates p42/p44 mitogen-activated protein kinases and p70 S6 kinase in neonatal and adult rat ventricular myocytes and cardiac microvascular endothelial cell. *Circulation* 1996; 94: I-552.
71. Baliga RR, Simmons WW, Kelly RA. Phosphatidyl-3-kinase and p70S$^6$K put not MEK-ERK-RSK pathway affect actin reorganization and protein synthesis in neuropeptide-Y induced cardiac myocyte hypertrophy. *Circulation* 1997; 96: I-445.
72. Maisel AS, Scott NA, Motulsky HJ *et al.* Elevation of plasma neuropeptide Y levels in congestive heart failure. *Am J Med* 1989; 86: 43–8.
73. Hulting J, Sollevi A, Ullman B *et al.* Plasma neuropeptide Y on admission to a coronary care unit: raised levels in patients with left heart failure. *Cardiovasc Res* 1990; 24: 102–8.
74. Edvinsson L, Ekman R, Hedner P, Valdemarsson S. Congestive heart failure: involvement of perivascular peptides reflecting activity in sympathetic, parasympathetic and afferent fibres. *Eur J Clin. Invest* 1990; 20: 85–9.
75. Ullman B, Jensen UM, Hulting J, Lundberg JM. Neuropeptide Y, noradrenaline and invasive haemodynamic data in mild to moderate chronic congestive heart failure. *Clin Physiol* 1993; 13: 409–18.
76. Ullman B, Londvall K, Lundberg JM *et al.* Response of plasma neuropeptide Y and noradrenaline to dynamic exercise and rampipril treatment in patients with congestive heart failure. *Clin Physiol* 1994; 14: 123–34.
77. Kaye DM, Lambert GW, Lefkovits J *et al.* Neurochemical evidence of cardiac sympathetic activation and increased central nervous system norepinephrine turnover in severe congestive heart failure. *J Am Coll Cardiol* 1994; 23: 570–8.
78. Anderson FL, Port J, Reid BB *et al.* Myocardial catecholamine and neuropeptide Y depletion in failing ventricles of patients with idiopathic dilated cardiomyopathy. Correlation with $\beta$-adrenergic receptor down-regulation. *Circulation* 1992; 85: 46–53.
79. Schunkert H, Dzau VJ, Tang SS *et al.* Increased rat cardiac angiotensin converting enzyme activity and mRNA expression in pressure overload left ventricle hypertrophy. Effects on coronary resistance, contractility and relaxation. *J Clin Invest* 1990; 86: 1913.
80. CONSENSUS Trial Study Group. Effects of enalapril on mortality in severe congestive heart failure: results of the Cooperative North Scandinavian Enalpril Study Group. *N Engl J Med* 1987; 316: 1429–35.
81. SOLVD Investigators. Effects of enalapril on mortality and development of heart failure in asymptomatic patients with reduced left ventricular ejection fraction. *N Engl J Med* 1992: 327: 685–91.
82. Dzau VJ. Tissue renin–angiotensin system in myocardial hypertrophy and failure. *Arch Intern Med* 1993; 89: 493.
83. Dazu VJ, Re R. Tissue angiotensin system in cardiovascular medicine. A paradigm shift? *Circulation* 1994; 89: 493.
84. Huang H, Arnal J-F, Llorens-Cortes C *et al.* Discrepancy between plasma and lung angiotensin-converting enzyme activity in experimental congestive heart failure. A novel aspect of endothelium dysfunction. *Circ Res* 1994; 75: 454.
85. Urata H, Healy B, Stewart RW *et al.* Angiotensin-II forming pathways in normal and failing human hearts. *Circ Res* 1990; 66: 683.
86. Lindpaintner K, Lu W, Niedermajer N *et al.* Selective activation of cardiac angiotensinogen gene expression in post-infarction ventricular remodeling in the rat. *J Mol Cell Cardiol* 1993; 25: 133.
87. Hirsch AT, Talsness CE, Schunkert H *et al.* Tissue-specific activation of cardiac angiotensin converting enzyme in experimental heart failure. *Circ Res* 1991; 69: 475.
88. Anversa P, Hillier B, Ricci *et al.* Myocyte cell loss and myocyte hypertrophy in the aging rat heart. *J Am Coll Cardiol* 1986; 8: 1441–8.
89. Pierzchalski P, Reiss K, Cheng W *et al.* p53 induces myocyte apoptosis via the activation of the renin–angiotensin system. *Expl Cell Res* 1997; 234: 57–65.
90. Kajstura J, Cigola E, Malhotra A *et al.* Angiotensin II induces apoptosis of adult ventricular myocytes *in vitro*. *J Mol Cell Cardiol* 1997; 29: 859–70.
91. Yamada T, Horiuchi M, Dzau VJ. Angiotensin II type 2 receptor mediates programmed cell death. *Proc Natl Acad Scri USA* 1996; 93: 156–60.
92. Horiuchi M, Yamada T, Hayashida W, Dzau VJ. Interferon regulatory factor-1 upregulates angiotensin II type 2 receptor and induces apoptosis. *J Biol Chem* 1997; 272: 11 952–8.
93. Horiuchi M, Hayashida W, Kambe T *et al.* Angiotensin type 2 receptor dephosphorylates Bcl-2 by activating mitogen-activated protein kinase phosphatase-1 and inducess apoptosis. *J Biol Chem* 1997; 272: 19 022–6.
94. Goussev A, Sharov VG, Shimoyama H *et al.* Effects of ACE inhibition on cardiomyocyte apoptosis in dogs with heart failure. *Am J Physiol* 1998; 275: H626–31.
95. Cody RJ, Haas GJ, Binkley PF *et al.* Plasma endothelin correlates with the extent of pulmonary hypertension in patients with chronic congestive heart failure. *Circulation* 1992; 85: 504–9.

96. Lerman A, Kubo SH, Tschumperlin LK, Burnett JC Jr. Plasma endothelin concentrations in humans with end-stage heart failure and after heart transplantation. *J Am Coll Cardiol* 1992; 20: 849–53.
97. McMurray JJ, Ray SG, Abdullah I *et al*. Plasma endothelin in chronic heart failure. *Circulation* 1992; 85: 1374–9.
98. Stewart DJ, Cernacek P, Costello KB, Rouleau JL. Elevated endothelin-1 in heart failure and loss of normal response to postural change. *Circulation* 1992; 85: 510–17.
99. Wei CM, Lerman A, Rodeffer RJ *et al*. Endothelin in human congestive heart failure. *Circulation* 1994; 89: 1580–6.
100. Cavero PG, Miller WL, Heublein DM *et al*. Endothelin in experimental congestive heart failure in the anesthetized dog. *Am J Physiol* 1990; 259(2 Pt 2): F312–7.
101. Margulies KB, Hildebrand FL Jr., Lerman A *et al*. Increased endothelin in experimental heart failure. *Circulation* 1990; 82(6): 2226–30.
102. Underwood RD, Aarhus LL, Heublein DM *et al*. Endothelin in thoracic inferior vena caval constriction model of heart failure. *Am J Physiol* 1992; 263(3 Pt 2): H951–5.
103. Loffler BM, Roux S, Kalina B *et al*. Influence of congestive heart failure in endothelin levels and receptors in rabbits. *J Mol Cell Cardiol* 1993; 25: 407–16.
104. Teerlink JR, Loffler BM, Hess P *et al*. Role of endothelin in the maintenance of blood pressure in conscious rat with chronic heart failure: acute effects of endothelin receptor antagonist Ro 47-0203 (bosentan). *Circulation* 1994; 90: 2510–18.
105. Sakai S, Miyauchi T, Kobayashi M *et al*. Inhibition of myocardial endothelin pathway improves long term survival in heart failure. *Nature* 1996; 384: 353–5.
106. Shimoyama H, Sabbah HN, Borzak S *et al*. Short-term hemodynamic effects of endothelin receptor blockade in dogs with chronic heart failure. *Circulation* 1996; 94: 779–85.
107. Sakai S, Miyauchi T, Sakurai T *et al*. Endogenous endothelin-1 participates in the maintenance of cardiac function in rats with congestive heart failure: marked increase in endothelin-1 production in the failing heart. *Circulation* 1996; 93: 1214–22.
108. Mulder P, Richard V, Derumeaux G *et al*. Role of endogenous endothelin in chronic heart failure. *Circulation* 1997; 96: 1976–82.
109. Arai M, Yoguchi A, Iso T *et al*. Endothelin-1 and its binding sites are upregulated in pressure overload cardiac hypertrophy. *Am J Physiol* 1995; 268: H2084–91.
110. Brown LA, Nunez DJ, Brookes CJ, Wilkins MR. Selective increase in endothelin-1 and endothelin A receptor subtype in the hypertrophied myocardium of the aorto-venocaval fistula rat. *Cardiovasc Res* 1995; 29: 768–74.
111. Schomisch-Moravec C, Reynolds EE, Stewart RW, Bond M. Endothelin is a positive inotropic agent in humans and rat heart *in vitro*. *Biochem Biophys Res Commun* 1989; 159: 14–18.
112. Kramer BK, Smith TW, Kelly RA. Endothelin and increased contractility in adult rat ventricular myocytes. *Circ Res* 1991; 68: 269–79.
113. Shubeita HE, McDonough PM, Harris AN *et al*. Endothelin induction of inositol phospholipid hydrolysis, sarcomere assembly, and cardiac gene expression in ventricular myocytes: a paracrine mechanism for myocardial cell hypertrophy. *J Biol Chem* 1990; 265: 20 555–62.
114. Okazawa M, Shiraki T, Ninomiya H *et al*. Endothelin-induced apoptosis of A375 human melanoma cells. *J Biol Chem* 1998; 273: 12 584–92.
115. Thomas T, Kurihara H, Yamagishi H *et al*. A signaling cascade involving endothelin-1, dHAND and msxl regulates development of neural-crest-derived branchial arch mesenchyme. *Development* 1998; 125: 3005–14.
116. Nakahashi T, Fukuo K, Nishimaki H *et al*. Endothelin-1 enhances nitric oxide-induced cell death in cultured vascular smooth-muscle cells. *J Cardiovasc Pharmacol* 1998; 31 Suppl 1: S351–3.
117. Yoshimura M, Yasue H, Okumura K *et al*. Different secretion patterns of atrial natriuretic peptide and brain natriuretic peptide in patients with congestive heart failure. *Circulation* 1993; 87(2): 464–9.
118. Wei CM, Heublein DM, Perrella MA *et al*. Natriuretic peptide system in human heart failure. *Circulation* 1993; 88(3): 1004–9.
119. Wu CF, Bishopric NH, Pratt RE. Atrial natriuretic peptide induces apoptosis in neonatal rat cardiac myocytes. *J Biol Chem* 1997; 272: 14 860–6.
120. Kapadia S, Lee JR, Torre-Amione G *et al*. Tumor necrosis factor gene and protein expression in adult feline myocardium after endotoxin administration. *J Clin Invest* 1995; 96: 1042–52.
121. Kapadia S, Torre-Amione G, Yokoyama T, Mann DL. Soluble tumor necrosis factor binding proteins modulate the negative inotropic effects of TNF-α *in vitto*. AM *J Physiol* 1995; 37: H517–25.
122. Torre-Amione G, Kapadia S, Lee J *et al*. Tumour necrosis factor-α and tumour necrosis factor receptors in the failing heart. *Circulation* 1996; 93: 704–11.
123. Habib FM, Springall DR, Davies GJ *et al*. Tumor necrosis factor and inducible nitric oxide synthase in dilated cardiomyopathy. *Lancet* 1996; 347: 1151–5.
124. Torre-Amione G, Kapadia S, Lee J *et al*. Expression and functional significance of tumour necrosis factor receptors in human myocardium. *Circulation* 1995; 92: 1487–93.
125. Krown KA, Page MT, Nguyen C *et al*. Tumour necrosis factor-α induced apoptosis in cardiac myocytes: involvement of the sphingolipid signaling cascade in cardiac cell death. *J Clin Invest* 1996; 98: 2854–65.
126. Levine B, Kalman J, Mayer L *et al*. Elevated circulating levels of tumour necrosis factor in severe chronic heart failure. *N Engl J Med* 1990; 223: 236–41.
127. Munger MA, Johnson B, Amber IJ *et al*. Circulating concentrations of proinflammatory cytokines in mild or moderate heart failure secondary to ischemic or idiopathic dilated cardiomyopathy. *Am J Cardiol* 1996; 723–7.
128. Testa M, Yeh M, Lee P *et al*. Circulating levels of cytokines and their endogenous modulators in patients with mild to severe congestive heart failure due to coronary heart disease or hypertension. *J Am Coll Cardiol* 1996; 28: 964–71.
129. Milani RV, Mehra MR, Endres S *et al*. The clinical relevance of circulating tumour necrosis factor-α in acute decompensated chronic heart failure without cachexia. *Chest* 1996; 110: 992–7.
130. McMurray J, Abdullah I, Dargie HJ, Shapiro D. Increased concentrations of tumour necrosis factor in cachectic patients with severe chronic heart failure. *Br Heart J* 1991; 66: 356–8.
131. Wiedermann CJ, Beimpoid H, Herold M *et al*. Increased levels of serum neopterin and decreased production of neutrophil superoxide anions in chronic heart failure with elevated levels of tumor necrosis factor-α. *J Am Coll Cardiol* 1993; 22: 1897–901.
132. Dutka DP, Elborn JS, Delamere F *et al*. Tumour necrosis factor-α in severe congestive cardiac failure. *Br Heart* 1993; 70: 141–3.

133. Katz SD, Rao R, Berman JW *et al.* Pathophysiological correlates of increased serum tumour necrosis factor in patients with congestive heart failure: relation to nitric oxide dependent vasodilation in the forearm circulation. *Circulation* 1994; 90: 12–16.
134. Matsumori A, Yamada T, Suzuki H *et al.* Increased circulating cytokines in patients with myocarditis and cardiomyopathy. *Br Heart J* 1994; 72(6): 561–6.
135. Ferrari R, Bachetti T, Confortini R *et al.* Tumor necrosis factor soluble receptors in patients with various degrees of congestive heart failure. *Circulation* 1995; 15: 92(6): 1479–86.
136. Torre-Amione G, Kapadia S, Benedict C *et al.* Proinflammatory cytokine levels in patients with depressed left ventricular ejection fraction: a report from the studies of left ventricular dysfunction (SOLVD). *J Am Coll Cardiol* 1996; 27: 1201–6.
137. Suffredini AF, Fromm RE, Parker MM *et al.* The cardiovascular response of normal humans to the administration of endotoxin. *N Engl J Med* 1989; 321: 280–7.
138. Hegewisch S, Weh HJ, Hossfeld DK. TNF-α induced cardiomyopathy. *Lancet* 1990; ii: 294–5.
139. Millar AB, Singer M, Meager A *et al.* Tumour necrosis factor in bronchopulmonary secretions of patients with adult respiratory distress syndrome. *Lancet* 1989; ii: 712–13.
140. Bozkurt B, Kribbs SB, Clubb FJ Jr *et al.* Pathophysiologically relevant concentration of tumor necrosis factor-α promote progressive left ventricular dysfunction and remodeling in rats. *Circulation* 1998; 97: 1382–91.
141. Kubota T, Miyagishima M, Bounoutas GS *et al.* Overexpression of tumor necrosis factor-α activates the expression of multiple members of apoptosis pathway in transgenic mice. *Circulation* 1998; Suppl 1: I-462.
142. De Moissac D, Mustapha S, Greenberg AH, Kirshenbaum LA. Bcl-2 activates the transcription factor NFκB through the degradation of the cytoplasmic inhibitor IκBα. *J Biol Chem* 1998; 273: 23 946–51.
143. Ing DJ, Dzau VJ, Webster KA, Bishoporic NH. Modulation of cytokine-induced cardiac myocyte apoptosis by nitric oxide, Bak, and Bcl-x. *Circ Res* 1999; 84: 21–33.
144. McMurray J, McLay J, Chpra M *et al.* Evidence for enhanced free-radical activity in chronic congestive heart failure secondary to coronay artery disease. *Am J Cardiol* 1990; 65: 1261–2.
145. McMurray J, Chopra M, Abdullah I *et al.* Evidence for oxidative stress in chronic heart failure in humans. *Eur Heart J* 1993; 14: 1493–8.
146. Diaz-Velez CR, Garcia-Castineiras S, Mendoza-Ramos E, Hernandez-Lopez E. Increased malondialdehyde in peripheral blood of patients with congestive heart failure. *Am Heart J* 1996; 131: 146–52.
147. Keith M, Geranmayegan A, Sole MJ *et al.* Increased oxidative stress in patients with congestive heart failure. *J Am Coll Cardiol* 1998; 31(6): 1352–6.
148. Mallat Z, Phillip I, Lebret M *et al.* Elevated levels of 8-isoprostaglandin F2α in pericardial fluid of patients with heart failure: a potential role for *in vivo* oxidant stress in ventricular dilatation and progression to heart failure. *Circulation* 1998; 97: 1536–9.
149. Dhalla AK, Singal PK. Antioxidant changes in hypertrophied and failed guinea pig hearts. *Am J Physiol* 1994; 266: H1280–5.
150. Hill MF, Singal PK. Antioxidant and oxidative stress changes during heart failure subsequent to myocardial infarction in rats. *Am J Pathol* 1996; 148: 291–300.
151. Tzortis JD, Siwik DA, Chang DL *et al.* Chronic oxidative stress induces a hypertrophic phenotype and apoptosis in neonatal rat cardiac myocytes *in vitro*. *Circulation* 1997; 961: I-60.
152. Ide T, Tsutsui, Kinugawa S *et al.* Enhanced myocardial generation of oxygen radicals in heart failure. *Circulation* 1990; Suppl 1: I-419.
153. Roberg K, Ollinger K. Oxidative stress causes relocation of the lysosomal enzyme cathepsin D with ensuing apoptosis in neonatal cardiomyocytes. *Am J Pathol* 1998; 152: 1151–6.
154. DeBelder AJ, Radomski MW, Why HJF *et al.* Nitric oxide activities in human myocardium. *Lancet* 1993; 341: 84–5.
155. Hare JM, Loh E, Creager MA, Colucci WS. Nitric oxide inhibits the positive inotropic response to β-adrenergic stimulation in humans with left ventricular dysfunction. *Circulation* 1995; 92: 2198–203.
156. Haywood GA, Tsao PS, von der Leyen HE *et al.* Expression of inducible nitric oxide synthase in heart failure. *Circulation* 1996; 93: 1087–94.
157. Brady AJ, Warren CB, Poole-Wilson PA *et al.* Nitric oxide attenuates cardiac myocyte contraction. *Am J Physiol* 1993; 265: H176–82.
158. Balligand JL, Kelly RA, Marsden PA *et al.* Control of cardiac muscle cell function by an endogenous nitric oxide signaling system. *Proc Natl Acad Sci USA* 1993; 90: 347–51.
159. Kawaguchi H, Shim WS, Wang Y *et al.* *In vivo* gene transfection of human endothelial cell nitric oxide synthase in cardiomyocytes causes apoptosis-like cell death. *Circulation* 1997; 95: 2441–7.
160. Stein B, Eschenhagen T, Rudiger J *et al.* Increased expression of contitutive nitric oxide synthase III, but not inducible nitric oxide synthase II, in human heart failure. *J Am Coll Cardiol* 1998; 32: 1179–86.
161. Zang J, Ing D, Dzau VJ *et al.* Nitric oxide activation of cardiomyocyte apoptosis, MAPK/ERK and Jun kinases exhibit differential dose-dependence and cGMP sensitivity. *Circulation* 1998; Suppl 1: I-742.
162. Mannick JB, Asano K, Izumi K *et al.* Nitric oxide produced by human B lymphocytes inhibits apoptosis and Epstein–Barr virus reactivation. *Cell* 1994; 79: 1137–46.
163. Kim Y-M, Bombeck CA, Billiar TR. Nitric oxide as a bifunctional regulator of apoptosis. *Circ Res* 1990; 84: 253–6.
164. Lembo G, Hunter JJ, Chien KR. Recent advances and prospects for growth factor therapy. *Ann NY Acad Sci* 1995; 752: 115.
165. Kelly RA, Smith TW. de Modulatione Cordis. *Circulation* 1996; 94: 2361–3.
166. Lee W-L, Chen J-W, Ting C-T *et al.* Mechanisms of the therapeutic effects of IGF-1 on dilated cardiomyopathy. *Circulation* 1998; Suppl 1: I-696.
167. Sheng Z, Knowlton K, Chen J *et al.* Cardiotrophin 1 (CT-1) inhibition of cardiac myocyte apoptosis via a mitogen-activated protein kinase-dependent pathway. Divergence from downstream CT-1 signals for myocardial cell hypertrophy. *J Biol Chem* 1997; 28: 272(9): 5783–91.
168. Zhu H, Qi M, McElwee-Witmer S *et al.* The relationship between hypertrophy and apoptosis in cultured neonatal ventricular myocytes. *Circulation* 1998; Suppl 1: I-344.
169. Zhao YY, Sawyer DR, Baliga RR *et al.* Neuregulins promote survival and growth of cardiac myocytes. Persistence of ErbB2 and ErbB4 expression in neonatal and adult ventricular myocytes. *J Biol Chem* 1998; 273: 10 261–9.
170. Guerra S, Kajstura J, Wang X *et al.* Myocyte apoptosis affects differently the male and female human heart in end-stage cardiac failure. *Circulation* 1998; Suppl 1: I-118.

171. Stephanou A, Brar B, Heads R *et al.* Cardiotrophin-1 induces heat shock protein accumulation in cultured cardiac cells and protects them from stressful stimuli. *J Mol Cell Cardiol* 1998; 30(4): 849–55.
172. Sawyer DB, Baliga RR, Schneider J *et al.* Neuregulin stimulates ErB4 receptor phosphorylation in neonatal rat ventricular myocytes. *Circulation* 1996; 94: I-644.
173. Baliga RR, Simmons WW, Sawyer DB *et al.* The role of MEK-MAPK-RSK pathway, PI3 kinase pathway and p70S$^6$K in neuregulin induced growth of cardiac myocytes. *Circulation* 1997; 96: I-362.
174. Baliga RR, Pimental DR, Simmons WW *et al.* Neuregulin-1 induced hypertrophy of cardiac myocytes: roles of MEK-ERK-MAPK, p70$^{S6}$ kinase and PI-3 kinase. *Am J Physiol* 1999; in press.
175. Sadoshima J, Izumo S. Rapamycin selectively inhibits angiotensin-II induced increase in protein synthesis in cardiac myocytes. *Circ Res* 1995; 77: 1040.
176. Cuevas P, Reimers D, Carcellar F *et al.* Fibroblast growth factor-1 prevents myocardial apoptosis triggered by ischemia–reperfusion injury. *Eur J Med Res* 1997; 28: 465–8.
177. Anand V, Chen W, Miyamoto T *et al.* Dominant negative receptor inhibition of FGF signaling provokes cardiomyocyte apoptosis *in vivo*. *Circulation* 1998; Suppl 1: I-345.
178. Schieffer B, Schieffer E, Fehse F *et al.* Protection from oxidative stress by leukemia inhibitory factor in adult ventricular myocytes. *Circulation* 1998; Suppl 1: I-247.
179. Williams RS. Cell cycle control in the terminally differentiated myocyte: a platform for myocardial repair? *Cardiol Clin* 1998; 16: 739–54.
180. Bunz F, Dutriaux A, Lengauer C *et al.* Requirement for p53 andp21 to sustain G2 arrest after DNA damage. *Science* 1998; 282: 1497–501.
181. Ambrosini G, Adida C, Altieri DC. A novel anti-apoptosis gene, *survivin*, expressed in cancer and lymphoma. *Nature Med* 1997; 3: 917–21.
182. Li F, Ambrosini G, Chu EY *et al.* Control of apoptosis and mitotic spindle checkpoint by survivin. *Nature* 1998; 396: 580–4.
183. Setoguchi M, Wang S, Leri A *et al.* Pacing-induced heart failure in dog: cyclins, cyclin-dependent kinases (cdks), DNA replication and myocyte proliferation. *Circulation* 1998; Suppl 1: I-608.
184. Burton PB, Barton PJ. Reversion to the fetal pattern of cyclin dependent kinase inhibitor expression is seen in acute and end-stage heart failure. *Circulation* 1998; Suppl 1: I-360.
185. DeRosa C, Skopicki HA. *In vivo* appearance of a cyclin-dependent kinase inhibitor in myocyte precursor cells is not sufficient to render the anti-apoptotic phenotype. *Circulation* 1998; Suppl 1: I-743.
186. Kiyokawa H, Kineman RD, Manova-Todorova KO *et al.* Enhanced growth of mice lacking cyclin-dependent kinase inhibitor function of p27$^{Kip1}$. *Cell* 1996; 85: 721–32.
187. Agah R, Kirshenbaum LA, Abdellatif M *et al.* Adenoviral delivery of E2F-1 directs cell cycle entry and p53-independent apoptosis in postmitotic adult myocardium *in vivo*. *J Clin Invest* 1997; 100: 2722–8.
188. Liu Y, Kistsis RN. Induction and DNA synthesis and apoptosis in cardiac myocytes by E1A oncoprotein. *J Cell Biol* 1996; 133: 325–34.
189. Jan YN, Jan LY. Asymmetric cell division. *Nature* 1998; 392: 775–8.
190. Fleckenstein A. Calcium antagonism: history and prospects for a multifaceted pharmacodynamic principle. In LH Opie (ed). *Calcium antagonists and cardiovascular diseases*. New York: Raven, 1984; 9–28.
191. Chen SJ, Bradley ME, Lee TC. Chemical hypoxia triggers apoptosis of cultured neonatal rat cardiac myocytes: modulation by calcium-regulated proteases and protein kinases. *Mol Cell Biochem* 1998; 178: 141–9.
192. Yano S, Tokumitsu H, Soderling TR. Calcium promotes cell survival through CaM-K kinase activation of the protein-kinase-B pathway. *Nature* 1998; 396: 584–7.
193. Makrigiannis AP, Blay J, Hoskin DW. Cyclosporin A inhibits 2-chloroadenosine-induced DNA cleavage in mouse thymocytes. *Int J Immunopharmacol* 1994; 16: 995–1001.
194. Bonnefoy-Berard N, Genestier L, Flacher M, Revillard JP. The phosphoprotein phosphatase calcineurin controls calcium-dependent apoptosis in B cell lines. *Eur J Immunol* 1994; 24: 325–9.
195. Yazdanbakhsh K, Choi JW, Li Y *et al.* Cyclosporin A blocks apoptosis by inhibiting the DNA binding activity of the transcription factor Nur77. *Proc Natl Acad Sci USA* 1995; 92: 437–41.
196. Molkentin JD, Lu JR, Antos CL *et al.* A calcineurin-dependent transcritptional pathway for cardiac hypertrophy. *Cell* 1998; 93: 215–28.
197. Mende U, Kagen A, Cohen A *et al.* Transient cardiac expression of contitutively active G$\alpha$q leads to hypertrophy and dilated cardiomyopathy by calcineurin-dependent and independent pathways. *Proc Natl Acad Sci* 1998; 95: 13 893–8.
198. Donehower LA, Harvey M, Slagle BL *et al.* Mice deficient for p53 are developmentally normal but susceptible to spontaneous tumors. *Nature* 1992; 356: 215–21.
199. Leri A, Liu Y, Malhotra A *et al.* Pacing induced heart failure in dogs enhances the expression of p53 and p53-dependent genes in ventricular myocytes. *Circulation* 1998; 97: 194–203.
200. Bialik S *et al.* Myocyte apoptosis during acute myocardial infarction in the mouse localizes to hypoxic regions but occurs independently of p53. *J Clin Invest* 1997; 100: 1363–72.
201. Bishopric NH, Kaiser S, Discher *et al.* p53-independent induction of apoptosis by hypoxia-reoxygenation of isolated cardiac myocytes. *Circulation* 1998; Suppl 1: I-743.
202. El-Diery WS *et al.* Killer/DR5 is a DNA damage inducible p53-regulated death receptor gene. *Nature Genet* 1997; 17: 141–3.
203. Schumann H, Bartling B, Rueckschloss *et al.* Expression of the apoptosis-mediating ligand TRAIL and its death domain receptors DR4, DR5 and decoy receptor DcR1 in normal and failing human myocardium. *Circulation* 1998; Suppl 1: I-361.
204. Jost CA, Marin MC, Kaelin WG. p73 is a human p53-related protein that can induce apoptosis. *Nature* 1997; 389: 191–4.
205. Osada M, Ohba M, Kawahara C *et al.* Cloning and functional analysis of human p51, which structurally and functionally resembles p53. *Nature Med* 1998; 4: 839–43.
206. Trink B, Okami K, Wu L *et al.* A new human p53 homologue. *Nat Med* 1998; 4(7): 747–8.
207. Yang A, Kaghad M, Wang Y *et al.* p63, a p53 homolog at 3q27-29, encodes multiple products with transactivating, death-inducing, and dominant negative activites. *Mol Cell* 1998; 2: 305–16.
208. Dell'Acqua G, Mann MJ, Dzau VJ. p53 alternative splicing in rat cardiomyocytes. *Circulation* 1998; Suppl 1: I-743.
209. Williams RS. Heat shock proteins and ischemic injury to the myocardium. *Circulation* 1997; 96: 4138–40.
210. Benjamin IJ, McMillan DR. Stress (heart shock) proteins: molecular chaperones in cardiovascular biology and disease. *Circ Res* 1998; 83: 117–32.
211. Hartl F. Molecular chaperones in cellular protein folding. *Nature* 1996; 381: 571–9.

212. Lindquist S, Craig EA. The heat-shock proteins. *Annu Rev Genet* 1988; 22: 631–77.
213. McMillian DR, Xiao X, Shao L *et al.* Targeted disruption of heat shock transcrition factor 1 abolishes thermotolerance and protection against heat-induced apoptosis. *J Biol Chem* 1998; 273: 7523–8.
214. Sharma HS, Stahl J, Weisensee D, Low-Friedrich I. Cytoprotective mechanisms in cultured cardiomyocytes. *Mol Cell Biochem* 1996; 160–1: 217–24.
215. Gabai V, Meriin A, Mosser D *et al.* Hsp70 prevents activation of stress kinases. *J Biol Chem* 1997; 272: 18 033–7.
216. Mehlen P, Schultze-Osthoff K, Arrigo AP. Small stress proteins as novel regulators of apoptosis: heat shock protein27 blocks Fas/APO-1 and staurosporine-induced cell death. *J Biol Chem* 1996; 271: 16 510–14.
217. Locke M, Tanguay RM. Diminished heat shock response in the aged myocardium. *Cell Stress Chaperones* 1996; 1: 251–60.
218. Knowlton AA, Kapadia S, Torre-Amione G *et al.* Differential expression of heat shock proteins in normal and failing human hearts. *J Mol Cell Cardiol* 1998; 30: 811–18.
219. Hockenberg D, Nunez G, Milliman C *et al.* Bcl-2 is an inner mitochondrial membrane protein that blocks programmed cell death. *Nature* 1990; 348: 334–6.
220. Allsopp T, Wyatt S, Paterson HF *et al.* The proto-oncogene Bcl-2 can selectively rescue neutrotrophic factor-dependent neurons from apoptosis. *Cell* 1993; 73: 295–307.
221. Cheng W, Kajstura J, Nitahara JA *et al.* Programmed myocyte cell death affects the viable myocardium after infarction in rats. *Expl Cell Res* 1996; 226: 316–27.
222. Kirshenbaum LA, de Moissac D. The Bcl-2 gene product prevents programmed cell death of ventricular myocytes. *Circulation* 1997; 96: 1580–5.
223. Misao J, Hayakawa Y, Ohno M *et al.* Expression of Bcl-2 protein, an inhibitor of apoptosis, and Bax, an accelerator of apoptosis, in ventricular myocytes of human hearts with myocardial infarction. *Circulation* 1996; 94: 1506–12.
224. Kirshenbaum LA, Greenberg AH, de Moissac D. Bel-2 activates the transcription factor NEκβ through the degradation of the cytoplasmic inhibitor Iκβ-α in ventricular myocytes. *Circulation* 1998; Suppl 1: I-743.
225. Green DR, Reed JC. Mitochondria and apoptosis. *Science* 1998; 281: 1309–12.
226. Wang Y, Huang S, Sah VP *et al.* Cardiac muscle cell hypertrophy and apoptosis induced by distinct members of the p38 mitogen-activated protein kinase family. *J Biol Chem* 1998; 273: 2161–8.
227. Zechner D, Craig R, Hanford DS *et al.* MKK6 activates myocardial cell NF-kB and inhibits apoptosis in a p38 mitogen-activated protein kinase-dependent manner. *J Biol Chem* 1998; 273: 8232–9.
228. Kharbanda S, Arbustini E, Kologie FD *et al.* Release of cytochrome c form mitochondria, activation of caspases and apoptosis in explanted cardiomyopathic hearts from cardiac allograft recipients. *Circulation* 1997; 96: I-115.
229. Yonehara S, Ishii A, Yonehara M. A cell-killing monoclonal antibody (anti-Fas) to a cell surface antigen co-downregulated with the receptor of tumor necrosis factor. *J Exp Med* 1989; 169: 1747–56.
230. Itoh N, Yonehara S, Ishii A *et al.* The polypeptide encoded by the cDNA for human cell surface antigen Fas can mediate apoptosis. *Cell* 1991; 66: 233–43.
231. Smith CA, Farrah T, Goodwin RG. The TNF receptor superfamily of cellular and viral proteins: activation, costimulation and death. *Cell* 1994; 76: 959–62.
232. Krammer PH, Behrmann I, Daniel P *et al.* Regulation of apoptosis in the immune system. *Curr Opin Immunol* 1994; 6: 279–89.
233. Nagata S, Golstein P. The Fas death factor. *Science* 1995; 267: 1449–56.
234. Suda T, Takahashi T, Golstein P, Nagata S. Molecular cloning and expression of the Fas ligand, a novel member of the tumor necrosis factor family. *Cell* 1993; 75: 1169–78.
235. Chinnaiyan AM, O-Rourke K, Tewari M, Dixit VM. FADD, a novel death-domain-containing protein, interacts with death domain of Fas and initiates apoptosis. *Cell* 1995; 81: 505.
236. Cohen G. Caspases: executioners of apoptosis. *Biochem J* 1997; 326: 1–6.
237. Cahill MA, Peter ME, Kischhkel FC *et al.* CD95 (APO-1/Fas) induces activation of SAP kinases downstream of ICE-like proteases. *Oncogene* 1996; 13: 2087–96.
238. Cheng J, Zhou T, Liu C *et al.* Protection from Fas-mediated apoptosis by a soluble form of the Fas molecule. *Science* 1994; 263: 1759–62.
239. Kayagaki N, Kawasaki A, Ebata T *et al.* Metalloproteinase-mediated release of human Fas ligand. *J Exp Med* 1995; 182: 1777–83.
240. Tanaka M, Suda T, Haze K *et al.* Fas ligand in human serum. *Nature Med* 1996; 2: 317–22.
241. Suda T, Okazaki T, Naito Y *et al.* Expression of the Fas ligand in cells of T cell lineage. *J Immunol* 1995; 154: 3806–3.
242. Watanabe-Fukunaga R, Brannan CI, Itoh N *et al.* The cDNA structure expression and chromosomal assignment of the mouse Fas antigen. *J Immunol* 1992; 148: 1274–9.
243. Tanaka M, Ito H, Adachi S *et al.* Hypoxia induces apoptosis with enhanced expression of Fas antigen messenger RNA in cultured neonatal rat cardiac myocytes. *Circ Res* 1994; 75: 426–33.
244. Nishigaki K, Minatoguchi S, Seishima M *et al.* Plasma Fas ligand, an inducer of apoptosis, and plasma soluble Fas, an inhibitor of apoptosis, in patients with congestive heart failure. *J Am Coll Cardiol* 1997; 29: 1214–20.
245. Toyozaki T, Hiroe M, Tanaka M *et al.* Levels of soluble Fas ligand in myocarditis. *Am J Cardiol* 1998; 15; 82(2): 246–8.
246. Ishiyama S, Hiroe M, Nishikawa T *et al.* The Fas/Fas ligand system is involved in the pathogenesis of autoimmune myocarditis in rats. *J Immunol* 1998; 161: 4695–701.
247. Schumann H, Morawietz H, Hakim K *et al.* Alternative splicing of the primary Fas transcript generating soluble Fas antagonists is suppressed in the failing human ventricular myocardium. *Biochem Biophys Res Commun* 1997; 239: 794–8.
248. Felzen B, Shilkrut M, Less H *et al.* Fas (CD95/Apo-1)-mediated damage to ventricular myocytes induced by cytotoxic T lymphocytes from perforin-deficient mice. *Circ Res* 1998; 82: 438–50.
249. Pan G, Bauer JH, Haridas V *et al.* Identification and functional characterization of DR6, a novel death-domain containing TNF receptor. *FEBS Lett* 1998; 431: 351–6.
250. Pabla R, Rees SA, Know KA *et al.* Apoptosis is mediated by ICE-like proteases in ventricular myocardium. *Circulation* 1996; 94: I-282.
251. Long X, Crow MT, Lakatta EG. ICE-related proteases are involve in hypoxia-induced apoptosis in cardiac myocytes. *Circulation* 1997; 96: I-737.

252. Bialik S, Cryns V, Drincic A *et al*. Cytochrome c release from the mitochondria precedes caspase activation in apoptotic myocytes during ischemia. *Circulation* 1998; Suppl 1: I-462.
253. Oh H, Kunisda K, Funamoto M, Yamauchi-Takihara K. Activation of gp130 inhibits doxorubicin induced cell death by Bcl-xL/caspase-3 interaction and PI 3-kinase/Akt pathway in cardiac myocytes. *Circulation* 1998; Suppl 1: I-462.
254. Bialik S, Geenen DL, Sasson IE *et al*. The caspase family of cyteine proteases mediate cardiac myocyte apoptosis during myocardial infarction. *Circulation* 1997; 96: I-552.
255. Thornberry NA. Caspases: key mediators of apoptosis. *Chem Biol* 1998; 5(5): R97–103.
256. Yaoita H, Ogawa K, Maehara K, Maruyama Y. Attenuation of ischemia/perfusion injury in rats by a caspase inhibitor. *Circulation* 1998; 97: 276–81.
257. Koseki T, Inohara N, Chen S, Nunez G. ARC, an inhibitor of apoptosis expressed in skeletal muscle and heart that interacts selectively with caspases. *Proc Natl Acad Sci USA* 1998; 95: 5156–60.
258. Iizuka K, Kawaguchi H, Kitabatake A. Effects of thiol protease inhibitors on fodrin degradation during hypoxia in cultured myocytes. *J Mol Cell Cardiol* 1993; 25: 1101–9.
259. Yoshida K, Inui M, Harada K *et al*. Reperfusion of rat heart after brief ischemia induces proteolysis of calspectin (nonthyroid spectrin or fodrin) by calpain. *Circ Res* 1995; 77: 603–10.
260. Astma DE, Bastiaanse EM, Jerzewski A *et al*. Role of calcium-activated neutral protease (calpain) in cell death in cultured neonatal rat cardiomyocytes during metabolic inhibition. *Circ Res* 1995; 76: 1071–8.
261. Field ML, Clark JF. Inappropriate ubiquitin conjugation: a proposed mechanism contributing to heart failure. *Cardiovasc Res* 1997; 33: 8–12.
262. Hilenski LL, Terracio L, Haas AL, Borg TK. Immunolocalization of ubiquitin-conjugates at Z-bands and intercalated discs of rat cardiac myocytes *in vitro* and *vivo*. *J Histochem Cytochem* 1992; 40: 1037–42.
263. Lopes UG, Erhardt P, Yao R, Cooper GM. p53-dependent induction of apoptosis by proteasome inhibitors. *J Biol Chem* 1997; 272: 12 893–6.

# Myocellular and myocardial extracellular matrix remodelling 

C. G. BRILLA AND H. RUPP

## Introduction

Arterial hypertension and coronary artery disease are the most frequent aetiological factors for congestive heart failure (CHF) [1]. To understand the progression of CHF, the interrelationship between underlying causes and regulatory systems needs to be addressed. In addition to cardiac growth and associated altered gene expression, neurohumoral regulatory mechanisms appear to be critically involved in the progressive deterioration of cardiac function. Despite recent advances in the management of CHF, the prognosis of patients with chronically overloaded hypertrophied hearts remains poor [2]. Therefore, the question arises as to whether appropriate drug targets have been chosen for current interventions. One of the problems involved in choosing a drug target relates to the fact that the heart is composed of various tissue compartments, i.e. myocyte and non-myocyte compartments. It appears that current drug targets mainly interact with cardiac myocytes and neurohumoral regulatory systems. In this chapter, the remodelling of the myocellular and extracellular compartments during the progression of CHF is described and potential additional drug targets are identified.

The non-myocyte compartment, the cardiac interstitium, contains blood- and lymph- carrying vessels, an amorphous intercellular substance, fibroblasts, macrophages and other leucocytes, fibrillar collagen, and various extracellular matrix proteins. Under certain circumstances structural abnormalities within the cardiac interstitium serve as the primary mechanism responsible for myocardial failure [3]. Fibrillar collagen, which is an essential component of the cardiac interstitium, maintains the alignment of cardiac myocytes throughout the cardiac cycle. Collagen fibres, which interconnect myocytes, facilitate the transmission of the myocyte-generated force to the ventricular chambers. In addition, energy stored in coiled collagen fibres during myocyte contraction contributes to myocardial relaxation and myocyte relengthening [4]. Recently, particular progress has been achieved in the treatment of patients with an adverse remodelling of the myocardial extracellular matrix [5]. For instance, angiotensin-converting enzyme (ACE) inhibitors have proven to be efficient in reversing deleterious processes due to reactive fibrosis. This type of therapy has been termed cardioreparation [6] since myocardial structure and function are pathologically altered when treatment starts. The structural remodelling of the myocardial collagen network in hypertensive heart disease and its relationship to diastolic and/or systolic myocardial failure are particularly important. The primary regulatory mechanism that appears to be responsible for the excessive accumulation of collagens or myocardial fibrosis is the renin–angiotensin–aldosterone system (RAAS) [7]. Therefore, ACE inhibitors or competitive aldosterone antagonists are of major clinical interest when targeting the structural cause of hypertensive heart disease and myocardial failure.

Myocardial failure has, however, been associated with the common presumption that the primary defect must reside within myocytes. There is accumulating evidence that the myocyte in addition, represents a drug target for the prevention of early progression of ventricular dysfunction. Primary abnormalities in myocyte contraction are known in certain conditions, particularly those associated with a critical reduction in coronary blood flow [8]. The question arises of whether the initiating events in myocellular remodelling that lead to reactive fibrosis via stimulation of neurohumoral systems could represent a logical pharmacological target. Since the effector hormones of the RAAS, angiotensin II (AngII) and aldosterone, are critically involved in the development of reactive fibrosis in chronically overloaded hearts, it is attractive to search for processes upstream to the neurohumoral activation. Of particular interest are mechanisms that represent turning points for the onset of neuroendocrine activation. The elucidation of those mechanisms is considered a prerequisite for developing drugs that not only are appropriate for cardioreparation but could prevent adverse reactions. The following sections delineate the links between impaired myocyte function and neurohumoral activation that lead to an adverse remodelling of myocardial structure associated with further impairment of cardiac function.

## Cardiac growth

The growth of cardiac myocytes, which are terminally differentiated cells, leads to myocyte hypertrophy [9] and an increase in mass and thickness of the myocardium, resulting in the left ventricular hypertrophy (LVH) seen in hypertensive heart disease, dilated cardiomyopathy or postmyocardial infarction. However, it should not be assumed that irrespective of its aetiological basis, LVH is always accompanied by non-myocyte cell growth. Non-myocyte cell growth is expressed as a structural remodelling of the cardiac interstitium. In ischaemic heart disease, the capillary density and the development of collateral vessels (neoangiogenesis) are regulated by various growth factors, particularly vascular endothelial growth factor (VEGF). VEGF promotes chemotaxis of endothelial cells and stimulates their proliferation and attachment to the extracellular matrix by inducing the expression of integrin surface receptors [10]. The accumulation of fibrillar collagen by increased collagen synthesis and/or decreased collagen degradation is secondary to the activation and proliferation of cardiac fibroblasts [7]. Collagen synthesis may be increased either per cell in the presence or absence of fibroblast proliferation or by primary proliferation of cardiac fibroblasts while per cell production remains unchanged. The regulation of collagen degradation may occur at various steps in the collagenolytic system: degradation of intracellular collagen may be decreased by the activation of prolyl-4-hydroxylase, the key enzyme required for proper folding of newly synthesized procollagen polypeptides, while degradation of extracellular collagen is dependent on interstitial collagenase or matrix metalloproteinase-1 (MMP-1) expression and activation. Tissue inhibitors of metalloproteinase (TIMP) may also be involved in the remodelling process.

It has been suggested that the growth of myocyte and non-myocyte cells takes place independently [11]. Coronary vasculitis and radiation-induced myocardial fibrosis are examples of non-myocyte cell growth and the remodelling of the interstitium that occurs without myocyte growth. The hypertrophy seen in primary volume overload states, e.g. an arteriovenous fistula [12] or chronic anaemia [13], or the administration of thyroxine or growth hormones [14], is an example of myocyte growth that occurs without the disproportionate involvement of fibroblasts and in which the myocardial collagen concentration remains normal. The growth of myocytes and the increase in fibroblasts can, however, be associated. In various forms of arterial hypertension, congenital and acquired aortic valvular stenosis, and coarctation of the aorta, LVH is accompanied by a reactive fibrosis that is not secondary to myocyte necrosis [15–19], representing examples of myocyte hypertrophy and disproportionate non-myocyte cell growth.

The hypertrophic remodelling of the myocardium is either a homogeneous or a heterogeneous process, based on whether or not there is a proportionate or disproportionate growth of myocyte and non-myocyte cells, respectively (Fig. 19.1) [20]. When tissue homogeneity is preserved, the proportion of muscular, vascular, and interstitial compartments is maintained and hypertrophy appears to be adaptive, as seen in the athlete's heart. In contrast, a heterogeneity in myocardial structure, based on disproportionate non-myocyte cell growth and loss of intercompartmental proportionality, causes a severely impaired pump performance that is associated with diastolic and/or systolic heart failure. Trophic factors that promote disproportionate non-myocyte cell growth or collagen gene expression leading to abnormal myocardial structure represent a decisive determinant of pathological hypertrophy with subsequent myocardial dysfunction. It therefore appears to be essential to view the hypertrophic process of the myocardium as more than the mere growth of cardiac myocytes. The entire cell population of the myocardium, as well as various proteins and enzymes and the expression of corresponding genes, need to be considered potentially recruitable into the growth process during the progression of CHF.

## Myocyte growth and phenotype

One of the key issues in the management of CHF is related to the intriguing finding that LVH mediated by the growth of heart muscle due to chronic overload may be a

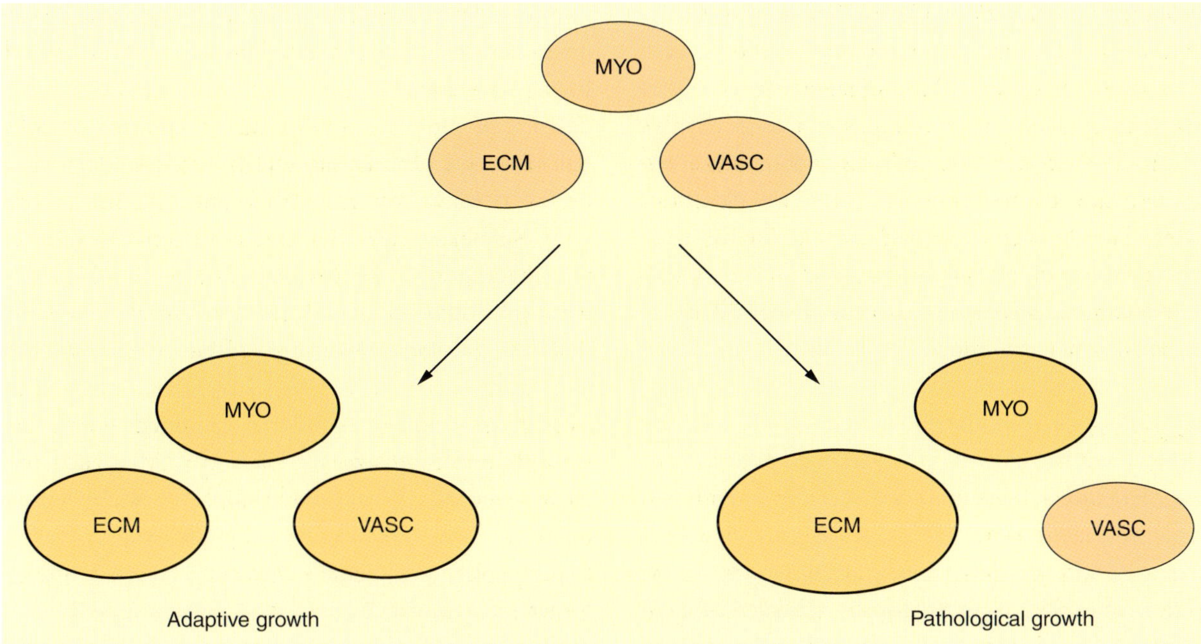


**Figure 19.1** *Adaptive versus pathological growth of myocardial tissue compartments. MYO = myocyte compartment; ECM = extracellular matrix; VASC = vascular compartment.*

predictor of CHF [1]. This epidemiological finding is paradoxical since myocellular growth is required for coping with overload states in order to keep wall stress within a normal range. Therefore, the mechanical load is the major physiological stimulus for myocyte hypertrophy [21, 22]. In addition to mechanical conditions, growth hormones and catecholamines stimulate the growth of cardiomyocytes (Fig. 19.2) [14, 23, 24]. The growth of overloaded skeletal muscle is associated with a redirected gene expression [21] but failure has not been observed. Taking into account the basic similarities between striated cardiac and skeletal muscle, the different outcome of work overload points to either specific defects or phenotypic changes in hypertrophied cardiomyocytes or associated adverse changes within the extracellular matrix. In hypertensive heart disease, myocyte hypertrophy, as determined by myocyte diameter

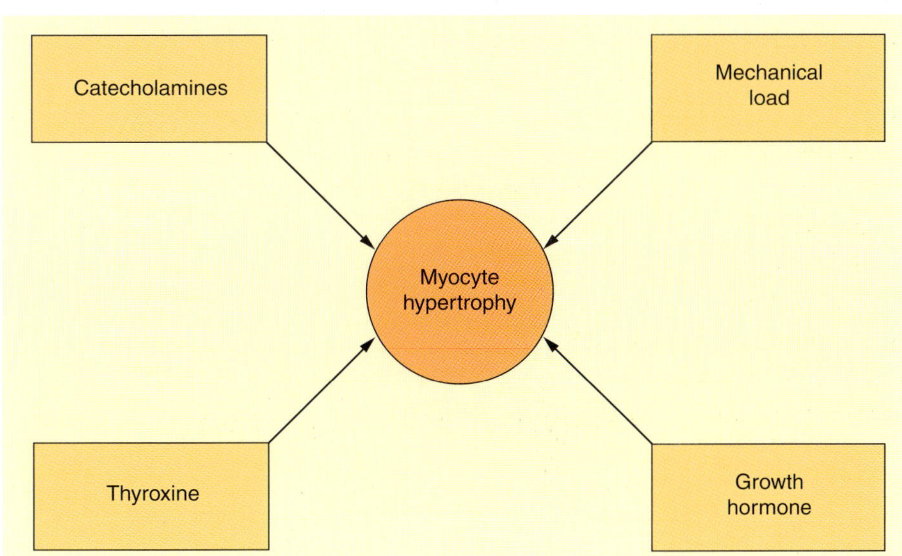


**Figure 19.2** *Stimuli of cardiac myocyte growth.*

is associated with myocardial fibrosis when measured morphometrically by collagen volume fraction of the left ventricular myocardium obtained by endomyocardial biopsies [5]. Thus, in hearts subjected to chronic overload, distinct changes need to occur which render the muscle performance inadequate. If these processes could be identified, pharmacological intervention could prevent the development of progression of heart failure.

There is increasing evidence that in the chronically overloaded heart the protein phenotype of cardiac muscle is altered in a distinct manner, in which both gene transcription and translation appear to be involved. One key feature associated with cardiac growth is the increased diffusion distances for myoplasmic ions involved in various signalling pathways. Any growth that is not associated with an appropriate increase in the density of membrane-bound receptors or cellular ion-handling systems can be regarded as maladapted. Based on this hypothesis, deficits in signal pathways need to be identified so that they can be used as pharmacological targets.

In CHF, chronic activation of the adrenergic system may cause β-adrenergic desensitization with downregulation of $\beta_1$-adrenergic receptors and uncoupling $\beta_2$-adrenoceptors (Table 19.1) [26]. The latter mechanism has been related to increased activity and gene expression of β-adrenoceptor kinase in failing myocardium, leading to phosphorylation and uncoupling of receptors. The $\beta_3$-adrenoceptors are known to mediate negative inotropic effects, but alterations in these receptors in CHF are not known. In addition, an increase in inhibitory G protein α-subunits (Giα) has been suggested to be causally linked to adenylyl cyclase desensitization in heart failure. In contrast, the catalytic subunits of adenylyl cyclase, the stimulatory G protein α-and βγ-subunits, remain unchanged. Recent evidence shows that increases in Giα also depress adenylyl cyclase in compensated cardiac hypertrophy in monogenic, polygenic, and secondary hypertension. These increases of Giα can suppress adenylyl cyclase in the absence of β-adrenergic receptor downregulation. Since cardiac hypertrophy due to chronic pressure overload is a strong predictor of cardiac failure, these observations indicate that adenylyl cyclase desensitization by Giα may be a pathophysiologically relevant mechanism contributing to the transition from compensated cardiac hypertrophy to heart failure [26]. For all these reasons, antiadrenergic treatment is currently an emerging and very promising approach to the treatment of CHF [27].

A great number of other pathomechanisms may be involved in chronically overloaded hypertrophied hearts. In view of the very limited knowledge, particularly on signals involved in gene expression, concentration is on genes that can be pharmacologically affected. The pharmacological target may not necessarily be a certain gene but a signal pathway modulating gene expression in which genes are often affected in a co-ordinated manner. Currently, the best characterized genes are those coding for myosin heavy chains (MHC) and the proteins of the sarcoplasmic reticulum (SR). The α- and β-MHC isoforms, i.e. V1 and V3, respectively, have differential effects on the kinetics of cross-bridge cycling [28]. An increased proportion of α-MHC (V1) results in an increased speed of contraction not only of skinned fibres [29] but also of isolated myosin–actin complexes [30]. The SR is crucially involved in regulating myoplasmic $Ca^{2+}$ fluxes during diastole and systole. An inadequately low density of SR $Ca^{2+}$ pumps leads to impaired relaxation and reduced systolic force due to insufficient $Ca^{2+}$ release.

It is well documented that the expression of SR $Ca^{2+}$-ATPase is decreased in overloaded failing hearts (Table 19.1) [31–33]. An inadequate expression of SR $Ca^{2+}$-ATPase is a representative example of genes that are not expressed in a manner that would be adequate for

**Table 19.1** Phenotype changes in cardiomyocytes in chronic heart failure

| Change | Results |
|---|---|
| Downregulation of $\beta_1$-adrenoceptors | Reduced capacity to respond to inotropic stimuli of the adrenergic system |
| Upregulation of β-adrenoceptor kinase | Uncoupling of $\beta_2$-adrenoceptors |
| Increase in inhibitory G protein α-subunits | Desensitization of adenylyl cyclase |
| Reduced expression of SR $Ca^{2+}$-ATPase | Impaired relaxation and reduced systolic force development |
| Reduced expression of myosin isozyme V1 | Impaired relaxation and reduced systolic force development |

SR = sarcoplasmic reticulum.

enlarged hearts. There is increasing evidence that in chronically pressure overloaded hearts and CHF, MHC expression or the corresponding change in myosin isozyme population is altered in a functionally co-ordinated manner. This is demonstrated by the correlation of the intermediary enzyme phosphate (E-P) of the SR $Ca^{2+}$-ATPase with myosin V1 in rat left and right ventricles [34, 35]. E-P represents an active SR $Ca^{2+}$ pump and is affected not only by transcription but also by translation. To assess whether an altered protein phenotype affects myocardial function, the rate of isovolumic relaxation of *in situ* hearts was examined. Both the rate of relaxation and the rate of contraction were linearly correlated with the proportion of myosin V1 [36]. In the absence of left heart failure with pulmonary congestion, rats with 6 weeks of supravalvular aortic constriction exhibited a reduced proportion of myosin V1 and a reduced rate of relaxation (Table 19.1), while myocardial hydroxyproline concentration as a measure of fibrosis was not increased. It appears that in this early chronic pressure overload model, altered myocardial function was primarily determined by changes in SR $Ca^{2+}$-ATPase associated with altered MHC expression. Any mismatch between sinus node activity and subcellular organelle structures is most probably the cause of the negative force–frequency relation observed in failing hearts. [37–39]. An inadequately high heart rate due to pacing leads to CHF [40]. Although the observed changes in the protein phenotype of chronically overloaded hearts have unfavourable consequences for overall myocardial function, particularly at high heart rates, they are unlikely to be responsible for the onset of acute pump failure. Instead, they represent early events which initiate secondary deleterious processes. The adverse remodelling of the extracellular matrix with development of reactive myocardial fibrosis appears to be of primary importance.

## Myocardial collagen matrix

In contrast to the load-dependent growth of cardiac myocytes, mechanical factors do not appear to account for the disproportionate accumulation of collagen that occurs with LVH in some conditions and not others, despite comparable elevations in wall stress due to chronic pressure or volume overload of the left ventricle [11–13, 15]. Moreover, types I and III collagen gene expression and collagen synthesis are temporally dissociated from the onset of myocyte growth [41, 42]. Thus, trophic factors that mediate myocyte and non-myocyte (i.e. cardiac fibroblast) cell growth of the myocardium can be independent of one another.

The myocardial collagen matrix is a structural continuum that includes the valve leaflets, chordae tendineae, and an interstitial collagen network, which is segregated into various components termed epimysium, perimysium, and endomysium (Fig. 19.3) [7, 43, 44]. Myocytes are connected to one another and to their neighbouring vascular and lymphatic capillaries by endomysial collagen fibres, which maintain myocyte alignment and prevent their slippage [45] ensuring the maintenance of myocardial architecture throughout the dynamic forces of the cardiac cycle. The most abundant structural proteins of the myocardial collagen matrix are fibrillar types I and III collagen [19], which usually coexist in common collagen fibres. The ratio of type I to III collagen in the normal non-human primate myocardium is 7.4:1 [19]. Type I has the highest tensile strength of all collagens and is not equalled by any protein in the body. Other collagen proteins present in the myocardium include types IV, V and VI, but only very small amounts of these collagens are found in the myocardium. Type IV collagen is associated with basal laminae, type V is found in the pericellular space, and type VI coats types I and III collagen fibres and appears to determine their thickness. The various geometrical features of collagen fibres, together with collagen phenotype, cross-linking, and concentration, determine the stiffness of the intact myocardium. Owing to the enormous tensile strength of type I collagen any disproportionate expansion of the myocardial matrix impairs myocardial function. Therefore, humoral regulatory systems that control myocardial collagen metabolism in CHF are of primary interest.

## Neurohumoral activation in heart failure

Various regulatory mechanisms are active during the progression of heart failure. It is often assumed that the Frank–Starling mechanism, which is reflected by the linear relationship between stroke volume and end-diastolic volume of either ventricle, can balance myocardial or circulatory failure. This may be applicable during acute heart failure if the heart does not already operate at its ideal sarcomeric length. However, hearts of patients with CHF have most of their fibres already chronically extended to the top of their force–length curve [46]. These hearts are unable to respond significantly to increased preload. Thus, the

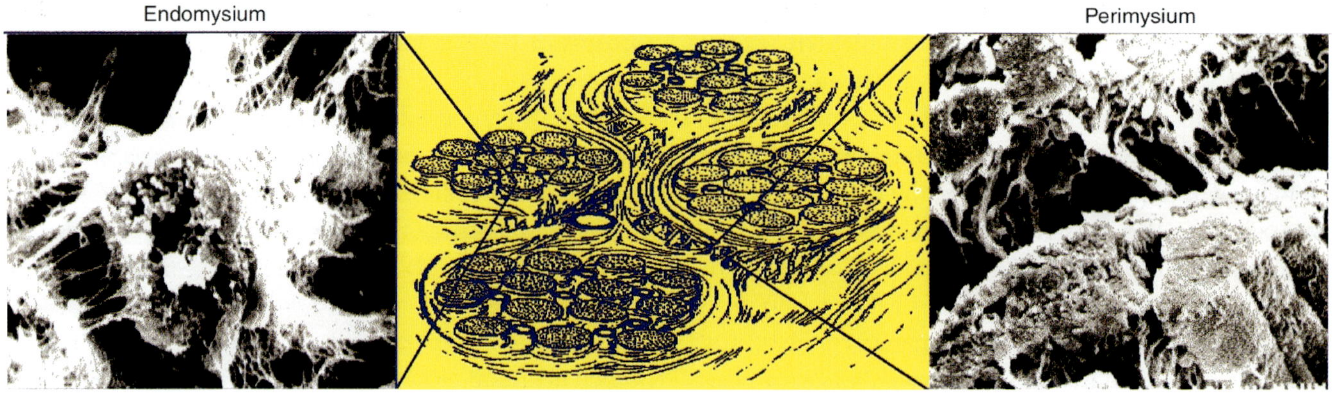


**Figure 19.3** *Myocardial collagen matrix: scanning electron micrographs (×3000) of endomysium showing weave of collagen fibres surrounding an individual myocyte and providing support between myocytes (left), and perimysium showing perimysial strands of collagen located between groups of myocytes (right).*

major physiological role of the Frank–Starling law is in synchronizing the stroke output of the two ventricles, which may vary considerably from beat to beat.

Of greater importance is the neurohormonal activation in acute or chronic heart failure (Fig. 19.4) [47]. The adrenergic system, which includes the sympathetic nervous system and circulating catecholamines released from the adrenal glands, raises both heart rate and myocardial contractility to provide sufficient cardiac output. However, if the underlying cause of acute heart failure cannot be eliminated, the rise in heart rate and myocardial contractility causes further deterioration of overall cardiac function due to increased myocardial oxygen consumption, which is particularly detrimental in ischaemic heart disease. Any activation of the adrenergic system is associated with increased renin release and followed by activation of the RAAS [48, 49]. The adrenergic system and the RAAS are interconnected. The most important interaction appears to

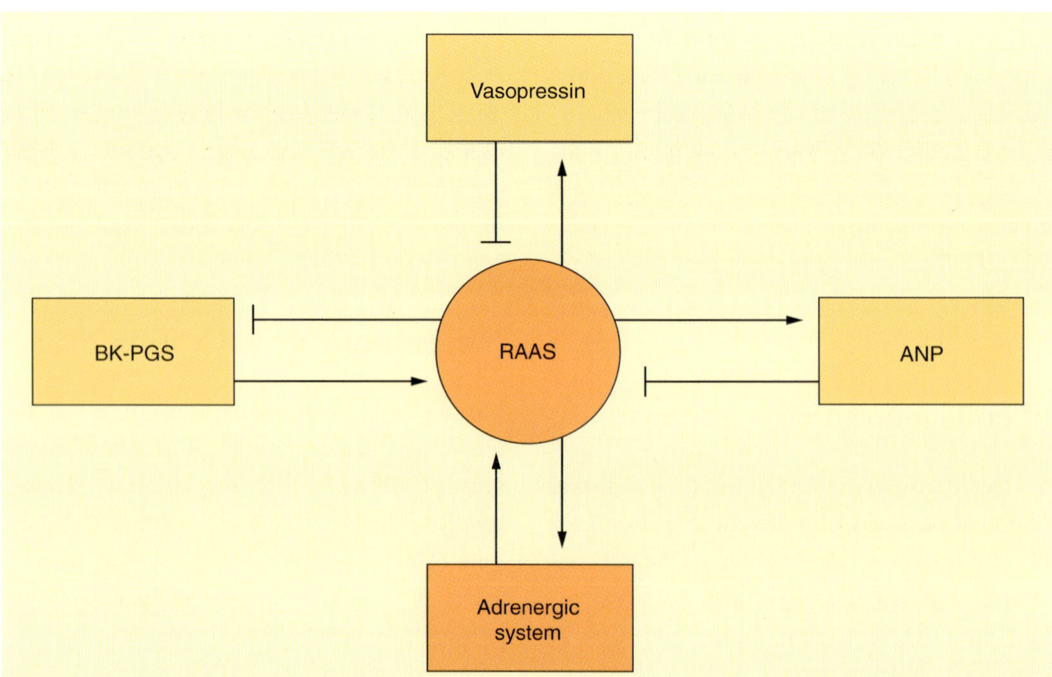


**Figure 19.4** *Interaction of neurohumoral regulatory systems in chronic heart failure. RAAS = renin–angiotensin–aldosterone system; ANP = atrial natriuretic peptide; BK-PGS = bradykinin–prostaglandin system; ↑ = stimulation; = ⊥ inhibition.*

be the direct stimulation of the adrenal glands by AngII to release catecholamines to the circulating blood and the stimulation of the juxtaglomerular apparatus of the kidneys by catecholamines to release renin, resulting in a vicious cycle between the RAAS and the adrenergic system in heart failure, in which the effector hormones of the RAAS are involved in the adverse structural remodelling of the myocardium.

Activation of neuroendocrine systems results in an array of physiological compensatory mechanisms in the kidney as a response to inappropriately low arterial blood volume. Although the ensuing vasoconstriction and retention of water and salt counteract inadequate perfusion pressure, they have detrimental consequences for long-term cardiac function as a result of progressive volume and pressure overload in the failing left ventricle. In the present context, emphasis is placed on activation of the RAAS to promote progressive myocardial fibrosis, although the enhanced influences of noradrenaline, arginine vasopressin, prostaglandins, endothelin, and atrial natriuretic peptide are also involved (Fig. 19.4) [50].

## Regulation of cardiac fibroblast function

A key element in the process of fibrosis is the cardiac fibroblast, which is responsible for the formation of types I and III collagen in the heart [51]. Collagen synthesis of cardiac fibroblasts is stimulated by either of the effector hormones of the RAAS, aldosterone and AngII, in a dose-dependent manner (Fig. 19.5) [52, 53]. Aldosterone stimulates collagen synthesis in concentrations similar to those found in plasma of patients with renovascular hypertension or CHF, and this response occurs via type I corticoid receptors since the competitive aldosterone receptor antagonist spironolactone abolishes the aldosterone mediated increase in collagen synthesis [54]. AngII stimulates collagen synthesis at concentrations that could be generated locally within the myocardium. The AngII-mediated increase in collagen synthesis can be antagonized by AngII type 1 ($AT_1$) receptor blockade [54]. To characterize signal transduction mechanisms of AngII, changes in intracellular calcium concentration of Fura-2-loaded cultured adult rat cardiac fibroblasts were examined by fluorescence photometry [55]. The intracellular calcium concentration was increased by AngII via $AT_1$ receptors in a dose-dependent manner [median effective concentration ($EC_{50}$) = $2.4 \times 10^{-8}$ mol/1)] involving two distinct phases: an initial calcium peak and a sustained elevated plateau phase. The initial calcium peak occurred transiently and independently of the duration of AngII application. While the magnitude of the transient calcium peak did not differ in a nominally $Ca^{2+}$-free solution, the AngII-mediated sustained plateau phase of intracellular calcium concentration was dependent on extracellular calcium. Thus, the initial transient calcium peak appears to arise from intracellular calcium stores, whereas the plateau phase involves an external calcium influx. The AngII-mediated dose-dependent increase in intracellular calcium transients was abolished by treatment with the $AT_1$ receptor antagonist candesartan, which also blunted the AngII-mediated increase in collagen synthesis

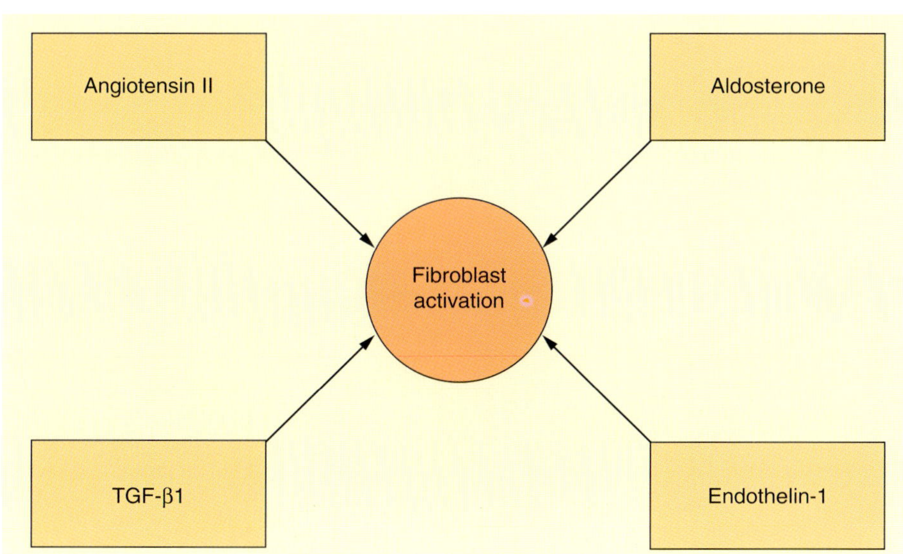


**Figure 19.5** *Humoral mediators stimulating collagen synthesis in cardiac fibroblasts.*

normalized to total protein synthesis [56]. Thus, AngII stimulates collagen synthesis in cultured adult rat cardiac fibroblasts via $AT_1$ receptors, probably using calcium as a second messenger (Fig. 19.6).

Collagen synthesis is also stimulated by various growth factors, e.g. endothelin-1 (ET-1) and transforming growth factor-$\beta_1$ (TGF-$\beta_1$) [57]. While AngII stimulates the expression of TGF-$\beta_1$, aldosterone increases the expression of ET-1 in cardiac fibroblasts and thus leads to an increase in collagen synthesis in an autocrine manner [58–60]. The release of TGF-$\beta_1$ may provide the initial trigger leading to fibrosis whenever neuroendocrine activation occurs [61] because the expression of TGF-$\beta_1$ is stimulated by any inadequate myocyte performance. This is controlled by autocrine effects on cardiac myocytes and paracrine effects on other myocardial cells including cardiac fibroblasts. For instance, mechanical stretch or ischaemic injury induce expression of TGF-$\beta_1$ in the heart, which potentiates c-*fos* mRNA expression [62]. The finding that intravenous infusion of TGF-$\beta_1$ did not result in collagen accumulation in the myocardium [63] demonstrates, however, that additional mediators such as AngII or aldosterone are important. In contrast to AngII, aldosterone, ET-1, and TGF-$\beta_1$, prostaglandin $E_2$ inhibits collagen synthesis of adult cardiac fibroblasts in a dose-dependent manner in addition to its antiproferative effects on cardiac fibroblasts [64].

Since the collagen network is in a dynamic state involving not only synthesis but also degradation, recent work has focused on the regulation of collagenolytic enzymes. This is exemplified by the crucial influence of MMPs on tissue remodelling during cardiac morphogenesis [65]. Adult rat myocardium contains uniformly distributed MMPs 1, 2, and 9 in an inactive or latent form (proMMP) [66]. The activation of proMMP involves mainly serine proteases, such as trypsin and neutrophil elastase, on which oxidized glutathione has synergistic effects. [66]. The activity of MMP is also controlled by TIMP, which maintain extracellular MMP in their inactive form [66, 67]. Processes in inflammatory cells that

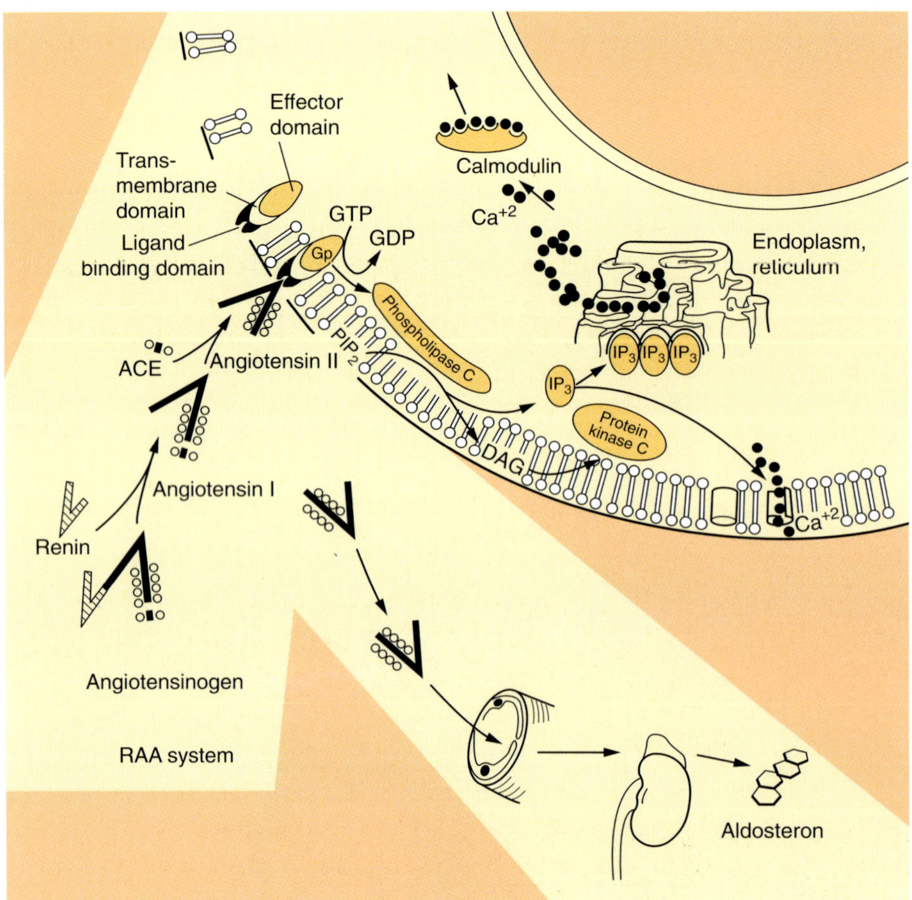


**Figure 19.6** *Schematic representation of the interaction between angiotensin II (Ang II) and cardiac fibroblasts. AngII attaches to the ligand binding domain of the membrane-bound $AT_1$ receptor of the fibroblast. The signal transduction probably includes a Gp protein, representing the effector domain of the receptor and which is driven by the conversion of GTP to GDP, and the activation of phospholipase C which converts membrane phospholipids for their participation in second-messenger pathways. In this case, $PIP_2$ is converted to inositol triphosphate ($IP_3$) and diacylglycerol (DAG). $IP_3$ diffuses through the cytosol and subsequently binds to the endoplasmic reticulum. The binding of three $IP_3$ molecules is considered necessary to open $Ca^{2+}$ channels in the endoplasmic reticulum and release $Ca^{2+}$ from this intracellular $Ca^{2+}$ storage site. A dose-dependent increase in intracellular $Ca^{2+}$ concentration has been found in cultured cardiac fibroblasts incubated with AngII. (From ref. 7 with permission.)*

involve the release of serine proteases not only activate proMMP but also inactivate TIMP [68]. AngII but not aldosterone decreased the activity of collagenase, i.e. MMP-1 which is the key enzyme for interstitial collagen degradation (Fig. 19.7) [54]. The inhibition of MMP-1 activity by AngII was attenuated by AngII type 2 receptor blockade [54]. The formation of fibronectin, which forms a scaffold on which collagen fibrils are organized [69], was also stimulated by AngII via $AT_1$ receptors [70]. Since the pump performance of the heart relies on the elastic recoil of the myocardium [71], a loss of the normal structure of the extracellular matrix is deleterious. Reduced elastic recoil may cause additional impairment of myocyte performance. Further key factors of extracellular matrix remodelling arise from the macrophages, which are required throughout the tissue repair process [72]. Activated macrophages secrete interleukine-1 (IL-1), IL-6, and tumour necrosis factor-α (TNF-α), which stimulate collagen production [73]. Monocytes express TGF-$\beta_1$ which induces the gene expression of IL-1 and TNF-α. Furthermore, IL-1 is a potent inducer of MMP expression [65]. Thus, few trigger events exist but a multitude of amplifying autocrine or paracrine processes with self-perpetuating actions leads to myocardial fibrosis.

## Renin–angiotensin–aldosterone system and myocardial fibrosis

The physiological role of the RAAS on the development of myocardial fibrosis is confirmed by *in vivo* studies [11, 74]. In various models of hypertension with a comparable degree of elevated systolic arterial pressure and a similar degree of LVH, myocardial fibrosis was found only in the presence of stimulated circulating RAAS, i.e. in renovascular hypertension or when aldosterone was chronically infused via subcutaneously implanted osmotic minipumps to raise plasma aldosterone levels, as seen in CHF. In this model, myocardial fibrosis was found in either ventricle: the pressure-overloaded, hypertrophied left ventricle or the non-overloaded, not hypertrophied right ventricle. In contrast, myocardial fibrosis was absent in both ventricles when the RAAS was not activated, although LVH was present (Fig. 19.8). Thus, the adverse remodelling of the extracellular matrix is not a necessary consequence of cardiac hypertrophy or chronic pressure overload [11]. Experimental models of arterial hypertension associated with the activation of local or systemic RAAS are characterized by progressive myocardial fibrosis [11, 52]. Low-output heart failure models, like rapid pacing in dogs, were associated

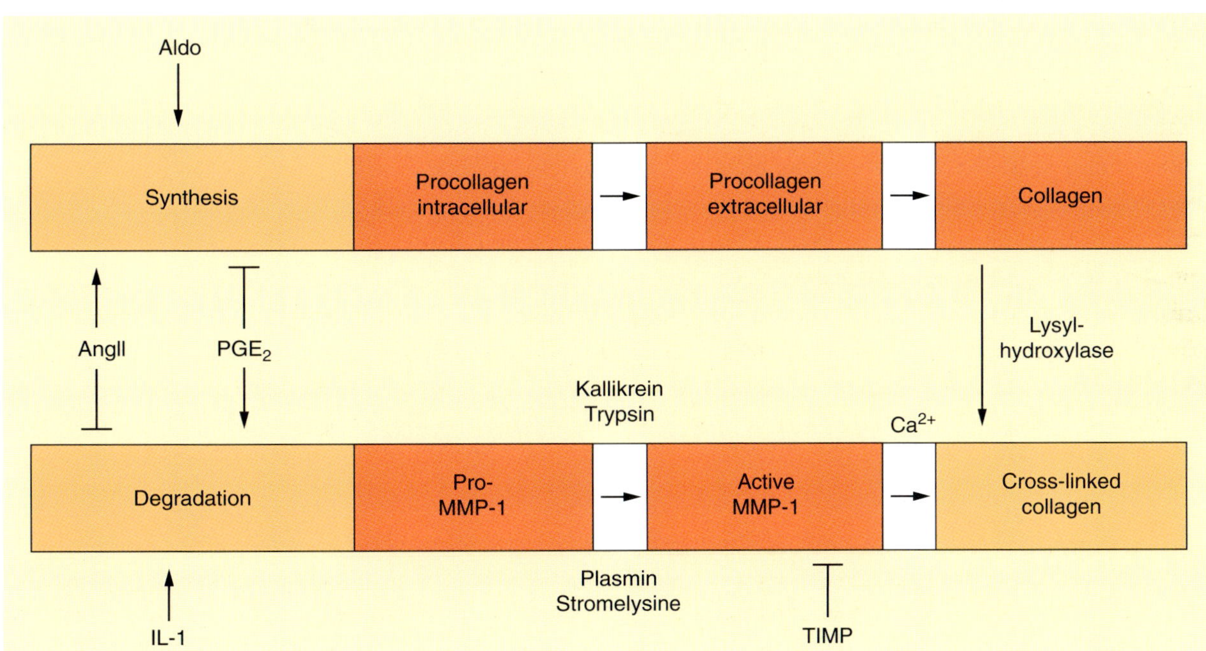


**Figure 19.7** *Myocardial collagen metabolism balanced by fibroblast-mediated collagen synthesis and interstitial degradation by matrix metalloproteinase-1 (MMP-1) and modulated by aldosterone (Aldo), angiotensin II (AngII), prostaglandin $E_2$ ($PGE_2$), interleukin-1 (IL-1), and tissue inhibitors of metalloproteinase (TIMP); ↑ = stimulation; = ⊥ inhibition.*

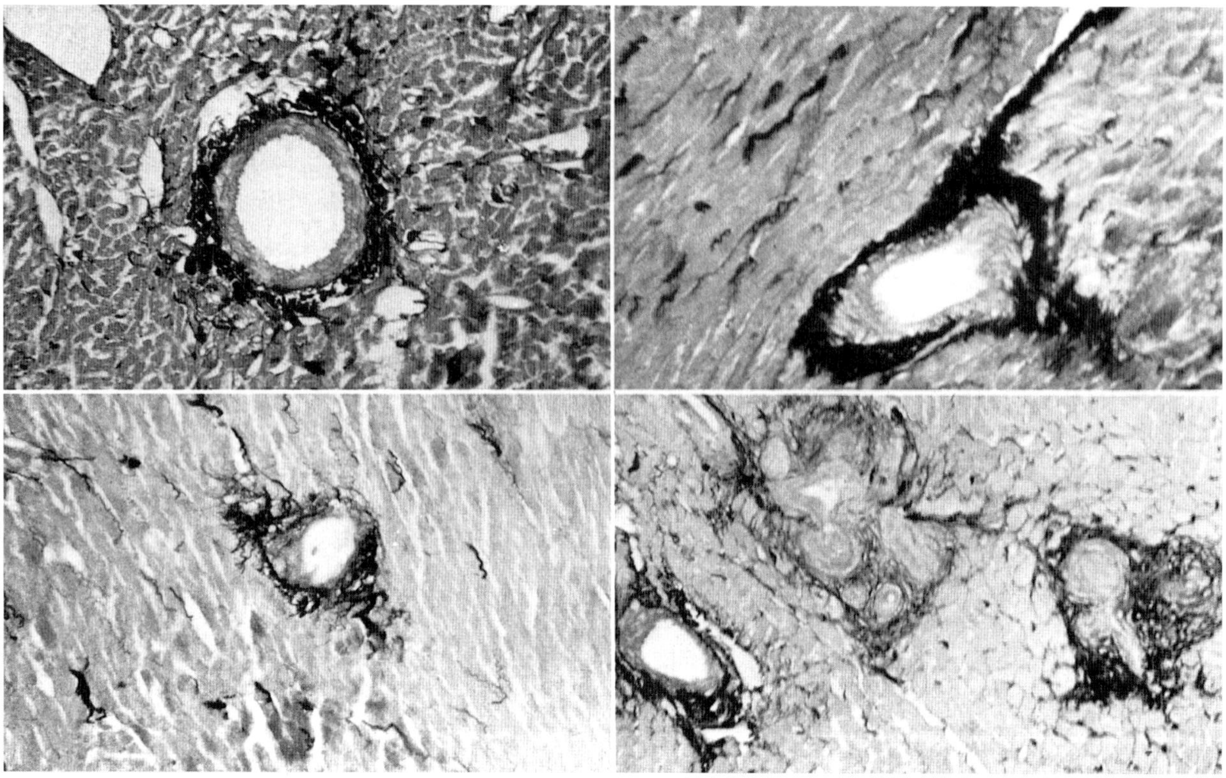

**Figure 19.8** *Photomicrographs of left and right* (next page) *ventricular rat myocardium stained with the collagen-specific dye Sirius Red. Collagen fibres appear black while the media of intramural coronary arteries and myocytes are grey. Unoperated control* (upper left *of each panel*), *renovascular hypertension* (upper right *of each panel*), *infrarenal aortic banding* (lower left *of each panel*), *and chronic aldosterone administration via subcutaneously implanted minipumps* (lower right *of each panel*) *are shown. The normal interstitial collagen and meshwork of collagen surrounding an intramyocardial coronary artery for each ventricle are shown in the upper left sections of each panel. With renovascular hypertension, the interstitial and perivascular accumulation of fibrillar collagen, or fibrosis, is evident in the hypertrophied, pressure-overloaded left ventricle and in the non-hypertrophied, non-overloaded right ventricle. Following chronic aldosterone administration, an interstitial and perivascular fibrosis was also seen in either ventricle. No such remodelling of the myocardium was found with infrarenal banding when the renin–angiotensin–aldosterone system was not stimulated. (From ref. 11 with permission.)*

with the activation of RAAS and progressive increases in preload. In this model, myocardial fibrosis was seen in either ventricle [75], while in states of increased preload and high cardiac output, e.g. arteriovenous fistula, fibrosis does not occur [12]. In arterial hypertension or heart failure, reactive myocardial fibrosis was associated with RAAS activation irrespective of the haemodynamic load. The haemodynamic load of the right or left ventricles does not appear to be the primary stimulus for interstitial collagen accumulation. These findings suggest that the development of myocardial fibrosis is preceded by neuroendocrine activation involving mainly the RAAS.

The development of myocardial fibrosis follows a distinct time-course. Best suited for assessing the detrimental influence of the RAAS on myocardial collagen matrix remodelling is the two-kidney–one-clip model of renovascular hypertension in the rat, which is associated with a marked release of renin, the key enzyme of the RAAS. Within days of inducing renovascular hypertension by unilateral renal ischaemia, expression of the types I and III collagen gene is increased [41]. During the first week after suprarenal abdominal aorta banding [42], a bilateral renal ischaemia model, an increase in protocollagen prolyl-4-hydroxylase activity occurs, which is followed by enhanced proline incorporation into collagen. Fibroblast proliferation is also seen during the first week in this model [76]. These findings suggest that collagen metabolism rises within existing fibroblasts while fibroblast proliferation may also contribute to the elevation of collagen synthesis. At 8 weeks of renovascular hypertension, a perivascular fibrosis of the intramural arteries becomes evident, with collagen fibres that emanate from the adventitia, radiating outwards for considerable distances between neighbouring muscle fibres, casting interstitial space, and creating an interstitial

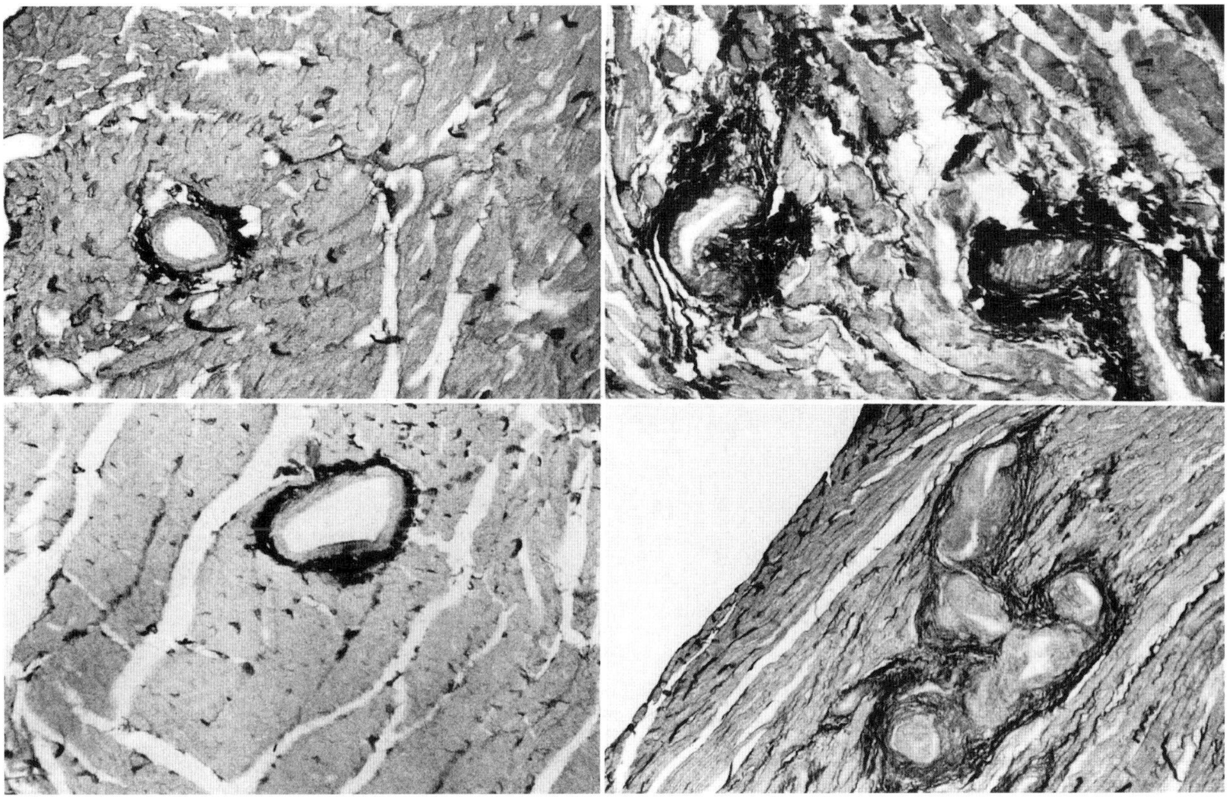

**Figure 19.8** *(Continued)*

fibrosis [17, 18]. The density of perimysial collagen fibres increases progressively and perimysial tendons and strands become thicker, often isolating myocytes from one another [17]. The collagen volume fraction of the left ventricle increases two- to three-fold [17, 18]. Myocardial diastolic stiffness and contractility are each increased at this stage of renovascular hypertension. At 12 weeks, foci of replacement fibrosis, secondary to myocyte necrosis, appear predominantly within the endomyocardium [77, 78]. The mechanism responsible for parenchymal cell loss is not clear, but given the prevalence of these scars within the endomyocardium, it appears that impaired coronary perfusion may be operative and is likely to be the result of an adverse remodelling of intramyocardial coronary arteries mediated by chronically elevated arterial pressure and AngII, with subsequent impairment of myocardial blood flow. With the appearance of these scars, the collagen volume fraction is now increased four-fold above control levels. This reparative fibrosis becomes even more pronounced at 32 weeks, where the overall collagen volume fraction is now increased six-fold above control and accounts for nearly 25% of the myocardial structural space [79]. Such pronounced perimuscular fibrosis may reduce myocyte-generated force causing a progressive atrophy of myocytes [80]. The functional consequence is a downward shift of the systolic stress–strain relationship, together with a marked elevation in diastolic stiffness [81]. Thus, combined diastolic and systolic dysfunction of the left ventricle appears in this late remodelling stage of hypertensive heart disease [79, 82]. In patients with primary hypertension and hypertensive heart disease, collagen volume fraction is increased by about 700% and associated with diastolic left ventricular dysfunction [5]. In these patients, the myocardial stiffness constant, i.e. the slope of the linear relationship between tangent elastic modulus and end-diastolic wall stress of the left ventricle, correlates with collagen volume fraction, but not with myocyte hypertrophy as determined morphometrically by myocyte diameter and obtained by left ventricular endomyocardial biopsies [5]. Thus, pathologically increased myocardial diastolic stiffness, impaired coronary reserve, and symptomatic heart failure are the functional consequences of interstitial and perivascular fibrosis, and medial thickening of intramyocardial coronary resistance vessels [15–18, 83].

## Modulation of cardiomyocyte gene expression by thyroid hormone analogues

The best characterized promoters of the cardiac myocyte are thyroid hormone-responsive elements (TREs) [84, 85]. Three TREs were identified and each was found to be active in transient transfection assays. [85]. The 3,5,3′-triiodothyronine ($T_3$) signal cascade depends on deiodination of thyroxine ($T_4$) to $T_3$, which is sensitive to the nutritional and general health status of the body. Since many proteins are affected by thyroid hormones [86–88], the thyroid-dependent modulation of gene expression represents an approach which influences the protein composition of the heart muscle cell in a co-ordinated manner. A complex antithetic regulation has been described for MHC, where α-MHC expression is stimulated by thyroid hormone at the expense of β-MHC (Fig 19.9) [84, 89]. It has been suggested that a $T_3$ response element is located near the start of β-MHC transcription and the $T_3$-receptor binding at this site interferes with the formation of the transcriptional initiation complex [89]. Thus, a pharmacological approach involving thyroid hormones or analogues may not only increase the expression of thyroid-dependent genes such as MHC [84] or SR $Ca^{2+}$-ATPase [90, 91], but also inhibit the expression of genes that are characteristic of functional states associated with hypothyroidism. Since a failing heart is subjected to influences resembling the euthyroid sick syndrome associated with reduced $T_3$, a therapeutic approach involving thyroid signalling appears attractive. Treatment of infarcted rat hearts with $T_4$ had initially beneficial effects which, however, could not be maintained when treatment was prolonged, most likely as a result of increased myocardial oxygen consumption [92]. Attempts have been made to develop thyroid analogues which retain their effect on gene transcription but ideally have no peripheral effects and do not induce tachycardia. A promising compound is DITPA (3,5-diiodothyropropionic acid), which binds to the $T_3$ receptors $\alpha$-$_1$ and $\beta$-$_1$ but has fewer systemic effects than thyroid hormones [93]. Further defining the structural elements of DITPA resulted in a simpler compound, DIHPA (3,5-diiodo-4-hydroxyphenylpropionic acid) [94]. When combined with captopril DITPA improved the function of infarcted rat hearts and the adverse effects of endogenous thyroid hormones were not observed [92, 93, 95]. Of particular importance was the finding that rate of relaxation improved, probably in relation to the increased expression of SR $Ca^{2+}$-ATPase (Fig. 19.9).

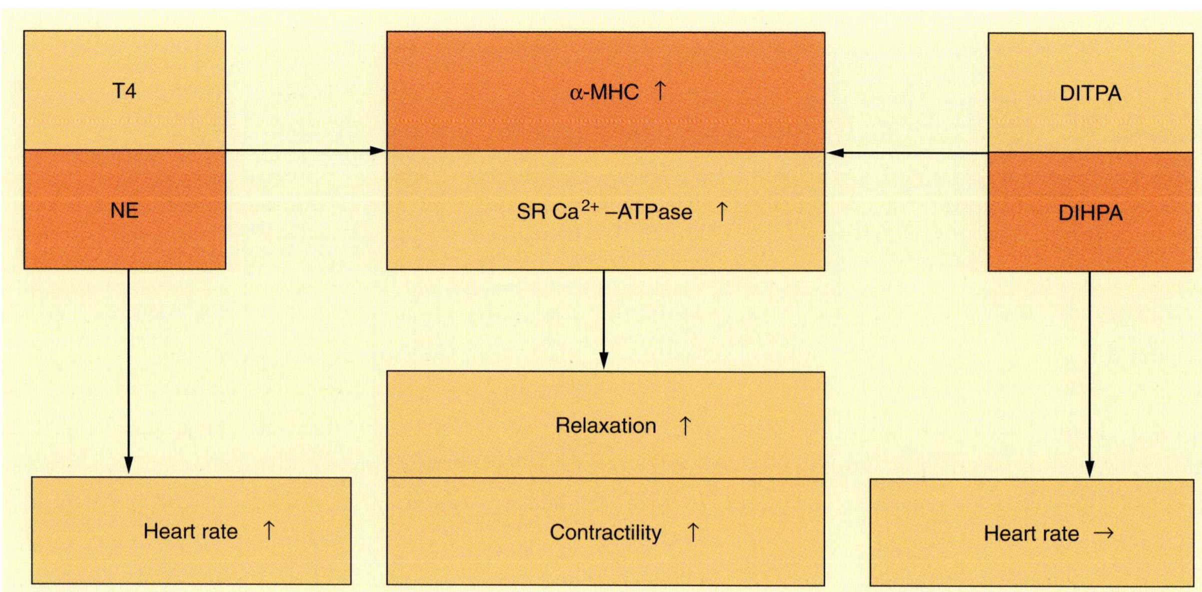


**Figure 19.9** *Effects of thyroxine ($T_4$), catecholamines [e.g. noradrenaline, NE], 3,5-diiodothyropropionic acid (DITPA), and 3,5-diiodo-4-hydroxyphenylpropionic acid (DIHPA) on α-myosin heavy chain (α-MHC), sarcoplasmic reticulum (SR) $Ca^{2+}$-ATPase, and heart rate. While thyroxine, DITPA, or DIHPA increases the expression of both α-MHC and SR $Ca^{2+}$-ATPase, catecholamines stimulate the expression of α-MHC but not clearly that of SR $Ca^{2+}$-ATPase. Instead, catecholamines increase the activity of SR $Ca^{2+}$-ATPase by phosphorylation of phospholamban. ↑ = increase; → = no change.*

## Regulation of cardiomyocyte gene expression by catecholamine-linked signals

Promoters mediating the influence of catecholamines on the heart muscle cell have only been partly characterized. The catecholamine-linked approach originated from the observation that α-MHC expression is increased after intermittent swimming of rats [96] and was independent of circulating thyroid hormones [97]. Further evidence for adrenergic influences was provided by the observation that the β-adrenoceptor-blocking drug atenolol had a greater effect on the proportion of α-MHC in swimming rats than in sedentary rats [97]. Injection of the β-agonists dobutamine or isoproterenol increased the proportion of α-MHC [98]. In cultured neonatal rat heart muscle cells, catecholamines induced similar changes in myosin expression (Fig. 19.9). In independent studies, catecholamines increased the abundance of α-MHC mRNA in cultured heart muscle cells [99, 100]. To observe the catecholamine-induced α-MHC transcription, cells had to be pre-exposed to serum, suggesting that the serum-inducible zinc finger protein Egr-1 may be involved [99, 100]. Catecholamines have comparable effects on cardiac myocytes in cell culture and in the intact organism. The difference in α-MHC expression between denervated and β-agonist-stimulated hearts is about 40%. Recently, important aspects of the intracellular signalling pathway of catecholamines have been characterized. A rise in cyclic adenosine monophosphate (cAMP) not only results in phosphorylation of the cAMP response element binding protein (CREB-P), which leads to phosphoCREB-P, but also induces an increased abundance of CREB-P mRNA [101]. Since the effects of cAMP were also observed in the presence of 2,3-butanedione monoxime, they appear to be independent of the contractile activity of the cardiomyocyte [101].

The cAMP-dependent signal pathway affecting gene expression could be relevant for the human heart. In patients with CHF, treatment with large doses of catecholamines increased the proportion of α-MHC to about 35% [102]. This demonstrates that α-MHC can be upregulated in the human heart with a predominance of β-MHC. An important observation is that catecholamines affect not only MHC expression but also SR $Ca^{2+}$-ATPase. In rabbits, surgical sympathectomy resulted in a depressed expression of the $Ca^{2+}$-ATPase gene [102]. Intermittently increased sympathetic activity would increase the potential of the heart muscle for fast contraction and relaxation. This mechanism is associated with phosphorylation of phospholamban, which results in stimulation of SR $Ca^{2+}$-ATPase by reducing the inhibitory influences of unphosphorylated phospholamban [34].

The intermittent administration of catecholamines may help chronically failing hearts, which exhibit a greatly reduced response to catecholamines, by changing the phenotype of cardiomyocytes and increasing the expression of α-MHC and SR $Ca^{2+}$-ATPase [103]. As in the case of thyroid hormones, the undesirable side-effects of catecholamines are tachycardia and increased oxygen consumption.

## Cardiomyocyte gene expression and energy metabolism-linked signals

In contrast to interventions linked to defined receptors, much less is known about molecular events associated with mechanisms modulating the intracellular metabolism of cardiomyocytes which are termed metabolic modulators. The use of metabolic modulators originated from the intriguing observation that α-MHC expression of normal [104] and particularly chronically overloaded hearts [105] can be increased by providing drinking water containing low amounts of sucrose. A comparison of chronically overloaded hearts and hearts of intermittently fasted rats revealed similar molecular abnormalities in the myocardium [105, 106]. Based on these finding, extensive studies were carried out to assess the therapeutic potential of drugs that increase glucose utilization [107–111]. The effect of sucrose could be mimicked by etomoxir, a drug that increases glucose oxidation at the expense of fatty acid oxidation (Fig. 19.10) [110]. Since this action mimics an anabolic state, i.e. carnitine palmitoyltransferase (CPT)-1 inhibition due to high malonyl-coenzyme A abundance [34, 112–114], it is not unexpected that high etomoxir doses are associated with homogeneous growth of the myocardium [109]. Etomoxir-induced cardiac growth was associated with increased α-MHC and a higher rate of SR $Ca^{2+}$ uptake [28, 110, 111]. Treatment with etomoxir resulted in an increased abundance of the SR intermediary enzyme phosphate E-P and an increased rate of relaxation of heart muscle. Increased myocardial expression of α-MHC in etomoxir-treated rats resembles that observed after a high caloric intake, which is also associated with enhanced

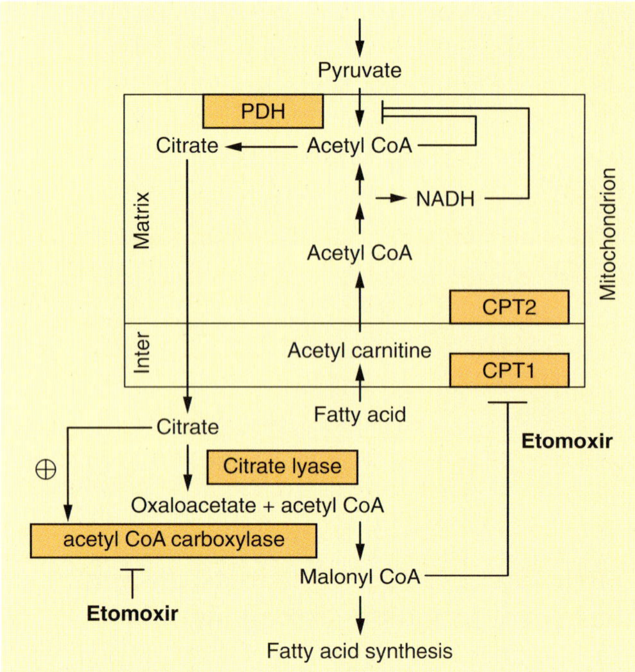


**Figure 19.10** *Drug targets of the carnitine palmitoyltransferase(CPT)-1 inhibitor etomoxir: inhibition of CPT-1 by etomoxir results in reduced fatty acid oxidation and subsequent activation of pyruvate dehydrogenase (PDH) and thus increased glucose oxidation; inhibition of acetyl coenzyme A (CoA) carboxylase results in reduced de novo fatty acid synthesis. NADH = reduced nicotinamide adenive dinucleotide.*

cardiac growth [111]. These changes are opposed to those observed after intermittent fasting [106]. It appears that etomoxir-induced growth of the heart represents a prototype of homogeneous growth as found in the athlete's heart. The left ventricle, which bears a higher load than the right ventricle, exhibits a lower proportion of α-MHC and a lower density of $Ca^{2+}$-ATPase. Etomoxir seems to interfere preferentially with processes dependent on workload, since its effect was greater in the left than in the right ventricle [34]. This view is supported by the finding that in overloaded ventricles due to aortic constriction, etomoxir had a pronounced effect on α-MHC [110, 115]. An important question arose as to whether a dissociation between cardiac growth and induction of desirable alterations in subcellular organelles could be achieved. In a recent rat study with chronically pressure-overloaded hearts due to supravalvular aortic constriction, it was shown that the proportion of α-MHC can be increased by low-dose etomoxir treatment without inducing additional myocardial growth [115]. Furthermore, rate parameters of ventricular contraction and relaxation improved [115]. Since etomoxir had no acute effect on cardiovascular parameters, e.g. heart rate as assessed by radiotelemetry, it does not induce responses typical of thyroid hormones or catecholamines. It remains to be shown whether intracellular mechanisms which are common to pathways of established receptor agonists are recruited. Although the molecular mechanisms involved in the treatment with etomoxir remain to be established, the drug offers the advantage of selectively affecting chronically overloaded hearts. No major side-effects have been observed in clinical trials focusing on the antidiabetic effects of etomoxir in patients with non-insulin-dependent diabetes [116–118]. Further work is required to examine whether alternative metabolic modulators or drugs acutely improving SR function [119] have etomoxir-like effects on the subcellular organelles of cardiac muscle.

## Interventions for controlling myocardial fibrosis

The effector hormones of the RAAS, AngII and aldosterone, are logical targets for the prevention or regression of myocardial fibrosis since either hormone stimulates collagen synthesis in cardiac fibroblasts. In the rat with renovascular hypertension, myocardial fibrosis was prevented by chronic ACE inhibition with captopril treatment [120]. In the same experimental model, myocardial fibrosis regressed with the ACE inhibitor zofenopril. In contrast, myocardial fibrosis increased by antihypertensive treatment with the combined α–β-receptor blocking agent labetalol, although blood pressure was normal and LVH minimized [121]. In related studies, rats with either renovascular hypertension or primary hyperaldosteronism were pretreated with small or large doses of the competitive aldosterone antagonist spironolactone. The smaller dose did not prevent hypertension or LVH, while the larger dose did. With either dose of spironolactone, however, the interstitial and perivascular fibrosis due to stimulation of the RAAS in renovascular hypertension or due to chronic aldosterone infusion was not seen [74]. The aldosterone-mediated fibrotic response of the myocardium has been confirmed in other laboratories [122, 123]. In genetic hypertension of spontaneously hypertensive rats (SHR), where local myocardial tissue levels of AngII are upregulated, the ACE inhibitor lisinopril was able to regress myocardial fibrosis irrespective of its antihypertensive effects by normalizing the myocardial AngII concentration and ameliorating myocardial stiffness [52, 83]. In the same model but with advanced hypertensive heart disease in aged animals, lisinopril removed fibrotic tissue from the myocardium, improving diastolic left ventricular function and preventing the occurrence of systolic left ventricular dysfunction as measured by the slope of the systolic stress–strain relationship of isolated hearts under isovolumic conditions [124]. In related studies with SHR, aortic fibrosis could be prevented by treatment with the aldosterone receptor antagonist spironolactone [125], which can be only explained by the presence of a local RAAS that includes the local generation of Aldo [126, 127]. These agents have cardioprotective and cardioreparative [6] properties because myocardial fibrosis could be either prevented or regressed.

This approach interrupts the hormone-mediated response that leads to fibroblast activation at the onset. One could also argue that the fibrous tissue response could be interrupted within the cardiac fibroblast at any point beginning with the signal-transduction pathway and beyond. Given the potential importance of calcium as an intracellular signal in promoting AngII-mediated cardiac fibroblast collagen synthesis, calcium-channel blockers may prove to have also cardioprotective or cardioreparative properties. The latter could be shown by regression of myocardial fibrosis using the calcium-channel blocker nifedipine, in the two-kidney–one-clip model of renovascular hypertension [121]. However, this needs to be examined more systematically.

Regression of interstitial and perivascular fibrosis represents a means by which myocardial failure due to collagen accumulation would be reversible. The premise of this approach is based on either inhibiting the stimulus to fibrous tissue formation, while retaining the myocardium's proteolytic enzyme system [128] for continued gradual collagen degradation, or actively invoking proteolytic digestion for more rapid degradation. At present, little is known about the regulation of the active or inactive forms of cardiac MMP-1, which is the key enzyme of interstitial collagen degradation. However, in pioneering studies using the SHR as a model for primary hypertension in humans, myocardial MMP-1 activity could be enhanced by chronic ACE inhibition with lisinopril, resulting in significant regression of myocardial fibrosis [124]. Laurent [129] underscored the fact that it is no longer tenable to view collagen as an inert protein and that its turnover may be more rapid than previously appreciated. In the heart, he estimates that collagen degradation may be as high as 5% per day.

One should, however, take into account that myocyte size declines more rapidly than the involution of collagen, a stable protein with a half-life of 80–120 days in the normal myocardium [129], and that not all antihypertensive agents can induce regression of myocardial fibrosis in hypertensive heart disease (Table 19.2).

## Clinical implications

It is widely recognized that the survival of patients with advanced, symptomatic heart failure is severely compromised despite widely used treatment with diuretics, digoxin, and vasodilators. These agents are prescribed to

**Table 19.2** Effects of antihypertensive drugs on myocardial structure

| Effect | Drugs |
|---|---|
| No regression of LVH | Hydralazine<br>Minoxidil |
| Regression of LVH, but no regression of myocardial fibrosis | α-Methyldopa<br>Clonidine<br>Reserpine<br>α-Receptor blockers<br>β-Receptor blockers<br>Diuretics |
| Regression of LVH and regression of myocardial fibrosis | ACE inhibitors<br>Spironolactone<br>$AT_1$ receptor antagonists<br>$Ca^{2+}$ channel blockers? |

LVH = left ventricular hypertrophy; ACE = angiotensin-converting enzyme; $AT_1$ = angiotensin II type 1.

attenuate the consequences of heart failure and therefore are palliative. More remedial therapy, with the objective of restoring the adverse structural remodelling and attendant functional abnormalities of the hypertrophied myocardium to normal, is needed. Drug with prognostic relevance in chronic heart failure include:

- a combination of isosorbidedinitrate and hydralazine;
- ACE inhibitors;
- β-receptor blockers;
- spironolactone;
- possibly, $AT_1$ receptor antagonists.

ACE inhibitors play a dominant role in the treatment of CHF. In addition to their beneficial effects on preload and afterload of chronically pressure and/or volume overloaded hearts, their favourable effects on the adverse structural remodelling of the myocardium include regression of myocyte hypertrophy, medial wall thickening of coronary resistance vessels, and myocardial fibrosis. The prognostic relevance of ACE inhibitors in patients with CHF may be partly explained by their pronounced antifibrotic effects, which were confirmed in a prospective, randomized, double-blind trial in which patients with LVH due to primary hypertension and left ventricular diastolic dysfunction were treated with either the ACE inhibitor lisinopril or the diuretic agent hydrochlorothiazide [5]. In this controlled trial, it was shown for the first time in humans that myocardial fibrosis can be regressed by chronic ACE inhibition, resulting in a significant improvement in left ventricular diastolic function [5].

The nature of the desired cardioreparative process will vary according to the aetiological basis of remodelling and hypertrophy of the myocardium. In this connection, the search for pathogenetic mechanisms must continue, including the identification of trophic factors that mediate myocyte and non-myocyte growth. Not surprisingly, antialdosterone treatment with spironolactone, in addition to basic therapy with ACE inhibitors, proved to be efficient, further reducing overall mortality by 30% in patients with severe CHF [130]. These prognostic effects of spironolactone may also be partly dependent on their proven antifibrotic effects on the myocardium. Phase III clinical trials are underway using the highly corticoid type I receptor-specific compound eplerenone.

These beneficial interventions are directed against the RAAS. In addition, the adrenergic system plays a major role in CHF. Although the adrenergic system can be pharmacologically inhibited at multiple levels, it is the use of receptor-blocking agents that has generated the most interest and provided the most data for this approach. From a large body of evidence [131], it is now clear that β-receptor blockade leads to a further reduction in total mortality of patients with CHF irrespective of the cause of heart failure. Whether treatment of failing hearts with negative-inotropic agents might have beneficial effects on protein phenotype has not been fully recognized. It has been suggested that interventions that reduce ventricular afterload will improve the function of subcellular organelles by reducing influences that lead to an adverse alteration of cardiac protein phenotype. Although this aspect of drug treatment has not been examined in detail, it is likely that several drug interventions act at least partially via this mechanism and may explain the beneficial effects of β-receptor-blocking agents in addition to their important effect on heart rate reduction, which leads to a more economical working condition with decreased oxygen consumption.

The response of the heart to pathological overload involves necessarily enhanced growth of the myocardium while maintaining wall stress in a normal range. If this growth would be associated with the appropriate protein composition of the heart muscle cell, pump failure would not a priori be expected. If, however, an imbalance occurs in the crucial proteins, a deterioration of cardiac function is likely to occur. Efforts are needed to develop drugs targeted at gene expression of the heart muscle cell. One potential approach could involve thyroid hormone analogues. In rats with left ventricular dysfunction after myocardial infarction, administration of the thyroid hormone analogue DITPA, combined with ACE inhibition by captopril, resulted in improvement of the resting and stressed cardiac index and left ventricular filling pressure [132]. Similar improvement of cardiac function was obtained when DITPA was administered to rabbits following myocardial infarction. Thus, a thyroid hormone analogue with inotropic selectivity may be a useful adjunct to ACE inhibition and antialdosterone therapy in the treatment of heart failure [132]. In an alternative approach, a drug-induced shift in the energy metabolism of the myocardium in favour of glucose utilization could be used. Chronic CPT-1 inhibition by treatment with etomoxir may represent such an approach for developing drugs that are useful in the prevention of undesirable consequences of pressure overload-induced LVH [115]. There is increasing evidence that etomoxir also has beneficial effects in patients with CHF. An open clinical pilot study showed that etomoxir administered on top of standard therapy (ACE inhibitors, diuretics, digitalis, and β-receptor blockers) improved the clinical status and myocardial function at maximum exercise in patients with CHF [133]. It should be pointed out that phenotype modulators would not acutely improve myocardial function but act via a chronically altered gene transcription or translation. Such an approach requires a certain amount of time to improve cardiac function, depending on the half-life of the various proteins of the cardiomyocyte. If treatment could be started before stimulation of the neuroendocrine system, with its detrimental effects on cardiac growth, one could envisage an approach with real preventive power.

## References


1. Kannel WB, Cobb J. Left ventricular hypertrophy and mortality — results from the Framingham Study. *Cardiology* 1992; 81: 291–8.
2. Beamish RE. Heart failure: the ironic failure of success. *Can J Cardiol* 1994; 10: 603.
3. Weber KT. Cardiac interstitium in health and disease: the fibrillar collagen network. *J Am Coll Cardiol* 1989; 13: 1637–52.
4. Factor SM, Robinson TF. Comparative connective tissue structure-function relationships in biologic pumps. *Lab Invest* 1988; 58: 150–6.
5. Brilla CG, Funck R, Rupp H. Lisinopril-mediated regression of myocardial fibrosis in patients with hypertensive heart disease. *Circulation* 2000; 102: 1388–93.
6. Brilla CG, Janicki JS, Weber KT. Cardioreparative effects of lisinopril in rats with genetic hypertension and left ventricular hypertrophy. *Circulation* 1991; 83: 1771–9.
7. Weber KT, Brilla CG. Pathological hypertrophy and cardiac interstitium. Fibrosis and renin–angiotensin–aldosterone system. *Circulation* 1991; 83: 1849–65.
8. Reimer KA, Jennings RB. Myocardial ischemia, hypoxia, and infarction. In: HA Fozzard, RB Jennings, E Haber, AM Katz (eds) *The heart and cardiovascular system*. New York: Raven Press, 1986, 1133–202.
9. Anversa P, Loud AV, Giacomelli F, Wiener J. Absolute morphometric study of myocardial hypertrophy in experimental hypertension. II. Ultrastructure of myocytes and interstitium. *Lab Invest* 1978; 38: 597–609.
10. Senger DR, Claffey KP, Benes JE *et al*. Angiogenesis promoted by vascular endothelial growth factor: regulation through α1β1 and α2β1 integrins. *Proc Natl Acad Sci USA* 1997; 94: 13 612–17.
11. Brilla CG, Pick R, Tan LB *et al*. Remodelling of the rat right and left ventricles in experimental hypertension. *Circ Res* 1990; 67: 1355–64.
12. Michel JB, Salzmann JL, Ossondo Nlom M *et al*. Morphometric analysis of collagen network and plasma perfused capillary bed in the myocardium of rats during evolution of cardiac hypertrophy. *Basic Res Cardiol* 1986; 81: 142–54.
13. Bartosova D, Chvapil M, Korecky B *et al*. The growth of the muscular and collagenous parts of the rat heart in various forms of cardiomegaly. *J Physiol* 1969; 200: 185–95.
14. Gilbert PL, Siegel RJ, Melmed S *et al*. Cardiac morphology in rats with growth hormone-producing tumors. *J Mol Cell Cardiol* 1985; 17: 805–11.
15. Hess OM, Schneider J, Koch R *et al*. Diastolic function and myocardial structure in patients with myocardial hypertrophy. Special reference to normalized viscoelastic data. *Circulation* 1981; 63: 360–71.
16. Pearlman ES, Weber KT, Janicki JS *et al*. Muscle fiber orientation and connective tissue content in the hypertrophied human heart. *Lab Invest* 1982; 46: 158–64.
17. Doering CW, Jalil JE, Janicki JS *et al*. Collagen network remodelling and diastolic stiffness of the rat left ventricle with pressure overload hypertrophy. Cardiovasc Res 1988; 22: 686–95.
18. Jalil JE, Doering CW, Janicki JS *et al*. Fibrillar collagen and myocardial stiffness in the intact hypertrophied rat left ventricle. *Circ Res* 1989; 64: 1041–50.
19. Weber KT, Janicki JS, Shroff SG *et al*. Collagen remodelling of the pressure-overloaded, hypertrophied nonhuman primate myocardium. *Circ Res* 1988; 62: 757–65.
20. Weber KT, Clark WA, Janicki JS, Shroff SG. Physiologic versus pathologic hypertrophy and the pressure-overloaded myocardium. *J Cardiovasc Phamacol* 1987; 10 (Suppl 6): S37–50.
21. Mann DL, Kent RL, Cooper G IV. Load regulation of the properties of adult feline cardiocytes: growth induction by cellular deformation. *Circ Res* 1989; 64: 1079–90.
22. Komuro I, Kaida T, Shibazaki Y *et al*. Stretching cardiac myocytes stimulates proto-oncogene expression. *J Biol Chem* 1990; 265: 3595–8.
23. Zimmer HG. Catecholamine-induced cardiac hypertrophy: significance of proto-oncogene expression. *J Mol Med* 1997; 75: 849–59.
24. Simpson P, McGrath A, Savion S. Myocyte hypertrophy in neonatal rat heart cultures and its regulation by serum and by catecholamines. *Circ Res* 1982; 51: 787–801.
25. Gregory P, Gagnon J, Essig DA *et al*. Differential regulation of action and myosin isoenzyme synthesis in functionally overloaded skeletal muscle. *Biochem J* 1990; 265: 525–32.
26. Böhm M, Flesch M, Schnabel P. Beta-adrenergic signal transduction in the failing and hypertrophied myocardium. *J Mol Med* 1997; 75: 842–8.
27. Bristow MR. Mechanism of action of beta-blocking agents in heart failure. *Am J Cardiol* 1997; 80: 26–40L.
28. Alpert NR, Hasenfuss G, Mulieri LA *et al*. The reorganization of the human and rabbit heart in response to hemodynamic overload. *Eur Heart J* 1992; 13 (Suppl D): 9–16.
29. Ebrecht G, Rupp H, Jacob R. Alterations of mechanical parameters in chemically skinned preparations of rat myocardium as a function of isoenzyme pattern of myosin. *Basic Res Cardiol* 1982; 77: 220–34.
30. Harris DE, Work SS, Wright RK *et al*. Smooth, cardiac and skeletal muscle myosin force and motion generation assessed by cross-bridge mechanical interactions *in vitro*. *J Muscle Res Cell Motil* 1994; 15: 11–19.
31. Limas CJ, Olivari MT, Goldenberg IF *et al*. Calcium uptake by sarcoplasmic reticulum in human dilated cardiomyopathy. *Cardiovasc Res* 1987; 21: 601–5.
32. Mercadier JJ, Lompre AM, Duc P. Altered sarcoplasmic reticulum Ca-ATPase gene expression in the human ventricle during end-stage heart failure. *J Clin Invest* 1990; 85: 305–9.
33. Takahashi T, Allen PD, Izumo S. Expression of A-, B-, and C-type natriuretic peptide genes in failing and developing human ventricles. Correlation with expression of the Ca ATPase gene. *Circ Res* 1992; 71: 9–17.

34. Vetter R, Rupp H. CPT-1 inhibition by Etomoxir has a chamber-related action on cardiac sarcoplasmic reticulum and isomyosins. *Am J Physiol* 1994; 267: H2091–9.
35. Rupp H, Schulze W, Vetter R. Dietary medium-chain triglycerides can prevent changes in myosin and SR due to CPT-1 inhibition by etomoxir. *Am J Physiol* 1995; 269: R630–40.
36. Turcani M, Rupp H. Etomoxir improves left ventricular performance of pressure-overloaded rat heart *Circulation* 1997; 96: 3681–6.
37. Hamilton N, Ianuzzo CD. Contractile and calcium regulating capacities of myocardia of different sized mammals scale with resting heart rate. *Mol Cell Biochem* 1991; 106: 133–41.
38. Pieske B, Hasenfuss G, Holubarsch C *et al.* Alterations of the force–frequency relationship in failing human heart depend on the underlying cardiac disease. *Basic Res Cardiol* 1992; 87 (Suppl I): 213–21.
39. Holubarsch C, Pieske B, Hasenfuss G. Pathologic versus adaptational alterations of hypertrophied and failing human myocardium. In: M Nagano, N Takeda, NS Dhalla (eds) *The adapted heart*. New York: Raven Press, 1994, 3–14.
40. O'Brien PJ, Ianuzzo CD, Moe GW *et al.* Rapid ventricular pacing of dogs to heart failure: biochemical and physiological studies. *Can J Physiol Pharmacol* 1990; 68: 34–9.
41. Chapman D, Weber KT, Eghbali M. Regulation of fibrillar collagen types I and III and basement membrane type IV collagen gene expression in pressure overloaded rat myocardium. *Circ Res* 1990; 67: 787–94.
42. Lindy S, Turto H, Uitto J. Protocollagen proline hydroxylase activity in rat heart during experimental cardiac hypertrophy. *Circ Res* 1972; 30: 205–9.
43. Caulfield JB, Borg TK. The collagen network of the heart. *Lab Invest* 1979; 40: 364–72.
44. Brilla CG, Maisch B, Weber KT. Myocardial collagen matrix remodelling in arterial hypertension. *Eur Heart J* 1992; 13 (Suppl D): 24–32.
45. Factor SM, Flomenbaum M, Zhao MJ *et al.* The effects of acutely increased ventricular cavity pressure on intrinsic myocardial connective tissue. *J Am Coll Cardiol* 1988; 12: 1582–9.
46. Jacob R, Gulch RW. Functional significance of ventricular dilatation. Reconsideration of Linzbach's concept of chronic heart failure. *Basic Res Cardiol* 1988; 83: 461–75.
47. Brilla CG, Krämer B, Hoffmeister HM *et al.* Low-dose enalapril as additional medication in severe chronic heart failure. *Dtsch Med Wochenschr* 1990; 115: 283–9.
48. Harris P. Evolution, cardiac failure, and water metabolism. Presidential address. *Adv Myocardiol* 1985; 5: 1–11.
49. Packer M. Neurohormonal interactions and adaptations in congestive heart failure. *Circulation* 1988; 77: 721–30.
50. Riley DJ, Weir M, Bakris GL. Renal adaptaion to the failing heart. Understanding the cascade of responses. *Postgrad Med* 1994; 95: 141–6.
51. Eghbali M, Weber KT. Collagen and the myocardium: fibrillar structure, biosynthesis and degradation in relation to hypertrophy and its regression. *Mol Cell Biochem* 1990; 96: 1–14.
52. Brilla CG, Reams GP, Maisch B, Weber KT. Renin–angiotensin system and myocardial fibrosis in hypertension: regulation of the myocardial collagen matrix. *Eur Heart J* 1993; 14 (Suppl J): 57–61.
53. Villarreal FJ, Kim NN, Ungab GD *et al.* Identification of functional angiotensin II receptors on rat cardiac fibroblasts. *Circulation* 1993; 88: 2849–61.
54. Brilla CG, Zhou G, Matsubara L, Weber KT. Collagen metabolism in cultured adult rat cardiac fibroblasts: response to angiotensin II and aldosterone. *J Mol Cell Cardiol* 1994; 26: 809–20.
55. Brilla CG, Scheer C, Rupp H. Angiotensin II and intracellular calcium of adult cardiac fibroblasts. *J Mol Cell Cardiol* 1998; 30: 1237–46.
56. Brilla CG, Scheer C, Rupp H. Renin-angiotensin system and myocardial collagen matrix: modulation of cardiac fibroblast function by angiotensin II type 1 receptor antagonism. *J Hypertens* 1997; 15: S13–19.
57. Eghbali M, Tomek R, Sukhatme VP *et al.* Differential effects of transforming growth factor-beta 1 and phorbol myristate acetate on cardiac fibroblasts. Regulation of fibrillar collagen mRNAs and expression of early transcription factors. *Circ Res* 1991; 69: 483–90.
58. Lee AA, Dillmann WH, McCulloch AD, Villarreal FJ. Angiotensin II stimulates the autocrine production of transforming growth factor-beta 1 in adult rat cardiac fibroblasts. *J Mol Cell Cardiol* 1995; 27: 2347–57.
59. Campbell SE, Katwa LC. Angiotensin II stimulated expression of transforming growth factor-beta1 in cardiac fibroblasts and myofibroblasts. *J Mol Cell Cardiol* 1997; 29: 1947–58.
60. Katwa LC, Weber KT. Aldosterone-induced expression of $ET_1$, $ET_3$ and $ET_B$ receptors by cultured adult rat cardiac fibroblasts. (Abstract). *Circulation* 1996; 94: I–146.
61. Chua CC, Diglio CA, Siu BB, Chua BH. Angiotensin II induces TGF-beta 1 production in rat heart endothelial cells. *Biochim Biophys Acta* 1994; 1223: 141–7.
62. Miki N, Hamamori Y, Hirata K *et al.* Transforming growth factor-beta 1 potentiated alpha 1-adrenergic and stretch-induced c-fos mRNA expression in rat myocardial cells. *Circ Res* 1994; 75: 8–14.
63. Sigel A, Douglas JA, Eghbali-Webb M. Regulation of mRNA transcripts and DNA synthesis in the rat heart following intravenous injection of transforming growth factor-beta1. *Mol Cell Biochem* 1994; 141: 145–51.
64. Brilla CG, Zhou G, Rupp H *et al.* Role of angiotensin II and prostaglandin $E_2$ in regulating cardiac fibroblast collagen turnover. *Am J Cardiol* 1995; 76: 8–13D.
65. Nakagawa M, Terracio L, Carver W *et al.* Expression of collagenase and IL-1 alpha in developing rat hearts. *Dev Dyn* 1992; 195: 87–99.
66. Tyagi SC, Ratajska A, Weber KT. Myocardial matrix metalloproteinase(s): localization and activation. *Mol Cell Biochem* 1993; 126: 49–59.
67. Marshall BC, Santana A, Xu QP *et al.* Metallo-proteinases and tissue inhibitor of metalloproteinases in mesothelial cells. Cellular differentiation influences expression. *J Clin Invest* 1993; 91: 1792–9.
68. Okada Y, Watanabe S, Nakanishi I *et al.* Inactivation of tissue inhibitor of metalloproteinases by neutrophil elastase and other serine proteinases. *FEBS Lett* 1988; 229: 157–60.
69. McDonald JA, Kelly DG, Broekelmann J. Role of fibronectin in collagen deposition: Fab, to the gelatin-binding domain of fibronectin inhibits both fibronectin and collagen organization in fibroblast extracellular matrix. *J Cell Biol* 1982; 92: 485.
70. Crawford DC, Chobanian AV, Brecher P. Angiotensin II induces fibronectin expression associated with cardiac fibrosis in the rat. *Circ Res* 1994; 74: 727–39.
71. Robinson TF, Factor SM, Sonnenblick EH. The heart as a suction pump. *Sci Am* 1986; 254: 84–91.

72. Wong HL, Wahl SM. Inflammation and repair. In: MB Sporn, AB Roberts (eds) *Peptide growth factors and their receptors II*. New York: Springer, 1991, 509–48.
73. Agelli M, Wahl SM. Collagen production by fibroblasts. *Methods Enzymol* 1988; 163: 642–56.
74. Brilla CG, Matsubara LS, Weber KT. Anti-aldosterone treatment and the prevention of myocardial fibrosis in primary and secondary hyperaldosteronism. *J. Mol Cell Cardiol* 1993; 25: 563–75.
75. Weber KT, Pick R, Silver MA *et al.* Fibrillar collagen and remodelling of dilated canine left ventricle. *Circulation* 1990; 82: 1387–401.
76. Morkin E, Ashford TP. Myocardial DNA synthesis in experimental cardiac hypertrophy. *Am J Physiol* 1968; 215: 1409–13.
77. Silver MA, Pick R, Brilla CG *et al.* Reactive and reparative fibrillar collagen remodelling the hypertrophied rat left ventricle: two experimental models of myocardial fibrosis. *Cardiovasc Res* 1990; 24: 741–7.
78. Brilla CG, Weber KT. Reactive and reparative myocardial fibrosis in arterial hypertension in the rat. *Cardiovasc Res* 1992; 26: 671–7.
79. Weber KT, Janicki JS, Pick R *et al.* Myocardial fibrosis and pathologic hypertrophy in the rat with renovascular hypertension. *Am J Cardiol* 1990; 65: 1–7G.
80. Jalil JE, Janicki JS, Pick R *et al.* Fibrosis-induced reduction of endomyocardium in the rat after isoproterenol treatment. *Circ Res* 1989; 65: 258–64.
81. Carroll EP, Janicki JS, Pick R, Weber KT. Myocardial stiffness and reparative fibrosis following coronary embolization in the rat. *Cardiovasc Res* 1989; 23: 655–61.
82. Capasso JM, Palackal T, Olivetti G, Anversa P. Left ventricular failure induced by long-term hypertension in rats. *Circ Res* 1990; 66: 1400–12.
83. Brilla CG, Janicki JS, Weber KT. Impaired diastolic function and coronary reserve in genetic hypertension. Role of interstitial fibrosis and medial thickening of intramyocardial coronary arteries. *Circ Res* 1991; 69: 107–15.
84. Morkin E. Regulation of myosin heavy chain genes in the heart. *Circulation* 1993; 87: 1451–60.
85. Hartong R, Wang N, Kurokawa R *et al.* Delineation of three different thyroid hormone-response elements in promoter of rat sarcoplasmic reticulum $Ca^{2+}$ ATPase gene. Demonstration that retinoid X receptor binds 5′ to thyroid hormone receptor in response element 1. *J Biol Chem* 1994; 269: 13 021–9.
86. Müller MJ, Seitz HJ. Thyroid hormone action on intermediary metabolism. *Klin Wochenschr* 1984; 62: 97–102.
87. Dillmann WH. Cardiac function in thyroid disease: clinical features and management considerations. *Ann Thorac Surg* 1993; 56: S9–14.
88. Dillmann WH. Biochemical basis of thyroid hormone action in the heart. *Am J Med* 1990; 88: 626–30.
89. Edwards JG, Bahl JJ, Flink IL *et al.* Thyroid hormone influences beta myosin heavy chain (beta MHC) expression. *Biochem Biophys Res Commun* 1994; 199: 1482–8.
90. Rohrer D, Dillmann WH. Thyroid hormone markedly increses the mRNA coding for sarcoplasmic reticulum $Ca^{2+}$-ATPase in the rat heart. *J Biol Chem* 1988; 263: 6941–4.
91. Arai M, Otsu K, MacLennan DH *et al.* Effect of thyroid hormone on the expression of mRNA encoding sarcoplasmic reticulum proteins. *Circ Res* 1991; 69: 266–76.
92. Morkin E, Pennock GD, Raya TE *et al.* Studies on the use of thyroid hormone and a thyroid hormone analogue in the treatment of congestive heart failure. *Ann Thorac Surg* 1993; 56: S54–60.
93. Pennock GD, Raya TE, Bahl JJ *et al.* Combination treatment with captopril and the thyroid hormone analogue 3,5-diiodothyropropionic acid. A new approach to improving left ventricular performance in heart failure. *Circulation* 1993; 88: 1289–98.
94. Pennock GD, Milavetz JJ, Raya TE *et al.* Identification of simple substituted phenols with thyromimetic activity: cardiac effects of 3.5-diiodo-4-hydroxyphenylpropionic acid. *J Pharmacol Exp Ther* 1994; 268: 216–23.
95. Pennock GD, Raya TE, Bahl JJ *et al.* Cardiac effects of 3,5-diiodothyropropionic acid, a thyroid hormone analog with inotropic selectivity. *J Pharmacol Exp Ther* 1992; 263: 163–9.
96. Rupp H. The adaptive changes in the isoenzyme pattern of myosin from hypertrophied rat myocardium as a result of pressure overload and physical training. *Basic Res Cardiol* 1981; 76: 79–88.
97. Rupp H, Wahl R. Influence of thyroid hormones and catecholamines on myosin of swim-exercised rats. *J Appl Physiol* 1990; 68: 973–8.
98. Rupp H, Berger HJ, Pfeifer A, Werdan K. Effect of positive inotropic agents on myosin isozyme population and mechanical activity of cultured rat heart myocytes. *Circ Res* 1991; 68: 1164–73.
99. Gupta MP, Gupta M, Stewart A, Zak R. Activation of alpha-myosin heavy chain gene expression by cAMP in cultured fetal rat heart myocytes. *Biochem Biophys Res Commun* 1991; 174: 1196–203.
100. Gupta MP, Gupta M, Zak R. The dynamic state of cardiac phenotype. Modulation by the beta-adrenergic system. In: M Nagano, N Takeda, NS Dhalla (eds) *The adapted heart*. New York: Raven Press, 1994, 65–83.
101. Goldspink PH, Russell B. The cAMP response element binding protein is expressed and phosphorylated in cardiac myocytes. *Circ Res* 1994; 74: 1042–9.
102. Kawana M, Kimata S, Hosoda S. The change in expression of cardiac myosin isozymes by the stimulation of the sympathetic nerve and thyroxine. In: M Nagano, N Takeda, NS Dhalla (eds) *The adapted heart*. New York: Raven Press, 1994, 393–401.
103. Rupp H, Takeda N. Sympathetic nervous system activity and regulation of cardiac gene expression. In: PK Ganguly (ed.) *Catecholamines and heart disease*. Boca Raton: CRC Press, 1991, 217–29.
104. Rupp H, Jacob R. Ventricular myocardium as a fast- or slow-type muscle. The influence of stressors and the preventive action of intense exercise. In: RE Beamish, V Panagia, NS Dhalla (eds) *Pathogenesis of stress-induced heart disease*. Boston, MA: Martinus Nijhoff, 1985, 147–58.
105. Rupp H, Elimban V, Dhalla NS. Sucrose feeding prevents changes in myosin isoenzymes and sarcoplasmic reticulum $Ca^{2+}$-pump ATPase in pressure-loaded rat heart. *Biochem Biophys Res Commun* 1988; 156: 917–23.
106. Rupp H, Elimban V, Dhalla NS. Diabetes-like action of intermittent fasting on sarcoplasmic reticulum $Ca^{2+}$-pump ATPase and myosin isoenzymes can be prevented by sucrose. *Biochem Biophys Res Commun* 1989; 164: 319–25.
107. Rupp H, Elimban V, Dhalla NS. Modification of myosin isozymes and SR Ca(2+)-pump ATPase of the diabetic rat heart by lipid-lowering interventions. *Mol Cell Biochem* 1994; 132: 69–80.

108. Dhalla NS, Elimban V, Rupp H. Paradoxical role of lipid metabolism in heart function and dysfunction. *Mol Cell Biochem* 1992; 116: 3–9.
109. Rupp H, Jacob R. Metabolically-modulated growth and phenotype of the rat heart. *Eur Heart J* 1992; 13 (Suppl D): 56–61.
110. Rupp H, Elimban V, Dhalla NS. Modification of subcellular organelles in pressure-overloaded heart by etomoxir, a carnitine palmitoyltransferase I inhibitor. *FASEB J* 1992; 6: 2349–53.
111. Rupp H, Wahl R, Hansen M. Influence of diet and carnitine palmitoyltransferase I inhibition on myosin and sarcoplasmic reticulum. *J Appl Physiol* 1992; 72: 352–60.
112. Chen S, Ogawa A, Ohneda M *et al.* More direct evidence for a malonyl-CoA-carnitine palmitoyltransferase I interaction as a key event in pancreatic beta-cell signaling. *Diabetes* 1994; 43: 878–83.
113. Kerner J, Zaluzec E, Gage D, Bieber LL. Characterization of the malonyl-CoA-sensitive carnitine palmitoyltransferase (CPTo) of a rat heart mitochondrial particle. Evidence that the catalytic unit is CPTi. *J Biol Chem* 1994; 269: 8209–19.
114. Belloiu DD. Biochemical considerations regarding cellular regulation through messenger and allosteric systems. Antagonism between catabolic oxidation of free fatty acids and anabolic aerobic glycolysis in the liver. *Endocrinologie* 1990; 28: 3–13.
115. Turcani M, Jacob R, Rupp H. Inhibition of carnitine palmitoyltransferase-1 by etomoxir increases relaxation parameters and working capacity of overloaded rat hearts. Abstract. *Pflügers Arch* 1994; 426 (Suppl): R150.
116. WolfHP. Possible new therapeutic approach in diabetes mellitus by inhibition of carnitine palmitoyltransferase 1 (CPT1). *Horm Metab Res* 1992; 26 (Suppl): 62–7.
117. Hubinger A, Weikert G, Wolf HP, Gries FA. The effect of etomoxir on insulin sensitivity in type 2 diabetic patients. *Horm Metab Res* 1992; 24: 115–18.
118. Ratheiser K, Schneeweiss B, Waldhausl W *et al.* Inhibition by etomoxir of carnitine palmitoyltransferase I reduces hepatic glucose production and plasma lipids in non-insulin-dependent diabetes mellitus. *Metabolism* 1991; 40: 1185–90.
119. Rupp H. Diastolic dysfunction of the heart: pharmacological strategies for modulating calcium sequestration of the sarcoplasmic reticulum. In: B Ostadal, NS Dhalla (eds) *Heart function in health and disease.* Boston, MA: Kluwer Academic, 1993, 251–71.
120. Jalil JE, Janicki JS, Pick R, Weber KT. Coronary vascular remodelling and myocardial fibrosis in the rat with renovascular hypertension: response to captopril. *Am J Hypertens* 1991; 4: 51–5.
121. Brilla CG. Regression of myocardial fibrosis in hypertensive heart disease: diverse effects of various antihypertensive drugs. *Cardiovasc Res* 2000; 46: 342–31.
122. Young M, Fullerton M, Dilley R, Funder J. Mineralocorticoids, hypertension, and cardiac fibrosis. *J Clin Invest* 1994; 93: 2578–83.
123. Robert V, Silvestre JS, Charlemagne D *et al.* Biological determinants of aldosterone-induced cardiac fibrosis in rats. *Hypertension* 1995; 26: 971–8.
124. Brilla CG, Matsubara L, Weber KT. Advanced hypertensive heart disease in spontaneously hypertensive rats: Lisinopril-mediated regression of myocardial fibrosis. *Hypertension* 1996; 28: 269–75.
125. Benetos A, Lacolley P, Safar ME. Prevention of aortic fibrosis by spironolactone in spontaneously hypertensive rats. *Arterioscler Thromb Vasc Biol* 1997; 17: 1152–6.
126. Brilla CG, Zhou G, Myers PR, Weber KT. Angiotensin II-mediated aldosterone synthesis in cultured bovine aortic endothelial cells. *J Hypertens* 1992; 10 (Suppl 4): S75.
127. Silvestre JS, Robert V, Hymes C *et al.* Myocardial production of aldosterone and corticosterone in the rat. Physiological regulation. *J Biol Chem* 1998; 273: 4883–91.
128. Montfort I, Perez-Tamayo R. The distribution of collagenase in normal rat tissues. *J Histochem Cytochem* 1975; 23: 910–20.
129. Laurent GJ. Dynamic state of collagen: pathways of collagen degradation *in vivo* and their possible role in regulation of collagen mass. *Am J Physiol* 1987; 252: C1–9.
130. Pitt B, Zannad F, Remme WJ *et al.* For the Randomized Aldactone Evaluation Study Investigators. The effect of spironolactone on morbidity and mortality in patients with severe heart failure. *N Engl J Med* 1999; 341: 709–17.
131. The MERIT-HF Investigators. Effect of metoprolol CR/XL in chronic heart failure: Metoprolol CR/XL randomised intervention trial in congestive heart failure (MERIT-HF). *Lancet* 1999; 353: 2001–7.
132. Morkin E, Pennock GD, Raya TE *et al.* Development of a thyroid hormone analogue for the treatment of congestive heart failure. *Thyroid* 1996; 6: 521–6.
133. Schmidt-Schweda S, Holubarsch C. First clinical trial with etomoxir in patients with chronic heart failure II–III. Abstract. *J Mol Cell Cardiol* 1997; 29: A55.

# SECTION III

# Pathogenetic basis of secondary cardiomyopathic disorders

# Myocardial involvement in ischaemic heart disease: role of hibernating myocardium

20

S. H. RAHIMTOOLA

## Introduction

An editorial in *American Heart Journal* in 1989 [1] stated:

The term *hibernating myocardium* was coined to describe a state of persistently impaired myocardial and LV [left ventricular] function at rest due to reduced coronary blood flow that can be partially or completely restored to normal if the myocardial oxygen supply/demand relationship is favourably altered, either by improving blood flow and/or by reducing demand [Fig. 20.1] [3, 4]. It likely results from a relatively uncommon response to reduced MBF [myocardial blood flow] at rest whereby the heart downgrades its myocardial function to the extent that blood flow and function are once again in equilibrium, and as a result, neither myocardial necrosis nor ischaemic symptoms are present. Obviously, if the myocardial oxygen supply/demand balance is subsequently altered unfavourably either temporarily or permanently, then symptoms and signs of ischaemia and/or of necrosis again occur. Repeated episodes of ischaemia may

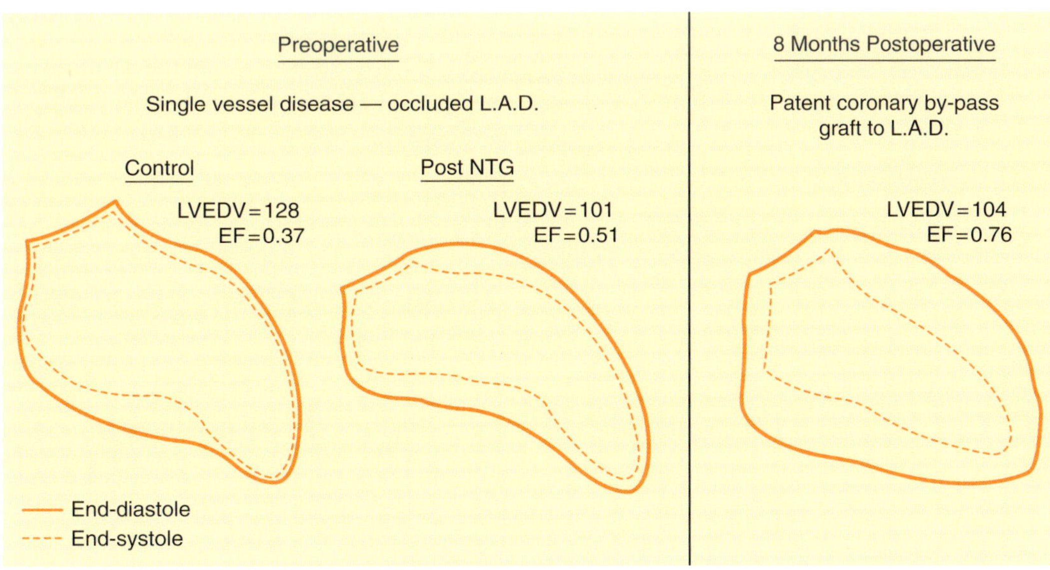


**Figure 20.1** *End-diastolic and end-systolic silhouettes of the left ventricle from the right anterior oblique ventriculogram. (A) In the preoperative studies the ejection fraction (EF) in the control state was 0.37 and there was a large akinetic area involving the anteroapical wall. After nitroglycerin (NTG), there was an improvement in wall motion in the akinetic zone, and EF improved to 0.51. The patient had no history of myocardial infarction. Coronary arteriography showed one-vessel disease with a totally occluded left anterior descending coronary artery (LAD). The distal LAD was filled by collaterals from the circumflex coronary artery and the posterior descending coronary artery. (B) At 8 months postoperatively on routine study, the graft was fully patent and there was good filling of the LAD. The patient now shows normal left ventricular wall motion function and a normal EF of 0.76. (From ref. 2 with permission.)*

lead to necrosis [5] and therefore are undesirable; thus the hibernating response of the heart, namely, a reduction of function to cope with a reduced MBF, could be considered an act of self preservation (little blood, little work) and the heart could be considered to be a 'smart heart.

Some earlier work and many subsequent studies have confirmed that most, if not all, of these initial postulates were correct. For example, short-term or acute hibernation results from both an adaptation [6–9] and a downregulation [10] to reduced myocardial blood flow (MBF), and hibernating myocardium (HM) in the clinical setting is associated with reduced MBF [11]. It was shown in 1974 [12] that in some patients with an occluded graft after coronary by pass surgery (CBS), the resting preoperative left ventricular (LV) systolic dysfunction improved and in some, even global LV systolic dysfunction had normalized, because other grafts in the patient were patent and provided adequate collateral circulation to the myocardial segments usually supplied by the occluded graft.

In the 1970s, attention was focused on proving the reversibility of resting LV dysfunction with CBS and on detecting it preoperatively [13–28]. In the 1980 Consensus Development Conference on Coronary Artery Bypass Surgery [29], the present author failed to convince people about the presence of abnormal LV function that was due to chronic, painless, persistent, severe myocardial 'ischaemia' at rest, and which was reversible [2, 30]. This concept was not accepted because: (1) chronic, persistent, low-flow ischaemia was not thought possible; (2) painless ischaemia was not generally accepted as an entity, particularly in the USA; and (3) there were no experimental studies documenting its occurrence. At that time it was generally believed that persistent abnormal LV function at rest was due to irreversible myocardial necrosis and that prolonged 'ischaemia' with or without pain was not possible. Even though painless ischaemia had been described in the 1970s, only in the 1980s did it become accepted as being quite common in patients with a variety of anginal syndromes [31, 32].

In 1979 it was shown that 'fixed' perfusion defects, as seen by thallium-201 ($^{201}$Tl) imaging on stress and redistribution, improved and even normalized after bypass surgery [33]. This was confirmed in 1983 in a larger number of patients [34]. These 'fixed' defects were considered to be the result of irreversible myocardial damage until Dilsizian *et al.* [35] documented in 1990 that on reinjection of $^{201}$Tl after the redistribution images had been obtained, many segments with 'fixed' defects had uptake of the tracer and were therefore viable. It is possible that a very large number of patients were denied revascularization because of these 'fixed' defects, emphasizing the need for caution in applying incomplete knowledge about tests to all patients. In 1979 Gewirtz *et al.* [36] documented that $^{201}$Tl could be taken up on redistribution after rest, but the clinical significance of this observation was initially not fully appreciated.

From 1983 to 1985, the author was unable to convince his colleagues that it was worth dedicating research funds to the study of chronic painless ischaemia and the associated LV dysfunction. A short, less complex term was needed to describe this phenomenon (abnormal LV function at rest due to chronic painless, resting, persistent myocardial ischaemia, which was reversible) before it would gain more widespread recognition and acceptance. Therefore, the author used the term 'hibernating myocardium' in 1984 [4] in a National Heart, Lung, and Blood Institute (NHLBI) Workshop on the Treatment of Coronary Artery Disease [37]. It was more readily accepted than at the 1980 Conference, probably because painless ischaemia was being more widely recognized, and attention was focused on the other more important statements about CBS. Bashour's editorial [38] in August 1986 drew attention to HM and the concept of 'electrical stunning' (transient Q waves from profound myocardial ischaemia). Braunwald and Rutherford's subsequent editorial [39] in December 1986 endorsed the concept of HM, believed that it was an appropriate use of the term, and confirmed its occurrence in patients.

## Advantages and definition of the term hibernating myocardium

The concept and the term HM have been accepted [11] because during the 1990s there has been a great deal of basic and clinical research in this area, a reassessment of the definition of ischaemia [40], the development and assessment of tests for the diagnosis of HM, and better treatment of patients with heart disease. Much work still needs to be done in this field.

HM is described by the clinical situation: impaired LV function at rest that is reversible by revascularization. Ross [41] described HM as perfusion–contraction matching which it is; however, in the normal heart and probably also in one with myocardial infarction (MI), a high degree of interstitial fibrosis, and with myocytes with myolysis or loss of sarcomeres, there is also a match between perfusion and contraction [42, 43]. Ross also suggested that the sustained perfusion–contraction matching seen in acute experimental studies and some clinical settings be termed 'short-term hibernation' and that the chronic perfusion–contraction matching seen in clinical syndromes be called 'chronic hibernation' [41]. Some of the differences between short-term and chronic hibernation are shown in Table 20.1.

Hearse [40] has defined HM as: 'exquisitely regulated tissue successfully adapting its activity to prevailing circumstances'.

## Hibernation and ischaemia

The question of whether HM is ischaemia or not is to some extent semantic, depending on the definition of ischaemia. Amazingly, even in 1994 there was no clear accepted definition of ischaemia [40]. If ischaemia is defined as just a reduction in MBF, then HM is a form of ischaemia. However, if one defines ischaemia as reduced MBF with evidence of an associated effect (apart from reduced LV contraction), then HM is probably not ischaemic myocardium. The definition of ischaemia as an imbalance between supply and demand may be too simplistic; at a minimum, 'demand' should be changed to 'need' [42].

One definition of ischaemia [42] could be: a reduction in MBF associated with perturbations of cardiac function(s) and/or structure. The definition could be modified or expanded to include special situations, such as 'absolute' versus 'relative' reduction in flow, anaemia, specific biochemical abnormalities, removal of metabolites, release of cytokines, or alteration of cardiac genes and gene products. One could also subcategorize myocardial ischaemia into physiological or biochemical, as suggested by Hearse [40].

Clinically, significant myocardial ischaemia is assumed to be present when there is some abnormality that can be demonstrated with the ischaemic episode. Therefore, it was postulated that HM may not represent ischaemia 'in the strict sense' [1].

Indeed, HM may be a unique pathophysiological state that we may not be able to characterize or define perfectly at present [44]; more research and data are needed. Hearse suggests that it may be more appropriately viewed as an example of: (1) an 'exquisitely regulated tissue successfully adapting its activity to prevailing circumstances' [40]; and (2) 'a process of controlled active down-regulation' [43].

**Table 20.1** Some characteristics of various manifestations of hibernating myocardium

| | | |
|---|---|---|
| Terminology | | |
| Experimental | Short term | Chronic |
| Clinical | Acute | Subacute |
| | Subacute | Chronic |
| Myocardium | | |
| Hibernating | Normal | Near normal |
| | Some structural changes | Some structural changes |
| | | Marked structural changes[a] |
| Adjacent | Infarcted | Infarcted |
| | Fibrotic | Fibrotic |
| | Normal | Normal |
| Prior to hibernation | Acute ischaemic Episode(s) | Acute ischaemic episode(s) |
| | Gradual reduction of blood flow | Gradual reduction of blood flow |
| | Stunning? | Stunning? |
| Recovery from hibernation | Rapid/slow | Rapid/slow/very slow |
| | Stunning may occur | Stunning? |
| | LV function: normal or less abnormal | LV function: normal or less abnormal |

[a]'De-differentiation' or 'disuse atrophy/wasting from prolonged inactivity and unloading of muscle' and varying degrees or degeneration/fibrosis from infarction.
LV = left ventricular.

## Some characteristics of hibernating myocardium

### Evidence of reduced myocardial blood flow

There is a large number of studies showing that there is reduced MBF in HM [11, 44, 45]. These include: (1) documentation of reduced MBF using inert gas techniques, position emission tomography (PET) using [$^{12}$N]ammonia (Table 20.2, and PET using [$^{13}$]acetate; (2) documentation of reduced perfusion by radionuclide studies rest–redistribution and of stress–redistribution–reinjection; (3) documentation of reduced perfusion by PET showing a 'mismatch' between perfusion and metabolism (reduced perfusion but normal metabolism); and (4) myocardial revascularization resulting in improvement in or normalization of both MBF (measured by PET or radionuclide uptake at rest) and LV dysfunction.

### Recovery of hibernating myocardium

The rate of recovery of resting LV dysfunction after revascularization and the morphological changes in the dysfunctional myocardium have allowed HM to be classified as acute, subacute, or chronic (Fig. 20.2) [53].

#### *Acute recovery*

When HM recovers 'immediately' or very rapidly after revascularization (Fig. 20.3) [55–57], it is presumptive evidence that the myocardium is normal or almost normal. This has been confirmed by electron-microscopic studies of transmural myocardial biopsies in patients undergoing CBS [58] or at autopsy [59]. Studies on acute hibernation confirm this observation.

#### *Chronic recovery*

The recovery time of HM after revascularization may be quite long, up to 1 year (Table 20.3). Electron-microscopic studies of transmural myocardial biopsies at the time of CBS have demonstrated marked abnormalities, the most striking of which are loss of myofibrillar content and excessive accumulation of glycogen [46, 61, 62]; normalization can be expected to take time after revascularization. Animal models of a longer duration of reduced coronary blood flow are being developed [16, 63–67].

#### *Subacute recovery*

Data from Matsuzaki *et al.* [68] showed that recovery of LV function after 5 h of reduced perfusion, reduced contraction, and little or no MI (hibernation) was gradual over a 7 day period; this is likely to represent stunning following reperfusion of HM. In a patient with HM reported by Baker *et al.* [69], recovery of LV dysfunction was gradual over 10–60 weeks. Some patients whose HM was revascularized by CBS [70] and percutaneous transluminal coronary angioplasty (PTCA) [71] showed a similar slow recovery of LV function. Since hibernation was likely to have been present for a prolonged period before reperfusion, this represents subacute hibernation. In patients whose ventricular function normalized months after revascularization, the myocardium may have undergone changes similar to those that may be present with early chronic hibernation (see

**Table 20.2** Myocardial blood flow at rest by positron emission tomography using [$^{13}$N] ammonia in hibernating myocardium (HM)

| Authors [ref.] | No. pts | Myocardial blood flow[a]: Areas with normal LV function[b] | Areas with HM[b] | *p*-Value |
|---|---|---|---|---|
| Vanoverschelde *et al.* [46] | 17 | 95.5 ± 26.7 | 77.1 ± 24.6 | < 0.001 |
| Czernin *et al.* [47] | 22 | 83 ± 20 | 57 ± 20 | < 0.05 |
| Marzullo *et al.* [48] | 14 | 100 ± 24 | 42 ± 12 | [c] |
| Shivalkar *et al.* [49] | 18 | 93.4 ± 12.6 | 63.8 ± 12.8 | < 0.005[d] |
| Sun *et al.* [50] | 5 | 80.8 ± 26 | 59.2 ± 25 | 0.004 |

[a]Mean ± SD ml/min per 100 g).
[b]In the same patients in each study.
[c]In each patient myocardial blood flow (mBF) was > 2SD below the mean in normals.
[d]Prof. W. Flameng, personal communication.
pts = patients; LV = left ventricular
NB. Sambuceti *et al.* [51] described six patients with LV dysfunction, all had MBF > 2SD below normal values. (From ref. 11 with permission.)

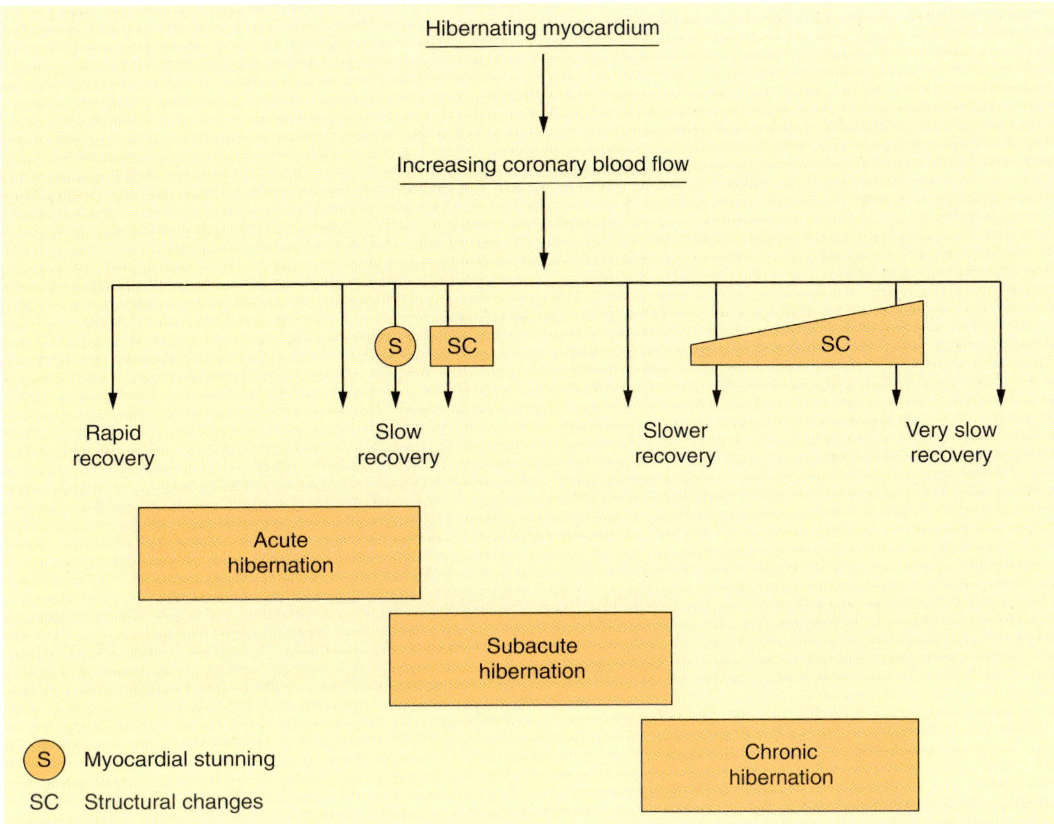


**Figure 20.2** *Rates of recovery (rapid to very slow) of left ventricular (LV) function after increasing coronary blood in hibernating myocardium (HM). The role of stunned myocardium and of structural changes in the myocardium is shown. The possible range of acute, subacute, and chronic HM based on rate of recovery of LV function is illustrated. (Adapted from ref. 52 with permission.)*

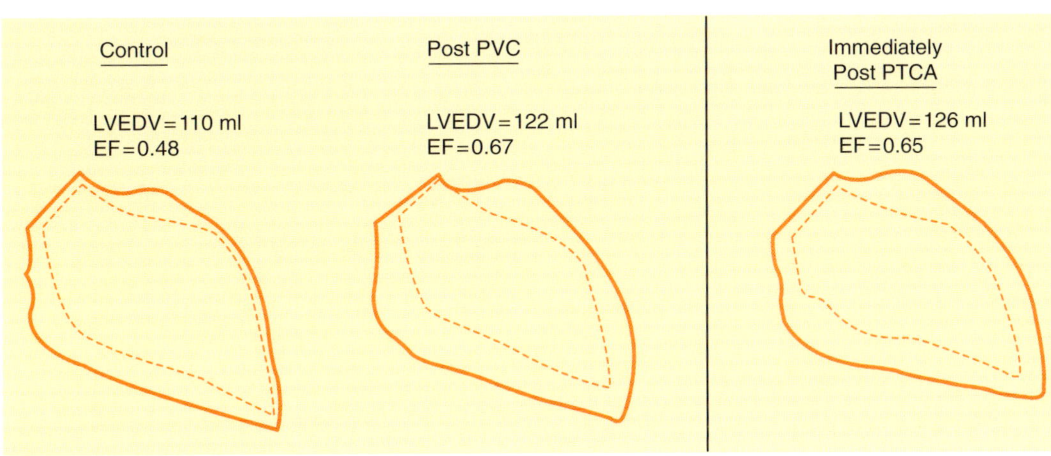


**Figure 20.3** *Example of hibernating myocardium. The patient had severe (95–99%) stenosis of the proximal left anterior descending coronary artery. At rest, the anterior left ventricular (LV) wall is severely hypokinetic or akinetic and the LV ejection fraction (EF) is 0.48. In the post-premature ventricular beat, the wall motion function and EF are normal. Immediately after successful percutaneous transluminal coronary angioplasty, LV wall motion and EF are normal. (From ref. 54 with permission.)*

**Table 20.3** Left ventricular (LV) function before and after coronary artery bypass grafting

| Time-point | LV end-diastolic dimension (mm) | Doppler mitral regurgitation | Radionuclide ejection fraction (%) | |
|---|---|---|---|---|
| | | | Rest | Exercise |
| Initial | 66 | Severe | 16 | 15 |
| 4 weeks postoperatively | 68 | Moderate | 26 | 24 |
| 6 weeks postoperatively | 52 | Mild | 33 | 34 |
| 1 year postoperatively[a] | 50 | — | 52 | — |

[a]L.W. Stevenson, personal communication (1992). (From ref. 60 with permission.)

above), which takes longer to recover. The delayed recovery of function could represent either stunning following hibernation [72] or subacute hibernation that takes time to recover (Fig. 20.2). It is likely that both can occur; in some patients reperfusion of HM is followed by stunning, and in others myocardial abnormalities associated with subacute hibernation take time to recover after reperfusion.

## From coronary artery disease to heart failure

LV dysfunction is an important consequence of coronary artery disease (CAD) and results from acute myocardial ischaemia, HM, or MI. Myocardial stunning, which is a short-term phenomenon, may be superimposed on any of these situations and may eventually lead to heart failure (Fig. 20.4). Occasionally, however, CAD produces a mechanical defect (e.g. mitral regurgitation, ventricular septal defect) that may result in clinical heart failure without significant LV systolic dysfunction. LV dysfunction from any cause results in or contributes to myocardial ischaemia by increasing myocardial oxygen need and reducing coronary blood flow [74]. Structural changes commonly

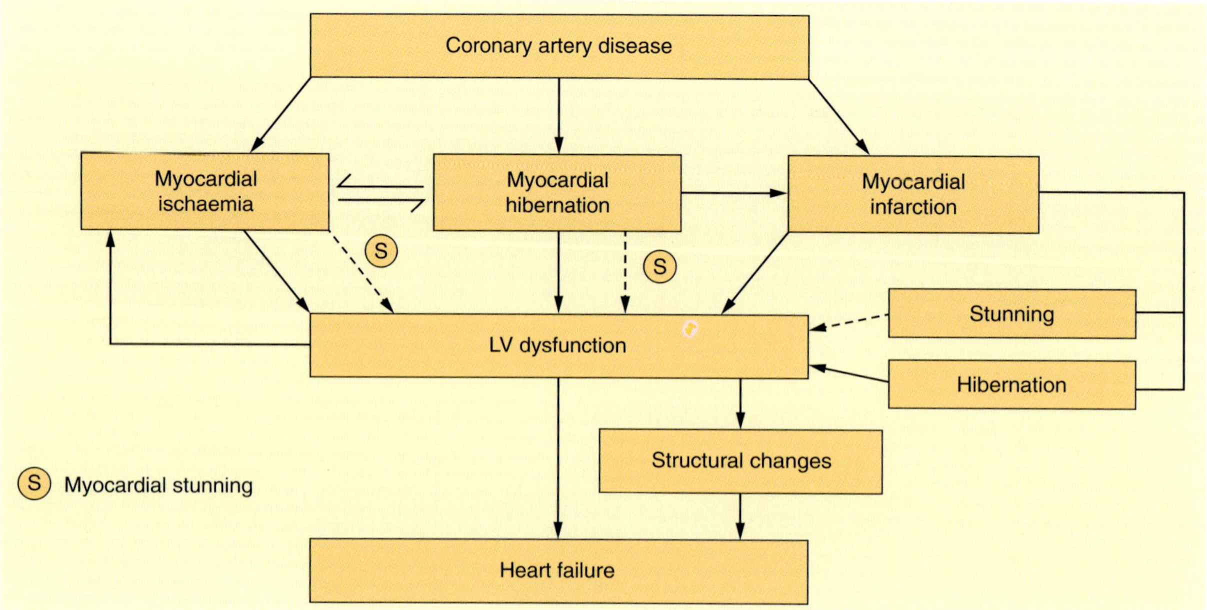


**Figure 20.4** *Coronary artery disease may result in myocardial ischaemia, hibernation, or infarction, all of which are associated with left ventricular (LV) dysfunction. Hibernation may also be associated with subsequent acute ischaemia or infarction. Stunning may be superimposed on ischaemia or hibernating myocardium on reperfusion. Both hibernating and stunned myocardium can be present in patients who have myocardial infarction. By definition, stunning usually improves spontaneously over time. LV dysfunction with or without associated structural changes may produce clinical heart failure. Except for infarcted myocardial tissue, all other states are potentially reversible with appropriate and timely treatment. (From ref. 73 with permission.)*

occur in LV dysfunction, and if it persists, may lead to heart failure. HM can be partially or completely restored to normal with therapy, and LV systolic dysfunction may normalize or improve. The extent of and the time to improvement of LV function is dependent of the adequacy of revascularization and the extent and severity of myocardial changes that were present prior to the revascularization. LV dysfunction or heart failure caused or exacerbated by HM can be improved with appropriate therapy. However, if the HM is not appropriately treated in a timely manner, it may be associated with progressive cellular damage, recurrent myocardial ischaemia, MI, heart failure, and death [73].

## Clinical picture

### Spectrum

Initially, the two clinical entities diagnosed in patients with CAD were angina and MI. Subsequently, it was recognized that these two conditions could be painless, and so the terms unstable angina and non-Q-wave MI were introduced. HM is one of three new ischaemic myocardial states that fit between angina and MI (Fig. 20.5) [75].

### Viable myocardium

Areas of LV myocardium that are viable are those that have: (1) normal LV function at rest; (2) LV dysfunction at rest but with irreversible damage, stunned myocardium, and HM; and (3) LV dysfunction from ischaemia, due to increased myocardial needs for, or a reduced supply of oxygen, substrates, etc.

The combinations of various myocardial states that may be present in patients with LV dysfunction at rest are shown in Table 20.4.

### Clinical conditions and hibernating myocardium

HM has thus far been documented in chronic stable and unstable angina, acute, MI, heart failure, and a nomylous left coronary artery from the pulmonary artery (ALCAPA) [75].

The angina associated with HM is either chronic stable or unstable. With acute MI, HM is known to occur in a region of the LV wall at a distance from the area of the MI (Fig. 20.6) [1]. LV dysfunction away from the area of a first infarct is presumptive evidence of HM in that area until

**Table 20.4** Myocardial states frequently present in patients in areas of left ventricular (LV) dysfunction at rest

| State of myocardium | Combinations of various myocardial states in patients with LV dysfunction at rest | | | | | |
|---|---|---|---|---|---|---|
| Irreversibly damaged | + | + | + | + | – | – |
| Viable and at risk | | | | | | |
| Hibernating | – | + | – | + | + | + |
| Ischaemic on 'stress' | – | – | + | + | – | + |

+ = yes; – = no. (From ref. 75 with permission.)

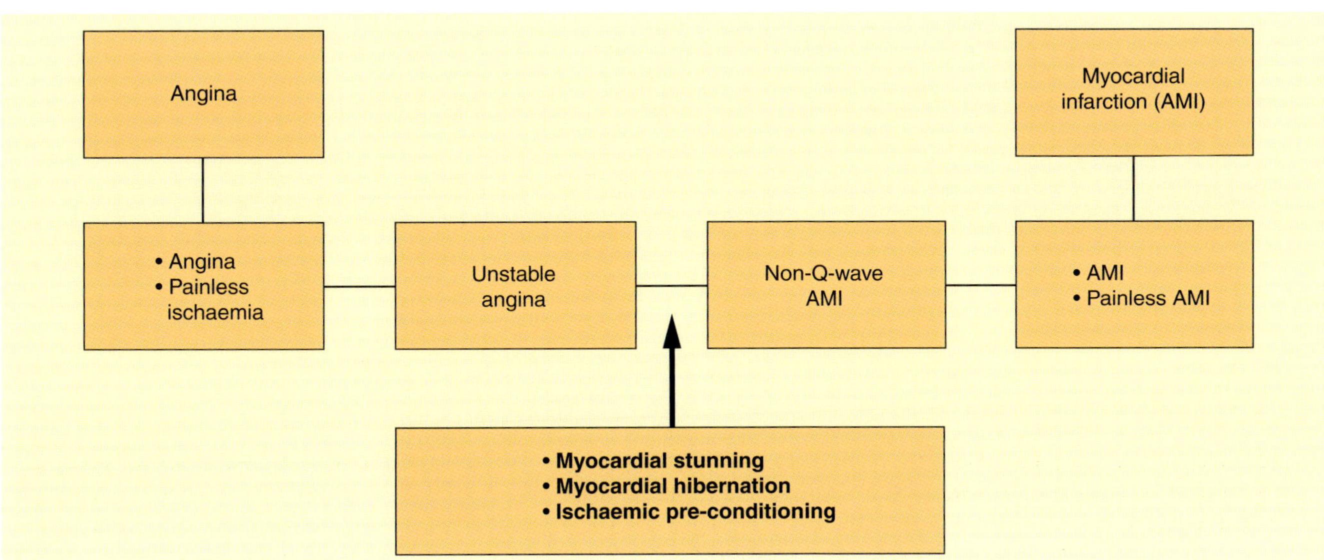


**Figure 20.5** *Evolution of the various clinical syndromes in patients with coronary artery disease. (From ref. 75 with permission.)*

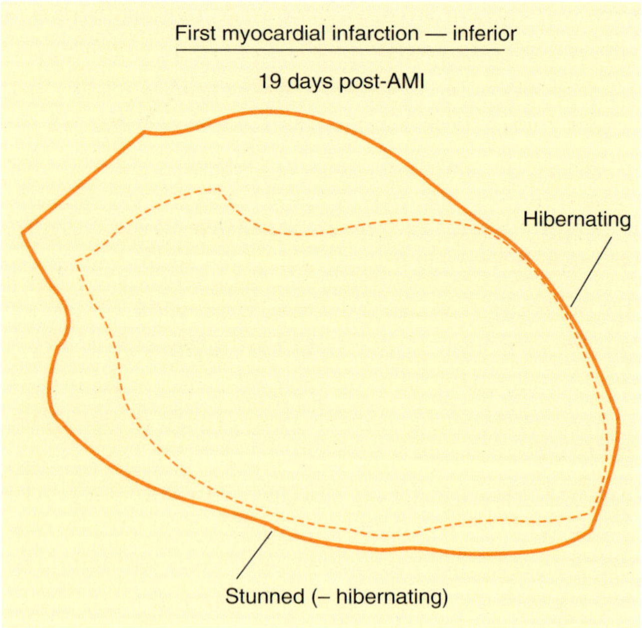


**Figure 20.6** *Preoperative ventriculogram of a patient with severe four-vessel coronary artery disease and a left ventricular ejection fraction (LVEF) of 0.45. After coronary bypass surgery, LV function was normal (LVEF = 0.63). This patient provides a good example of the demonstration of the difference between the hibernating and stunned myocardium. The anterior wall is hibernating and the inferior wall is stunned. However, since it is possible that blood flow may not have been fully restored to the posterior descending artery, the inferior wall could have been hibernating as well. (From ref. 1 with permission.)*

proven otherwise. HM is also known to occur in the LV wall in the area of the MI (Fig. 20.7) [76].

Adams *et al.* documented the frequency of HM in the setting of acute MI after thrombolytic therapy [77]. They studied 41 patients an average of 8 days after a first acute MI, all of whom had received thrombolytic therapy. Using PET they demonstrated mismatch (HM) in 78% of the patients, 31% of whom had a large area of mismatch.

Using PET, Tamaki *et al.* [78] showed increased [$^{18}$F]fluorodeoxyglucose (FDG) uptake, indicating HM in 48 of 84 (57%) patients after MI. At follow-up, a cardiac event (cardiac death, non-fatal MI, unstable angina, or late revascularization) occurred in 3% of patients with no increase in FDG and in 33% of patients who had increased FDG uptake. An increase in FDG was seen 16 of 17 patients who had a subsequent event. Multivariate analysis showed that an increase in FDG uptake was the most significant predictor of a subsequent cardiac event ($p = 0.0006$), followed by the number of diseased vessels ($p = 0.008$). This study demonstrates that HM occurs in many patients after MI and is associated with a high incidence of subsequent cardiac events.

Montalescott *et al.* [79] performed a randomized trial of PTCA versus no PTCA of the infarct-related artery 6 weeks after an acute MI in patients who had single-vessel disease with no clinical or exercise-induced evidence of myocardial ischaemia. Patients who were randomized to PTCA

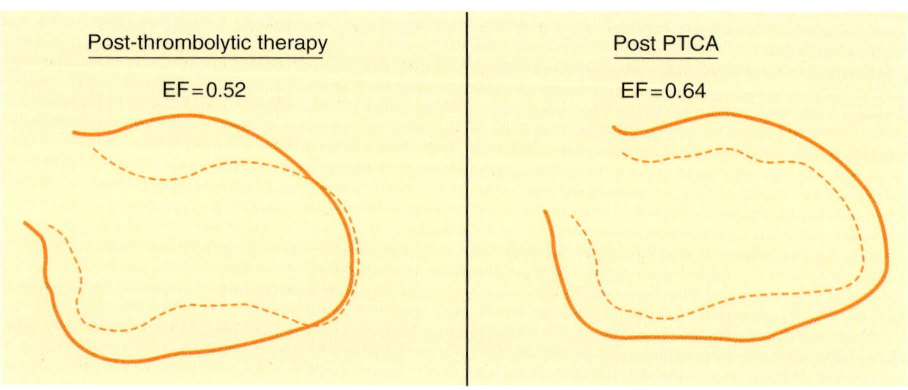


**Figure 20.7** *A 48-year-old woman who sustained an acute anterior wall myocardial infarction was treated with tissue plasminogen activator 2 h after the onset of chest pain. Twenty-four hours later, the patient had recurrent angina and underwent emergency cardiac catheterization and coronary angioplasty. A tracing of the right antero-oblique left ventriculogram is shown. Left: anterior akinesis/dyskinesis after thrombolytic therapy. The patient underwent percutaneous transluminal coronary angioplasty of a high-grade stenosis of the left anterior descending and circumflex coronary arteries. Right: repeat ventriculography 1 week later demonstrating dramatic recovery of abnormal wall motion and improvement in global left ventricular systolic function. (From ref. 76 with permission.)*

had increased coronary blood flow, an improvement in the $^{201}Tl$ pathological/normal ratio after exercise, and improved LV wall motion. The left ventricular ejection fraction (LVEF) did not change significantly (0.51 ± 0.03 to 0.52 ± 0.04) in the group randomized to no PTCA, whereas it increased from 0.48 ± 0.03 to 0.51 ± 0.04 ($p < 0.04$) in the PTCA group. This study demonstrates the occurrence of HM in the infarcted area or in an area that was presumed to be infarcted, as well as the improvement in LV function after revascularization of HM.

Brunken *et al.* studied 20 patients with chronic Q waves on the electrocardiogram (ECG). Of 31 dysfunctional LV segments, six (20%) had perfusion–metabolism mismatch (HM) on PET [80]. This study suggests that some patients with an old MI and chronic Q waves on the ECG may have HM.

HM is also documented in heart failure or severe LV dysfunction. Akins *et al.* [81] studied two patients with heart failure but without angina, who had severe CAD and stress-induced ischaemia. CBS improved the abnormal resting LV function and the clinical heart failure. Shanes *et al.* [82] described a patient with heart failure and a presumed dilated left ventricle. The patient had severe CAD with stress-induced ischaemia and the LV dysfunction returned to normal after bypass surgery.

Data from patients referred for cardiac transplantation to the present author's department have been very interesting. One patient, in whom revascularization instead of transplantation was carried out, had a gradual improvement in LV function over the 1 year postoperative period (Table 20.3) [60]. Among 207 patients evaluated for heart transplantation from 1984 to 1990, 22 (11%) underwent CBS instead of transplantation and their 40 month actuarial survival rate was 72%; almost all of the deaths were perioperative [83]. More recently, 112 patients with a diagnosis of idiopathic dilated cardiomyopathy (IDCM) were referred for cardiac transplantation [84]. The LVEF was < 0.35 and on PET studies 38 (34%) had perfusion–metabolism mismatch (HM). With CBS, hospital mortality was 10% and the 5 year survival was 71.4%. These studies document that patients with chronic resistant heart failure due to CAD or to presumed IDCM may have HM, which should be diagnosed early and treated appropriately.

Lee *et al.* [85] studied 50 patients with perfusion–metabolism mismatch (HM) who were revascularized; they had a 4% mortality and a 4% incidence of angina/MI, whereas 21 patients who were not revascularized had a mortality of 14% and angina/MI occurred in 62%. Using PET, Eitzman *et al.* [86] studied 82 patients with an LVEF of 0.34 ± 0.13. HM, indicated by a mismatch on PET, was present in 54% (44 of 82). On follow-up, death or MI occurred in 5% (two of 38) of patients who had no HM, in 4% (one of 26) of patients who had HM and were revascularized, and in 50% (nine of 18) of patients who had HM but were not revascularized. DiCarli *et al.* [87] studied patients with severe LV dysfunction (LVEF 0.25 ± 0.07) who had angina or were referred for cardiac transplantation. HM, demonstrated by PET, was present in 46% (43 of 93). Patients with HM who were revascularized had a much lower incidence of cardiac death than those who were not revascularized (4% vs 33%; 2 year actuarial survival 88% vs 50%; $p = 0.03$).

These studies demonstrate the presence of HM in many patients with severe LV dysfunction with or without heart failure; the incidence of death or MI was high in patients who were not revascularized. As mentioned earlier, Ragosta *et al.* [88] showed that postrevascularization improvement in LVEF could be predicted, using multivariate analysis, by the number of viable, asynergic myocardial segments per patient, that is, the number of myocardial segments that were hibernating. Angina has not been correlated.

ALCAPA [89–95] is a congenital anomaly associated with HM. The clinical picture is varied; LV dysfunction is common but LV function may be normal in myocardial ischaemia and MI may occur. The HM may be present because of chronic reduction of MBF. Detailed pathological and ultrastructural changes have been documented [94]. After reimplantation of the coronary artery into the aorta, LV function improves and even normalizes [76, 89–93] (Fig. 20.8). The improvement in LV function may be rapid or slow (12 or more months) and is dependent on the severity of structural changes of the HM. The extent of irreversibly damaged myocardium will determine the extent of postoperative LV dysfunction. LV dilatation occurs as a result of LV dysfunction and MI. Associated mitral regurgitation is due to the LV dilatation and MI. Surgery consists of excising a button of the pulmonary artery surrounding the ostium of the left coronary artery and anastomosing the button with the left coronary artery into the aorta. The mitral regurgitation may or may not need surgical attention. Early diagnosis and surgery are important.

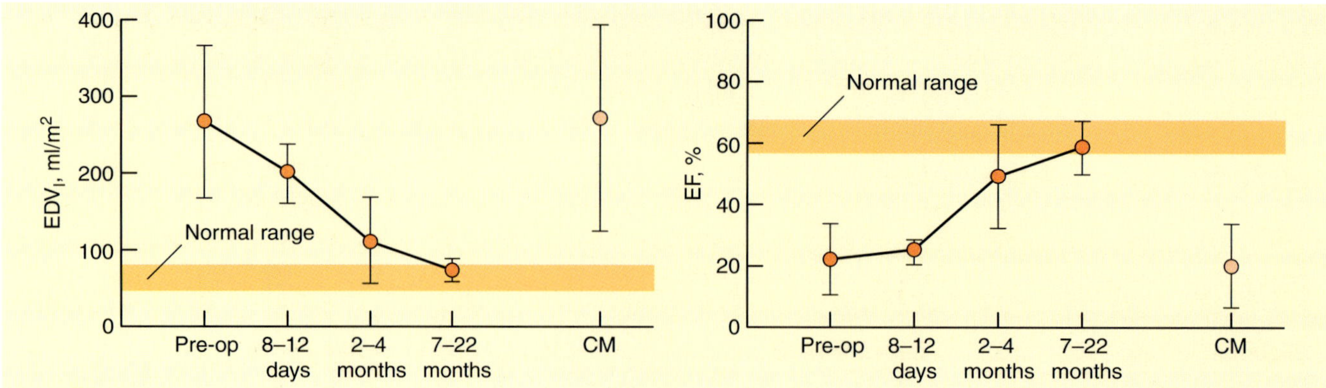


**Figure 20.8** *Preoperative and postoperative left ventricular end-diastolic volume (LVEDV) index (left) and left ventricular ejection fraction (LVEF) (right) in five patients aged 2–8.5 years who underwent surgical correction for anomalous left coronary artery from the pulmonary artery (ALCAPA). d = days after surgery; mos = months after surgery; CM = data on patients with idiopathic dilated cardiomyopathy at the author's institution. (From ref. 90 with permission.)*

## Why diagnose hibernating myocardium?

HM in patients with angina, acute MI, and ALCAPA has been shown to improve or normalize after myocardial revascularization. HM, if revascularized, is associated with a lower cardiovascular event rate [4]. CBS, if it increases or normalizes MBF, reduces or eliminates the frequency and severity of angina and the need for pharmacological treatment [30]. Randomized trials in selected patients with left main CAD, three-vessel CAD with normal LV function left anterior descending coronary artery [4], and two-vessel CAD if one of the vessels was the proximal have documented better survival in those assigned to CBS than in those assigned to medical treatment. In patients with LV dysfunction at rest, CBS has resulted in improved survival [4], particularly in patients with three-vessel CAD [4]. As a result, the conventional wisdom developed that patients with LV dysfunction at rest and with unstable angina or stable chronic angina and left main or three-vessel CAD should undergo revascularization by interventional techniques, without the need for documenting the presence of HM.

However, two recent studies have shown the advantages of documenting HM in patients with three-vessel CAD and an LVEF of $< 0.35$. Pagley *et al.* [96] documented, by a retrospective review of 70 patients undergoing CBS for 'ischaemic cardiomyopathy', that 33 patients with a myocardial viability index $> 0.67$ (determined by $^{201}$Tl scintigrams) had a significantly better short- and long-term cardiac event-free survival ($p = 0.019$) than 37 patients with a viability index $\leq 0.67$. The two subgroups were similar with regard to age, gender, presenting clinical syndrome, ECG, haemodynamic variables, number of diseased coronary arteries and LVEF. The viability index was the only independent predictor of a 3 year survival free of a cardiac event and was a better index than LVEF (Fig. 20.9).

The other study, by Haas *et al.* [97], described 35 patients who had CBS on the basis of clinical presentation and angiographic data (group A), and 34 patients who had CBS on the basis of PET findings of HM in addition to the clinical presentation and angiographic data (group B). Group B patients (those with HM) had a lower hospital mortality rate (0% vs 11.4%, $p = 0.04$), a lower rate of complicated postoperative recovery (33% vs 67%, $p = 0.05$), and a lower incidence of low-output syndrome (3% vs 17%, $p = 0.05$), and fewer patients needed catecholamine support (0% vs 29%, $p = 0.002$). Furthermore, the 1 year survival rate was better (97 $\pm$ 8% vs 79 $\pm$ 8%, $p < 0.01$) (Fig. 20.10). The LVEF increased from 26% to 35% ($p = 0.003$) in group B, but the change in group A was not significant. Testing for HM is important for determining outcome in patients with three-vessel CAD and severe LV dysfunction (LVEF $\leq 0.35$).

The studies of Pagley and Haas are important because they provide data that question the conventional wisdom. It is reasonable that an assessment of HM allows better assessment of the risks and benefits in patients with LV dysfunction who are to undergo revascularization, as well as allowing better selection of patients who should undergo revascularization. This is further supported by studies in

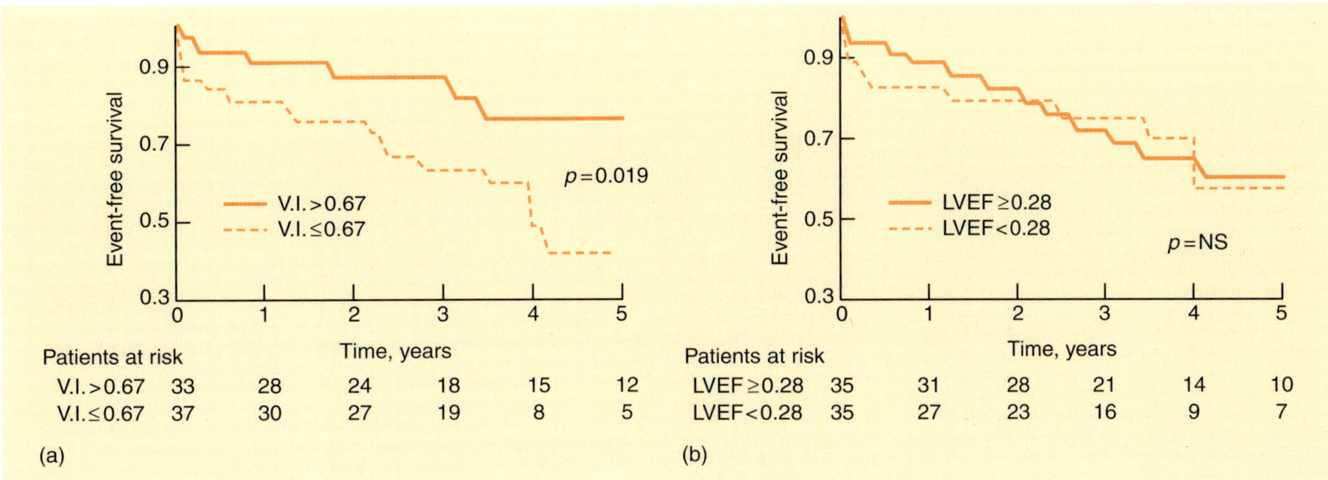


**Figure 20.9** *Kaplan–Meier survival analysis demonstrating survival free from cardiac events (cardiovascular death or heart transplantation). (A) Comparison of event-free survival among patients in group 1 [viability index (V.I.) > 0.67; solid line] and group 2 (V.I. ≤ 0.67; broken line). (B) Comparison of event-free survival among patients with left ventricular ejection fraction (LVEF) greater than or equal to the median of 0.28 (solid line) and those with LVEF less than the median of 0.28 (dotted line). (From ref. 96 with permission.)*

patients with severe chronic heart failure and patients being considered for heart transplantation [60, 83–86, 98]. Documentation of HM in such patients has allowed the choice of appropriate therapy, i.e. revascularization rather than transplantation.

## Diagnostic tests

A number of tests can be used to diagnose HM. LV dysfunction at rest is determined by two-dimensional echocardiography and radionuclide or contrast ventriculography. The most commonly used tests for documenting viable myocardium in the segments that are dysfunctional at rest (HM) include dobutamine echocardiography, thallium and Sestamibi, single-photon emission computed tomography (SPECT), myocardial perfusion imaging, and PET.

The sensitivity, specificity, and predictive accuracies of these tests are shown in Table 20.5 [99, 100].

## Whom should be tested?

It is not yet possible to provide a definite answer for several reasons. First, it is not known which test or combination of tests is best, that is, with a very high positive and negative

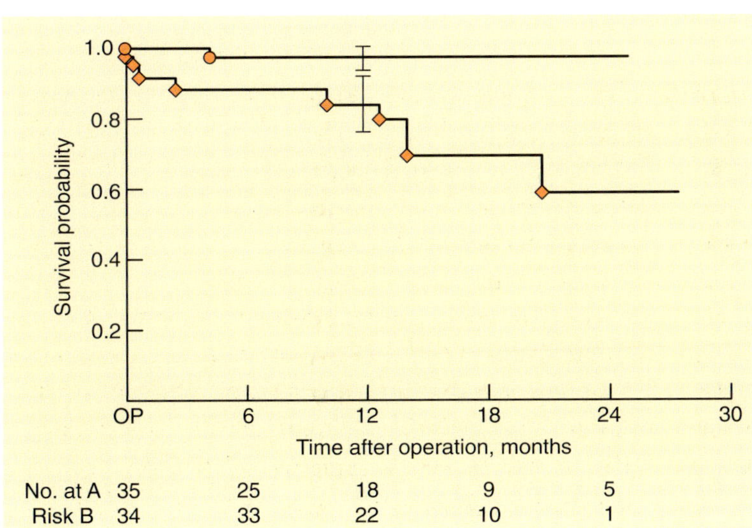


**Figure 20.10** *Actuarial survival curve (± SE) with the hospital mortality included. Diamonds = group A, in which hibernating myocardium (HM) was not documented; circles = group B, in which HM was documented (p < 0.01). (From ref. 97 with permission.)*

**Table 20.5** Diagnostic tests for hibernating myocardium

| | Dobutamine echocardiography | Thallium-201 | | [$^{99m}$Tc]MIBI | PET |
|---|---|---|---|---|---|
| | | Rest/redist. | Reinjection | | |
| Sensitivity [a] | 84 | 86 | 90 | 83 | 88 |
| Specificity [a] | 81 | 47 | 54 | 69 | 73 |
| Predictive accuracy [b] | | | | | |
| Positive test | 83 | 69 | | — | 82 |
| Negative test | 81 | 90 | | — | 83 |

Data are percentages.
Redist = redistribution; [$^{99m}$Tc]MIBI = technetium - 99m-??
PET = positron emission tomography. (From [a]ref. 99 and [b]ref. 100, with permission.)

predictive accuracy, for the diagnosis of HM. In an individual centre, any two tests may have similar accuracy [101, 102], and the sensitivity and specificity of a test can be altered, depending on the criteria used [103]. There are few data on the accuracy of these tests in any one of the several clinical conditions in which HM has been documented. Moreover, frequently the protocol for performing the test or tests is not standardized, the data obtained are evaluated subjectively and not quantified, and the standards for assessing the accuracy may be inadequate. Newer tests, for example, PET imaging with carbon-11 acetate alone or in combination with other tracers and advances in SPECT imaging, also need to be evaluated. Finally, the amount of HM and the amount of irreversibly damaged myocardium cannot be diagnosed reliably, although some initial data are promising.

Diagnostic tests are not perfect. Nevertheless, it is possible to provide some guidelines based on the assessment and consideration of the severity of LV dysfunction, the extent and severity of CAD and the state of the distal coronary arteries, and the clinical conditions in which HM has been documented so far.

Patients with normal LV function and those with coronary arteries that are not suitable for revascularization do not need to be tested (Table 20.6) [75]. Transmyocardial laser revascularization is still an experimental procedure. Diagnostic testing for HM is needed in the following patients: [75] (1) those known to have significant CAD and those with suspected CAD or suspected IDCM who are being considered for heart transplantation; (2) those with significant CAD and severe LV dysfunction (i.e. LVEF < 0.35); and (3) those with CAD and LV dysfunction who are asymptomatic, those who have symptoms due to heart failure or LV dysfunction, and those with only mild or minimal angina.

**Table 20.6** Diagnostic testing for hibernating myocardium[a]

| | |
|---|---|
| Usually not needed[b] | Normal LV function |
| | Coronary arteries not suitable for revascularization |
| Usually needed[b] | Suspected CAD/suspected IDCM, being considered for heart transplantation |
| | CAD plus severe LV dysfunction (LVEF ≤ 0.35) |
| | CAD plus dysfunction in patients who are asymptomatic or have heart-fallure symptoms: mild/minimal angina |
| Individualized[c] | Unstable angina/severe stable angina |
| | Acute myocardial infarction |
| | ALCAPA |

[a]Only needed in patients with left ventricular (LV) dysfunction at rest.
[b]Clinical judgement may be needed.
[c]Clinical judgement frequently needed.
CAD = coronary artery disease; IDCM = idiopathic dilated cardiomyopathy; LVEF = left ventricular ejection fraction; ALCAPA = anomalous left coronary artery from the pulmonary artery. (From ref. 75 with permission.)

If patients do not fit into these subgroups, that is, mainly those with mild to moderate LV dysfunction (LVEF 0.36–0.49), one may need to consider the clinical condition with which they present. Diagnostic testing is probably not indicated in patients with unstable angina, that is, angina at rest, progressively increasing angina despite medical therapy, angina $\leq$ 2 weeks after MI, and in most patients with severe, chronic, stable angina, because revascularization is often undertaken in these patients for relief of symptoms. However, one must recognize that: (1) the severity of angina may not be related to the extent of myocardium at risk, extent and severity of CAD, and LV function [103]; (2) in patients with angina (if unstable angina is excluded), the extent of CAD and LV function and the extent and severity of ischaemia are predictors of outcome but angina is not [104, 105]; and (3) documentation of the amount of HM may allow better assessment of the risks and benefits of revascularization.

Post-MI patients pose a more difficult problem because of the complexity and variety of clinical situations that may be present. These include the clinical state of the patient, the location of the current and previous MI, the extent and severity of the CAD, the extent and severity of LV dysfunction, and the feasibility of revascularizing all dysfunctional myocardial segments; thus, the need to revascularize some or all dysfunctional LV segments may require evaluation by testing for HM.

ALCAPA is a congenital disorder that often presents with LV dysfunction or heart failure with or without mitral regurgitation. The severe LV dysfunction and dilatation improve or normalize after surgical correction [75, 90]. Patients with ALCAPA should be diagnosed early and have early reimplantation of the left coronary artery into the aorta. In all the above subgroups of patients, assessment of HM may allow better assessment of the risks and benefits of revascularization.

## Treatment of hibernating myocardium

The most definitive evidence of improvement of HM has been with revascularization by either percutaneous catheter techniques or [1–4, 12, 18, 27, 30, 33–35, 39, 43, 44, 50, 55–57, 60, 76, 89–95, 106–112]. The aim is to obtain complete myocardial revascularization or, alternatively, as complete a revascularization as possible. The decision to perform revascularization is made and the technique chosen after considering several factors: (1) the suitability of the coronary arteries for revascularization; (2) the severity of LV dysfunction; (3) the extent of HM; (4) the risks of revascularization; and (5) the estimation of functional recovery after revascularization, including the extent of irreversibly damaged myocardium and the skill of the revascularization team. Symptoms are of secondary consideration. The greater the severity of angina, the greater the need for revascularization. Heart-failure symptoms also may signify a significant need for revascularization. Since all the factors to be considered in recommending revascularization cannot be accurately quantitated at the present time, clinical judgement becomes important in the decision to recommend revascularization.

## Importance to clinicians

The outcome of patients with CAD is determined not only by the extent and severity of the CAD but also by the amount of LV myocardium that is or can be irreversibly damaged. The myocardium that may become irreversibly damaged (the amount of myocardium that is at risk) is the myocardium that is hibernating or at risk from acute ischaemic episodes. In patients with LV dysfunction at rest, several combination of irreversibly damaged myocardium and HM may be present in a patient (Table 20.4).

One of the goals in clinical practice is to reduce the amount of irreversibly damaged myocardium and, therefore, to salvage HM and protect the ischaemic myocardium. HM results in LV dysfunction at rest. In clinical practice when one sees a patient with Lv dysfunction at rest one should ask whether there is HM (viable myocardium) in the area of the LV dysfunction. The need to assess the presence and extent of HM in patients is shown in Table 20.6. At present, successful revascularization of the HM will reduce the LV dysfunction and reduce the amount of myocardium at risk. It may prolong life, reduce or correct clinical heart failure, and improve the symptomatic state of the patient.

## References


1. Rahimtoola SH. The hibernating myocardium. *Am Heart J* 1989; 117: 211–21.
2. Rahimtoola SH. Coronary bypass surgery for chronic angina — 1981: a perspective. *Circulation* 1982; 65: 225–41.

3. Rahimtoola SH. Unstable angina: current status. *Mod Concepts Cardiovasc Dis* 1985; 54: 19–23.
4. Rahimtoola SH. A perspective on the three large multicenter randomized clinical trials of coronary bypass surgery for chronic stable angina. *Circulation* 1985; 72 (Suppl. V): 123–35.
5. Geft IL, Fishbein Mc, Ninomiya K *et al.* Intermittent brief periods of ischaemia have a cumulative effect and may cause myocardial necrosis. *Circulation* 1982; 66: 1150–53.
6. Pantely GA, Malone SA, Rhen WS *et al.* Regeneration of myocardial phosphocreatine in pigs despite continued moderate ischaemia. *Circ Res* 1990; 67: 1481–93.
7. Arai AE, Pantely GA, Anselone CG *et al.* Active down-regulation of myocardial energy requirements during prolonged moderate ischaemia in swine. *Circ Res* 1991; 69: 1458–69.
8. Schulz R, Guth BD, Pieper K *et al.* Recruitment of an inotropic reserve in moderately ischaemic myocardium at the expense of metabolic recovery: a model of short-term hibernation. *Circ Res* 1992; 70: 1282–95.
9. Schulz R, Rose J, Martin C *et al.* Development of short-term myocardial hibernation. Its limitation by the severity of ischaemia and inotropic stimulation. *Circulation* 1993; 88: 684–95.
10. Arai AE, Grauer SE, Anselone CG *et al.* Metabolic adaptation to a gradual reduction in myocardial blood flow. *Circulation* 1995; 92: 244–52.
11. Rahimtoola SH. Hibernating myocardium has reduced blood flow at rest that increases with low-dose dobutamine (Editorial). *Circulation* 1996; 94: 3055–61.
12. Bonchek LI, Rahimtoola SH, Chaitman BR *et al.* Vein graft occlusion: immediate and late consequences and therapeutic implications. *Circulation* 1974; 50 (Suppl II): 84–97.
13. Anderson RP. Effects of coronary bypass graft occlusion on left ventricular performance. *Circulation* 1972; 46: 507–13.
14. Banka VS, Bodenheimer MM, Shah R, Helfant RH. Intervention ventriculography: comparative value of nitroglycerin, post-extrasystolic potentiation and nitroglycerin plus post-extrasystolic potentiation. *Circulation* 1976; 53: 632–7.
15. Bodenheimer MM, Banka VS, Fooshee C *et al.* Relationship between regional myocardial perfusion and the presence, severity and reversibility of asynergy in patients with coronary heart disease. *Circulation* 1978; 58: 789–95.
16. Bolukoglu H, Liedtke J, Nellis S *et al.* An animal model of chronic coronary stenosis resulting in hibernating myocardium. *Am J Physiol* 1992; 263: H20–9.
17. Bourrassa M, Lesperance J, Campeau J *et al.* Fate of left ventricular contraction following aortocoronary venous grafts: early and late post-operative modifications. *Circulation* 1972; 46: 724–30.
18. Chatterjee K, Swan HJC, Parmley WW *et al.* Influence of direct myocardial revascularization on left ventricular asynergy and function in patients with coronary heart disease. *Cricíulation* 1973; 47: 276–86.
19. Chesebro JH, Ritman EL, Frye RL *et al.* Regional myocardial wall thickening response to nitroglycerin. A predictor of myocardial response to aortocoronary bypass surgery. *Circulation* 1978; 57: 952–7.
20. Dyke SH, Cohn PF, Gorlin R, Sonnenblick EJ. Detection of residual myocardial function in coronary artery disease using post-extrasystolic potentiation. *Circulation* 1974; 50: 694–9.
21. Helfant RH, Pine R, Meister SG *et al.* Nitroglycerin to unmask reversible asynergy. Correlation with post-coronary bypass ventriculography. *Circulation* 1974; 50: 108–13.
22. Horn HR, Teicholz LE, Cohn PF *et al.* Augmentation of left ventricular contraction pattern in coronary artery disease by an inotropic catecholamine: the epinephrine ventriculogram. *Circulation* 1974; 49: 1063–71.
23. Klausner SC, Ratshin RA, Tybert JV *et al.* The similarity of changes in segmental contraction patterns induced by post-extrasystolic potentiation and nitroglycerin. *Circulation* 1976; 54: 615–23.
24. Massie B, Botvinick EH, Brundage BH *et al.* Relationship of regional myocardial perfusion to segmental wall motion. Physiological basis for understanding the presence and the reversibility of asynergy. *Circulation* 1978; 58: 1154–63.
25. McAnulty JH, Hattenhauer MT, Rösch J *et al.* Improvement in left ventricular wall motion following nitroglycerin. *Circulation* 1975; 51: 140–5.
26. Popio KA, Gorlin R, Bechtel D, Levine JA. Postextrasystolic potentiation as a predictor of potential myocardial viability: preoperative analyses compared with studies after coronary bypass surgery. *Am J Cardiol* 1977; 39: 944–53.
27. Rees G, Bristow JD, Kremkau EL *et al.* Influence of aortocoronary bypass surgery on left ventricular performance. *N Engl J Med* 1971; 284: 1116–20.
28. Stadius M, McAnulty JH, Culter J *et al.* Specificity, sensitivity and accuracy of the nitroglycerin ventriculogram as a predictor of surgically reversible wall motion abnormalities (Abstract). *Am J Cardiol* 1980; 45: 399.
29. Frye RL, Frommer PL (eds) Consensus Development Conference on Coronary Artery Bypass Surgery. Medical and scientific aspects. NIH, December 3–5, 1980. *Circulation* 1982; 65 (Suppl II): I-129.
30. Rahimtoola SH. Postoperative exercise response in the evaluation of the physiologic status after coronary bypass surgery. *Circulation* 1982; 65 (Suppl II): 106–14.
31. Deanfield J, Maseri A, Selwyn AP *et al.* Myocardial ischaemia during daily life in patients with stable angina: its relation to symptoms and heart rate changes. *Lancet* 1983: ii: 753–8.
32. Maseri A. The changing face of angina pectoris: practical implications. *Lancet* 1983; i: 746–9.
33. Berger BC, Watson DD, Burwell LR *et al.* Redistribution of thallium at rest in patients with stable and unstable angina and the effect of coronary artery bypass surgery. *Circulation* 1979; 60: 1114–25.
34. Gibson RS, Watson DD, Taylor GJ *et al.* Prospective assessment of regional myocardial perfusion before and after coronary revascularization surgery by quantitative thallium-201 scintigraphy. *J Am Coll Cardiol* 1983; 1: 804–15.
35. Dilsizian V, Rocco TP, Freedman NMT *et al.* Enhanced detection of ischaemic but viable myocardium by the reinjection of thallium after stress redistribution imaging. *N Engl J Med* 1990; 323: 141–6.
36. Gerwirtz H, Beller GA, Strauss HW *et al.* Transient defects of resting thallium scans in patients with coronary artery disease. *Circulation* 1979; 59: 707–13.
37. Braunwald E, Hollingsworth C, Passamani E (eds) NHLBI Workshop on Surgery in the Treatment of Coronary Artery Disease, September 6 and 7, 1984. Bethesda, Maryland. *Circulation* 1985; 72 (Suppl V): 1–168.
38. Bashour TT. Of myocardial life, hibernation and death. *Am Heart J* 1986; 112: 427–8.

39. Braunwald E, Rutherford JD. Reversible ischaemic left ventricular dysfunction: evidence for the 'hibernating myocardium'. *J Am Coll Cardiol* 1986; 8: 1467–70.
40. Hearse JD. Myocardial ischaemia: can we agree on a definition for the 21st century? *Cardiovasc Res* 1994; 28: 1737–44.
41. Ross J Jr. Myocardial perfusion-contraction matching: implications for coronary heart disease and hibernation. *Circulation* 1991; 83: 1076–82.
42. Rahimtoola SH. Commentary on 'The definition of ischaemia'. *Cardiovas Res* 1994; 28: 1745.
43. Hearse DJ. Myocardial hibernation: a form of endogenous protection? *Eur Heart J* 1997; 18 (Suppl A): A2–7.
44. Takeishi Y, Tono-ka I, Kubota I *et al.* Functional recovery of hibernating myocardium after coronary bypass surgery: does it coincide with improvement in perfusion? *Am Heart J* 1991; 122: 665–70.
45. Rahimtoola SH. Hibernating myocardium is hypoperfused. *Basic Res Cardiol* 1997; 92 (Suppl 1.2): 9–11.
46. Vanoverschelde JL, Wijns W, Depre C *et al.* Mechanisms of chronic regional postischemic dysfunction in humans: new insights from the study of noninfarcted collateral-dependent myocardium. *Circulation* 1993; 87: 1513–23.
47. Czernin J, Porenta G, Brunken R *et al.* Regional blood flow, oxidative metabolism, and glucose utilization in patients with recent myocardial infarction. *Circulation* 1993; 88: 884–95.
48. Marzullo P, Parodi O, Sambuceti G *et al.* Residual coronary reserve identifies segmental viability in patients with wall motion abnormalities. *J Am Coll Cardiol* 1995; 26: 342–50.
49. Shivalkar B, Maes A, Borgers M *et al.* Only hibernating myocardium shows early recovery after coronary revascularization. *Circulation* 1996; 94: 308–15.
50. Sun KT, Czernin J, Krirokapich J *et al.* Effects of Dobutamine stimulation on myocardial blood flow, glucose metabolism and wall motion in normal and dysfunctional myocardium. *Circulation* 1996; 74: 3146–54.
51. Sambuceti G, Parodi O, Giorgetti A *et al.* Microvascular dysfunction in collateral-dependent myocardium. *J Am Coll Cardiol* 1995; 26: 615–23.
52. Rahimtoola SH. *Basic Res Cardiol* 1995; 90: 38–40.
53. Rahimtoola SH. The hibernating myocardium in ischaemic and congestive heart failure. *Eur Heart J* 1993; 14 (Suppl A): A22–6.
54. Rahimtoola SH. *Circulation* 1991; 84 (Suppl I): 81–4.
55. Topol EJ, Weiss JL, Guzman PA *et al.* Immediate improvement of dysfunctional myocardial segmetns after coronary revascularization: detection by intraoperative transesophageal echocardiography. *J Am Coll Cardiol* 1984; 4: 1123–34.
56. Cohen M, Chainey R, Hershman R *et al.* Reversal of chronic ischaemic myocardial dysfunction after transluminal coronary angioplasty. *J Am Coll Cardiol* 1988; 12: 1193–8.
57. La Canna G, Alfieri O, Giubbini R *et al.* Echocardiography during infusion of dobutamine for identification of reversible dysfunction in patients with chronic coronary artery disease. *J Am Coll Cardiol* 1994; 23: 617–26.
58. Flameng W, Vanhaecke J, Van Belle H *et al.* Relation between coronary artery stenosis and myocardial purine metabolism, histology and regional function in humans. *J Am Coll Cardiol* 1987; 9: 1235–42.
59. Cabin HS, Clubb KS, Vita H, Zaret BL. Regional dysfunction by equilibrium radionuclide angiocardiography: a clinicopathological study evaluating the relation of degree of dysfunction to the presence and extent of myocardial infarction. *J Am Coll Cardiol* 1987; 10: 743–7.
60. Luu M, Stevenson LW, Brunken RC *et al.* Delayed recovery of revascularized myocardium after referral for cardiac transplantation. *Am Heart J* 1990; 119: 668–70.
61. Flameng W, Suy R, Schwartz F *et al.* Ultrastructural correlates of left ventricular contraction abnormalities in patients with chronic ischaemic heart disease: determinants of reversible segmental asynergy postrevascularization surgery. *Am Heart J* 1981; 102: 846–57.
62. Borgers M, Thone F, Wonters L *et al.* Structural correlates of regional myocardial dysfunction in patients with critical coronary artery stenosis: chronic hibernation? *Cardiovasc Pathol* 1993; 2: 237–45.
63. Fedele FA, Gerwitz H, Capone RJ *et al.* Metabolic response to prolonged reduction of myocardial blood flow distal to a severe coronary artery stenosis. *Circulation* 1988; 78: 729–35.
64. Fallavollita JA, Perry BJ, Canty JM Jr. F-2-Deoxyglucose deposition and regional flow in pigs with chronically dysfunctional myocardium. Evidence for transmural variations in chronic hibernating myocardium. *Circulation* 1997; 95: 1900–9.
65. Chen C, Ma L, Linfert DR *et al.* Myocardial cell death and apoptosis in hibernating myocardium. *J Am Coll Cardiol* 1997; 30: 1407–17.
66. Ma L, Chen L, Gillam L *et al.* Nitroglycerin enhances the ability of dobutamine stress echocardiography to detect hibernating myocardium. *Circulation* 1997; 96: 3992–4001.
67. McFalls EO, Baldwin D, Palmer B *et al.* Regional glucose uptake within hypoperfused swine myocardium as measured by positron emission tomography. *Am J Physiol* 1997; 272: H343–9.
68. Matsuzaki M, Gallagher KP, White F, Ross J Jr. Sustained regional dysfunction produced by prolonged coronary stenosis: gradual recovery after reperfusion. *Circulation* 1983; 68: 170–82.
69. Baker WB, Klein MS, Reardon MJ *et al.* Reversible cardiac dysfunction (hibernation) from ischaemia due to compression of the coronary arteries by a pseudoaneurysm. *N Engl J Med* 1991; 325: 1858–61.
70. Marwick TH, MacIntyre WJ, Lafont A *et al.* Metabolic responses of Hibernating and infarcted myocardium to revascularization. A follow-up study of regional perfusion, function, and metabolism. *Circulation* 1992; 85: 1347–53.
71. Nienaber CA, Brunken RC, Sherman CT *et al.* Metabolic and functional recovery of ischaemic human myocardium after coronary angioplasty. *J Am Coll Cardiol* 1991; 18: 966–78.
72. Kloner RA, Przyklenk K. Hibernation and stunning of the myocardium. *N Engl J Med* 1991; 325: 1877–9.
73. Rahimtoola SH. From coronary artery disease to heart failure: role of the hibernating myocardium. *Am J Cardiol* 1995; 75: 16–22E.
74. Knight C, Fox KM. The vicious circle of ischaemic left ventricular dysfunction. *Am J Cardiol* 1995; 76: 4–7B.
75. Rahimtoola SH. Importance of diagnosing hibernating myocardium: how and in whom? *J Am Coll Cardiol* 1997; 30: 1701–6.
76. Kulick D, Rahimtoola SH. Assessment of the survivors of acute myocardial infarction: the case for coronary angiography. In: B Gersh, SH Rahimtoola (eds) *Acute myocardial infarction*. Amsterdam: Elsevier, 1991; 448–68.

77. Adams JN, Norton M, Trent R *et al.* Hibernating myocardium after acute myocardial infarction treated with thrombolysis. *Heart* 1996; 75: 422–6.
78. Tamaki N, Kawamoto M, Takahashi N *et al.* Prognostic value of an increase in fluorine-18 deoxyglucose uptake in patients with myocardial infarction: comparison with stress thallium imaging. *J Am Coll Cardiol* 1992; 22: 1621–7.
79. Montalescott G, Faraggi M, Drobinski G *et al.* Myocardial viability in patients with Q were myocardial infarction and no residual ischaemia. *Circulation* 1992; 86: 47–55.
80. Brunken R, Tillisch J, Schwaiger M *et al.* Regional perfusion, glucose metabolism, and wall motion in patients with chronic electrocardiographic Q wave infarction. Evidence for persistence of viable tissue in some infarct regions by positron emission tomography. *Circulation* 1986; 73: 951–63.
81. Akins CW, Pohost GM, DeSanctis RW, Block PC. Selection of angina-free patients with severe left ventricular dysfunction for myocardial revascularization. *Am J Cardiol* 1980; 46: 695–700.
82. Shanes JG, Kondos GT, Levitsky S *et al.* Coronary artery obstruction: a potentially reversible cause of dilated cardiomyopathy. *Am Heart J* 1985; 110: 173–8.
83. Louie HW, Laks H, Milgalter E *et al.* Ischaemic cardiomyopathy: criteria for coronary revascularization and cardiac transplantation. *Circulation* 1991; 84 (Suppl III): 290–5.
84. Duong TH, Hendi P, Fonarow G *et al.* Role of positron emission tomographic assessment of myocardial viability in the management of patients who are referred for cardiac transplantation (Abstract). *Circulation* 1995; 92: I–123.
85. Lee KS, Marwick TH, Cook SA *et al.* Prognosis of patients with left ventricular dysfunction, with and without viable myocardium after myocardial infarction. Relative efficacy of medical therapy and vascularization. *Circulation* 1994; 90: 2687–94.
86. Eitzman D, Al-Aonar Z, Kanter HL *et al.* Clinical outcome of patients with advanced coronary artery disease after viability studies with positron emission tomography. *J Am Coll Cardiol* 1992; 20: 559–65.
87. DiCarli M, Davidson M, Little R *et al.* Value of metabolic imaging with positron emission tomography for evaluating prognosis in patients with coronary artery disease and left ventricular dysfunction. *Am J Cardiol* 1994; 73: 527–33.
88. Ragosta M, Beller GA, Watson DD *et al.* Quantitative planar rest-redistribution thallium 201 imaging in detection of myocardial viability and prediction of improvement in left ventricular function after coronary bypass surgery in patients with severely depressed left ventricular function. *Circulation* 1993; 87: 1630–41.
89. Levitsky S, van de Horst RL, Hastreiter AR, Fisher EA. Anomalous left coronary artery in the infant. Recovery of ventricular function following early direct aortic implantation. *J Thorac Cardiovasc Surg* 1980; 79: 598–602.
90. Rein AJJ, Colan SD, Parness IA, Sanders SP. Regional and global left ventricular function in infants with anomalous origin of the left coronary artery from the pulmonary trunk: preoperative and postoperative assessment. *Circulation* 1987; 75: 115–23.
91. Hurwitz RA, Caldwell RL, Girod DA *et al.* Clinical and hemodynamic course of infants and children with anomalous left coronary artery. *Am Heart J* 1989; 118: 1176–81.
92. Carvalho JS, Redington AN, Oldershaw PJ *et al.* Analysis of left ventricular wall movement before and after reimplantation of anomalous left coronary artery in infancy. *Br Heart J* 1991; 65: 218–22.
93. Jin Z, Berger F, Uhlemann F *et al.* Improvement in left ventricular dysfunction after aortic reimplantation in 11 consecutive paediatric patients with anomalous origin of the left coronary artery from the pulmonary artery. Early results of a serial echocardiographic follow-up. *Eur Heart J* 1994; 15: 1044–9.
94. Shivalkar B, Borgers M, Daenen W *et al.* ALCAPA syndrome: An example of chronic myocardial hypoperfusion? *J Am Coll Cardiol* 1994; 23: 772–8.
95. Lambert V, Touchot A, Losay J *et al.* Midterm results after surgical repair of the anomalous origin of the coronary artery. *Circulation* 1996; 94 (Suppl II): 38–43.
96. Pagley PR, Beller GA, Watson DD *et al.* Improved outcome after coronary bypass surgery in patients with ischaemic cardiomyopathy and residual myocardial viability. *Circulation* 1997; 97: 793–800.
97. Haas F, Haehnel CJ, Picker W *et al.* Preoperative positron emission tomographic viability assessment and perioperative risk in patients with advanced ischaemic heart disease. *J Am Coll Cardiol* 1997; 30: 1693–700.
98. Dreyfuss GD, Dubec D, Blasco A *et al.* Myocardial viability assessment in ischaemic cardiomyopathy: benefits of coronary revascularization. *Ann Thorac Surg* 1994; 57: 1402–8.
99. Bax JJ, Wijns W, Cornell JH *et al.* Accuracy of currently available techniques for prediction of functional recovery after revascularization in patients with left ventricular dysfunction due to chronic coronary artery disease: comparison of pooled data. *J Am Coll Cardiol* 1997; 30: 1451–60.
100. Bonow RO. Identification of viable myocardium. *Circulation* 1996; 94: 2674–80.
101. Vanoverschelde JL, D'Hondt AM, Marwick T *et al.* Head-to-head comparison of exercise-redistribution-reinjection thallium single-photon emission computed tomography and low dose dobutamine echocardiography for prediction of reversibility of chronic left ventricular ischaemic dysfunction. *J Am Coll Cardiol* 1996; 28: 432–42.
102. Qureishi U, Nagueh SF, Afridi I *et al.* Dobutamine echocardiography and quantitative rest-redistribution $^{210}$Tl tomography in myocardial hibernation. Relation of contractile reserve to $^{201}$Tl uptake and comparative prediction of recovery of function. *Circulation* 1997; 95: 626–35.
103. Hultgren HN, Peduzzi P. For the Participants of the Veternas Administration Cooperative Study of Surgery for Coronary Arterial Occlusive Disease. Relation of severity of symptoms to prognosis in stable angina pectoris. *Am J Cardiol* 1984; 54: 988–93.
104. Kaul S, Lilly DR, Gascho JA *et al.* Prognostic utility of the exercise thallium-201 test in ambulatory patients with chest pain: comparison with cardiac catheterization. *Circulation* 1988; 77: 745–58.
105. Califf RM, Mark DB, Harrell FE Jr *et al.* Importance of clinical measures of ischaemia in the prognosis of patients with documented coronary artery disease. *J Am Coll Cardiol* 1988; 11: 20–6.
106. Brundage BH, Massie BM, Botvinick EH. Improved regional ventricular function after successful surgical revascularization. *J Am Coll Cardiol* 1984; 3: 902–8.

107. Cigarroa CG, deFilippi CR, Brickner ME *et al.* Dobutamine stress echocardiography identifies hibernating myocardium and predicts recovery of left ventricular function after coronary revascularization. *Circulation* 1993; 88: 430–6.
108. Elefteriades JS, Tolis G Jr, Levi E *et al.* Coronary artery bypass grafting in severe left ventricular dysfunction, excellent survival with improved ejection fraction and function state. *J Am Coll Cardiol* 1993; 22: 1411–17.
109. Ferrari R, LaCanna G, Giubbini R *et al.* Hibernating myocardium in patients with coronary artery disease: identification and clinical importance. *Cardiovasc Drugs The* 1992; 6: 287–93.
110. Mizuno K, Arakawa K, Shibuya T *et al.* Improved regional and global diastolic performance in patients with coronary artery disease after percutaneous transluminal coronary angioplasty. *Am Heart J* 1988; 115: 302–6.
111. Tillisch J, Brunken R, Marshall R *et al.* Reversibility of cardiac wall motion abnormalities predicted by positron tomography. *N Engl J Med* 1986; 314: 884–8.
112. Van den Berg EK Jr, Popma JJ, Dehmer GJ *et al.* Reversible segmental left ventricular dysfunction after coronary angioplasty. *Circulation* 1990; 81: 1210–16.

# Hypertensive heart disease and progressive myocellular loss



G. PONS-LLADÓ, M. BALLESTER AND I. CARRIÓ

## Introduction

Systemic hypertension is a leading cause of congestive heart failure [1–3]. Because of the high prevalence of hypertension in the community [3], the problem of heart failure attributable to hypertension constitutes an important issue in public health. The relationship among hypertension, cardiac hypertrophy, and the development of overt heart disease was enunciated by Sir William Osler, who described the progression from 'full compensation' to a state of 'broken compensation' [4]. Experimental studies by Meerson [5], illustrated these stages, paving the way towards understanding the deletereous effects of hypertension on the structure and function of the heart. Essential in the pathogenesis of decompensation is the concept that ventricular hypertrophy may itself be a pathological process and that, although initially compensatory for an excessive load, the hypertrophied myocardium is functionally abnormal [6]. Increasing levels of systolic blood pressure have been reported to be associated with progressively increasing left ventricular (LV) mass, as seen echocardiographically [7]. Although LV hypertrophy may be associated with supernormal ventricular ejection phase indices [8], in a large proportion of these patients the exercise-induced depression in systolic function [9, 10] and depressed mid-wall fractional shortening/end-systolic stress relationship [11] suggest that LV hypertrophy may actually result in systolic dysfunction. Loss of cardiomyocytes is likely to precede the deterioration of ventricular systolic function, which may occur late in the natural history of hypertension [12, 13]. Myocardial degeneration associated with LV hypertrophy has indeed been demonstrated in necropsy specimens wherein the degree of hypertrophy correlated with the extent of myocardial damage [12, 13]. The intriguing sequence of events by which the hypertrophied heart leads to progressive deterioration and myocellular loss has been referred to as 'cardiomyopathy of overload' [14].

## Assessment of hypertensive heart disease

LV hypertrophy was believed to occur in between 3 and 8% of hypertensive patients in studies using electrocardiography [15]. The clinical introduction of echocardiography in the late 1960s demonstrated that the prevalence is in fact higher, between 12 and 30% [16]. LV hypertrophy occurs even in ambulatory patients with uncomplicated and well-controlled hypertension. M-mode echocardiography is usually used to measure LV mass [17, 18] (Fig. 21.1), which is the ultimate criterion for the diagnosis and assessment of severity of hypertrophy. Although two-dimensional echocardiography determinations are theoretically superior to M-mode techniques and provide a complete view of the left ventricle in real time [19] (Fig. 21.2), suboptimal definition of endocardial and epicardial borders, particularly in still-frame images, limits the applicability and accuracy of this technique [20]. Serial echocardiographic studies have

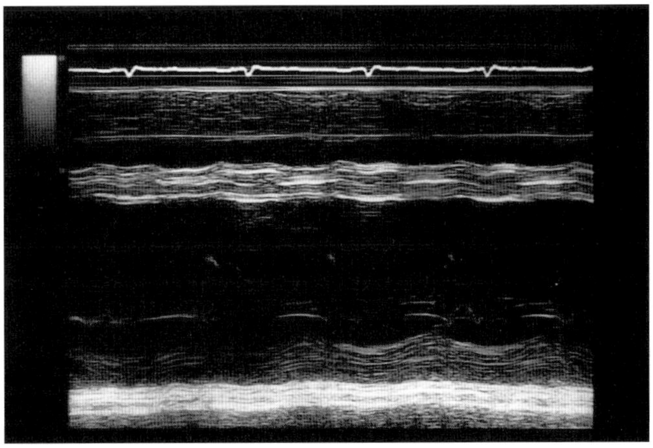

**Figure 21.1** *M-mode echocardiographic recording obtained at the level of the left ventricle. Measurements of the septal and posterior wall thickness and the internal left ventricular (LV) diameter in diastole can be integrated in a formula [17, 18] derived from the volume calculation of a prolate ellipsoid that allows the obtention of LV mass.*

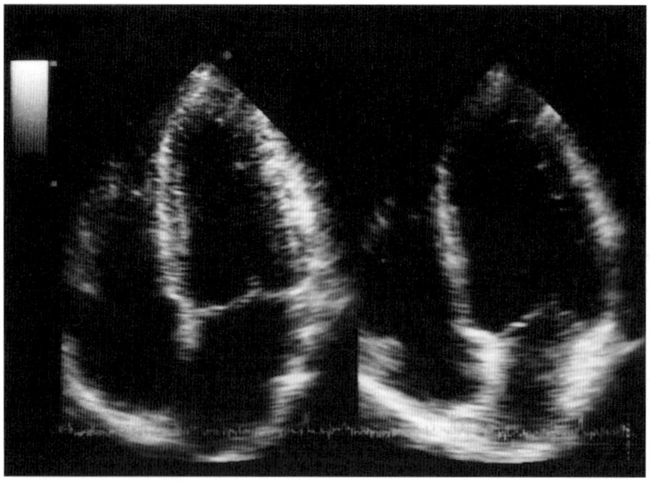

**Figure 21.2** *Systolic and diastolic frames from a two-dimensional echocardiographic study obtained from an apical four-chamber view. Although useful for chamber volume calculations by planimetry of the endocardial border, left ventricular mass estimation requires an accurate measurement of both the endocardial and epicardial limits, which is far more hazardous owing to frequent uncertainties in delineating these borders.*

demonstrated the efficacy of antihypertensive treatment in reducing LV mass [21]. In addition to the study of LV structure, ultrasound methods provide useful information about systolic [8, 10, 11] and diastolic LV function [22].

Magnetic resonance imaging (MRI) has proved to be extremely accurate in the estimation of LV mass [23], by virtue of its excellent definition, wide field of view, and the lack of interference from the surrounding structures. Since it allows a true anatomical calculation from the summation of short-axis slices [24], independent of geometrical assumptions (Fig. 21.3), it has an advantage over other contemporary methods. The estimation of myocardial mass by MRI is highly reproducible [25], which is particularly desirable in longitudinal studies of regression of hypertrophy. Echocardiography in serial studies has shown large confidence intervals, precluding its application in the individual patient [26].

A complete non-invasive cardiac assessment may be accomplished in hypertensive patients by echocardiography and MRI, and both may contribute significantly to clinical management. However, the progressive loss of cardiomyocytes, which may determine the phase of decompensation in hypertensive heart disease, is not specifically addressed by these methods. Such a technique would be of enormous interest in the assessment and staging of patients and in the evaluation of the efficacy of interventional strategies in hypertensive heart disease.

## *In vivo* detection of myocardial damage in hypertensive patients

Non-invasive assessment of cardiomyocyte injury has been clinically determined by the serum concentration of various intramyocytic constituents. These cytoplasmic substances are released into the bloodstream when the myocyte membrane becomes leaky after diverse forms of insult. They include contractile proteins (e.g. troponin light myosin chains), enzymes (e.g. creatine kinase, lactic dehydrogenase, glutamic oxyltransferase), or pigments (e.g. myoglobin). During ongoing and diffuse but minimal myocardial necrosis, the serum concentration of the washed out cytoplasmic constituents is not sufficient for the diagnosis of or staging of myocardial damage.

Based on the principle that loss of sarcolemmal integrity demonstrations myocyte necrosis, antimyosin scintigraphy was used in mid-1980s for the diagnosis of myocarditis [27]. Imaging with radiolabelled monoclonal antimyosin antibodies targets heavy chains of myosin, which are not soluble in blood, through sarcolemmal breaches. Normal myocytes with intact sarcolemma do not permit entry of antimyosin antibody. This technique has since been used for the non-invasive detection of various cardiovascular diseases that are characterized by diffuse myocardial necrosis such as allograft rejection [28], cardiomyopathies [29], or adriamycin cardiotoxicity [30]. In numerous studies, antimyosin scintigraphy has provided highly reproducible and accurate results. The sensitivity of antimyosin uptake has often exceeded that of histological examination of endomyocardial biopsy. Furthermore, assessment of myocardial uptake of antimyosin antibody by calculation of the heart-to-lung ratio (HLR) [31] allows quantitation of the severity of myocardial damage (Fig. 21.4). In the normal population, the upper normal limit for HLR is 1.55 (mean ± 2 SD) [31].

Antimyosin scintigraphy was employed in a series of patients with varying degrees of long-standing primary hypertension to elucidate the prevalence and distribution of myocardial damage and its potential relationship with the morphological and functional status of the left ventricle as assessed by echocardiography. The 39 patients (14 male and 25 female) had a mean age of 55 ± 11 years. Thirty consecutive asymptomatic patients were from the outpatient clinics of the hypertension unit: 16 had normal echocardiograms and did not show evidence of LV hypertrophy (group I); the other 14 demonstrated echocardiographic evidence of LV hypertrophy based on an indexed LV mass

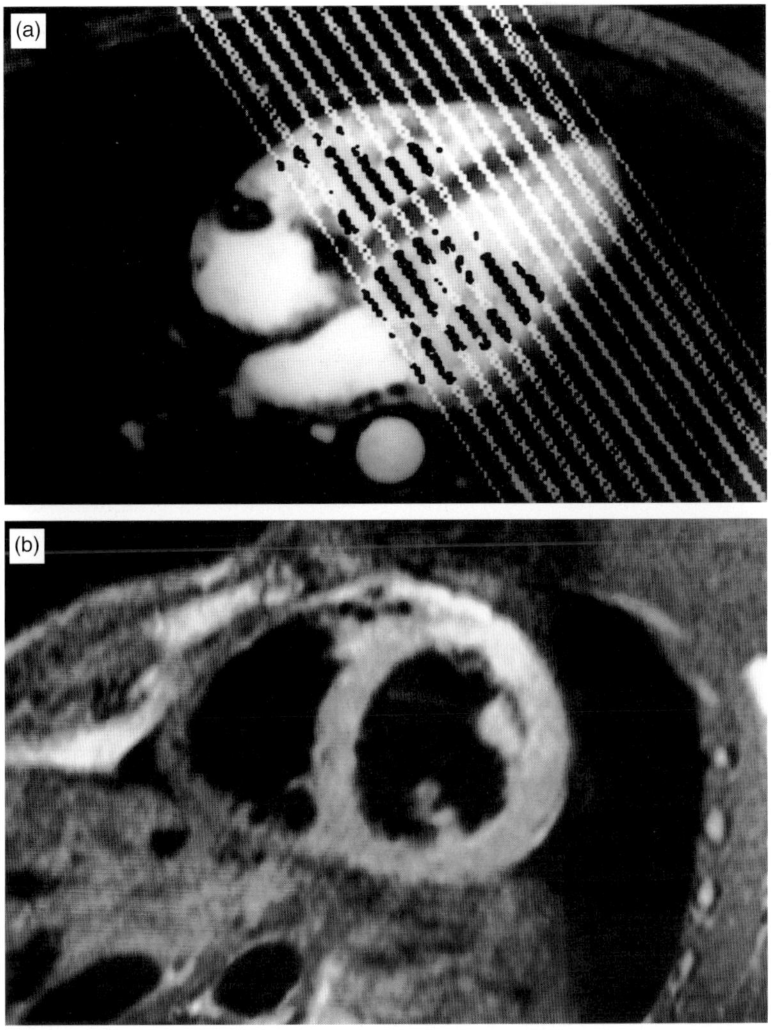


**Figure 21.3** *Calculation of left ventricular (LV) mass by magnetic resonance imaging. (a) Horizontal long-axis view of the heart where a series of transverse contiguous slices has been planned encompassing the left ventricle from base to apex. (b) One of the series of short-axis LV slices obtained where the endocardial and epicardial borders of the chamber are clearly visualized, allowing an accurate measurement of the myocardial area by planimetry, the volume of the slice being obtained by multiplying the resultant area by the slice thickness. The summation of volumes from all slices in the series gives an accurate estimation of LV mass free from geometrical assumptions.*

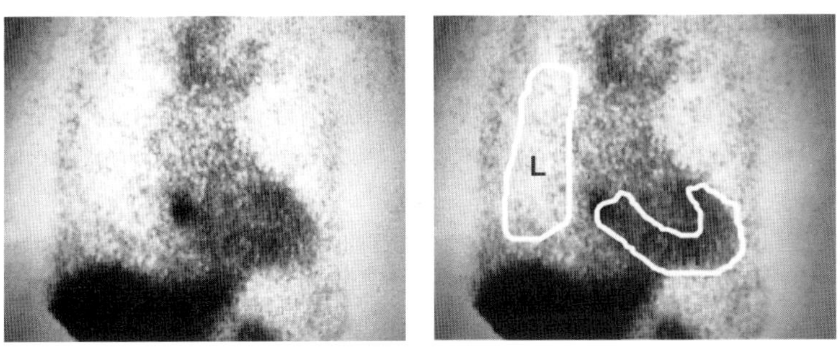


**Figure 21.4** *Indium-111 antimyosin scintigraphy from a patient with extensive myocardial cell lesion. In the right panel the method of quantification based on the calculation of the heart-to-lung ratio of uptake is shown. H = heart; L = lung.*

over the upper normal limits in the laboratory (> 123 g/m$^2$ in men and >109 g/m$^2$ in women) (group II). Coronary artery disease was deemed unlikely in these 30 patients because of a lack of history of chest pain. Hypertension was adequately controlled in all patients at the time of the study: six were receiving a β-blocker alone, 11 were on calcium channel blockers, and the remaining 13 were receiving combined therapy including these drugs and, in some cases, also thiazide diuretics. The remaining nine of the 39 patients (group III), had a history of long-term hypertension poorly controlled at the time of presentation. They were hospitalized for evaluation of chest pain (three patients) or heart failure (six patients); all had normal coronary arteries at a subsequent angiographic examination. All of these nine patients were receiving combination therapy of two or more of these agents: diuretics, digoxin, calcium channel blockers, nitrates, and vasodilators; none received angiotensin-converting enzyme (ACE) inhibitors.

All nine patients of group III had an abnormal antimyosin scan indicating a significant degree of myocar-

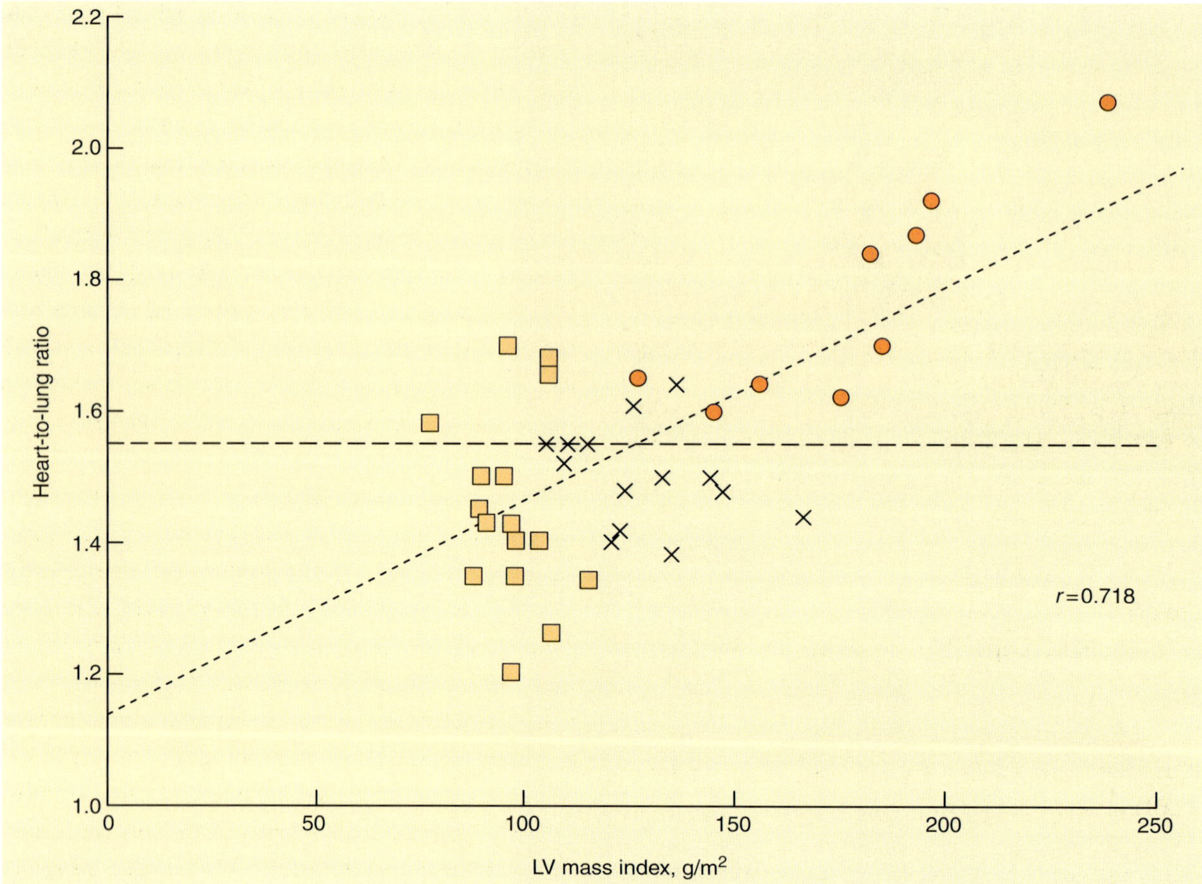


**Figure 21.5** *Correlation between indexed left ventricular (LV) mass and the severity of myocardial damage detected by antimyosin antibody heart-to-lung uptake ratio (HLR) in 39 patients with hypertension. Open squares = patients without LV hypertrophy; crosses = asymptomatics with increased LV mass; solid circles = patients with advanced hypertensive heart disease and cardiac decompensation. The horizontal line indicates the normal limit of antimyosin uptake (HLR < 1.55). There is a significant positive correlation between LV mass index and HLR (r = 0.718).*

dial damage (mean HLR of antimyosin uptake 1.77 ± 0.16). The mean antimyosin uptake was normal in patients of group I (HLR 1.45 ± 0.14) and group II (HLR 1.50 ± 0.07), although abnormal antimyosin scans were observed in four patients (25%) of group I and two patients (15%) of group II ($p = 0.0007$, compared with group III).

Bivariate and multivariate regression analyses were performed to evaluate clinical and echocardiographic determinants of myocardial damage. A significant correlation was observed between antimyosin uptake and age ($p = 0.017$). Systolic blood pressure showed a positive, although nonsignificant, correlation with the severity of myocardial damage ($p = 0.086$). Various echocardiographic parameters such as end-diastolic ($p = 0.003$) and end-systolic ($p = 0.000$) diameters, LV posterior wall thickness ($p = 0.000$), and LV mass ($p = 0.000$) (Fig. 21.5) correlated significantly with HLR by bivariate regression analysis. Left ventricular ejection fraction (LVEF) inversely correlated ($p = 0.000$).

Multivariate regression analysis of all significant variables demonstrated that indexed LV mass was the main independent predictor of antimyosin uptake in the LV myocardium ($r = 0.813$). A minor contribution was observed upon stepwise addition of LVEF ($r = 0.895$) and age (0.915). This *in vivo* demonstration that myocardial damage in hypertensive patients is largely dependent on LV mass substantiates the large body of evidence claiming that the loss of cardiomyocytes forms the basis of the progressive LV deterioration in patients with chronic pressure overload. Evidence of myocyte degeneration was observed in a small proportion of ambulatory patients (groups I and II) who had either no or only mild LV hypertrophy, whereas all patients with advanced hypertensive heart disease (group III) demonstrated evidence of myocardial damage. Once the myocardial hypertrophy has

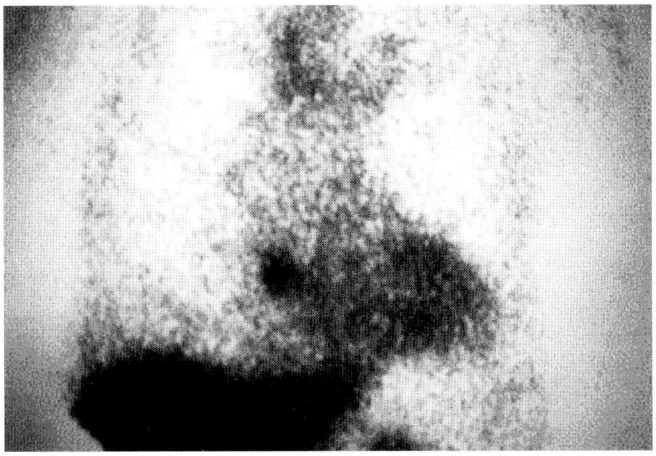

**Figure 21.6** *Antimyosin scan showing myocardial uptake of labelled antibodies, thus revealing the presence of active myocardial damage.*

started to occur, the LV mass strongly correlates with, and becomes the main independent predictor of, myocardial damage.

## Possible mechanisms of myocyte loss in hypertensive heart disease

The mechanisms leading to the death of myocytes are not well understood. Increased LV mass and systolic pressure significantly augment intramyocardial tension and oxygen demand but are not accompanied by a proportional increase in vascular density per unit area of hypertrophied myocardium. The discordance between oxygen demand and supply may result in relative myocardial ischaemia and myocellular death [32–34]. Recently, it has been proposed that apoptosis or programmed cell death may also contribute to myocardial damage in hypertrophic hearts [14, 35]. Apoptosis is a form of cell death distinct from myocyte necrosis and does not result in an inflammatory response [36, 37]. Growth response to pressure overload in terminally differentiated cells such as cardiomyocytes results in increased protein synthesis and myocyte hypertrophy. Although there is significant expression of foetal cardiac genes, cell division cannot be induced [14]. In hypertension, haemodynamic load to myocytes via stretch receptors [38] or integrin-mediated [39] mechanisms, and paracrine or autocrine stimulation of various neurohumoral receptors [40–42] including angiotensin are likely to initiate the cascade of compensatory ventricular hypertrophy. The induction of various immediate-early response proto-oncogenes, such as c-*myc* and c-*fos*, and early growth factors such as transforming growth factor-β (TGF-β) and erg-1, results in numeric growth of sarcomeres and provides a short-term adaptive measure [43–47]. The persistence of a growth stimulus should normally result in cell division, but since the cardiac myocytes have little or no ability to re-enter the cell cycle, programmed cell death may ensue [14, 35]. Indeed, apart from the growth response, the proto-oncogenes have also been shown to be involved in the induction of programmed cell death [48]. It is likely that a more severe hypertrophic response will be associated with more severe programmed cell death and therefore with more intense antimyosin uptake. It is also possible that repetitive ischaemia not sufficient to result in necrosis may induce apoptosis.

Hypertensive heart disease is a progressive myocardial disorder that may eventually lead to gradual myocellular loss and heart failure. In the light of evidence of myocardial damage, especially in patients who are apparently well controlled medically, the goal of antihypertensive treatment should be reconsidered. If progressive loss of myocytes determines the development of cardiomyopathy, then the optimum treatment of hypertension will have to be based on alleviation of myocardial damage rather than only the control of blood pressure. It is also desirable to evaluate the role of pharmacological agents such as ACE inhibitors [49, 50] or the newer generation of β-blockers [51] which are likely to inhibit the long-term neurohumoral or autocrineparacrine effects leading to progression of LV dysfunction and ventricular remodelling.

## References

1. Vasan RS, Levy D. The role of hypertension in the pathogenesis of heart failure: a clinical mechanistic overview. *Arch Intern Med* 1996; 156: 1789–96.
2. McKee PA, Castelli WP, McNamara PM, Kannel WB. The natural history of congestive heart failure: The Framingham Heart Study. *N Engl J Med* 1971; 285: 1441–6.
3. Burt VL, Culter JA, Higgins M, Horan MJ, Labarthe D, Whelton P, Brown C, Roccella EJ. Trends in the prevalence, awareness, treatment and control of hypertension in the adult US population: data from the health examination surveys, 1960–1991. *Hypertension* 1995; 26: 60–69.
4. Osler W. *The principles and practice of medicine: designed for the use of practitioners and students of medicine*. New York: Appleton, 1892: 634.
5. Meerson FZ. On the mechanism of compensatory hyperfunction and and insufficiency of the heart. *Cor Vasa*. 1961; 3: 161–77.
6. Grossman W. Cardiac hypertrophy : useful adaptation or pathologic process. *Am J Med* 1980; 69: 576–84.
7. Prineas RJ, Castle CH, Curb JD, Harrist R, Lewin A, Stamler J. Hypertension Detection and Follow-up Program: baseline electrocardiographic characteristics of the hypertensive participants. *Hypertension*. 1983; 5: 160–89.

8. Devereux RB, Savage DD, Drayer JIM, Laragh JH. Left ventricular hypertrophy and function in high, normal and low renin forms of hypertension. *Hypertension* 1982; 4: 524–31.
9. Wasserman AG, Katz RJ, Varghese PJ, Leiboff RH, Bren GG, Schlesselman S, Varma VM, Reba RC, Ross AM. Exercise radionuclide ventriculographic responses in hypertensive patients with chest pain. *N Engl J Med* 1984;311: 1276–80.
10. Blake J, Devereux RB, Borer JS, Szulc M, Pappas TW, Laragh JH. Relation of obesity, high sodium intake, and eccentric left ventricular hypertrophy to left ventricular exercise dysfunction in essential hypertension. *Am J Med* 1990; 88: 477–85.
11. de Simone G, Devereux RB, Roman MJ, Ganau A, Saba PS, Alderman MH, Laragh JH. Assessment of left ventricular function by midwall fractional shortening/end-systolic stress relationship in human hypertension. *J Am Coll Cardiol* 1994; 23: 1444–51.
12. Ferrans VJ, Rodríguez EN. Morphology of the heart in left ventricular hypertrophy. In: Messerli FH, ed. *The heart and hypertension*. New York: York Medical Books, 1987: 75–84.
13. Maron BJ, Ferrans VJ, Roberts WC. Ultrastructral features of degenerated cardiac muscle cells in patients with cardiac hypertrophy. *Am J Pathol.* 1975; 79: 387–434.
14. Katz AM. Cardiomyopathy of overload. A major determinant of prognosis in congestive heart failure. *N Engl J Med* 1990; 322: 100–10.
15. Hypertension Detection and Follow-up Program Cooperative Group. Five years findings of the Hypertension Detection and Follow-up Program: reduction of mortality of persons with high blood pressure, including mild hypertension. *JAMA* 1979; 242: 2562–71.
16. Hammond IW, Devereux RB, Alderman MH, Lutas EM, Spitzer MC, Crowley JS, Laragh JH. The prevalence and correlates of echocardiographic left ventricular hypertrophy among employed patients with uncomplicated hypertension. *J Am Coll Cardiol* 1986; 7: 639–50.
17. Devereux RB, Reichek N. Echocardiographic determination of left ventricular mass in man. Anatomic validation of the method. *Circulation* 1977; 55: 613–18.
18. Devereux RB, Alonso DR, Lutas EM, Gottlieb GJ, Campo E, Sachs I, Reichek N. Echocardiographic assessment of left ventricular hypertrophy: comparison to necropsy findings. *Am J Cardiol* 1986; 57: 450–8.
19. Schiller NB, Skioldebrand CG, Schiller EJ, Mavroudis CC, Silverman NH, Rahimtoola SH, Lipton MJ. Canine left ventricular mass estimation by two-dimensional echocardiography. *Circulation* 1983; 68: 210–61.
20. Devereux RB. Detection of left ventricular hypertrophy by M-mode echocardiography: anatomic validation, standardization, and comparison to other methods. *Hypertension* 1987; 9 (Suppl. II): II-19-II-26.
21. Dahlof B, Pennert K, Hansson L. Reversal of left ventricular hypertrophy in hypertension patients: a meta-analysis of 109 treatment studies. *Am J Hypertens* 1992; 5: 95–110.
22. Shepherd RFJ, Zachariah PK, Shub C. Hypertension and left ventricular diastolic function. *Mayo Clin Proc* 1989; 64: 1521–32.
23. Katz J, Milliken MC, Stray-Gundersen J, Buja LM, Parkey RW, Mitchell JH, Peshock RM. Estimation of human myocardial mass with MR imaging. *Radiology* 1988; 169: 495–8.
24. Pons-Lladó G, Carreras F, Borrás X, Llauger J, Palmer J, Bayés de Luna A. Left ventricular mass by echocardiography and magnetic resonance (abstract). *J Cardiovasc Magn Reson* 1999; 1: 91–2.
25. Bottini PB, Carr AA, Prisant LM, Flickinger FW, Allison JD, Gottdiener JS. Magnetic Resonance imaging compared to echocardiography to assess left ventricular mass in the hypertensive patient. *Am J Hypertension* 1995; 8: 221–8.
26. Gottdiener JS, Livengood SV, Meyer PS, Chase GA. Should echocardiography be performed to assess efects of antihypertensive therapy? Test-retest reliability of echocardiography for measurement of left ventricular mass and function. *J Am Coll Cardiol* 1995; 25: 424–30.
27. Yasuda T, Palacios IF, Dec GW, Fallon JT, Gold HK, Leinbach RC, Strauss HW, Khaw BA, Haber E. Indium 111-monoclonal antimyosin antibody imaging in the diagnosis of acute myocarditis. *Circulation* 1987; 76: 306–11.
28. Ballester M, Bordes R, Tazelaar HD, Carrio I, Marrugat J, Narula J, Billingham ME. Evaluation of biopsy classification for rejection: relation to detection of myocardial damage by monoclonal antimyosin antibody imaging. *J Am Coll Cardiol* 1998; 31: 1357–61.
29. Obrador D, Ballester M, Carrio I, Berna L, Pons-Llado G. High prevalence of myocardial monoclonal antimyosin antibody uptake in patients with chronic idiopathic dilated cardiomyopathy. *J Am Coll Cardiol* 1989; 13: 1289–93.
30. Narula J, Strauss HW, Khaw BA. Antimyosin positivity in doxorubicin cardiotoxicity: earlier than the conventional evidence. *J Nucl Med* 1993; 34: 1507–9.
31. Carrio I, Berna L, Ballester M, Estorch M, Obrador D, Cladellas M, Abadal L, Ginjaume M. Indium 111 antimyosin scintigraphy to assess myocardial damage in patients with suspected myocarditis and cardiac rejection. *J Nucl Med* 1988; 29: 1893–900.
32. Parodi O, De Maria R, Oltrona L, Testa R, Sambuceti G, Roghi A, Merli M, BelingherL, Accinni R, Spinelli F, Pellegrini A, Baroldi G. Myocardial blood flow distribution in patients with ischemic heart disease or dilated cardiomyopathy undergoing heart transplantation. *Circulation* 1993; 88: 509–522.
33. Marcus ML, Mueller TB, Eastham CL. Effects of short- and long-term left ventricular hypertrophy on coronary circulation. *Am J Physiol* 1981; 241: H358–362.
34. Anversa P, Capasso JM. Cardiac hypertrophy and ventricular remodeling. *Lab Invest* 1991; 64: 441–5.
35. Narula J, Haider N, Virmani R, DiSalvo TG, Kolodgie FD, Hajjar RJ, Schmidt U, Semigran MJ, Dec GW, Khaw BA. Apoptosis in myocytes in end-stage heart failure. *N Engl J Med* 1996; 335: 1182–9.
36. James T. Apoptosis in normal and abnormal heart. *Circulation* 1994; 90: 556–73.
37. Komura I, Kaida T, Shibazaki Y, Kurabayashi M, Katoh Y, Hoh E, Takaku F, Yazaki Y. Stretching cardiomyocytes stimulates protooncogene expression. *J Biol Chem* 1990; 265: 3595–8.
38. Hynes RO. Integrins: versatality, modulation and signaling in cell adhesion. *Cell* 1992; 69: 11–25.
39. Aceto JF, Baker KM. [$Sar^1$] angiotensin-II receptor-mediated stimulation of protein synthesis in chick heart cells. *Am J Physiol* 1990; 258: H806–H813.
40. Beinlich CJ, White GJ, Baker KM, Morgan HE. Angiotensin II and left ventricular growth in newborn pig heart. *J Mol Cell Cardiol* 1991; 23: 1031–8.
41. Sadoshima J, Xu Y, Slayter HS, Izumo S. Autocrine release of Angiotensin II mediates stretch-induced hypertrophy of cardiac myocytes in vitro. *Cell* 1993; 75: 977–84.
42. Lee YA, Lindpaintener K. Role of cardiac renin-angiotensin system in hypertensive cardiac hypertrophy. *Eur J Med* 1993; 14 (Suppl. J): 42–8.

43. Izumo S, Nadal-Ginard B, Madhavi V. Proto-oncogene induction and reprograming of cardiac gene expression produced by pressure overload. *Proc Natl Acad Med Sci USA* 1988; 85: 339–43.
44. Khairalla PA, Robertson AL, Davila D. Effect of angiotensin II on DNA, RNA and protein synthesis. In Genest J, Koiw E, Eds. Hypertension '72. New York, Springer-Verlag, 1972: 212–20.
45. Chien KR, Zhu H, Knowlton KU, Miller-Hance W, van-Bilsen M, O'Brien TX, Evans SM. Transcriptional regulation during cardiac growth and development. *Annu Rev Physiol* 1993; 55: 77–95.
46. Francis GS, Carlyle WC. Hypothetical pathways of cardiac myocyte hypertrophy: response to myocardial injury. *Eur Heart J* 1993; 14 (Suppl. J): 49–56.
47. Evan GI, Wyllie AH, Gilbert CS, Littlewood TD, Land H, Brooks M, Waters CM, Penn LZ, Hancock DC. Induction of apoptosis in fibroblasts by c-Myc protein. *Cell* 1992; 69: 119–28.
48. The CONSENSUS Trial Study Group. Effects of Enalapril on mortality in severe congestive heart failure: results of the Cooperative North Scandanavian Enalapril Survival Study (CONSENSUS). *N Engl J Med* 1987; 316: 1429–35.
49. The SOLVD investigators: effects of Enalapril on survival in patients with reduced left ventricular ejection fractions and congestive heart failure. *N Engl J Med* 1991; 325: 293–302.
50. Packer M, Bristow MR, Cohn JN, Colucci WS, Fowler MB, Gilbert EM, Shusterman NH; for the US Carvedilol Heart Failure Study Group. Effect of Carvedilol on mortality and morbidity in chronic heart failure. *N Engl J Med* 1996; 334: 1349–55.
51. Eichorn EJ, Bristow MR. Medical therapy can improve the biological properties of the chronically failing heart: a new era in the treatment of heart. *Circulation* 1996; 94: 2285–96.

# The myocardium in diabetes mellitus 22

Y. CHANDRASHEKHAR, J. NARULA AND A. E. ISKANDRIAN

## Introduction

Diabetes mellitus (DM) is a major health problem in almost all parts of the world [1, 2]. The global prevalence is estimated to be at least 100 million patients and is projected to increase to 215 million in the next 10–12 years [3]. The incidence of DM appears to be increasing in the USA, as well as in other developed countries [4, 5] and is therefore rapidly becoming one of the leading causes of morbidity and mortality in these populations (Fig. 22.1). DM is frequently underdiagnosed: various estimates suggest that there is at least one undiagnosed patient for every patient diagnosed correctly. There is often a latent period of 4–7 years between the onset of the disease and its clinical recognition [6]. Despite underdiagnosis, the prevalence of DM is projected to be 6–7% in persons between 45 and 64 years of age and to increase to 10–12% in older individuals. In addition, about 40 million individuals have impaired glucose tolerance and some of these will end up with overt disease and its complications. Thus, the total estimated burden of DM-related complications is enormous.

DM is associated with significant morbidity and mortality. It shortens the average life span by about 7–10 years [7] and patients with DM have a mortality rate two to four times higher than non-diabetics [8]. While DM affects a number of organ systems, cardiovascular complications are the most common cause of death. Patients with DM are six times more likely to be hospitalized in a given year compared with non-diabetics, and myocardial infarction (MI) and strokes account of 80% of deaths and hospitalizations in diabetics [8–14]. In fact, diabetics without a previous MI have as bad a prognosis as non-diabetic patients with a previous MI (Fig. 22.2) [11]. Cardiovascular disease appears earlier in life in diabetics, negates the protection against coronary artery disease (CAD) seen in premenopausal women, and is more often fatal [14].

Diabetics have a high prevalence of traditional cardiovascular risk factors. However, DM continues to be a potent risk factor for adverse cardiovascular events even after adjustment for other risk factors [9, 11–13]. The Multiple Risk Factor Intervention Trial (MRFIT) showed that diabetics had a three-fold excess of adverse events over a 12 year period of follow-up, even when corrected for demographics and other risk factors (smoking, hypertension, and increased lipids).

Direct myocardial involvement, affecting both the myocytes and the interstitium, is also frequently seen in the diabetic patient and heart failure is an important complication. The myocardium is involved very early in the disease, and many of the subtle indices of myocardial involvement are present even before overt impaired glucose intolerance.

This chapter will review the current evidence about the pathogenic factors and prognostic implications of the myocardial involvement in diabetic patients. Studies of various interventions aimed at reducing the adverse cardiovascular effects of myocardial structural and functional changes in diabetic patients are presented. The discussion focuses on type II DM but with suitable comparisons with the less common type I.

## Myocardial involvement secondary to coronary artery disease

Coronary vascular disease is a major determinant of myocardial dysfunction in diabetic patients. Vascular involvement in the diabetic heart is commonly due to obstructive epicardial coronary artery involvement. However, small-vessel CAD and endothelial dysfunction are also common and contribute significantly to myocardial dysfunction in the diabetic patient. Although many of these conditions coexist in the same patient, each is discussed

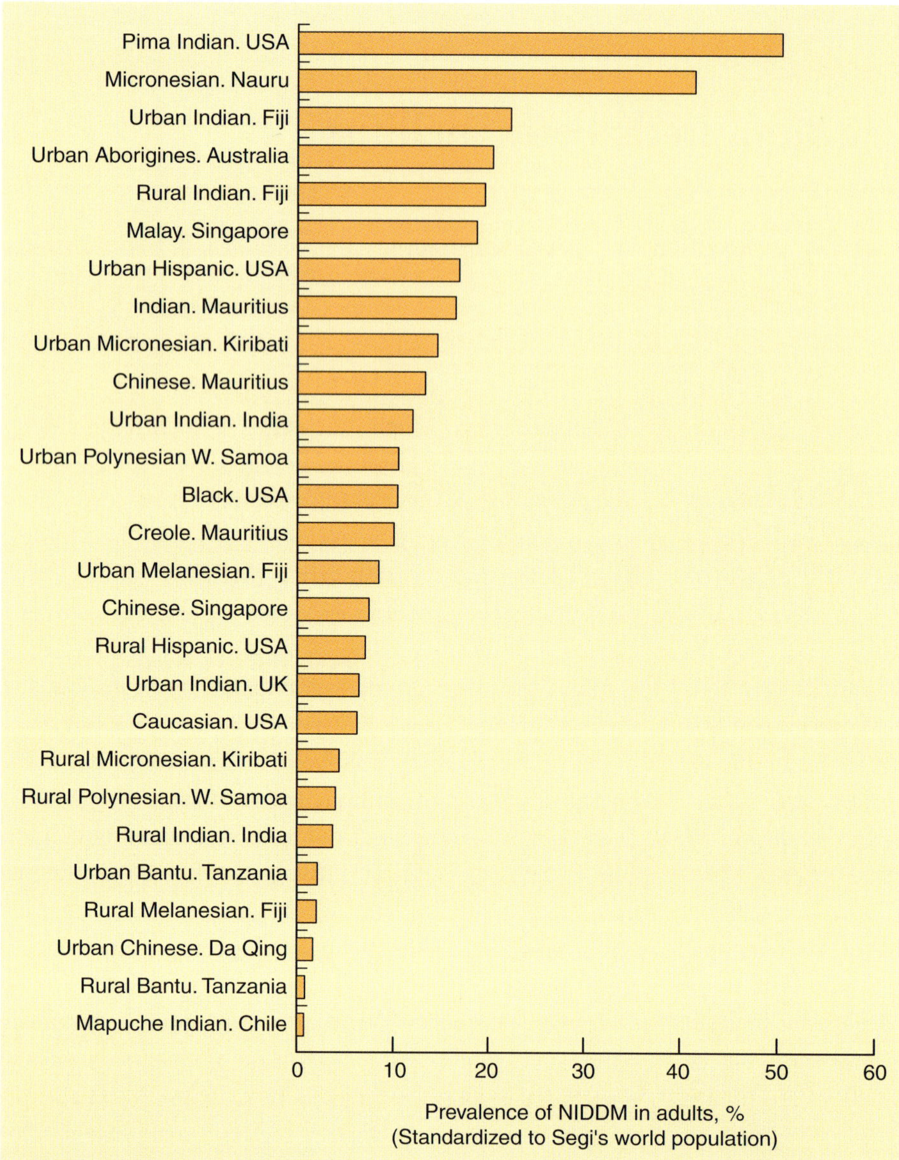


**Figure 22.1** *Prevalence of non-insulin diabetes worldwide. (From ref. 5.)*

separately to evaluate their contribution to myocardial failure in the diabetic patient, and their pathogenesis is outlined to clarify the role of prevention and treatment.

## Epidemiology of macrovascular coronary artery disease in diabetes

DM is associated with a very high incidence and prevalence of CAD: the age-adjusted prevalence in patients with DM is between 30 and 51% [14%]. Diabetics have more extensive CAD, the stenosis is more severe, and the residual vessel size is smaller than in non-diabetics. There is a higher prevalence of ulcerated plaques, more vessel clot burden, greater progression of atheroma, and a higher incidence of total occlusions [15–17]. The vessel morphology is less amenable to revascularization [18–20]. This is seen consistently in both antemortem [15, 17, 18] and postmortem studies [21]. Angiographic studies have confirmed these findings in the setting of all varieties of coronary syndromes [15, 17, 18].

There is also an excess of CAD-related heart disease in diabetic patients [14, 22, 23]. More than three-quarters of the deaths and hospital admissions in diabetic patients are for cardiovascular complications [23]. Although microvascular complications are very often cited as major adverse events in patients with DM, fatal macrovascular complications, especially those due to CAD, are 70 times more

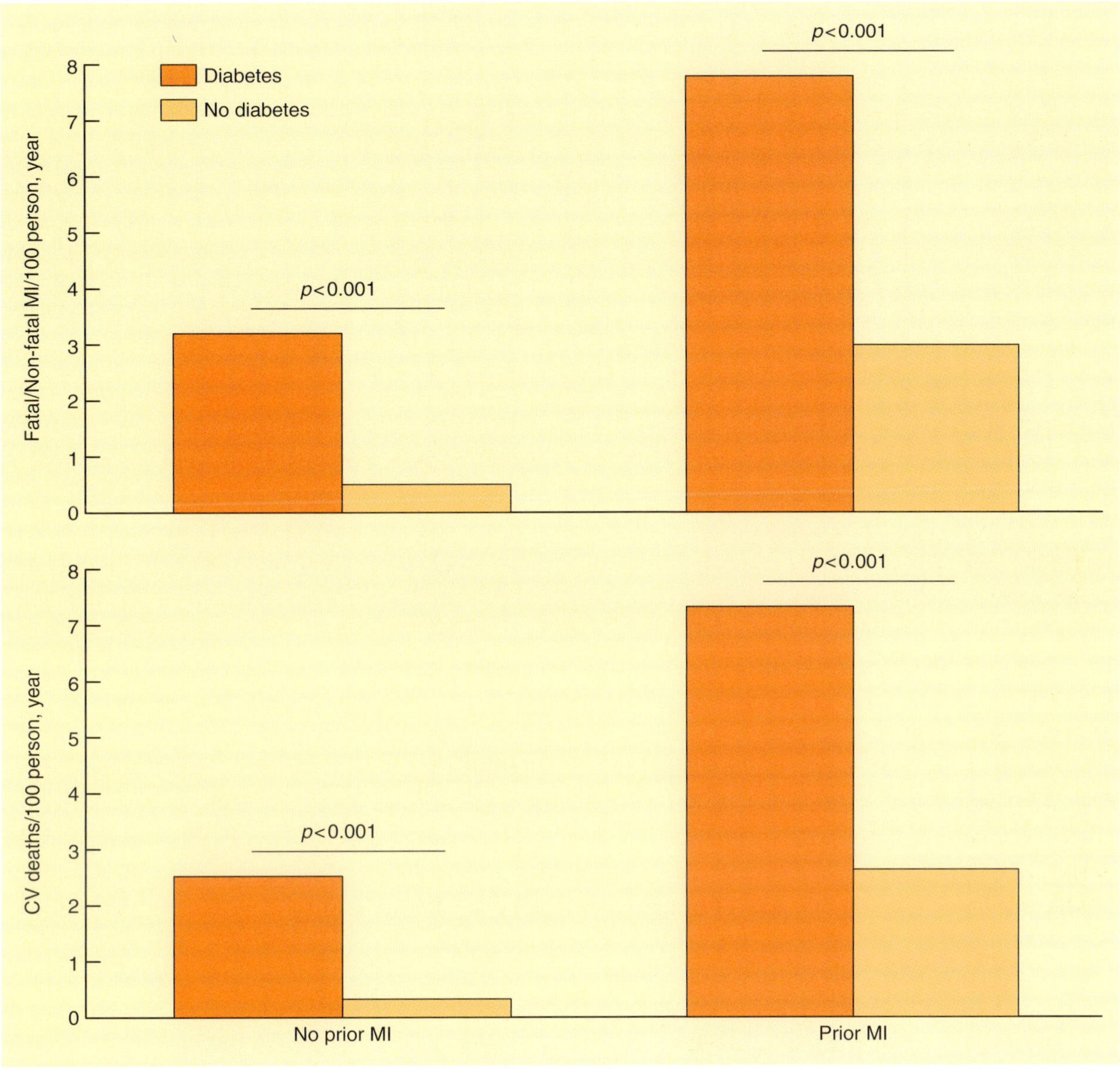


**Figure 22.2** *Adverse prognosis in diabetics. Diabetics without a known myocardial infarction (MI) have a prognosis as bad as non-diabetics with a previous MI. Diabetics with a previous MI have one of the highest cardiovascular event rates on follow-up. (Data from ref. 11.)*

common [14, 24, 25]. Better control of DM has resulted in a reduction in some major microvascular complications; this has occurred at a time when there have been no major advances in preventing macrovascular complications. Diabetic patients are likely to present with excessive cardiovascular morbidity in the future [25]. MI and congestive heart failure (CHF) are the two most common clinical conditions associated with myocardial involvement in diabetics.

The risk of diabetic cardiovascular complications in not the same in all ethnic populations. There is a higher risk in Western Europe (Switzerland, Germany, and the UK) and the Far East [26, 27]. There is an overlapping relationship between nature (genes) and nurture (environment). Thus, populations with a low incidence of CAD, such as in Japan and Africa, have a low incidence of diabetic vascular disease, unless they migrate to areas with a population with a high prevalence of CAD. It appears that there needs to be an inherent tendency in the population to develop atheromatous lesions before DM can accelerate their occurrence [28, 29]. There are many unresolved issues in the relationship between ethnicity and diabetic heart disease, as exemplified by the Pima Indians. They have one of the highest incidences of DM in the world but have a low incidence of fatal diabetic heart disease [30]. The Pima people, however, remain at risk for microvascular complications. In addition, the same people living in the mountains of Mexico have a different epidemiological pattern, suggesting a mixture of nature and nurture in the pathogenesis. The cause of this anomaly is unclear. A similar pattern of a high incidence of DM with a relatively low incidence of vascular involvement has been noted in Navajo tribes in the USA [31].

Compared with men, women with DM seem to have greater adverse cardiovascular effects [32], especially premenopausal women. While the prevalence of CAD is extremely low in non-diabetic premenopausal women [33], several studies [32–34] have shown that this protection is lost in premenopausal diabetic women, although the reason for this remains unknown. Many studies have shown that the risk imposed by DM in women persists even after adjustment for smoking, hypertension, and hypercholesterolaemia [14, 23, 35]. In the Framingham Study, DM remained a risk factor for cardiovascular mortality in women, even after adjustment for lipids [36]. However, other studies have confirmed the pathogenetic importance of the typical hyperlipidaemia pattern [increased very low-density lipoprotein (VLDL) and decreased high-density lipoprotein (HDL)] seen in diabetics [34]. Lipoprotein profiles are more abnormal in diabetic women compared with non-diabetic women and all men (diabetic and non-diabetic) [37], and this is believed to be important in reducing the protection against atherosclerosis in diabetic women. Smoking has been shown to be particularly hazardous in women with diabetes, much more so than in men [38].

One fundamental, unanswered question is whether the degree of glycaemic control affects the risk of developing CAD and its complications. It is surprising that there are few data on this issue. In patients with type I DM, there is evidence that the risk of CAD is proportional to the degree of hyperglycaemia, and this risk can be reduced with aggressive blood sugar control [39]. The data for type II DM are a little less clear. Some epidemiological studies have suggested that the risk is proportional to the degree of hyperglycaemia [40] but other data do not clearly support this. The effect of aggressively managing hyperglycaemia in patients with type II DM is uncertain.

The relationship between the duration of DM and the risk of microvascular complications is well established. However, this relation is uncertain with regard to macrovascular complications. In some studies, the duration of DM was not an important indicator of CAD risk when age was factored into the equation, while other studies showed an increased incidence of cardiac complications with increasing duration of DM [41]. In patients with type I DM, the deaths due to CAD begin to occur in the fourth decade of life, which is similar to those seen in non-diabetic populations. However, between the ages of 30 and 55 years, CAD mortality is much higher in the DM group [42]. Onset of DM before the age of 20 years has a smaller, impact on CAD risk than DM that occurs later in life. It has been suggested that the occurrence of DM during the early stages of atheromatous plaque formation might accelerate the atheromatous process and contribute to the risk of progression of CAD [42]. Type II DM is diagnosed later than type I and therefore type II diabetics have a higher mortality rate than controls right from the time of diagnosis. Similar to the type I DM population, the risk of CAD-related events increases with the duration of the diabetes [42–44].

### Pathogenesis of coronary artery disease in diabetes

Several theories about the pathogenesis of diabetic cardiovascular complications have been proposed. Most of these are conjectural and need additional proof. The main issue is whether hyperglycaemia or hyperinsulinaemia is responsible for the pathogenesis of cardiovascular injury. There is no consensus on this issue and the evidence is discussed in brief below.

### Association of hyperinsulinaemia and coronary artery disease

Although DM is primarily recognized by hyperglycaemia and increased blood glucose levels correlate well with diabetic complications, there is some evidence that insulin per se may be pathogenetic in cardiovascular complications associated with DM. Insulin resistance and hyperinsulinaemia are two major features of type II DM. It is not known whether insulin resistance by itself or the hyperinsulinaemia that it invokes mediates the excess risk of CAD. Insulin resistance is seen years before the overt development of DM [45] and low insulin sensitivity is associated with atherosclerosis in diabetic individuals, independent of insulin levels [46]. Insulin resistance is also a central component of the metabolic syndrome, which brings together a constellation of adverse cardiovascular risk factors [47].

It has been proposed that insulin resistance may be the more important independent marker for CAD in diabetics and that insulin levels may not reflect insulin resistance accurately [46]. One of the problems with clarifying the individual, separate role for each of these entities is the difficulty in measuring insulin resistance. No major trial has looked at the role of insulin resistance independently of the associated hyperinsulinaemia.

Since hyperinsulinaemia and insulin resistance are present decades before the onset of overt DM [47], CAD is often seen in patients with increased insulin but without overt hyperglycaemia [43]. Similarly, CAD is often seen in those with newly diagnosed DM who could not have had a prolonged period of hyperglycaemia [48]. Hyperinsulinaemia can accelerate atherosclerosis [49] and there is some evidence that insulin may contribute to the risk of CAD [50, 51]. It is not clear whether this is due to a direct effect or because of an association with other risk factors. Hyperinsulinaemia is consistently clustered with other risk factors in the insulin resistance syndrome or syndrome X, or Reaven's syndrome [47] and this could be one way by which it mediates increased cardiovascular risk in diabetic patients. Some studies suggest that insulin acts independently of other risk factors, while others could not demonstrate an independent effect after controlling for other antecedent risk factors [52, 53].

### *Putative mechanisms of hyperinsulinaemia as a factor for coronary artery disease*

Despite the lack of evidence for a direct role of insulin in CAD, there is a number of postulated mechanisms by which increased insulin can mediate CAD. Insulin has several haemodynamic effects, including vasodilatation and activation of the sympathetic nervous and renin–angiotensin systems [54, 55]. It has been shown to be directly atherogenic [49]. Insulin receptors are found in the vasculature and control gene expression in vascular cells [56]. These mitogenic effects require very high levels of insulin, while its antiproliferative (increased nitric oxide) and vasodilatory actions are seen at physiological insulin levels [56]. It is postulated that the mitogenic actions predominate during insulin resistance in diabetics and this may promote atherogenesis and plaque instability.

### *Evidence against the hyperinsulinaemia hypothesis*

There are some reasons to believe that this hypothesis is far from proven [52]. Several prospective studies have questioned an association between hyperinsulinaemia and the risk of CAD [57]. The relationship between hyperinsulinaemia and CAD is weak in women and in the elderly. Furthermore, the endogenous hyperinsulinaemia seen with insulin-producing tumours is not associated with increased cardiovascular risk [58]. Moreover, progressive β-cell dysfunction results in a reduction in circulating insulin levels in the later stages of DM at a time when CAD events are high. This confounds the relationship between insulin and CAD-related events. Others have suggested that pro-insulin molecules may be more important in the insulin hypothesis [59]. This issue has not yet been resolved.

### *Cardiovascular risk of exogenous insulin administration*

In the USA, 43% of patients are treated with insulin alone and another 10% take it in addition to oral hypoglycaemics; the proportion of patients using insulin increases with the duration of DM [60]. It is therefore important to have adequate information on the cardiovascular effects of insulin use. There is a high risk for CAD and CAD-related events among patients with type II DM treated with insulin. This has been used as support for the insulin hypothesis. One cannot, however, exclude the possibility that the metabolic or cellular abnormalities that underlie insulin resistance and produce the hyperglycaemia that requires insulin treatment are the true risk factors for accelerated atherosclerosis [57, 61]. There are insufficient data to clarify whether exogenous insulin administration is a risk factor for cardiovascular disease.

The secondary Prevention Reinfarction Israeli Nifedipine Trial (SPRINT) study [62] prospectively looked at 5839 consecutive patients with acute MI. Insulin-treated DM was seen in 2% of the men and 6% of the women. Another 8% of men and 12% of women were on oral hypoglycaemic drugs. Insulin treatment increased in-hospital mortality [odds ratio (OR) 2.24 in men and 1.8 in women]. Diabetic patients treated with oral drugs had a lower risk ratio (1.26 in men and 1.46 in women). Similar effects were seen over a 10 year period of follow-up: women on insulin seemed to have the greatest risk of long-term mortality [risk ratio (RR) 2.59; 95% confidence interval (CI) 1.89–3.56]. A similar adverse prognosis for insulin-treated diabetics was noted in other data, including the Global Utilization of Streptokinase and Tissue Plasminogen Activator for Occluded Coronary Arteries (GUSTO) trial [17, 20]. The 30 day mortality was highest among diabetic patients treated with insulin (12.5%) compared with non-insulin-treated diabetics (9.7%) and non-diabetic (6.2%) patients ($p < 0.001$). It is whether the high mortality not clear is due to insulin or to the underlying severity of DM which necessitated the use of insulin. An association between insulin use and increased CAD risk has been described in Pima Indians and some other populations [30].

Two long-term, randomized clinical trials compared cardiovascular outcomes in patients given exogenous insulin as part of their treatment regimens. The University Group Diabetes Program (UGDP) [63] compared the effects of a fixed-dose standard insulin regimen, a variable-dose insulin regimen, and a diet plus oral placebo regimen in over 600 patients with type II DM. These patients were followed up for 13 years (1962–1975). While the variable-dose insulin regimen (mean insulin dose of 47 IV/day by the end of the trial) reduced plasma glucose more than the other two regimens, the prevalence of total deaths, cardiovascular deaths, and MI was similar in all three treatment groups. This trial was conducted many years ago and there have been significant changes in DM and risk-factor management since then. It is not clear whether these data are applicable today. The Diabetes Control and Complications Trial (DCCT) [64] compared intensive insulin treatment with conventional insulin treatment in over 1400 patients with DM followed for up to 10 years (1983–1993). Intensive treatment resulted in better glycaemic control [mean haemoglobin AIc ($HbA_{Ic}$) level was 7.2% vs 9.0%, respectively] and a better lipid profile, but the total insulin dose used in both groups was approximately similar. There were fewer cardiovascular events in the intensive treatment group. However, this trial has not clarified the adverse impact, if any, of insulin. A preliminary analysis of the UK Prospective Diabetes (UKPD) study, which looked at the effect of intensive glycaemic control using oral drugs or insulin, showed that while all of the pharmacological therapies were better than diet, there was no difference in the risk factor levels or cardiovascular events over a 6 year period [64]. Finally, the pilot project in the Veteran's Administration (VA) Cooperative study prospectively compared the effects of intensive and standard insulin therapy in patients with type II DM. This study found that intensive insulin therapy was associated with an increase in cardiovascular events [65]. This issue therefore remains unresolved. However, various authorities continue to recommend that insulin should be used where needed without fear of worsening atheromatous events [66].

## Association of hyperglycaemia with coronary artery disease

Since the insulin hypothesis accounts for only a small proportion of risk of CAD in diabetics [10], other factors may also be important. Hyperglycaemia is predictive for adverse coronary heart disease (CHD)-related events [67]. The DCCT highlighted the adverse role of hyperglycaemia in microvascular disease in type I DM patients [68]. However, the independent adverse role of hyperglycaemia is less well proven in patients with macrovascular complications [68, 69] and in patients with type II DM.

A few epidemiological studies have suggested that the risk of CAD-associated mortality is proportional to the degree of hyperglycaemia [40]. There is also some evidence that increased glucose levels, but far below those needed to diagnose impaired glucose tolerance (dysglycaemia) may be harmful [70]. Hyperglycaemia, like cholesterol, acts as a continuous variable for the risk of CAD [70]. The lower level at which hyperglycaemia poses no cardiovascular risk is unknown, but it may be much lower than that traditionally measured as impaired glucose tolerance [70]. The glycaemic threshold for macrovascular complications may be lower than that for microvascular complications [70]. Finally, more precise measurements of glycaemia, e.g. $HbA_{Ic}$, show a better correlation of DM with CAD and other vascular complications than measurement of the hyperglycaemia itself [71].

### *Putative mechanisms of hyperglycaemia as a factor for coronary artery disease*

An increase in the activity of the sorbitol pathway has been postulated to be important in the genesis of diabetic complications. A minor pathway of normal glucose metabolism (< 5% in the euglycaemic state), the aldose reductase or sorbitol pathway, changes glucose to fructose in the cell through an intermediate, sorbitol. This pathway becomes increasingly significant in periods of uncontrolled hyperglycaemia [72] and can mediate tissue damage. The mechanism by which sorbitol causes tissue damage is unclear and inhibiting this pathway does not seem to influence macrovascular disease [73]. Hyperglycaemia increases oxidative species and changes the cellular redox state, which could change vascular permeability [74], influence intracellular signalling [75], alter gene and protein expression [76], and impair contractility. There are few direct data to show that changing cellular oxidant status influences diabetic macrovascular complications, but it may reduce some microvascular complications.

Hyperglycaemia causes non-enzymatic modification of macromolecules to form compounds known as advanced glycation end-products (AGEs) [77], which are increased in DM proportional to its severity. Various tissues have AGE receptors [78] and activating them alters protein function, signal transduction pathways, extracellular matrix molecules, and gene expression [78]. For example, AGEs on type IV collagen prevent normal matrix formation [79], interfere with matrix–cell interactions, and reduce cell adhesion [80]. AGEs also decrease the elasticity of large vessels, increase fluid filtration across the vessel, and reduce vasodilatory and antiproliferative responses to nitric oxide [77]. Hyperglycaemia also affects the endothelial structure and function, increases adhesion molecule expression, and impairs endothelial-dependent vasodilatation [81]. The clinical significance of these changes is unclear. In one study, inhibition of AGE formation improved arterial elasticity, reduced aortic impedance, and improved left ventricular (LV) function.

#### *Evidence against hyperglycaemia and coronary artery disease*

Not all data are clearly supportive of the hyperglycaemic hypothesis. Several cross-sectional and prospective studies do not support the hypothesis when adjusted for other risk factors [10]. The association between the level and duration of hyperglycaemia [40, 82], measures of control [83], and the effect of intensive glycaemic control [69] and cardiovascular disease in diagnosed type II DM is inconsistent. It is critical to resolve this issue given the fact that major recommendations now encourage aggressive glycaemic control [84].

### Miscellaneous mechanisms and genesis of diabetic myocardial complications

Various growth factors have been postulated to be important in the genesis of the vascular complications of DM [84] and these affect both the vasculature and the myocardium. Hyperglycaemia and hyperinsulinaemia also affect the hormonal systems, including angiotensin II and endothelins [55, 84, 85], and this could be another way by which diabetes can be cardiotoxic and vasculotoxic. Angiotensin II levels are increased in obese diabetics, probably related to angiotensinogen production in adipocytes and the existence of renin-independent pathways for angiotensin II production in these cells [86, 87]. Angiotensin II is a potent growth factor, is atherogenic, can cause direct vascular and myocyte injury [88, 89], and increases expression of coagulation factors, all of which can accelerate myocardial injury. Furthermore, angiotensin II can inhibit insulin signalling pathways and contribute to insulin resistance [90]. While these are attractive hypotheses, more work is needed to clarify the role of hormones and growth factors in diabetic heart disease.

### Role of conventional coronary risk factors in myocardial complications of diabetes

The traditional risk factors are important in the genesis of CAD even in patients with diabetes (Fig. 22.3). For every conventional risk factor, diabetics have a three- to six-fold increase in cardiovascular risk [13, 92]. The contributions of conventional risk factors to CAD in DM are not similar in all populations. One example is the Asian Indians, who have a high prevalence of heart disease both in their native lands and more so when they settle in prosperous countries [93]. In these populations, as well as in Pima Indians [30], conventional risk factors do not seem to explain the high risk of CAD adequately. Similarly, Mexican Americans in the USA have a worse risk factor profile, but for unclear reasons have a lower rate of CAD events [94]. These examples emphasize the variable contribution of conventional risk factors in diabetes. This also suggests that DM-specific factors, such as diabetic vascular dysfunction and effects of advanced glycation products, may be important in diabetic heart disease [95].

An excess of conventional risk factors is seen in diabetic patients [61, 96, 97]; however, some studies do not show an excess of smoking or hypercholesterolaemia [97]. Multiple risk factors are common in individual with DM [13, 96], which adds to the risk associated with each factor alone [13]. Persons with impaired glucose tolerance have a level of risk factors intermediate between those with DM and non-diabetics. One common cluster of rise factors is associated with the multiple metabolic syndrome [61].

### Multiple metabolic syndrome (syndrome X) and myocardial complications

A typical cluster of risk factors is associated with insulin resistance, hyperinsulinaemia, and eventually frank diabetes. This clustering occurs more often than by chance and has been variously termed syndrome X, multiple metabolic syndrome, or insulin resistance syndrome [47, 61]. Components of this syndrome have been shown to occur even in childhood [98] and predict a later occurrence of

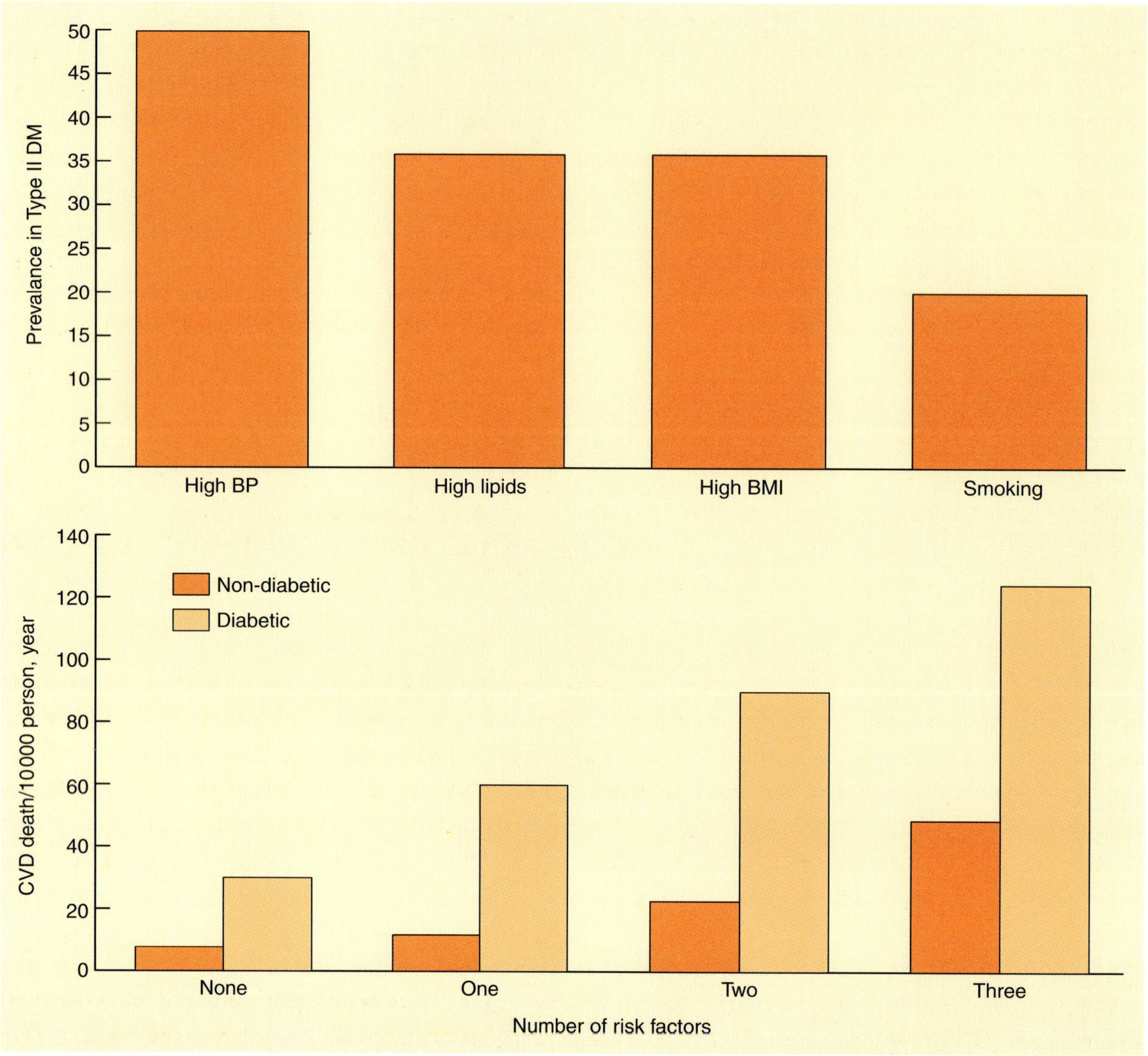


**Figure 22.3** (Top) *Prevalence of risk factors in patients with diabetes. (Data from ref. 91.)* (Bottom) *Risk of adverse events increases non-linearly as the number of risk factors increases in a given patient. (Data from ref. 13.)*

DM. The components of this entity include obesity (chiefly central, visceral, fat increase), hypertension, hyperinsulinaemia and impaired glucose tolerance, dyslipidaemia [increased triglycerides and small, dense low-density lipoprotein [LDL], decreased HDL], and various coagulation abnormalities. Other entities are being continually added. Some of the components antedate the onset of frank glucose intolerance. The pathogenesis of this syndrome is debated and may be a combination of genetic and environmental factors [99]. Visceral obesity has been implicated to have a central role [100] and since obesity can be modulated, this suggests that the occurrence of the syndrome could be reduced. There is an excess of fixed [101] and dynamic [102] coronary obstruction in these patients. The importance of this syndrome lies in the fact that the cardiovascular morbidity in these diabetics may be dependent on many or all of these components. Since these factors are brought into play long before clinically detectable glucose intolerance (the ticking clock phenomenon), prevention, early detection, and treatment of the factors that initiate and drive this metabolic pathway may reduce the subsequent cardiac involvement.

### *Hypertension in myocardial complications of diabetes*

Hypertension is common in patients with hyperinsulinaemia and occurs more often than expected in diabetic patients [103]; conversely, hypertensive patients have a somewhat excess occurrence of DM [104]. The latter could be due to an increased risk of type II DM in hypertensive patients, an adverse risk factor profile, or the use of antihypertensive drugs, chiefly β-blockers or thiazides [105]. DM is not associated with secondary forms of hypertension [106]. Unlike patients with type I DM, in whom hypertension is a late complication and related to kidney disease, type II DM patients often present with hypertension. The hypertension is volume dependent, and associated with increased sympathetic activity and low renin activity.

The combined effect of hypertension and hyperinsulinaemia is synergistic [107] and this is believed to be important for the progression of atheromatous lesions. Hypertension is a major risk factor even when adjustment has been made for other factors. It also plays a role in diabetic cardiomyopathy, as discussed later. Data on the benefits of treating hypertension in the diabetic patient are scarce and derived primarily from subgroup analysis of trials looking at treatment of hypertension in general [108]. The Cochrane database recently reviewed these data. It was found that in the primary prevention trials ($n = 2$), treatment of hypertension caused a significant reduction in cardiovascular mortality (or 0.64; 95% CI 0.5–0.84) but did not reduce the all-cause mortality. There was a reduction in total mortality in short- and long-term secondary prevention trials but the benefit of a reduction in cardiovascular mortality was difficult to demonstrate given the paucity of data and the non-uniform nature of the studies. There was no evidence that any one drug was superior and the studies could not establish appropriate cut-off levels for blood-pressure control. A target blood pressure in diabetic patients in unclear. Since the effects on end-organ protection, especially the kidney, are dependent on a significant reduction in pressure, a target of 130/85 mmHg has been suggested [109].

The choice of antihypertensive drugs is difficult in diabetic patients because many drugs have adverse metabolic effects. Thiazide diuretics can reduce intracellular potassium, worsen glucose tolerance, and increase lipids [110]. However, these effects are not sustained and may marginally influence the course of DM [110]. There is a suggestion that diuretics might increase glycosylated haemoglobin values even when the blood glucose is unchanged [111]. None of these changes has been proven to have clinical significance, especially at lower doses of the hydrochlorthiazides. One retrospective study showed an increase in mortality with diuretic use [112]. β-blockers, especially the non-β-selective ones, may increase blood glucose [113], worsen lipid profiles [114], and influence the hypoglycaemic awareness in diabetics. However, β-blockers have been safely used in diabetics and are desired in the post-MI period. Angiotensin-converting enzyme (ACE) inhibitors are safe and even advantageous in the diabetic patient. Apart from providing renal protection, they may improve insulin resistance [115]. Calcium channel blockers are frequently used in hypertension [116] but their safety has been recently questioned. The (ABCD) study [117] was a prospective, randomized, blinded study in a population of patients with type II DM and hypertension, randomized to either a calcium channel blocker (nisoldipine) or an ACE inhibitor (enalapril). The 470 patients were randomly allocated to the drugs but the enalapril group ended up with a more adverse baseline risk profile. Treatment with enalapril for a mean of 5 years was associated with a lower incidence of MI (RR for nisoldepine 9.5; 95% CI 2.3–21.4) as well as an increased time to first adverse event compared with nisoldipine. Although this arm of the trial was looking at a secondary endpoint and did not definitely prove that calcium blockers increase adverse events, these data suggest that ACE inhibitors may be the first line of choice in diabetic patients.

### *Obesity and cardiac complications in diabetes*

Obesity is commonly found in patients with type II DM and has pathogenetic implications as well [100]. Obesity is also a central component of syndrome X [100] and correlates strongly with other CAD risk factors. An increase in adipocyte mass is associated with increased sympathetic activity [118], increased tumour necrosis faction (TNF) alpha levels [119], and increased tissue angiotensinogen production; in addition, adipocytes can convert angiotensinogen to angiotensin independently of renin [86, 87]. The body mass index is not an accurate indicator of visceral fat accumulation and hence does not correlate well with cardiovascular risk implications. An increase in intra-abdominal fat, determined by computed tomography (CT) or, as a surrogate, an increase in waist: hip ratio, has high predictive accuracy for adverse events [120]. Visceral fat accumulation has the greatest adverse implications [121]. Some of these changes are reversed with weight loss.

### *Lipid abnormalities and cardiac complications in diabetes*

Several abnormalities in lipid metabolism have been found in patients with DM. A characteristic pattern of lipid abnormalities is seen in patients with syndrome X, including increased triglycerides and VLDL, low HDL cholesterol levels, increased small, dense forms of LDL [122], and apolipoprotein E increased (apoE) [123]. The greater proportion of large, triglyceride-laden VLDL particles and excess of small, dense LDL particles [124] is a highly atherogenic profile. Not surprisingly, triglyceride levels are independently associated with CAD in diabetics [125], unlike the situation in non-diabetics where its independent role is less certain. Total cholesterol levels [126] and LDL cholesterol levels [127] are not remarkably abnormal in diabetics, with even modest control of hyperglycaemia. Lipoprotein (a) [Lp(a)], usually a strong determinant of CAD risk, has not been shown to be predictive of CAD in diabetic patients. Several other biochemical abnormalities contribute to the characteristic profile in diabetes: a reversible reduction in lipoprotein lipase (which increases circulating VLDL), impaired insulin-mediated suppression of hepatic VLDL secretion, reduced amount of HDL containing apolipoproteins $A_1$ and $A_2$, and increased activity of CETP, which is proatherogenic [127, 128].

The mechanism by which DM influences lipid profiles is nuclear. VLDL is increased owing to a combination of increased production (mediated by increased synthesis because of hyperglycaemia, and mobilization of free fatty acids due to a non-suppression of insulin-sensitive lipase activity) and reduced clearance (impaired lipoprotein lipase activity). Impaired lipoprotein lipase activity reduces the production of HDL, and the hypertriglyceridaemia results in triglyceride-rich HDL particles, which are efficiently metabolized in the liver. Both of these actions result in low HDL levels in the diabetic patient [126–128].

How does altered lipid metabolism influence the risk of CAD in the diabetic patient? There is an excess of LDL glycosylation in these patients [129], in proportion to the degree of hyperglycaemia; and the glycosylated LDL has a greater susceptibility to oxidative modification [130]. Small, dense LDL particles, which are also more susceptible to oxidation, are common in diabetics. Thus, there is increased proclivity to the formation of oxidized LDL [131], which increases atherogenecity [132]. The combination of glycosylation and oxidation of LDL is highly proatherogenic [133]. AGEs also perturb lipid metabolism in diabetic patients and contribute to accelerated vascular injury. Glycation of the apoB fraction prevents LDL clearance [134], while glycation of HDL increases its catabolism. This in part mediates the adverse risk-factor profile seen in diabetic patients.

The abnormal lipid profile improves significantly with control of DM and this should first be addressed before treating the hyperlipidaemia [135]. The decrease in lipids is related to the degree of hyperglycaemic control, independently of the type of therapy used [136]. In contrast to type I DM, lipid abnormalities are more difficult to control in patients with type II DM. The NCEP guidelines are generally applicable also to diabetic subjects, but there may be a role for more aggressive therapy even in patients without obvious CAD [11]. The hypertriglyceridaemia should be addressed vigorously since it remains a major risk factor. VLDL changes significantly after therapy, while the change in HDL is often disappointing [136]. The choice of drugs is complicated by the fact that a number of antilipid agents, such as niacin, while effective, worsen diabetic control. Moreover, bile acid-binding resins can worsen VLDL levels and fibric acid derivatives can increase LDL while reducing high triglyceride levels. The significance of the latter effect is unknown, but it may be the result of a reduction in the highly atherogenic, small, dense LDL particles; therefore, fibric acid derivatives that are particularly effective in reducing hypertriglyceridaemia may play an important role in the diabetic patient. The best choice, however, seems to be the 3-hydroxy-3-methylglutaryl-coenzyme A (HMG-CoA) reductase inhibitors. They have a much greater beneficial effect on mortality and other endpoints in diabetic patients compared with non-diabetic subjects. One problem with using statins is that most diabetics do not have major perturbations in the total cholesterol level and hypertriglyceridaemia is of major concern. The newer agents have significant effects on triglyceride metabolism and may become the drugs of choice.

### *Coagulation abnormalities and cardiac complications in diabetes*

Many changes occur in diabetic patients which result in an adverse balance between prothrombotic and antithrombotic processes [137]. Endothelial injury, reduced nitric oxide (NO) production, hyperhomocysteinaemia, and reduced endothelial function reduce vasodilatation, decrease flow reserve, and provide for a prothrombotic endothelial milieu in patients with DM. There is an increase in factors in the coagulation cascade (including fibrinogen, factors XII, XI, and VIII, and von Willebrand factor), a reduction in endogenous anticoagulant activity (reduced antithrombin III, protein C), and an inhibition of endogenous fibrinolysis [reduced plasmin and tissue plasminogen activator (tPA) [138] levels and an increase in plasminogen activator inhibitor and LP(a) activity]. Abnormal platelet function adds to the prothrombotic state: platelets show greater aggregation with endogenous and exogenous stimuli, and platelet-dependent thrombin generation is increased [139]. These phenomena may explain the high incidence of acute coronary episodes and somewhat reduced efficacy of aspirin in patients with diabetes. However, thrombolytic therapy is effective and many of these changes are reversed with glycaemic control [139], suggesting that it is possible to modify a number of adverse risk factors in diabetes.

### Association of diabetic kidney disease and cardiac complications in diabetes

Diabetic nephropathy, both overt proteinurea and microalbuminurea, is one of the most potent predictors for CAD and related deaths in patients with type I and type II DM [140]. In one study, overt proteinurea increased the risk of CAD mortality by 37-fold in patients with type I DM, and by four- to five-fold in patients with type II DM [141]. The reason for this association is unclear. Diabetic proteinurea may be an obvious and easily recognized marker of widespread vascular injury, or it may be due to the other risk factors in patients with diabetic nephropathy: a poor family history, hypertension, greater lipid abnormalities, and higher levels of advanced glycation products [142, 143]. However, the risk of CAD in patients with microalbuminurea is over and above that of other risk factors.

## Microvascular disease, endothelial dysfunction, and cardiac complications in diabetes

The endothelium is a common target in diabetes. The microcirculation, especially the coronary bed, has been shown to be abnormal in both clinical and experimental DM, independent of large-vessel atheromatous disease [144]. This evidence has been obtained from morphological [145, 146] and functional studies of the coronary circulation in experimental animals [147] and humans (Fig. 22.4) [148]. Vascular and endothelial dysfunction is common with hyperglycaemia and insulin resistance [149]. Endothelial dysfunction occurs early in the natural history of the disease and is predictive of vascular complications [150]. Microcirculatory function has been assessed in a number of ways. Clinically, vascular function has been commonly evaluated by studying endothelial-dependent and-independent vasodilation or metabolic vasodilatation, or measuring coronary flow reserve. Impairment in endothelium-dependent vasodilation has been shown in conduit [151] and elastic [152] arteries in animals. There are similar data for humans in both the peripheral [153] and coronary [148, 154, 155] circulation. The non-endothelial-dependent circulatory function [155], reactive hyperaemia [156], and demand-mediated vasodilation [157, 158] are also frequently abnormal, suggesting widespread vascular problems in diabetics. There appears to be some correlation between glycaemic control, end-organ damage, and microvascular dysfunction in humans with DM [158]. One of the major problems with these kinds of data is that it is impossible to exclude other causes of abnormal endothelial function, including subclinical atherosclerosis [159]. Similarly, the confounding effects of abnormal ventricular haemodynamics, hyperlipidaemia, LV hypertrophy, and hypertension are difficult to factor in [160, 161].

The exact reasons for these changes are unclear. Hyperglycaemia causes abnormalities in endothelial structure and function in cells under culture conditions [162], increases adhesion molecule expression, and increases endothelial monocyte–macrophage adhesion [163, 164]. Permanent structural changes [145], increased production or an increased sensitivity to [165, 166] vasoconstrictor substances, reduced vasodilation [167], and effects of hyperlipidaemia [168] might also explain these changes. Moreover, acute hyperglycaemia can reduce endothelial-dependent vasodilatation [169] independently of insulin levels, and oral diabetic agents of the sulfonylurea class increase coronary resistance [170] and reduce ischaemic hyperaemia [171]. These are other possible mechanisms for impaired small-vessel function in diabetes. The abnormal endothelial function does not improve with L-arginine supplementation or with ACE inhibition [172], but some studies suggest a positive role for antioxidants [173, 174]; pancreatic transplantation also improves endothelial function in diabetics [175].

The clinical significance of abnormal endothelial function is uncertain. Endothelial function measured in the periphery using flow- or endothelial-dependent

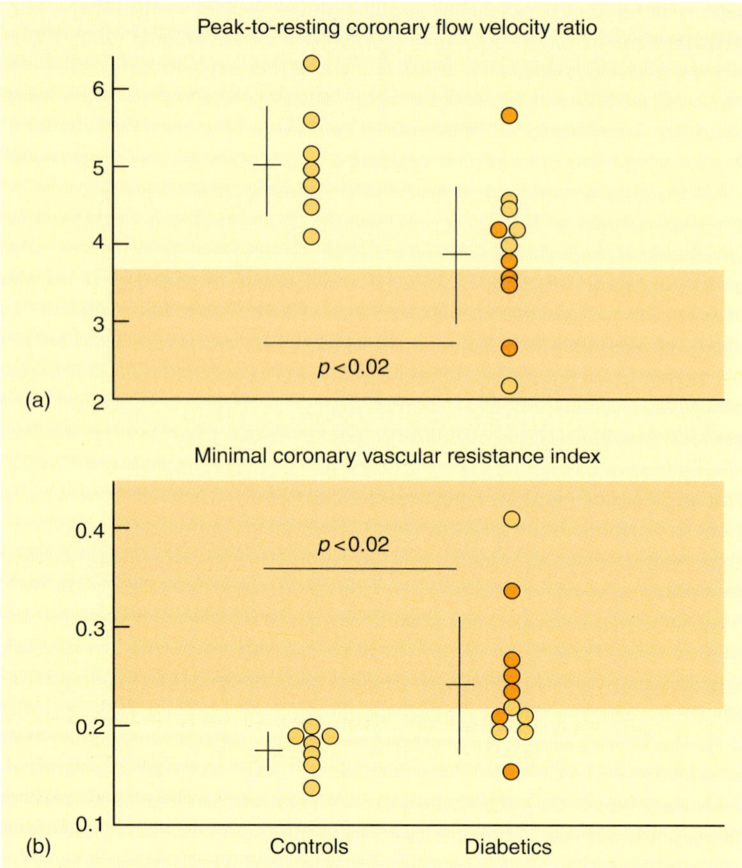


**Figure 22.4** *Coronary vascular endothelial dysfunction in diabetics with normal left ventricular function and normal coronary angiogram. (Data from ref. 148.)*

(acetylcholine) vasodilatory agents may be an important marker for diabetic coronary vascular dysfunction [168, 169] and adverse cardiovascular events [176]. Abnormal endothelial function may reduce coronary flow reserve and worsen myocardial inschaemia. Repeated ischaemia or inadequate metabolic vasodilatation during periods of increased demand may cause cardiac dysfunction. Abnormal endothelial function may be a factor in the poor prognosis and high incidence of heart failure following MI. No study has yet demonstrated a direct relationship between abnormal endothelial function and heart failure.

## Myocardial involvement unrelated to vascular disease

### Diabetic cardiomyopathies

Myocardial involvement can often present as heart failure. Patients with DM have an increased risk of congestive heart failure with [177] and without [178] coexisting CAD (Fig. 22.5). It has long been known that women with diabetes have the highest risk of developing CHF even without associated CAD [179]. Some of the early studies showed that patients with CHF also had a higher incidence of diabetes and this led to the hypothesis that diabetes may be responsible for left ventricular dysfunction in a subset of patients [180]. There is also an increased incidence of idiopathic cardiomyopathy in diabetics [181]. In the Framingham studies [178], men with diabetes had a two-fold increase and diabetic women a five-fold increase in compared with CHF non-diabetic subjects; these changes persisted even when normalized for other factors, including the presence of CAD. Diabetes, treated with insulin, was responsible for the excess risk of CHF in this study.

Patients with DM also have an increased incidence of heart failure following an acute ischaemic event. The MILIS study [182] evaluated 85 diabetic and 415 non-diabetic patients after an MI and found that the former did worse than the latter despite similar infarct size and ejection fraction. The diabetic patients had more heart failure (30% vs 10.1% at 6 months) and increased mortality (26% vs 14.5%, $p < 0.01$) compared with non-diabetic subjects. Up to half of women and one-quarter of men develop sig-

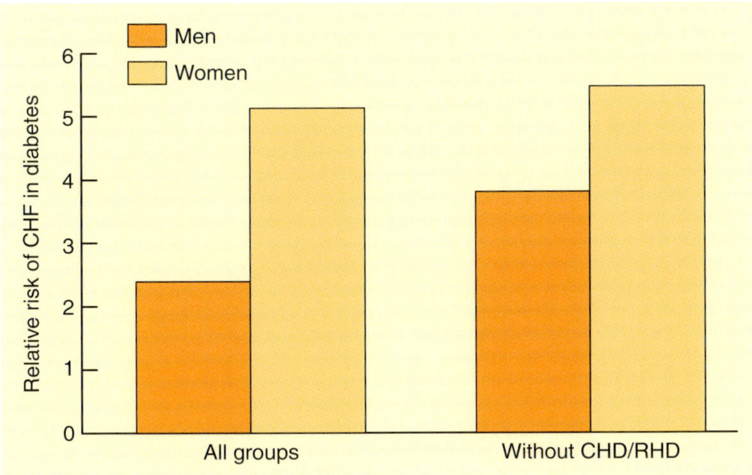


**Figure 22.5** *Prevalence of congestive heart failure in the Framingham cohort, followed for 18 years.*

nificant CHF after an MI, and heart failure accounts for up to 22% of deaths in diabetic women [183]. Most of the early deaths are due to heart failure, while late deaths are due to a combination of heart failure and recurrent ischaemic events [184]. The common causes of heart failure in patients with DM are extensive CAD, hypertensive heart disease, and diabetic cardiomyopathy that occurs in presence of normal coronary arteries.

While CAD (both microvascular and macrovascular) is the predominant mechanism of myocardial involvement and heart failure in patients with DM [177, 185, 186], a number of other entities can result in myocardial dysfunction, independently of small- and large-vessel disease. These include non-ischaemic diabetic diastolic dysfunction, non-ishaemic subclinical diabetic systolic dysfunction, non-ischaemic diabetic cardiomyopathy, and non-ischaemic diabetic LV hypertrophy and hypertrophic cardiomyopathy. Some of these conditions coexist with obstructive CAD and with each other. They can influence reparative mechanisms and function in patients with CAD and affect prognosis in the diabetic patient.

## Non-ischaemic diabetic diastolic dysfunction

Experimental studies show that DM commonly impairs diastolic function in the whole heart [187, 188], in isolated cardiac muscle preparations [189], and in isolated cardiomyocytes [190]. The diastolic defect appears much earlier than systolic dysfunction [190] and can be induced even in cardiomyocytes in a high glucose–low insulin culture medium [191]. Diastolic dysfunction is manifested as prolonged duration of action potential [192], prolonged calcium transient decay [190], prolonged myocardial relaxation, reduced peak velocity of relaxation [188, 190, 191], reduced diastolic compliance [193], and increased chamber stiffness. Diastolic function is affected early in the disease course [194–197] and is more commonly abnormal than systolic function [186]. Indeed, in some studies diastolic dysfunction occurred even when contractility and contractile reserve (after stimulation with dobutamine) were normal.

Diastolic dysfunction can be a part of ischaemic heart disease; however, there are convincing data that DM can cause diastolic dysfunction in the absence of critical CAD or inducible ischaemia [198–200]. Hypertension commonly coexists with DM and the presence of both induces morphological changes in the myocardium [201], significantly increasing the possibility of diastolic dysfunction [201]. However, there are ample data to show that DM by itself can induce diastolic dysfunction [195–198]. The classic presentation includes a patient with small ventricles, increased filling pressures, and normal systolic function [202]; other changes include impaired LV relaxation and reduced ventricular filling rates (Fig. 22.6).

Newer echocardiographic techniques such as tissue backscatter and tissue echo density have revealed changes consistent with early structural abnormalities in the interstitium [203, 204]. It is important to note that in the most quoted study [203], there was no independent confirmatory evidence of either increased interstitial structural changes or diabetic dysfunction. Diastolic dysfunction has been thought to result from abnormalities in the myocyte or the interstitium. Abnormal intracellular calcium handling is thought to be important [190, 205] but, as discussed below, the results have been inconsistent,

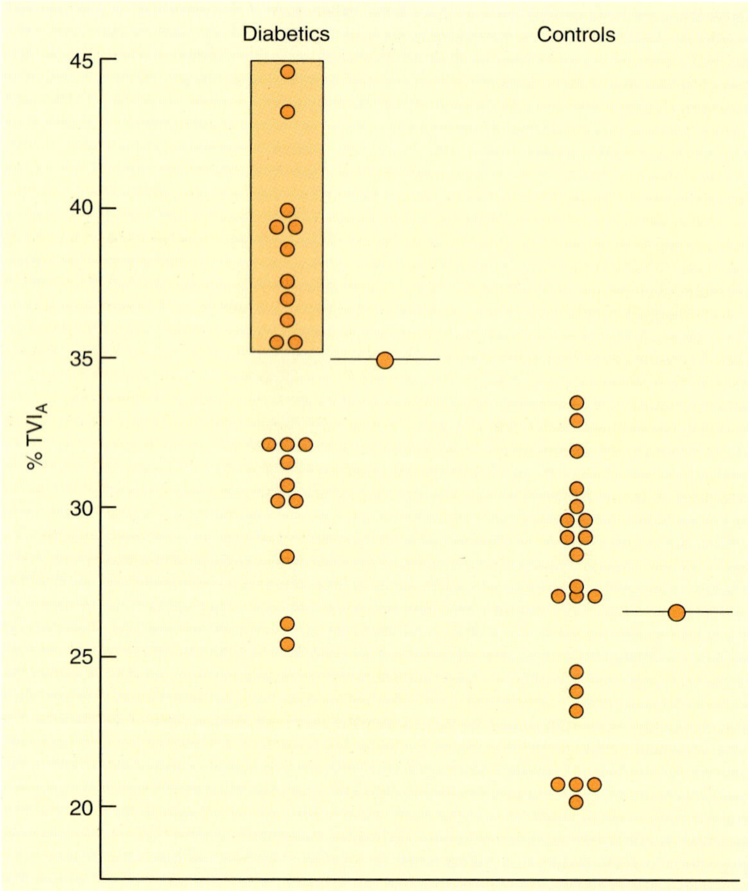


**Figure 22.6** *Echo-Doppler evidence of diastolic dysfunction in the diabetic patient. Atrial contraction contributes to a greater extent towards stroke volume in patients with diabetes. None of the patients had evidence of heart disease. (Data from ref. 198.)*

especially when not classified according to the type of diabetes. There is significant cellular hypertrophy in diabetic hearts, which is worse when associated with hypertension [201]. DM is associated with increased LV hypertrophy and increased LV mass, especially in women [206]. Interstitial abnormalities include an excess of collagen [207], which could change the diastolic properties of the left ventricle. An abnormal interstitium is the result of a number of changes. Increased vascular permeability in the diabetic vasculature can be associated with increased interstitial tissue formation [85, 186]. The effects of AGE include an increase in collagen synthesis and an increase in growth factor activity [208]. All of these changes alter diastolic function in the diabetic heart, and reversing some of these biochemical changes may improve compliance [209].

Clinical data on diastolic dysfunction in DM need to be interpreted cautiously. The prevalence of pure diastolic dysfunction is unknown. In various studies, echocardiographic diastolic dysfunction was recorded in 30–53% of diabetic subjects without evidence of any overt cardiac disease [198]. Most of the data come from small case series, which have severe selection bias. Ischaemia was excluded using indirect measures, LV hypertrophy was a confounding factor in some studies [195], and autonomic function was not always quantitated. The latter has been shown to influence significantly LV relaxation indices [210]. In addition, patients with type II DM in these studies were older than those with type I DM. A number of entities can influence diastolic dysfunction in the middle-aged and elderly population and many studies did not carefully exclude these cofactors. Most of the data for diastolic dysfunction in diabetic patients come from an evaluation of E/A ratios during Doppler echocardiography. No study has extensively investigated multiple aspects of ventricular filling. Pulmonary vein filling patterns, which would have strengthened the diagnosis of diastolic dysfunction, were not determined. Finally, the E/A ratio is highly sensitive to loading conditions, which were not clearly delineated in the clinical studies.

It is not clear whether aggressive treatment of hyperglycaemia improves diastolic dysfunction. Some cross-sectional studies in type I [199] or both type I and II DM

[211] suggest that there is little correlation between metabolic control and changes in diastolic dysfunction. Diastolic dysfunction has not been shown to change significantly with treatment of DM [212] except in some studies in animals [213] and humans without retinopathy [197]. The clinical significance of many of these subtle changes in myocardial function are also uncertain. Very few studies have correlated diastolic dysfunction with clinical indices of well-being, exercise tolerance, or other measures of heart failure. There are experimental data [186] and a clinical belief [177, 214] that the effects of an ischaemic event are greater in patients with significant diastolic dysfunction. In the MILIS study, diabetic and non-diabetic patients had a similar LV ejection fraction (EF) but diabetics had a higher incidence of heart failure. This would suggest that diastolic dysfunction is important in the causation of clinical heart failure in diabetic subjects [182].

## Non-ischaemic subclinical diabetic systolic dysfunction

Studies have shown that DM affects both systolic and diastolic function of the whole heart [193, 213, 215], the papillary muscle [216], and the isolated cardiomyocytes (Fig. 22.7) [190, 191, 217]. However, while studies of whole heart systolic function in diabetic animals consistently show abnormal function [188], those of isolated muscle preparations have less uniform results [189]. These changes are time dependent: systolic dysfunction appears much later than diastolic function [190, 191].

Early abnormalities in myocardial function have been demonstrated in diabetic patients using physiological measurements [218, 219], cardiac catheter measurements [220], radionuclide studies [196, 200, 210, 221–224], and echocardiography [195, 199, 225, 226). In the hope of avoiding latent CAD or the effects of other systemic diseases, most of the studies have been in patients with type I DM or in a mixture of patients with type I on II; only a few have been done in patients with only type II DM [195, 196].

These studies show that diabetic patients have a normal or depressed EF at rest. The resting EF may even be increased in some patients [226, 227], especially women with type II DM [196]. Thus, resting EF is not a useful parameter for determining abnormal LV function in diabetics. Various forms of stress have been used to unmask latent systolic dysfunction. Changes in EF with exercise have been primarily used to diagnose systolic dysfunction [196, 220, 222–224, 227]. Diabetic patients with normal systolic function at rest show no increase in EF during exercise, suggesting an impaired contractile reserve. An abnormal response to exercise is seen in 35–71% of diabetic patients, and more often in women with type II DM [196]. There is an increased prevalence of abnormal systolic function with increasing duration of the disease [186, 226]. The relationship with indices of metabolic control is not very certain [196, 220, 222]: there is some correlation between systolic dysfunction and the presence of microvascular disease in some studies [224] but not in others [196]. Autonomic neuropathy has been related to systolic dysfunction in some studies [228] but not in others [196]. Systolic dysfunction progresses rather quickly in the diabetic: in one study [229] in which patients with type II DM had a starting resting EF similar to that of controls, the EF deteriorated significantly during 4 years of follow-up.

Although unclear, the mechanisms of impaired systolic function may include abnormalities in calcium handling at rest or stress [230, 231], impaired calcium sensitivity in single [232] and multicellular situations [233], and abnormal energy [234]. Reduced β-adrenergic receptors and an impaired response to catecholamines could also be contributory [235].

The clinical significance of subclinical systolic dysfunction is unclear. Unlike diastolic dysfunction, there is evidence that systolic function improves with diabetic control [236, 237]. Impaired contractile reserve, which can be demonstrated using LV function indices during exercise, could be important during stress and ischaemia. In major thrombolytic therapy trials, the non-infarct segments seemed to contract less than expected and this was thought to be important in the higher morbidity in patients with DM [20, 177]. Impaired contractile reserve could explain why diabetic patients with heart failure are more symptomatic and require more frequent hospitalizations.

As with most literature in this field, the clinical studies need careful interpretation. Even though asymptomatic diabetic patients show evidence of systolic and diastolic dysfunction using sensitive indices, these are uncommon in absence of associated aggravating factors such as hypertension [238]. Not all studies find the existence of impaired contractile reserve in asymptomatic diabetic patients, and those that do are subject to significant methodological problems, which make them far from satisfactory. Carefully performed studies have not found evidence of systolic dysfunction either at rest or during stress. An important

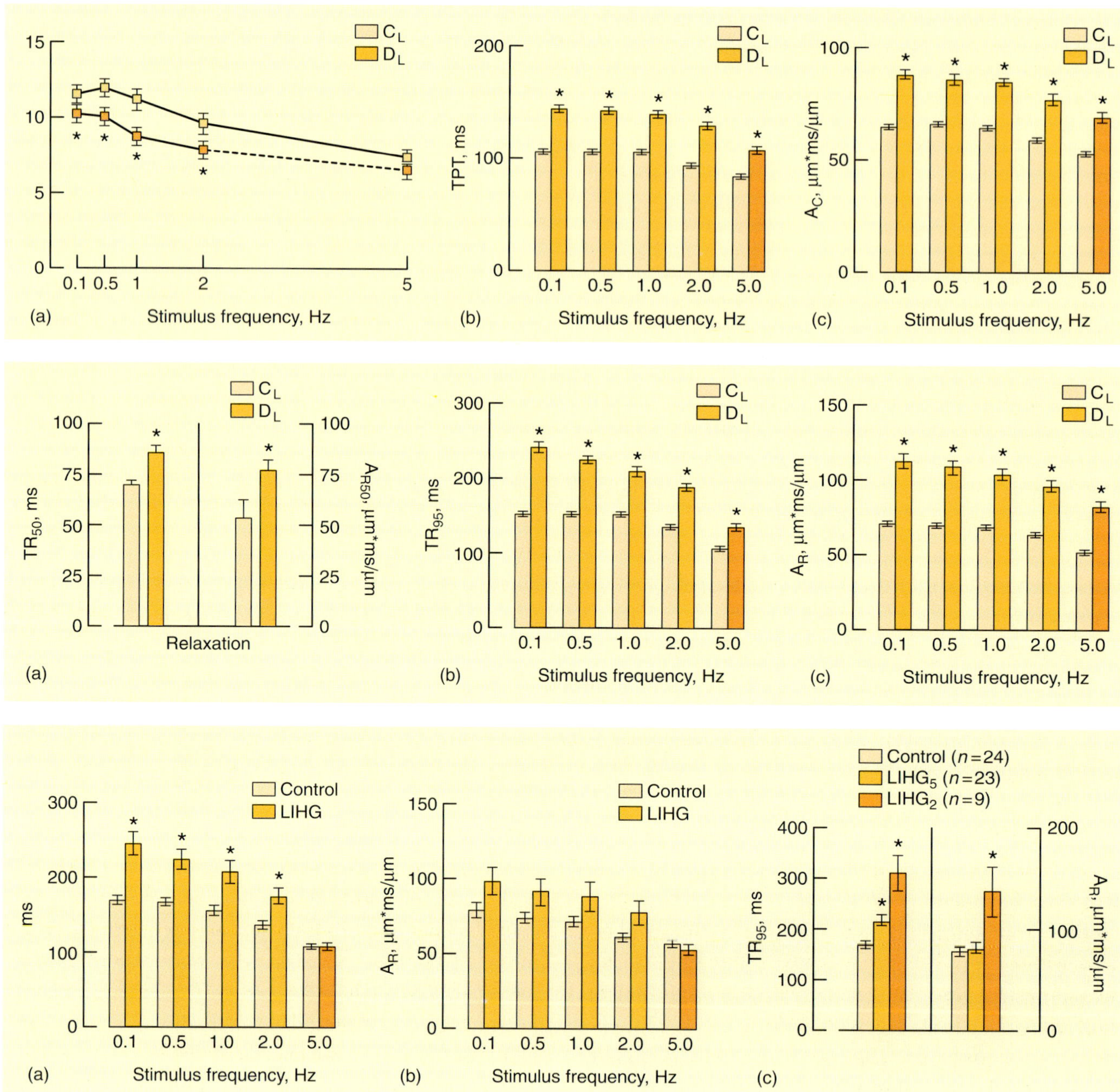


**Figure 22.7** *Systolic and diastolic dysfunction can be shown in cardiomyocytes isolated from diabetic animals* (Top) *or in myocytes exposed to low insulin and high glucose media* (Bottom) *(Data from refs. 190, 191.)*

study by Borow *et al.* [227] showed that young diabetics, without evidence of hypertension or exercise-induced ischaemia, had a normal to increased EF at rest; 45% of diabetics failed to increase their EF with exercise despite normal measures of contractility at rest and normal response to afterload manipulation (Fig. 22.8). Patients whose EF did not increase had a greater resting EF. This well-conducted study seriously questioned the existence of subclinical systolic dysfunction in longstanding DM and postulated that an abnormal response to exercise was not related to impaired myocardial reserve. Changes in peripheral control of the circulation and reduced preload on standing may have played a part in preventing an exercise-induced rise in EF. This study also showed that the lack of rise in EF with exercise was not related to autonomic dysfunction. In other studies, patients who showed improvement in LV function

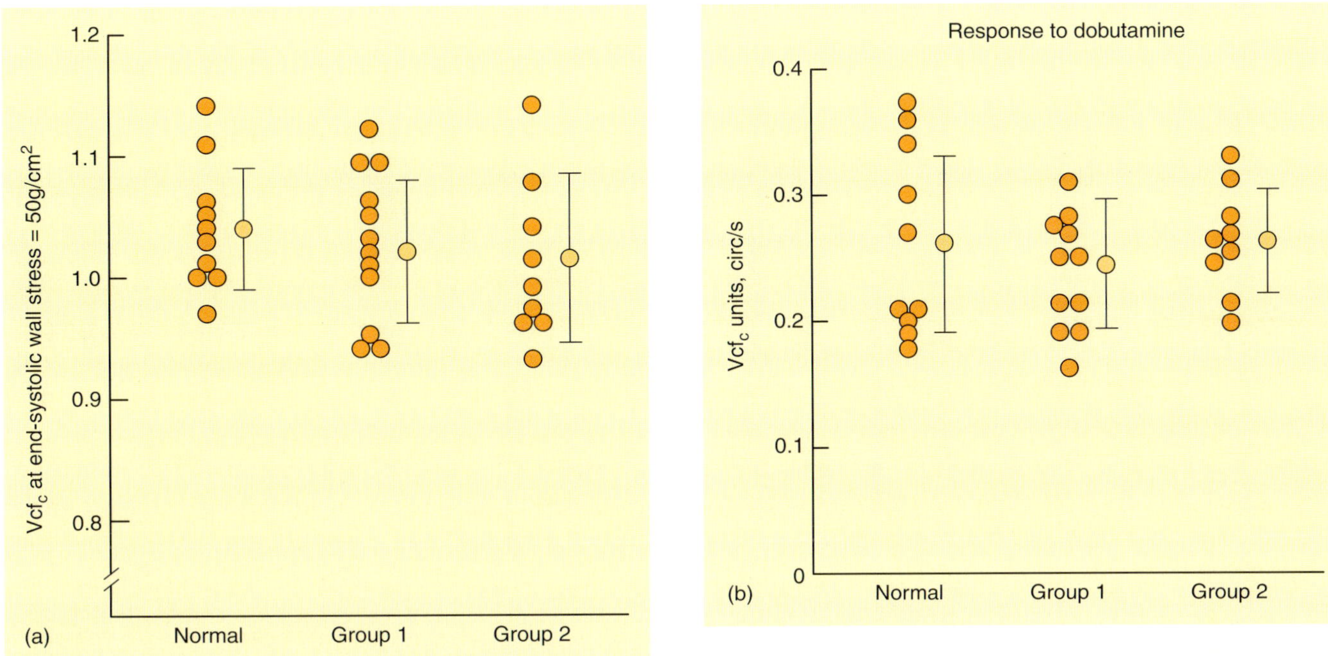


**Figure 22.8** *Not all investigators find evidence for systolic dysfunction in diabetics. Here, normal young adult diabetic subjects had normal velocity of circumferential fibre shortening at rest* (left) *and after dobutamine* (right). *Group I = Patients who increased ejection fraction (EF) on exercise; Group II = patients who had a fall in EF with exercise. (Data from ref. 227.)*

with diabetic control did not have significant impairment of systolic function to begin with, and both patients with and without heart disease were included. In one study, most of the abnormalities in cardiac function seemed to be in the group with pre-existing heart disease [195]. A significant proportion of patients fails to achieve adequate maximum exercise heart rates in studies reporting a lack of increase in EF with exercise [196]. Thus, factors other than impaired myocardial function may be responsible for a lack of increase in EF during exercise. Studies have often used methods that are too insensitive to avoid inclusion of patients with CAD [195]. In the study by Mustonen *et al.* [196] 28% of patients with an inadequate exercise EF and who were thought to be free of CAD clinically had reversible ischaemia on perfusion imaging studies. Finally, there is a significant selection bias in most of these studies and the final study groups form a tiny proportion of the original cohort [195, 196].

## Left ventricular hypertrophy and hypertrophic cardiomyopathy in diabetes mellitus

Diabetic patients have increased LV hypertrophy even in the early stages of the disease [239]. In the Framingham study [206], DM was an independent risk factor for LV hypertrophy in women but not in men. The degree of hypertrophy can be significant, sometimes as much as that seen with hypertrophic cardiomyopathy [240]. Significant LV hypertrophy is also found in the rare diabetic patient with a point mutation affecting the tRNA leucine mitochondrial gene [241]. In patients with significant DM-induced LV hypertrophy, histological examination shows cardiomyocyte hypertrophy, little necrosis, but an excess of interstitial fibrosis [186]. This could be one reason for the high incidence of diastolic dysfunction and diastolic heart failure in patients with DM.

Up to 50% of patients with type II DM have hypertension either alone or in combination with the multiple metabolic syndrome. Many studies suggest that the coexistence of DM and hypertension in the same patient is deadly [201, 242–244], as it changes the natural history of DM and is pivotal in the genesis of diabetic heart disease [242]. Patients with both DM and hypertension have greater degrees of LV hypertrophy and interstitial fibrosis than that seen with either disease alone in pathological [243, 244] and echocardiographic [239] studies, even when factored for the degree of blood pressure elevation. There is also an excess of echocardiographic [239] and clinical heart failure. Both impaired diastolic [245] and systolic function [239] have been described in diabetic–hypertensive patients.

It is difficult to identify the individual contribution of either hypertension or DM to the genesis of myocardial involvement and heart failure. Hypertension can result in a form of cardiomyopathy similar to that seen with DM alone, which is associated with impaired systolic [246] and diastolic [247] cardiac function. The diastolic dysfunction is due to a combination of both impaired ventricular relaxation and reduced compliance due to an increase in myocardial wall thickness. The stiff ventricle also impairs LV systolic performance during tachycardia and exercise. These findings may significantly contribute to heart failure in the diabetic. Hypertension increases the prevalence and speeds the progression of CAD, as well as influencing coronary perfusion [248] in patients with DM. In one large study [107], the combination of hypertension and DM resulted in a three times greater increase in CAD prevalence than that with either alone, possibly contributing to heart failure.

While more common when DM coexists with hypertension [240], LV hypertrophy can occur even without obvious hypertension, especially in women [206]. While LV dysfunction is more common in diabetic patients with an increase in LV mass, significant diastolic dysfunction has been described in hypertensive patients who do not have hypertrophy [245], even when adjusted for blood pressure elevation. These data suggest that heart failure in the diabetic could be due to the cardiac effects of diabetes, hypertension, or both.

## Non-ischaemic diabetic cardiomyopathy

Diabetics have a high incidence of heart failure, a fact not totally explained by CAD. Some studies, both angiographic [185] and at autopsy [21], showed that the prevalence and severity of CAD are not much worse in diabetics with heart failure than in those without heart failure. Diabetic cardiomyopathy, first described in 1972 by Rubler *et al.* [249] in four patients with diabetic nephropathy, is an entity that may explain the occurrence of heart failure in this situation. Despite some doubts as to its existence, diabetic cardiomyopathy has been shown to be a distinct entity [186]. It is diagnosed when CHF exists in diabetic patients without obvious evidence of epicardial CAD. Many believe that this entity is also independent of any microvascular disease [250] or inducible ischaemia [251].

Histological studies show myocyte necrosis with some amount of cellular hypertrophy [145, 146, 243, 244]. Interstitial fibrosis is a prominent component. There is an infiltration of periodic acid–schiff (PAS) positive material in the interstitium. Some studies have shown involvement of small intramyocardial coronary arteries (Fig. 22.9). The changes include basement membrane thickening, microaneurysm formation [252], and focal microvascular stenosis. These changes are more prominent when hypertension and DM coexist [186, 201].

Microvascular disease and consequent ischaemia cannot be totally excluded in patients with diabetic cardiomyopathy. In one of the original studies on diabetic cardiomyopathy by Hamby *et al.* [180, 181], some of the patients with normal epicardial coronary arteries showed evidence of microvascular disease, including intimal thickening and perivascular fibrosis at autopsy. Such microvascular changes were not seen in non-diabetic subjects. In a study of 116 patients with DM with or without heart failure, there were extensive small vessel changes which resulted in areas with luminal narrowing [253]. There are several other structural changes in the microvasculature, including increased thickness of the capillary basement membrane [254] and microaneurysm formation [252], especially in areas with myocyte degeneration. These changes may be involved in the causation of diabetic cardiomyocyte injury. Apart from structural changes, functional abnormalities at the microvascular level can contribute to heart failure. Some investigators have postulated that microvascular spasm in a hypertensive diabetic model can contribute to cardiomyopathy [255]. The microvasculature in diabetic patients may be more sensitive to catecholamine-induced vasoconstriction [214]. However, not all studies have found major structural changes at pathological examination [256] or in endocardial biopsies [250], and most studies noting microvascular abnormalities have not shown them to have functional significance [202, 251].

## Cellular mechanisms for diabetic myocardial involvement

DM results in several functional changes at the muscle and cellular level which could contribute to the high incidence of heart failure, and these are summarized in Table 22.1. Some of these changes may not be applicable to humans. For example, a shift in myosin isoforms from the fast V1 to the slower V3 isoform is thought to explain abnormal contraction in rats. However, humans naturally have an excess of the slower form and so this phenomenon may not be important to humans [257]. A number of changes in intracellular calcium handling has been documented in the

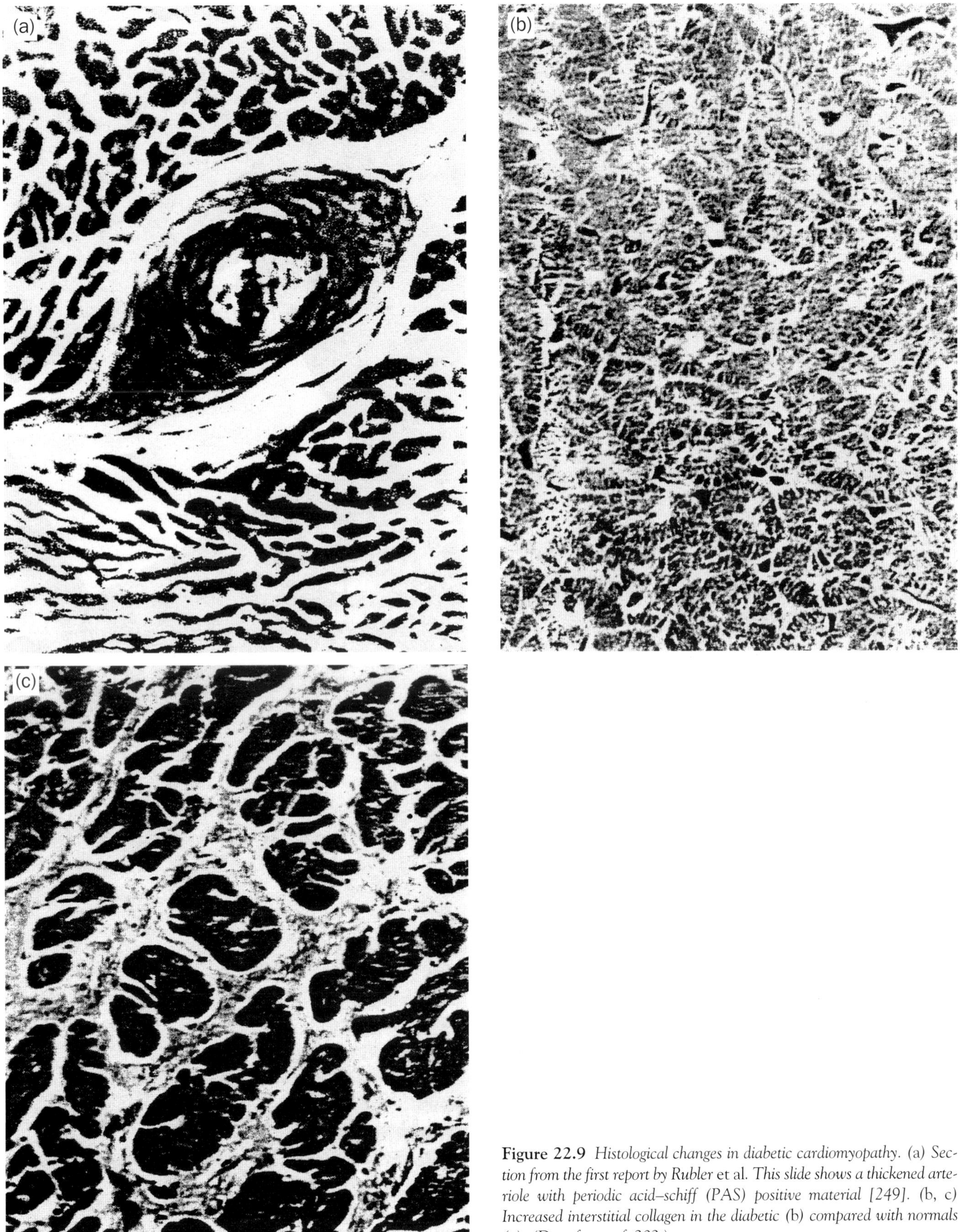


**Figure 22.9** *Histological changes in diabetic cardiomyopathy. (a) Section from the first report by Rubler* et al. *This slide shows a thickened arteriole with periodic acid–schiff (PAS) positive material [249]. (b, c) Increased interstitial collagen in the diabetic (b) compared with normals (c). (Data from ref. 202.)*

**Table 22.1** Alterations in the diabetic heart: implications for heart failure

| |
|---|
| General abnormalities |
| Reduced protein synthesis |
| Reduced glucose uptake |
| Reduced rate of glucose oxidation |
| Reduced L-carnitine levels |
| Abnormal calcium handling |
| Increased intracellular calcium |
| Increase in size of intracellular poor of $Ca^{2+}$ in type II DM, normal in type I DM |
| Prolonged intracellular $Ca^{2+}$ transient |
| Prolonged action potential |
| Reduced extrusion of $Ca^{2+}$ |
| Both type I DM and type II DM: reduced $Na^{+}/Ca^{2+}$ exchanger activity |
| Reduced $Na^{+}/K^{+}$-ATPase activity |
| Sarcoplasmic reticulum $Ca^{2+}$ pump activity reduced only in type I DM |
| Depressed mitochondrial calcium uptake |
| Increased intracellular $Na^{+}$ level |
| Altered receptor states |
| Reduced number of β-receptors |
| Reduced response to adrenergic stimulation which is restored by insulin |
| Reduced cAMP response |
| Reduced response to ouabain and reduced ouabain binding sites |
| Dysfunction of contractile apparatus or coupling |
| Calcium overload induced changes in kinase activity |
| V1 to V3 isoenzyme shift in animals, which is reversed with insulin |
| Changes in troponin T to the T3 isoform |
| Reduced calcium sensitivity in papillary muscles and myocytes |
| Impaired activation of PKC reversed with glycaemic control |

This table summarizes the commonly reported abnormalities, especially for type II diabetes mellitus (DM). Many of the changes are controversial and not fully proven. A several of these changes differ depending on the diabetic syndrome under study.
PKC = protein kinase C.

diabetic heart [190, 191, 230–233]. Once again, the significance of these abnormalities is unclear, especially since changes are variable when classified according to the type of diabetes. Finally, it is not known which changes are primary or secondary epiphenomena.

The type II diabetic heart in general shows an increase in the intracellular calcium pool, chiefly due to reduced extrusion. A prominent abnormality is impaired sarcolemmal $Na^{+}/Ca^{2+}$ exchanger activity. Sarcolemmal and sarcoplasmic reticular calcium pump function is not significantly altered. Some of the defects in cellular calcium transport can be reversed with verapamil [258, 259]. In one study with diabetic–hypertensive rats [260], diltiazem prevented the progression of heart failure without reducing the blood pressure, suggesting a role for altered calcium handling in the genesis of heart failure in this model. Abnormal substrate metabolism and energetics may be important in the genesis of diabetic cardiomyopathy [261, 262]. Other theories such as excessive sorbitol production or glycosylation, which are important for diabetic injury in other organ systems, are not particularly relevant in the heart [261]. Abnormal lipid metabolism and toxic lipid intermediates or triacylglycerol were once thought to be important. However, despite some evidence that experimental heart failure in diabetics is associated with increased myocardial lipids [186], there are few data showing that lipids are directly involved. Other miscellaneous postulated mechanisms include changes in cellular membranes (such as N-methylation and protein phosphorylation), and the inhibitory effects of cytokines. TNF-α is increased in obese diabetics [119] and the muscle produces TNF in type II DM [263]. Apart from worsening insulin sensitivity [264], TNF has a direct depressive effect on cardiac contraction [265] and can increase cardiac apoptosis [266]. This could play a role in cardiac dysfunction. The role of neurohormones in the genesis of diabetic cardiomyopathy is also unclear. Hyperglycaemia and hyperinsulinaemia affect the hormonal system, including angiotensin II, the sympathetic system, and endothelins [267], and this could be another way by which DM can be cardiotoxic and vasculotoxic. Insulin stimulates the sympathetic nervous system, increases the pressure response to angiotensin II, and enhances angiotensin II-mediated production of aldosterone [47, 55, 118]. The latter has been shown to increase myocardial fibrosis in other situations [268]. As discussed before, angiotensin II levels are increased in obese diabetics, probably related to angiotensinogen production in adipocytes and the existence of renin-independent pathways for angiotensin II production in these cells [86, 87]; angiotensin II has significant haemodynamic effects and can cause direct vascular and myocyte injury [89]. There have not been any major investigations in this regard.

There are some major unresolved issues in diabetic cardiomyopathy. It is a diagnosis of exclusion and many clinical studies have not been very rigorous in this. In addition, idiopathic dilated cardiomyopathy is not an uncommon entity [269] and given the extensive prevalence of diabetes, it is likely that they occur in the same patient. There are no pathognomonic changes in diabetic cardiomyopathy (even at histology) and it may be impossible to separate the two entities. One major problem is that there have been no systematic studies evaluating the prevalence and natural history of pure diabetic cardiomyopathy. It is not clear whether the widely prevalent minor functional abnormalities (systolic and diastolic dysfunction) seen in asymptomatic diabetic patients progress to frank cardiomyopathy or whether the entity occurs by itself. It is therefore difficult to be certain about its clinical impact and significance in general.

## Impact of treatment of diabetes on evolution of left ventricular dysfunction

It is not known why these changes occur in the diabetic heart. The relative role of hyperglycaemia and hyperinsulinaemia in the pathogenesis of diabetic cardiomyopathy is unclear. It is not clear whether aggressive treatment of DM changes the incidence of diabetic cardiac dysfunction. In experimental studies, insulin improves diabetic cardiomyopathy [258, 270–273], while oral sulphonylurea drugs may not [274], despite similar glycaemic control. Other studies have not shown any major improvement in myocardial structural changes following the control of experimentally induced hyperglycaemia [274, 275]. There are insufficient data at present for interpretation of this evidence. The data in humans are more sketchy. Many of the cardiac abnormalities, especially those in asymptomatic patients, are not always related to the duration or severity of DM, or the presence of other complications [186, 198, 200, 221, 222, 228]. There is minimal correlation with the presence autonomic neuropathy [210] and retinopathy [197]. The less studied effect of diabetic control has shown both improvement [195, 197, 276] and no improvement (especially in groups with end-organ damage [197, 229, 277]) in cardiac dysfunction with treatment. It is therefore impossible to conclude whether aggressively treating DM influences cardiomyopathy.

## Cardiac autonomic neuropathy and myocardial complications in diabetics

Autonomic neuropathy involving both the parasympathetic and sympathetic nervous systems is a frequent accompaniment of DM [278, 279]. It occurs early [280], but the prevalence is dependent on the duration of the diabetes; nearly all patients coming for pancreatic transplantation have autonomic dysfunction [281]. Diabetic patients with autonomic neuropathy show reduced LV function and sudden death [282, 283]. Thus, the occurrence of autonomic neuropathy results in a poor prognosis and reduced survival in diabetic patients [282]. Data on the temporal sequence of changes during the course of autonomic neuropathy are limited but seem to suggest that reduced parasympathetic activity is more frequent and occurs earlier than abnormalities in sympathetic function [283, 284]. Autonomic neuropathy has other pathophysiological implications. Unlike normal subjects, diabetic patients have higher sympathetic tone during waking hours, as well as a loss of parasympathetic tone during both day and night [283]. This alters the circadian occurrence of myocardial ischaemia and MI [285]. There is evidence that silent ischaemia in diabetic patients may be related to autonomic neuropathy [284].

Autonomic neuropathy may be important in the LV dysfunction seen in diabetic patients. The sympathetic system is important for enhancing inotropy and lusitropy in the normal and abnormal heart. Diabetic animals show cardiac denervation on histology [286] and abnormal catecholamine turnover [287]. This could contribute to diabetic cardiomyopathy [288]. Uptake of iodine-123-meta-iodobenzylguanidine ([$^{123}$I]MIBG) (an index of innervation), diastolic function, and indices of autonomic neuropathy are interrelated, suggesting a role for the autonomic nervous system in the control of LV function [289]. One study found that diastolic dysfunction, but not systolic dysfunction, correlated with reduced cardiac MIBG uptake in diabetic subjects.

Diabetic autonomic neuropathy also causes changes in myocardial blood flow and may influence myocardial function. Stevens *et al.* [279] studied myocardial innervation and blood flow with position emission tomography. They found patchy areas of innervation: innervation was preserved in the proximal LV wall even in presence of advanced neuropathy. While resting myocardial blood flow was higher in the neuropathic patients, adenosine-induced blood flow was lower than the non-neuropathic diabetic group or in the patients without diabetes. Surprisingly, regions with persistent sympathetic innervation showed a greater reduction in coronary flow reserve. The role of innervation or the lack of it in the diabetic myocardium needs more clarification.

## Effects of ischaemic syndromes on myocardium in diabetes

Even though a proportion of diabetic patients shows asymptomatic myocardial dysfunction and an even smaller subset shows clinically recognizable non-ischaemic cardiomyopathy, the majority has an acute ischaemic event related to myocardial involvement. The pathophysiology and therapeutic options in modifying progressive myocardial dysfunction in these patients are discussed below.

### Influence of silent ischaemia

Diabetic patients have a reduced pain perception during ischaemic episodes which could result in progressive myocardial dysfunction that is not clinically recognized. Reduced pain perception is thought to result in a high prevalence of painless ischaemic syndromes, including silent myocardial ischaemia at rest or during exercise [290, 291]. In one study [291], only 28% of the diabetic patients with positive thallium scintigraphy experienced angina pectoris during the treadmill test compared with 68% of non-diabetic patients. Diabetic patients also have less pain during an MI [292, 293]. Not surprisingly, diabetic patients have a greater incidence of unrecognized MI than do non-diabetic subjects in clinical [292, 294] and autopsy studies [295]. Diabetic patients often present with atypical symptoms which delay the diagnosis of CAD. The cause of the reduced perception of pain is believed to be the high prevalence of autonomic neuropathy in diabetic patients [284]. More recent studies have shown that these patients also have a significantly reduced MIBG uptake, even when corrected for myocardial perfusion defects, suggesting sympathetic cardiac denervation [296]. Patients with autonomic dysfunction also have a loss of the circadian pattern of ischaemia, unlike normal subjects or patients with no autonomic dysfunction [285]. However, not all studies have agreed that diabetics have more episodes of silent ischaemia. The ACIP trial [297], which looked at patients with abnormal exercise treadmill tests and single averaged electrocardiograms, could not find any difference in the prevalence or severity of silent ischaemia in diabetic patients. The cause of these variable results may depend on the population being studied.

This lack of a clinical warning system may contribute to the increased adverse events in diabetic patients. One study showed that diabetic patients without an anginal warning system had longer and more severe ischaemia [298]. Whether this puts them in greater danger is unclear at present.

### Unstable ischaemic syndromes

Diabetic patients also have a high incidence of acute ischaemic syndromes. Angioscopic studies [15] as well as data from autopsies [299] show a high prevalence of unstable plaques with thrombus formation in diabetic patients with chest pain (Fig. 22.10) [15]. The abnormal haematological, rheological, and metabolic milieu also results in a worse short- and long-term prognosis. Fava *et al.* [300], in a prospective, case–control study, compared the outcome of unstable angina in patients with type II DM and non-diabetic controls. There were 162 diabetic patients and 162 non-diabetic control patients with unstable angina in the study. The 3 month mortality in diabetic patients ($n = 162$) was 8.6% (95% CI 4.4–12.9%) compared with 2.5% (95% CI 0.1–4.9%) in control patients ($p = 0.014$). The 1 year mortality was 16.7% (95% CI 10.9–22.4%) in diabetic patients and 8.6% (95% CI 4.4–12.9%) in non-diabetic patients ($p = 0.029$). However, by 1 year, the frequency of recurrent ischaemic events and coronary artery bypass grafting was similar, suggesting that most of the differences are accounted for in the early follow-up period. The adverse effect of DM on ischaemic heart disease is also evident in patients with chest pain being evaluated for MI. In a study of 2058 consecutive hospitalized patients, Karlson *et al.* [301] showed that diabetic patients had a 28% 1 year

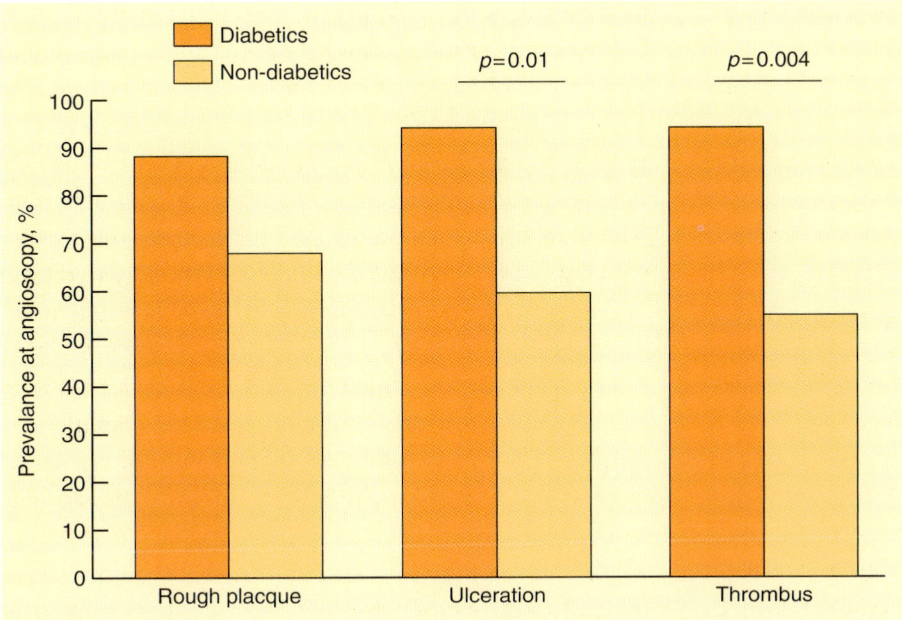


**Figure 22.10** *Diabetic subjects have more unstable lesions at angioscopy, which could account for their high event rates and worse prognosis. (Data from ref. 15.)*

mortality (twice of that seen in non-diabetics) and a 20% incidence of reinfarction. The prognosis of diabetic patients presenting with myocardial-related chest pain is poor irrespective of whether they sustain an MI.

## Acute myocardial infarction

In the diabetic, acute MI is one of the most common causes of myocardial damage, is the main mechanism of heart failure, and accounts for a majority of the deaths [10, 82, 177, 182–184, 302–304]. In general, diabetics have a complicated course after MI [177, 303, 304], including an increased incidence recurrent MI [304] and heart failure [177, 182, 183, 305], and this results in a higher short- [306] and long-term mortality rate [307–316]. Women with DM have approximately twice the mortality rate of men with DM [306, 308] and the prognosis is worst in obese women [309]. The duration of DM does not seem to influence hospital mortality after MI. Presentation is often atypical, manifesting as sudden heart failure, cardiac shock, arrhythmia, or sudden death [182–184, 292]. During hospitalization, patients with DM and acute MI have more heart failure, more mechanical complications, and a higher mortality than those without diabetes. This difference persists even after adjusting for LV function and risk-factor profile [126]. The adverse prognosis in patients with DM and MI continues over the long term [177, 182, 304, 310, 311]: there is a higher mortality rate, greater morbidity, and a greater need for intervention. This is primarily due to recurrent ischaemic events and increased pump failure.

The cause of this poor outcome is not totally clear [177, 304]. DM does not increase infarct size and does not reduce the prevalence of patent infarct-related arteries following thrombolysis [17, 20, 317]. Arrhythmic events are not affected significantly by DM [306, 311]. The risk is only partially related to an increased rate of infarct extension, recurrent ischaemia, and mechanical complications [177, 182–185, 310, 312, 313]. The most important determinant for adverse prognosis in patients with MI is an excess of heart failure [182, 183, 314–316]. In one study [315], LV regional EF was evaluated using radionuclide studies in 20 patients with type II DM and 29 non-diabetic patients 3 weeks after an acute MI. There was no difference in the extent of myocardial necrosis and CAD in the two groups. However, diabetic patients had a lower regional EF in the non-infarcted area and a lower ratio of systolic blood pressure to LV end-systolic volume in the remodelled myocardium. As expected, female diabetic patients fared the worst. Iwasaka *et al.* [179] performed radionuclide angiography at 3 weeks and 1 year after MI in 21 women and 29 men with DM and compared the findings with those in 62 non-diabetic subjects. In diabetic patients, the LV end-diastolic volume (LVEDV) increased between 3 months and 1 year, while the LV global and regional EF in the non-infarct area and the ratio of systolic blood pressure to LV end-systolic volume (pressure:volume ratio) decreased. The degree of remodelling was greater in diabetic women than in diabetic men.

The excess of heart failure in patients with DM is probably dependent on a number of factors. Aronson *et al.* [177] tried to evaluate why diabetics do poorly after an MI. It appears that abnormalities in the remote non-infarct wall are critical for the adverse prognosis. In the GUSTO trial [20, 317] the admission and 7 day global and regional EF were no different in patients with and without diabetes. However, the remote non-infarct segment did not show compensatory hyperkinesis in diabetics. As expected, these patients had more heart failure and shock, with worse outcome than those without DM, despite similar rates of successful thrombolysis [317]. Silent remote wall MI [294, 295, 312], diastolic dysfunction [177, 182, 183], reduced vasodilatory reserve due to the presence of multivessel disease [18–21, 317, 318], small-vessel disease, endothelial dysfunction [148, 155], and abnormal cellular metabolism may contribute to remote non-infarct wall dysfunction. Diabetics have more multivessel disease, with a more pronounced distribution of moderately sized lesions and more unstable plaques with ulceration [15]. Abnormal coagulation and reduced fibrinolysis with the increased tendency to plaque rupture may increase the chance of reinfarction, while autonomic abnormalities favour sudden cardiac death. Diabetic patients have more remodelling in the post-MI period [179]. Several other basic mechanisms may also be operative in diabetics. The benefits of the preconditioning of the myocardium may be inhibited by the influence of hypoglycaemic drugs that inhibit the ATPase-sensitive potassium channels [319]. Abnormalities in endothelial vasodilator mechanisms, including defective NO production may compromise endothelial cell function [320]. A higher incidence of silent ischaemia, plaque disruption, and thrombosis in diabetic patients [321] may help to explain the increased rate of acute coronary syndromes and MI observed in the post-MI period. It is therefore not surprising that despite equal efficacy of thrombolytic therapy, diabetic patients with acute MI continue to have a higher mortality rate than non-diabetic patients.

## Preserving the diabetic myocardium

### Acute myocardial infarction in a diabetic

#### *Importance of angiotensin-converting enzyme inhibition*

The GISSI-3 study group [322] recently published a retrospective analysis to determine the effects of early ACE inhibition (<24 h) in diabetic patients in the post-MI period. Since this is the largest (although not prospective) database of diabetics with an MI it will be considered in some depth. Treatment was started within 24 h and continued for 6 weeks; 15.2% of patients had DM, mostly type II. The main endpoint of the study was all-cause mortality at 6 weeks, and the secondary endpoint was the number of patients who died plus the number of survivors who had late (beyond day 4 of hospital stay) clinical heart failure or extensive LV damage in the absence of clinical heart failure (a combined end point). Echocardiographic data were available in 66% of the diabetic patients alive at follow-up.

Lisinopril decreased the 6 week mortality in diabetic patients (8.7% vs 12.4%; OR 0.68, 95% CI 0.53–0.86), which was much greater than that in non-diabetic patients (5.6% vs 5.9%; OR 0.95, 95% CI 0.83–1.09). This corresponded to 37 ± 12 lives saved per 1000 diabetics compared with 3 ± 4 lives saved per 1000 non-diabetics. The benefit was maintained at 6 months, despite stopping treatment at 6 weeks after MI (mortality at 6 months: 12.9% vs 16.1%, OR 0.77, 95% CI 0.62–0.95) and was consistent across all subgroups. The combined endpoint was also much lower in diabetic patients than in non-diabetics (incidence at 6 weeks: 21.6% vs 24.5%; OR 0.85, 95% CI 0.71–1.01 in diabetics, and 14.3 vs 15.5%; OR 0.91, 95% CI 0.83–1.00 in non-diabetics). This benefit in diabetics persisted even at 6 months but was not significant. There was an excess of heart failure in the lisinopril-treated diabetic group which reduced the benefit seen for combined endpoints. Thus, early ACE inhibition is critical in the treatment of diabetic patients with an MI. A similar benefit was seen in the subgroup analysis in the SAVE [323] and Trandolapril Cardiac Evaluation (TRACE) trials [324]. Free wall rupture is increased in diabetic patients with MI [325] and may be modified by ACE inhibition [326], giving diabetics an important benefit.

#### *Importance of blood sugar control*

Acute MI is associated with hyperglycaemia for a number of reasons, including the effects of increased stress hormones and a change in GLUT transporters. Blood glucose levels strongly correlate with short- and long-term mortality in diabetic patients with an MI [327]. Fava *et al.* [328] compared blood glucose levels on admission with long-term mortality (3.5 years) in 333 diabetic and 565 non-diabetic patients with MI. There was a significant association between mortality and blood glucose levels on admission in diabetic patients ($r = 0.92$) but not in non-diabetic individuals. The DIGAMI study [329] looked at the effect of insulin–glucose infusion (24 h) followed by multidose insulin treatment and compared it with standard treatment in 620 patients with DM and acute MI. There were 102 (33%) deaths in the treatment group compared with 138 (44%) deaths in the control group (relative risk 0.72, 95% CI 0.55–0.92; $p = 0.011$). Approximately one life was saved for every nine patients treated with insulin. The most pronounced effects were seen in patients who were at a low risk to start with. These data are very intriguing and suggests that intensive metabolic control at the start of MI may somehow protect patients from the adverse effects of MI. Not studied was the role of short-term (immediate post-MI) versus long-term glycaemic control. More studies are needed before widespread acceptance of this protocol.

***Importance of thrombolysis***

Despite initial fears that thrombolysis may be associated with an increased risk and reduced success in diabetic patients, there is evidence that thrombolytic therapy is useful in patients with MI who also have DM.

*Profile of patients coming for thrombolysis* The GUSTO study [17, 20], which enrolled 41 021 patients with acute MI, 944 of whom had diabetes, helped to create the profile of the type of diabetic patient coming for thrombolytic therapy in clinical practice. Patients with DM were more likely to be older women with an anterior wall MI, and to have triple-vessel CAD and a greater number of previous revascularization procedures. They presented later to the hospital than non-diabetic patients. They had a higher mortality rate despite effective thrombolysis. Patients on insulin were twice as likely to die as those not on insulin. tPA was better than streptokinase. Diabetic patients had a higher incidence of strokes (1.9 vs 1.4, $p < 0.001$, but intracranial hemorrhage was not different), CHF, cardiogenic shock, and arrhythmias. Revascularization rates were not different. All this suggests that part of the reason why diabetics do poorly after MI is that they present as a high-risk group and are sicker at presentation.

*Number of patients eligible* Some data show that diabetic patients receive thrombolysis less often than non-diabetic patients [330–332]. This may be related to poor pain perception, delay in presentation, and reluctance in medical personal to use the drug for fear of increased complications. One study [330] found that, over a 3 year period, only 35% of patients with DM received thrombolysis compared with 47% of patients without diabetes; 60% of the diabetics arrived at the hospital more than 12 h after onset of symptoms. Fortunately, it appears that the use of thrombolytic therapy in DM is slowly increasing [333].

Proliferative, haemorrhagic retinopathy has been considered a contraindication to thrombolysis and fears of increased complications may have limited the number of patients with DM who have been eligible for thrombolytic therapy. This fear appears to be unfounded. In the GUSTO study [20], of the 6,011 patients with DM, ocular haemorrhage occurred in 0.05% compared with 0.006% of patients without diabetes. Diabetic retinopathy should not be considered a contraindication to thrombolysis in patients with acute MI.

*Angiographic results of thrombolysis* Given the abnormal procoagulant state that exists in diabetic patients, it is natural to question whether the high mortality rate in these patients is related to inadequate reperfusion. Woodfield *et al.* [317] looked at the data from the GUSTO subset to answer this question. Even though the diabetic cohort was sicker and presented much later, the 90 min patency rates (TIMI-3 flow, 40% vs 38%), reocclusion rates (9.2% vs 5.3%), and immediate and 7 day regional and global LV functions were no different from those of the non-diabetic population. Despite this, the 30-day mortality rate was 11.3% in diabetic vs 5.9% in non-diabetic patients ($p <$ OR $= 0.0001$), which persisted after adjusting for clinical and angiographic variables.

*Magnitude of benefits* Thus, despite an increase in prothrombotic factors, reduced endogenous thrombolytic mechanisms, and extensive CAD, patients with DM have similar reperfusion rates [177, 317] but greater benefit from thrombolysis than non-diabetic patients (Fig. 22.11). In the overview by the Fibrinolytic Therapy Trialists (FTT) [334], there was a 21.7% reduction in cardiac events (13.6% vs 17.3%) in diabetics compared with a 14% reduction (8.7% vs 10.2%) in the non-diabetic population. In the FTT analysis, diabetic patients had benefits second only to those obtained in patients with left bundle branch block in terms of lives saved. This benefit was greater than that in all patients or those with anterior MI. Lynch *et al.* [333] compared the mortality of patients before (1984–1987) and

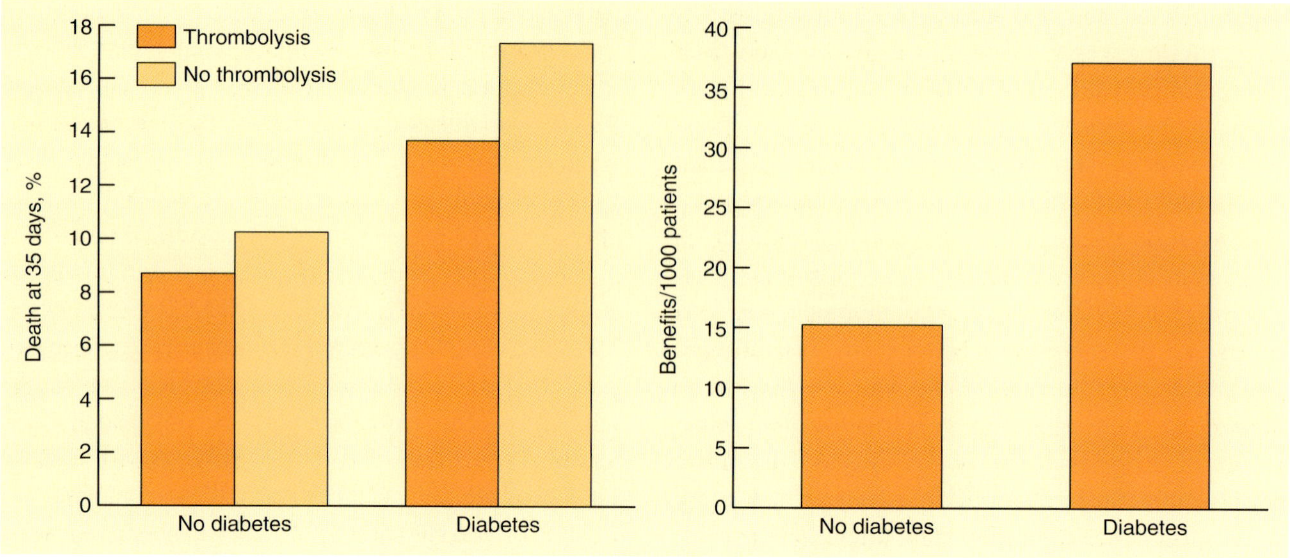


**Figure 22.11** *Given the high-risk nature of a myocardial infarction in diabetics, thrombolytic therapy benefits diabetics much more than non-diabetic subjects. (Data from ref. 334.)*

during the thrombolytic era (1990–1992) at one hospital in the UK. Thrombolytic therapy caused a 45% reduction in mortality and a 52% reduction in heart failure in non-diabetic patients, and a 42% reduction in mortality and a 45% reduction in heart failure in diabetic patients compared with the prethrombolytic period.

## Chronic coronary artery disease

DM is a recognized risk factor for poor outcome after either percutaneous [18, 19, 335] or surgical [318, 336, 337] revascularization, yet the proportion of diabetic patients who have such procedures continues to increase and now constitutes 25% of the total. Since these procedures address active ischaemia, they may be effective in reducing DM-related morbidity and mortality. Although data in this regard are limited, the following section will try to synthesize some current information.

### *Effectiveness of percutaneous coronary angiography in diabetic patients*

Diabetic patients have greater morbidity than their non-diabetic counterparts with every mode of non-surgical revascularization, including balloon angioplasty [18, 19, 318, 335, 338, 339], intracoronary stents [340], atherectomy [341], and percutaneous laser angioplasty [342]. Up to 20% of patients undergoing percutaneous coronary angiography (PTCA) are diabetic. PTCA can be successfully done in patients with MI [343] or in patients with more chronic forms of CAD [18, 338, 344]. Diabetic patients undergoing angioplasty or stenting have similar procedural success rates in the post-MI period or with elective procedures to non-diabetics. However, diabetic patients have worse long-term outcomes than non-diabetic patients, including higher rates of repeated interventions and lower survival rates [18, 338, 339, 344].

The effectiveness of PTCA in patients with chronic stable CAD has been summarized from an analysis of the National Heart, Lung, and Blood Institute (NHLBI) Registry [18]. The analysis compared baseline clinical and angiographic characteristics and short- and long-term outcomes of PTCA in 281 diabetic and 1833 non-diabetic patients between 1985 and 1986. Compared with the non-diabetic patients, the diabetic patients were older, were more likely to be female, and had more comorbid baseline conditions. They were more likely to have diffuse, extensive, triple-vessel disease. Angiographic success and completeness of revascularization were similar in both groups, yet diabetic patients experienced more in-hospital deaths and more procedural non-fatal MI. Long-term mortality, non-fatal MI, and need for repeat revascularization procedures were higher in diabetics.

While PTCA is effective in diabetic CAD, it is associated with an increase in restenosis [18, 19, 318, 344], both after the initial PTCA and after repeat procedures [335, 345–348]. There is evidence that diabetics requiring insulin fare the worst [344, 345]. A large proportion of patients has asymptomatic or silent restenosis. The high incidence of restenosis is due to an increase in risk factors, endothelial hyperplasia due to an excess of growth factors, and abnormal coagulation cascades [348]. There is an increased need for repeat interventions even after atherectomy [349] and laser angioplasty [342]. Data on the restenosis rates with coronary stenting are few but some studies suggest increased intimal hyperplasia even following stent implantation [350] and increased restenosis [340, 351]. The use of IIb/IIIa-receptor blockade has significantly improved the safety and efficacy of coronary interventions. However, some data show that owing to complex interactions in diabetics, the degree of benefit from these interventions may be different to that in non-diabetic subjects [352, 353]. In the EPIC study [352], while abciximab significantly reduced the 3 year composite ischaemic endpoint (MI, repeat revascularization, death) in non-diabetic subjects, this benefit was not as marked in diabetics.

### *Surgical revascularization in diabetic patients*

Approximately 15–20% of patients coming for coronary artery bypass graft (CABG) have DM [354]. Owing to more extensive disease, diabetics often end up with a greater number of bypass grafts [355]. CABG is effective in diabetic patients with CAD. In a subanalysis of the Coronary Artery Surgery Study (CASS) data, diabetic patients (> 65 years of age) derived a similar degree of benefit with CABG to the non-diabetic cohort [354]. While DM does not significantly affect surgical mortality in most series [355–357], it results in higher postoperative morbidity, reduces the long-term event-free interval, and decreases long-term survival after CABG [356, 358–360]. These adverse effects persist even after factoring in the poorer angiographic anatomy and LV function seen in these patients [356, 358–360], and are probably related, amongst other things, to accelerated CAD in non-grafted vessels and a reduced incidence of complete revascularization [16, 361]. DM is an independent risk factor for lesion progression and graft occlusion after CABG [361, 362].

### *Choice of revascularization by percutaneous coronary angiography versus coronary artery bypass graft*

Long-term data comparing PTCA and CABG for multivessel CAD are now available from randomized prospective trials. The BARI tual [363] compared the 5 year cardiac mortality and MI rates in 1829 patients with multivessel disease randomized to CABG or PTCA. The 353 treated diabetic patients (19% of a total 1829 subjects in the trial) with multivessel disease and objective evidence of ischaemia were randomly assigned to CABG or PTCA and followed for an average of 5.4 years. The patients with DM were more often women. African–Americans had a worse risk factor profile, and a greater prevalence of heart failure, chronic renal failure, and peripheral vascular disease. They also had a higher prevalence of three-vessel disease with more significant lesions which were more distally located. They had less complete revascularization with either CABG or PTCA, with a smaller minimum lumen diameter after PTCA. This profile has been confirmed in other studies [18, 338]. Among those with DM, the in-hospital mortality was 1.2% for CABG and 0.6% for PTCA. Among the DM patients receiving PTCA, 7.1% required emergency CABG, 2.9% underwent non-emergency CABG, and 2.4% required emergency PTCA during the initial hospitalization. Diabetic patients assigned to surgery (receiving at least one internal mammary artery graft) had better survival (all-cause mortality CABG vs PTCA, 19% vs 35%, $p = 0.003$) and reduced mortality (5.8% vs 20.6% $p = 0.0003$) rates compared with 4.8% and 4.7%, respectively, for other patients. Results of PTCA and surgery were similar in the non-diabetic group even when stratified according to LV function or number of diseased vessels (Fig. 22.12). A similar benefit was seen in the CABRI study, which only included 122 diabetic patients [364]. These data seem to support the use of CABG in diabetic patients with multivessel disease.

Not everyone totally agrees that CABG is a better option in those diabetic patients who can be offered revascularization. Subsequent analysis of small numbers of diabetic patients in other randomized trials of revascularization have provided conflicting results [365, 366], while observational studies in diabetic patients with multivessel disease [367, 368] could not confirm the BARI findings. The Duke University database [368] analysed data from 3220 patients with symptomatic two- or three-vessel CAD who underwent PTCA or CABG between 1984 and 1990, 24% of whom were diabetic. They found that the 5 year unadjusted as well as adjusted survival rate was lower in diabetics (74% and 86% for CABG; 76% and 88% for PTCA) than in non-diabetics. However, diabetics offered PTCA did not seem to be worse off than those offered CABG. In another study [367], the outcome of PTCA ($n = 279$) or CABG ($n = 246$) was analysed in a cohort of 525 consecutive, medically treated, comparable diabetic patients

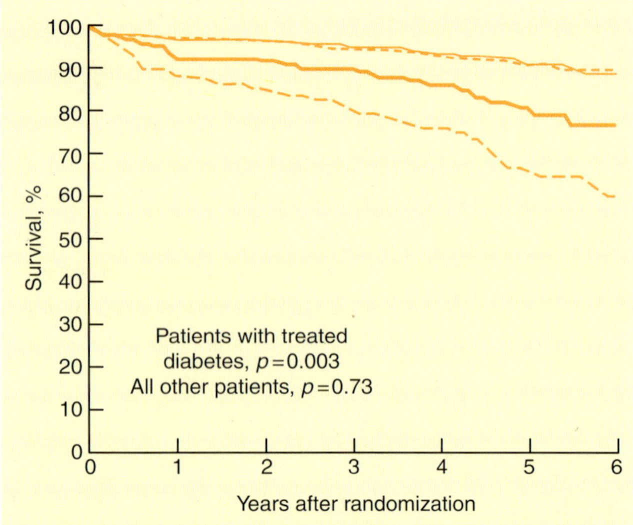


| | | | |
|---|---|---|---|
| Patients with treated diabetes | | | |
| CABG | 180 | 161 | 93 |
| PTCA | 173 | 139 | 69 |
| All other patients | | | |
| CABG | 734 | 696 | 449 |
| PTCA | 742 | 701 | 468 |

**Figure 22.12** *The BARI trial showed that diabetics did worse after multivessel percutaneous coronary angiography than patients undergoing coronary artery bypass surgery. (Data from ref. 344.)*

followed up for over 55 months. Complete revascularization was accomplished more often in the surgery group (79%) than in the angioplasty group (42%; $p < 0.001$); repeat revascularization (8% vs 64%; $p = 0.001$), cardiac events (32% vs 41%; $p = 0.04$), and death (30% vs 37%; $p = 0.08$) occurred less frequently in the bypass patients. Importantly, incomplete revascularization, but not mode of revascularization, correlated with late mortality.

The results for diabetic patients in the BARI trial [363] do not necessarily apply to all patients with diabetes. It has been suggested that the BARI trial showed the benefits of using internal mammary artery graft in diabetics rather than any specific diabetic-related adverse event with PTCA. This, together with the higher incidence of the need for repeat procedures in the diabetic patient, may be more important in determining outcome. Treated diabetics in the BARI trial who refused randomization were selected for treatment with PTCA without apparent compromise in survival compared with those having CABG [369]. This suggests that PTCA can be selectively offered to diabetics with multivessel disease, depending on the technical factors associated with the case.

## Will stenting change the implications of the BARI trial?

The BARI trial [361] was conducted in the pre-stent era and its results may not be totally applicable today. Diabetes increases the rate of restenosis after balloon angioplasty, with reported restenosis rates ranging from 47 to 69% [18, 335, 370]. Stents have been shown to improve significantly the results of coronary interventions [371, 372], chiefly through the reduction of restenosis [373] and reduced chronic occlusion [370]. Thus, coronary stenting would be expected to be useful in diabetics, although data are as yet insufficient. Initial studies, especially in vein grafts, suggest that diabetics have increased intimal hyperplasia [340, 350] and thus increased restenosis despite stents. There have been no controlled trials comparing PTCA and stenting in diabetics; however, observational studies have evaluated the efficacy of stenting in these patients. Abizaid *et al.* [374] compared the results of stenting in 248 patients with diabetes (151 on oral drugs and 97 on insulin) and in 706 non-diabetic patients. This study also carefully evaluated the intravascular ultrasound findings before and after intervention and further subclassified patients based on the type of diabetes. Patients with type I DM had smaller vessels by both angiography and intravascular ultrasound before and after stenting; the vessels of non-insulin-dependent diabetics did not differ from those of non-diabetic subjects. Patients with type I DM also had a slightly higher in-hospital mortality rate, more repeat procedures, and a higher event rate on follow-up for 1 year. Non-insulin-dependent diabetics behaved similarly to non-diabetics following stenting except for a minor increase in repeat procedures due to disease progression in other arterial segments (Fig. 22.13). Van Belle *et al.* [370] studied 300 patients (84% males, one-third with unstable angina) receiving single-vessel stenting, 19% of whom were diabetics and who had a 6 month follow-up angiogram. They compared these data with results in 300 patients receiving simple balloon angioplasty. The diabetics had significantly greater restenosis with balloon angioplasty than non-diabetic patients (63% vs 36%) and late vessel occlusion (14% vs 3%), despite similar preprocedural and postprocedural vessel morphology. Diabetics treated with insulin had the highest restenosis rate (81%). However, the rates of restenosis (25% vs 27%) and chronic occlusion (2% vs 1%) following stenting were similar in both groups. This suggests that stenting essentially abolishes the adverse influence of diabetes. Subanalysis of the STRESS trial

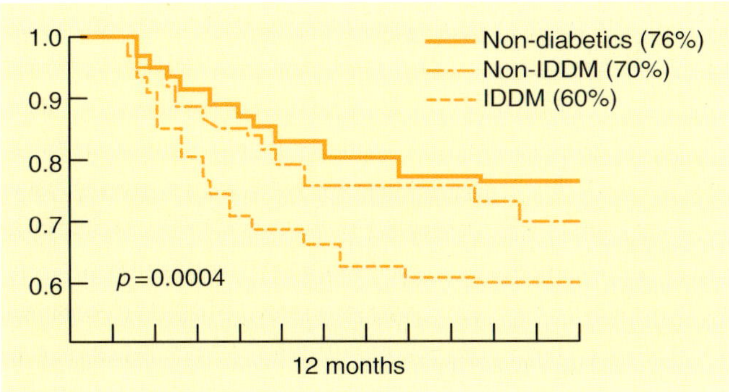


**Figure 22.13** *Although there are no randomized trials looking to see whether stents may make multivessel percutaneous coronary angiography useful in the diabetic patients, observational studies show that diabetics subjects, especially those with non-insulin-dependent diabetes mellitus, do as well as non-diabetic subjects with stents. (Data from ref. 374.)*

[375] also points to a reduction in restenosis with coronary stenting in diabetic patients.

The theoretical arguments to support the use of stents are unsettled since the mechanism of restenosis in diabetics is unclear. Two common mechanisms account for restenosis following PTCA: intimal hyperplasia and arterial remodelling. The relative contribution of each of these, especially in diabetic patients, is unknown. A number of growth factors is abnormally increased in diabetes and intimal–medial proliferation has been postulated to be important for restenosis in this group [340, 348]. Stenting may not influence this mechanism significantly. However, there is increasing evidence that vascular remodelling and not intimal hyperplasia is the important determinant in restenosis [376–378]. Atherectomy specimens from restenotic lesions in diabetic patients show minimal smooth-muscle proliferation [378], suggesting that remodelling may be more important. Stenting significantly influences the process of remodelling and is therefore likely to be useful in diabetics. This issue is complicated by data using intravascular ultrasound [350] which suggest that while non-stented segments show significant remodelling following coronary intervention in both normal and diabetic subjects, stented segments in diabetic patients shows an excess of intimal hyperplasia, and intimal hyperplasia remains an important issue even with coronary stenting. This is supported by other recent data showing an excess of restenosis in diabetic patients following stenting [379, 380]. While some authorities believe that multivessel PTCA should be proscribed in the diabetic patient [381], stents may change this scenario.

## Secondary prevention strategies in diabetic patients

The protocols for secondary prevention of MI are the same for patients with and without diabetes. However, data on the efficacy of various drugs for secondary prevention are lacking in patients with diabetes. There have been no randomized, prospective studies which specifically evaluate the effect of pharmacological treatment on the prognosis of diabetic patients during an acute MI. Even in the major studies, diabetic groups were not randomized a priori and most of the data are from post hoc analyses.

There is some preliminary evidence that the benefits of low-dose aspirin in secondary prevention are similar for diabetic and non-diabetic patients [382], although the dose needed to be effective is unknown. Biochemical studies suggest that a higher dose of aspirin may be needed to inhibit platelet aggregation [383]. Hyperglycaemia may inhibit the action of aspirin [384]; in the ISIS-2 study, aspirin in a dose of 150 mg/day given during an MI was of no benefit in diabetic patients [385]. Similarly, aspirin has not been shown to be useful in the primary prevention of MI in diabetic patients [386]. Thus, the underlying condition may affect the utility of aspirin therapy. Concern that diabetic patients may be at an increased risk of bleeding after antiplatelet therapy was countered by one study, in which aspirin at 750 mg/day in patients with diabetic retinopathy did not increase intraocular bleeding [386]. It is important to note in addition to the usual adverse effects of aspirin (gastrointestinal bleeding and increased renal failure), recent data suggest that aspirin prevents the beneficial effects of ACE inhibition in patients with heart failure [387]. In addition, patients with DM have a smaller benefit with oral anticoagulants than non-diabetic subjects in the post-MI period [388].

Unlike aspirin, there is extensive evidence that β-blockers are very effective in reducing post-MI mortality [389–393]. Given the high risk of adverse events in the post-MI period in diabetic patients, it is not surprising that these patients benefit the most with post-MI β-blocker therapy. Pooled data [394] from three randomized studies looking at β-blocker use during an MI [391–393] and three studies of β-blockade in the post-MI period in diabetic patients [389, 390, 395] suggest that the in-hospital mortality is reduced by 37% in diabetic patients treated with β-blockers compared with 13% in non-diabetics so treated. A similar difference exists for the long-term post-MI mortality rate (48% vs 33%) when β-blockade was initiated in the post-MI period. There is significant underusage of β-blockade in patients with MI [396] and there is an extra, but unfounded, fear [397] that β-blockers may mask hypoglycaemia or worsen metabolic parameters. β-Blockade should therefore be used in diabetic patients with acute MI unless severely contraindicated.

As discussed previously, ACE inhibitors have also been shown to be useful in secondary prevention. In the GISSI-3 study [322], lisinopril reduced the 6 week mortality rate in patients with type I DM (11.8% vs 21.1; 44% reduction, $p < 0.05$) and non-type I DM (8.0% vs 10.6%; 25% reduction; $p < 0.05$). The SOLVD study (approximately 70% subjects had CAD and previous MI) showed similar effects of ACE inhibition in patients with and without DM II [398].

Data suggest that diabetic patients respond well to cholesterol reduction, either as primary or as secondary prevention. Three major trials studied the effect of treating hyperlipidaemia in diabetic patients. Analysis of a study [399] of 202 diabetic and 4242 non-diabetic patients with previous MI or angina pectoris and a total serum cholesterol of 5.5–8.0 mmol/l and triglycerides < 2.5 mmol/l showed that the clinical benefits of lipid lowering were greater in diabetic patients than in those without diabetes. Simvastatin was equally effective in both groups. However, total mortality (RR 0.57 vs 0.71), major cardiovascular events (RR 0.45 vs 0.68), and atherosclerotic events (RR 0.63 vs 0.74) at follow-up of 5.4 years were lower in patients with diabetes. These effects were independent of concomitant aspirin or β-blocker use [399]. The CARE trial [400] also showed that the combined coronary events were lower in diabetic patients ($n = 586$) treated with pravastatin, suggesting that lowering cholesterol is effective in these patients; diabetic patients had a 25% risk reduction compared with 23% in non-diabetic subjects. A secondary analysis in this study showed that entry levels of blood glucose influenced event rates but did not affect the effectiveness of risk reduction with lipid lowering. Similar data are available from the Helsinki Heart Study [401], which included 135 diabetic patients among the 4081 subjects in the trial.

### Antidiabetic drugs and risk of adverse events

There has been some concern that oral antidiabetic agents may increase the risk of CAD-related events in patients with diabetes. In 1970, the UGDP trial [63], showed that tolbutamide, a first-generation sulphonylurea, increased the risk of major cardiovascular events. However, there was no increase in cardiovascular events in patients treated with sulphonylurea in the UK prospective DM study [64] over a 6 year follow-up period. The reasons for these discrepant results are unclear. There was a number of shortcomings in the UGDP trial which may have something to do with these results. Sulphonylureas inhibit $K^+$ ATP channels [402, 403] and this may reduce ischaemic preconditioning, worsen ischaemia, and cause arrhythmias [402]. There is evidence that these drugs can abolish preconditioning in humans [402, 404]. Current recommendations suggest using the smallest dose of short-acting agents from the sulphonylurea subgroup of oral antidiabetic drugs, since the risk is unknown.

### Can the natural history of coronary artery disease and diabetic cardiomyopathy be changed?

It is not clear whether primary or secondary prevention of CAD is effective in changing the natural history in patients with diabetes. Some investigators believe that, given the high event rates in the diabetic group, risk-factor modification can reduce CAD-related mortality to a greater extent (four times greater) than that possible in non-diabetic patients [405]. This has not been rigorously tested and others believe that these measures have a smaller impact in diabetic patients. Several treatment options have detrimental effects on metabolic parameters in patients with DM and some drugs may increase CAD mortality [112].

There have been no studies evaluating the benefits of intensive glycaemic control and aggressive management of risk factors. Eastman *et al.* [25] tried to calculate mathematically the extent of this benefit using epidemiological data (Table 22.2). They found that DM reduced the life expectancy by about 9–11 years and that the effects of standard versus intensive glycaemic control did not change this result. Modifying multiple risk factors was more effective in reducing mortality than controlling a single risk factor. The disease itself accounted for half the mortality in patients with diabetes. Even so, with the data available, intensive glycaemic control and aggressive risk-factor modification increased life expectancy by 0.2 years.

## Conclusions

DM is a significant problem worldwide and cardiovascular involvement is its principal complication. Cardiac involvement can be due to coronary vascular disease or to primary myocardial dysfunction. Both entities can present as heart

**Table 22.2** Model predictions of survival and lifetime cumulative incidence of cardiovascular events after diagnosis of diabetes

| | Years of life remaining | Stroke (%) | Myocardial infarction (%) | CHD (%) | CVD (%) | Fatal CHD (%) | Fatal CVD (%) |
|---|---|---|---|---|---|---|---|
| Standard care | 18.3 | 5.3 | 14.3 | 27.1 | 47.2 | 6.3 | 16.2 |
| Stop smoking | 18.3 | 5.0 | 11.9 | 25.3 | 43.5 | 5.2 | 14.7 |
| Treat SBP to <120 mmHg | 18.5 | 2.7 | 12.0 | 24.6 | 41.4 | 4.4 | 14.1 |
| Treat total serum cholesterol to <5.2 mmol/l | 18.4 | 5.8 | 13.8 | 26.7 | 46.5 | 6.0 | 15.9 |
| Increase HDL cholesterol to non-diabetic range | 18.3 | 5.4 | 13.4 | 25.1 | 44.9 | 4.6 | 15.0 |
| Do all of the above | 18.5 | 2.2 | 8.1 | 19.7 | 35.9 | 2.6 | 12.6 |
| Do all of the above and eliminate excess non-CVD mortality risk | 24.3 | 3.7 | 11.2 | 28.1 | 50.6 | 4.1 | 20.3 |
| Standard care with diabetes coefficients eliminated from CVD model | 18.5 | 2.6 | 7.5 | 20.3 | 34.0 | 3.2 | 13.3 |
| Intensive care | 20.0 | 6.1 | 15.5 | 26.0 | 45.0 | 7.1 | 9.7 |
| All risk factors treated as above | 20.2 | 2.7 | 8.8 | 18.1 | 32.7 | 2.9 | 5.4 |
| All risk factors treated as above and excess non-CVD mortality rate eliminated | 28.1 | 5.1 | 12.8 | 27.1 | 47.6 | 5.3 | 9.8 |
| Intensive care with diabetes coefficients eliminated from CVD model | 20.3 | 3.0 | 7.8 | 18.8 | 29.7 | 3.8 | 6.0 |
| Person without diabetes | 29.3 | 2.3 | 5.7 | 18.1 | 27.3 | 2.5 | 3.6 |

Mathematical model to quantify the benefits of risk factor intervention in patients with diabetes (assumed to be diagnosed at the age of 51 years in this model). Modification of single risk factors causes only small changes in outcome. Modifying all factors reduces the risk by half. This also suggests that diabetes itself (and its non-cardiovascular morbidity) accounts for about half of the adverse effect. The effect of intensive control of diabetes affects non-cardiovascular events favourably and hence may reduce total mortality.
SBP = systolic blood pressure; CVD = cardiovascular disease; CHD = coronary heart disease.
(From ref. 25.)

failure and, not surprisingly, diabetics have an excess of subclinical and clinical heart failure. While there are widespread abnormalities in small vessels and the endothelial structure and function in diabetic patients, it is not clear to what extent these contribute to heart failure. Primary myocardial systolic and diastolic dysfunction is commonly recognized in diabetics. Since diabetics, even without obvious CAD, have a poorer prognosis, it is important that every effort be made to preserve the diabetic myocardium. Aggressive risk-factor modification is vital and there is a sense that these patients need a greater degree of risk factor modification than non-diabetic subjects. Many of the risk factors are present years before the manifestation of DM, so risk-factor intervention needs to be started before obvious hyperglycaemia in high-risk subjects. It is not clear whether tight glycaemic control prevents heart failure or even modifies existing myocardial dysfunction. Thrombolytic therapy is very effective in diabetics should be used to a maximum. Revascularization is feasible in the diabetic but incurs a higher rate of suboptimal short- and long-term results; surgical revascularization using an internal mammary graft is the most ideal therapy when feasible. Despite suboptimal results in diabetics compared with non-diabetics, catheter revascularization, especially coronary stenting, has an important role. Secondary prevention strategies have not been evaluated in diabetics in a focused manner. However, indirect data suggest that these measures have a more significant impact on diabetic than on non-diabetic patients. It is not clear whether the natural history of DM and diabetic heart disease can be modified to a significant extent, but projections from available data suggest that this should be eminently feasible. One limitation is the lack of clear data on the pathogenetic factors involved in the genesis of diabetic heart disease. This needs to be clarified so that therapies targeted at pathogenetic mechanisms are available in future.

## References

1. Harris MI. NIDDM – epidemiology and scope of the problem. *Diabetes Spectrum* 1996; 9: 26–34.
2. Harris MI, Cowie CC, Reiber G. *Diabetes in America*. 2nd edn. Washington DC: US Government Printing Office, 1995.
3. McCarty D, Zimmet P. *Diabetes 1994 to 2010: global estimates and projections*. Melbourne: International Diabetes Institute, 1994.

4. Kenny SJ, Aubert RE, Geiss LS. Prevalence and incidence of non insulin dependent diabetes mellitus. In: MI Harris, CC Cowie, G Reiber (eds). *Diabetes in America*. 2nd edn. Washington DC: US Government Printing Office, 1995, 47.
5. Zimmet PZ, McCarty DJ, de Courten MP. The global epidemiology of non-insulin-dependent diabetes mellitus and the metabolic syndrome. *J Diabetes Complications* 1997; 11: 60–8.
6. Harris MI, Klein RE, Welborn TA *et al.* Onset of NIDDM occurs at least 4–7 years before clinical diagnosis. *Diabetes Care* 1992: 15: 815–19.
7. Geiss LS, Herman WH, Smith PJ. Mortality in NIDDM. In: MI Harris, CC Cowie, G Reiber (eds). *Diabetes in America*. 2nd edn. Washington DC: US Government Printing Office, 1995, 233–45.
8. Roman SH, Harris MI. Management of diabetes mellitus from a public health perspective. *Endocrinol Metab Clin North Am* 1997; 26: 443–74.
9. American Diabetes Association. Consensus Statement: role of cardiovascular risk factors in prevention and treatment of macrovascular disease in diabetes. *Diabetes Care* 1993; 16: 72–8.
10. Pyorala K, Laskso M, Uunistupa M. Diabetes and antherosclerosis: an epidemiological view. *Diabetes Metab Rev* 1987; 3: 463–524.
11. Haffner SM, Lehto S, Ronnemma T *et al.* Mortality from coronary heart disease in subjects with type 2 diabetes and in non diabetic subjects with and without prior myocardial infarction. *N Engl J Med* 1998; 339: 229–34.
12. Kannel W, McGee D. Diabetes and cardiovascular risk factors: the Framingham Study. *Circulation* 1979; 59: 8–15.
13. Stamler J, Vaccaro O, Neaton J *et al.* Diabetes, other risk factors, and 12 yr cardiovascular mortality for men screened in the Multiple Risk Factor Intervention Trial. *Diabetes Care* 1993; 16: 434–44.
14. Wingard DL, Barrett-Connor E. Heart disease and diabetes. In: MI Harris, CC Cowie, G Reiber (eds). *Diabetes in America*. 2nd edn. Washington DC: US Government Printing Office, 1995, 429–48.
15. Silva JA, Escobar A, Collins TJ *et al.* Unstable angina: a comparison between diabetic and nondiabetic patients. *Circulation* 1995; 92: 1731–6.
16. Alderman EL, Corley SD, Fisher LD *et al.* Five year angiographic follow-up of factors associated with progression of coronary artery disease in the coronary artery surgery study (CASS). *J Am Coll Cardiol* 1993; 22: 1141–54.
17. Granger C, Califf R, Young S *et al.* Outcome of patients with diabetes mellitus and acute myocardial infarction treated with thrombolytic agents. *J Am Coll Cardiol* 1993; 21: 920–5.
18. Kip KE, Faxon DP, Detre KM *et al.* for the Investigators of the NHLBI PTCA Registry. Coronary angioplasty in diabetic patients: the National Heart, Lung, and Blood Institute Percutaneous Transluminal Coronary Angioplasty Registry. *Circulation* 1996; 94: 1818–25.
19. Stein B, Weintraub W, Gebhart SSP *et al.* Influence of diabetes mellitus on early and late outcome after percutaneous transluminal coronary angioplasty. *Circulation* 1995; 91: 979–89.
20. Mak KH, Moliterno DJ, Granger CB *et al.* Influence of diabetes mellitus on clinical outcome in the thrombolytic era of acute myocardial infarction. GUSTO-I Investigators. Global Utilization of Streptokinase and Tissue Plasminogen Activator for Occluded Coronary Arteries. *J Am Coll Cardiol* 1997; 30: 171–9.
21. Waller B, Palumbo P, Roberts W. Status of the coronary arteries at necropsy in diabetes mellitus with onset after age 30 years. *Am J Med* 1980; 69: 498–506.
22. Haffner SM. The prediabetic problem: development of non insulin dependent diabetes mellitus and related abnormalities. *J Diabetes Complications* 1997; 11: 69–76.
23. Kleinman JC, Donahue RP, Harris MI *et al.* Mortality among diabetics in a national sample. *Am J Epidemiol* 1988; 28: 389–401.
24. Turner R, Cull C, Holman R. United Kingdom Prospective Diabetes Study 17: a 9 year update of a randomized, controlled trial on the effect of improved metabolic control on complications in non-insulin dependent diabetes mellitus. *Ann Intern Med* 1996; 124: 136–45.
25. Eastman RC, Keen H. The impact of cardiovascular disease on people with diabetes: the potential for prevention. *Lancet* 1997; 350: si29–32.
26. Diabetes Drafting Group. Prevalence of small vessel and large vessel disease in diabetic patients from 14 centers: the WHO Multinational Study of Vascular Disease in Diabetics. *Diabetologia* 1985; 28: 615–40.
27. Fuller JH, Stevens LK, Wang SL. International variations in cardiovascular mortally associated with diabetes mellitus: the WHO Multinational Study of Vascular Disease in Diabetes. *Ann Med* 1996; 28: 319–22.
28. Krolewski AS, Warram JH, Valsania P *et al.* Evolving natural history of coronary artery disease in diabetes mellitus. *Am J Med* 1991; 90 (Suppl 2A): 56–61S.
29. Matsumoto T, Ohashi Y, Yamada N *et al.* Coronary artery disease mortality is actually low in diabetic Japanese by direct comparison with the Joslin cohort. *Diabetes Care* 1994; 17: 1062–3.
30. Nelson RG, Sievers ML, Knowler WC *et al.* Low incidence of fatal coronary disease in Pima Indians despite high prevalence of non-insulin dependent diabetes. *Circulation* 1990; 81: 987–95.
31. West KM. Diabetes in Americans Indians and other native populations of the new world. *Diabetes* 1974; 23: 841–55.
32. Barrett-Connor E, Cohn B, Wingard D, Edelstein SL. Why is diabetes mellitus a stronger risk factor for fatal ischemic heart disease in women then in men? The Rancho Bernardo Study. *JAMA* 1991; 265: 627–31.
33. Castelli WP. Cardiovascular disease in women. *Am J Obstet Gynecol* 1988; 158: 1553–60.
34. Goldschmid MG, Barrett-Connor E, Edelstein SL *et al.* Atherosclerosis in coronary heart disease: dyslipidemia and ischemic heart disease mortality among men and women with diabetes. *Circulation* 1994; 89: 991–7.
35. Pan WH, Cedres LB, Liu K *et al.* Relationship of clinical diabetes and asymptomatic hyperglycemia to risk of coronary heart disease mortality in men and women. *Am J Epidemiol* 1986; 123: 504–16.
36. Lerner DJ, Kannel WB. Patterns of coronary heart disease morbidity and mortality in the sexes: a 26-year follow-up of the Framingham population. *Am Heart J* 1986; 111: 383–90.
37. Walden CE, Knopp RH, Wahl PW *et al.* Sex differences in the effect of diabetes mellitus on lipoprotein triglyceride and cholesterol concentrations. *N Engl J Med* 1984; 311: 953–9.
38. Moy CS, LaPorte RE, Dorman JS *et al.* Insulin-dependent diabetes mellitus mortality. The risk of cigarette smoking. *Circulation* 1990; 82: 37–43.
39. Diabetes Control and Complications Trial (DCCT) Research Group. Effect of intensive diabetes management on macrovascular events and risk factors in the diabetes control and complications trial. *Am J Cardiol* 1995; 75: 894–903.

40. Moss SE, Klein R, Klein BEK *et al.* The association of glycemia and cause specific mortality in a diabetic population. *Arch Intern Med* 1994; 154: 2473–9.
41. Nathan DM. Long term complications of diabetes mellitus. *N Engl J Med* 1993; 328: 1676–85.
42. Krolewski AS, Kosinski EJ, Warram JH *et al.* Magnitude and determinants of coronary artery disease in juvenile onset, insulin dependent diabetes mellitus. *Am J Cardiol* 1987; 59: 750–5.
43. Jarrett RJ, Shipley MJ. Type 2 (non insulin dependent) diabetes mellitus and cardiovascular disease—putative association via common antecedents: further evidence from the Whitehall Study. *Diabetologia* 1988; 31: 737–40.
44. Manson JE, Colditz GA, Stampfer MJ *et al.* A prospective study of maturity onset diabetes mellitus and risk of coronary heart disease and stroke in women. *Arch Intern Med* 1991; 151: 1141–7.
45. Haffner SM, Stern MP, Hazuda HP *et al.* Cardiovascular risk factors in confirmed prediabetic individuals. does the clock for coronary heart disease start ticking before the onset of clinical diabetes? *JAMA* 1990; 263: 2893–8.
46. Howard G, O'Leary D, Ayad M *et al.* Lower insulin sensitivity is related to atherosclerosis in non diabetics: the Insulin Resistance Atherosclerosis Study (IRAS). *Diabetes* 1994; 43 (Suppl 1): 60A.
47. Reaven GM. Role of insulin resistance in human disease. *Diabetes* 1988; 37: 1595–607.
48. Fontbonne A, Charles MA, Thibult N *et al.* Hyperinsulinemia as a predictor of coronary heart disease mortality in a healthy population: the Paris Prospective Study 15 year follow up. *Diabetologia* 1991; 34: 356–61.
49. Stout RW. Insulin and atheroma: a 20 yr perspective. *Diabetes Care* 1990; 13: 631–54.
50. Hillson RM, Hockaday TDR, Mann JI *et al.* Hyperinsulinemia is associated with development of electrocardiographic abnormalities in diabetics. *Diabetes Res* 1984; 1: 143–9.
51. Janka HU, Ziegler AG, Standl E *et al.* Daily insulin dose as a predictor of macrovascular disease in insulin treated non insulin dependent diabetics. *Diabetes Metab* 1987; 13: 359–64.
52. Wingard DL, Barrett-Connor EL, Ferrara A. Is insulin really a heart disease risk factor? *Diabetes Care* 1995; 18: 1299–304.
53. Orchard TJ, Eichner J, Kuller LH *et al.* Insulin as a predictor of coronary heart disease: interaction with apo E phenotype; a report from MRFIT. *Ann Epidemiol* 1994; 4: 40–5.
54. Tack CJ, Smits P, Willemsen JJ *et al.* Effects of insulin on vascular tone and sympathetic nervous system in NIDDM. *Diabetes* 1996; 45: 15–22.
55. Velloso LA, Folli F, Sun XJ *et al.* Cross-talk between the insulin and angiotensin signaling systems. *Proc Natl Acad Sci USA* 1996; 93: 12490–5.
56. King GL, Davidheiser S, Banskota N *et al.* Insulin receptors and actions on vascular cells. In: U Smith, NE Brunn, T Hedner *et al.* (eds) *Novo Nordisk Foundation Symposium No. 5*, Novo Foundaton: Stockholm, 1991; 183.
57. Jarrett RJ. Why is insulin not a risk factor for coronary heart disease? *Diabetologia* 1994, 37: 945–7.
58. Leonetti F, Iozzo P, Giaccari A *et al.* Absence of clinically overt atherosclerotic vascular disease and adverse changes in cardiovascular risk factors in 70 patients with insulinoma. *J Endocrinol Invest* 1993; 16: 875–80.
59. Yudkin JS. Coronary heart disease in diabetes mellitus: three new risk factors and a unifying hypothesis. *J Intern Med* 1995; 238: 21–30.
60. Harris MI. Medical care for patients with diabetes. Epidemiologic aspects. *Ann Intern Med* 1996; 124: 117–22.
61. Reaven GM, Laws A. Insulin resistance, compensatory hyperinsulinemia, and coronary heart disease. *Diabetologia* 1994; 37: 948–52.
62. Behar S, Boyko V, Reicher-Reiss H, Goldbourt U. Ten-year survival after acute myocardial infarction: comparison of patients with and without diabetes. SPRINT Study Group. Secondary Prevention Reinfarction Israeli Nifedipine Trial. *Am Heart J* 1997; 133: 290–6.
63. Klimt CR, Knatterud GL, Meinert CL, Prout TE. The University Group Diabetes Program. a study of the effect of hypoglycemic agents on vascular complications in patients with adult onset diabetes.1. Design, methods and baseline characteristics. II. Mortality results. *Diabetes* 1970; 19 (Suppl 2): 747–830.
64. UK Prospective Diabetes Study Group. UK Prospective Diabetes Study 16. Overview of 6 years therapy of type II diabetes. *Diabetes* 1995; 44: 1249–58.
65. Abraira C, Colwell JA, Nuttall FO *et al.* and VA CSDM Group. Veterans affairs cooperative study on glycemic control and complications in type II diabetes (VA CSDM). Results of the feasibility trial. *Diabetes Care* 1995, 18: 1113–23.
66. Davidoff F. Control, complications, confidence: the Regenstrief Conference on the risks and benefits of intensive management in NIDDM. Editorial. *Ann Intern Med* 1996; 124: 65–6.
67. Laakso M. Glycemic control and the risk for coronary heart disease in patients with non-insulin dependent diabetes mellitus. *Ann Intern Med* 1996; 124: 127–30.
68. Diabetes Control and Complications Trial Research Group. The effect of intensive treatment of diabetes on the development and progression of long-term complications in insulin-dependent diabetes mellitus. *N Engl J Med* 1993; 329: 977–86.
69. Nathan DM. The pathophysiology of diabetes complications: how much does the glucose hypothesis explain: *Ann Intern Med* 1996; 124: 86–9.
70. Gerstein HC, Yusuf S. Dysglycemia and risk of cardiovascular disease. *Lancet* 1996; 347: 949–50.
71. Singer DE, Nathan DM, Anderson KM *et al.* Association of Hb A1c with prevalent cardiovascular disease in the original cohort of the Framingham heart study. *Diabetes* 1992; 41: 202–8.
72. Kinoshita JH, Nishimura C. The involvement of aldose reductase in diabetic complications. *Diabetes Metab Rev* 1988; 4: 323–37.
73. Engerman RL, Kern TS, Garment MB. Capillary basement membrane in retina, kidney, and muscle of diabetic dogs and galactosemic dogs and its response to 5 years aldose reductase inhibition. *J Diabetes Complications* 1993; 7: 241–5.
74. Williamson JR, Chang K, Frangos M *et al.* Hyperglycemic pseudohypoxia and diabetic complications. *Diabetes* 1993; 42: 801–13.
75. Xia P, Kramer RM, King GL. Identification of the mechanism for the inhibition of Na,K-adenosine triphosphatase by hyperglycemia involving activation of protein kinase C and cytosolic phospholipase A2. *J Clin Invest* 1995; 96: 733–40.
76. King GL, Shiba T, Oliver J *et al.* Cellular and molecular abnormalities in the vascular endothelium of diabetes mellitus. *Annu Rev Med* 1994; 45: 179–88.
77. Bierhaus A, Hofmann MA, Ziegler R, Nawroth PP. AGEs and their interaction with AGE receptors in vascular disease and diabetes mellitus. The AGE concept. *Cardiovasc Res* 1988; 37: 586–600.

78. Neeper M, Schmidt AM, Brett J *et al.* Cloning and expression of RAGE: a cell surface receptor for advanced glycosylation end products of proteins. *J Biol Chem* 1992; 267: 14998–5004.
79. Charonis AS, Reger LA, Dege JE *et al.* Laminin alterations after *in vitro* nonenzymatic glucosylation. *Diabetes* 1990; 39: 807–14.
80. Haitoglou CS, Tsilibary EC, Brownlee M *et al.* Altered cellular interactions between endothelial cells and nonenzymatically glucosylated laminin/type IV collagen. *J Biol Chem* 1992; 267: 12404–7.
81. Lin SJ, Hong CY, Chang MS *et al.* Increased aortic endothelial cell death enhanced transendothelial macromolecular transport in streptozotocin diabetic rats. *Diabetologia* 1993; 36: 926–30.
82. Morrish NJ, Stevens LK, Head J *et al.* A prospective study of mortality among middle-aged diabetic patients (the London cohort of the WHO Multinational Study of Vascular Disease in Diabetics) 1: causes and death rates. *Diabetologia* 1990; 33: 538–41.
83. Meigs JB, Singer DE, Sullivan L *et al.* Metabolic control and prevalent cardiovascular disease in non-insulin-dependent diabetes mellitus: the NIDDM Patient Outcomes Research Team. *Am J Med* 1997; 102: 38–47.
84. American Diabetes Association. Standards of medical care for patients with diabetes mellitus. *Diabetes Care* 1994; 6: 616–23.
85. Williamson JR, Kilo C. Extracellular matrix changes in diabetes mellitus. In DG Scarpelli, G Migahi (eds) *Comparative pathobiology of major age-related diseases*. New York: Liss, 1984, 269.
86. Harp JB, DiGirolamo M. Composition of the renin angiotensin system in adipose tissue: changes with maturation and adipose mass enlargement. *J Gerontol Biol Sci Med Sci* 1995; 50: B270–6.
87. Saye JA, Ragsdale NV, Crey RM, Peach MJ. Localisation of angiotensin peptide forming enzymes of 3T3 F442A adipocytes. *Am J Physiol* 1993; 263: C1570–6.
88. Malik FS, Lavie CJ, Mehra MR *et al.* Renin–angiotensin system: genes to bedside. *Am Heart J* 1997; 134: 514–26.
89. Tan LB, Jalil JE, Pick R *et al.* Cardiac myocyte necrosis induced by angiotensin II. *Circ Res* 1991; 69: 1185–95.
90. Feener EP, Hansen H, Folli F. Angiotensin inhibits insulin signaling in rat aortic smooth muscle cells (Abstract) *Diabetes* 1997; 46 (Suppl) 212.
91. Harris MI. Epidemiologic studies on the pathogenesis of non-insulin-dependent diabetes mellitus (NIDDM). *Clinical and Investigative Medicine* 1995; 18: 231–9.
92. Resengren A, Welin L, Tsipogianni A, Wilhelmsen L. Impact of cardiovascular risk factors on coronary heart disease and mortality among middle aged diabetic men: a general population study. *BMJ* 1989; 288: 1127–31.
93. McKeigue PM, Miller GJ, Marmot MG. Coronary heart disease in South Asians overseas: a review. *Clin Epidemiol* 1989; 42: 597–609.
94. Mitchell BD, Stern MP, Haffner SM *et al.* Risk factors for cardiovascular mortality in Mexican Americans and non-Hispanic whites. *Am J Epidemiol* 1990; 131: 423–33.
95. Semenkovich CF, Heinecke JW. The mystery of diabetes and atherosclerosis. *Diabetes* 1997; 46: 327–34.
96. Wingard DL, Barrett-Connors E, Criqui MH, Suarez L. Clustering of heart disease risk factors in diabetic compared to nondiabetic adults. *Am J Epidemiol* 1983; 117: 19–26.
97. Ford ES, DeStefano F. Risk factors for mortality from all causes and from coronary heart disease among persons with diabetes. *Am J Epidemiol* 1991; 133: 1220–30.
98. Myers L, Coughlin SS, Weber LS *et al.* Prediction of adult cardiovascular multifactorial risk status from childhood risk factor levels. The Bogalusa heart study. *Am J Epidemiol* 1995; 142: 918–24.
99. Reaven GM, Lithell H, Landsberg L. Hypertenstion and associated metabolic abnormalities — the role of insulin resistance and the sympthoadrenal system. *N Engl J Med* 1996; 334: 374–81.
100. Hopkins PN, Hunt SC, Wu LL, Williams GH, Williams RR. Hypertension, dyslipidemia, and insulin resistance: links in a chain or spokes on a wheel? *Curr Opin Lipidol* 1996; 7: 241–53.
101. Despres JP, Marette A. Relation of components of insulin resistance syndrome to coronary disease risk. *Curr Opin Lipidol* 1994; 5: 274–89.
102. Shinozaki K, Suzuki M, Ikebuchi M *et al.* Insulin resistance associated with compensatory hyperinsulinemia as an independent risk factor for vasospastic angina. *Circulation* 1995; 92: 1749–57.
103. Fuller JH, Stevens LK, Wang S. Epidemiology of hypertension in diabetic patients. *J Cardiovasc Pharmacol* 1996; 28 (Suppl 28): S1–5.
104. Morales PA, Mitchell BD, Valdez RA *et al.* Incidence of NIDDM and impaired glucose tolerance in hypertensive subjects: the San Antonio Heart Study. *Diabetes* 1993; 42: 154–61.
105. Lithell H. Effect of anti-hypertensive drugs on insulin, glucose and lipid metabolism. *Diabetes Care* 1991; 14: 203–9.
106. Shamiss A, Carroll J, Rosenthal T. Insulin resistance in secondary hypertension. *Am J Hypertens* 1992; 5: 26–8.
107. Assmann G, Schulte H. The Prospective Cardiovascular Muenster (PROCAM) Study: prevalence of hyperlipidemia in persons with hypertension and/or diabetes mellitus and their relationship to coronary heart disease. *Am Heart J* 1988; 116: 1713–24.
108. Fuller J, Stevens LK, Chaturvedi N, Holloway JF. Antihypertensive therapy in diabetes mellitus (Cochrane Review). In: *The Cochrane Library*. Issue 2. Oxford: Update Software, 1998.
109. Grossman E, Messerli FH. Diabetic and hypertensive heart disease. *Ann Intern Med* 1996; 125: 304–10.
110. Moser M, Ross H. The treatment of hypertension in diabetic patients. *Diabetes Care* 1993; 16: 542–7.
111. Bloomgarden Z, Ginsburg-Fellner F, Rayfield E *et al.* Elevated hemoglobin A1c and low density lipoprotein cholesterol levels in thiazide treated diabetic patients. *Am J Med* 1984; 77: 823–7.
112. Warram JH, Laffel L, Valsania P *et al.* Excess mortality associated with diuretic therapy in diabetes mellitus. *Arch Intern Med* 1991; 151: 1350–6.
113. Holm G, Johannson S, Verdin A *et al.* The effect of beta blockade on glucose tolerance and insulin release in adult diabetics. *Acta Med Scand* 1980; 208: 187–91.
114. Weidmann P, Ferrier C, Saxenhofer H *et al.* Serum lipoproteins during treatment with antihypertensive drugs. *Drugs* 1988; 35 (Suppl 2): 118–34.
115. Pollare T, Lithell H, Berne C. A comparison of the effects of hydrochorthiazide and captopril on glucose and lipid metabolism in patients with hypertension. *N Engl J Med* 1989; 321: 868–73.
116. Manolio TA, Cutler JA, Furberg CD *et al.* Trends in pharmacologic management of hypertension in the United States. *Arch Intern Med* 1995; 155: 829–37.
117. Estacio RO, Jeffers BW, Hiatt WR *et al.* The effect of nisoldipine as compared with enalapril on cardiovascular outcomes in patients with non-insulin-dependent diabetes and hypertension. *N Engl J Med* 1998; 338: 645–52.
118. Macdonald IA. Advances in our understanding of the role of the sympathetic nervous system in obesity. *Int J Obes* 1995; 19: S2–7.

119. Hotamisligil GS, Amer P, Caro JF *et al.* Increased adipose tissue expression of tumor necrosis factor alpha in human obesity and insulin resistance. *J Clin Invest* 1995; 95: 2409–15.
120. Sjostrom CD, Hakangard AC, Lissner L, Sjostrom L. Body compartment and subcutaneous adipose tissue distribution risk patterns in obese subjects. *Obes Res* 1995; 3: 9–22.
121. Freedman DS, Williamson DF, Croft JB *et al.* Relation of body fat distribution to ischemic heart disease. The national health and nutrition examination survey I (NHANES I) epidemiologic follow up study. *Am J Epidemiol* 1995; 142: 53–63.
122. Tchernof A. Larnarche B, Prud'Homme D *et al.* The dense LDL phenotype: association with plasma lipoprotein levels, visceral obesity, and hyperinsulinemia in men. *Diabetes Care* 1996; 19: 629–37.
123. Bierman E. Atherogenesis in diabetes. *Atheroscler Thromb* 1992; 12: 647–56.
124. Austin MA, King MC, Vranizan KM, Krauss RM. Atherogenic lipoprotein phenotype: a proposed genetic marker for coronary heart disease risk. *Circulation* 1990; 82: 495–506.
125. Fontbonne A, Eschwege E, Cambien F *et al.* Hypertriglycendemia as a risk factor for coronary heart disease mortality in subjects with impaired glucose tolerance or diabetes: results from the 11 year follow-up of the Paris Prospective Study. *Diabetologia* 1989; 32: 300–4.
126. Kannel W. Lipids, diabetes, and coronary heart disease: insights from the Framingham Study. *Am Heart J* 1985; 110: 1100–7.
127. Tashnen MR. Hyperlipidaemia in diabetes. *Baillieres Clin Endocrinol Metab* 1990: 4: 743–75.
128. Syvanne M, Kahri J, Virtanen KS, Tashnen MR. HDL containing apolipoproteins A-1 and A-11 (LpA-1:A-II) as markers of coronary artery disease in men with non-insulin dependent diabetes mellitus. *Circulation* 1995; 92: 364–70.
129. Bucala R, Makita Z, Vega G *et al.* Modification of low density lipoprotein by advanced glycosylation end products contributes to the dyslipidemia of diabetes and renal insufficiency. *Proc Natl Acad Sci USA* 1994; 91: 9441–5.
130. Bowie A, Owens D, Collins P *et al.* Glycosylated low density lipoprotein is more sensitive to oxidation: implications for the diabetic patient: *Atherosclerosis* 1993; 102: 63–7.
131. Chisolm G, Irwin K, Penn M. Lipoprotein oxidation and lipoprotein-induced cell injury in diabetes. *Diabetes* 1992; 41 (Suppl 2): 61–6.
132. Sobinen IA, Tertov VV, Kochinsky T *et al.* Modified low density lipoproteins from diabetic patients causes cholesterol accumulation in human intimal aortic cells. *Atherosclerosis* 1993; 100: 41–54.
133. Lyons TJ. Glycation and oxidation: a role in the pathogenesis of atherosclerosis. *Am J Cardiol* 1993; 71: 26–31B.
134. Steinbrecher UP, Witztum JL. Glycosylation of low density lipoproteins to an extent comparable to that seen in diabetics slows their catabolism. *Diabetes* 1984; 33: 130–4.
135. American Diabetes Association. Consensus statement: detection and management of lipid disorders in diabetes. *Diabetes Care* 1993; 16: 828–39.
136. Nathan DM, Roussell A, Godine JE. Glyburide or insulin for metabolic control in non insulin dependent diabetes mellitus. *Ann Intern Med* 1988; 108: 334–40.
137. Kwaan H. Changes in blood coagulation, platelet function, and plasminogen-plasmin system in diabetes. *Diabetes* 1992; 41 (Suppl 2): 32–5.
138. Juhan-Vague I, Alessi MC, Vague P. Increased plasminogen activator inhibitor levels. A possible link between insulin resistance and atherothrombosis. *Diabetologia* 1991; 34: 457–62.
139. Aoki I, Shimoyama K, Aoki N *et al.* Platelet-dependent thrombin generation in patients with diabetes mellitus: effects of glycemic control on coagulability in diabetes. *J Am Coll Cardiol* 1996; 27: 560–6.
140. Gall MA, Borch-Johnsen K, Nielsen FS *et al.* Albuminuria and poor glycemic control predict mortality in NIDDM. *Diabetes* 1995; 44: 1303–9.
141. Borch-Johnsen K, Kreiner S. Proteinuria: value as predictor of cardiovascular mortality; in insulin dependent diabetes mellitus. *BMJ* 1987; 294: 1651–4.
142. Earle K, Walker J, Hill C *et al.* Familial clustering of cardiovascular disease in patients with insulin-dependent diabetes and nephropathy. *N Engl J Med* 326: 673–7.
143. Makita Z, Radoff S, Rayfield EJ *et al.* Advanced glycosylation end products in patients with diabetic nephropathy. *N Engl J Med* 1991; 325: 836–42.
144. Factor SM, Segal BH, van Hoeven KH. Diabetes and coronary artery disease. *Caron Artery Dis* 1992; 3: 4–10.
145. Sutherland CG, Fisher BM, Frier BM *et al.* Endomyocardial biopsy pathology in insulin-dependent diabetic patients with abnormal ventricular function. *Histopathology* 1989; 14: 593–602.
146. Yarom R, Zirkin H, Stammler G, Rose AG. Human coronary microvessels in diabetes and ischaemia: morphometric study of autopsy material. *J Pathol* 1992; 166: 265–70.
147. Durante W, Sunahara FA, Sen AK. Effect of diabetes on metabolic coronary dilatation in the rat. *Cardiovasc Res* 1989; 23: 40–5.
148. Nitenberg A, Valensi P, Sachs R *et al.* Impairment of coronary vascular reserve and ACh-induced coronary vasodilation in diabetic patients with angiographically normal coronary arteries and normal left ventricular systolic function. *Diabetes* 1993; 42: 1017–25.
149. Cohen RA, Dysfunction of vascular endothelium in diabetes mellitus *Circulation* 1993; 87 (Suppl 5): 67–76.
150. Stehouwer CDA, Nauta JJP, Zeldenrust GC *et al.* Urinary albumin excretion, cardiovascular disease, and endothelial dysfunction in non-insulin dependent diabetes mellitus. *Lancet* 1992; 340: 319–23.
151. Fujii K, Heistad DD, Faraci FM. Effect of diabetes mellitus on flow-mediated and endothelium-dependent dilatation of the rat basilar artery. *Stroke* 1992; 23: 1494–8.
152. Meraji S, Jayakody L, Senaratme P *et al.* Endothelium-dependent relaxation in aorta of BB rats. *Diabetes* 1987; 36: 978–81.
153. Calver A, Collier J, Vallance P. Inhibition and stimulation of nitric oxide synthesis in the human forearm arterial bed of patients with insulin-dependent diabetes mellitus. *J Clin Invest* 1992; 90: 2548–54.
154. Quyyumi AA, Cannon RO, Panza JA *et al.* Endothelial dysfunction in patients with chest pain and normal coronary arteries. *Circulation* 1992; 86: 1864–71.
155. Nahser PJ, Brown RE, Oskarsson H *et al.* Coronary heart disease/myocardial infarction: maximal coronary flow reserve and metabolic coronary vasodilation in patients with diabetes mellitus. *circulation* 1995; 91: 635–40.
156. Koltai MZ, Wagner M, Pogatsa G. Altered hyperemic response of the coronary arterial bed in alloxan diabetes. *Experientia* 1983; 39: 738–40.
157. Yokoyama I, Momomura S, Ohtake T *et al.* Reduced myocardial flow reserve in non-insulin-dependent diabetes mellitus. *J Am Coll Cardiol* 1997; 30: 1472–7.
158. Akasaka T, Yoshida K, Hozumi T *et al.* Retinopathy identifies marked restriction of coronary flow reserve in patients with diabetes mellitus. *J Am Coll Cardiol* 1997; 30: 935–41.

159. Vogel RA Coronary risk factors, endothelial function, and atherosclerosis. *Clin Cardiol* 1997; 20: 426–32.
160. De Meyer GR, Herman AG. Vascular endothelial dysfunction. *Prog Cardiovasc Dis* 1997; 39: 325–42.
161. Mattei P, Virdis A, Ghiadoni L *et al*. Endothelial function in hypertension. *J Nephrol* 1997; 10: 192–7.
162. Lorenzi M, Cagliero E, Toledo S. Glucose toxicity for human endothelial cell culture; delayed replication, disturbed cell cycle, and accelerated death. *Diabetes* 1985; 34; 621–7.
163. Richardson M, Hadcock SJ, DeReske M, Cybulsky MI. Increased expression *in vivo* of VCAM-I and E-selectin by aortic endothelium of normalipidemic and hyperlipidemic diabetic rabbits. *Atheroscler Thromb* 1994; 14: 760–76.
164. Hadcock S, Richardson M, Winocour PH, Hutton MW. Intimal alterations in rabbits aortas during the first 6 months of alloxan-induced diabetes. *Atheroscler Thromb* 1991; 11: 517–29.
165. Downing SE, Lee JC, Fripp RR. Enhanced sensitivity of diabetic hearts to alpha-adrenergic stimulation. *Am J Physiol* 1983; 245: H808–13.
166. Ren-Ming HU, Levin ER, Pedram A, Frank HJL. Insuline stimulates production and secretion of endothelin from bovine endothelial cells. *Diabetes* 1993; 42: 351–8.
167. Umeda F, Inoguchi T, Nawata H. Reduced stimulatory activity on prostacyclin production by cultured endothelium cells in serum from aged diabetic patients. *Atherosclerosis* 1989; 75: 61–6.
168. Clarkson P, Celermajer DS, Donald AK *et al*. Impaired vascular reactivity in insulin-dependent diabetes mellitus is related m disease duration and low density lipoprotein cholesterol levels. *J Am Coll Cardiol* 1996; 28: 573–9.
169. Williams SB, Goldfine AB, Timimi FK *et al*. Acute hyperglycemia attenuates endothelium dependent vasodilation in humans *in vivo*. *Circulation* 1998; 97: 1695–701.
170. Samaha FF, Heineman FW, Ince C *et al*. ATP-sensitive potassium channel is essential to maintain basal coronary vascular tone *in vivo*. *AM J Physiol* 1992; 262: C1220–7.
171. Aversano T, Ouyang P, Silverman H. Blockade of the ATP-sensitive potassium channel modulates reactive hyperemia in the canine coronary circulation. *Circ Res* 1991; 69: 618–22.
172. Mullen MJ, Clarkson P, Donald AE *et al*. Effect of enalapril on endothelial function in young insulin-dependent diabetic patients: a randomized, double-blind study. *J Am Coll Cardiol* 1998; 31: 1330–5.
173. Timimi FK, Ting HH, Haley EA *et al*. Vitamin C improves endothelial dependent vasodilation in patients with diabetes mellitus. *J Am Coll Cardiol* 1998; 31: 552–7.
174. Nitenberg A, Paycha F, Ledoux S *et al*. Coronary artery responses to physiological stimuli are improved by desferoxamine but not by L arginine in non insulin dependent diabetic patients with angiographically normal coronary arteries and no other risk factors. *Circulation* 1998; 97: 736–43.
175. Pieper GM, Adams MB, Roza AM. Pancreatic transplantation reverses endothelial dysfunction in experimental diabetes mellitus. *Surgery* 1998; 123: 89–95.
176. Goodfellow J, Ramsey MW, Luddmgron LA *et al*. Endothelium and inelastic arteries: an early marker of vascular dysfunction in non-insulin dependent diabetes. *BMJ* 1996; 312: 744–5.
177. Aronson D, Rayfield EJ, Chesebro JH. Mechanisms determining course and outcome of diabetic patients who have had acute myocardial infarction. *Ann Intern Med* 1997; 126: 296–306.
178. Kannel WB, Hjortland M, Castelli WP. Role of diabetes in congestive heart failure: the Framingham Study. *Am J Cardiol* 1974; 34: 29–34.
179. Iwasaka T, Sugiura T, Abe Y *et al*. Residual left ventricular pump function following acute myocardial infarction in postmenopausal diabetic women. *Coron Artery Dis* 1994; 5: 237–42.
180. Hamby R, Sherman L, Mehta J, Aintablian A. Reappraisal of the role of the diabetic state in coronary artery disease. *Chest* 1976; 70: 251–7.
181. Hamby RL, Zoneraich S, Sherman L. Diabetic cardiomyopathy. *JAMA* 1974; 229: 1749–54.
182. Stone PH, Muller JE, Hanwell T *et al*. The effect of diabetes mellitus on prognosis and serial left ventricular function after acute myocardial infarction: contribution of both coronary disease and left ventricular dysfunction to the adverse prognosis. The MILIS Study Group. *J Am Coll Cardiol* 1989; 14: 49–57.
183. Savage MP, Krolewski AS, Kenien GG *et al*. Acute myocardial infarction in diabetes mellitus and significance of congestive heart failure as a prognostic factor. *Am J Cardiol* 1988; 62: 665–9.
184. Ulvenstam G, Aberg A. Bergstrand R *et al*. Long-term prognosis after myocardial infarction in men with diabetes. *Diabetes* 1985; 34: 787–92.
185. Wilson CS, Gau GT, Fulton RE, Davis GD. Coronary artery disease in diabetic and non diabetic patients: a clinical and angiographic comparison. *Clin Cardiol* 1983; 6: 440–6.
186. Zarich SW, Nesto RW. Diabetic cardiomyopathy. *Am Heart J* 1989; 118: 1000–12.
187. Davidoff AJ, Pinault FM, Rodgers RL. Ventricular relaxation of diabetic spontaneously hypertensive rat. *Hypertension* 1990; 15: 643–51.
188. Rodgers RL. Depressor effect of diabetes in the spontaneously hypertensive rat: associated changes in heart performance. *Can J Physiol Pharmacol* 1986; 64: 1177–84.
189. Brown RA, Robinson E, Dunbar JC. Inotropic effects of ethanol on the isolated papillary muscle of diabetic rats. *Alcohol* 1993; 10: 231–5.
190. Ren J, Davidoff AJ. Diabetes rapidly induces contractile dysfunction in isolated ventricular myocytes. *Am J Physiol* 1997; 272: H148–58.
191. Davidoff AJ, Ren J. Low insulin and high glucose induce abnormal relaxation in cultured adult rat ventricular myocytes. *Am J Physiol* 1997; 272: H159–67.
192. Jourdon P, Feuvray D. Calcium and potassium currents in ventricular myocytes isolated from diabetic rats. *J Physiol Lond* 1993; 470: 411–29.
193. Regan TJ, Ettinger PO, Kahn MI *et al*. Altered myocardial function and metabolism in chronic diabetes mellitus without ischemia in dogs. *Circ Res* 1974; 35: 222–7.
194. Raev DC. Which left ventricular function is impaired earlier in the evolution of diabetic cardiomyopathy? An echocardiographic study of young type I diabetic patients. *Diabetes Care* 1994; 17: 633–9.
195. Vanninen E, Mustonen J, Vainio P *et al*. Left ventricular function and dimensions in newly diagnosed nor-insulin dependent diabetes mellitus. *Am J Cardiol* 1992; 70: 371–8.
196. Mustonen JN, Uusitupa M, Tahvanainen K *et al*. Impaired left ventricular systolic function during exercise in middle-aged insulin-dependent and non-insulin dependent diabetic subjects without clinically evident cardiovascular disease. *Am J Cardiol* 1988; 62: 1273–9.

197. Hiramatsu K, Ohara N, Shigematsu S *et al.* Left ventricular filling abnormalities in non-insulin dependent diabetes mellitus and improvement by a short term glycemic control. *Am J Cardiol* 1992; 70: 1185–9.
198. Zarich SW, Arbuckle BE, Cohen LR *et al.* Diastolic abnormalities in young asymptomatic diabetic patients assessed by pulsed Doppler echocardiography. *J Am Coll Cardiol* 1988; 12: 114–20.
199. Uusitupa M, Mustonen J, Laskso M *et al.* Impairment of diastolic function in middle-aged type 1 (insulin-dependent) and type 2 (non-insulin dependent) diabetic patients free of cardiovascular disease. *Diabetologia* 1988; 31: 783–91.
200. Mildenberger RR, Bar-Shlomo B, Druck MN *et al.* Clinically unrecognized ventricular dysfunction in young diabetic patients. *J Am Coll Cardiol* 1984; 4: 234–8.
201. Fein FS, Zola BE, Malhotra A *et al.* Hypertensive diabetic cardiomyopathy in rats. *Am J Physiol* 1990; 258: H793–805.
202. Regan TJ, Lyons MM, Ahmed SS *et al.* Evidence for cardiomyopathy in familial diabetes mellitus. *J Clin Invest* 1977; 60: 884–99.
203. Perez JE, McGill JB, Santiago JV *et al.* Abnormal myocardial acoustic properties in diabetic patients and their correlation with the severity of disease. *J Am Coll Cardiol* 1992; 19: 1154–62.
204. Bibello V, Talarico L, Picano E *et al.* Increased echo density of myocardial wall in the diabetic heart: an ultrasound tissue characterization study. *J Am Coll Cardiol* 1995; 25: 1408–15.
205. Pierce GN, Russell JC. Regulation of intracellular calcium in the heart during diabetes. *Cardiovasc Res* 1997; 34: 41–7.
206. Galderisi M, Anderson KM, Wilson PW, Levy D. Echocardiographic evidence for the existence of a distinct diabetic cardiomyopathy (the Framingham Heart Study). *Am J Cardiol* 1991; 68: 85–9.
207. Regan TJ, Wu CF, Yeh CK *et al.* Myocardial composition and function in diabetes. The effects of chronic insulin use. *Circ Res* 1981: 49: 1268–77.
208. Brownlee M. Glycation and diabetic complications. *Diabetes* 1994; 43: 836–41.
209. Norton GR, Candy G, Woodiwiss AJ. Aminoguanidine prevents the decreased myocardial compliance produced by streptozotocin-induced diabetes mellitus in rats. *Circulation* 1996; 93: 1905–12.
210. Kahn JK, Zola B, Juni JE, Vinik AI. Radionuclide assessment of left ventricular diastolic filling in diabetes mellitus with and without cardiac autonomic neuropathy. *J Am Coll Cardiol* 1986; 7: 1303–9.
211. Jermendy G, Khoor S, Koltai MZ, Pogatsa G. Left ventricular diastolic dysfunction in type I (insulin-dependent) diabetic patients during dynamic exercise. *Cardiology* 1990; 77: 9–16.
212. Fein FS. Diabetic cardiomyopathy. *Diabetes Care* 1990; 13: 1169–79.
213. Litwin SE, Raya TE, Anderson PG *et al.* Abnormal cardiac function in the streptozotocin-diabetic rat. Changes in active and passive properties of the left ventricle. *J Clin Invest* 1990; 86: 481–8.
214. Fein FS, Sonnenblick EH. Diabetic cardiomyopathy. *Prog Cardiovasc Dis* 1985; 27: 255–70.
215. Schaffer SW, Mozaffri MS, Artman M, Wilson GL. Basis for mechanical defects associated with non insulin dependent diabetes. *Am J Physiol* 1989; 256: E25–30.
216. Fein FS, Kornstein LB. Strobeck JE *et al.* Altered myocardial mechanics in diabetic rats. *Circ Res* 1980; 47: 922–33.
217. Okayama H, Hamada M, Hiwada K. Contractile dysfunction in the diabetic rat heart is an intrinsic abnormality of the cardiac myocyte. *Clin Sci* 1994; 86: 257–62.
218. Seneviratne BI. Diabetic cardiomyopathy: the preclinical phase. *BMJ* 1977; i: 1444–6.
219. Shapiro LM, Howat AP, Calter MM. Left ventricular function in diabetes mellitus. 1: Methodology and prevalence and spectrum of abnormalities. *Br Heart J* 1981; 45: 122–8.
220. Fisher BM, Gillen G, Lindop GBM *et al.* Cardiac function and coronary arteriography in asymptomatic type I (insulin-dependent) diabetic patients: evidence for a specific diabetic heart disease. *Diabetologia* 1986; 29: 706–12.
221. Airakesinen KEJ, Ikaheimo M, Kaila J *et al.* Impaired left ventricular filling in young female diabetics. An echocardiographic study. *Acta Med Scand* 1984; 216: 509–16.
222. Vered A, Battler A, Segal P *et al.* Exercise-induced left ventricular dysfunction in young men with asymptomatic diabetes mellitus (diabetic cardiomyopathy). *Am J Cardiol* 1984; 54: 633–7.
223. Fisher BM, Gillen G, Ong-Tone L *et al.* Cardiac function and insulin-dependent diabetes: radionuclide ventriculography in young diabetics. *Diabetic Med* 1985: 2: 251–6.
224. Margonato A, Gerundini P, Vicedomini G *et al.* Abnormal cardiovascular response to exercise in young asymptomatic diabetic patients with retinopathy. *Am Heart J* 1986: 112: 554–60.
225. Paillole C, Dahan M, Paycha F *et al.* Prevalence and significance of left ventricular filling abnormalities determined by Doppler echocardiography in young type 1 (insulin dependent) diabetes mellitus. *Am J Cardiol* 1989; 64: 1010–16.
226. Theusen L, Cristiansen JS, Falstie-Jensen N *et al.* Increased myocardial contractility in short term type 1 diabetic patients: an echocardiographic study. *Diabetologia* 1985; 28: 822–6.
227. Borow KM, Jaspan JB, Williams KA *et al.* Myocardial mechanics in young adult patients with diabetes mellitus: effects of altered load, inotropic state and dynamic exercise. *J Am Coll Cardiol* 1990; 15: 1508–17.
228. Zola B, Kahn JK, Juni JE, Vinik AI. Abnormal cardiac function in diabetic patients with autonomic neuropathy in the absence of ischemic heart disease. *J Clin Endocrinol Metab* 1986; 63: 208–14.
229. Mustonen JN, Uusitupa MI, Laakso M *et al.* Left ventricular systolic function in middle-aged patients with diabetes mellitus. *Am J Cardiol* 1994; 73: 1202–8.
230. Yu, Z, Quamme GA, McNeill JH. Depressed [$Ca^{2+}$] responses to isoproterenol and cAMP in isolated cardiomyocytes from experimental diabetic rats. *Am J Physiol* 1994; 266: H 2334–42.
231. Yu Z, Tibbits GF, McNeill JH. Cellular functions of diabetic cardiomyocytes: contractility, rapid-cooling contracture, and ryanodine binding: *Am J Physiol* 1994; 266: H2082–9.
232. Hoffman PA, Menon V, Gannaway KF. Effects of diabetes on isometric tension as a function of [$Ca^{2+}$] and pH in skinned cardiac myocytes. *Am J Physiol* 1995; 269: H1656–63.
233. Khandoudi N, Guo AC, Chesnais M, Feuvray D. Skinned cardiac fibers of diabetic rats contractile activation and effects of 2,3-butanedione monoxime (BDM) and caffeine. *Cardiovasc Res* 1993; 27: 447–52.
234. Pierce GN, Dhalla NS. Heart mitochondrial function in chronic experimental diabetes in rats. *Can J Cardiol* 1985; 1: 48–54.
235. Fein FS, Scheuer J. Heart disease in diabetes. In D Porte Jr, RS Sherman (eds) *Diabetes mellitus*. 5th edn. Connecticut: Appleton-Lange, 1997, 1105–25.
236. Uusitupa M, Siitonen O, Aro A *et al.* Effect of correction of hyperglycaemia on left ventricular function in non-insulin dependent (type 2) diabetics. *Acta Med Scand* 1983; 213: 363–8.

237. Mustonen I, Laaxso M, Uusitupa M *et al.* Improvement of left ventricular function after starting insulin treatment in patients with non-insulin dependent diabetes. *Diabetes Res* 1988; 9: 27–30.
238. Bell DS. Diabetic cardiomyopathy. A unique entity or a complication of coronary artery disease. *Diabetes Care* 1995; 18: 708–14.
239. Grossman E, Shemesh J, Shamiss A *et al.* Left ventricular mass in diabetes-hypertension. *Arch Intern Med* 1992; 152: 1001–4.
240. Venco A, Grandi A, Barzizza F, Finardi G. Echocardiographic features of hypertensive diabetic heart muscle disease. *Cardiology* 1994; 74: 28–34.
241. Yoshida R, Ishida Y, Hozumi T *et al.* Congestive heart failure in mitochondrial diabetes mellitus. *Lancet* 1994; 344: 1375.
242. Barnett AH. Diabetes and hypertension. *Br Med Bull* 1994; 50: 397–407.
243. Factor SM, Minase T, Sonnenblick EH. Clinical and morphological features of human hypertensive-diabetic cardiomyopathy. *Am Heart J* 1980; 99: 446–58.
244. van Hoeven KH, Factor SM. A comparison of the pathological spectrum of hypertensive, diabetics, and hypertensive-diabetic heart disease. *Circulation* 1990; 82: 848–55.
245. Nagano N, Nagano M, Yo Y *et al.* Role of glucose intolerance in cardiac diastolic function in essential hypertension. *Hypertension* 1994; 23: 1002–5.
246. Grossman E, Oren S, Messerli FH. Left ventricular mass and cardiac function in patients with essential hypertension. *J Hum Hypertens* 1994; 8: 417–21.
247. Inouye I, Massie B, Loge D *et al.* Abnormal left ventricular filling: an early finding in mild to moderate systemic hypertension. *Am J Cardiol* 1984: 53: 120–6.
248. Arora GD, Reeves WC, Movahed A. Alteration of coronary perfusion reserve in hypertensive patients with diabetes. *J Hum Hypertens* 1994; 8: 51–7.
249. Rubler S, Dlugash J, Yucheogly Y. New types of cardiomyopathy associated with diabetic glomerulosclerosis. *Am J Cardiol* 1972: 30: 595–602.
250. Shirey EK, Proudfit WL, Hawk WA. Primary myocardial disease: correlation with clinical findings, angiographic and biopsy diagnosis: follow-up of 139 patients. *Am Heart J* 1980; 62: 251–4.
251. Genda A, Mizuno S, Nunoda S *et al.* Clinical studies on diabetic myocardial disease using exercise testing with myocardial scintigraphy and endomyocardial biopsy. *Clin Cardiol* 1986; 9: 375–82.
252. Factor SM, Okun EM, Minase T. Capillary microaneurysms in the human diabetic heart. *N Engl J Med* 1980; 302: 384–8.
253. Blumenthal HT, Alex M, Goldenberg S. A study of lesions of the intramural coronary artery branches in diabetes mellitus. *Arch Pathol* 1960; 70: 27–42.
254. Fischer VW, Barner HB, Larose LS. Pathomorphologic aspects of muscular tissue in diabetes mellitus. *Hum Pathol* 1984; 15: 1127–36.
255. Factor SM, Sonnenblick EH. Hypothesis: is congestive cardiomyopathy caused by a hyperactive myocardial microcirculation (microvascular spasm)? *Am J Cardiol* 1982: 50: 1149–52.
256. Sunni S, Bishop SP. Kent SP, Geer JC. Diabetic cardiomyopathy. A morphological study of intramyocardial arteries. *Arch Pathol Lab Med* 1986; 110: 375–81.
257. Schaub MC, Hefti MA, Zuellig RA, Morano I. Modulation of contractility in human cardiac hypertrophy by myosin essential light chain isoforms. *Cardiovasc Res* 1998; 37: 381–404.
258. Fein FS, Strobeck JE, Malhotra A *et al.* Reversibility of diabetic cardiomyopathy with insulin in rats. *Circ Res* 1981; 49: 1251–61.
259. Afzal X, Ganguly PK, Dhalla KS *et al.* Beneficial effects of verapamil in diabetic cardiomyopathy. *Diabetes* 1988: 37: 93–4.
260. Fein FS, Cho S, Malhotra A *et al.* Beneficial effects of diltiazem on the natural history of hypertensive diabetic cardiomyopathy in rat. *J Am Coll Cardiol* 1991; 18: 1406–17.
261. Schaffer SW. Cardiomyopathy associated with non insulin dependent diabetes mellitus. *Mol Cell Biochem* 1991; 107: 1–20.
262. Rodrigues B, Cam MC, McNeill JH. Myocardial substrate metabolism. Implications for diabetic cardiomyopathy. *J Mol Cell Cardiol* 1995; 27: 169–79.
263. Saghizade M, Ong JM, Barvey WT *et al.* The expression of TNF alpha by human muscle. Relationship to insulin resistance. *J Clin Invest* 1996; 97: 1111–16.
264. Hotamisligil GS,Budavari A, Murray D, Speilgelman BM. Reduced tyrosine kinase activity of the insulin receptor in obesity diabetes. Central role of TNF alpha. *J Clin Invest* 1994; 94: 1543–9.
265. Kelly RA, Smith TW. Cytokines and cardiac contractile function. *Circulation* 1997; 95: 778–81.
266. Meldrum DR. Tumor necrosis factor in the heart. *Am J Physiol* 1998; 274: R577–95.
267. Takahashi K, Ghatei MA, Larn HC, Bloom SR. Elevated plasma endothelin in patients with diabetes mellitus. *Diabetologia* 1990; 33: 306–10.
268. Weber KT, Brilla CG, Campbell SE *et al.* Myocardial fibrosis: role of angiotensin II and aldosterone. *Basic Res Cardiol* 1993; 88 (Suppl 1): 107–24.
269. Killip T. Epidemiology of congestive heart failure. *Am J Cardiol* 1985; 56: 2–6A.
270. Tahiliani AG, Vadlamudirv SV, McNeill JH. Prevention and reversal of altered myocardial function in diabetic rats by insulin treatment. *Can J Physiol Pharmacol* 1983; 61: 516–23.
271. Fein FS, Miller Green B, Dola B, Sonnenblick EH. Reversibility of diabetic cardiomyopathy in rabbits. *Am J Physiol* 1986; 250: H108–13.
272. Fein F, Strobeck JE, Malhotra A *et al.* Reversibility of diabetic cardiomyopathy with insulin in rats. *Circ Res* 1981; 49: 1251–61.
273. Baandrup E, Ledet T, Rasch R. Experimental diabetic cardiomyopathy preventable by insulin treatment. *Lab Invest* 1991: 45: 169–73.
274. Wu CF, Haider B, Ahmed SS *et al.* The effect of tolbutamide on the myocardium in experimental animals. *Circulation* 1973; 55: 200–55.
275. Haider B, Yeh CK, Thomas G *et al.* Influence of diabetes on the myocardium and coronary arteries of rhesus monkeys fed an atherogenic diet. *Circ Res* 1981; 49: 1278–88.
276. Carlstrom S, Karlefors T. Haemodynamic studies on diagnosed diabetics before and after adequate insulin treatment. *Br Heart J* 1970; 32: 355–8.
277. Lababidi Z, Goldstein DE. High prevalence of echocardiographic abnormalities in diabetic youths. *Diabetes Care* 1983; 6: 18–22.
278. Low PA. Diabetic autonomic neuropathy. *Semin Neurol* 1996; 16: 143–51.
279. Stevens MJ, Dayanikli F, Raffel DM *et al.* Scintigraphic assessment of regionalized defects in myocardial sympathetic innervation and blood flow regulation in diabetic patients with autonomic neuropathy. *J Am Coll Cardiol* 1998; 31: 1575–84.

280. Pfeifer MA, Weinberg CR, Cook D *et al.* Autonomic neural dysfunction in recently diagnosed diabetic patients. *Diabetes Care* 1984; 7: 447–53.
281. Kennedy WR, Navuro X, Sutherland DE. Neuropathy profile of diabetic patients in a pancreas transplantation program. *Neurology* 1995; 45: 773–80.
282. Ziegler D. Diabetic cardiovascular autonomic neuropathy: prognosis, diagnosis and treatment. *Diabetes Metab Rev* 1994; 10: 339–83.
283. Oikawa N, Umetsu M, Toyota. T'Goto Y. Quantitative evaluation of diabetic autonomic neuropathy by using heart rate variations: Relationship between cardiac parasympathetic or sympathetic damage and clinical conditions. *Tohuku J Exp Med* 1986: 148: 125–33.
284. Acharya DU, Shekhar YC, Aggarwal A. Anand IS. Lack of pain during myocardial infarction in diabetics — autonomic dysfunction responsible? *Am J Cardiol* 1991; 68: 793–6.
285. Bernardi L, Ricordi L, Lazzari P *et al.* Impaired circadian modulation of sympathetic activity in diabetes: a possible explanation for altered temporal onset of cardiovascular disease. *Circulation* 1992; 86: 1443–52.
286. Faerman I, Faccio E, Milei J *et al.* Autonomic neuropathy and painless myocardial infarction in diabetic patients: histologic evidence of their relationship. *Diabetes* 1979; 6: 1147–58.
287. Ganguly PK, Dhalla KS, Innes IR *et al.* Altered norepinephrine turnover and metabolism in diabetic cardiomyopathy. *Circ Res* 1986; 59: 684–93.
288. Mantysaari M, Kuikka I, Mustonen I. *et al.* Impaired ventricular repolarization association with disturbed left ventricular sympathetic function and diastolic filling in diabetes. *Am Heart J* 1993; 125: 1458–60.
289. Mustonen J, Mantysaari M, Kuikka J *et al.* Decreased myocardial $^{123}$I-meta-iodobenzylguanidine uptake is associated with disturbed left ventricular diastolic filling in diabete. *Am Heart J* 1992; 123: 804–5.
290. Murray D, O'Brein T, Muirooney R, O'Sullivan D. Autonomic dysfunction and silent myocardial ischaemia on exercise testing in diabetes mellitus. *Diabetic Med* 1990; 7: 580–4.
291. Nesto R, Phillips R, Kett K *et al.* Angina and exertional myocardial ischemia in diabetic and non diabetic patients: assessment by exercise thallium scintigraphy. *Ann Intern Med* 1988; 108: 170–5.
292. Margolis JR, Kannel WS, Feinleib M *et al.* Clinical features of unrecognized myocardial infarction: silent and asymptomatic: eighteen-year follow-up study: the Framingham Study. *Am J Cardiol* 1973; 32: 1–7.
293. Kannel WB, Abbott RD. Incidence and prognosis of unrecognized myocardial infarction: an update on the Framingham Study. *N Engl J Med* 1984; 311: 1144–7.
294. Niakan E, Harati Y, Rolak L. Comstock J. Rokey R. Silent myocardial infarction and diabetic cardiovascular autonomic neuropathy. *Arch Intern Med* 1986; 146: 2229–30.
295. Cabin HS, Robens WC. Quantitative comparison of extent of coronary narrowing and size of healed myocardial infarct in 33 necropsy patients with clinically recognized and in 28 with clinically unrecognized (silent) previous acute myocardial infarction. *Am J Cardiol* 1982; 50: 677–81.
296. Langer A, Freeman MR, Josse RG, Armstrong PW. Metaiodobenzylguanidine imaging in diabetes mellitus: assessment of cardiac sympathetic denervation and its relation to autonomic dysfunction and silent myocardial ischemia. *J Am Coll Cardiol* 1995; 25: 610–18.
297. Caracciolo EA, Chaitman BR, Forman SA *et al.* For the ACIP Investigators. Diabetics with coronary disease have a prevalence of asymptomatic ischemia during exercise treadmill testing and ambulatory ischemia monitoring similar to that of nondiabetic patients: an ACIP database study. *Circulation* 1996; 93: 2097–105.
298. Ranjadayalan K, Umachandran V, Ambepityia G *et al.* Prolonged anginal perceptual threshold in diabetes: effects on exercise capacity and myocardial ischemia. *J Am Coll Cardiol* 1990; 16: 1120–4.
299. Davis M, Bland J, Hangartner J *et al.* Factors influencing the presence or absence of acute coronary artery thrombi in sudden ischemic death. *Eur Heart J* 1989; 10: 203–8.
300. Fava S, Azzopardi J, Agius-Muscat H. Outcome of unstable angina in patients with diabetes mellitus. *Diabetic Med* 1997; 14: 209–13.
301. Karlson BW, Strombom U, Ekvall HE, Herlitz J. Prognosis in diabetics in whom the initial suspicion of acute myocardial infarction was not confirmed. *Clin Cardiol* 1993; 16: 559–64.
302. Bell DS. Diabetes mellitus and coronary artery disease. *Coronary Artery Dis* 1996; 7: 715–22.
303. Smith JW, Marcus FI, Serokman R, the Multicentre Postinfarction Research Group. Prognosis of patients with diabetes mellitus after acute myocardial infarction. *Am J Cardiol* 1984; 54: 718–21.
304. Jacobv RM, Nesto RW. Acute myocardial infarction in the diabetic patient: pathophysiology, clinical course and prognosis. *J Am Coll Cardiol* 1992; 20: 736–44.
305. Jaffe AS, Spadaro JJ, Schectman K *et al.* Increased congestive heart failure after myocardial, infarction of modest extent in patients with diabetes mellitus. *Am Heart J* 1984; 108; 31–7.
306. Yudkin JS, Oswald GA. Determinants of hospital admission and case fatality in diabetic patients with myocardial infarction. *Diabetes Care* 1988; 11: 351–8.
307. Abbott RD, Donahue RP, Kannel WB, Wilson PWF. The impact of diabetes on survival following myocardial infarction in men vs. women. The Framingham Study. *JAMA* 1988; 260: 3456–60.
308. Donahue RP, Goldberg RJ, Chen Z *et al.* The influence of sex and diabetes mellitus on survival following acute myocardial infarction: a community wide perspective. *J Clin Epidemiol* 1993; 46: 245–52.
309. Tansey M, Opie L, Kennelly B. High mortality in obese women diabetics with acute myocardial infarction. *BMJ* 1977; i: 1624–7.
310. Miettinen H, Lehto S, Salomaa V *et al.* Impact of diabetes on mortality after the first myocardial infarction. The FINMONICA Myocardial Infarction Register Study Group. *Diabetes Care* 1998; 21: 69–75.
311. Karlson BW, Herlie J, Hjelmarson A. Prognosis of acute myocardial infarction in diabetic and non-diabetic patients. *Diabetic Med* 1993; 10: 449–54.
312. Malmberg K, Ryden L. Myocardial infarction in patients with diabetes mellitus. *Eur Heart J* 1998; 9: 259–64.
313. Fava S, Azzopardi J, Muscat HA, Fenech FF. Factors that influence outcome in diabetic subjects with myocardial infarction. *Diabetes Care* 1993; 17: 1615–18.
314. Melchior T, Gadsboll N, Hildebrandt P *et al.* Clinical characteristics, left and right ventricular ejection fraction, and long-term prognosis in patients with non-insulin-dependent diabetes surviving an acute myocardial infarction. *Diabetic Med* 1996; 13: 450–6.
315. Iwasaka T, Takahashi N, Nakamura S *et al.* Residual left ventricular pump function after acute myocardial infarction in NIDDM patients. *Diabetes Care* 1992; 15: 1522–6.

316. Yudkin JS, Blauth C, Drury P *et al*. Prevention and management of cardiovascular disease in patients with diabetes mellitus: an evidence base. *Diabetic Med* 1996; 13 (Suppl 4): S101–21.
317. Woodfield S, Lundergan C, Reiner I *et al*. Angiographic findings and outcome in diabetic patients treated with thrombolytic therapy for acute myocardial infarction: the GUSTO experience. *J Am Coll Cardiol* 1996; 28: 1661–9.
318. Weintraub WS, Stein B, Kosinski A *et al*. Outcome of coronary bypass surgery versus coronary angioplasty in diabetic patients with multivessel coronary artery disease. *J Am Coll Cardiol* 1998; 31: 10–19.
319. Tomai F, Crea F, Gaspardone A *et al*. Ischemic preconditioning during coronary angioplasty is prevented by glibenclamide, a selective ATP-sensitive $K^+$ channel blocker. *Circulation* 1994: 90: 700–5
320. Cohen RA, Vanhoutte PM. Endothelium-dependent hyperpolarization: beyond nitric oxide and cyclic GMP. *Circulation* 1995; 92: 3337–49.
321. Sobel BE. Altered fibrinolysis and platelet function in the development of vascular complications of diabetes. *Curr Opin Endocrinol Diabetes* 1996; 3: 355–60.
322. Zuanetti G, Latini R, Maggioni AP *et al*. Effect of the ACE inhibitor lisinopril on mortality in diabetic patients with acute myocardial infarctionh: data from the GISSI-3. *Circulation* 1997; 96: 4239–45.
323. Moye LA, Pfeffer MA, Wun CC *et al*. For the SAVE Investigators. Uniformity of captopril benefit in the SAVE study: subgroup analysis. *Eur Heart J* 1994; 15: 2–8.
324. Torp-Pedersen C, Kober L, Carlsen J, on behalf of the TRACE Study Group. Angiotensin-converting enzyme inhibition after myocardial infarction: Trandolapril Cardiac Evaluation study. *Am Heart J* 1996; 132: 235–43.
325. Kereiakes D. Myocardial infarction in the diabetic patient. *Clin Cardiol* 1985; 8: 446–50.
326. GISSI-3 Investigators. Causes of early in-hospital mortality of patients with acute myocardial infarction: the impact of ACE-inhibitor treatment. *Circulation* 1995; 92 (Suppl 1): I-673.
327. Malmberg K, Ryden L, Hamsten A *et al*. Mortality prediction in diabetic patients with myocardial infarction: experiences from the DIGAMI study. *Cardiovasc Res* 1997; 34: 248–53.
328. Fava S, Aquilina O, Azzopardi J *et al*. The prognostic value of blood glucose in diabetic patients with acute myocardial infarction. *Diabetic Med* 1996; 13: 80–3.
329. Malmberg K, Rydin L, Efendic S *et al*. Randomized trial of insulin–glucose infusion followed by subcutaneous insulin treatment in diabetic patients with acute myocardial infarction (DIGAMI study): effects on mortality at 1 year. *J Am Coll Cardiol* 1995; 26: 57–65.
330. Hansen HHT, Kjaergaard SC, Bulow I *et al*. Thrombolytic therapy in diabetic patients with acute myocardial infarction. *Diabetes Care* 1996; 19: 1135–7.
331. Pieffer MA, Moye LA, Braunwald E *et al*. for the SAVE Investigators. Selection bias in the use of thrombolytic therapy in acute myocardial infarction. *JAMA* 1991; 266: 528–32.
332. French IK, Williams BF, Hart HH *et al*. Prospective evaluation of eligibility for thrombolytic therapy in acute myocardial infarction. *BMJ* 1996; 312: 1637–41.
333. Lynch M, Gammage M, Lamb P *et al*. Acute myocardial infarction in diabetic patients in the thrombolytic era. *Diabetic Med* 1994; 12: 162–5.
334. Fibrinolytic Therapy Trialists (FTT) Collaborative Group. Indications for fibrinolytic therapy in suspected acute myocardial infarction: collaborative overview of early mortality and major morbidity results from all randomized n of more than 1000 patients. *Lancet* 1994; 343: 311–22.
335. Ellis SG, Narins CR. Problem of angioplasty in diabetics. *Circulation* 1997; 96: 1707–10.
336. James TW, Quinton HB, Birkmeyer JD *et al*. Diabetes and coronary artery bypass graft surgery risk (Abstract). *Circulation* 1996; 94(Suppl I): I-412.
337. Fietsam RJ, Bassett J, Glover JL. Complications of coronary artery surgery in diabetic patients. *Am Surg* 1996; 57: 551–7.
338. Ellis SG, Vandormael MG, Cowley MJ *et al*., the multivessel Angioplasty Prognosis Study Group. Coronary morphologic and clinical determinants of procedural outcome with angioplasty for multivessel coronary disease: implications for patient selection. *Circulation* 1990; 82: 1193–202.
339. Weintraub WS, Kosinski AS, Brown CL, King SB III. Can restenosis after coronary angioplasty be prediected from clinical variables? *J Am Coll Cardiol* 1993; 21: 6–14.
340. Carrozza JP Jr. Kuntz RE, Fishman RF, Baim DS. Restenosis after arterial injury caused by coronary stenting in patients with diabetes mellitus. *Ann Intern Med* 1993; 118: 344–9.
341. Levine GN, Jacobs AK, Keeler GP *et al*. Impact of diabetes mellitus on percutaneous revascularization (CAVEAT-I). CAVEAT-I Investigators. Coronary Angioplasty Versus Excisional Atherectomy. *Am J Cardiol* 1997; 79: 748–55.
342. Rabbani LE, Edelman ER, Ganz P *et al*. Relation of restenosis after excimer laser angioplasty of fasting insulin levels. *Am J Cardiol* 1994; 73: 323–7.
343. Baim D, Diver D, Feit F *et al*., for the TIMI II Investigators: coronary angioplasty performed within the Thrombolysis in Myocardial Infarction II Study. *Circulation* 1992; 85: 93–8.
344. Bypass Angioplasty Revascularization Investigation (BARI) Investigators. Comparison of coronary bypass surgery with angioplasty in patients with multivessel disease. *N Engl J Med* 1996; 335: 217–25.
345. Quigley PJ, Hlatky MA, Hinohara T *et al*. Repeat percutaneous transluminal coronary angioplasty and predictors of recurrent stenosis. *Am J Cardiol* 1989; 63: 409–13.
346. Deligonul U, Vandormeal M, Kern MJ, Galan KL. Repeat coronary angioplasty for restenosis: results and predictors of follow-up clinical events. *Am Heart J* 1989; 117: 997–1002.
347. Hollman J, Badhwar K, Beck GJ *et al*. Risk factors for recurrent stenosis following successful coronary angioplasty. *Cleve Clin J Med* 1989; 56: 517–23.
348. Aronson D, Bloomgarden Z, Rayfield EJ. Potential mechanisms promoting restenosis in diabetic patients. *J Am Coll Cardiol* 1996; 27: 528–35.
349. Wuth DC, Leon MB, O'Neill W *et al*. Rotational atherectomy multicenter registry: acute results, complications and 6-month angiographic follow-up in 709 patients. *J Am Coll Cardiol* 1994; 24: 641–8.
350. Kornowski R, Mintz GS, Kent KM *et al*. Increased restenosis in diabetes mellitus after coronary interventions is due to exaggerated intimal hyperplasia. A serial intravascular ultrasound study. *Circulation* 1997; 95: 1366–9.
351. Wong SC, Baim DS, Schatz RA *et al*. Immediate results and late outcome after stent implantation in saphenous vein graft lesions: the multicenter U.S. Palmaz-Schatz experience. *J Am Coll Cardiol* 1995; 26: 704–12.

352. Molitemo DJ, Califf RM, Anderson K *et al.*, for the EPIC Study Investigators. Special considerations in diabetics receiving platelet IIb/IIIa antagonists during coronary interventions: results from the EPIC Trial (Abstract). *J Am Coll Cardiol* 1995; 25: 155A.
353. Kleiman NS, Lincoff AM, Kereiakes DJ *et al.* Diabetes mellitus, glycoprotein IIb/IIIa blockade, and heparin: evidence for a complex interaction in a multicenter trial. EPILOG Investigators. *Circulation* 1998; 97: 1912–20.
354. Barzilay J, Kronmal RA, Bittner V *et al.* Coronary artery disease and coronary artery bypass grafting in diabetic patients aged > 65 years (report from the Coronary Artery Surgery Study (CASS) registry). *Am J Cardiol* 1994; 74: 334–9.
355. Salomon N, Page U, Okies J *et al.* Diabetes mellitus and coronary artery bypass. *J Thorac Cardiovasc Surg* 1983; 68: 264–71.
356. Adler D, Goldman L, O'Neil A *et al.* Long-term survival of more than 2000 patients after coronary artery bypass grafting. *Am J Cardiol* 1986; 58: 195–201.
357. Smith L, Harrell F, Rankin J *et al.* Determinants of early versus late cardiac death in patients undergoing coronary artery bypass graft surgery. *Circulation* 1991; 84 (Suppl 3): 245.
358. Morris J, Smith R, Jones R *et al.* Influence of diabetes and mammary artery grafting on survival after coronary bypass. *Circulation* 1991; 84 (Suppl 3): 275–81.
359. Weintraub W, Wenger N, Jones E *et al.* Changing clinic characteristics of coronary surgery patients. *Circulation* 1993; 88: II79–II86.
360. Higgins T, Estafanous F, Loop F *et al.* Stratification of morbidity and mortality outcome by preoperative risk factors in coronary artery bypass patients. *JAMA* 1992; 267: 2344–8.
361. Manske CL, Wang Y, Wilson RF, White CW. Coronary revascularization may improve short term survival in insulin-dependent diabetics considered for renal transplantation. *Circulation* 1991; 84 (Suppl II): II-516.
362. McLaughlin P, Morton B, McLaughlin M *et al.* Long-term effect of hyperlipidemia, diabetes and smoking on graft patency and progression of disease following aorto-coronary bypass. *Circulation* 1974; 49 (Suppl III): III-191.
363. Anonymous. Influence of diabetes on 5-year mortality and morbidity in a randomized trial comparing CABG and PTCA in patients with multivessel disease: the Bypass Angioplasty Revascularization Investigation (BARI). *Circulation* 1997; 96: 1761–9.
364. CABRI. Long-term follow-up of European Revascularization Trials (Abstract). *Circulation* 1995; 93: II.
365. Weintraub WS, Mauldin PD, Becker E *et al.* A comparison of the costs of and quality of life after coronary angioplasty or coronary surgery for multivessel coronary artery disease: results from the Emory Angioplasty versus Surgery Trial (EAST). *Circulation* 1995; 92: 2831–40.
366. Weintraub WS, King SB III, Guyton RA, Kosinski AS. Coronary surgery and PTCA in diabetics with multivessel disease: can the BARI results be generalized? *Circulation* 1996; 94 (Suppl I): I-435.
367. Gum PA, O'Keefe JH Jr, Borkon AM *et al.* Bypass surgery versus coronary angioplasty for revascularization of treated diabetic patients. *Circulation* 1997; 96 (9 Suppl): II-7–10.
368. Barsness GW, Peterson ED, Ohman EM *et al.* Relationship between diabetes mellitus and long-term survival after coronary bypass and angioplasty. *Circulation* 1997; 96: 2551–6.
369. Detre K, Rosen A, Jones R *et al.* and the BARI Investigators. Is five-year mortality different for treatment by choice vs. random assignment in the Bypass Angioplasty Revascularization Investigation (BARI)? (Abstract) *J Am Coll Cardiol* 1996; 29 (Suppl): 243A.
370. Van Belle E, Bauters C, Hubert E *et al.* Restenosis rates in diabetic patients: a comparison of coronary stenting and balloon angioplasty in native coronary vessels. *Circulation* 1997; 96: 1454–60.
371. Fischman DL, Leon MB, Baim DS *et al.* A randomized comparsion of coronary-stent placement and balloon angioplasty in the treatment of coronary artery disease. *N Engl J Med* 1994; 331: 496–501.
372. Serruys PW, de Jaegere P, Kiemeneij F *et al.* A comparison of balloon-expandable-stent implantation with balloon angioplasty in patients with coronary artery disease. *N Engl J Med* 1994; 331: 489–95.
373. Hoffmann R, Mintz GS, Dussaillant GR *et al.* Patterns and mechanisms of in-stent restenosis: a serial intravascular ultrasound study. *Circulation* 1996; 94: 1247–54.
374. Abizaid A, Karnowski R, Mintz GS *et al.* The influence of diabetes mellitus on acute and late clinical outcome following coronary stent implantation. *J Am Coll Cardiol* 1998; 32: 584–9.
375. Savage MP, Fischman DL, Slota P *et al.* Coronary intervention in the diabetic patient: improved outcome following stent implantation versus balloon angioplasty. *J Am Coll Cardiol* 1997; 29 (Suppl A): 188.
376. Lafont A, Gusman LA, Whitlow PL *et al.* Restenosis after experimental angioplasty: intimal, medial and adventitial changes associated with constrictive remodeling. *Circ Res* 1995; 76: 996–1002.
377. Kakuta T, Currier JW, Haudenschild CC *et al.* Differences in compensatory vessel enlargement and not intimal formation account for restenosis after angioplasty in the hypercholesterolemic rabbit model. *Circulation* 1994; 89: 2809–15.
378. Murcia AM, Fallon JT, Fuster V. Smooth muscle cell proliferation does not account for restenosis in diabetic patients (Abstract). *Circulation* 1996; 94 (Suppl I): I-619.
379. Yoke H, Nosaka T, Kimura T *et al.* Coronary stenting in diabetic patients: early and follow-up results (Abstract). *J Am Coll Cardiol* 1997; 29: 455A.
380. Elezi S, Schuhlen H, Wehinger A *et al.* Stent placement in diabetic versus non-diabetic patients: six month angiographic follow-up (Abstract). *J Am Coll Cardiol* 1997; 29: 188A.
381. O'Neill WW. Multivessel balloon angioplasty should be abandoned in diabetic patients. *J Am Coll Cardiol* 1998; 31: 20–2.
382. Antiplatelet Trialists Collaboration. Collaborative overview of randomized trials of anti platelet therapy: prevention of death, myocardial infarction, and stroke by prolonged antiplatelet therapy in various categories of patients. *BMJ* 1994; 308: 81–106.
383. Barbash GI, White HD, Modan M, Van de Werf F. Significance of diabetes mellitus in patients with acute myocardial infarction: data from the GISSI study. *J Am Coll Cardiol* 1993; 22: 707–13.
384. Davi G, Catalano I, Averna M *et al.* Thromboxane biosynthesis and platelet function in type II diabetes mellitus. *N Engl J Med* 1990; 332: 1769–74.
385. ISIS 2 Collaborative Group. Randomized trial of intravenous streptokinase, oral aspirin, both, or neither among 17,187 cases of suspected acute myocardial infarctions: ISIS 2. *Lancet* 1988; ii: 349–60.
386. ETDDRS Investigators. Aspirin effects on mortality and morbidity in patients with diabetes mellitus. Early treatment diabetic retinopathy study report 14. *JAMA* 1992; 268: 1292–300.

387. Nguyen KN, Aursnes I, Kjekshus J. interaction between enalapril and aspirin on mortality after acute myocardial infarction: subgroup analysis of the Cooperative Scandinavian Enalapril Survival Study (CONSENSUS II). *Am J Cardiol* 1997; 79: 115–19.
388. van Bergen PFMM, Deckers JW, Jonker JJC *et al.* Efficacy of long term anticoagulant treatment in subgroups of patients after myocardial infarction. *Br Heart J* 199; 73: 117–21.
389. Beta Blocker Heart Attack Trial Research Group. A randomized trial of propranolol in patients with acute myocardial infarction. 1. Mortality results. *JAMA* 1982; 247: 1707–14.
390. Gundersen T, Kjekshus J. Timolol treatment after myocardial infarction in diabetic patients. *Diabetes Care* 1983; 6: 285–90.
391. ISIS-1 (First International Study of Infarct Survival) Collaborative Group. Randomized trial of intravenous atenolol among 16027 cases of suspected acute myocardial infarction. *Lancet* 1986; ii: 57–66.
392. Malmberg K, Herlitz J, Hjalmarson A *et al.* Effects of metoprolol on mortality and late infarction in diabetics with suspected acute myocardial infarction: retrospective data from two large studies. *Eur Heart J* 1989; 10: 423–8.
393. Roberts R, Rogers W, Mueller H *et al.* Immediate versus deferred beta-blockade following thrombolytic therapy in patients with acute myocardial infarction: Results of the Thrombolysis in Myocardial Infarction (TIMI) II-B study. *Circulation* 1991; 83: 422–37.
394. Zuanetti G, Latini R. Impact of pharmacological treatment on mortality after myocardial infarction in diabetic patients. *J Diabetes Complications* 1997; 11: 131–6.
395. Australian and Swedish Pindolol Study Group. The effect of pindolol on the two year mortality after complicated myocardial infarction. *Eur Heart J* 1983; 4: 367–75.
396. Viskin S, Barron HV. Beta blockers prevent cardiac death following a myocardial infarction; so why are so many infarct survivors discharged without beta blockers? *Am J Cardiol* 1996; 78: 821–2.
397. Burris JF. Beta blockers, dyslipidemia, and coronary artery disease: a reassessment. *Arch Intern Med* 1993; 153: 2085–92.
398. ASPIRE Steering Group. A British Cardiac Society survey of the potential for the secondary prevention of coronary disease: ASPIRE (Action on Secondary Prevention through Intervention to Reduce Events) principal results. *Heart* 1996; 75: 334–42.
399. Kjekshus J, Pedersen TR, for the Scandinavian Simvastatin Survival Study Group. Reducing the risk of coronary events: evidence from the Scandinavian Simvastatin Survival Study. *Am J Cardiol* 1995; 76: 64–8C.
400. Sacks FM, Pfeffer MA, Moye LA *et al.* The effect of pravastatin on coronary events after myocardial infarction in patients with average cholesterol levels. *N Engl J Med* 1996; 335: 1001–9.
401. Koskinen P, Manrtari M, Manninen V *et al.* Coronary heart disease incidence in NIDDM patients in the Helsinki Heart Study. *Diabetes Care* 1992; 15: 820–5.
402. Engler RL, Yellon DM. Sulfonylurea KATP blockade in type II diabetes and preconditioning in cardiovascular disease. Time for reconsideration. *Circulation* 1996; 94: 2297–301.
403. Smits P, Thien T Cardiovascular effects of sulphonylurea derivatives implications for the treatment of NIDDM? *Diabetologia* 1995, 38: 116–21.
404. Brady PA, Terzic A. The sulphonylurea controversy. More questions from the heart. *J Am Coll Cardiol* 1998; 31: 950–6.
405. Yudkin JS. How can we best prolong life? Benefits of coronary risk factor reduction in non-diabetic and diabetic subjects. *BMJ* 1993; 306: 1313–18.

# Infective diseases of the myocardium



R. VIRMANI AND A. P. BURKE

## Introduction

Infectious diseases of the heart may result in inflammation of the endocardium, myocardium, or pericardium. There may be isolated involvement of each of the three layers of the heart, or any combination thereof. The most common cardiac site of infection by an infectious agent (other than viruses) is the endocardium, resulting in endocarditis or valvulitis. Myocarditis may involve, in addition to the cardiac myocytes, the interstitium and blood vessels, often with contiguous inflammation of the epicardium and pericardium. There are three mechanisms by which infectious agents cause myocardial damage: direct invasion of the myocardium; production of a myocardial toxin, e.g. diphtheria; and immune-mediated myocardial damage [1, 2]. Myocarditis may be the direct result of an autoimmune process in the absence of prior infection; in addition, autoimmune processes play an important role in the pathogenesis of infectious, especially bacterial and viral, myocarditis.

A host of infectious agents may invade the myocardium, including viruses, bacteria (including rickettsia), protozoa, and metazoa (Table 23.1). By far the most common agents causing myocarditis in North America are viruses, especially enteroviruses. In the developing world, parasitic diseases are most prevalent; for example, in South America, Chagas' cardiomyopathy (caused by *Trypanosoma cruzi*) is endemic.

**Table 23.1** Principal infectious agents associated with myocarditis

| | |
|---|---|
| **Bacterial infections** | |
| Streptococcal | Brucellosis |
| Staphylococcal | Diphtheria |
| Pneumococcal | Salmonellosis |
| Meningococcal | Tuberculosis |
| Haemophilus | Tularemia |
| Gonococcal | Psittacosis |
| **Spirochaetal infections** | |
| Leptospirosis | Relapsing fever |
| Lyme disease | Syphilis |
| **Fungal infections** | |
| Aspergillosis | Coccidiomycosis |
| Actinomycosis | Cryptococcosis |
| Blastomycosis | Histoplasmosis |
| Candidiasis | |
| **Parasitic infections** | |
| Cysticercosis | Trichinosis |
| Schistosomiasis | Trypanosomiasis |
| Toxoplasmosis | Visceral larva migrans |
| **Rickettsial infections** | |
| Rocky Mountain spotted fever | Scrub typhus |
| Q fever | Typhus |
| Mycoplasma pneumoniae | |
| **Viral infections** | |
| Adenovirus | |
| Arbovirus | Poliomyelitis |
| Coxsackievirus | |
| Cytomegalovirus | Respiratory syncytial virus |
| Echovirus | Rabies |
| Encephalomyocarditis virus | Rubella |
| Hepatitis | Rubeola |
| Human immunodeficiency virus | Vaccinia |
| Infectious mononucleosis | Varicella |
| Influenza | Variola |
| Mumps | Yellow fever |

(Adapted from ref. 3.)

### Inflammatory subtypes of myocarditis and aetiology

The type of inflammation may provide a clue to the underlying aetiology of the myocarditis. A predominance of lymphocytes (lymphocytic myocarditis) is the most common histological type of myocarditis, and is usually due to an idiopathic process, a presumed viral or postviral process, or an autoimmune disease (Fig. 23.1; Table 23.1). However, bacteria, fungi, protozoa, and toxic agents may occasionally elicit a lymphocytic response, and must be ruled out before an idiopathic or viral cause is diagnosed. Conversely, lymphocytic myocarditis may contain polymorphonuclear leucocytes as well as plasma cells with a few macrophages, especially in chronic myocarditis. In children with viral myocarditis, the inflammatory infiltrate may be predominantly neutrophilic, especially in the early phases of illness, although lymphocytes generally predominate.

Lymphocytic myocarditis may heal with scars (Fig. 23.2), resulting in dilated cardiomyopathy. Chida *et al.* [4] have shown that in elderly patients with insidious or healed myocarditis and unexplained congestive heart failure (CHF), the fibrous and focal lesions at autopsy are located predominantly in the subepicardial and middle layers of the left ventricle and focally in the right ventricle as well.

When the infiltrate is predominantly neutrophilic, it is more likely to be bacterial, an early phase of viral myocarditis or, in children, persistent viral myocarditis. Ischaemic myocardial damage manifests as groups of necrotic myocytes with a polymorphonuclear infiltration. Macrophage giant cells are usually a component of well-formed granulomas in sarcoidosis (Fig. 23.3), and are associated with myocyte necrosis in giant cell myocarditis (Fig. 23.4); they are rarely present in the interstitium in hearts with hypersensitivity myocarditis (Fig. 23.5). When eosinophils are seen, one must rule out parasitic infections, idiopathic hypereosinophilic syndrome (Fig. 23.6), giant cell myocarditis, and hypersensitivity myocarditis (Table 23.2).

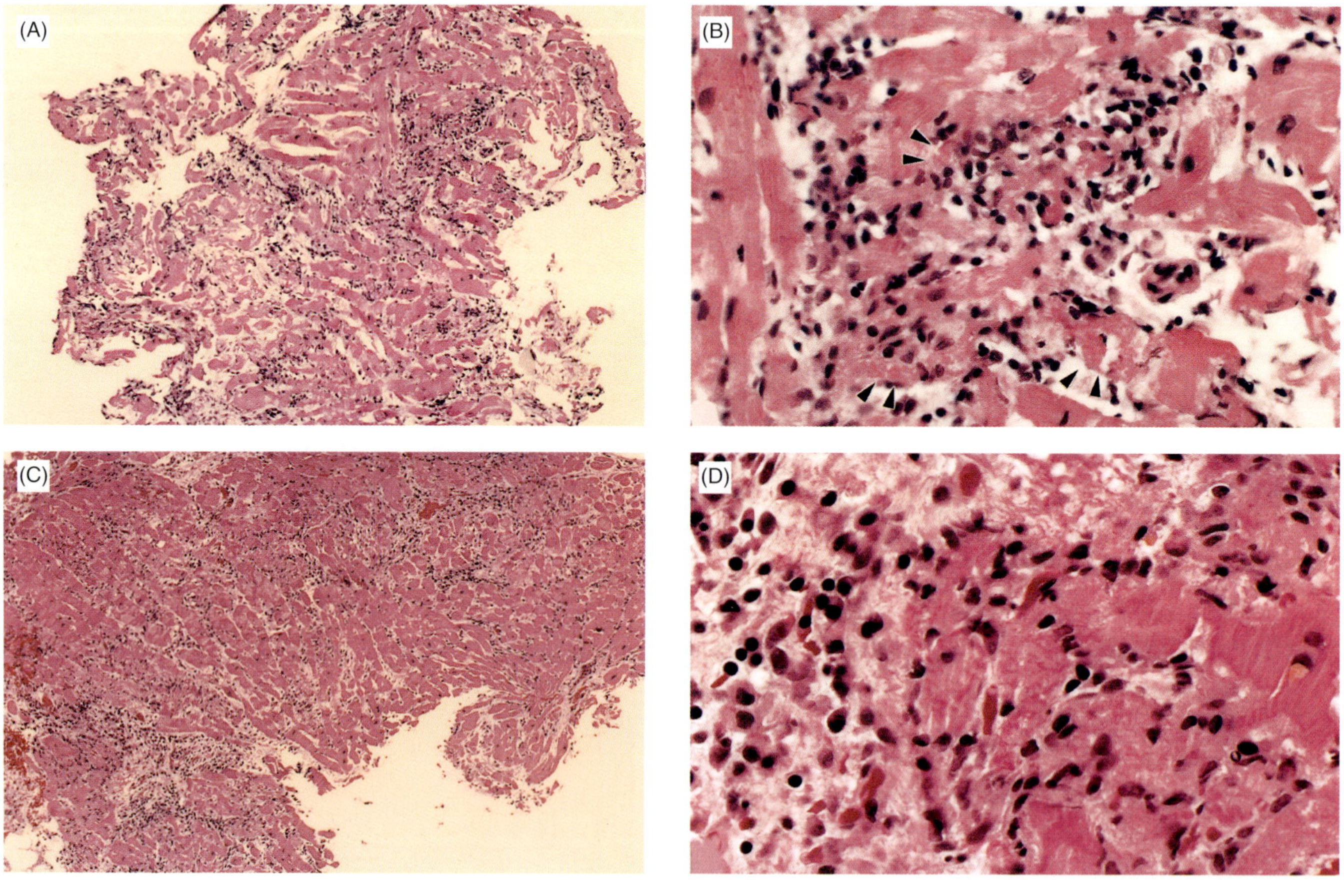


**Figure 23.1** *Lymphocytic myocarditis in a 45-year-old white female who presented with sudden onset of dyspnoea at rest. Clinical examination revealed severe congestive heart failure. A right ventricular biopsy was performed. (A) Low-power view showing diffuse lymphocytic infiltrate. (B) High-power view showing myocyte necrosis* (arrowheads) *in areas of lymphocytic infiltrate. The patient was treated with high doses of corticosteroids and remained on low-dose corticosteroid therapy until 2 months before her second episode, which was 2.5 years after the first biopsy. (C, D) The right ventricular biopsy showed a similar picture to the first biopsy, with diffuse lymphocytic infiltration and focal myocyte necrosis.*

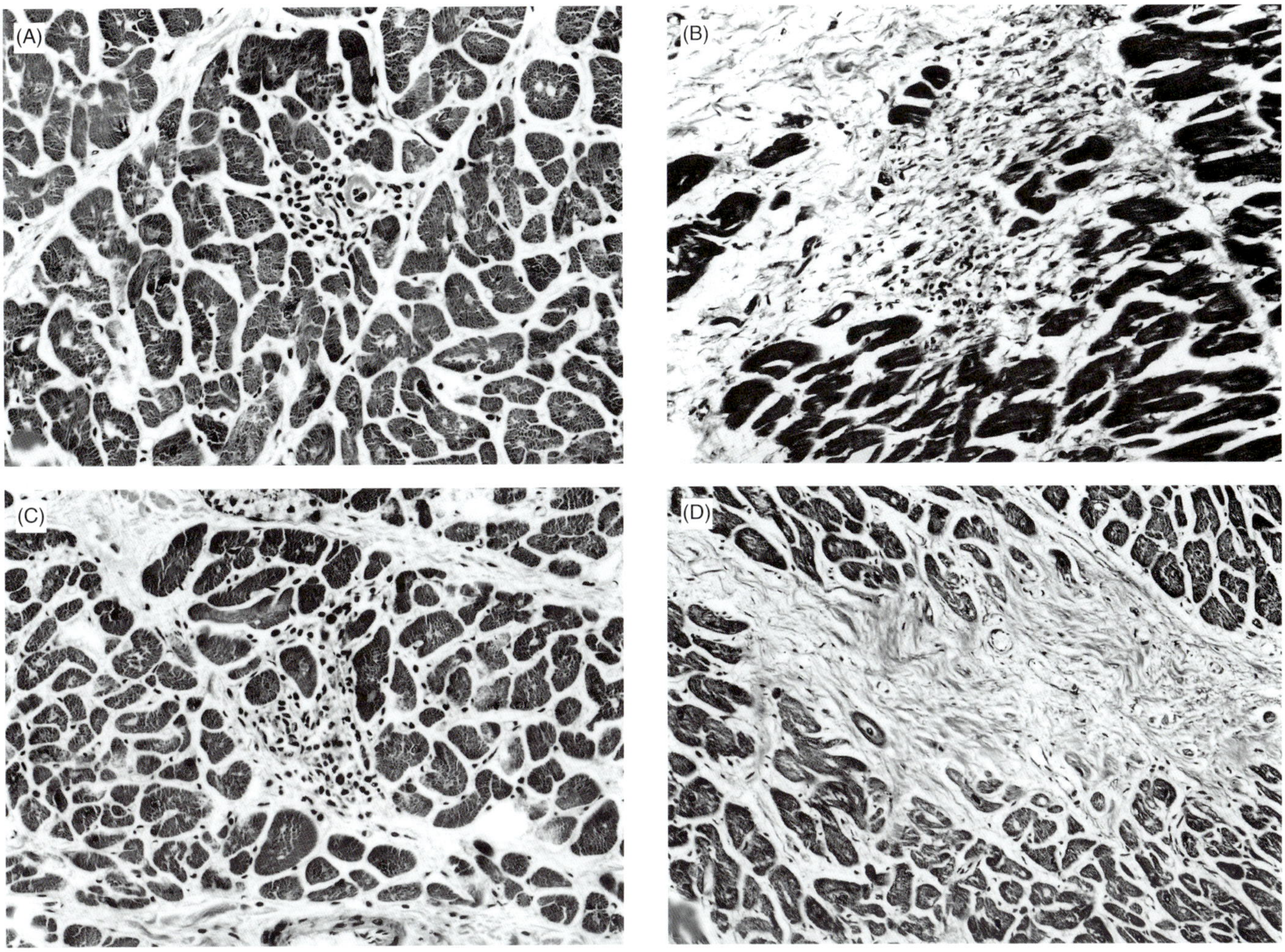


**Figure 23.2** *Ongoing myocarditis. (A) Inflammation can be focal and ongoing. Note a single focus in this field showing myocyte necrosis and surrounding lymphocytic infiltrate. (B) In the same heart other areas show healed and healing myocarditis. Note the sparse lymphocytic infiltrate with interstitial fibrosis. (C, D) Other areas in the same heart showing borderline myocarditis (C) and scarring (D).*

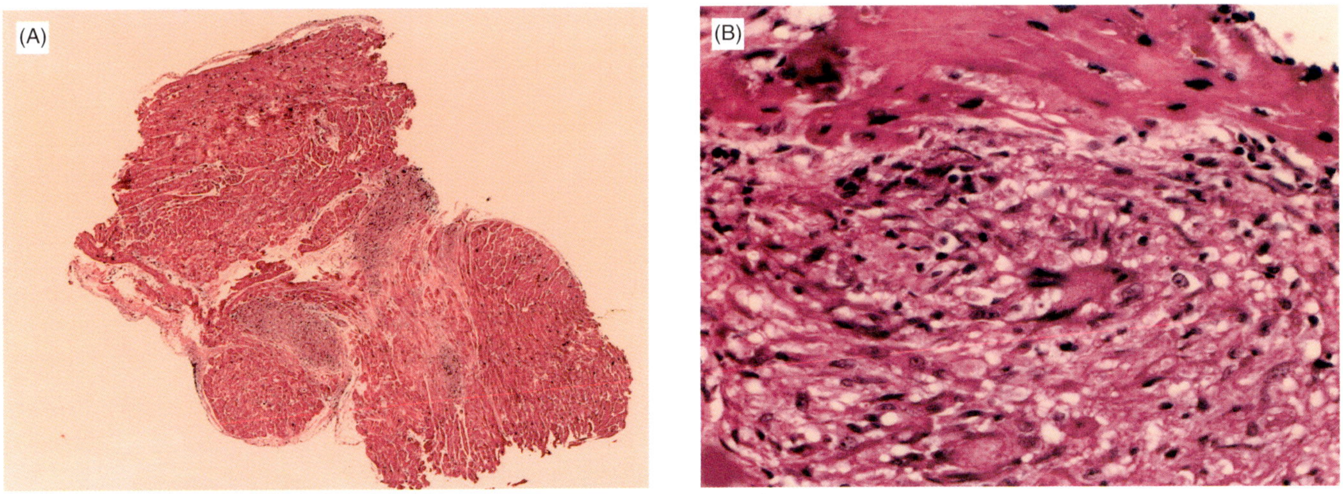


**Figure 23.3** *Sarcoidosis in a 35-year-old black male with dilated cardiomyopathy (ejection fraction 36%). There was no known lymphadenopathy or interstitial lung disease. (A) Endomyocardial biopsy demonstrating two well-formed granulomas. (B) Higher magnification of one of the granulomas demonstrating well-formed non-caseating granuloma consisting of giant cells and histiocytes with scattered lymphocytes.*

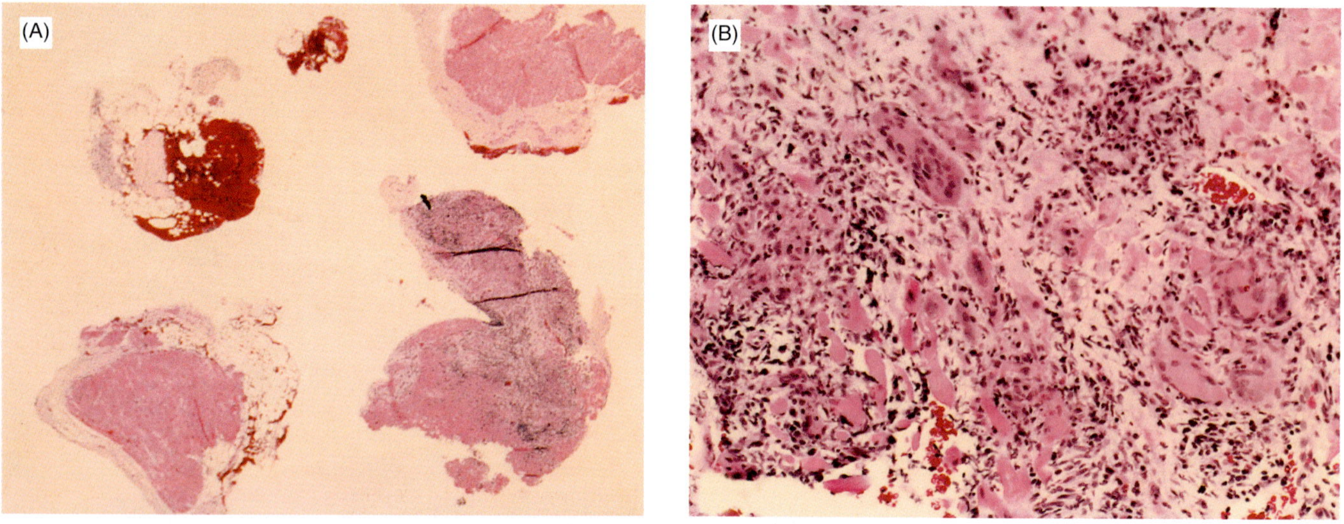


**Figure 23.4** *Giant-cell myocarditis. A 50-year-old male with a 2-week history of congestive heart failure and a clinical diagnosis of dilated cardiomyopathy (ejection fraction 35%) underwent right heart endomyocardial biopsy. (A) Four pieces of myocardium, one of which shows extensive inflammatory infiltrate. High power view showing a dense inflammatory infiltrate of lymphocytes, macrophages, and a large number of giant cells. Scattered eosinophils are also seen within the inflammatory infiltrate.*

## Lymphocytic myocarditis

### Incidence of myocarditis in acute-onset congestive heart failure

In Western countries, the most prevalent form of myocarditis presenting as CHF is idiopathic lymphocytic myocarditis, which in many patients follows a recent viral infection or flu-like illness. In order to determine the prevalence of symptomatic myocarditis in patients with CHF, most authorities agree that recent onset, an ejection fraction of < 45%, and an exclusion of coronary and valvular disease be used as entry criteria into any study of myocarditis. Prior to 1987, there was a wide variation in the incidence of myocarditis in patients with acute onset of CHF, i.e. 15–63% [6–8]. Since the use of immunosuppressive therapy for biopsy-proven myocarditis, pathologists needed a more uniform definition. Often, interstitial fibroblasts or endothelial nuclei of capillaries are mistaken for lymphocytes. Until the early 1980s, only haematoxylin and eosin (H&E)-stained sections were used to establish the presence of myocarditis; immunological markers for the distinction of lymphocytes were not in general use. A few lymphocytes may be normally present in the interstitium, without any destruction of adjoining myocytes.

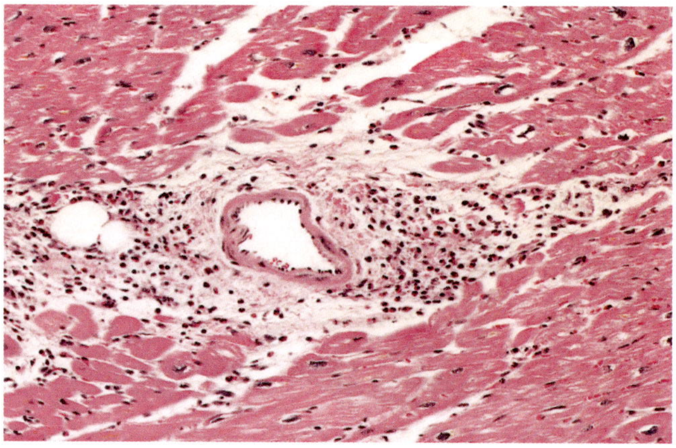

**Figure 23.5** *Hypersensitivity myocarditis. The inflammation is perivascular and composed of histiocytes, lymphocytes, and eosinophils.*

Cognizant of the need for establishing reliable diagnostic criteria before a multicentre National Institutes of Health (NIH) myocarditis treatment trial could be initiated, several cardiac pathologists met in conjunction with the American College of Cardiology meeting in Dallas, Texas. Their goal was to define myocarditis from a morphological standpoint in endomyocardial biopsies. Using their criteria (the Dallas criteria, outlined below), the incidence of lymphocytic myocarditis on endomyocardial biopsy has varied from 9.1 to 26% [9–12]. Although the range is smaller than that published prior to the institution of the Dallas criteria, the rate of myocarditis in patients with acute-onset CHF is still dependent on criteria used to define the population in which the endomyocardial biopsies are being performed.

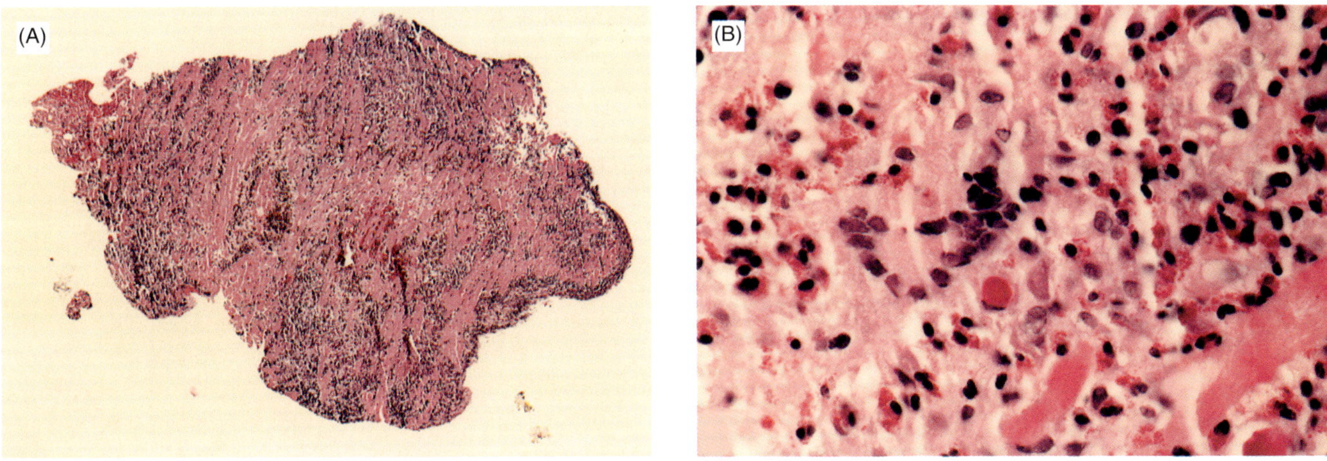


**Figure 23.6** *Hypereosinophilic syndrome. A 27-year-old man who presented with upper respiratory tract infection was found clinically to be in florid congestive heart failure with peripheral eosinophilia. An endomyocardial biopsy was performed. (A) Note extensive myocardial inflammation along with marked destruction of myocytes. (B) High-power view showing predominant eosinophil infiltration, macrophages, and a rare giant cell.*

## Dallas criteria

The Dallas criteria for diagnosing myocarditis are based on inflammation of the myocardium with necrosis and/or degeneration of adjacent myocytes (Fig. 23.1A–D). This definition emphasizes the importance of myocyte damage, which may be in the form of necrosis or vacuolization, and manifested by irregular cellular outlines, cellular disintegration with lymphocytes, or macrophages within the sarcolemma [13]. Contraction bands, which are a very common artefact in endomyocardial biopsies, must not be mistaken for vacuolization or necrosis. As mentioned above, the inflammatory infiltrate is primarily lymphocytic, but may contain macrophages or plasma cells and, in childhood cases of myocarditis, neutrophils. Occasionally, a biopsy may demonstrate interstitial eosinophilic infiltrates, diagnostic of hypersensitivity myocarditis [14]; this entity should be considered distinct from lymphocytic myocarditis, as the treatment and prognosis are different.

The Dallas criteria classifications (Table 23.3) are based on whether the first biopsy or subsequent biopsies are examined. If the first biopsy is examined, the diagnoses that can be rendered are myocarditis with or without fibrosis, borderline myocarditis, and no myocarditis. Myocarditis can occur in the presence of fibrosis, which is dependent on the duration of the illness. The diagnosis of borderline myocarditis is rendered when the inflammatory infiltrate is mild and there is absence of myocardial degeneration.

Subsequent biopsies in patients with a previous biopsy diagnosis of myocarditis are used to follow up the myocarditis and evaluate the treatment. Myocarditis that persists without much change from the previous biopsy is considered

**Table 23.2** Inflammatory infiltrates and differential diagnosis in myocarditis

| Lymphocytic | Neutrophilic | Eosinophilic | Giant cells |
|---|---|---|---|
| Idiopathic | Bacterial infections | Hypersensitivity | Sarcoidosis |
| Viral | Ischaemic | Parasitic infestations | Giant cell myocarditis |
| Sarcoidosis | Idiopathic | Hypereosinophilic syndrome | Hypersensitivity |
| Toxic | Viral (early, especially in children) | Idiopathic | Rheumatoid diseases |
| Collagen vascular | Pressor agents | | Rheumatic fever |
| Right ventricular dysplasia | | | Tuberculosis |
| Kawasaki disease | | | Fungal infections |
| Lymphoma | | | |

(Adapted from ref. 5.)

**Table 23.3** Classification of myocarditis (Dallas criteria)

| |
|---|
| **First biopsy** |
| Myocarditis with or without fibrosis |
| Borderline myocarditis (repeat biopsy may be indicated) |
| No myocarditis |
| **Subsequent biopsies** |
| Ongoing (persistent) myocarditis with or without fibrosis |
| Resolving (healing) myocarditis with or without fibrosis |
| Resolved (healed) myocarditis with or without fibrosis |

'ongoing myocarditis' or 'persistent myocarditis' (Fig. 23.2A, B). If the myocarditis is less than in the previous biopsy and there are changes of healing identified, then the term 'resolving myocarditis' or 'healing myocarditis' is used. If the myocarditis is fully healed with only areas of fibrosis and absence of inflammation, then the diagnosis is 'healed myocarditis' or 'resolved myocarditis'. If, following a symptom-free interval and a diagnosis of fully resolved myocarditis, the patient develops another episode of myocarditis, the consequent biopsy is treated as a first biopsy.

Infectious aetiologies may masquerade as lymphocytic myocarditis and should be excluded before the Dallas criteria for lymphocytic myocarditis are applied. In addition, the myocyte damage must not be typical of ischaemic injury secondary to coronary artery disease. Ischaemic infiltrates are often accompanied by haemosiderin deposits. Endocardial and adjoining myocardial involvement is common in myocarditis, whereas in ischaemic injury a layer of subendocardial myocytes is spared from ischaemic damage.

### *Treatment of myocarditis*

There are many published studies showing that immunosuppressive therapy may be useful in the treatment of myocarditis. However, the most definitive study by Mason *et al.* [15] failed to show the benefit of azothiaprine and prednisone or cyclosporine and prednisolone over conventional drugs for the treatment of heart failure. All three groups showed a similar improvement in the ejection fraction with time and survival did not improve with immunosuppressive therapy. It has been suggested that the performance of endomyocardial biopsy in patients suspected of myocarditis is not indicated, since patients with idiopathic dilated cardiomyopathy and myocarditis have an identical outcome and myocarditis progresses to idiopathic dilated cardiomyopathy [16].

### *Limitations of the Dallas criteria*

Regardless of the histopathological criteria used, the inherent limitation of biopsy size results in foci of acute or ongoing myocarditis being missed. Partly because of small sample size, the authors of the Dallas criteria did not agree on the quantitation of myocarditic lesions, as has been applied to the diagnosis of myocarditis at autopsy [13] or to the diagnosis of acute allograft rejection on biopsy. In the authors' opinion, myocarditic lesions should be readily apparent and recognizable at low magnification. A single focus of cell necrosis in autopsy hearts does not constitute clinically significant myocarditis. Whether this also applies in cases of endomyocardial biopsy, as per the Dallas criteria, is questionable.

Experience with myocarditis in autopsy hearts shows that the inflammatory lesions are usually quite extensive, surrounding at least five to eight myocytes that have a moth-eaten, necrotic appearance. In unquestionable cases of death due to myocarditis, the inflammatory foci are never single, but are diffuse within a given area of myocardium, and sometimes involve large areas of the myocardium ($>0.5\ mm^2$) in the left and right ventricles, with or without atrial involvement. Therefore, the absence of myocarditis on endomyocardial biopsy ('no myocarditis' by Dallas criteria) may be more reliable in ruling out significant clinical myocarditis than previously believed.

In contrast, myocardial lymphocytic infiltration is not unusual in persons dying of non-cardiac causes. One study reported that 42% of autopsy hearts (ten of 24 hearts) in patients dying secondary to trauma showed lymphocyte infiltration, and necrosis was documented only in one patient (4%) [17]. The finding of focal collections of lymphocytes in the myocardium is not surprising, as lymphocytes occur focally in all organs, including lung, liver, and brain.

Because of the range of inflammation present in normal hearts, a category of 'borderline myocarditis' may not be helpful and should not be used. Instead, the amount of inflammatory infiltrate should be quantitated as being mild, moderate, or severe and focal, confluent, or diffuse. The extent of myocyte necrosis should also be quantitated, whether groups of myocytes are involved or only one or two myocytes. The amount and distribution of the fibrosis, when present, should be characterized as endocardial, replacement, or interstitial in location, and the extent mentioned [13].

## Specific aetiological agents and myocarditis

### Viral myocarditis

Enteroviruses, especially Coxsackie viruses, are common infections in children, and cause up to 50% of cases of myocarditis [18, 19]. The diagnosis of a viral aetiology is problematic, however. Viral cultures give a low yield because of transient infection, and serological diagnosis based on rising serum titres is not specific and requires follow-up study. Recently, the polymerase chain reaction (PCR) has been used to detect viral nucleic acid in endomyocardial biopsies. Martin *et al.* [20] studied 38 infants and children with suspected acute viral myocarditis, and detected the viral genome in 26 of 38 (68%) biopsies by PCR [20]. The viral types were varied and, surprisingly, enteroviruses were not the most prevalent organism. There were 15 cases of adenoviral infection, eight enteroviruses, two herpes simplex virus, and one cytomegalovirus (CMV). There was disagreement with the histopathological finding of myocarditis in 13 of the 26 (50%) PCR-positive specimens, and the discrepancy was usually associated with adenovirus, suggesting that the amplification of adenoviral DNA is not necessarily associated with the patient's illness.

Other viral infections infrequently cause sporadic cases of usually fatal myocarditis. There have been reports of myocarditis due to influenza, Lassa fever (arenavirus), Epstein–Barr virus, poliomyelitis, rubella (German measles), rubeola (measles), varicella (chicken pox), variola, and vaccinia viruses. Myocardial involvement in influenza is rare, but cardiac symptoms occur in 5–10% of patients during an epidemic [21]. Cardiac involvement occurs within 1–2 weeks of the onset of the illness [22]. The cellular infiltrate is predominantly lymphocytic with some macrophages; rarely, the infiltration is neutrophilic. Lassa fever is a major cause of morbidity in West Africa, but cardiac symptoms, although frequent, do not play a significant role in mortality [23, 24]. Childhood viral diseases such as mumps, rubeola, rubella, and varicella have all been complicated, rarely, by lymphocytic myocarditis [25–28].

Immunosuppressed patients infected with the human immunodeficiency virus (HIV) and transplant recipients are prone to the development of myocarditis. In patients with the acquired immunodeficiency syndrome (AIDS), idiopathic myocarditis is more frequent than myocarditis caused by a specific organism, by nearly a 2:1 ratio [29]; however, in cases of infectious myocarditis, CMV is the most common viral organism demonstrated and second only to *Toxoplasma gondii* [29]. CMV is diagnosed by demonstrating the typical nuclear and cytoplasmic inclusions of viral particles.

The mechanisms involved in the induction of inflammation and myocyte necrosis in viral myocarditis are poorly understood. In the immunocompetent murine model, Coxsackievirus can be cultured from the heart only in the first few days postinoculation (myocardial cultures are positive consistently up to day 7). However, the morphological lesions of myocarditis are small and infrequent prior to 2 weeks, are most numerous thereafter, and largely regress by 8 weeks. In contrast, myocardial cultures of immunodeficient mice may be positive more than 100 days postinoculation, and the myocarditis lesions increase as the duration of the viraemia increases; they are most numerous and largest 92 days following inoculation [30]. Thus, immune factors in immunocompetent patients may induce and enlarge the lesions of myocarditis. In acute myocarditis, there is prominent infiltration of the myocardium by natural killer (NK) cells. Instead of inducing myocardial damage by direct cell-mediated cytotoxicity, T-cells and NK cells, when activated, secrete cytokines, some of which have the ability to cause myocyte cell death [31]. In experimental animals, human tumour necrosis factor-$\alpha$ and interleukin-1$\beta$ have been shown to induce myocarditis in the B.10 A strain of mouse, which is genetically resistant to coxsackievirus B infection [32]. Cytokines may therefore play a role in human myocarditis which is probably triggered by an autoimmune mechanism following a viraemia. Circulating antimyocardial autoantibodies have been demonstrated in sera of patients with documented myocarditis, substantiating this hypothesis.

### Bacterial myocarditis

Haematogenous spread to the myocardium is possible in any patient with systemic bacteraemia. The myocardium shows areas of polymorphonuclear leucocyte infiltration around and within intramyocardial small vessels. The surrounding myocytes undergo necrosis as the suppurative inflammatory response extends into the interstitium. Grossly, areas of acute inflammation appear as small abscesses within the myocardium. Often, bacteria can be identified in areas of suppuration (Fig. 23.7). Tissue Gram stains, such as the Brown and Hopps or Brown and Brenn stains, are helpful in suggesting the shape and characteristics of the bacterium.

In cases of haematogenously acquired bacterial myocarditis, there is often infective endocarditis of the aortic, mitral, or both valves. The myocardial suppuration is exacerbated by contiguous spread from the valvular infection and by septic emboli. The frequency of myocardial involvement in infective endocarditis is high, and the detection of myocarditis increases if multiple sections of the myocardium are examined. The most common organisms that cause infection of the myocardium are staphylococci, streptococci, pneumococci, and meningococci.

*Mycobacterium tuberculosis* may cause myocarditis, which generally results from contiguous spread of pericarditis, or haematogenous and lymphatic spread. In salmonella infection, non-specific electrocardiographic (ECG) abnormalities are not unusual [33]. Myocarditis is rare, but has been reported as a fatal complication, consisting histologically of lymphocytes and monocytes with myocardial necrosis [34]. Similarly, in atypical *Mycoplasma pneumoniae* infection, ECG abnormalities are common but myocarditis is not [25].

Infections secondary to spirochaetes include Weil's disease (leptospirosis), syphilis (*Treponema pallidum*), Lyme disease (*Borrelia burgdorferi*) and relapsing fever (*Borrelia recurrentis*) (Fig. 23.8). Most patients with mild leptospirosis have no evidence of heart involvement; however, in fatal infections the heart is involved in over 50% of cases [35]. The ECG abnormalities include first-degree heart block and transient ST and T wave changes, which may be secondary to the presence of myocarditis. Morphological changes consist of petechiae or areas of haemorrhage, most often in the subepicardial regions [36]. Microscopically, the myocardium shows foci of necrosis with mononuclear cell infiltration and rare neutrophils. Syphilitic involvement of the myocardium is rare and is only seen in cases of gumma formation [39, 40].

Myocardial involvement in Lyme disease is seen in 4–10% of cases, but is not well documented [41]. Cardiac involvement usually occurs 4–8 weeks after the initial manifestation. Atrioventricular (AV) block is the most common cardiac complication, occurring in 87% of symptomatic patients [42]. Histologically, fatal cases show a transmural inflammatory infiltrate, which is polymorphous. Lymphocytes show a predilection for the endocardial surface [43], and the myocardium demonstrates clusters of macrophages and neutrophils with adjacent myocyte necrosis [43–45]. Spirochaetes can be seen in the area of the inflammatory infiltrates and between myocytes [46]. It is unclear whether continued disease activity requires the persistence of spirochaetes in the myocardium or whether it results from an immune-mediated mechanism. The number of spirochaetes usually seen is small compared with the extent of the inflammation, suggesting a combined effect of local spirochaetal presence with an immunological reaction [44, 46]. Eventually, in the course of infection, there may be endocardial and interstitial fibrosis [44]. When examining myocardial tissue from a patient with known or suspected Lyme disease, causes other than Lyme myocarditis must be considered. The cardiac involvement

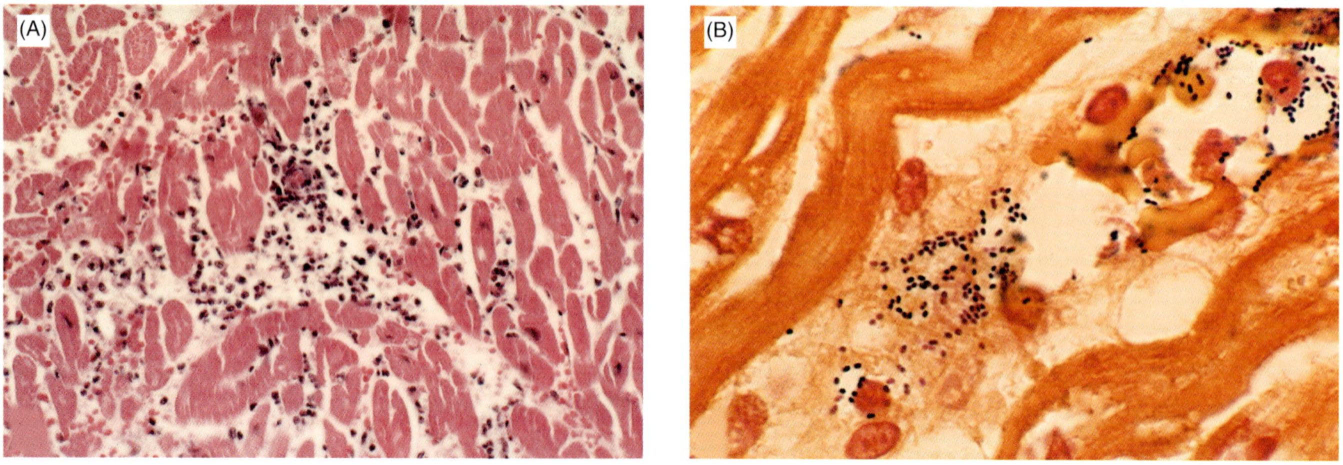


**Figure 23.7** *Bacterial myocarditis. A middle-aged woman died from meningococcal myocarditis following fever of unknown origin and sudden collapse. (A) At autopsy, there was a neutrophilic infiltrate of small vessels, within the surrounding interstitial space, and myocardium with myocyte necrosis (B) Brown and Hopps stain showing Gram-positive organisms in pairs from a patient dying from pneumococcal sepsis.*

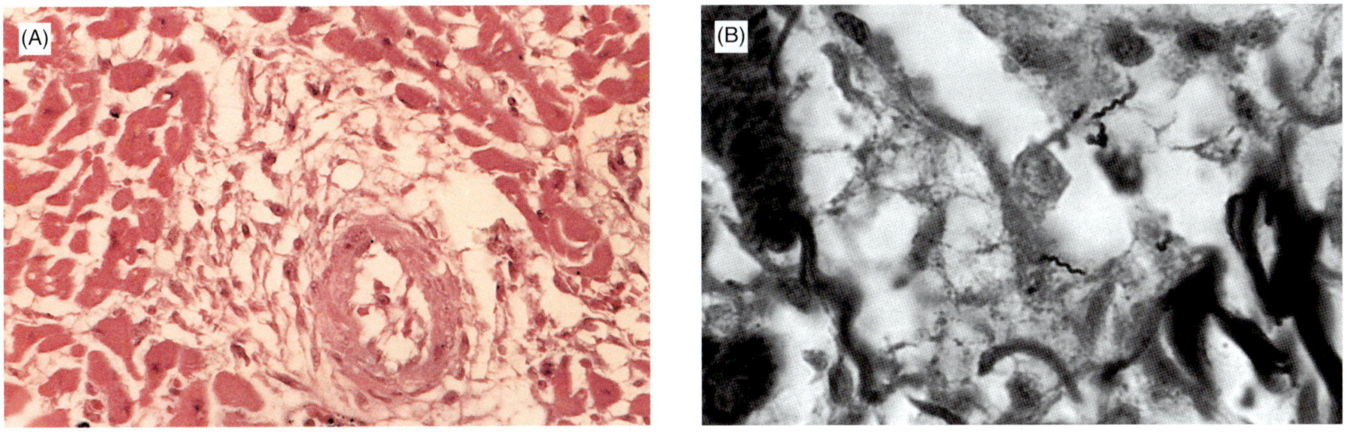


**Figure 23.8** *Relapsing fever. (A) Note perivascular chronic mild inflammatory infiltrate on H&E stain. (B) Warthin–Starry stain showing sparse infiltration by spirochetes* (Borrelia recurrentis)*.*

in Lyme disease is considered to be benign, as most patients recover without any sequelae [41].

Relapsing fever is a tick- or louse-borne disease caused by a Gram-negative, helical spirochaete, *B. recurrentis*, measuring 0.2–0.5 $\mu$m by 3–20 $\mu$m (Fig. 23.8). It is characterized by episodes of fever separated by apyrexial intervals. Cardiac complications are common, and include AV conduction defects, sudden death, and tachyarrhythmias [37, 38]. The heart may exhibit perivascular chronic myocarditis, which is predominantly histiocytic. Organisms may be identified by Warthin–Starry stains (Fig. 23.8).

Myocardial damage due to bacteria may be entirely indirect, from either autoimmunity or bacterial toxins. The most common cardiac finding following β-haemolytic streptococcal infection is rheumatic fever, resulting in valvulitis and myocarditis with or without the presence of Aschoff nodules. The latter is considered the hallmark of the hypersensitivity reaction to β-haemolytic streptococci. The myocardium may be injured by bacterial toxins, the best example being *Corynebacterium diphtheriae*. Myocardial involvement in diphtheria was reported to occur in one-quarter of cases [47, 48], and was the most common cause of death. Morphological findings of toxic myocarditis due to diphtherial toxin consist of a flabby and dilated heart with fatty infiltration of the myocytes, and granular and hyaline degeneration of myocytes. Interstitial infiltration by inflammatory cells is not common, but when present consists of mononuclear cells. In the late stages there are areas of fibrosis and myocyte hypertrophy [48]. The toxin, which inhibits protein synthesis, has an affinity for the conduction system of the heart, resulting in partial or complete AV heart block [47].

## Rickettsial myocarditis

Rickettsial diseases that may cause cardiac complications are Q fever, Rocky Mountain spotted fever, and Scrub typhus [49]. The myocardial involvement consists of a perivasculitis composed of lymphocytes and macrophages. Myocardial necrosis is not prominent, except in scrub typhus. Rocky Mountain spotted fever is characterized by a systemic vasculitis that may involve the myocardium with inflammation and myocarditis (Fig. 23.9). In the USA, Rocky Mountain spotted fever is reported predominantly in the eastern states, especially along the Atlantic costs. The disease is transmitted by infected ticks. The organisms grow in the endothelial and smooth muscle cells of the vessels [50, 51].

## Myocarditis in Whipple's disease

The original description of Whipple's disease, affecting the intestine and mesenteric lymphatic tissues, appeared in 1907. It was not until 1963 that Enzinger and Helwig described involvement of the heart, characterized by periodic acid–Schiff (PAS)-positive macrophages among the myocardial fibres within areas of interstitial fibrosis [52]. In 1975, MacAllister and Fenoglio reviewed the autopsy findings in 19 patients dying with Whipple's disease [53]: 58% had clinical cardiac findings and 79% had gross cardiac lesions. Histologically, they observed PAS-positive macrophages in the pericardium, myocardium, and valves of each patient with cardiac disease. The myocardium showed focal interstitial fibrosis in 89% of cases, with interspersed PAS-positive macrophages, scattered lymphocytes, and Anitschkow cells. Occasionally, the areas of fibrosis and macrophage infiltrates were perivascular in location, but no

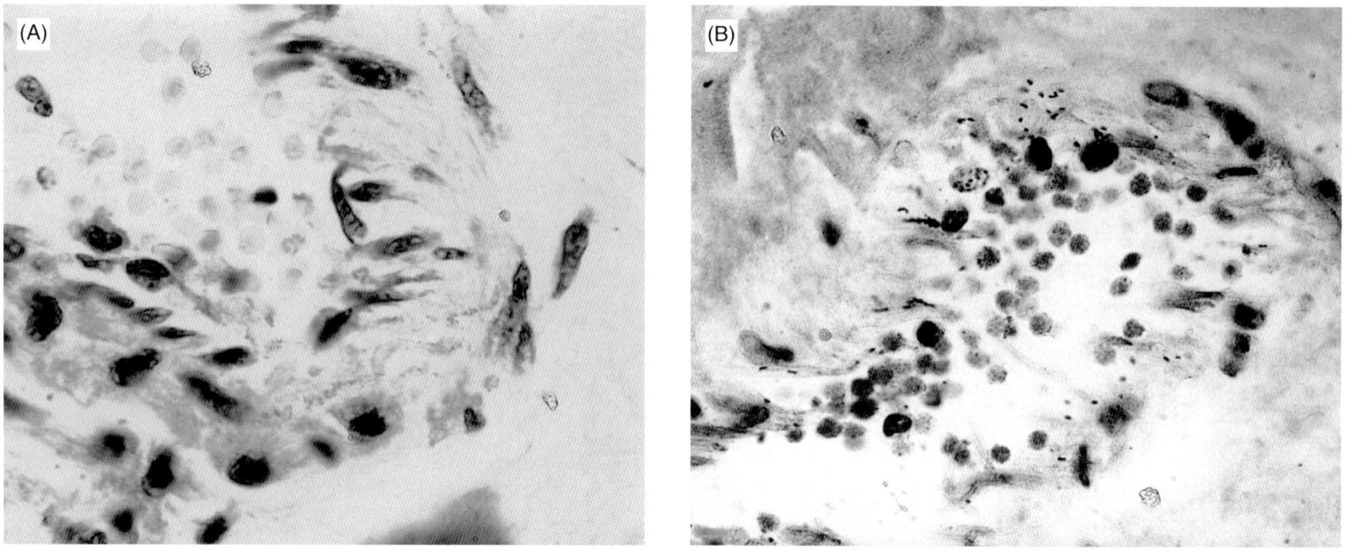


**Figure 23.9** *(A) The rickettsial organisms causing Rocky mountain spotted fever* (Rickettsia rickettsii) *infect endothelial cells, resulting in swelling of intramyocardial capillaries. (B) Silver impregnation stains demonstrating the small, intracellular organisms.*

Aschoff nodules were identified. Lie and Davis [54] reported a case of Whipple's disease with myocardial lesions consisting of lymphocytes, histiocytes, and plasma cells [52]. Southern *et al.* [55] described a 44-year-old man with a long prodromal period characterized by granulomatous lymphadenitis and progressive lymphoedema of the extremities without any gastrointestinal involvement. This patient's clinical condition deteriorated with the onset of lymphocytic myocarditis; at autopsy, a diagnosis of Whipple's disease was made. This case demonstrates that Whipple's disease should be considered in the differential diagnosis of a patient presenting with granulomatous disease. The diagnosis is confirmed by ultrastructural demonstration of rod-shaped bodies that are 1.5–2.0 $\mu$m long and 0.2–0.4 $\mu$m in diameter within macrophages and sometimes in the extracellular tissues. These organisms were identified as *Tropheryma whippelii* in 1992 [56]. Currently, the diagnosis may be confirmed by PCR techniques on tissue or blood [57].

## Fungal myocarditis

Fungal infections involving the heart are rare; they usually occur in immunocompromised patients such as those with malignancies or receiving chemotherapy, steroids, radiation, or immunosuppressive therapy. Patients after recent cardiac surgery, intravenous drug abusers, and those with AIDS are also at risk. The overall incidence of fungaemia is increasing, probably as a consequence of the prolonged use of antibiotics in surgical patients and patients surviving longer with malignancies [58]. Blood cultures are not always rewarding, and only approximately 40–50% are positive. The most common organisms are *Candida* species (Fig. 23.10), *Aspergillus* species, *Phycomycetes*, and *Cryptococcus*. Less common organisms are *Histoplasma capsulatum*, *Curvularia lunato*, and *Helminthosporum* [58]. Overall, the heart is the most frequent organ involved in fatal cases of systemic fungal infection, and is affected in 45% of autopsies. Endocardial involvement is seen in 29%, both myocardial and endocardial in 15%, myocardial and pericardial in 8%, and isolated pericardial involvement in 3% of patients with fungaemia. Myocardial involvement is most frequently seen secondary to systemic *Candida* infection. Often, these patients have received antibiotics for a prolonged period, or have an underlying neoplasm. Fungal infections in patients recovering from cardiac surgery are caused by *Candida* species in over 50% of cases, with *Aspergillus* and *Cryptococcus* in the remainder.

Morphological recognition of fungal organisms is not always possible on H&E-stained sections, and special stains such as methenamine silver and PAS are required. Histologically, *Candida* species are identified by observing blastospores (yeast cells) in association with pseudohyphae or hyphae. *Aspergillus* can be seen in H&E-stained sections; however, fungal stains increase the detection rate of the organism. *Aspergillus* shows distinct dichotomous branching

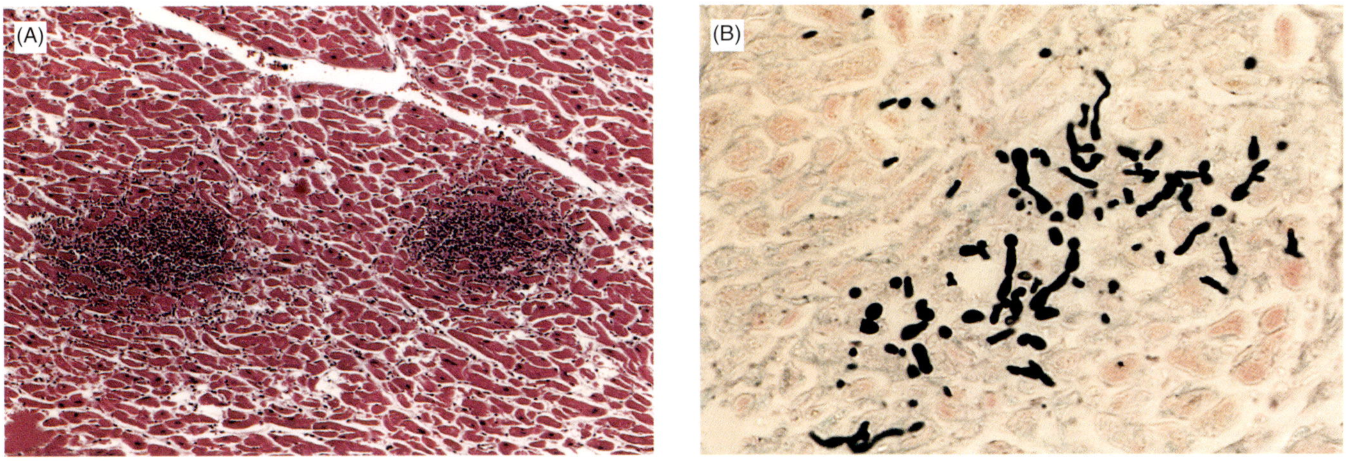


**Figure 23.10** *(A) H&E-stained section in a case with fungal myocarditis; note two microabscesses with neutrophil infiltration. (B) Gomori methenamine silver stain showing blastospores and pseudohyphae, characteristic of* Candida *species.*

of hyphae, advancing in the same direction. However, individual species cannot be determined without culture. *Phycomycetes*, such as *mucormycosis*, have, in contrast to *Aspergillus*, broad, haphazardly branching hyphae best appreciated in H&E sections (Fig. 23.11). The hyphae are mostly 10–15 μm in diameter, are partially collapsed, and often appear twisted. *Cryptococcus neoformans* has a thick cell wall, stains blue in H&E stain, and has a thick, mucinous capsule that appears clear. The thick wall demonstrates carminophilic material when stained with the mucicarmine stain.

Fungal endocarditis is often a result of infection by *Candida albicans*, other candidal species, *Torulopsis glabrata* and *Arpergillus* sp. By far the most common underlying predisposing conditions are prior valve surgery and intravenous drug abuse. The most common fungal infections in prosthetic valve endocarditis are *C. albicans* and *Aspergillus* species, while intravenous drug abuse patients are most frequently infected by species of *Candida* other than *C. albicans* [59]. The frequency of fungal cardiac involvement is greater in men than in women and the survival rate is less than 50% [59].

## Protozoal myocarditis

### *Background*

Most of the parasitic diseases involving the myocardium occur in the hot and humid climate of the tropics. However, because of travel and population migration, it is not unusual to see parasitic diseases in the USA and Europe; therefore, they should be considered in the differential diagnosis of myocarditis.

### *Trypanosomiasis (Chagas' disease)*

The protozoan *Trypanosoma cruzi*, a unicellular flagellate, is the agent of Chagas' disease, which is a major public health problem in Latin America. It has been reported that 16–18 million people worldwide are infected with the organism and about 90 million are at risk [60]. It is estimated that more than 100 000 infected people are currently residing in the USA [61].

The disease is transmitted to humans, usually before the age of 20 years, through the bite of the reduvidi bug or through the deposition of the animal's faeces on the abraded skin or conjunctiva. The animal carries the parasites in the gastrointestinal tract. Conjunctival entry results in conjunctivitis and periorbital oedema, forming the Romana sign [62], whereas entry through the skin results in chagomas.

The natural history of Chagas' disease is divided into three phases: an acute phase, lasting for 1–3 months; a latent, asymptomatic phase; and, after 10–20 years, a symptomatic or an asymptomatic chronic phase. In the acute phase the parasite multiplies by binary fission in the blood and then resides in the host cells of the skeletal muscle and myocardium, where it forms pseudocysts [63]. The residence of the parasite inside the host cells results in its protection against host immune defences. When the pseudocysts rupture, there is parasitaemia, followed by lymphadenopathy, hepatosplenomegaly, and myocarditis. The intracellular parasites in the myocardium elicit a marked inflammatory infiltrate, especially around the fibres that have ruptured [64]. When rupture occurs close to

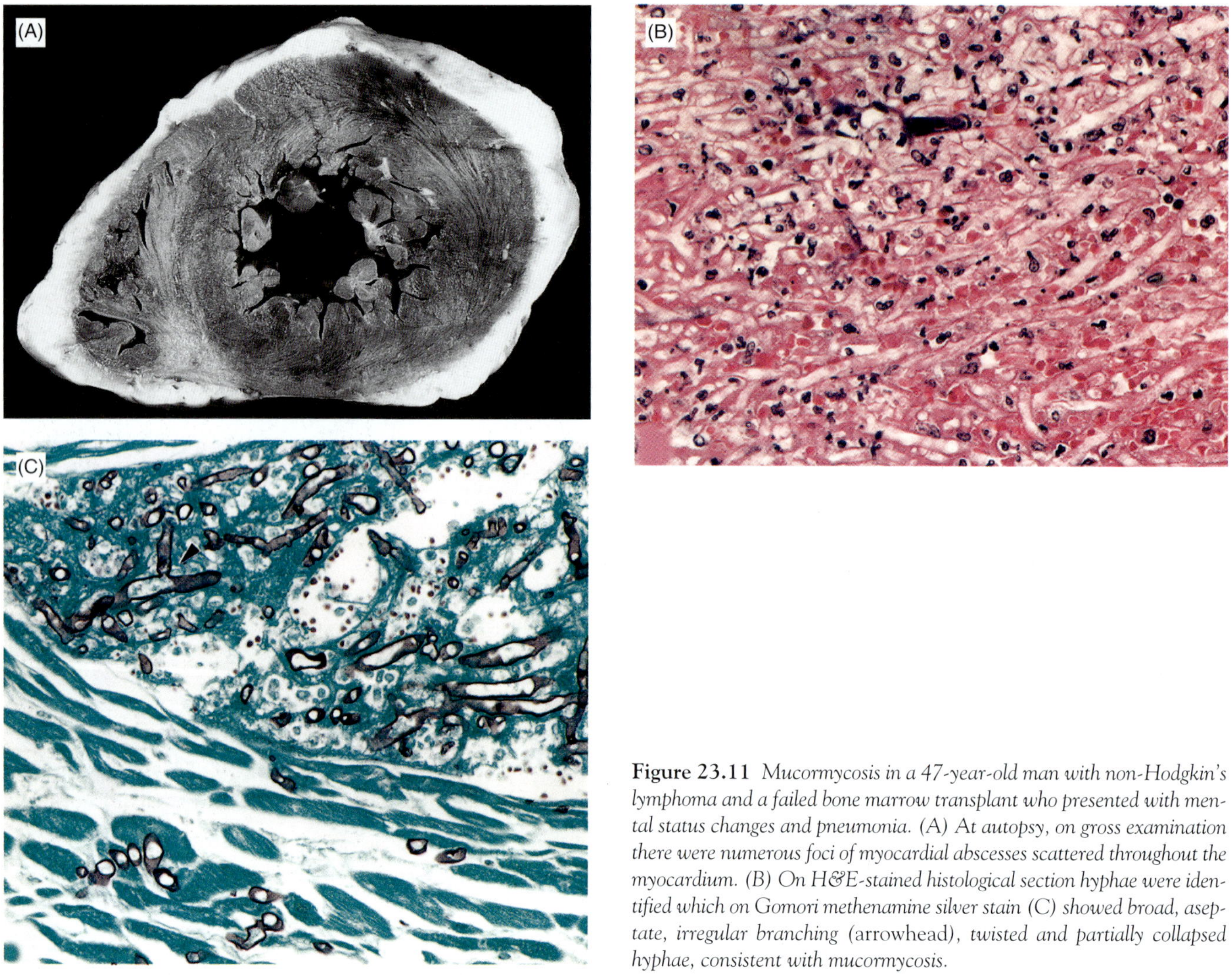


**Figure 23.11** *Mucormycosis in a 47-year-old man with non-Hodgkin's lymphoma and a failed bone marrow transplant who presented with mental status changes and pneumonia. (A) At autopsy, on gross examination there were numerous foci of myocardial abscesses scattered throughout the myocardium. (B) On H&E-stained histological section hyphae were identified which on Gomori methenamine silver stain (C) showed broad, aseptate, irregular branching* (arrowhead), *twisted and partially collapsed hyphae, consistent with mucormycosis.*

endocardium, spillage into the cavity results in a mural thrombus, and when it involves the epicardial surface, pericarditis and pericardial effusion ensue. Clinically, the patient presents with fever, muscle pains, sweating, lymphadenopathy, and hepatosplenomegaly. Acute myocarditis, CHF, and rarely meningoencephalitis may also occur in the acute phase [65]. Overall, acute illness is seen in less than 10% of patients and, of these, is fatal in 10% [62].

In the latent phase of the disease the patient is asymptomatic; however, there may be an underlying cardiomyopathy. Histological abnormalities have been reported in endomyocardial biopsies in 60% of patients in the latent phase [66]. The chronic phase develops in 30% of infected patients, and is the cause of death in up to 70% of these [67–70]. Two types of dysfunction are recognized: a myogenic form and a neurogenic form [70–72]. The myogenic form gives rise to cardiomyopathy characterized by an enlarged and a dilated heart weighing 500–600 g. The ventricles and the atria are dilated, especially on the right side, which is thin-walled. In approximately 50% of hearts, an apical aneurysm of the left ventricle is present (Fig. 23.12), and in another 25% the aneurysm is located in the posterior wall underneath the posterior mitral leaflet [73]. The aneurysms often contain a thrombus; the right atrium also frequently contains a thrombus. Microscopically, there is extensive scarring, especially in the left ventricle. There are focal cellular infiltrates consisting of lymphocytes, plasma cells, and macrophages [62]. The basement membrane of the capillaries, vascular smooth muscle cells, and myocytes is thickened [68, 71, 74–76]. Parasites are not usually found in the myocardium [71].

The neurogenic form of the chronic phase of Chagas' disease is characterized by conduction system involvement manifest as right bundle branch block, complete or

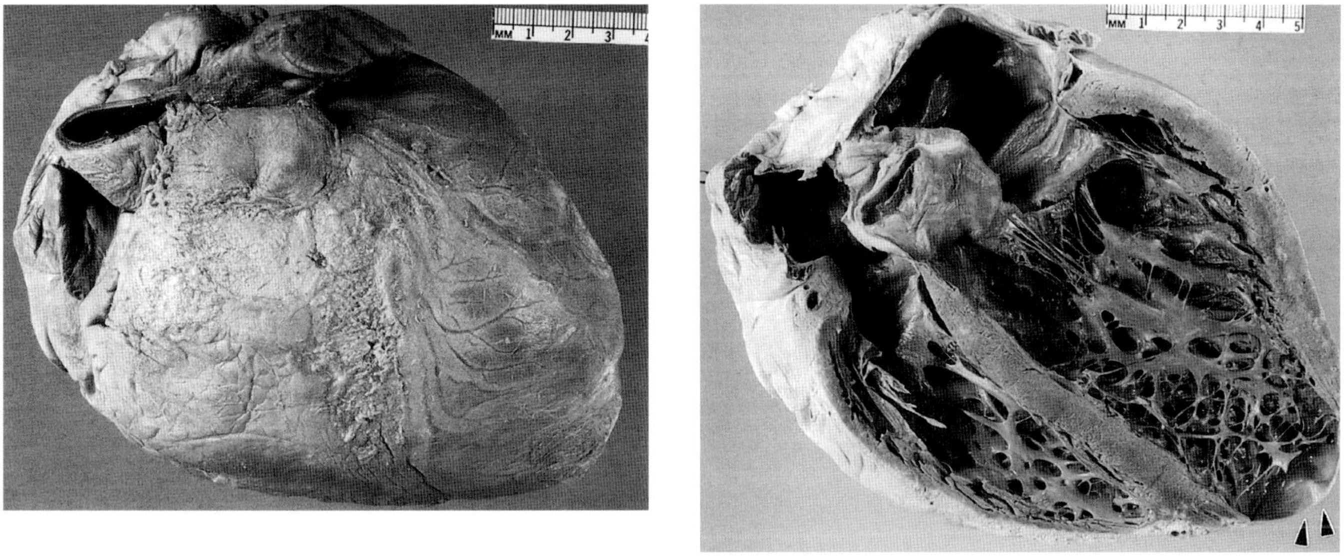

**Figure 23.12** *Chagas' disease. Four-chamber view of the heart showing more marked dilatation of the ventricles than of the atria. Note the apical aneurysm* (arrowheads)*, which is characteristic of chronic Chagas' disease and is seen in 50% of cases.*

incomplete left anterior hemiblock, nodal dysfunction, QRS abnormalities, and sudden death [62]. Pathologically, the nerves and ganglia are frequently abnormal, and there is evidence of parasympathetic denervation [62, 76]. 'Tissue tropism' of various strains results in different expressions in different geographical locations. Cardiac disease is common in Argentina and Venezuela, while involvement of the gastrointestinal tract is more frequent in Brazil and leads to megaoesophagus, megastomach, and megacolon [77].

The congenital form of Chagas' disease is due to transplacental migration of the trypanosomes. The infant may die within a few days of birth from myocarditis. The complement-fixation test (the Machado–Guerreiro test) is used for diagnosis; a positive test is indicated by a reaction with a dilution of serum at or above 1:8. This test has a sensitivity of 90% and a specificity of 98%. Other tests that help to establish the diagnosis are immunohaemagglutination (positive reaction, at or above a 1:64 dilution of serum), and indirect immunofluorescence (positive reaction, at or above a 1:32 dilution) [62].

### *Toxoplasmosis*

The causative organism of toxoplasmosis is *Toxoplasma gondii*, an obligate intracellular parasite. This organism has a crescentic or pyriform nucleated structure, 4–6 $\mu$m in length and 2–3 $\mu$m in width, and a cone-shaped tip on one end which it uses to penetrate the host. The parasite is harboured in the cat and is passed in the faeces, which are ingested by animals that act as the intermediate host. Humans are infected by the ingestion of uncooked or partially cooked meat, or by close contact with pets. Congenital and acquired forms of the disease occur. Involvement of the heart is unusual, but may occur in immunosuppressed patients with malignancies, individuals with AIDS, or following cardiac or bone-marrow transplantation (Fig. 23.13) [78, 79].

The prevalence of cardiac disease has been difficult to assess, as the disease is masked by neurological symptoms [78]. Cardiac involvement usually occurs during the course of multivisceral dissemination, but isolated cases have been reported without cerebral involvement and may reflect reactivation of *T. gondii* as a result of immune compromise [78, 80]. Cardiac symptoms consist of atrial and ventricular arrhythmias, AV block, pericarditis, and heart failure. The diagnosis is made antemortem by endomyocardial biopsy [81].

In order to determine the prevalence of toxoplasmosis at autopsy, Hofman *et al.* [79] evaluated 182 patients with HIV, and toxoplasmosis was diagnosed in 21 (12%). Toxoplasmic encephalitis occurred in 86% of these patients, with isolated cardiac involvement in the remaining 14%. The cardiac lesions consisted of acute myocarditis (29%), rare foci of myocarditis (38%), and intramyocyte toxoplasmic cysts without inflammation (19%). Antibody labelling against *Toxoplasma* identified organisms in only half of the cases of

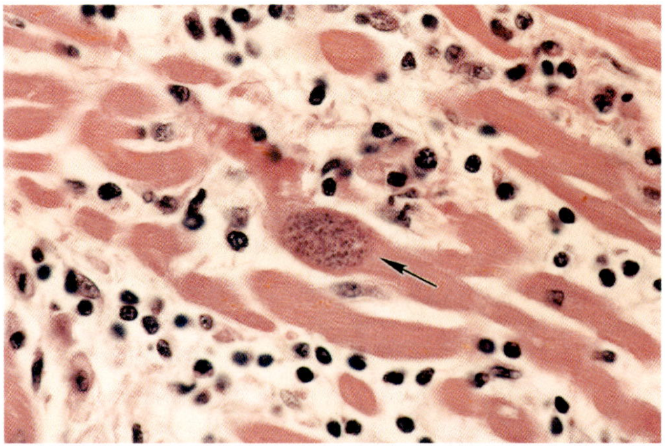

**Figure 23.13** *Toxoplasmosis. Note the lymphocytic myocarditis with an intramyocyte* Toxoplasma *cyst* (arrow) *with barely discernible tachyzoites.*

lymphocytic myocarditis. Six patients (approximately 30%) presented with cardiac symptoms (fever, global heart failure of sudden onset, and biventricular hypokinesia) and, of these, computed tomographic (CT) brain scan suggested toxoplasmosis in four, while the other two were suspected of having viral myocarditis. The diagnosis of myocarditis was missed in 11 (50%) patients, probably because of the focal nature of the myocardial involvement. Cardiac toxoplasmosis can be treated effectively with a combination of sulfadiazine and pyromethamine prior to the development of extensive irreversible myocardial lesions [79].

#### *Miscellaneous protozoal myocarditis*

Other protozoan diseases that may rarely involve the heart are African trypanosomiasis and malaria. The African sleeping sickness is caused by *Trypanosomiasis gambinese* or *T. rhodesiense*, which usually do not cause severe cardiac symptoms as seen in Chagas' disease [82]. Malaria does not cause specific myocardial changes; however, when cardiac symptoms occur, the aetiological organism is *Plasmodium falciparum*. Cardiac pathological changes secondary to malaria, which is especially prevalent in India, result from parasitized red cells blocking myocardial capillaries, leading to secondary myocardial ischaemia [83, 84].

### Metazoal myocardial disease

#### *Echinococcosis (hydatid cyst)*

Echinococcosis is an infection caused by the larval tapeworm of the genus *Echinococcus*. It is an endemic disease in many sheep-raising regions of the world, especially Australia, New Zealand, and Iceland. It usually causes hydatid cysts in the liver (60%) and lung (20%). Cardiac involvement is uncommon, occurring in 0.5–2% of cases [85–87]. The adult *E. granulosus* is a small (3–6 mm long) tape worm. The scolex (head) has four suckers and a double crown of 28–50 hooklets. The adult lives in the dog intestine and the egg is passed in the faeces, which are ingested. Humans may serve as the intermediate host, rather than the usual host, the sheep.

In the intermediate host, the oncospheres pass through the intestine and lodge in the capillaries of various organs. When the heart is involved, the embryo passes from the liver via the subclavian vein from the thoracic duct into the right ventricle, escaping the pulmonary circulation which usually acts as a filter. The most common site of involvement in the heart is the left ventricular free wall. However, the right atrium and ventricle, and the pericardium may also be involved [85–87]. The cyst in the heart may degenerate and calcify without causing symptoms, rupture into the pericardium causing acute pericarditis, or rupture into the ventricle with resultant systemic or pulmonary emboli. The hydatid cyst is usually single but multiple cysts have been reported occasionally [86]. The symptoms depend on the location, size, and integrity of the cyst wall, and patients may be asymptomatic. When the cyst ruptures into a cavity, hydatid fluid is liberated into the circulation, causing profound circulatory collapse from an anaphylactic reaction to the protein in the fluid [86]. Of 269 cases of hydatid cysts reported by DiBello and Menondez [88], 35% were located in the left ventricle, of which 37% had ruptured; whereas of the 13% located in the right ventricle, 80% had ruptured.

Echocardiography is the best imaging tool for establishing the diagnosis of myocardial echinococcal cysts, and CT scans and magnetic resonance imaging are also useful. Laboratory tests are generally unrewarding, although peripheral eosinophilia is often present and may be a useful adjunct finding.

The hydatid cysts may occasionally be excised surgically, and vary in size from 0.5 to 12 cm. When the cyst has ruptured, the centre of the mass shows the presence of necrotic matter containing membrane residues (finely laminated and amphophilic), with a foreign-body inflammatory reaction of a granulomatous type with an eosinophilic infiltrate [86]. When the cyst is intact the diagnosis is established by the laminated and amphophilic appearance of the cyst wall or by the scolices and hooklets in the cyst aspirate. There is a fibrotic wall around the hydatid cyst which arises from the host.

### *Visceral larva migrans*

Visceral larva migrans is an infection of the human viscera by the migrating larvae of *Toxocara canis* and *T. cati*, which are common intestinal ascrid of the dog and cat, respectively. Children 1–3 years of age, because of the habit of crawling and putting various objects in the mouth, are most susceptible to visceral larva migrans [89]. The organs most frequently involved are the lung and the liver. Only rarely has the heart been reported to be involved. Myocarditis may occur from the invasion of the myocardium by the larvae (Fig. 23.14). The myocardial lesions show an intense eosinophilic infiltrate with focal areas of necrosis and a granulomatous reaction, especially around the larvae [89]. CHF and death may occur, but patients with cardiac involvement may be asymptomatic [89].

## Idiopathic giant cell myocarditis

Giant cell myocarditis is a rare condition of unknown aetiology that usually follows an acute course characterized by progressive CHF, refractory ventricular arrhythmias, and a high mortality rate [90]. Although not currently believed to be due to an infection, this entity is briefly described here as a particularly lethal variant of lymphocytic myocarditis. The disease has been reported in patients 16–69 years of age (mean 43 ± 13 years), is equally distributed in men and women, and mostly affects whites (90%). It is uncommon in blacks and Asians (5% each) and rare in patients of Middle Eastern origin. Autoimmune disorders are reported in 19% of patients and are usually those of Crohn's disease and ulcerative colitis. Other rare associations include Hashimoto's thyroiditis, rheumatoid arthritis, myasthenia gravis, and Takayasu's arteritis [91].

The majority of patients presents with CHF (75%) and a smaller percentage (14%) has palpitations, syncope, or sudden death secondary to ventricular tachycardia. Sustained, refractory ventricular tachycardia is a frequent finding during the course of the disease. Rarely, patients may present with chest pain and ECG findings suggestive of acute myocardial infarction [91].

The heart weight at autopsy is usually within normal limits or is mildly increased. The inflammatory infiltrate involves the epicardial, mid-myocardial, and endocardial surfaces of the heart. All patients have left ventricular involvement, with diffuse, yellow–brown, circumferential discoloration that is concentrated in the mid-myocardium without sharp demarcation from the surrounding uninvolved tissue. The gross appearance mimics an acute myocardial infarction when the lesion is transmural or subendocardial [90].

Histologically, there is an extensive inflammatory infiltrate composed mainly of lymphocytes, macrophages, eosinophils, and giant cells in the presence of prominent myocyte necrosis. The giant cells are usually in close apposition to the advancing edge of the lesion, and are macrophage in origin as demonstrated by KP-1 positivity. The nuclei in the giant cells vary in number from two to 20 and are ovoid with inconspicuous nucleoli. Giant cells are usually present in areas of active inflammation and necro-

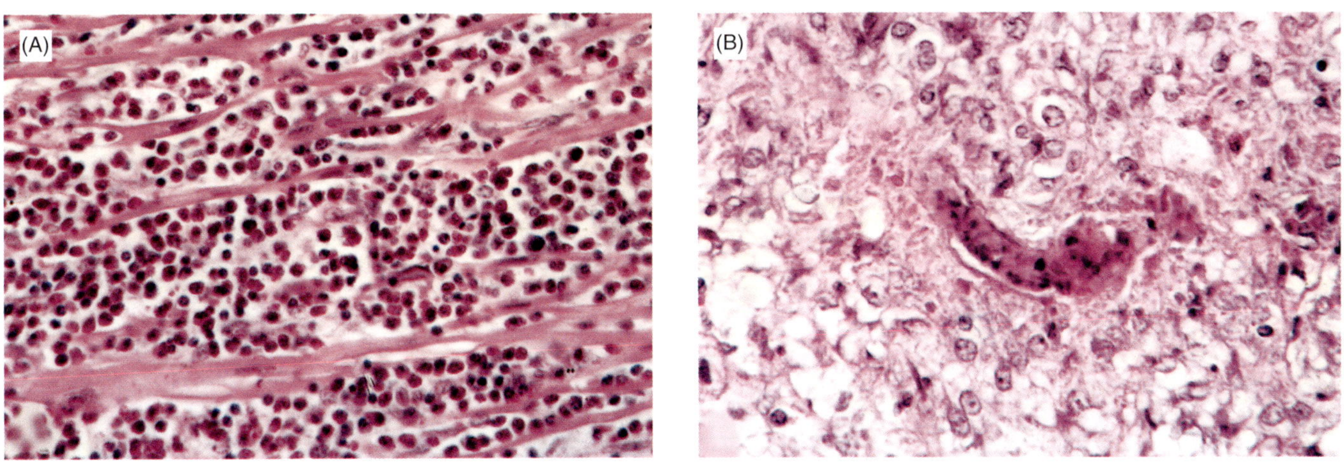


**Figure 23.14** *Visceral larva migrans (*Toxocara canis*). A 2.5-year-old girl underwent repair of tetralogy of Fallot. During surgery the surgeon noted a white nodule in the right atrial wall which was biopsied. (A) Histological examination showed several granulomas within the myocardium and diffuse eosinophiloic infiltrate. Remnants of a nematode larva were found in the centre of one granuloma. (B) Note the cylindrical body with a chitinous cuticle still visible.*

sis, but are not evenly distributed. The giant cells are not present in the epicardial fat, although inflammation may be present. Immunophenotying of the lymphocytes shows that T-lymphocytes outnumber B-cells by at least a ten-fold margin, and that the majority of the T-cells are CD8 cells. Hearts with acute lesions may have areas of healing as well as areas of scarring, and only rarely is there an absence of active lesions [90].

The median survival period or time until transplantation is 5.5 months in 89% of cases. No differences have been noted in the duration of survival in men and women or between younger and older patients. The survival rate of patients with giant cell myocarditis is lower than for patients with lymphocytic myocarditis. Patients treated with corticosteroids and cyclosporine, azathioprine, or both survive longer (12.3 months) than patients who received no treatment (3.0 months, $p = 0.001$). Of the patients who underwent heart transplantation, 26% had a giant cell myocarditis in the transplanted heart and one died of recurrent disease. Recurrences are seen an average of 3.0 years after transplantation [91].

## References


1. Peters NS, Poole-Wilson PA. Myocarditis — continuing clinical and pathologic confusion. *Am Heart J* 1991; 121: 942–7.
2. Herzum M, Maisch B. Humoral and cellular immune reactions to the myocardium in myocarditis. *Herz* 1992; 17: 91–6.
3. Marboe CC, Fenoglio JJ Jr. Pathology and natural history of human myocarditis. *Pathol Immunopathol Res* 1988; 7: 226–39.
4. Chida K, Ohkawa S, Esaki Y. Clinicopathologic characteristics of elderly patients with persistent ST segment elevation and inverted T waves: evidence of insidious or healed myocarditis? *J Am Coll Cardiol* 1995; 25: 1641–9.
5. Aretz HT. Myocarditis: the Dallas criteria. *Hum Pathol* 1987; 18: 619–23.
6. Nippoldt TB, Edwards WD, Holmes DR Jr *et al.* Right ventricular endomyocardial biopsy: clinicopathologic correlates in 100 consecutive patients. *Mayo Clin Proc* 1982; 57: 407–18.
7. Fenoglio JJ Jr, Ursell PC, Kellogg CF *et al.* Diagnosis and classification of myocarditis by endomyocardial biopsy. *N Engl J Med* 1983; 308: 12–18.
8. Parrillo JE, Aretz HT, Palacios I *et al.* The results of transvenous endomyocardial biopsy can frequently be used to diagnose myocardial diseases in patients with idiopathic heart failure. Endomyocardial biopsies in 100 consecutive patients revealed a substantial incidence of myocarditis. *Circulation* 1984; 69: 93–101.
9. Kasper EK, Agema WR, Hutchins GM *et al.* The causes of dilated cardiomyopathy: a clinicopathologic review of 673 consecutive patients. *J Am Coll Cardiol* 1994; 23: 586–90.
10. Rizeq MN, Rickenbacher PR, Fowler MB, Billingham ME. Incidence of myocarditis in peripartum cardiomyopathy. *Am J Cardiol* 1994; 74: 474–7.
11. Herskowitz A, Vlahov D, Willoughby S *et al.* Prevalence and incidence of left ventricular dysfunction in patients with human immunodeficiency virus infection. *Am J Cardiol* 1993; 71: 955–8.
12. Lieberman EB, Hutchins GM, Herskowitz A *et al.* Clinicopathologic description of myocarditis. *J Am Coll Cardiol* 1991; 18: 1617–26.
13. Aretz H, Billingham M, Edwards W *et al.* Myocarditis: a histologic definition and classification. *Am J Cardiovasc Pathol* 1987; 1: 3–14.
14. Beghetti M, Wilson GJ, Bohn D, Benson L. Hypersensitivity myocarditis caused by an allergic reaction to cefaclor. *J Pediatr* 1998; 132: 172–3.
15. Mason JW, O'Connell JB, Herskowitz A *et al.* A clinical trial of immunosuppressive therapy for myocarditis. The Myocarditis Treatment Trial Investigators. *N Engl J Med* 1995; 333: 269–75.
16. Martino TA, Liu P, Sole MJ. Viral infection and the pathogenesis of dilated cardiomyopathy. *Circ Res* 1994; 74: 182–8.
17. Anderson DW, Virmani R, Reilly JM *et al.* Prevalent myocarditis at necropsy in the acquired immunodeficiency syndrome. *J Am Coll Cardiol* 1988; 11: 792–9.
18. Archard LC, Richardson PJ, Olsen EG *et al.* The role of Coxsackie B viruses in the pathogenesis of myocarditis. *Biochem Soc Symp* 1987; 53: 51–62.
19. Kandolf R, Ameis D, Kirschner P *et al.* *In situ* detection of enteroviral genomes in myocardial cells by nucleic acid hybridization: an approach to the diagnosis of viral heart disease. *Proc Natl Acad Sci USA* 1987; 84: 6272–6.
20. Martin A, Webber S, Fricker F *et al.* Acute myocarditis. Rapid diagnosis by PCR in children. *Circulation* 1994; 90: 330–9.
21. Herskowitz A, Campbell S, Deckers J *et al.* Demographic features and prevalence of idiopathic myocarditis in patients undergoing endomyocardial biopsy. *Am J Cardiol* 1993; 71: 982–6.
22. Chan KY, Iwahara M, Benson LN *et al.* Immunosuppressive therapy in the management of acute myocarditis in children: a clinical trial. *J Am Coll Cardiol* 1991; 17: 458–60.
23. Cummins D, Bennett D, Fisher-Hoch SP *et al.* Electrocardiographic abnormalities in patients with Lassa fever. *J Trop Med Hyg* 1989; 92: 350–5.
24. Cummins D. Lassa fever. *Br J Hosp Med* 1990; 43: 186–8, 190, 192.
25. Saiman L, Prince A. Infections of the heart. *Adv Pediatr Infect Dis* 1989; 4: 139–61.
26. Ozkutlu S, Soylemezoglu O, Calikoglu AS *et al.* Fatal mumps myocarditis. *Jpn Heart J* 1989; 30: 109–14.
27. Waagner DC, Murphy TV. Varicella myocarditis. *Pediatr Infect Dis J* 1990; 9: 360–3.
28. Frustaci A, Abdulla AK, Caldarulo M, Buffon A. Fatal measles myocarditis. *Cardiologia* 1990; 35: 347–9.
29. Anderson DW, Virmani R. Patterns of heart disease in human immunodeficiency virus infection. *Hum Pathol* 1990; 21: 253–9.
30. Sato S, Tsutsumi R, Burke *et al.* Persistence of replicating coxsackievirus B3 in the athymic murine heart is associated with development of myocarditic lesions. *J Gen Virol* 1994; 75: 2911–24.
31. Ansari AA, Sundstrom JB, Runnels H *et al.* The absence of constitutive and induced expression of critical cell-adhesion molecules on human cardiac myocytes. Its role in transplant rejection. *Transplantation* 1994; 57: 942–9.

32. Lane JR, Neumann DA, Lafond-Walker A *et al.* Role of IL-1 and tumor necrosis factor in coxsackie virus-induced autoimmune myocarditis. *J Immunol* 1993; 151: 1682–90.
33. Singh S, Singhi S. Cardiovascular complications of enteric fever. *Indian Pediatr* 1992; 29: 1319–22.
34. Burt CR, Proudfoot JC, Roberts M, Horowitz RH. Fatal myocarditis secondary to *Salmonella* septicemia in a young adult. *J Emerg Med* 1990; 8: 295–7.
35. Dixon AC. The cardiovascular manifestations of leptospirosis. *West J Med* 1991; 154: 331–4.
36. Watt G, Padre LP, Tuazon M, Calubaquib C. Skeletal and cardiac muscle involvement in severe, late leptospirosis. *J Infect Dis* 1990; 162: 266–9.
37. Wengrower D, Knobler H, Gillis S, Chajek-Shaul T. Myocarditis in tick-borne relapsing fever. *J Infect Dis* 1984; 149: 1033.
38. Mekasha A. Louse-borne relapsing fever in children. *J Trop Med Hyg* 1992; 95: 206–9.
39. Jackman JD Jr, Radolf JD. Cardiovascular syphilis. *Am J Med* 1989; 87: 425–33.
40. Chino M *et al.* Ruptured ventricular aneurysm in secondary syphilis. *Lancet* 1993; 342: 935–6.
41. Cox J, Krajden M. Cardiovascular manifestations of Lyme disease. *Am Heart J* 1991; 122: 1449–55.
42. McAlister HF, Klementowicz PT, Andrews C *et al.* Lyme carditis: an important cause of reversible heart block. *Ann Intern Med* 1989; 110: 339–45.
43. Duray PH. The surgical pathology of human Lyme disease. An enlarging picture. *Am J Surg Pathol* 1987; 11 (Suppl 1): 47–60.
44. Duray PH, Steere AC. Clinical pathologic correlations of Lyme disease by stage. *Ann NY Acad Sci* 1988; 539: 65–79.
45. van der Linde MR, Crijns HJ, Lie KI. Transient complete AV block in Lyme disease. Electrophysiologic observations. *Chest* 1989; 96: 219–21.
46. de Koning J, Hoogkamp-Korstanje JA, van der Linde MR, Crijns HJ. Demonstration of spirochetes in cardiac biopsies of patients with Lyme disease. *J Infect Dis* 1989; 160: 150–3.
47. Stockins BA, Lanas FT, Saavedra JG, Opazo JA. Prognosis in patients with diphtheric myocarditis and bradyarrhythymias: assessment of results of ventricular pacing. *Br Heart J* 1994; 72: 190–1.
48. Havaldar PV, Patil VD, Siddibhavi BM *et al.* Fulminant diphtheretic myocarditis. *Indian Heart J* 1989; 41: 265–9.
49. Ganjoo RK, Sharma SN, Roy AK. Typhus myocarditis. *J Assoc Physicians India* 1989; 37: 357.
50. Marin-Garcia J. Left ventricular dysfunction in Rocky Mountain spotted fever. *Clin Cardiol* 1983; 6: 501–6.
51. Marin-Garcia J, Mirvis DM. Myocardial disease in Rocky Mountain spotted fever: clinical, functional, and pathologic findings. *Pediatr Cardiol* 1984; 5: 149–54.
52. Enzinger FM, Helwig EB. Whipple's disease: a review of the literature and report of 15 patients. *Virchow Arch A Pathol Anat Histopathol* 1963; 336: 238–69.
53. McAllister HA, Fenoglio JJ. Cardiac involvement in Whipple's disease. *Circulation* 1975; 52: 152–6.
54. Lie JT, Davis JS. Pancarditis in Whipple's disease: electronmicroscopic demonstration of intracardiac bacillary bodies. *Am J Clin Pathol* 1976; 66: 22–30.
55. Southern JF, Moscicki RA, Magro C *et al.* Lymphedema, lymphocytic myocarditis, and sarcoidlike granulomatosis. Manifestations of Whipple's disease. *JAMA* 1989; 261: 1467–70.
56. Relman Da, Schmidt TA, MacDermott RP, Falkow S. Identification of the uncultured bacillus of Whipple's disease. *N Engl J Med* 1992; 327: 293–301.
57. Mooney EE, Kenan DJ, Sweeney EC, Gaede JT. Myocarditis in Whipple's disease: an unsuspected cause of symptoms and sudden death. *Mod Pathol* 1997; 10: 524–9.
58. Atkinson JB, Connor DH, Robinowitz M *et al.* Cardiac fungal infections: review of autopsy findings in 60 patients. *Hum Pathol* 1984; 15: 935–42.
59. Rubinstein E, Lang R. Fungal endocarditis. *Eur Heart J* 1995; 16(Suppl B): 84–9.
60. Hagar JM, Rahimtoola SH. Chagas' heart disease in the United States. *N Engl J Med* 1991; 325: 763–8.
61. Kirchhoff LV, Neva FA. Chagas' disease in Latin American immigrants. *JAMA* 1985; 254: 3058–60.
62. Hagar JM, Rahimtoola SH. Chagas' heart disease. *Curr Probl Cardiol* 1995; 20: 825–924.
63. Palacios-Pru E, Carrasco H, Scorzs C, Espinoza R. Ultrastructural characteristics of different stages of human chagasic myocarditis. *Am J Trop Med Hyg* 1989; 41: 29–40.
64. Morris SA, Tanowitz HB, Wittner M, Bilezikian JP. Pathophysiological insights into the cardiomyopathy of Chagas' disease. *Circulation* 1990; 82: 1900–9.
65. Sadigursky M, von Kreuter BF, Ling PY, Santos-Buch CA. Association of elevated anti-sarcolemma, anti-idiotype antibody levels with the clinical and pathologic expression of chronic Chagas myocarditis. *Circulation* 1989; 80: 1269–76.
66. Mady C, Barretto AC, Stolf N *et al.* (Endomyocardial biopsy in the indeterminate form of Chagas' disease). *Arq Bras Cardiol* 1981; 36: 387–90.
67. Bestetti RB, Freitas OC, Muccillo G, Oliveira JS. Clinical and morphological characteristics associated with sudden cardiac death in patients with Chagas disease. *Eur Heart J* 1993; 14: 1610–14.
68. Rossi MA, Bestetti RB. The challenge of chagasic cardiomyopathy. The pathologic roles of automonic abnormalities, autoimmune mechanisms and microvascular changes, and therapeutic implications. *Cardiology* 1995; 86: 1–7.
69. Carrasco HA, Guerrero L, Parada H *et al.* Ventricular arrhythmias and left ventricular myocardial function in chronic chagasic patients. *Int J Cardiol* 1990; 28: 35–41.
70. Casado J, Davila DF, Donis JH *et al.* Electrocardiographic abnormalities and left ventricular systolic function in Chagas' heart disease. *Int J Cardiol* 1990; 27: 55–62.
71. Rossi MA. Comparison of Chagas' heart disease to arrhythmogenic right ventricular cardiomyopathy. *Am Heart J* 1995; 129: 626–9.
72. Pimenta J, Miranda M, Pereira CB. Electrophysiologic findings in long-term asymptomatic chagasic individuals. *Am Heart J* 1983; 106: 374–80.
73. Puigbo JJ, Valecillos R, Hirschhaut E *et al.* Diagnosis of Chagas' cardiomyopathy. Non-invasive techniques. *Postgrad Med J* 1977; 53: 527–32.
74. Rossi MA. Microvascular changes as a cause of chronic cardiomyopathy in Chagas' disease. *Am Heart J* 1990; 120: 233–6.
75. Rossi MA. The pattern of myocardial fibrosis in chronic Chagas' heart disease. *Int J Cardiol* 1991; 30: 335–40.
76. Rossi MA, Ramos SG. Coronary microvascular abnormalities in Chagas' disease. *Am Heart J* 1996; 132: 207–10.

77. Gallo Junior L, Morelo Filho J, Maciel BC *et al.* Functional evaluation of sympathetic and parasympathetic system in Chagas' disease using dynamic exercise. *Cardiovasc Res* 1987; 21: 922–7.
78. Roldan EO, Moskowitz L, Hensley GT. Pathology of the heart in acquired immunodeficiency syndrome. *Arch Pathol Lab Med* 1987; 111: 943–6.
79. Hofman P, Drici MD, Gibelin P *et al.* Prevalence of toxoplasma myocarditis in patients with the acquired immunodeficiency syndrome. *Br Heart J* 1993; 70: 376–81.
80. Adair OV, Randive N, Krasnow N. Isolated toxoplasma myocarditis in acquired immune deficiency. *Am Heart J* 1989; 118: 856–7.
81. Albrecht H, Stellbrink HJ, Fenske S *et al.* Successful treatment of *Toxoplasma gondii* myocarditis in AIDS. *Eur J Clin Microbiol Infect Dis* 1994; 13: 500–4.
82. Poltera AA. Pathology of human African trypanosomiasis with reference to experimental African trypanosomiasis and infections of the central nervous system. *Br Med Bull* 1985; 41: 169–74.
83. Franzen D, Curtius JM, Heitz W *et al.* Cardiac involvement during and after malaria. *Clin Invest* 1992; 70: 670–3.
84. Sharma SN, Mohapatra AK, Machave YV. Chronic falciparum cardiomyopathy . *J Assoc Physicians India* 1987; 35: 251–2.
85. Russo G, Tamburino C, Cuscuna S *et al.* Cardiac hydatid cyst with clinical features resembling subaortic stenosis. *Am Heart J* 1989; 117: 1385–7.
86. Oliver JM, Sotillo JF, Dominguez FJ *et al.* Two-dimensional echocardiographic features of echinococcosis of the heart and great blood vessels. Clinical and surgical implications. *Circulation* 1988; 78: 327–37.
87. Akhtar MJ. Hydatid disease of the right ventricle and role of tomographic scanning in its diagnosis. *Int J Cardiol* 1991; 33: 432–4.
88. DiBello R, Menondez H. Intracardiac rupture of hydatid cysts of heart. *Circulation* 1963; 27: 366–408.
89. Dao AH, Virmani R. Visceral larva migrans involving the myocardium: report of two cases. *Pediatr Pathol* 1986; 6: 449–56.
90. Litovsky SH, Burke AP, Virmani R. Giant cell myocarditis: an entity distinct from sarcoidosis characterized by multiphasic myocyte destruction by cytotoxic T cells and histiocytic giant cells. *Mod Pathol* 1996; 9: 1126–34.
91. Cooper LT Jr, Berry GJ, Shabetai R. Idiopathic giant-cell myocarditis — natural history and treatment. Multicenter Giant Cell Myocarditis Study Group Investigators. *N Engl J Med* 1997; 336: 1860–6.

# Molecular basis of postinfectious autoimmune myocardial disorders

24

E. CUNHA-NETO, L. GUILHERME, A. C. GOLDBERG AND J. KALIL

## Introduction

There is a category of heart disorders that occurs years after infection by pathogenic microorganisms, where the tissue damage to the heart, usually secondary to inflammation, occurs in the absence, or near absence, of the relevant pathogen. Rheumatic heart disease (RHD; from *Streptococcus pyogenes*), chronic Chagas' disease cardiomyopathy (CCC; from *Trypanosoma cruzi*) and 'idiopathic' (postviral) dilated cardiomyopathy (DCM; from coxsackievirus B3 and other enteroviruses) are life-threatening heart disorders for which surgical treatment is only partially effective. Evidence from experimental models and patients indicates the involvement of autoimmune mechanisms in heart tissue damage from the above disorders. The heart is an immunocompetent organ, with lymph-node drainage, and thus is under the surveillance of recirculating 'experienced' lymphocytes; moreover, it is relatively rich in histiocytes/dendritic cells capable of presenting antigens to T-cells [1]. Autoimmune diseases are characterized by immune responses to self components which lead to inflammatory target organ damage. The establishment of CCC, RHD, and DCM as organ-specific autoimmune diseases depends on matching several of the criteria for autoimmune disease recently revisited by Rose and Bona [2]. Elucidation of the pathogenesis of autoimmune diseases at the molecular level could lead to improved treatment as a result of the identification of relevant self-antigens and disease-inducing pathogenic antigens involved in molecular mimicry.

### Molecular basis of autoimmunity

One of the basic roles of the immune system is to fight invasion by pathogens, by directing a powerful artillery against them while attempting to spare self tissues. Self–non-self discrimination is thus a key feature of the immune system, achieved by incompletely understood mechanisms. The failure to discriminate leads to autoimmune disorders. Organ-specific autoimmune diseases rely on T-cell recognition of organ-specific self antigens, either by T-cell-dependent autoantibody-mediated autoimmunity or T-cell-mediated autoimmune diseases. T-cells recognize antigens via the variable regions of the clonotypic T-cell antigen receptor molecule (TCR). Antigens are recognized as peptide fragments embedded into the antigen-binding groove of major histocompatibility complex (MHC) molecules. The highly polymorphic nature of the amino acid sequence in the region lining the antigen-binding groove selects for the binding of antigenic peptide fragments (epitopes) that share discrete sequence motifs capable of interacting with that particular antigen-binding groove. Thus, a distinct set of epitopes from a given protein antigen is presented to the T-cells in each individual bearing a different MHC molecule. Furthermore, the MHC-driven thymic selection process trims away most (but not all) undesirable autoaggressive T-cells at early development stages in the thymus, releasing mature T-cells with a distinct antigen recognition repertoire. On the whole, this implies that each individual may be able to recognize different antigenic peptides from a given protein. Since there are hundreds of different human leucocyte antigen (HLA; the human MHC) alleles/molecules in the human species, a wide diversity of different recognition repertoires is expected to occur. The presentation of a self epitope by a given HLA molecule allows the recognition by self epitope-specific T-cells, the necessary conditions for an autoimmune response. In organ-specific T-cell-dependent autoimmune diseases, tissue damaging or effector mechanisms include T-cell-mediated cytotoxicity towards cells expressing the target antigen, usually carried out by $CD8^+$ T-cells, or delayed-type hypersensitivity, usually carried by inflammatory or

Th1 $CD4^+$ T-cells capable of secreting inflammatory or $T_1$-type cytokines [interferon-γ (IFN-γ) and tumour necrosis factor (TNF)] after recognition of its target epitope, activating macrophages and other lymphocytes. The triggering mechanisms of autoimmune diseases are still largely unknown, but always involve the loss of control of self-recognizing, potentially autoaggressive B- or T-cells, many times secondary to polyclonal activation or antigenic mimicry (structural similarity between foreign and self antigens), along with a transition to full pathogenic potential, leading autoreactive T-cells to cause tissue damage. Environmental (e.g. infections) as well as genetic (familial occurrence, HLA association) factors are known to play a role.

### Infection and autoimmunity

Infectious agents are important environmental triggers of autoimmune disease owing to their self-replicating nature and persistence into the host, leading to chronic immune stimulation. Infection may trigger autoimmunity in a variety of ways. The ability to stimulate the innate immunity, which is shared by most infectious agents, triggers a danger signal in the mammalian host, inducing the expression of costimulatory molecules in antigen-presenting cells and inflammatory cytokines in tissue. Pathogen-induced tissue damage, with release of self-antigens in inflamed tissue, can also cause autoimmune recognition. Moreover, molecular mimicry, the ability of a pathogen to cover itself with molecules antigenically similar to self-antigens as a means of escaping immune detection, is a frequent survival strategy that is thought often to lead to immunological cross-reactions, autoimmune recognition, and target organ destruction among susceptible individuals [3]. Molecular mimicry can occur between two epitopes with little amino acid sequence homology: as few as three identical amino acid residues are enough for cross-reactive recognition of two peptide epitopes by a single T-cell or immunoglobulin molecule. Thus, immunological cross-reactivity can occur between completely unrelated proteins.

## Rheumatic heart disease

Rheumatic fever (RF) is a sequel of throat infection by group A streptococci, affecting 3–4% of non-treated children. RHD develops 4–8 weeks or more after. Infection with *pyogenes* in about 30% of individuals with RF. The clinical signs of RF, as established by Jones [4], include major criteria to diagnose initial attacks of RF, such as polyarthritis, carditis, and chorea, along with minor criteria.

The pathogenic mechanisms involved in the development of RF and RHD remain unclear; however, an array of evidence indicates that an abnormal humoral and cellular immune response occurs. This section focuses on recent concepts regarding streptococcal antigenicity, humoral and cellular cross-reactive immune responses, and MHC–peptide–TCR interactions.

### Infectious component

Lancefield classified haemolytic streptococci into two major serogroups based on their cell-wall carbohydrate antigens [5]. M protein is the major antigen in *S. pyogenes*. This protein has antiphagocytic properties and shares structural homology with α-helical coiled-coil human proteins such as cardiac myosin, tropomyosin, keratin, laminin, and vimentin [6–9]. Over 85 different M-protein serotypes of group A streptococci have been recognized [10] and it has been consistently found that some serotypes are more frequently associated with RF ('rheumatogenic' serotypes), while others are more often associated with acute glomerulonephritis ('nephritogenic' serotypes) [11–13]. The M protein extends from the cell wall and contains multiple repeat regions that are conserved in the COOH-terminal half. Some antigenic variations are seen on the $NH_2$-terminal among different serotypes, usually at the first 11 amino acid residues that define these serotypes [10].

### Genetic susceptibility

The existence of a genetic pattern of susceptibility to RF and RHD was pointed out by Cheadle in the late nineteenth century [14]. Some authors have found that the pattern of inheritance fits a mendelian autosomic recessive model [15, 16]. Discordance for susceptibility to RF and RHD among identical twins suggested that if a mendelian pattern of inheritance is present, penetrance must be incomplete [17]. In search of genetic associations, a correlation with blood groups or secretor status was observed in of patients with RF: children with RF had a decreased frequency of O blood group and an increased frequency of non-secretor phenotype [18]. Patarroyo *et al.* [19] reported that a B-cell alloantigen (no. 883) was present in 75% of RF patients from Bogotá and 71% of RF patients from New York, compared with less than 15% of controls. However, indirect evidence suggested that the 883 alloantigen may be associated with HLA class II molecules [20, 21].

**Table 24.1** HLA class II antigens and rheumatic fever

| HLA | Country | Population | Refs. |
|---|---|---|---|
| DR4, DR9, DR2 | USA | American Caucasian Afro-American | [23, 24] |
| DR 4 | Saudi Arabia | Arabian | [25] |
| DR3, DQW2, D8/17 | India | Indian | [26] |
| DR7, DR53 | Brazil | Mulatto | [27] |
| Allogenotope TaqI DRbeta 13.81 kb | Brazil | Mulatto | [28] |
| DR1, DR6 | South Africa | African | ]29] |
| DR11 | Turkey | Turkish | [30] |

The D8/17 monoclonal antibody [22] identifies a similar B-cell alloantigen present in 90–100% of RF patients [21]. No consistent association with HLA class I antigens was found; however, association with different HLA class II antigens has been described in several populations (Table 24.1) [23–30]. Owing to the lack of concordance as to the RF-associated HLA class II haplotype in different regions of the world, a collaborative multicentre study was performed and no homogeneous association was found [31]. The different regional associations may be due to the prevalence of different rheumatogenic serotypes of *S. pyogenes* in the studied countries, causing different HLA class II molecules to present different M-protein epitopes. Alternatively, different frequencies in HLA antigens among different ethnic groups may lead to HLA presentation of 'promiscuous' streptococcal immunodominant epitopes, resulting in different HLA associations.

## Autoimmunity and molecular mimicry in rheumatic fever and heart disease

### *Autoantibodies and cross-reactive antibodies*

Antigenic mimicry between streptococcal antigens, mainly M-protein epitopes, and heart components has been proposed as the triggering factor for autoimmunity in individuals with a genetic predisposition. Molecular mimicry was first demonstrated at the antibody level. Heart-reactive antibodies were first described in the sera of patients with RF in 1945 [32]. Streptococcal antibodies cross-react with several human tissues including heart, skin, brain, glomerular basement membrane, and striated and smooth muscles [33]. Studies by Kaplan [34, 35] showed that rabbits immunized with streptococcal cell wall developed antibodies that bound mammalian heart tissue; furthermore, he was the first to demonstrate the presence of *S. pyogenes*–heart cross-reactive antibodies in the sera of patients with RF and RHD as well as to identify myocardium-bound immunoglobulins and complement in patients with acute RF. After these pioneering reports, several studies demonstrated the presence of cross-reactive antibodies in sera from animal models and humans or using monoclonal antibodies (mAb), as shown in Table 24.2 [36–60]. The role of these antibodies remains unclear, and it is possible that they appear secondary to the activation of streptococcal peptide-specific Th cells on the periphery.

### *Role of cellular immunity: autoreactive and cross-reactive T-cells*

Histological studies of heart valve tissue from RHD patients showed an intense infiltration of lymphomononuclear cells, basically plasma cells and T-cells, which were in close apposition to the fibroblasts [61]. Immunohistochemical studies demonstrated that T-cells in valve tissue are $CD4^+$, the 'helper' T-cell phenotype, suggesting a direct role for these cells in the pathogenesis of RHD [62, 63]. The Aschoff nodule, a pathognomonic histopathological feature of RF, is an angglomerate of monocytes and macrophages [63–66] which probably present antigen to $CD4^+$ T-cells infiltrating heart tissue. Valvular fibroblasts from RHD patients also present HLA-DR antigens [67] and may act as antigen-presenting cells (APC). Studies of human tonsils and peripheral blood from RF patients and controls showed a higher CD4/CD8 T-cell ratio among patients [68, 69]. It was also demonstrated that peripheral T-cells recognize streptococcal cell wall and mammalian tissue antigens [70–75]. Furthermore, peripheral T-lymphocytes from RHD patients recognize a 50 000–54 000 mol.wt myocardial protein. Reactivity was increased after priming patient cells with *S. pyogenes*, suggesting that this protein fraction may contain a target of molecular mimicry associated with the pathogenesis of RHD [76]. Human T-cells stimulated with streptococcal antigens display cytotoxic activity towards immortalized human heart cells [77, 78]. Peripheral blood T-cells from patients with acute RF, or T-cells lines derived from RHD heart valve specimens, did not cross-react with myosin or other mammalian cytoskeletal proteins after stimulation with streptococcal cell wall or the T-cell mitogen phytohaemagglutinin, and peripheral blood lymphocytes of RF patients [79].

**Table 24.2** M protein cross-reactive autoantibodies

| M protein | Epitope position | Nature of antibody | Human tissue cross-reactivity | Refs. |
|---|---|---|---|---|
| M1 | 13–19 | Human | 43 000 mol. wt/kidney protein | [52] |
| | 23–26 | | 56 000 mol. wt/kidney protein (vimentin) | |
| | 1–12 | Murine mAb | None | [56] |
| | 13–19 | | 43 000 mol. wt/protein (kidney/heart) | |
| M5 | ? | Rabitt | Sarcolemma | [36, 44] |
| | ? | Human | ND | [38] |
| | 1–20, 1–40 | Rabbit | None | [40] |
| | ? | Rabbit | Cardiac myosin | [44] |
| | 1–35 | Rabbit | None | [45] |
| | 84–116 | Rabbit | Cardiac myosin | [47] |
| | 164–197 | Rabbit | 40 000 mol. wt/heart protein | [48] |
| | 84–116, 117–134, 164–197 | Murine mAb | Vimentin | [60] |
| | ? | Human mAb | Skeletal muscle myosin; myosin actin and/or keratin | [50] |
| | 184–197 | Murine and human mAb | Cardiac myosin | [54] |
| | ? | Murine mAb | Tropomyosin | [55] |
| | ? | Murine mAb | Valvar proteins | [57] |
| M6 | ? | Human | ND | [38] |
| | ? | Human | ND | [39] |
| | 1–20, 10–20, 12–31 | Rabbit | None | [46] |
| | ? | Murine mAb | 53 000 mol. wt/glomerular protein | [49] |
| | ? | Human mAb | Skeletal muscle myosin; myosin actin and/or keratin | [50] |
| | ? | Murine mAb | Tropomyosin | [55] |
| | 223–245, 256–277, 240–260, | Rabbit | Denatured forms of myosin] | [58] |
| | 272–292 | Rabbit, human | Human brain | [59] |
| | B repeat region | | | |
| M12 | ? | Murine mAb | 53 000 mol. wt/glomerular protein | [49] |
| | 1–25 | Rabbit | Vimentin (mesangial cells) | [53] |
| M19 | 1–24 | Rabbit | 60 000 mol. wt/myocardial protein | [51] |
| M24 | ? | Human, rabbit | Brain | [37] |
| | S-CB7 | Human, rabbit | None | [41] |
| | 23–35, 18–35, 13–35 | Rabbit | None | [43] |

ND = not determined.

On studying the peripheral T-cell response to streptococcal M-protein peptides, it was observed that peptide M5(81–96) was frequently recognized, especially by DR53-positive patients with severe RHD [96a]. The T-cells infiltrating heart lesions of these patients also recognize immunodominant M5 protein peptides including M5(81–96), and such clones cross-reactively recognize myocardial and valve proteins [80, 81]. This report was the first to demonstrate human infiltrating T-cell cross-reactivity between a bacterial product and human tissue in established postinfectious autoimmune disease, providing strong evidence for the participation of molecular mimicry in the generation of heart tissue damage in patients with RHD. Table 24.3 summarizes literature data on T-cell cross-reactive M5 epitopes [80–84]. Some immunodominant cross-reactive M-protein T-cell epitopes, M5(81–96) and M5(163–177), were recognized both by human T-cell clones infiltrating RHD lesions [80] and T-cells from immunized mice [84, 87].

Recognition of streptococcal M-protein epitopes seems to play a central role in protection and immunopathology.

**Table 24.3** Heart cross-reactive T-cell epitopes of streptococcal M5 protein

| M5 epitope | Sequence | Nature of T-lymphocytes | Tissue cross-reactivity | Refs. |
|---|---|---|---|---|
| 1–20 | TVTRGTISDPQRAKEALDKY | Human intralesional T-cell clones from RHD patients | 24 000–30 000 mol. wt myocardium protein | [80] |
| 11–25 | QRAKEALDKYELENH | | 150 000–65 000 mol. wt myocardium protein | |
| 81–96 | DKLKQQRDTLSTQKET | | 90 000–150 000 mol. wt aortic valve protein | |
| 83–103 | LKQQRDTLSTQKETLEREVQN | | 150 000–30 000 mol. wt aortic valve protein | |
| 163–177 | ETIGTLKKILDETVK | | 24 000–44 000 mol. wt myocardium protein and 90 000–150 000 mol. wt aortic valve protein | |
| 347–366 | AKKQVEKALEEANSKLAALE | Murine T-cell clones and human normal peripheral T-cell lines | Porcine heart myosin, human myosin peptides, and human mitral extract | [82, 83] |
| 337–356 | LRRDLDASREAKKQVEKAL | Human normal peripheral T-cell lines and mouse lymph-node cells | Porcine heart myosin, human myosin peptides, and human mitral extract | [83] |
| 397–416 | LKEQLAKQAEELAKLRAGKA | RHD peripheral T-cell lines | Human cardiac and skeletal muscle myosin peptides | |
| 40–58 | GLKTENEGLKTENEGLKTE | Murine lymph-node cells | Human cardiac myosin peptides | [84] |
| 59–76 | KKEHEAENDKLKQQRDTL | | | |
| 137–154 | VKDKIAKEQENKETIGTL | | | |
| 150–167 | TIGTLKKILDETVKDKIA | | | |
| 254–271 | EASRKGLRRDLDASREAK | | | |
| 293–308 | KGLRRDLDASREAKKQ | | | |

M5 protein peptides were numbered according to the sequence of M5 protein used in Refs. 80, 82 and 83, based on Manjula *et al.* [85], and the numbering used in Ref. 84 was based on Miller *et al.* [86]. RHD = rheumatic heart disease.

Recently, it was reported that the pepsin-cleaved fragment of M5 protein had superantigenic activity for human T-cells, stimulating those expressing the TCR Vβ 2, 4, and 8 families [88–92]. Superantigens are proteins that polyclonally activate T-cells by an HLA class-II-dependent, but haplotype-unrestricted, mechanism. Proliferative responses to superantigens are limited to T-cells expressing particular TCR Vβ gene families and are independent of antigen specificity, but can expand tissue-damaging cells possessing that Vβ gene family. Other groups, however, found no evidence of superantigenicity using recombinant M5 protein or recombinant pepM5 [93] and it was also reported that the superantigenicity of purified pepM1 and pepM5 was due to contamination with pyrogenic exotoxins [94, 95]. Studies by the present authors on TCR Vβ in PBMC from six patients with severe RHD and infiltrating T-cell lines derived from the myocardium and/or mitral valve from four patients showed no expansion of any particular Vβ family. However, CDR3 length profiles showed an altered distribution; several oligoclonal profiles were found in infiltrating T-cell lines. Some VβJβ families were shared by myocardium and mitral valve T-cell lines derived from the same patient, and the sequences of the CDR3 region were homologous, but not identical [95a]. These results suggest that antigen-driven clonal expansion, rather than superantigenicity of M protein, influences the expansion of pathogenic T-cells in RHD patients.

The inflammatory process that occurs in patients with acute RF and RHD is driven by cytokines produced at the site of the lesions. The increased number of $CD4^+$ T-cells in peripheral blood is associated with a rise in serum levels of interleukin-1 (IL-1), TNF-α, and IL-2 [96–98]. Tonsillar and blood mononuclear cells from RF patients stimulated *in vitro* by pokeweed mitogen displayed different cytokine profiles: tonsillar cells produced significantly less IL-1, TNF, and IL-2, while blood mononuclear cells produced more IL-2 and TNF than controls, suggesting an abnormal regulation of cytokine production in patients with RF and RHD [99].

There is no ideal animal model for RF and RHD, but some investigators have developed models suitable for testing limited aspects of RHD pathogenesis. In the 1960s, a murine model was developed in which injection of a non-biodegradable polysaccharide component of the streptococcal cell wall into mice induced cardiac inflammation [61]. Another report showed that immunization of mice with *S. pyogenes* extracts induced a specific proliferative response to syngeneic heart extracts *in vitro*; furthermore, the transfer of spleen cells from mice immunized with *S. pyogenes* extracts induced the appearance of heart lesions in syngeneic recipients [100]. In one study [101], inflammatory heart disease was induced in mice injected with certain M-protein synthetic peptides; in another [82], peptide immunization induced strong *in vitro* proliferative responses after imunization, but no heart lesions.

### Conclusion: towards immunological intervention

The knowledge acquired since the 1940s gives us a better understanding of the mechanisms of tissue damage and protection. This knowledge may allow the development of a safe and effective vaccine, devoid of heart corss-reactive epitopes. Synthetic peptide and recombinant vaccines are being developed that induce specific immune responses and protect mice from infectious challenge by *S. pyogenes* without inducing tissue cross-reactions [102–108]. The transition of such vaccines to humans depends on further study of the mechanism inducing heart tissue damage in RHD.

## Chronic Chagas' disease cardiomyopathy

CCC is the most important clinical consequence of infection by the protozoan intracellular parasite *T. cruzi*, which affects 20 million individuals in the Americas. *Trypanosoma cruzi* replicates in the cytoplasm of host cells and establishes a chronic infection. There is no known 'sterile immunity'. CCC is an inflammatory dilated cardiomyopathy that may be fatal. It is seen in 25–30% of individuals unaffected with *T. cruzi* 5–30 years after the primary infection [109] and represents about 20% of hospital admissions for congestive heart failure (CHF) in São Paulo, Brazil [110]. CCC occurs with increased severity in males, for yet unknown reasons [111]. The remaining 60–70% of chronically *T. cruzi*-infected individuals either remain asymptomatic ('indeterminate' patients) or develop denervation of parietal smooth muscle in the digestive tract (5–10%). As there is no vaccine for Chagas' disease, and treatment with anti-*T. cruzi* drugs may not abort the progression towards CCC [112], heart disorders are treated only symptomatically. Histopathologically, there is a diffuse myocarditis with focal aspects [113] and a lymphomononuclear infiltrate rich in $CD8^+$ T-cells [114]. Given the scarcity of *T. cruzi* parasites *in situ* [115], infiltrating T-cells have been implicated as the ultimate effectors of heart tissue damage. The pathogenesis of CCC is still under intense debate. A direct role for heart parasitism has been proposed by Higuchi *et al.* [115] and Jones *et al.* [116], who found *T. cruzi* antigen and DNA in CCC hearts by immunohistochemical and polymerase chain reaction (PCR) techniques, respectively. However, PCR identification of *T. cruzi* DNA on cardiomyopathy-free hearts from asymptomatic patients as well as CCC hearts [116a], and the finding of low-grade parasitism in organs other than the heart, which nevertheless do not develop a tissue-damaging inflammatory infiltrate [117, 118], argue against the notion that parasitism per se is necessary and sufficient for tissue damage. Such evidence suggested the possible involvement of autoimmunity in the pathogenesis of CCC and prompted early investigators to postulate that lymphocytes in the heart recognize and mount delayed-type hypersensitivity responses towards tissue-specific heart components as a result of chronic *T. cruzi* infection, the autoimmune hypothesis of pathogenesis [119].

### Autoimmunity and molecular mimicry in chronic Chagas' disease cardiomyopathy: in search of defined antigenic targets

An antiheart autoimmune response can be triggered either by molecular mimicry with some *T. cruzi* antigen homologous to heart proteins, or by the display of intracellular sequestered heart proteins secondary to parasite-driven myocarditis during acute infection. Since molecular mimicry is the most established autoimmunity-inducing mechanism, investigators have been searching since the 1970s for

**Table 24.4** Molecular mimicry in Chagas' disease: cross-reactive antibodies

| *Trypanosoma cruzi* molecule | Host component | Host | Disease-related | Refs. |
|---|---|---|---|---|
| α-Gal residues | α-Gal EVI*<br>EVI* | A | No | [120, 121] |
| SRA | Skeletal muscle<br>SRA | A | NT | [122] |
| ? | Neurons, liver, kidney, testis | A | NT | [123] |
| ? | Neurons | A | NT | [124] |
| Sulphated glycolipids | Neurons | A | NT | [125] |
| Fl-160 | 47 000 mol. wt neuronal protein | A | No | [126] |
| Microtubule-associated proteins | Microtubule-associated proteins (brain) | A,H | No | [129] |
| Ribosomal P protein | Ribosomal P protein (HeLa cell line) | H | Yes | [127] |
| Ribosomal P0 protein | $\beta_1$-Adrenoreceptor | H | No | [130] |
| 23 000 mol. wt ribosomal protein | 23 000 mol. wt ribosomal protein (HeLa cells, reticulocytes) | H | No | [128] |
| B13 protein | Human cardiac myosin heavy chain (human ventricle) | H | Yes | [131] |

SRA =
EVI = endothelial–vascular–interstitial pattern;
A = animal model; H = human; NT = not tested.

cross-reactive antibodies that recognize simultaneously *T. cruzi* and mammalian components. Table 24.4 lists the antibody-based molecular mimicry systems involving defined target antigens [120–131]. Most of the cross-reactive autoantibodies described were either present in symptom-free individuals, or the self-antigen recognized had ubiquitous expression, which seemed to indicate that most of the cross-reactive antibodies disclosed had limited clinical significance, not unlike the innocuous 'natural' autoantibodies found in sera from normal individuals [132].

## Cardiac myosin as a major heart-specific antigen in chronic Chagas' disease cardiomyopathy

$CD4^+$ T-cells from chronically *T. cruzi* infected BALB/c mice apparently can induce the production of heart lesions, suggesting a possible role for T-cell-mediated autoimmunity in murine models of CCC [133]. Myosin, the most abundant heart protein, is a major antigen in several instances of heart-specific autoimmunity; moreover, immunization with cardiac myosin in Freund's adjuvant induces severe myocarditis in mice [134]. Cardiac myosin is recognized by $CD4^+$ T-cells in murine models of CCC [135]. Anticardiac myosin antibodies [136] and delayed-type hypersensitivity responses to cardiac myosin (Leon and Engman, Northwestern University, Chicago, personal communication) have been found in *T. cruzi*-infected mice with intense myocarditis. These reports on cardiac myosin autoimmunity in murine models of Chagas' disease suggest the possible relevance of myosin recognition in the pathogenesis of human CCC. Affinity-selected, anticardiac myosin heavy-chain antibodies in sera from patients with Chagas' disease specifically recognized a defined *T. cruzi* antigen [131], the recombinant protein B13 [137]. Cardiac myosin B13-cross-reactive antibodies were present in sera from 100% of CCC patients but only 14% of asymptomatic patients [131]. Furthermore, T-cell clones derived from CCC heart lesions were reported to recognize cross-reactively cardiac myosin heavy chain and B13 *T. cruzi* protein, but not other recombinant or crude *T. cruzi* antigens [138]. As heart macrophages are known to present constitutively antigenic myosin peptides on HLA class II molecules, myosin-loaded macrophages rather than HLA class II-negative cardiomyocytes may trigger the pathogenic $CD4^+$ T-cells [1]. Such results suggest that autoimmunity and

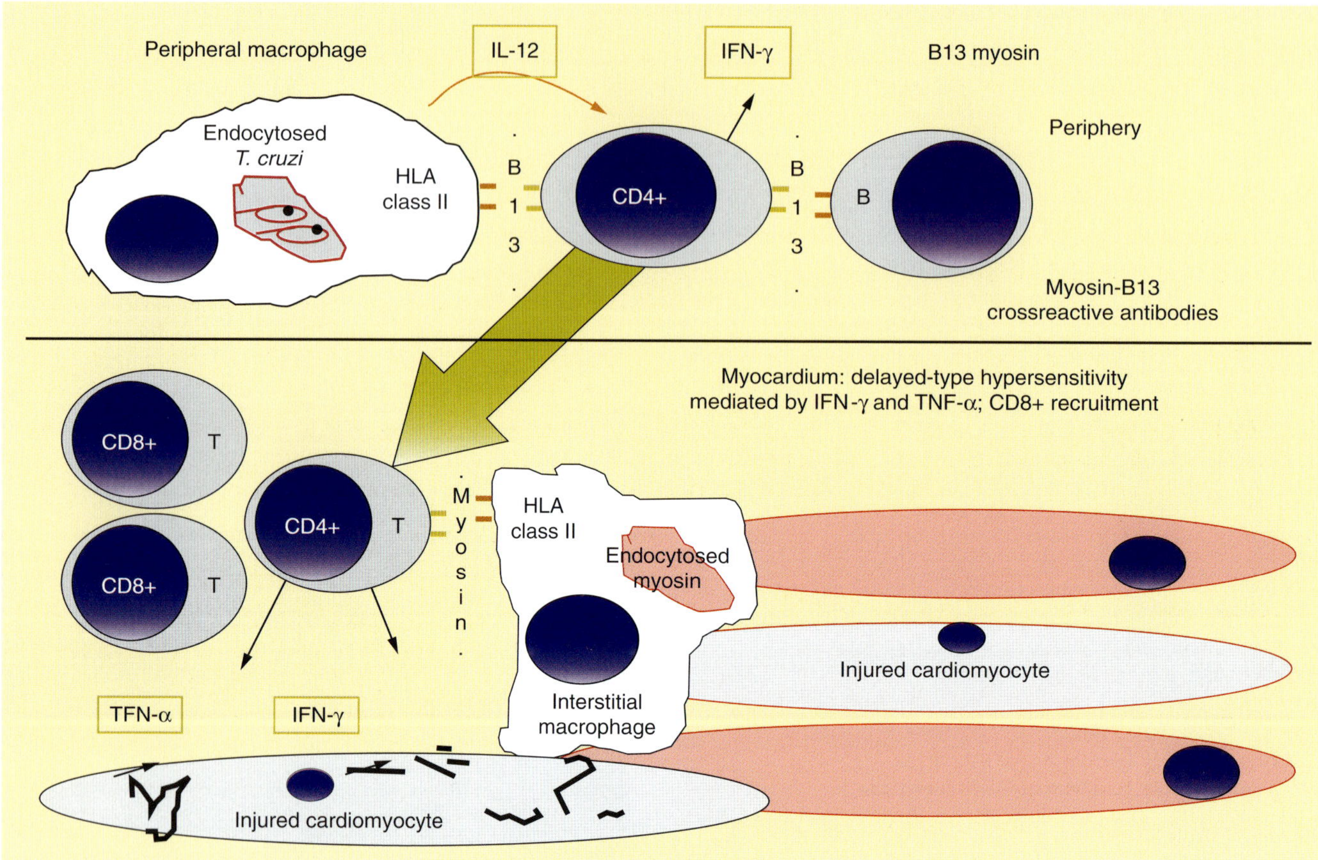


**Figure 24.1** *Pathogenesis of chronic Chagas' disease cardiomyopathy.*

molecular mimicry targets, rather than direct antigenic action of *T. cruzi*, are the primary stimuli of the heart tissue damaging T-cell infiltrate. Furthermore, *in vitro* sensitization of lymphocytes from a *T. cruzi* seronegative individual with B13 protein elicits cardiac myosin-cross-reactive T-cell clones [139]. In an analogous fashion, challenge with B13 antigen along with *T. cruzi* infection may break immunological tolerance towards cardiac myosin and elicit cardiac myosin-responsive T-cells *in vivo*.

Thus, in natural *T. cruzi* infection, cross-reactive $CD4^+$ T-cell clones that are sensitized in the periphery by macrophages presenting a heart cross-reactive *T. cruzi* antigen (e.g. B13 protein) after endocytosis of the parasite could become activated upon recirculation to the heart tissue, where heart antigen (e.g. cardiac myosin) epitopes are constitutively presented by class II MHC molecules on heart interstitial macrophages. From then on, $CD4^+$ T-cells might initiate and maintain a typical delayed-type hypersensitivity reaction in heart tissue by the release of inflammatory cytokines and cellular recruitment (Fig. 24.1).

## Cytokine production in Chagas' disease

Membrane components of *T. cruzi*, such as mucin-like glicoconjugates, are potent inducers of IL-12 *in vitro* [140]; this cytokine is abundantly produced during murine *T. cruzi* infection [141, 142]. This leads to increased production of IFN-γ in *T. cruzi*-infected mice [143, 144] which, in turn, stimulates macrophages to secrete TNF-α and nitric oxide (NO) via inducible nitric oxide synthase (iNOS), the final mediator of the protective anti-*T. cruzi* effect of this cytokine cascade [145, 146]. In humans, there seems to be a similar shift towards production of $T_1$-type cytokines such as IFN-γ among peripheral T-cells and CCC patients display increased numbers of IFN-γ producing cells [147–149]. As noted before, the inflammatory infiltrate in hearts of patients with Chagas' cardiomyopathy is rich in $CD4^+$ and $CD8^+$ T-cells with a 2:1 predominance of the $CD8^+$ subset [114]. There is little information on the functional role of heart-infiltrating $CD8^+$ T-cells. T-cells infiltrating heart lesions of CCC patients predominantly express IFN-γ and TNF-α but little or no IL-4 (Fig. 24.1) [147,

150–152]. Histiocytes and endothelial cells display increased expression of HLA class I and class II molecules, endothelial cells express intercellular adhesion molecule-1 (ICAM-1) and E-selectin, while CCC cardiomyocytes only display increased levels of HLA class I [153]. These phenotype changes are consistent with the *in situ* production of proinflammatory $T_1$-type cytokines. It seems likely that the dominant production of IFN-$\gamma$ and TNF-$\alpha$ in the heart lesions of patients with CCC is related to lifelong low-grade tissue infection with *T. cruzi*, secondary to its IL-12 inducing activity. The finding of predominantly $T_1$-type cytokine production by heart-infiltrating T-cells in human CCC also points to the concept that protection and pathology share the same underlying immunological effector mechanisms.

### Conclusion: pathogenesis of chronic Chagas' disease cardiomyopathy

Data in the literature are consistent with the view that *T. cruzi* infection may trigger potentially pathogenic T-cells, as has been postulated for other infectious agents in organ-specific autoimmune diseases [154]. The provision of the initial antigenic stimulus (*T. cruzi* B13 protein) in the presence of costimulatory signals [155] and IL -12 production, generates 'experienced', HLA-restricted, B13-specific, IFN-$\gamma$-producing $CD4^+$ T-cells in a large majority of infected individuals. These experienced T-cells are able to migrate to heart tissue, where myocardial protein (e.g. myosin) epitopes are constitutively presented by class II MHC molecules on heart interstitial macrophages, and potentially can start tissue damage [1]. However, the presence of potentially pathogenic B13-specific T-cells in the peripheral blood of *T. cruzi*-infected asymptomatic individuals without heart disease indicates that their presence may be necessary but not sufficient for the establishment of diffuse myocarditis and heart damage (Abel *et al.*, submitted for publication; Faé *et al.*, submitted for publication) [147]. The generation of a heart-damaging T-cell infiltrate may only occur in a subset of *T. cruzi*-infected individuals whose T-cell repertorie allows cross-reactive recognition of heart antigen (e.g. cardiac myosin) by *T. cruzi* (e.g. B13)-specific T-cells and are able to produce increased levels of inflammatory cytokines. Thus, molecular mimicry could be the link between low-grade persistence of *T. cruzi* in the chronically infected host and heart tissue damage in areas devoid of parasite antigens [114, 138]. The possession of such a cross-reactive T-cell repertoire could be the mechanism underlying differential susceptibility to CCC progression.

## Dilated cardiomyopathy

'Idiopathic' DCM is a disorder of the heart muscle presenting with ventricular dilation and impairment of left and/or right ventricular systolic pump function, often producing symptoms of CHF. Histopathological features include extensive fibrosis, myocyte necrosis, and mild mononuclear cell infiltration in some cases. DCM occurs mainly in adult males [156] and may be the late sequel of acute viral myocarditis, possibly mediated through an immunological mechanism. Reversible forms of DCM, possibly involving toxic or metabolic mechanisms, are associated with pregnancy, alcohol abuse, selenium deficiency, hypophosphataemia, hypocalcaemia, thyroid disease, cocaine use, and chronic uncontrolled tachycardia. Here, the discussion of pathogenic immune mechanisms is restricted to the 'viral-immune' hypothesis of 'idiopathic'/postviral DCM.

### Viral aetiology of acute myocarditis and dilated cardiomyopathy

Enterovirus was linked to myocarditis for the first time in 1956, when coxsackievirus B4 was isolated from the heart of an infant after a fatal infection [157]. Epidemiological studies show that the incidence of acute myocarditis increases after enteroviral epidemics [158]. However, only indirect evidence is available supporting a viral aetiology for DCM. Neutralizing antibodies [159] and immunoglobulin M (IgM) antibodies [160] against coxsackievirus B are increased in DCM patients when compared with controls from different towns, but not when compared with matched healthy subjects in the same neighbourhood. Several studies employed molecular biology techniques such as *in situ* hybridization and reverse transcription (RT)-PCR for the detection of the enteroviral genome in heart samples. Some studies reported negative findings, while others reported a high incidence of viral genome in control heart samples. A retrospective meta-analysis of 12 independent studies disclosed an overall higher frequency of enteroviral mRNA in heart samples from patients with acute myocarditis and DCM (10–75%; average 23%) than in control samples (6–7%) [161]. The apparent progression of some patients with a clinical diagnosis of acute myocarditis to CHF [162], and the progression of experimental models of virus-induced myocarditis to a chronic stage [163], are evidence of the involvement of prior enterovirus infection in DCM.

Indirect evidence indicates that coxsackievirus B3 is estimated to cause 7–30% of acute myocarditis, of which about 10% are estimated to progress to DCM [164, 165]. Other viruses have been implicated in myocarditis and DCM, such as adenovirus, influenza virus, cytomegalovirus, and human immune deficiency virus (HIV) but their role has not been thoroughly investigated [162, 166].

## Evidence for autoimmunity in myocarditis and dilated cardiomyopathy

Using the Dallas histological criteria, only 8% of patients with DCM display borderline myocarditis [167]. However, using immunohistochemistry to identify inflammatory mononuclear cells, up to 38% of biopsy samples reveal pathologically increased levels of lymphocytic infiltration with activation markers on lymphocytes, macrophages, and endothelial cells, suggesting that the immunopathological process is still active in a significant number of DCM patients [168]. Several studies have demonstrated circulating autoantibodies in the sera of patients with DCM, that are directed against heart proteins such as actin, cardiac myosin α- and β-chains, laminin, collagen, adenine nucleotide mitochondrial translocator, branched-chain α-ketoacid dehydrogenase, $\beta_1$-adrenergic receptor, and muscarinic receptor [169–173]. Even though some of the antireceptor or antienzyme antibodies may be functional (e.g. the anti-$\beta_1$-adrenoreceptor, antimuscarinic receptor, and antiadenine nucleotide translocator antibodies), only antibodies to human α-cardiac myosin heavy chain are considered to be organ and disease specific, since this protein is not expressed outside the myocardium and its autoantibodies are present in DCM patients but not in controls with ischaemic heart disease [174–176]. Cardiac myosin-specific autoantibodies were found in sera from 26% of DCM patients, and recognition was directed to α- and β-cardiac myosin heavy chains [177]. A murine anticoxsackievirus B4 monoclonal antibody identified a putative shared epitope in residues 1632–1647 of murine cardiac myosin heavy chain, suggesting a possible role for molecular mimicry in the genesis of the antiheart response [178].

The pathogenic importance in humans of humoral autoimmune responses in myocarditis and DCM remains to be established, as autoantibody generation may be secondary to tissue damage caused by another event. In any case, autoantibody generation in DCM signals the presence of potentially pathogenic $CD4^+$ T-cells of similar specificity. Cardiac myosin-specific T-cells were not detected in the peripheral blood of DCM patients, and the authors suggested that myosin-specific T-cells could be sequestered into the heart, or under the effect of suppression, associated to other antigens in DCM patients [179]. Nevertheless, it has been reported that passive transfer of peripheral blood lymphocytes from myocarditis patients can induce heart lesions in immunodeficient *SCID* mice [180].

Chronic myocarditis can be induced in susceptible mouse strains (sharing the A/J genetic background) by infection with coxsackievirus B3 [163]. This virus-induced chronic myocarditis resembles some features of DCM; specifically, susceptible mouse strains developing chronic myocarditis also have anticardiac myosin heavy-chain IgG autoantibodies [163]. The late myocarditis induced by coxsackievirus B3 in mice is characterized by a significant inflammatory response and infiltration of virus-specific inflammatory or $T_1$-type T-cells. Non-myocardiogenic viral strains induce $T_2$-type cytokine responses [181], but concomitant administration of IL-1 or IL-2 with the virus restores the susceptible phenotype. When coxsackievirus B3-infected mice with and without myocarditis received a syngeneic heterotopic cardiac transplant, hearts transplanted to myocarditis-positive recipients also developed myocarditis in the absence of viral RNA, further stressing the autoimmune nature of lesions [182]. Immunization of mouse strains susceptible to CB3-induced late myocarditis with cardiac myosin induces a similar late myocarditis [134]. $CD4^+$ T-cells, but not IgG antibodies from a myosin-immunized animal, can transfer myocarditis to a naive syngeneic mouse, thus defining myosin-induced myocarditis as a T-cell-mediated, organ-specific autoimmune disease [183]. Neu and colleagues [166] dissected the requirements for disease induction in the myosin-induced myocarditis-A/J mouse model. Using monoclonal antibody depletion or targeted gene disruption, it was found that $CD4^+$ and $CD8^+$ T-cells play a pathogenic role at the initiation phase, but $CD8^+$ T-cells cause significant tissue damage in established disease; $CD8^+$ T-cells also play a regulatory role. The development of myosin-induced myocarditis is under multigenic control by both MHC and non-MHC genes [134]. In the A/J and BALB/c murine models, immunization with peptides derived from α-cardiac myosin (which is heart specific) was more efficient in the induction of myocarditis than β-cardiac myosin peptides (which are also expressed in slow-twich striated muscle and are about 95% identical to α-cardiac myosin) [184, 185]. The applicability of these findings to humans is more difficult since α-cardiac myosin is the dominant isoform in ventricles of small mammals but is scarce in human ventricles [186].

Inflammatory cytokines, including TNF, seem to play important roles in inflammatory and autoimmune disease states. Blockade of TNF-α with monoclonal antibodies aborts myosin-induced myocarditis [166]. Mice lacking expression of the TNF receptor p55 (TNFR-p55) do not develop myocarditis after myosin immunization, and $CD4^+$ T-cells from a myosin-immunized animal cannot transfer myocarditis to syngeneic TNFR-p55-deficient mice [166]. Conversely, transgenic mice with heart-specific overexpression of TNF-α develop an inflammatory dilated cardiomyopathy, consistent with the known cardioinhibitory effect of this cytokine [187]. These data suggest that TNF-α blockade inhibits, and TNF-α hyperexpression exacerbates, the upregulation of MHC class II expression in heart macrophages, necessary for presentation of cardiac myosin peptides in the heart to $CD4^+$ T-cells in myosin-induced carditis. Moreover, TNF-α (along with other inflammatory cytokines) increases expression of iNOS in macrophages and cardiomyocytes, resulting in the synthesis of NO, which is cytotoxic to cardiomyocytes [188, 189]. In myosin-induced myocarditis, iNOS expression is high in the inflamed heart [190]. Macrophages from mice genetically deficient in IRF-1, the crucial transcription factor for iNOS, are unable to release NO and do not develop myosin-induced myocarditis [166]. These results may have a bearing on the pathogenesis of human DCM, since TNF-α is detectable in plasma and heart tissue of DCM patients [191–193], and iNOS can be detected in human DCM heart tissue [194, 195].

## Immunogenetic factors and susceptibility

Up to 25% of cases of DCM are familial. Clinical parameters such as gender, age of onset, and severity have been reported to be indistinguishable between familial and non-familial cases, antiheart and anticardiac myosin autoantibodies are also found in familial cases. The reported incidence of autoantibodies is higher among familial DCM (24%) than non-familial (15%) DCM [196].

Given the important role of the HLA system in the control of specific immune responses (see p. 423) several investigators studied a possible role of HLA polymorphism in the susceptibility to DCM, comparing the frequency of HLA alleles between patient and control groups. HLA-DR4 was more common in DCM patients from North America, France, and Northern Italy [197–203], but a geographical association was weak and several other studies did not confirm it [204, 205]. A British study reported that even though frequencies of HLA-DR4 among DCM patients and controls were similar, DR4 was significantly more common is familial than in non-familial cases, and was associated with two-thirds of the families at risk for DCM [206]. A role for HLA-DQ alleles was postulated by other studies in North America [207], Italy [204], and Japan [208]; the DR4-DQ4 haplotype was reported to be significantly associated with DCM [202]. It is likely that ethnic variation among different patient groups may have played a role in the different results reported. The relatively small sample number in most studies (below 50 patients) may also explain the discordant results. Other authors searched for a possible association between the presence of a given HLA allele or molecule and an antiheart immune response. Circulating antibodies against the β-adrenergic receptor have been associated with the presence of HLA-DR4 alleles [172], whereas no association has been found between circulating immunofluorescence-detected cardiac autoantibodies and HLA-DR antigens [175]. Immunogenetic studies in coxsackievirus B3-induced myocarditis and cardiac myosin-induced myocarditis have shown an important role for the polymorphisms at the MHC loci, TCR-α-chain, and cardiac myosin, which are the essential components of autoimmune recognition in experimental disease [185, 186, 209–211]. Results from experimental models, demonstrating other potentially important loci influencing susceptibility to murine myocarditis/DCM, should bring insights for research in human disease.

In distinct DCM families, disease segregates in autosomal-dominant, autosomal-recessive, or X-linked transmission patterns [212], even though some affected family members may be asymptomatic and only identified by echocardiographic investigation, which indicates incomplete penetrance. Several different gene loci that present mutational variants known to cause hereditary dilated cardiomyopathies have been identified, and this shows that different molecular phenotypes can generate a similar clinical syndrome [213]. It is possible that these 'dilated cardiomyopathy' loci also carry predisposing alleles, perhaps with a milder phenotype or a smaller penetrance, the partial molecular defects of which may generate a 'susceptible' state. According to this hypothesis, carriers of these alleles may have an increased sensitivity to inflammatory or autoimmune myocardial damage, leading to increased cardiomyocyte death or fibrosis after an otherwise trivial inflammatory insult, eventually overwhelming the cardiac reserve, and leading to overt CHF.

## Conclusion and hypothesis: pathogenesis of postinfectious autoimmune disease

Human CCC, RHD, and DCM fulfil many of the criteria for autoimmune diseases postulated by Rose and Bona [2]. The insights obtained from assigning postinfectious autoimmune disease status to such heart disorders may help to unravel the pathogenesis of classical autoimmune diseases in search of a triggering infectious agent. Results in the literature are consistent with the view that infection by *T. cruzi*, *S. pyogenes*, and enterovirus may trigger potentially pathogenic T-cells, as has been postulated for other infectious agents in organ-specific autoimmune diseases [155]. The provision of the initial antigenic stimulus (heart cross-reactive molecule in the pathogen) in the presence of costimulatory signals and IL-12 production, as expected in prototype responses to pathogens, may generate 'experienced', HLA-restricted, antigen-specific, IFN-$\gamma$-producing T-cells that are potentially able to migrate to heart tissue in a large majority of infected individuals. Beyond this stage comes an important checkpoint for the pathogenesis of chronic heart disease: either the pathogen is cleared effectively and the protective immune response refrains from targeting the heart tissue, or chronic inflammation and antibody production continue at a later stage as a consequence of the breakdown of T-cell immunological tolerance to heart antigens, in the presence of a small load of the pathogen or even in its complete absence. Latent viruses that could periodically be activated, systemic, low-grade

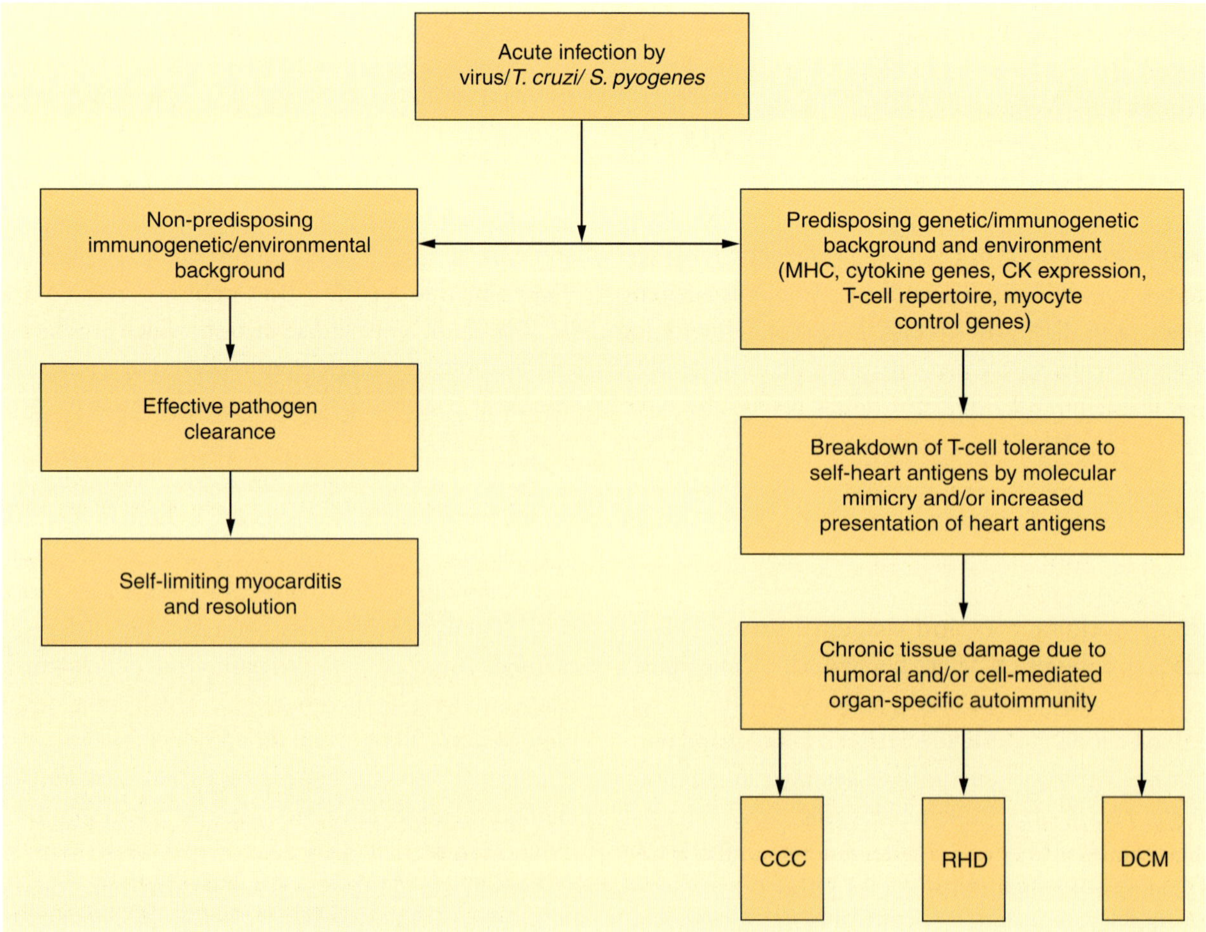


**Figure 24.2** *Final scheme of pathogenic events in postinfectious immunological disorders of the heart.*

*T. cruzi* infection, and streptococcal recolonization of upper respiratory tract are likely to play a role in the maintenance of immunological memory, maintaining the stimuli for the progression of autoimmunity [214]. It can be hypothesized that the generation of a T-cell infiltrate only occurs in a subset of infected individuals whose T-cell receptor repertoire allows cross-reactive recognition of pathogen antigens with immunodominant or major target organ autoantigens, e.g. cardiac myosin in Chagas' heart disease, DCM, and possibly RHD. Furthermore, progression to full pathogenic potential (tissue damage) may be dependent on the cytokine balance and genetic profile of the individual, including genes related to the immune system and heart function (e.g. cytokines, HLA, TCR, and gene loci that have mutational variants that cause dilated cardiomyopathy) [213]. The precise molecular characterization of those steps may allow the accurate diagnosis, prognosis, and therapy of such diseases. A scheme of the pathogenic events in postinfections immunological cardiac disorders is presented in Figure 24.2.

The identification of the relevant autoantigenic target in the three diseases may allow the use of antigen-specific tolerance induction therapy to block the heart lesion process without interfering with the protective immune response against the infectious agent. The $T_1$-type cytokine profile observed in CCC heart lesions, which is probably also present in RHD and DCM, is consistent with a delayed-type hypersensitivity mechanism of tissue damage. This may allow the possibility of using immune deviation therapy (in which cytokines produced in the target organ switch from inflammatory, $T_1$, to anti-inflammatory, $T_2$) in the control of tissue damage in all three diseases. Positive results in immunological blockade of pathogenic T-cell responses in human autoimmune diseases, such as rheumatoid arthritis and autoimmune uveitis, have already been reported using oral tolerance with organ-specific antigens to induce immune deviation [215–217].

## References


1. Smith S, Allen P. Expression of myosin-class II major histocompatibility complexes in the the normal myocardium occurs before induction of autoimune myocarditis. *Proc Natl Acad Sci USA* 1992; 89: 9131–5.
2. Rose NR, Bona C. Defining criteria for autoimmune diseases (Witebsky's postulates revisited). *Immunol Today* 1993; 14: 426–30.
3. Oldstone MBA. Molecular mimicry and autoimmune disease. *Cell* 1990; 50: 819–20.
4. Dajani AS, Ayoub E, Bierman FZ *et al.* Guidelines for the diagnosis of rheumatic fever: Jones criteria, updated 1992. *Circulation* 1993; 87: 302–7.
5. Lancefield RC. Specific relationships of cell composition to biologic activity of hemolytic streptococci. *Harvey Lectures* 1941; 36: 251–65.
6. Shikhman AR, Cunningham MW. Immunological mimicry between *N*-acetyl-β-D-glucosamine and cytokeratin peptides. *J Immunol* 1994; 152: 4375–87.
7. Shikhman AR, Greenspan NS, Cunningham MW. Cytokeratin peptide SFGSGFGGGY mimics *N*-acetyl-β-D-glucosamine in reaction with antibodies and lectins and induces *in vivo* anti-carbohydrate antibody response. *J Immunol* 1994; 153: 5593–606.
8. Manjula BN, Fischetti VA. Tropomyosin-like 7-residue periodicity in three immunologically distinct streptococcal M proteins and its implication for the antiphagocytic property of the molecule. *J Exp Med* 1980; 151: 695–708.
9. Manjula BN, Trus BL, Fischetti VA. Presence of two distinct regions in the coiled-coil structure of the streptococcal PepM5 protein: relationship to mammalian coiled-coil proteins and implications to its biological properties. *Proc Natl Acad Sci USA* 1985; 82: 1064–8.
10. Fishetti V. Streptococcal M protein. *Sci Am* 1991; 264: 32–9.
11. Wannamaker LW. Differences between streptococcal infections of the throat and skin (in two parts). *N Engl J Med* 1970; 282: 23–31, 78–85.
12. Stollerman GH. The changing face of rheumatic fever in the 20th century. *J Med Microbiol* 1998; 47: 1–3.
13. Kujala GA, Doshi H, Brick JE. Rheumatic fever and poststreptococcal glomerulonephritis: a case report (Letter). *Arthritis Rheum* 1989; 32: 236–9.
14. Cheadle WR. Harveian lectures on the various manifestations of the rheumatic state as exemplified in childhood and early life. *Lancet* 1889; 371: 821–7.
15. Wilson MG, Schweitzer M. Pattern of hereditary susceptibility in rheumatic fever. *Circulation* 1954; 10: 699–704.
16. Uchida IA. Possible genetic factors in the etiology of rheumatic fever. *Am J Hum Genet* 1953; 5: 61–9.
17. Taranta A, Torosdag S, Metrakos JD *et al.* Rheumatic fever in monozigotic and dizigotic twins (Abstract). *Circulation* 1959; 20: 788.
18. Glynn IE, Holborow EJ. Relation between blood groups, secretor status and susceptibility to rheumatic fever. *Arthritis Rheum* 1961; 4: 203–7.
19. Patarroyo ME, Winchester RJ, Vejerano A *et al.* Association of a B-cell alloantigen with susceptibility to rheumatic fever. *Nature* 1979; 278: 173–4.
20. Ayoub EM. The search for host determinants of susceptibility to rheumatic fever: the missing link. *Circulation* 1984; 69: 197–201.
21. Gibofsky A, Khanna A, Suh E, Zabriskie JB. The genetics of rheumatic fever: relationship to streptococcal infection and autoimmune disease. *J Rheumatol* 1991; 18 (Suppl 30): 1–13.
22. Zabriskie JB, Lavenchy D, Williams RC Jr *et al.* Rheumatic fever-associated B cell alloantigens as identified by monoclonal antibodies. *Arthritis Rheum* 1985; 28: 1047–51.
23. Ayoub EM, Barrett DJ, MacLaren NK, Krischen JP. Association of class II histocompatibility leukocyte antigens with rheumatic fever. *J Clin Invest* 1986; 77: 2019–26.

24. Anastasiou-Nana M, Anderson JL, Carquist JF, Nanas JN. HLA DR typing and lymphocyte subset evaluation in rheumatic heart disease: a search for immune response factors. *Am Heart J* 1986; 112: 992–7.
25. Rajapakse CNA, Halim K, Al-Orainey L *et al.* A genetic marker for rheumatic heart disease. *Br Heart J* 1987; 58: 659–62.
26. Jhinghan B, Mehra NK, Reddy KS *et al.* HLA, blood groups and secretor status in patients with established rheumatic fever and rheumatic heart disease. *Tissue Antigens* 1986; 27: 172–8.
27. Guilherme L, Weidebach W, Kiss MH *et al.* Association of human leukocyte class II antigens with rheumatic fever or rheumatic heart disease in a Brazilian population. *Circulation* 1991; 83: 1995–8.
28. Weidebach W, Goldberg AC, Chiarella J *et al.* HLA class II antigens in rheumatic fever: analysis of the DR locus by RFLP and oligotyping. *Hum Immunol* 1994; 40: 253–8.
29. Maharaj B, Hammond MG, Appadoo B *et al.* HLA-A, B, DR and DQ antigens in black patients with severe chronic rheumatic heart disease. *Circulation* 1987; 76: 259–61.
30. Olmez U, Turgay M, Ozenirler S *et al.* Association of HLA class I and class II antigens with rheumatic fever in a Turkish population. *Rheumatology* 1992; 22: 49–52.
31. Goldberg AC, Kalil J, Kotb M *et al.* HLA and rheumatic fever: 12th International Histocompatibility Workshop study. In: D Charron (ed.) *HLA: Genetic Diversity of HLA; functional and medical implication.* EDK: Sévres, France, 1997, 413–18.
32. Calveti PA. Autoantibodies in rheumatic fever. *Proc Soc Exp Biol Med* 1945; 60: 379–81.
33. Stollerman GH. Rheumatogenic streptococci and autoimmunity. *Clin Immunol Immunopathol* 1991; 61: 113–42.
34. Kaplan MH, Suchy ML. Immunological relation of streptococcal and tissue antigens. II. Cross-reactions of antisera to mammalian heart tissue with a cell wall constituent of certain strains of group A streptococci. *J Exp Med* 1964; 119: 643–50.
35. Kaplan MH, Svec KH. Immunologic relation of streptococcal antibody cross-reactive with heart tissue: association with streptococcal infection, rheumatic fever and glomerulonephritis. *J Exp Med* 1964; 119: 651–66.
36. Dale JB, Beachey EH. Protective antigenic determinant of streptococcal M protein shared with sarcolemmal membrane protein of human heart. *J Exp Med* 1982: 156: 1165–76.
37. Kingston D, Glynn LE. Anti-streptococcal antibodies reacting with brain tissue. I. Immunofluorescent studies. *Br J Exp Pathol* 1976; 57: 114–28.
38. Bisno AL, Berrios X, Quesney F *et al.* Type-specific antibodies to structurally defined fragments of streptococcal M proteins in patients with acute rheumatic fever. *Infect Immun* 1982; 38: 573–9.
39. Flores A, Johnson DR, Kaplan EL, Wannamaker LW. Factors influencing antibody responses to streptococcal M proteins in humans. *J Infect Dis* 1983; 147: 1–15.
40. Dale JB, Seyer JM, Beachey EH. Type-specific immunogenecity of a chemically synthesized peptide fragment of type 5 streptococcal M protein. *J Exp Med* 1983; 158: 1727–32.
41. Jolivet M, Audibert F, Beachey EH *et al.* Epitope specific immunity elicited by a synthetic streptococcal antigen without carrier or adjuvant. *Biochem Biophys Res Commun* 1983; 117: 359–66.
42. Beachey EH, Tartar A, Seyer JM, Chedid L. Epitope-specific protective immunogenicity of chemically synthesized 13-, 18-, and 23-residue peptide fragments of streptococcal M protein. *Proc Natl Acad Sci USA* 1984; 81(7): 2203–7.
43. Dale JB, Beachey EH. Multiple, heart-cross-reactive epitopes of streptococcal M proteins. *J Exp Med* 1985; 161: 113–22.
44. Dale JB, Beachey EH. Epitopes of streptococcal M proteins shared with cardiac myosin. *J Exp Med* 1985; 162: 583–91.
45. Dale JB, Beachey EH. Localization of protective epitopes of the amino terminus of type 5 streptococcal M protein. *J Exp Med* 1986; 163: 1191–202.
46. Dale JB, Seyer JM. Protective and nonprotective epitopes of chemically synthesized peptides of the $NH_2$-terminal region of type 6 streptococcal M protein. *J Immunol* 1986; 136(6): 2287–92.
47. Dale JB, Beachey EH. Sequence of myosin-crossreactive epitopes of streptococcal M proteins. *J Exp Med* 1986; 164: 1785–90.
48. Sargent SJ, Beachey EH, Corbett CE, Dale JB. Sequence of protective epitopes of streptococcal M proteins shared with cardiac sarcolemmal membranes. *J Immunol* 1987; 139: 1285–90.
49. Goroncy-Bermes P, Dale JB, Beachey EH, Opferkuch W. Monoclonal antibody to human renal glomeruli cross-reacts with streptococcal M protein. *Infect Immun* 1987: 55: 2416–19.
50. Cuningham MW, McCormack JM, Talaber LR *et al.* Human monoclonal antibodies reactive with antigens of the group. A *Streptococcus* and human heart. *J Immunol* 1988; 141: 2760–6.
51. Bronze M, Beachey EH, Dale JB. Protective and heart-crossreactive epitopes located within the $NH_2$ terminus of type 19 streptococcal M protein. *J Exp Med* 1988; 167: 1849–59.
52. Kraus W, Ohyama K, Snyder DS, Beachey EH. Autoimmune sequence of streptococcal M protein shared with the intermediate filament protein, vimentin. *J Exp Med* 1989; 169: 481–92.
53. Kraus W, Seyer JM, Beachey EH. Vimentin-cross-reactive epitope of type 12 streptococcal M protein. *Infect Immun* 1989; 57: 2457–61.
54. Cunningham MW, McCormack JM, Fenderson PG *et al.* Human and murine antibodies cross-reactive with streptococcal M protein and myosin recognize the sequence GLN-LYS-SER-LYS-GLN in M protein. *J Immunol* 1989; 143: 2677–83.
55. Fenderson PG, Fischetti VA, Cunningham MW. Tropomyosin shares immunologic epitopes with group A streptococcal M proteins. *J Immunol* 1989; 142: 2475–81.
56. Kraus W, Dale JB, Beachey EH. Identification of an epitope of type 1 streptococcal M protein that is shared with a 43kDa protein of human mocardium and renal glomeruli. *J Immunol* 1990; 145: 4089–93.
57. Gulizia JM, Cunningham MW, McManus BM. Immunoreactivity of anti-streptococcal monoclonal antibodies to human heart valves. Evidence for multiple cross-reactive epitopes. *Am J Pathol* 1991; 138: 285–301.
58. Vashishtha A, Fischetti VA. Surface-exposed conserved region of the streptococcal M protein induces antibodies cross-reactive with denatured forms of myosin. *J Immunol* 1993; 150: 4693–701.
59. Bronze MS, Dale JB. Epitopes of streptococcal M proteins that evoke antibodies that cross-react with human brain. *J Immunol* 1993; 151: 2820–8.
60. Baird RW, Bronze MS, Kraus W *et al.* Epitopes of group A streptococcal M protein shared with antigens of articular cartilage and synovium. *J Immunol* 1991; 146: 3132–7.

61. Williams RC Jr. Host factors in rheumatic fever and heart disease. *Hosp Pract* 1982; 17(8): 125–38.
62. Raizada V, Williams RC Jr, Chopra P *et al.* Tissue distribution of lymphocytes in rheumatic heart valves as defined by monoclonal anti-T cells antibodies. *Am J Med* 1983: 74: 225–37.
63. Kemeny E, Grieve T, Marcus R *et al.* Identification of mononuclear cells and T cell subsets in rheumatic valvulitis. *Clin Immunol Immunopathol* 1989; 52: 225–37.
64. Gunnar H, Arora R, Williams RC Jr *et al.* Immunofluorescence studies of florid rheumatic Aschoff lesions. *Arthritis Rheum* 1986; 29: 207–11.
65. Chopra P, Narula J, Kumar SA *et al.* Immunohistochemical characterization of Aschoff nodules and endomyocardial inflammatory infiltrates in left atrial appendages from patients with chronic rheumatic heart disease. *Int J Cardiol* 1988; 20: 99–105.
66. Assis RVC, Higuchi ML. New pathological aspects of rheumatic heart disease. *Cardiol Young* 1992; 2: 216–21.
67. Amoils B, Morrison RC, Wadee AA *et al.* Aberrant expression of HLA-DR antigen on valvular fibroblasts from patients with active rheumatic carditis. *Clin Exp Immunol* 1986; 66: 88–94.
68. Bathia R, Narula J, Reddy KS *et al.* Lymphocyte subsets in acute rheumatic fever and rheumatic heart disease. *Clin Cardiol* 1989; 12: 34–8.
69. Bhatnagar PK, Nijhawan R, Prakash K. T cell subsets in acute rheumatic fever, rheumatic heart disease and acute glomerulonephritis cases. *Immunol Lett* 1987; 15: 217–19.
70. Mclaughin JF, Paterson PY, Hartz RS, Embury SH. Rheumatic carditis: *in vitro* responses of peripheral blood leukocytes to heart and streptococcal antigens. *Arthritis Rheum* 1972; 15: 600–8.
71. Read SE, Fischetti VA, Utermohlen V *et al.* Cellular reactivity studies to streptococcal antigens. Migration inhibition studies in patients with streptococcal infections and rheumatic fever. *J Clin Invest* 1974; 54: 439–50.
72. Meric N, Berkel AI. Cellular immunity in children with acute rheumatic fever and rheumatic carditis. *Pediatr Res* 1979; 13: 16–20.
73. Read SE, Reid HFM, Fischetti VA *et al.* Serial studies on the cellular immune response to streptococcal antigens in acute and convalescent rheumatic fever patients in Trinidad. *J Clin Immunol* 1986; 6: 433–41.
74. Gray ED, Wannamaker LW, Ayoub E, El Kholy A. Cellular immune responses to extracellular streptococcal products in rheumatic heart disease. *J Clin Invest* 1981; 68: 665–71.
75. Gross WL, Schlaak M. Modulation of human lymphocyte functions by group A streptococci. *Clin Immunol Immunopathol* 1984; 32: 234–47.
76. El-Demellawy M, El-Ridi R, Guirguis NI *et al.* Preferential recognition of human myocardial antigens by T lymphocytes from rheumatic heart disease patients. *Infect Immun* 1997; 65: 2197–205.
77. Dale JB, Simpson WA, Ofek I, Beachey E. Blastogenic responses of human lymphocytes to structurally defined polypeptide fragments of streptococcal M protein. *J Immunol* 1981; 126: 1499–505.
78. Kotb M, Courtney HS, Dale JB, Beachey EH. Cellular and biochemical responses of human T lymphocytes stimulated with streptococcal M proteins. *J Immunol* 1989; 142: 966–70.
79. Yoshinaga M, Figueiroa F, Wahid MR *et al.* Antigenic specificity of lymphocytes isolated from valvular specimens of rheumatic fever patients. *J Autoimmun* 1995; 8: 601–13.
80. Guilherme L, Cunha-Neto E, Coelho V *et al.* Human — infiltrating T cell clones from rheumatic heart disease patients recognize both streptococcal and cardiac proteins. *Circulation* 1995; 92: 415–20.
81. Zabriskie JB. T-cells and T-cell clones in rheumatic fever valvulitis. Getting to the heart of the matter? *Circulation* 1995; 92: 281–2.
82. Pruksakorn S, Galbraith A, Houghten RA, Good MF. Conserved T and B cell epitopes on the M protein of group A streptococci. *J Immunol* 1992; 149: 2729–35.
83. Pruksakorn S, Currie B, Brandt E *et al.* Identification of T cell autoepitopes that cross-react with the C-terminal segment of the M protein of group A streptococci. *Intern Immunol* 1994; 6: 1235–44.
84. Cunningham MW, Antone SM, Smart M *et al.* Molecular analysis of human cardiac myosin-cross-reactive B and T-cell epitopes of the group A streptococcal M5 protein. *Infect Immun* 1997; 65: 3913–23.
85. Manjula BN, Acharya AS, Mische MS *et al.* The complete amino acid sequence of a biologically active 197-residue fragment of M protein isolated from type 5 group A streptococci. *J Biol Chem* 1984; 259: 3686–93.
86. Miller LC, Gray ED, Beachey EH, Kehoe MA. Antigenic variation among group A streptococcal M proteins: nucleotide sequence of the serotype 5 M protein gene and its relationship with genes encoding types 6 and 24 M proteins. *J Biol Chem* 1988; 263: 5668–73.
87. Robinson JH, Atherton MC, Goodacre JA *et al.* Mapping T-cell epitopes in group A streptococcal type 5 M protein. *Infect Immun* 1991; 59: 4324–31.
88. Tomai M, Kotb M, Majumdar G, Beachey EH. Superantigenicity of streptococcal M protein. *J Exp Med* 1990; 172: 359–62.
89. Tomai MA, Schlievert PM, Kotb M. Distinct T-cell receptor Vβ gene usage by human T lymphocytes stimulated with the streptococcal pyrogenic exotoxins and pep M5 protein. *Infect Immun* 1992; 60: 701–5.
90. Watanabe-Ohnishi R, Aelion J, Legros L *et al.* Characterization of unique human TCR Vb specificities for a family of streptococcal superantigens represented by rheumatogenic serotypes of M protein. *J Immunol* 1994; 152: 2066–73.
91. Tomai MA, Aelion J, Dockter ME *et al.* T cell receptor V gene usage by human T cells stimulated with the superantigen streptococcal M protein. *J Exp Med* 1991; 174: 285–8.
92. Wang B, Schlievert PM, Gaber AO, Kotb M. Localization of an immunologically functional region of the streptococcal superantigen pepsin-extracted fragment of type 5 M protein. J Immunol 1993; 151: 1419–29.
93. Degnan B, Taylor J, Hawkes C *et al.* Streptococcus pyogenes type 5M protein is an antigen, not a superantigen, for human T cells. *Hum Immunol* 1997; 53: 206–15.
94. Fleischer B, Schmidt KH, Gerlach D, Kohler W. Separation of T cell stimulating activity from streptococcal M protein. *Infect Immun* 1992; 1767–70.
95. Li PLL, Tiedemann RE, Moffat LS, Fraser JD. The superantigen streptococcal pyrogenic exotoxin C (SPE-C) exhibits a novel mode of action. *J Exp Med* 1997; 186: 375–91.

96. Morris K, Mohan C, Wahi PL *et al.* Enhancement of Il-1, Il-2 production and Il-2 receptor generation in patients with acute rheumatic fever and active rheumatic heart disease: a prospective study. *Clin Exp Immunol* 1993; 91: 429–36.

96a. Guiherme L, Oshiro SE, Faé KC *et al.* T cell reactivity against streptococcal antigens in the periphery mirrors reactivity of heart infiltrating T lymphocytes in rheumatic heart disease patients. *Infect Immun* (in press), 2001.

96b. Guiherme L, Dulphy N, Douay C *et al.* Molecular evidence for antigen-driven immune responses in cardiac lesions of rheumatic heart disease patients. *Int Immunol* 2000; 12: 1063–74.

97. Narin N, Kutukculer N, Ozyurek R *et al.* Lymphocyte subsets and plasma Il-1 alpha, Il-2 and TNF-alpha concentrations in acute rheumatic fever and chronic rheumatic heart disease. *Clin Immunol Immunopathol* 1995; 77: 172–6.

98. Samsonov MY, Tilz GP, Pisklakov VP *et al.* Serum soluble receptors for tumor necrosis factor-alpha and interleukin-2, and neopterin in acute rheumatic fever. *Clin Immunol Immunopathol* 1995; 74: 31–4.

99. Miller LC, Gray ED, Mansour M *et al.* Cytokines and immunoglobulin in rheumatic heart disease: production by blood and tonsilar mononuclear cells. *J Rheumatol* 1989; 16: 1436–42.

100. Dos Reis GA, Gaspar MIC, Barcinski MA. Immune recognition in the streptococcal carditis of mice: the role of macrophages in the generation of heart-reactive lymphocytes. *J Immunol* 1982; 128: 1514–21.

101. Huber AS, Cunningham MW. Streptococcal M protein peptide with similarity to myosin induces $CD4^+$ T cell-dependent myocarditis in MRL/++ mice and induces partial tolerance against coxsackieviral myocarditis. *J Immunol* 1996; 156: 3528–34.

102. Beachey EH, Seyer JM, Dale JB. Protective immunogenecity and T lymphocyte specificity of a trivalent hybrid peptide containing $NH_2$-terminal sequences of types 5, 6 and 24 M proteins synthesized in tandem. *J Exp Med* 1987; 166: 647–56.

103. Bessen D, Fischetti VA. Influence of intranasal immunization with synthetic peptides corresponding to conserved epitopes of M protein on mucosal colonization by goup A streptococci. *Infect Immun* 1988; 565: 2666–72.

104. Bessen D, Fischetti VA. Passive acquired mucosal immunity to group A streptococci by secretory immunoglobulin A. *J Exp Med* 1988; 167: 1945–9.

105. Bessen D, Fischetti VA. Synthetic peptide vaccine against mucosal colonization by group A streptococci. I. Protection against a heterologous M serotype with shared C repeated region epitopes. *J Immunol* 1990; 145: 1251–6.

106. Dale JB, Chang EC. Intranasal immunization with recombinant group A streptococcal M fragment fused to the B subunit of *Escherichia coli* labile toxin protects mice against systemic challenge infections. *J Infect Dis* 1995; 171: 1038–41.

107. Pruksakorn S, Currie B, Brandt ER *et al.* Towards a vaccine for rheumatic fever: identification of a conserved target epitope on M protein of group A streptococci. *Lancet* 1994; 344: 639–42.

108. Brandt ER, Hayman WA, Currie B *et al.* Human antibodies to the conserved region of the M protein: opsonization of heterologous strains of group A streptococci. *Vaccine* 1997; 15: 1805–12.

109. Macêdo V. Chagas' disease (American trypanosomiasis) In: JB Wyngaarden, LH Smith (eds) *Cecil textbook of medicine*. 16th edition. Philadelphia, PA: WB Saunders, 1982, 1728–31.

110. Barretto AC, Arteaga E, Mady C *et al.* Male sex. Prognostic factor in Chagas' disease. *Arq Bras Cardiol* 1993; 60: 225–7.

111. Freitas HFG, Mansur A, Cuoco MAR *et al.* Chagas' disease as an etiology of severe heart feilure with a worse prognosis. *Circulation* 1998: 94: 803.

112. Teixeira A, Cunha-Neto E, Rizzo LV, Silva R. Trypanocidal nitroarene treatment of experimental *T. cruzi* infection does not prevent progression of chronic heart disease. *J Infectious Dis* 1990; 162: 1420.

113. Higuchi ML, De Morais CF, Pereira Barreto AC *et al.* The role of active myocarditis in the development of heart failure in chronic Chagas' disease: a study based on endomyocardial biopsies. *Clin Cardiol* 1987; 10: 665–70.

114. Higuchi ML, Gutierrez PS, Aiello VD *et al.* Immunohistochemical characterization of infiltrating cells in human chronic chagasic myocarditis: comparison with myocardial rejection process. *Virchows Archiv A. Pathol Anat* 1993; 423: 157–60.

115. Higuchi ML, De Brito T, Reis MM *et al.* Correlation between *T. cruzi* parasitism and myocardial inflammatory infiltrate in human chronic chagasic myocarditis: light microscopy and immunohistochemical findings. *Cardiovasc Pathol* 1993; 2: 101–6.

116. Jones EM, Coley DG, Tostes S *et al.* Amplification of a *Trypanosoma cruzi* DNA sequence from inflammatory lesions in human chagasic cardiomyopathy. *Am J Trop Med Hyg* 1993; 48: 348–57.

116a. Anez N, Carrasco H, Parada H *et al.* Myocardial parasite persistence in chronic chagasic patients. *Am J Trop Med Hyg* 1999; 60: 726–32.

117. Chocair PR, Amato-Neto V, Sabbaga E, Torrecillas PH. Aspectos clinico-diagnósticos relativos à fase aguda da doenca de Chagas, em pacientes submetidos a transplante de rim e imunodeprimidos. *Rev Soc Bras Med Trop* 1985; 18: 43–5.

118. Vazquez MC, Riarte A, Pattin M, Lauricella M. Chagas' disease can be transmitted through kidney transplantation. *Transplant Proc* 1993; 25: 3259–60.

119. Andrade Z. Anatomia Patológica da Doença de Chagas. *Rev Goiana Med* 1958; 4: 103–19.

120. Cossio PM, Laguens RP, Diez C *et al.* Chagasic cardiopathy. Demonstration of a serum gamma globulin factor which reacts with endocardium and vascular structures. *Circulation* 1974; 50: 1252–9.

121. Khoury EL, Diez C, Cossio *et al.* Heterophil nature of EVI antibody in *Trypanosoma cruzi* infection. *Clin Immunol Immunopathol* 1983; 27: 283–8.

122. Santos-Buch CA, Acosta AM, Zweerink HJ *et al.* Primary muscle disease: definition of a 25 kDa polypeptide myopathic specific Chagas antigen. *Clin Immunol Immunopathol* 1985; 37: 334–50.

123. Snary D, Flint JE, Wood JN *et al.* A monoclonal antibody with specificity for *Trypanosoma cruzi*, central and peripheral neurons and glia. *Clin Exp Immunol* 1983; 54: 617–24.

124. Wood JN, Hudson L, Jessel TM *et al.* A monoclonal antibody defining antigenic determinants on subpopulations of human neurons and *Trypanosoma cruzi* parasites. *Nature* 1982; 296: 34–8.

125. Petry K, Eisen H. Chagas disease: a model for the study of autoimmune diseases. *Parasitol Today* 1989; 5: 111–16.

126. Van Voorhis W, Schelekewy L and Trong H. Molecular mimicry by *Trypanosoma cruzi*: the F1-160 epitope that mimics mammalian nerve can be mapped to a 12-aminoacid peptide. *Proc Natl Acad Sci USA* 1991; 88: 5993–7.

127. Levin MJ, Mesri E, Benarous R *et al.* Identification of major *Trypanosoma cruzi* antigenic determinants in chronic Chagas' heart disease. *Am J Trop Med Hyg* 1989; 41: 530–8.
128. Bonfá E, Viana VS, Barreto AC *et al.* Autoantibodies in Chagas' disease: an antibody cross-reactive with human and *Trypanosoma cruzi* ribosomal proteins. *J Immunol* 1993; 150: 3917–23.
129. Kerner N, Liegeard P, Levin MJ *et al. Trypanosoma cruzi*: antibodies to MAP-like protein in chronic Chagas' disease cross-react with mammalian cytoskeleton. *Exp Parasitol* 1991; 73: 451–9.
130. Ferrari I, Levin MJ, Wallukat G *et al.* Molecular mimicry between the immunodominant ribosomal protein PO of *Trypanosoma cruzi* and a functional epitope on the human β1-adrenergic receptor. *J Exp Med* 1995; 182: 59–65.
131. Cunha-Neto E, Duranti M, Gruber A *et al.* Autoimmunity in Chagas' disease cardiopathy: biological relevance of a cardiac myosin-specific epitope crossreactive to an immunodominant *Trypanosoma cruzi* antigen. *Proc Natl Acad Sci USA* 1995; 92: 3541–5.
132. Senecal JL, Ichiki S, Girard D, Raymond Y. Autoantibodies to nuclear lamins and to intermediate filament proteins: natural, pathologic or pathogenic? *J Rheumatol* 1993; 20: 211–19.
133. Ribeiro-dos-Santos R, Rossi MA, Laus JL *et al.* Anti-CD4 treatment abrogates rejection and reestablishes long-term tolerance to syngeneic newborn hearts grafted in mice chronically infected with *Trypanosoma cruzi*. *J Exp Med* 1992; 175: 29–39.
134. Neu N, Rose N, Beisel K *et al.* Cardiac myosin infuces myocaritios in genetically predisposed mice. *J Immunol* 1987; 139: 3630–6.
135. Rizzo LV, Cunha-Neto E, Teixeira A. Specific inhibition of reactivity of $CD4^+$ T cells against myosin in mice chronically infected with *Trypanosoma cruzi*. *Infect Immun* 1989; 57: 2640–4.
136. Tibbetts RS, McCormick TS, Rowland EC *et al.* Cardiac antigen-specific autoantibody production is associated with cardiomyopathy in *Trypanosoma cruzi*-infected mice. *J Immunol* 1994; 152: 1493–9.
137. Gruber A, Zingales B. *Trypanosoma cruzi*: characterization of two recombinant antigens with potential application in the diagnosis of Chagas' disease. *Exp Parastiol* 1993; 76: 1–12.
138. Cunha-Neto E, Coelho V, Guilherme L *et al.* Autoimmunity in Chagas' disease: identification of cardiac myosin-B13 *Trypanosoma cruzi* protein crossreactive T cell clones in heart lesions of a chronic Chagas' cardiomyopathy patient. *J Clin Invest* 1996; 98: 1709–12.
139. Abel LCJ, Kalil J, Cunha-Neto E. Molecular mimicry between cardiac-myosin and *Trypanosoma cruzi*-antigen B13: identification of a B13-driven human T cell clone that recognizes cardiac myosin. *Braz J Med Biol Res* 1997; 30: 1305–8.
140. Camargo MM, Almeida IC, Pereira ME *et al.* Glycoconjugates isolated from *Trypanosoma cruzi* but not from *Leishmania* species membranes trigger nitric oxide synthesis as well as microbicidal activity in IFN-gamma-primed macrophages. *J Immunol* 1997; 158: 5890–901.
141. Aliberti JC, Cardoso MA, Martins GA *et al.* Interleukin-12 mediates resistance to *Trypanosoma cruzi* in mice and is produced by murine macrophages in response to live trypomastigotes. *Infect Immun* 1996; 64: 2381–6.
142. Frosch S, Kraus S, Fleischer B. *Trypanosoma cruzi* is a potent inducer of interleukin-12 production in macrophages. *Med Microbiol Immunol (Berl)* 1996; 185: 189–93.
143. Torrico F, Heremans H, Rivera MT *et al.* Endogenous IFN-gamma is required for resistance to acute *Trypanosoma cruzi* infection in mice. *J Immunol* 1991; 146: 362–32.
144. Cardillo F, Voltarelli JC, Reed SG, Silva JS. Regulation of *Trypanosoma cruzi* infection in mice by gamma interferon and interleukin 10: role of NK cells. *Infect Immun* 1996; 64: 128–34.
145. Munoz-Fernandez MA, Fernandez MA, Fresno M. Synergism between tumor necrosis factor-alpha and interferon-gamma on macrophage activation for the killing of intracellular *Trypanosoma cruzi* through a nitric oxide-dependent mechanism. *Eur J Immunol* 1992; 22: 301–7.
146. Silva JS, Vespa GN, Cardoso MA *et al.* Tumor necrosis factor alpha mediates resistance to *Trypanosoma cruzi* infection in mice by inducing nitric oxide production in infected gamma interferon-activated macrophages. *Infect Immun* 1995; 63: 4862–7.
147. Abel LCJ, Rizzo LV, Ianni B *et al.* Chronic Chagas' disease cardiomyopathy patients display an increased γ-IFN response to *Trypanosoma cruzi* infection. Journal of Autoimmunity (in press), 2001.
148. Dutra WO, Gollob KJ, Pinto-Dias J *et al.* Cytokine mRNA profile of peripheral blood mononuclear cells isolated from individuals with *Trypanosoma cruzi* chronic infection. *Scand J Immunol* 1996; 45: 79–86.
149. Arnholdt ACV, Piuvezam MR, Russo DM *et al.* Analysis and partial epitope mapping of human T cell responses to *Trypanosoma cruzi* cysteinyl proteinase. *J Immunol* 1993; 351: 3171–9.
150. Reis MM, Higuchi ML, Benvenutti LA *et al.* An '*in situ*' quantitative immunohistochemical study of cytokines and IL-2R in chronic human chagasic myocarditis: correlation with the presence of myocardial *T. cruzi* antigens. *Clin Immunol Immunopathol* 1997; 83: 165–72.
151. Cunha-Neto E, Rizzo LV, Albuquerque F *et al.* Cytokine production Profile of heart-infiltrating T cells in Chagas' disease cardiomyopathy. *Braz J Med Biol Res* 1998; 31: 133–7.
152. Reis DD, Jones EM, Tostes S *et al.* Characterization of inflammatory infiltrate in chronic chagasic myocardial lesions: presence of tumor necrosis factor + cells and dominance of granzyme $A^+$, $CD8^+$ lymphocytes. *Am J Trop Med Hyg* 1993; 48: 637–44.
153. Reis DD, Jones EM, Tostes S *et al.* Expression of major histocompatibility complex antigens and adhesion molecules in hearts of patients with chronic Chagas' disease. *Am J Trop Med Hyg* 1993; 49: 192–200.
154. Matzinger P. Tolerance, danger, and the extended family. *Annu Rev Immunol* 1994; 12: 991–1045.
155. Frosch S, Kuntzlin D, Fleischer B. Infection with *Trypanosoma cruzi* selectively upregulates B7-2 molecules on macrophages and enhances their costimulatory activity. *Infect Immun* 1997; 65: 971–7.
156. De Maria R, Gavazzi A, Recalcati F *et al.* Italian Multicenter Cardiomyopathy Study Group: comparison of clinical findings in idiopathic dilated cardiomyopathy in women versus men. *Am J Cardiol* 1993; 72: 580–5.
157. Van Creveld S, DeJager H. Myocarditis in new-borns caused by Coxsackie virus. Clinical and pathological data. *Ann Pediatr* 1956; 48: 1–22.
158. Helin M, Savola J, Lapinleimu K. Cardiac manifestations during a Coxsackie BS epidemic. *BMJ* 1968; iii: 97–9.
159. Cambridge G, MacArthur CG, Waterson AP *et al.* Antibodies to Coxsackie B viruses in congestive cardiomyopathy. *Br Heart J* 1979; 41: 692–6.
160. Keeling PG, Lukaszyk A, Poldniecki J *et al.* A prospective case–control study of antibodies to Coxsackie-B virus in idiopathic dilated myocardiopathy. *J Am Coll Cardiol* 1994; 23: 593–8.

161. Baboonian C, Treasure T. Meta-analysis of association of enterovirus with human heart disease. *Heart* 1997; 78: 539–43.
162. Woodruff JF. Viral myocarditis: a review. *Am J Pathol* 1980; 101: 484.
163. Neu N, Beisel KW, Traystman MD *et al.* Autoantibodies specific for the cardiac myosin isoform are found in mice susceptible to coxsackie B3-induced myocarditis. *J Immunol* 1987; 138: 2488–92.
164. Cohen JI. Enteroviruses and reoviruses. In: Fauci, Braunwald, Isselbacher (eds) *Harrison's principles of internal medicine*. 14th edition. New York: McGraw Hill, 1997.
165. Liu P. Cardiomyopathies and myocarditis: the molecular era has arrived. *Curr Opin Cardiol* 1995; 10: 289–92.
166. Penninger JM, Neu N, Bachmaier K. A genetic map of autoimmune disease. *Immunologist* 1996; 4: 76.
167. Kawai C, Matsumori A, Fujiwara H. Myocarditis and dilated cardiomyopathy. *Ann Ver Med* 1987; 38: 221–39.
168. Kühl U, Noutsias M, Schultheiss H-P. Immunohistochemistry in dilated cardiomyopathy. *Eur Heart J* 1995; 16 (Suppl O): 100–6.
169. Maisch B. Autoreactivity to the cardiac myocyte, connective tissue and the extracellular matrix in heart disease and postcardiac injury. *Springer Semin Immunopathol* 1989; 11: 369–97.
170. Neumann DA, Burek CL, Baughman KL, Rose NR. Circulating heart-reactive antibodies in patients with myocarditis and cardiomyopathy. *J Am Coll Cardiol* 1990; 16: 839–46.
171. Fu LXM, Magnusson Y, Bergh C-H *et al.* Localization of a functional autoimmune epitope of second extracellular loop of the human muscarinic receptor in patients with idiopathic dilated cardiomyopathy. *J Clin Invest* 1993; 91: 1964–8.
172. Limas CJ, Limas C, Kubo SH, Olivari MT. Anti-beta-receptor antibodies in human dilated cardiomyopathy and correlation with HLA-DR antigens. *Am J Cardiol* 1990; 65: 483–7.
173. Magnusson Y, Marullo S, Hoyer S *et al.* Mapping of a functional autoimmune epitope on the beta 1-adrenergic receptor in patients with idiopathic dilated cardiomyopathy. *J Clin Invest* 1990; 86: 1658–63.
174. Caforio ALP, Baboonian C, McKenna WJ. Postviral autoimmune heart disease — fact or fiction? *Eur Heart J* 1997; 18: 1051–5.
175. Caforio ALP, Bauce B, Boffa GM *et al.* Autoimmunity in myocarditis and dilated cardiomyopathy: cardiac autoantibody frequency and clinical correlates in a patient series from Italy. *G Ital Cardiol* 1997; 27: 106–12.
176. Caforio ALP, Bonifacio E, Stewart JT *et al.* Novel organ-specific circulating cardiac autoantibodies in dilated cardiomyopathy. *J Am Coll Cardiol* 1990; 15: 1527–34.
177. Caforio ALP, Grazzini M, Mann JM *et al.* Identification of alpha and beta-cardiac myosin heavy chain isoforms as major autoantigens in dilated cardiomyopathy. *Circulation* 1992; 85: 1734–42.
178. Beisel KW, Srinivasappa J, Prabhakar BS. Identification of a putative shared epitope between Coxsackie virus B4 and alpha cardiac myosin heavy chain. *Clin Exp Immunol* 1991; 86: 49–55.
179. Bromelow KV, Souberbelle B, Alavi A *et al.* Lack of T cell response to cardiac myosin and a reduced T cell response to PPD in patients with idiopathic dilated cardiomyopathy. *J Autoimmun* 1997; 10: 219–27.
180. Schwimmbeck PL, Badorff C, Schultheiss HP, Strauer BE. Transfer of human myocarditis into severe combined immunodeficiency mice. *Circ Res* 1994; 75: 156–64.
181. Huber SA, Polgar J, Schultheiss P, Schwimmbeck P. Augmentation of pathogenesis of coxsackie B3 infections in mice by exogenous administration of interleukin-1 and interleukin-2. *J Virol* 1994; 68: 195–206.
182. Nakamura H, Yamamura T, Umemoto S *et al.* Autoimmune response in chronic ongoing myocarditis demonstrated by heterotopic cardiac transplantation in mice. *Circulation* 1996; 94: 3348–54.
183. Smith SC, Allen PM. Myosin-induced acute myocarditis is a T cell mediated disease. *J Immunol* 1991; 147: 2141–7.
184. Donermeyer DL, Beisel KW, Allen PM, Smith SC. Myocarditis-inducing epitope of myosin binds constitutively and stably to I-Ak on antigen-presenting cells in the heart. *J Exp Med* 1995; 182: 1291–300.
185. Pummerer CL, Luz K, Grässi G *et al.* Identification of cardiac myosin peptides capable of inducing autoimmune myocarditis in BALB/C mice. *J Clin Invest* 1996; 97: 2057–62.
186. Beisel KW. Immunogenetic basis of myocarditis: role of fibrillary antigens. *Springer Semin Immunopathol* 1989; 11: 31–42.
187. Kubota T, McTiernan CF, Frye CS *et al.* Cardiac-specific overexpression of tumor necrosis factor-alpha causes lethal myocarditis in transgenic mice. *J Cardiac Fail* 1997; 3: 117–24.
188. Finkel MS, Oddis CV, Jacob TD *et al.* Negative inotropic effects of cytokines on the heart mediated by nitric oxid. *Science* 1992; 257: 387–9.
189. Roberts AB, Vodovotz Y, Roche NS *et al.* Role of nitric oxide in antagonistic effects of transforming growth factor-beta and interleukin-1 beta on the beating rate of cultured cardiac myocytes. *Mol Endocrinol* 1992; 257: 387–9.
190. Bachmaier K, Neu N, Pummerer C *et al.* iNOS expression and nitrotyrosine formation in the myocardium in response to inflammation is controlled by the interferon regulatory transcription factor-1. *Circulation* 1997; 96: 585–91.
191. Torre-Amione G, Kapadia S, Lee J *et al.* Expression and functional significance of tumor necrosis factor receptors in human myocardium. *Circulation* 1995; 92: 1487–93.
192. Torre-Amione G, Kapadia S, Lee J *et al.* Tumor necrosis factor-$\alpha$ and tumor necrosis factor receptors in failing human heart. *Circulation* 1996; 93(4): 704–11.
193. Doyama K, Fujiwara H, Fukumoto M *et al.* Tumor necrosis factor is expressed in cardiac tissues of patients with heart failure. *Int J Cardiol* 1996; 54: 217–25.
194. DeBelder AJ, Radomski MW, Why HJ *et al.* Nitric oxid synthase activities in human myocardium. *Lancet* 1993; 341: 84–5.
195. DeBelder AJ, Radomski MW, Why HJ *et al.* Myocardial calcium-independent nitric oxid synthase activity is present in dilated myocardiopathy, myocarditis, and post-partum cardiomyopathy but not in ischemic or valvar heart disease. *Br Heart J* 1995; 74: 426–30.
196. Caforio ALP, Goldman JH, Haven AJ *et al.* Evidence for autoimmunity to myosin and other heart-specific autoantigens in patients with dilated cardiomyopathy and their relatives. *J Cardiol* 1995; 54: 157–63.
197. Grant SC, Sheldon S, Dyer PA *et al.* Do specific HLA antigens predispose to ischaemic heart disease or idiopathic dilated cardiomyopathy? *Br Heart J* 1994; 71: 76–8.
198. Carlquist JF, Ward RH, Husebye D *et al.* Major histocompatibility complex class II gene frequencies by serologic and deoxyribonucleic acid genomic typing in idiopathic dilated cardiomyopathy. *Am J Cardiol* 1994; 74: 918–20.

199. Limas CJ, Limas C. HLA antigens in idiopathic dilated cardiomyopathy. *Br Heart J* 1989; 62: 379–83.
200. Komajda M, Raffoux C, Salame E *et al*. HLA A-B and DR in dilated myocardiopathies. *Arch Mal Coeur Vaiss* 1987; 80: 1233–7.
201. Anderson JL, Carlquist JF, Lutz JR *et al*. HLA A, B and DR typing in idiopathic dilated cardiomyopathy: a search for immune response factors. *Am J Cardiol* 1984; 53: 1326–30.
202. Carlquist JF, Menlove RL, Murray MB *et al*. HLA class II (DR and DQ) antigen associations in idiopathic dilated cardiomyopathy. Validation study and meta-analysis of published HLA association studies. *Circulation* 1991; 83: 515–22.
203. Limas CJ. Autoimmunity in dilated cardiomyopathy and the major histocompatibility complex. *Int J Cardiol* 1996; 54: 113–16.
204. Lozano MD, Rubocki RJ, Wilson JE *et al*. Human leukocyte class II associations in patients with idiopathic dilated cardiomyopathy. Myocarditis Trial Investigators. *J Card Failure* 1997; 3: 97–103.
205. Agarwal AK, White AG, Ali M *et al*. HLA antigens in an Omani population with dilated cardiomyopathy. *Int J Cardiol* 1996; 55: 29–32.
206. McKenna CJ, Codd MB, McCann HA, Sugrue DD. Idiopathic dilated cardiomyopathy: familial prevalence and HLA distribution. *Heart* 1997; 77: 549–52.
207. Limas CJ, Limas C. HLA-DR antigen linkage of anti-beta receptor antibodies in idiopathic dilated and ischaemic cardiomyopathy. *Br Heart J* 1992; 67: 402–5.
208. Nishi H, Kimura A, Fukuta S *et al*. Genetic analysis of dilated cardiomyopathy — HLA and immunoglobulin genes may confer susceptibility. *Jpn Circ J* 1992; 56: 1054–61.
209. Liao L, Sindhwani R, Leinwand L *et al*. Cardiac α heavy chains differ in their induction of myocarditis. *J Clin Invest* 1993; 92: 2877–82.
210. Traystman MD, Chow LH, McManus BM *et al*. Susceptibility to Coxsackievirus B3-induced chronic myocarditis maps near the murine TCRα and Myhcα loci on chromosome 14. *Am J Pathol* 1991; 138: 721–6.
211. Malkiel S, Kuan AP, Diamond B. Autoimmunity in heart disease: mechanisms and genetic susceptibility. *Mol Med Today* 1996; 2: 336–42.
212. Goerss JB, Mitchels VV, Burnett J *et al*. Frequency of familial dilated cardiomyopathy. *Eur Heart J* 1995; 16 (Suppl O): 2–4.
213. Schowengerdt KO, Towbin JA. Genetic basis of inherited myocardiopathies. *Curr Opin Cardiol* 1995; 10: 312–21.
214. Zinkernagel RM, Ehl S, Aichele P *et al*. Antigen localisation regulates immune responses in a dose- and time-dependent fashion: a geographical view of immune reactivity. *Immunol Rev* 1997; 156: 199–209.
215. Nussenblatt RB, Gery I, Weiner HL *et al*. Treatment of uveitis by oral administration of retinal antigens: results of a phase I/II randomized masked trial. *Am J Ophthalmol* 1997; 123: 583–92.
216. Barnett ML, Kremer JM, St Clegg DO *et al*. Treatment of rheumatoid arthritis with oral type II collagen. Results of a multicenter, double-blind, placebo-controlled trial. *Arthritis Rheum* 1998; 41: 290–7.
217. Weiner HL. Oral tolerance for the treatment of autoimmune diseases. *Annu Rev Med* 1997; 48: 341–51.

# Alcohol-induced myocardial damage: reversibility and clinical implications



M. BALLESTER, V. MARTÍ, M. PUIG, M. CAMPRECIÓS AND V. BROSSA

## Introduction

The concept that heavy alcohol consumption *per se* can lead to myocardial disease is relatively recent. In Paul Dudley White's textbook, *Heart disease*, published in 1931, there is no mention of alcohol as an aetiological agent in the chapter on the diseases of the myocardium. Rather, alcohol was at that time deemed to be of immense help for the alleviation of angina [1]. In Paul Wood's 1968 textbook *Heart disease*, excessive alcohol consumption is regarded as a precipitating factor of heart failure, and the effects of chronic alcoholism are included in the section on Nutritional cardiomyopathy [2].

Early reports of patients with hyperkinetic heart failure who responded to thiamine administration led to the belief that alcohol exerted its deleterious effect through vitamin deficiency [3, 4]. However, it was only when the nutritional status of most patients with possible alcohol-induced cardiomyopathy was shown not to be impaired that alcohol *per se* started to be considered as a direct toxic agent to the myocardium [5, 6]. That chronic alcohol consumption can lead to depression of cardiac function has been shown by several investigators since the late 1960s [7–13].

Alcohol-induced myocardial disease is expressed in the form of a dilated cardiomyopathy indistinguishable from the morphological and functional features of other myocardial disease, such as idiopathic dilated cardiomyopathy. In fact, the term alcoholic cardiomyopathy was proposed by Brigden in 1977 to describe the possible association between important alcohol consumption and myocardial disease [14]. Alcoholic cardiomyopathy has become the most common cause of non-ischaemic dilated cardiomyopathy in the Western world [15, 16]. The clinical presentations include arrhythmias, hypertension, heart failure, and sudden death [5–13, 17]. Cardiac hypertrophy may be detected in alcoholic patients [18], and the reported association between chronic alcoholism and hypertension could be responsible for this finding [19–21].

Although the effects of alcohol consumption on the heart have been long suspected, no direct evidence that the human myocardium is susceptible to the adverse effects of alcohol is available. Since congestive cardiomyopathy has not been reproduced experimentally, the association between chronic alcoholism and myocardial disease is largely based on epidemiological data [22, 23]. Some authors have expressed their reluctance to admit that alcohol consumption induces cardiotoxicity. The widespread use of alcohol complicates the establishment of a causal relationship between excessive use and cardiac disease.

Analysis of cardiac function has been traditionally undertaken as a clinical and epidemiological research tool to evaluate the effects of acute and chronic consumption of alcohol on the human myocardium. Clinical evidence of the cardiotoxicity of alcohol has been reported in numerous clinical studies of acute alcohol consumption in normals [24–31] and after alcohol withdrawal in chronic drinkers [5, 6, 9–14, 32]. In 1972, Song and Rubin [34] produced muscle damage in healthy volunteers by feeding them daily doses of alcohol for several weeks and inferred that similarities between cardiac and peripheral muscles could make the former susceptible to the toxic effects of alcohol. An elegant clinical study conducted by DeMakis *et al.* in 1974 [32], showed that alcohol withdrawal in alcoholic patients presenting with heart failure was followed by a striking clinical improvement and increased survival rate compared with patients who had not refrained from alcohol, a phenomenon confirmed by other groups [35]. In fact, descriptions of the echocardiographic normalization of left ventricular dysfunction have subsequently been reported after alcohol withdrawal [36, 37]. A direct correlation was reported between the lifetime consumption of alcohol and the degree of impairment of systolic function [6].

Although these and other studies support the idea that alcohol exerts a toxic effect on the human myocardium, evidence of the deleterious effect of alcohol on the human myocardium is at best indirect.

## Detection of myocardial damage

Although no specific pathological features are linked to alcohol-induced heart disease [38], myofibrillar disruption has been described, suggesting the presence of myocardial damage [39, 40]. Non-invasive detection of myocardial damage has been recently become possible by the assessment of the myocardial uptake of the Fab fragments of indium-111-labelled monoclonal antimyosin antibodies injected intravenously. Uptake of these antibodies by the myocardium only occurs when the integrity of the sarcolemma is lost as a result of cell damage and the antibody fragments bind to the exposed myosin to which they have a selective affinity [41–44]. This technique, initially used to detect, locate, and quantitate an acute myocardial infarction [45], has been used for the detection of acute or chronic diffuse myocardial damage in several clinical settings, such as adriamycin-induced cardiotoxicity [46–48], acute myocarditis [49–52], idiopathic dilated cardiomyopathy [53–55], acute cardiac rejection after transplantation [56–60], or diseases secondary to myocardial involvement [61–65]. In some patients, antimyosin imaging allows detection of damage earlier than the myocardial biopsy, the only established invasive method for detecting myocardial cell damage [52, 59, 66]. Semiquantitation of myocardial antibody uptake through the heart-to-lung ratio (HLR) [55] has been shown to correlate directly with the severity of myocardial damage as assessed by endomyocardial biopsy [48, 58]. This method provides a means for assessing both the presence and intensity of myocardial damage *in vivo*, allows comparison between different groups of patients, and may be used to follow the course of cell damage in individual patients [48, 58].

In view of the efficacy of antimyosin antibodies in detecting diffuse myocyte damage, this method was evaluated in patients with possible alcohol-related dilated cardiomyopathy [55, 67]. In a recent series, 56 patients with dilated cardiomyopathy selected on the basis of their significant alcohol consumption (100 g/day of alcohol for over 10 years) were studied with antimyosin antibodies [67]; all were social drinkers and none required psychiatric support. All patients were subjected to gamma imaging 48 h after intravenous injection of antimyosin antibodies labelled with 2.0 mCi of [$^{111}$In]chloride. The magnitude of antimyosin uptake or severity of myocardial damage was determined by calculation of the HLR [50], which provides an estimation of the relative cardiac antibody uptake against the lung as background. A HLR of 1.55 obtained in normal volunteers was used as a cut-off point to differentiate normal from abnormal scans [50, 55, 67].

The 56 patients (mean age 46 years) had consumed a mean of 123 g/day of alcohol for 21 years, with a mean total cumulative lifetime intake of 914 kg. Thirty-six (64%) had a history of chronic (> 1 year) heart disease, whereas the remaining 20 had acute (< 3 months, nine patients) or subacute (3–12 months, 11 patients) disease. Functional class corresponded to the New York Heart Association (NYHA) class II in 27 patients and class III–IV in the remaining 29. The mean left ventricular diastolic diameter in these patients was 71 mm and the ejection fraction was 28%.

According to their drinking habit, these 56 patients were allocated to subgroup of active (28 patients) or past (28 patients) alcohol consumers. Those who admitted alcohol consumption up to the time of the antimyosin study or within the past 3 months were classified as active consumers. Table 25.1 compares the clinical and scintigraphic features of the two groups: antibody uptake was observed in 21 of 28 active alcohol consumers (75%) ver-

**Table 25.1** Clinical features of patients with alcoholic dilated cardiomyopathy according to their drinking habit

| | Active ($n$ = 28) | Past ($n$ = 28) | $p$ |
|---|---|---|---|
| Age (years) | 47 ± 11 | 45 ± 11 | NS |
| Duration of symptoms (months) | 54 ± 59 | 39 ± 37 | NS |
| Symptoms > 1 year | 61% | 68% | NS |
| NYHA | 2.7 ± 0.8 | 2.8 ± 0.8 | NS |
| Alcohol/day (g) | 117 ± 43 | 129 ± 75 | NS |
| Consumption (years) | 22 ± 10 | 22 ± 8 | NS |
| Cumulative alcohol (kg) | 927 ± 483 | 901 ± 480 | NS |
| LV end-diastolic diameter (mm) | 70 ± 10 | 72 ± 10 | NS |
| LV ejection fraction (%) | 28 ± 11 | 29 ± 12 | NS |
| Prevalence of AM uptake | 21/28 (75%) | 9/28 (32%) | < 0.001 |
| Heart-to-lung ratio | 1.75 ± 0.26 | 1.49 ± 0.17 | < 0.0001 |

(From ref. 67 with permission.) Data are means ± SD or $n$ (%). NYHA = New York Heart Association; LV = left ventricular; AM = antimyosin; NS = not significant.

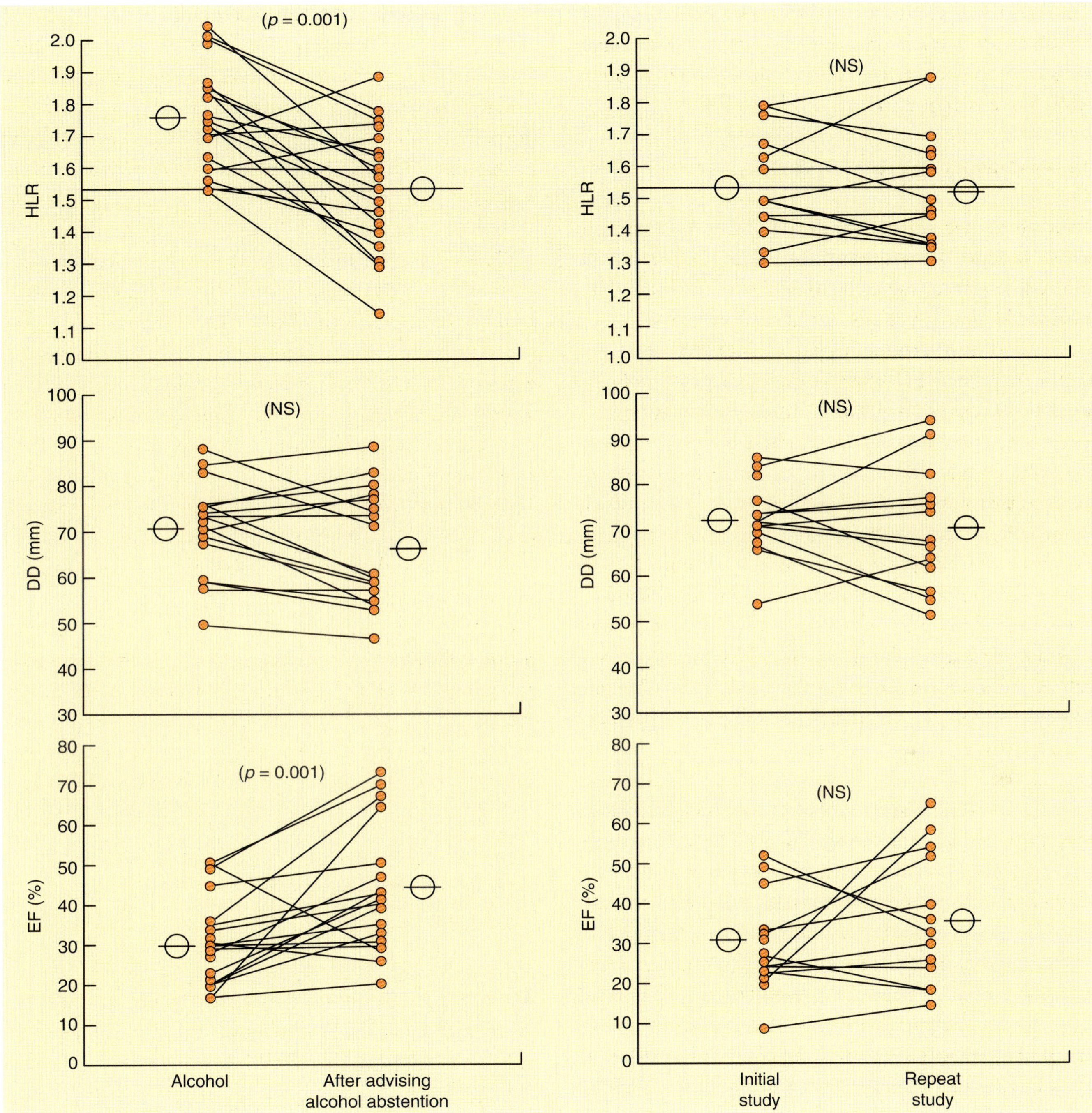


**Figure 25.1** *Repeat antimyosin and echocardiographic studies in patients with alcoholic dilated cardiomyopathy. Left column: patients with active alcohol consumption before and after cessation of drinking. Right column: patients with alcoholic dilated cardiomyopathy and past consumption. In the active group, decrease or disappearence of myocardial uptake of antimyosin antibodies is accompanied by improvement in the ejection fraction. In past consumers, no statistically significant modifications are noted in repeat antimyosin or echocardiographic studies. DD = end-diastolic left ventricular diameter by echocardiography; EF = echocardiographic left ventricular ejection fration; HLR = heart-to-lung ratio of antimyosin antibody uptake. (Reproduced from ref. 67 with permission.)*

sus nine of 28 (32%) past consumers ($p < 0.001$). The intensity of antibody uptake represented as HLR was 1.75 ± 0.26 and 1.49 ± 0.17 ($p < 0.0001$), respectively; an inverse correlation was noted between the interval between cessation of alcohol consumption and antimyosin uptake ($r = -0.37$; $p < 0.01$). The cumulative alcohol consumption did not correlate with left ventricular size, ejection fraction, the severity of myocardial damage.

Nineteen of the 28 active consumers were restudied after a mean of 9 months of cessation of alcohol consumption (Fig. 25.1). A reduction in HLR from 1.76 to 1.55 ($p < 0.001$) was associated with an improvement in the left ventricular ejection fraction (30–43%, $p < 0.001$) but no significant changes were seen in diastolic diameter (71–67 mm). In the 15 past alcohol consumers evaluated 19 months after the initial study, no significant changes were noted in the intensity of antibody uptake (HLR 1.55–1.54), left ventricular diastolic diameter (71–70 mm), or ejection fraction (31–35%).

These results show that, in chronic alcoholics who present with dilated cardiomyopathy, the prevalence and intensity of the myocardial damage are higher in active than in past alcohol consumers. Cessation of alcohol consumption in the former leads to a reduction in or disappearance of damage that parallels an improvement in ejection fraction, while no significant changes occur in patients with a past history of alcoholism and ventricular dysfunction. This suggests that alcohol consumption is the main cause of myocardial damage and ventricular dysfunction in some individuals.

## Idiopathic versus alcohol-related dilated cardiomyopathy

Several authors question whether the idiopathic and alcoholic forms of dilated cardiomyopathy are different entities. The presumed patients catalogued as having alcoholic dilated cardiomyopathy may in fact be individuals with the idiopathic form of the disease who happen to be heavy drinkers. McKenna *et al.* [68] recently presented the results of a case–control study of questionnaires comprising patients with dilated cardiomyopathy, and their findings were compared with a group of randomly selected control subjects. Results showed that significantly more patients with cardiomyopathy consumed alcohol above the recommended limits than the control group. In contrast, in a comparison between 88 patients with dilated cardiomyopathy and 29 patients with possible alcoholic dilated cardiomyopathy, both referred for heart transplantation and with a similar degree of left ventricular dilatation and decreased ejection fraction (Table 25.2), Obrador *et al.* [55] found a lower prevalence and intensity of antimyosin antibody uptake in the alcoholic group. Although phenotypically similar, the idiopathic and alcoholic forms of dilated cardiomyopathy may represent two different entities.

**Table 25.2** Myocardial damage in idiopathic and alcoholic dilated cardiomyopathy

| | Idiopathic ($n$ = 88) | Alcoholic ($n$ = 29) | $p$ |
|---|---|---|---|
| Age (years) | 43 ± 13 | 44 ± 10 | NS |
| Sex (male/female) | 63/25 | 29/0 | 0.001 |
| Onset of disease (months) | 40 ± 47 | 50 ± 54 | NS |
| Acute | 17 (19.3%) | 3 (10.3%) | NS |
| Subacute | 16 (18.1%) | 6 (20.6%) | NS |
| Chronic stable | 39 (44.3%) | 15 (51.7%) | NS |
| Chronic unstable | 16 (18.1%) | 5 (17.2%) | NS |
| NYHA (I–II/III–IV) | 47/41 | 15/14 | NS |
| Alcohol/day (g) | 19 ± 28 | 120 ± 73 | 0.0001 |
| Consumption (years) | 6.2 ± 9.5 | 20.4 ± 7.8 | 0.0001 |
| Cumulative alcohol intake (kg) | 100 ± 158 | 844 ± 451 | 0.0001 |
| LV diastolic diameter (mm) | 71.9 ± 12 | 72 ± 10 | NS |
| LV ejection fraction (%) | 29.3 ± 9 | 29.9 ± 13 | NS |
| Prevalence of AM uptake at initial study | 77% | 48% | 0.003 |
| Heart-to-lung ratio | 1.74 ± 0.27 | 1.62 ± 0.31 | 0.04 |
| | OUTCOME | | |
| Prevalence of AM uptake at initial study | 70% | 35% | 0.01 |
| Heart-to-lung ratio | 1.63 ± 0.19 ($n$ = 43) | 1.46 ± 0.17 ($n$ = 17) | 0.003 |
| Transplantation | 28 (31%) | 4 (13%) | 0.05 |
| Death CHF | 11 (12%) | 3 (10%) | NS |
| Sudden death | 3 (3.4%) | 1 (3.4%) | NS |
| Survivors | 46 (52%) | 21 (72%) | 0.05 |

(From ref. 55 with permission.) Data are means ± SD or $n$ (%).
NYHA = New York Heart Association; LV = left ventricular; AM = antimyosin; CHF = congestive heart failure; NS = not significant.

## Myocardial damage in alcoholic patients without clinical evidence of cardiac involvement

In a recent series, 15 consecutive patients referred to an alcohol detoxication unit who fulfilled the diagnostic criteria for alcoholism were studied with antimyosin antibody imaging [67]. These patients (mean age 36 years) had consumed 156 g/day of alcohol for a mean of 17 years, leading to a total cumulative lifetime consumption of 978 kg of alcohol. Echocardiographic examination disclosed normal left ventricular size and function in all subjects (mean left ventricular diastolic diameter 46 mm and ejection fraction 77%). Antimyosin studies in these patients showed that only 20% had evidence of myocardial uptake of antimyosin

**Table 25.3** Clinical features, alcohol consumption and myocardial damage in alcoholic patients active consuming alcohol with and without associated cardiac disease

| | Cardiomyopathy[a] ($n$ = 28) | Psychiatric ($n$ = 15) | $p$ |
|---|---|---|---|
| Age (years) | 47 ± 11 | 36 ± 4 | < 0.001 |
| Alcohol/day (g) | 117 ± 43 | 156 ± 59 | < 0.02 |
| Consumption (years) | 22 ± 10 | 17 ± 5 | = 0.07 |
| Cumulative doses (kg) | 927 ± 483 | 978 ± 537 | = 0.75 |
| Diastolic diameter (mm) | 70 ± 10 | 46 ± 6 | < 0.001 |
| Ejection fraction (%) | 28 ± 11 | 77 ± 5 | < 0.001 |
| Antimyosin uptake | 21/28 (75%) | 3/15 (20%) | < 0.01 |
| Heart-to-lung ratio | 1.74 ± 0.26 | 1.44 ± 0.17 | < 0.001 |

(From ref. 67 with permission.) Data are means ± SD or $n$ (%).
[a]Patients included are the 28 in group I who actively consumed alcohol at the time of evaluation with antimyosin antibodies.

antibodies; repeat antimyosin studies showed disappearance of antibody uptake in two who refrained from alcohol and its persistence in the remainder who did not.

These results suggest that, (1) myocardial damage can exist without conventional evidence of alcohol-induced heart disease or cardiomyopathy; and (2) not all individuals exposed to high doses of alcohol develop myocardial damage, as three-quarters of the very heavy drinkers had no cardiac damage, as shown by a normal antimyosin scan. A comparison of the clinical, echocardiographic, and isotopic features of active heavy drinkers with and without cardiomyopathy (Table 25.3) revealed a higher age of subjects in the cardiomyopathy group. Years of consumption and the calculated cumulative alcohol intake were similar in both groups, and the prevalence of antimyosin uptake was higher in the cardiomyopathic group ($p < 0.01$). It appears that while almost all patients with alcohol-related dilated cardiomyopathy who actively consume alcohol have myocardial damage, alcohol-related damage is observed in only 20% of patients exposed to similar doses of alcohol, years of consumption, and total cumulative alcohol intake. The explanation for this difference is probably that heavy alcohol consumption does not induce myocardial damage in all individuals. Genetic susceptibility could be responsible, as previously shown in other forms of alcohol-induced disease.

## Effects of acute alcohol ingestion on the myocardium

Studies undertaken to evaluate the effects of acute alcohol consumption on ventricular function in normal individuals have been conflicting. Some suggest that transient left ventricular impairment occurs after drinking alcohol, while others show the inability of acute alcohol ingestion to elicit functional changes [24–31]. The capability of an acute alcohol intake to elicit possible myocardial damage was explored in six young healthy individuals with a mean age of 24 years before and after acute ethanol exposure [67]. Baseline electrocardiogram (ECG), echo-Doppler, and antimyosin antibody studies were performed before and after 3 days of acute alcohol consumption (Table 25.4). The subjects were instructed to consume 1.2 g/kg of ethanol (whiskey diluted in juice to a total of 400 ml) in 30 min (total 3.6 g/kg) every day for 3 consecutive days. On the third day, and 60 min after consumption of the alcohol, ECG and echo-Doppler studies were performed, and antimyosin antibodies were injected.

Upon acute administration of alcohol every subject developed dizziness compatible with mild to moderate acute alcohol toxicity. After 60–109 g of alcohol administration (mean 86 g), blood ethanol concentrations were (mean ± 5D): 18 ± 10, 27 ± 7, 26 ± 4, 23 ± 5, and 22 ± 6 mmol/l at 30, 60, 90, 120, and 150 min, respectively. Creatine kinase, lactate dehydrogenase (LDH), and aldolase blood concentrations remained normal after acute alcohol exposure. No ECG or echo-Doppler changes were noted, except for an increase in the maximum pulmonary velocity ($p <$ 0.05) (Table 25.4). Antimyosin uptake was not detected after ethanol consumption, and HLR was unchanged (1.37 ± 0.1 vs 1.36 ± 0.1) ($p = 0.28$) (Table 25.4). In this study, acute alcohol ingestion was not associated with detectable antimyosin uptake or functional left ventricular changes. It may be that transient alcohol exposure is incapable of inducing such damage or that the individuals in this study were not susceptible to the effects of alcohol.

## Possible relationship of myocardial damage to ventricular systolic function in patients with alcoholic cardiomyopathy

Figure 25.2 shows the hypothetical relationship between myocardial damage and the status of the left ventricular function before and after cessation of alcohol [67]. These constructs are based on variable combinations of myocardial morbid states, including normal myocardium, myocardium that is actively and irreversibly damaged (detected by antimyosin antibodies), reversibly impaired

**Table 25.4** Echo-Doppler and antimyosin studies before and after acute alcohol intake for 3 consecutive days in six healthy volunteers

| | | Doppler parameters | | | | | | | | | | | | |
|---|---|---|---|---|---|---|---|---|---|---|---|---|---|---|
| | | Echocardiographic parameters | | | | Aortic and pulmonary flow parameters | | | | Diastolic parameters | | | | Antimyosin studies |
| Subject | Condition | Heart rate (beats/min) | LVDD (mm) | LVEF (%) | LV mass (g) | MAV (m/s) | MPV (m/s) | AAT (ms) | PAT (ms) | E/A ratio | IVRT (ms) | MDR ($m/s^2$) | TDR ($m/s^2$) | HLR |
| 1 | Basal | 65 | 50 | 69 | 242 | 1.2 | 1.0 | 80 | 110 | 1.33 | 60 | 6.5 | 3.0 | 1.40 |
| | Ethanol | 71 | 47 | 74 | 233 | 1.2 | 1.1 | 90 | 120 | 1.33 | 70 | 4.0 | 2.8 | 1.40 |
| 2 | Basal | 66 | 44 | 77 | 171 | 1.0 | 1.0 | 90 | 150 | 2.00 | 40 | 4.9 | 3.0 | 1.35 |
| | Ethanol | 78 | 42 | 76 | 158 | 1.1 | 1.1 | 90 | 150 | 1.25 | 50 | 5.0 | 3.9 | 1.35 |
| 3 | Basal | 68 | 50 | 82 | 226 | 1.1 | 0.9 | 105 | 140 | 1.40 | 65 | 4.3 | 3.0 | 1.20 |
| | Ethanol | 88 | 48 | 80 | 241 | 1.1 | 1.0 | 110 | 100 | 1.75 | 55 | 4.3 | 3.2 | 1.20 |
| 4 | Basal | 80 | 52 | 58 | 241 | 1.0 | 0.8 | 95 | 140 | 1.25 | 60 | 2.3 | 2.5 | 1.35 |
| | Ethanol | 75 | 52 | 67 | 258 | 1.2 | 0.9 | 110 | 130 | 1.50 | 70 | 2.8 | 2.7 | 1.30 |
| 5 | Basal | 65 | 54 | 70 | 192 | 1.3 | 0.9 | 90 | 130 | 1.40 | 60 | 4.6 | 2.2 | 1.44 |
| | Ethanol | 58 | 50 | 66 | 211 | 1.2 | 0.9 | 90 | 90 | 1.75 | 50 | 3.9 | 2.9 | 1.40 |
| 6 | Basal | 57 | 50 | 76 | 274 | 1.0 | 0.8 | 100 | 140 | 2.25 | 85 | 6.7 | 3.1 | 1.50 |
| | Ethanol | 68 | 51 | 80 | 266 | 1.4 | 1.2 | 100 | 150 | 2.00 | 50 | 4.5 | 3.3 | 1.52 |
| Mean | Basal | 65 | 50 | 72 | 224 | 1.1 | 0.9 | 93 | 135 | 1.60 | 61 | 4.9 | 2.8 | 1.37 |
| | Ethanol | 71 | 48 | 73 | 228 | 1.2 | 1.0* | 98 | 123 | 1.59 | 57 | 4.0 | 3.1 | 1.36 |
| SD | Basal | 10 | 3 | 8 | 37 | 0.1 | 0.8 | 8 | 13 | 0.41 | 14 | 1.6 | 0.3 | 0.10 |
| | Ethanol | 5 | 4 | 6 | 39 | 0.1 | 0.1 | 9 | 25 | 0.28 | 10 | 0.7 | 0.4 | 0.10 |

(From ref. 67 with permission.)

AAT = aortic acceleration time; E/A ratio = peak *E* velocity/peak *A* velocity ratio; HLR = heart-to-lung ratio; IVRT = isovolumetric relaxation time; LV mass = left ventricular mass; LVDD = left ventricular end-diastolic diameter; LVEF = left ventricular ejection fraction; MAV = maximum aortic velocity; MDR = mitral deceleration rate; MPV = maximum pulmonary velocity; PAT = pulmonary acceleration time; TDR = tricuspid deceleration rate. * $p < 0.05$ between basal and after acute alcohol intake values.

myocardium (no antimyosin uptake), and scar tissue due to the myocardial mass lost during ethanol injury. Examples A–D depict four possible outcomes during chronic active alcohol consumption: A, a subgroup of individuals with low susceptibility to alcohol, in whom despite heavy active alcohol intake the ventricular function is normal and no myocardial damage is detected; B, a subgroup of patients with scintigraphic evidence of myocardial damage but normal ventricular function, which could represent early or limited ethanol-induced myocardial damage; C and D, two possible constructs in patients with alcoholic dilated cardiomyopathy and antimyosin uptake which are clinically indistinguishable at the time of consumption. Both present with dilated cardiomyopathy and myocardial damage, but cessation of alcohol consumption reveals an evolution from C to pattern E (recovery of function and absent damage), or D to F (no antimyosin uptake but variable degrees of dysfunction due to previous myocardial mass loss), or G (persistent antimyosin uptake in addition to decreased left ventricular function).

The previous considerations suggest that in the evaluation of patients with alcoholic dilated cardiomyopathy, uptake of antimyosin antibodies may provide a marker of alcohol exposure. However, it is not useful to estimate the extent of the myocardial damage or to predict the presence or magnitude of functional ventricular recovery after cessation of alcohol.

## Residual alcoholic cardiomyopathy

Despite functional improvement after alcohol withdrawal in patients with alcoholic dilated cardiomyopathy, several sequelae may be observed. Left ventricular dilatation remains, which probably reflects the difficulty of the regres-

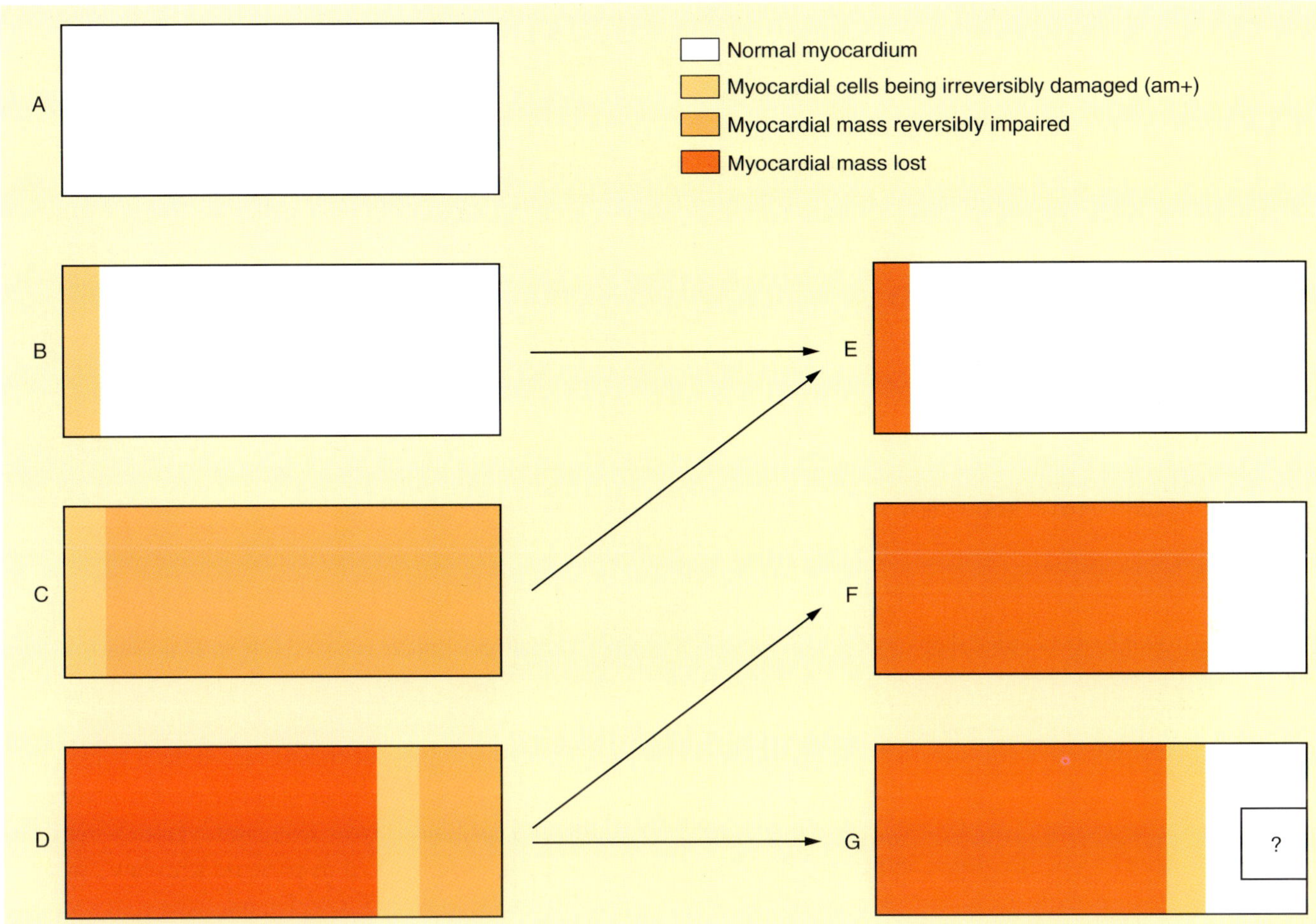


**Figure 25.2** *Possible constructs of the relationship between normally functioning myocardium, myocardial damage detected by antimyosin antibodies and undamaged but functionally impaired myocardium during alcohol consumption and after cessation of alcohol intake. Arrows indicate possible evolutions after cessation of alcohol consumption. (Reproduced from ref. 67 with permission.) (See text for explanation of the patterns.)*

sion of left ventricular remodelling in advanced stages of the disease. In one study [67], residual left ventricular dilatation (> 55 mm) was detected in 29 of the 34 patients with alcoholic dilated cardiomyopathy after cessation of consumption (85%). A low ejection fraction may be observed even after striking functional recovery; this is probably due to the loss of myocardial mass during the consumption of alcohol. In the above-mentioned study, 11 of 34 patients with alcoholic dilated cardiomyopathy restudied after alcohol withdrawal had an increased ejection fraction of over 50%, but in the remaining 23 variable degrees of impaired ventricular contraction. Ongoing active myocardial damage may be detected; this was shown by increased antimyosin uptake in 17 patients that persisted in an other 17 (ten former active and seven past consumers). The significance of this observation is not clear; it could be due to an undetected lack of compliance to alcohol abstention, inclusion of patients with idiopathic dilated cardiomyopathy, who show a high prevalence of antimyosin uptake [55], or to myocardial damage due to end-stage heart failure [69].

## Possible mechanisms of alcohol-related myocardial damage

Long-term intake of large amounts of alcohol affects several organs, including heart and skeletal muscle. The precise mechanism of the deleterious effect of alcohol is uncertain [70]. Alcohol and several of its metabolites have been implicated in the pathogenesis of organic disease. Although alcohol is not metabolized directly by the cardiac muscle, acetaldehyde and acetate, which occur in liver dysfunction, may play a role [71]. Alcohol has been shown experimentally to be directly toxic to sarcolemmal proteins

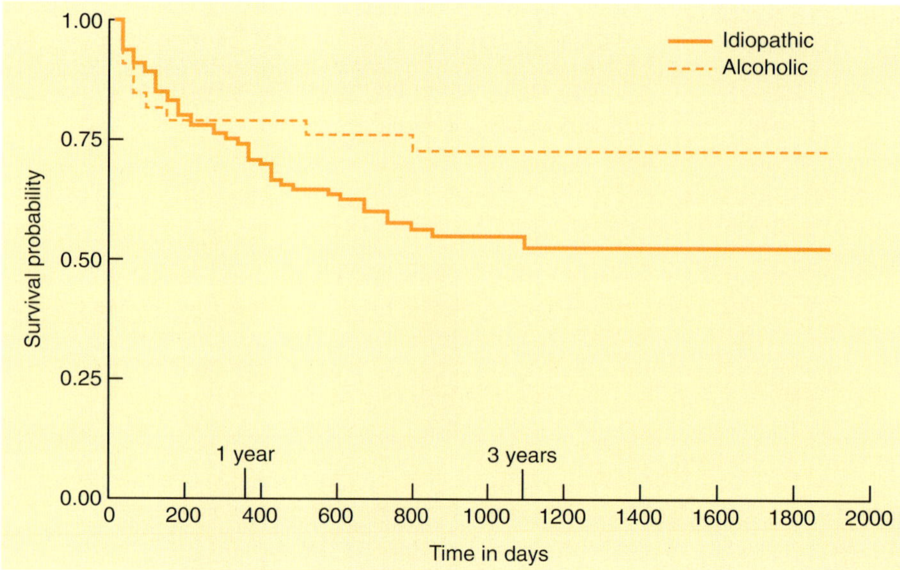


**Figure 25.3** *Survival curves in patients with idiopathic and alcoholic dilated cardiomyopathy. Note the improved survival in the latter. This could be ascribed to cessation in the destruction of myocardial cells after alcohol withdrawal as observed in repeat antimyosin antibody studies. (Reproduced from ref. 55 with permission.)*

and this may result in myocardial damage [33, 72]. In some cases, altered nutritional status may favour the development of heart failure, which in the case of beri-beri (thiamine deficiency) presents clinically as high-output heart failure [3, 4]. Fatty acid ethyl esters, the end-product of the myocardial metabolism of alcohol, may damage the myocardial cells [73–78]. Evidence indicates that myocardial metabolism in humans is non-oxidative and basically dependent on three enzymes, synthases I–III. These enzymes metabolize alcohol to produce different types of ethyl esters of fatty acids, which have been shown experimentally to interfere with mitochondrial function and could potentially account for the damaging effect on the myocardium [74].

## Importance of the detection of alcohol-induced cardiomyopathy

The importance of detecting alcohol-induced cardiomyopathy cannot be overemphasized because of the reversibility of this condition. The quest for its detection must be extremely active. Questionnaires must be given to patients with dilated cardiomyopathy, through which the most precise clinical history of alcohol abuse is illicited. Family and friends should be interviewed to detect abnormal drinking behaviour. Some patients presenting with alcohol-induced cardiomyopathy are neither addicted to alcohol nor aware that alcohol may be the cause of their illness; a large percentage is social drinkers who may be ready to give up their habit. In a recent series of 205 patients with dilated cardiomyopathy referred for heart transplantation, prospective questioning of their drinking habit revealed that 56 (27%) complied with the World Health Organization (WHO) definition of chronic alcoholism [67].

Although a large percentage of active alcohol consumers with dilated cardiomyopathy may improve, such improvement can also be observed in patients who have stopped drinking for more than 3 months, implying that recovery may take time to occur (see Fig. 25.1, repeat studies in former consumers). The physician must carefully observe the effects of drug withdrawal and vigorously prolong medical treatment with diuretics, digitalis, and peripheral vasodilators.

Actuarial survival curves in patients with idiopathic dilated cardiomyopathy show a progressive tendency to die or require transplantation as a result of heart failure during the first 3 or 4 years, after which a plateau is reached (Fig. 25.3) [55]. In alcoholic dilated cardiomyopathy, the probability of these events is lower, and plateaus 6 months after presentation (Table 25.2, Fig. 25.3). The better outcome in alcoholics than in patients with idiopathic dilated cardiomyopathy is ascribed to the cessation of active destruction of myocardial mass after alcohol withdrawal, as observed in the aforementioned negative antimyosin studies.

Myocardial damage is strongly related to heavy alcohol consumption. It is usually present in active consumers and less so in former consumers with dilated cardiomyopathy. In active drinkers, alcohol withdrawal is associated with the resolution of myocardial damage and an improvement in left ventricular systolic function. The lower prevalence of damage in subjects with a history of heavy alcohol consumption but no evidence of cardiomyopathy suggests the role of different myocardial susceptibilities to alcohol. Cessation of myocardial damage after alcohol withdrawal can account for the improved survival of alcoholic patients with dilated cardiomyopathy.

## References


1. White PD. *Heart disease*. London: Macmillan, 1931, 863.
2. Wood P. *Diseases of the heart and circulation*. 3rd edition. London: Eyre and Spottiswoode.
3. Blankerhorn MA, Vilter CF, Scinker IM *et al*. Occidental beri-beri heart disease. *JAMA* 1946; 131: 717.
4. Braunwald E, Wynne J. High output states: beri-beri heart disease. In: E Braunwald (ed.) *Heart disease*. Philadelphia, PA: WB Saunders, 1984, 1399.
5. Dancy M, Bland JM, Leech G *et al*. Preclinical left ventricular abnormalities in alcoholics are independent of nutritional status, cirrhosis and cigarette smoking. *Lancet* 1985: 1122–5.
6. Urbano–Marquez A, Estruch R, Navarro-López F *et al*. The effects of alcoholism on skeletal and cardiac muscle. *N Engl J Med* 1989; 320: 409–15.
7. Alexander CS. Idiopathic heart disease. I. Analysis of 100 cases with a special reference to chronic alcoholism. *Am J Med* 1966; 41: 213.
8. Tobin JR Jr, Driscoll JF, Lim MT *et al*. Primary myocardial disease and alcoholism. The clinical manifestations and course of the disease in a selected population of patients observed for three or more years. *Circulation* 1967; 35: 754–64.
9. Regan TJ, Levinson GE, Oldewurtel HA *et al*. Ventricular function in noncardiacs with alcoholic fatty liver: role of ethanol in the production of cardiomyopathy. *J Clin Invest* 1969; 48: 397–407.
10. Burch GE, Giles TD. Alcoholic cardiomyopathy. Concept of the disease and its treatment. *Am J Med* 1971; 50: 141–5.
11. Spodick DH, Pigott VM, Chirife R. Preclinical cardiac malfunction in chronic alcoholism. Comparison with matched normal controls with alcoholic cardiomyopathy. *N Engl J Med* 1972; 287: 677–80.
12. Kelbaek H, Nielsen BM, Eriksen J *et al*. Left ventricular performance in alcoholic patients without chronic liver disease. *Br Heart J* 1987; 58: 352–7.
13. Fuster V, Gersh BJ, Giuliani ER *et al*. The natural history of idiopathic dilated cardiomyopathy. *Am J Cardiol* 1981; 47: 525–31.
14. Brigden W. Alcoholic cardiomyopathy. *Br J Hosp Med* 1977; 18: 122–5.
15. Walsh TK, Vacek JL. Ethanol and heart disease. An understimated contributing factor. *Postgrad Med* 1986; 79: 60.
16. Regan TJ. Alcoholic cardiomyopathy. In: DP Zipes, Rowlands (eds) *Progress in cardiology*. Philadelphia, PA: Lea and Febiger, 1989, 129.
17. Vikhert AM, Tsiplenkova VG, Cherpachenko NM. Alcoholic cardiomyopathy and sudden cardiac death. *J Am Coll Cardiol* 1986; 8: 3–11A.
18. Mathews EC, Gardin JM, Henry WL *et al*. Echocardiographic abnormalities in chronic alcoholics with and without overt congestive heart failure. *Am J Cardiol* 1981; 47: 570–8.
19. Kannel WB, Sorlie P. Hypertension in Framingham. In: O Paul (ed.) *Epidemiology and control of hypertension*. New York: Station Intercontinental Medical Book Corp., 1974.
20. Klatsky AL, Friedman GD, Siegelaub AB *et al*. Alcohol consumption and blood pressure. Kaiser–Permanente Multiphasic Health Examinations data. *N Engl J Med* 1977; 296: 1194–200.
21. Wallace RB, Lynch CF, Pomrehn PR *et al*. Alcohol and hypertension: epidemiologic and experimental considerations. *Circulation* 1981; 64 (Suppl III): 41–7.
22. Dec GW, Fuster V. Medical progress: idiopathic dilated cardiomyopathy. *N Engl J Med* 1994; 331: 1564.
23. Segel L, Klaussner S, Gnadt JH, Amsterdam E. Alcohol and the heart. *Med Clin North Am* 1984; 68: 147.
24. Wendt V, Ajluni R, Bruce TA *et al*. Acute effect of alcohol on the human myocardium. *Am J Cardiol* 1966; 17: 804–12.
25. Juchems R, Klobe R. Hemodynamic effects of ethyl alcohol in man. *Am Heart J* 1969; 78: 133–5.
26. Riff DP, Jain A, Doyle JT. Acute hemodynamic effects of ethanol on normal human volunteers. *Am Heart J* 1969; 78: 592–7.
27. Gould L, Reddy CVR, Goswami K *et al*. Cardiac effects of two cocktails in normal man. *Chest* 1973; 63: 943–7.
28. Blomquist G, Salin B, Mitchell JH. Acute effects of ethanol ingestion on the response to submaximal and maximal exercise in man. *Circulation* 1970; 42: 263–70.
29. Delgado CE, Fortuin NJ, Ross RS. Acute effects of low doses of alcohol on left function by echocardiography. *Circulation* 1975; 51: 535–40.
30. Lang RM, Borow KM, Neumann A, Feldman T. Adverse cardiac effect of acute alcohol ingestion in young adults. *Ann Intern Med* 1985; 102: 742–7.
31. Kelbaek J, Gjorup T, Brynjolf I *et al*. Acute effects of alcohol on left ventricular function in healthy subjects at rest and during upright exercise. *Am J Cardiol* 1985; 55: 164–7.
32. Demakis JG, Proskey A, Rahimtoola SH *et al*. The natural course of alcoholic cardiomyopathy. *Ann Intern Med* 1974; 80: 293–7.
33. Rubin E. Alcoholic myopathy in heart and skeletal muscle. *N Engl J Med* 1979; 301: 28–33.
34. Song SK, Rubin E. Ethanol produces muscle damage in human volunteers. *Science* 1972; 175: 327.
35. Schwartz L, Sample KA, Wigle ED. Severe alcoholic cardiomyopathy reversed with abstention from alcohol. *Am J Cardiol* 1975; 36: 963–6.
36. Sacher ML, Siskind SJ, Boal BH. Gated radionuclide angiocardiography in the noninvasive evaluation of a partially reversible alcoholic cardiomyopathy. *Am J Med* 1986; 80: 1205–7.
37. Pavan D, Nicolosi GL, Lestuzzi C *et al*. Normalization of variables of left ventricular function in patients with alcoholic cardiomyopathy after cessation of excessive alcohol intake: an echocardiographic study. *Eur Heart J* 1987; 8: 535–40.
38. Pomerance A, Davis MJ. *The pathology of the heart*. Oxford: Blackwell Scientific, 1975.
39. Alexander CS. Idiopathic heart disease. Electron microscopic examination of myocardial biopsy specimens in alcoholic heart disease. *Am J Med* 1966; 41: 229.
40. Hibbs RG, Ferrans VJ, Black WC *et al*. Alcoholic cardiomyopathy — an electron microscopic study. *Am Heart J* 1965; 69: 766.
41. Khaw BA, Gold HK, Leinbach RC *et al*. Early imaging of experimental myocardial infarction by intracoronary administration of $^{131}I$-labeled anticardiac myosin (Fab′)2 fragments. *Circulation* 1978; 58: 1137–42.
42. Khaw BA, Falbn JT, Beller GA, Haber E. Specificity of localization of myosin-specific antibody fragments in experimental myocardial infarction: histologic, histochemical, autoradiographic and scintigraphic studies. *Circulation* 1979; 60: 1527–31.

43. Khaw BA, Scott J, Falbn JT *et al.* Myocardial injury: quantitation by cell sorting initiated with antimyosin fluorescent spheres. *Science* 1982; 217: 1050–3.
44. Khaw BA, Mattis JA, Melincoff G *et al.* Monoclonal antibody to cardiac myosin: imaging of experimental myocardial infarction. *Hybridoma* 1984; 3: 11–23.
45. Khaw BA, Gold HK, Yasuda T *et al.* Scintigraphic quantification of myocardial necrosis in patients after intravenous injection of myosin-specific antibody. *Circulation* 1986; 74: 501–8.
46. Estorch M, Carrió I, Bernà L, Martínez-Duncker C *et al.* 111-Indium antimyosin scintigraphy after doxorubicin therapy in patients with advanced breast cancer. *J Nucl Med* 1990; 31: 1965–9.
47. Carrió I, Estorch M, Bernà L *et al.* Assessment of anthracycline induced myocardial damage by quantitative 111-In-antimyosin monoclonal antibody studies. *Eur J Nucl Med* 1991; 18: 806–12.
48. Carrió I, López-Pousa A, Estorch M *et al.* Detection of doxorubicin cardiotoxicity in patients with sarcomas by indium-111-antimyosin monoclonal antibody studies. *J Nucl Med* 1993; 34: 1503–7.
49. Yasuda T, Palacios IF, Dec W *et al.* Indium 111-monoclonal antimyosin antibody imaging in the diagnosis of acute myocarditis. *Circulation* 1987; 76: 306–11.
50. Carrió I, Berná L, Ballester M *et al.* Indium-111 antimyosin scintigraphy to assess miocardial damage in patients with suspected myocarditis and cardiac rejection. *J Nucl Med* 1988; 29: 1893–900.
51. Dec GW, Palacios I, Yasuda T *et al.* Antimyosin antibody cardiac imaging: its role in the diagnosis of myocarditis. *J Am Coll Cardiol* 1990; 16: 97–104.
52. Narula J, Khaw BA, Dec GW Jr *et al.* Recognition of acute myocarditis masquerading as acute myocardial infarction. *N Engl J Med* 1992; 328: 100–4.
53. Obrador D, Ballester M, Carrió I *et al.* High prevalence of ongoing myocyte damage in patients with chronic dilated cardiomyopathy. *J Am Coll Cardiol* 1989; 13: 1289–93.
54. Obrador D, Ballester M, Carrió I *et al.* Active myocardial damage without attending inflammatory response in idiopathic dilated cardiomyopathy. *J Am Coll Cardiol* 1993; 21: 1667–71.
55. Obrador D, Ballester M, Carrió I *et al.* Presence, evolving changes, and prognostic implications of myocardial damage detected in idiopathic and alcoholic dilated cardiomyopathy by 111-In monoclonal antimyosin antibodies. *Circulation* 1994; 89: 2054–61.
56. Frist W, Yasuda T, Segall G *et al.* Noninvasive detection of human cardiac transplant rejection with In-111 antimyosin (Fab) imaging. *Circulation* 1987; 76 (Suppl V): 81–5.
57. Ballester M, Obrador D, Carrió I *et al.* 111-In-monoclonal antimyosin antibody studies after the first year of heart transplantation: identification of risk groups for developing rejection during long-term follow-up and clinical implications. *Circulation* 1990; 82: 2100–8.
58. Ballester M, Obrador D, Carrió I *et al.* Early postoperative reduction of monoclonal antimyosin antibody uptake is associated with absent rejection-related complications after heart transplantation. *Circulation* 1992; 85: 61–8.
59. Hosenpud JD. Noninvasive diagnosis of cardiac allograft rejection. Another of many searches for the grail. *Circulation* 1992; 85: 368–71.
60. Ballester M, Bordes R, Tazelaar T *et al.* Evaluation of biopsy classification for rejection: relation to the detection of myocardial damage by 111-In-monoclonal antimyosin antibody imaging. *J Am Coll Cardiol* 1998; 31: 1357–61.
61. Van Vlies B, Van Royen EA, Visser CA *et al.* Frequency of myocardial indium-111 antimyosin uptake after uncomplicated coronary artery bypass grafting. *Am J Cardiol* 1990; 66: 1191–5.
62. Narula J. Pathologic basis for the role of antimyosin imaging for the detection of cardiac involvement in systemic disorders. In: BA Khaw, J Narula, WH Strauss (eds) *Monoclonal antibodies in cardiovascular disease*. Philadelphia, PA: Lea and Febiger, 1994, 118–26.
63. Martí V, Ballester M, Udina C *et al.* Evaluation of myocardial cell damage by In-111 monoclonal antimyosin antibodies in patients under chronic tricyclic antidepressant drug treatment. *Circulation* 1995; 91: 1619–23.
64. Martí V, Ballester M, Obrador D *et al.* Active myocardial damage in hyperthyroidism: a concurrent mechanism of heart failure reversed by treatment. *Eur Heart J* 1995; 16: 1014–16.
65. Martí V, Ballester M, Rigla M *et al.* Myocardial damage does not occur in untreated hyperthyroidism unless associated with congestive heart failure. *Am Heart J* 1997; 134: 1133–7.
66. Narula J, Strauss HW, Khaw BA. Antimyosin positivity in doxorubicin cardiotoxicity: earlier than conventional evidence. *J Nucl Med* 1993; 34: 1503–7.
67. Ballester M, Martí V, Obrador D *et al.* Spectrum of alcohol-induced myocardial necrosis detected by 111-In-monoclonal antimyosin antibodies. *J Am Coll Cardiol* 1997; 29: 160–7.
68. McKenna CJ, Codd MB, McCann HA, Sugrue DD. Alcohol consumption and idiopathic dilated cardiomyopathy. *Am Heart J* 1998; 135: 833–7.
69. Katz AM. Cardiomyopathy of overload: a major determinant of prognosis in congestive heart failure. *N Engl J Med* 1990; 322: 100–10.
70. Richardson PJ, Wodak AD, Atkinson L, Saunders JB. Relation between alcohol intake, myocardial enzyme activity and myocardial function in dilated cardiomyopathy. Evidence for the concept of alcohol induced heart muscle disease. *Br Heart J* 1986; 56: 165–70.
71. Schreiber SS, Oratz M, Rothschild MA *et al.* Alcoholic cardiomyopathy. II. The inhibition of cardiac microsomal protein synthesis by acetaldehyde. *J Molec Cell Cardiol* 1974; 6: 207–13,
72. Rubin E, Rottenberg H. Ethanol induced injury and adaptation in biological membranes. *Fedn Proc* 1982; 42: 2465–71.
73. Lange LG, Bergmann SR, Sobel BE. Identification of fatty acid ethyl esthers as products of rabbit myocardial ethanol metabolism. *J Biol Chem* 1981; 256: 12 968–73.
74. Lange LG, Sobel BE. Mitochondrial dysfunction induced by fatty acids ethyl esters, myocardial metabolites of ethanol. *J Clin Invest* 1983; 72: 724–31.
75. Laposata EA, Lange LG. Presence of nonoxidative ethanol metabolism in human organs commonly damaged by ethanol abuse. *Science* 1986; 231: 497–9.
76. Bora PS, Spilburg CA, Lange LG. Purification and characterization of fatty acid ethyl ester synthase from human myocardium. *FEBS Lett* 1989; 258: 236–9.
77. Bora PS, Bora NS, Wu X, Lange LG. Molecular cloning, sequencing, and expression of human myocardial fatty acid ethyl ester synthase-III cDNA. *J Biol Chem* 1991; 266: 16 774–7.
78. Bora PS, Wu X, Spilburg CA, Lange LG. Purification and characterization of fatty acid ethyl ester synthase-III from human myocardium. *J Biol Chem* 1991; 267; 13 217–21.

# HIV-related cardiomyopathic disease 26

A. HERSKOWITZ

## Introduction

It is estimated that 42 million people worldwide have been infected with human immunodeficiency virus (HIV), the virus that causes acquired immunodeficiency syndrome (AIDS), and that almost 12 million people died from AIDS-related diseases up to 1997. In the USA, 641 086 patients have been diagnosed with AIDS up to 1997, and at least 385 000 have died [1]. As more effective anti-retroviral therapies have slowed the progression from HIV to AIDS and from AIDS to death, new non-infectious complications of late-stage HIV infection, including HIV-related heart disease, have emerged.

Early in the AIDS epidemic, cardiac disease was considered an unusual manifestation of advanced HIV infection. Cardiac disease as a primary cause of death in patients with AIDS was reported in 1.1% of autopsies performed from 1981 to 1985 and in 6.3% of autopsies performed from 1986 to 1988. This suggested that a growing population of HIV-infected patients was at risk for cardiac involvement [2]. Early autopsy studies noted abnormalities such as myocarditis secondary to opportunistic infections, neoplastic infiltration of the heart, particularly by Kaposi's sarcoma and lymphoma, non-bacterial thrombotic endocarditis, and pericardial effusions. Most of these post-mortem findings were not associated with clinically evident heart disease during life. In 1986, Cohen *et al.* [3] described the first cases of rapidly fatal dilated cardiomyopathy in AIDS patients. Subsequently, a growing number of prospective echocardiographic studies has described a high incidence of symptomatic cardiac disease in HIV-infected patients.

The most common and life-threatening cardiovascular complication of HIV infection appears to be the development of primary heart muscle disease associated with significant global left ventricular dysfunction (also termed cardiomyopathy). The finding of HIV-related cardiomyopathy has fuelled a growing concern that a significant subgroup of HIV-infected patients may be predisposed to the development of severe and progressive ventricular dysfunction. The goal of this chapter is to review the epidemiology of HIV-related cardiomyopathy and its clinical characteristics, describe the pathogenic mechanisms that may be responsible for heart involvement, and discuss potential therapeutic strategies. Fundamental questions regarding the aetiology of HIV-related cardiomyopathy remain, however, and require further intensive study. (1) Is this form of cardiomyopathy HIV related or is it related to some of the same lifestyle factors associated with increased risk of HIV infection? (2) What clinical, behavioural, and immunological risk factors and markers are associated with the development of left ventricular dysfunction? (3) If the cardiomyopathy is HIV related is it associated with direct HIV-1 infection of the heart or does HIV-1 facilitate infection with some other cardiotropic virus or viruses? (4) If cardiotropic viruses are involved in its pathogenesis, is cardiac injury caused directly by virus replication within myocardial cells or secondary to virus-induced autoimmunity?

The cardiac abnormalities that have been described in HIV-infected patients are listed in Table 26.1. The most common form of symptomatic heart disease in patients with HIV infection is congestive heart failure (CHF) associated with severe global left ventricular hypokinesis. Large pericardial effusions with cardiac tamponade, high-grade arrhythmias with sudden cardiac death, infectious and tumour involvement of the myocardium and pericardium, and systemic embolization caused by non-bacterial thrombotic endocarditis or infective endocarditis are less common but can likewise present as medical emergencies.

**Table 26.1** Various presentations and potential causes of HIV-related heart disease

| |
|---|
| **Heart muscle disease** |
| Primary (idiopathic) cardiomyopathy |
| Dilated |
| Non-dilated |
| Secondary cardiomyopathy |
| Myocarditis |
| Viral or due to other opportunistic infection |
| Postviral cardiac autoimmunity |
| Drug hypersensitivity |
| Drug-related cardiotoxicity |
| Iatrogenic (nucleoside analogues and pentamidine) |
| Illicit (cocaine) |
| Malignant infiltration (Kaposi's sarcoma, lymphoma) |
| Nutritional deficiency (selenium) |
| Autonomic dysfunction |
| Isolated right ventricular disease |
| Pulmonary hypertension |
| Secondary to pulmonary infection |
| Secondary to microvascular pulmonary emboli |
| Primary pulmonary hypertension |
| **Pericardial disease** |
| Pericardial effusion |
| Serous |
| Infectious (bacterial, myobacterial, opportunistic) |
| Malignant |
| **Endocarditis** |
| Non-bacterial thrombotic |
| Infective (left- and right-sided valves) |
| **Rhythm disturbances** |
| High-grade atrial and ventricular ectopy |
| Secondary to primary heart muscle disease |
| Secondary to iatrogenic medications (pentamidine) |
| Conduction disturbances (secondary to autonomic dysfunction) |

## Epidemiological characteristics of HIV-related cardiomyopathy

Recent prospective clinical and echocardiographic studies (Table 26.2) have shown that symptomatic cardiac disease is quite common in HIV-infected patients, particularly during late-stage infection [4–15]. In a review of reports from the USA and Europe of cardiac disease in HIV-seropositive patients, Anderson and Virmani [2] found that clinically significant cardiac disease occurs in 6–7%. Hsia and Ross [4] evaluated 343 HIV-seropositive patients by serial echocardiograms. These authors found left ventricular dysfunction in 9.3% of patients and a further 6% developed symptomatic heart disease each year thereafter, mainly CHF. In an echocardiographic study of randomly selected HIV-seropositive outpatients in Baltimore [3], the present authors found a prevalence and incidence of global left ventricular dysfunction in 14.5% and 18%, respectively, with 6% of patients per year developing progressive left ventricular dysfunction and CHF. The largest and most recent prospective echocardiographic study by Barbaro *et al.* [15] followed 952 asymptomatic HIV-infected patients in Italy over 5 years. An echocardiographic diagnosis of dilated cardiomyopathy was made in 76 patients (8%), equivalent to a rate of 1.6% of patients per year. The difference in the yearly rates of new cases of HIV-related dilated cardiomyopathy leading to symptomatic CHF ranged from 1.6 to 17% [4–15]; is likely to be a function of several factors, including the HIV risk group studied and the extent and severity of immunodeficiency. For example, the study by Barbaro *et al.* [15] excluded intravenous drug users (IVDUs), an HIV risk subgroup predisposed to develop cardiomyopathy. In addition, all study patients at baseline were asymptomatic ([Centers for Disease Control (CDC)] class II) with mean CD4 cell counts of 670 $mm^3$, and only 12 of the 952 patients developed AIDS over the 5 year follow-up period. Yet, despite the relative 'wellness' of the HIV population studied, depressed CD4 cell counts during follow-up were clearly associated with the development of significant left ventricular dysfunction and CHF: 71 of the 76 patients who developed dilated cardiomyopathy had CD4 cell counts $< 400/mm^3$. The association of severely depressed CD4 cell counts with the development of HIV-related cardiomyopathy in this cohort (asymptomatic at baseline) is consistent with findings in other studies in which approximately 80% of all patients diagnosed with HIV-related cardiomyopathy and CHF had either AIDS or an AIDS-related complex [4–14].

Cumulatively, the prospective echocardiographic studies summarized in Table 26.2 support the following consensus. (1) The two most common forms of HIV-related symptomatic cardiac disease are left ventricular dysfunction and large pericardial effusion. (2) Rapid onset of CHF and severe global left ventricular dysfunction are often associated with a poor short-term prognosis, with more than half of the patients dying from primary cardiac failure within 6–12 months of presentation. (3) A more chronic presentation of progressive left ventricular dysfunction leading to CHF is less frequently associated with a rapid downhill clinical course, and may be more amenable to standard heart

**Table 26.2** Summary data from prospective echocardiography studies in HIV-infected patients

| | Patients (*n*) | AIDS (%) | Male (%) | IVDU (%) | LV hypokinesis on presentation (%) | CHF (%) | Large pericardial effusion (%) |
|---|---|---|---|---|---|---|---|
| Hsia and Ross[4] | 343 | NA | NA | NA | 9 | 4 | 2 |
| Herskowitz *et al.*[5] | 69 | 79 | 83 | 56 | 14 | 6 | 1 |
| Levy *et al.*[6] | 60 | 58 | 100 | 0 | 23 | NA | NA |
| Kinney *et al.*[7] | 63 | 30 | 100 | 93 | 3 | NA | 2 |
| Monsuez *et al.*[8] | 86 | 50 | 91 | 34 | 7 | NA | 12 |
| Himelman *et al.*[9] | 70 | 73 | 97 | 4 | 11 | 6 | 1 |
| Blanchard *et al.*[10] | 70 | 71 | 99 | 0 | 11 | 7 | 3 |
| Corallo *et al.*[11] | 102 | 100 | 78 | 70 | 41 | 17 | 9 |
| Akhras *et al.*[12] | 124 | 81 | 100 | 0 | 16 | 6.5 | 2 |
| Currie *et al.*[13] | 296 | 34 | NA | 69 | 15 | 4.4 | NA |
| De Castro *et al.*[14] | 136 | 68 | 76 | 60 | 13 | 13 | NA |
| Barbaro *et al.*[15] | 952 | 0 | 72 | 0 | NA | 8 | NA |

HIV = human immunodeficiency virus; AIDS = acquired immunodeficiency syndrome; IVDU = intravenous drug user; LV = left ventricular; CHF = congestive heart failure; NA = not applicable.

failure therapy, compared with rapid-onset cardiac disease. (4) The majority of patients appears to have clinically silent abnormalities, such as small pericardial effusions, non-bacterial thrombotic endocarditis, and mild left ventricular dysfunction, the latter often demonstrating spontaneous resolution. (5) The majority of HIV-infected patients with severe cardiomyopathy has severely depressed CD4 cell counts (<200/mm$^3$). Thus, the severe form of HIV-related cardiomyopathy is largely associated with late-stage HIV infection, although IVDUs may develop severe cardiomyopathy with symptoms of CHF when CD4 counts are not severely depressed. (6) HIV-related cardiomyopathy is not related to any specific opportunistic infections, and approximately 40% of the patients have not experienced an opportunistic infection before their cardiac symptoms. (7) HIV-related cardiomyopathy is not a disease limited to any HIV risk group. In addition, while HIV-related cardiomyopathy does not appear to be associated with classic cardiac risk factors such as hypertension and diabetes mellitus, other clinical markers of susceptibility, such as dyslipidaemia and exposure to potential direct cardiotoxic effects of cocaine and alcohol, have not yet been well defined.

From a cardiac public-health perspective, HIV-related cardiomyopathy is already an epidemic. Estimates by the Public Health Service suggest that by the year 2000 the total number of cases of AIDS in the USA would have risen to 350 000. Initial estimates by Anderson and Virmani [2] of 5000 patients with AIDS per year developing clinically symptomatic cardiac disease appear to be overly conservative. Assuming a 6% per year rate of development of symptomatic heart disease in patients with AIDS, a total of 21 000 AIDS patients will require chronic cardiac care each year. Since there are an estimated 470 000 new cases per year of CHF in the USA, HIV-related cardiomyopathy may comprise almost 5% of these. Assuming a cost of $10 000 per year per patient with HIV-related cardiomyopathy, the health-care cost for this HIV-related complication is likely to exceed $210 million per year. Further cross-sectional prospective studies in all HIV risk groups are clearly required, in particular, new longitudinal studies in patients treated with the new-generation combination antiretroviral therapy. The impact of this relatively new form of HIV therapy, particularly in patient subgroups previously underrepresented in prospective echocardiographic studies (e.g. women and minorities), on the pathogenesis of HIV-related cardiomyopathy, is essentially unknown.

## Clinical characteristics of HIV-related cardiomyopathy

In 1986 Cohen *et al.* [3] described three HIV-seropositive patients who presented with signs and symptoms of CHF associated with severe left ventricular dysfunction. The typical signs and symptoms of heart failure can be mimicked by other common HIV-related conditions, and thus are easily missed or misdiagnosed. Symptoms of low cardiac output such as fatigue and malaise are commonly seen in patients with AIDS. Cough and dyspnoea associated with diffuse pulmonary rales are often considered to be due to *Pneumocystis carinii* pneumonia or some other opportunistic lung infection, as opposed to pulmonary congestion related to heart failure.

In an effort to gain some insight into potential risk factors or markers of HIV-related cardiomyopathy, numerous clinical variables were examined in 93 patients with HIV-related global left ventricular hypokinesis, with and without New York Heart Association (NYHA) class III or class IV CHF (Table 26.3). Most patients with NYHA class III or IV CHF have sinus tachycardia, S3 gallop, and pulmonary rales, while elevated jugular venous pressure and peripheral oedema are uncommon. In contrast to patients presenting with CHF patients with asymptomatic left ventricular hypokinesis found incidentally on echocardiography have no peripheral stigmata of vascular congestion. Only a small minority of these patients has resting tachycardia and dilated left ventricular cavities. No differences were noted between HIV-infected patients with and without congestive heart failure with respect to age, gender, risk groups, immunoglobulin levels, blood pressure, serum chemistries and antinuclear antibody levels, history of hypertension, cholesterol levels, diabetes, alcohol abuse, or recreational drug use. Electrocardiographic changes, such as QRS voltage indicative of left ventricular hypertrophy, ventricular ectopic beats, left atrial enlargement, bundle branch block, and non-specific ST-T wave abnormalities, were found equally in both groups.

**Table 26.3** Clinical and demographic characteristics of HIV-seropositive patients with global left ventricular hypokinesis on two-dimensional echocardiography

| | No CHF ($n$ = 43) | CHF ($n$ = 50) | $p$-Value |
|---|---|---|---|
| African–American | 62% | 78% | 0.09 |
| CD4 < 200/mm$^3$ | 61% | 82% | 0.06 |
| CD4 median/mm$^3$ | 120 | 23 | 0.04 |
| LV ejection fraction | 53% | 30% | < 0.0001 |
| LV dilation | 32% | 80% | 0.0002 |
| RV dilation | 13% | 63% | < 0.0001 |
| Pericardial effusion | 13% | 67% | < 0.0001 |
| S3 gallop rhythm | 3% | 78% | < 0.0001 |
| Heart rate > 100 beats/min | 16% | 62% | < 0.0001 |
| Peripheral oedema | 3% | 10% | NS |
| One or more OI | 35% | 53% | 0.15 |
| Body-surface area | 1.9 ± 0.2 | 1.8 ± 0.2 | 0.02 |
| Weight (median) (kg) | 73.5 | 63.5 | 0.005 |
| Weight loss over 1 year (kg) | 0.9 | 9.5 | 0.0001 |
| Platelet count (median) | 228K | 183K | 0.015 |
| Haematocrit (median) | 36.4 | 29.6 | 0.001 |
| Serum albumin (median) | 4.3 | 2.8 | < 0.0001 |
| Anti-heart antibodies (yes/no) | 50% | 53% | NS |
| Markedly elevated antibody titres | 23% | 61% | < 0.0001 |
| Any exposure to zidovudine | 63% | 59% | NS |
| h/o zidovudine-related toxicity[a] | 8% | 43% | 0.004 |

[a]Defined as either (1) anaemia (haemoglobin 7.5 g/dl), granulocytopenia (< 750/mm$^3$), changes in liver function tests or skeletal myositis; or (2) requiring discontinuation of drug or cotherapy with erythropoeitin.
LV = left ventricular; RV = right ventricular; OI = opportunistic infection; NS = not significant.

In a further attempt to identify predictive clinical markers of HIV-related heart disease, a retrospective analysis was performed of 180 consecutive HIV-infected inpatients who had a clinically indicated echocardiogram at The Johns Hopkins Hospital over a 3 year period. The purpose of the study was to identify the primary indications for echocardiography in patients hospitalized in an inner-city AIDS service and to describe the specific echocardiographic findings in these patients. Among patients in different HIV risk and stage-of-infection groups, the results revealed different clinical indications for echocardiography, as well as different patterns of echocardiographic abnormalities. A significantly increased proportion of non-AIDS patients was intravenous drug users, was admitted to rule out endocarditis, and was found to have valvular abnormalities including definite or possible vegetations on echocardiographic examination. Left-sided valvular abnormalities and endocarditis were uniquely found in IVDUs, which confirmed a previous report [16] in which a significant proportion (13%) of 85 HIV-seronegative IVDUs had left-sided valvular abnormalities. Among IVDU, left ventricular dysfunction was just as likely in patients without AIDS as it was in AIDS patients, suggesting that IVDUs may be independently at risk for left ventricular dysfunction. Given the demographics of this inpatient population, the findings in homosexual men and other non-IVDU risk groups are limited to those patients with AIDS. Essentially, it was found that ventricular dysfunction was more common among patients with more advanced HIV infection. Patients with mild left ventricular dysfunction were likely to have a clinical diagnosis of sepsis, although no single opportunistic infection was implicated. Moderate to severe global left ventricular dysfunction was not associated with any specific clinical diagnosis or opportunistic infection. Therefore, no clear clinical or demographic predisposition to serious cardiac manifestations of HIV infection was found in the majority of patients with AIDS, and thus the prospective identification of patients at increased risk for cardiac complications remains difficult.

## Pathology and immunopathogenesis of HIV-related cardiomyopathy

Current hypotheses concerning the aetiology of cardiomyopathy related to HIV infection include myocardial infection with HIV-1 or coinfection with other cardiotropic viruses [15, 17–19], postviral cardiac autoimmunity [20], selenium deficiency, autonomic dysfunction, and cardiotoxicity from alcohol and illicit drugs such as cocaine and heroin. A causal role for myocarditis in the development of HIV-related cardiomyopathy has recently become more likely. In early autopsy studies [12], lymphocytic myocarditis was a frequent finding in patients both with and without cardiac disease during life. More recent studies [15, 17, 22, 23] have clearly demonstrated a remarkably high prevalence of myocarditis (up to 83%) in endomyocardial biopsy specimens in patients with HIV-related cardiomyopathy and severe left ventricular dysfunction.

At The Johns Hopkins Hospital endomyocardial biopsies were performed on 37 consecutive HIV-seropositive patients with moderate to severe global left ventricular dysfunction. Patient clinical characteristics and biopsy findings are presented in Table 26.4. Of the 37 patients who underwent biopsy, 21 (57%) had either active or borderline myocarditis on histology (Fig. 26.1). Of the 28 patients who presented with signs and symptoms of CHF, 19 (68%) had either active or borderline myocarditis, suggesting a strong relationship between the presence of myocarditis on endomyocardial biopsy and the severity of left ventricular dysfunction. The high prevalence of myocarditis in patients with HIV-related cardiomyopathy was more recently confirmed by Barbaro *et al.* [15]. Of the 76 patients who underwent endomyocardial biopsy within 1 month of presentation of CHF symptoms, 63 (76%) had either active or borderline myocarditis. The pattern of histological findings in HIV-infected patients with myocarditis appears to be indistinguishable from typical cases of myocarditis in patients without HIV risk factors. Immunohistological studies, however, reveal some differences. HIV-related myocarditis is predominantly composed of $CD8^+$ lymphocytes and is associated with intense, induced major histocompatibility complex (MHC) antigen class I expression (Fig. 26.1). In contrast, non-HIV-related myocarditis is associated with a mixed $CD4^+$ $CD8^+$ lymphocytic infiltrate and both increased MHC class I and II myocyte expression [24].

Because many patients with HIV infection have markedly depressed circulating leucocyte counts, myocardial infiltrates on endomyocardial biopsy may be diminished and difficult to appreciate by routine histology. Of the 16 HIV-infected patients in a previous study [17] who showed no histological evidence of myocarditis, eight (50%) showed immunohistological evidence of increased numbers of CD45 (common leucocyte antigen)-positive cells. All eight patients had AIDS and presented with symptoms of CHF and markedly depressed left ventricular ejection fractions. These findings suggest that by using a more sensitive immunohistological method, a subgroup of patients with no histological evidence of myocarditis may be identified, and may have similar immune-mediated heart disease.

### Virus-associated myocarditis as a potential cause of HIV-related cardiomyopathy

#### *Non-HIV-1 viruses*

The association between myocarditis and symptomatic cardiomyopathy in HIV-infected patients with a low level of circulating CD4 cells may result from a predisposition to cardiotropic viral infection. Cytomegalovirus (CMV) is prevalent in patients with AIDS, and CMV-induced myocarditis has been demonstrated in HIV-infected patients with cardiomyopathy [17, 18]. In one study [17], 48% of patients who underwent endomyocardial biopsy had positive hybridization signals for the non-replicating form of CMW. Recently, coxsackievirus B (CVB) infection, perhaps the most common cardiotropic viral infection inducing myocarditis in the general population, as well as Epstein–Barr virus (EBV), have been described in endomyocardial biopsy samples from patients with HIV-related myocarditis [15].

#### *HIV-1 infection: background*

HIV is known to infect non-lymphoid organs including the brain, bowel, heart, kidney, liver, eyes, prostate, adrenal

**Table 26.4** Clinical characteristics of and biopsy findings in HIV-1 seropositive patients with and without myocardial inflammation on endomyocardial biopsy

| | | No myocarditis (Dallas criteria, $n$ = 16) | | |
|---|---|---|---|---|
| | Idiopathic active or borderline myocarditis (Dallas criteria, $n$ = 17) | Positive immunohistological findings ($n$ = 8) | Negative immunohistological findings ($n$ = 8) | $p$-Value |
| Clinical and demographic characteristics | | | | |
| Age (years) | 38 ± 9 | 37 ± 10 | 38 ± 11 | 0.95 |
| Race | | | | |
| Black | 88 | 63 | 63 | 0.23 |
| White | 12 | 37 | 37 | 0.23 |
| Male gender | 71 | 100 | 63 | 0.17 |
| IVDU | 59 | 13 | 50 | 0.09 |
| AIDS-defining opportunistic infection | 53 | 63 | 25 | 0.22 |
| Median CD4 T-cell count/mm$^3$ | 21 | 24 | 272 | 0.002 |
| CD4 T-cell count < 200/mm$^3$ | 89 | 100 | 38 | 0.004 |
| Congestive heart failure at presentation | 94 | 100 | 13 | < 0.0001 |
| Any exposure to zidovudine | 59 | 63 | 75 | 0.94 |
| Zidovudine-related non-cardiac toxicity | 65 | 50 | 38 | 0.42 |
| Echocardiographic findings | | | | |
| LV ejection fraction | 24 ± 12 | 29 ± 15 | 41 ± 13 | 0.007 |
| Dilated LV cavity | 65 | 88 | 25 | 0.03 |
| Dilated RV cavity | 71 | 88 | 13 | 0.002 |
| Pericardial effusion | 65 | 75 | 25 | 0.01 |
| Immunohistochemical findings | | | | |
| Increased MHC class I staining | 65 | 100 | 0 | 0.0002 |
| CD8-predominant myocardial Infiltrate | 77 | 75 | 0 | 0.0008 |
| *In situ* hybridization findings | | | | |
| Myocyte CMV IE-2 gene transcripts | 64 | 66 | 0 | 0.008 |
| Myocyte HIV-1 gene transcripts | 7 | 66 | 0 | 0.002 |

Data presented are means ± SD or percentage of patients.
IVDU = intravenous drug users; LV = left ventricular; RV = right ventricular; MHC = major histocompatibility complex; CMV = cytomegalovirus; IE-2 = immediate-early.

gland, joints, and skin [25]. In many instances, while confirmation of infection with HIV is needed, studies indicate that this agent is polytropic and not solely T-lymphotropic. The preferential infection and growth of HIV in T-lymphoid cells is dependent on the surface CD4 molecule. However, many types of cell that have been shown to be infected by HIV, including human skin, muscle, bone-derived fibroblasts, brain-derived glial cells, and capillary endothelial cells are CD4$^-$ [26]. Like cardiac myocytes, these cell types lack detectable CD4 mRNA. While the nature of the cell-surface molecules responsible for viral entry into a CD4$^-$ cell is unknown, the presence of fusion proteins such as cell-surface chemokine receptors (e.g. CCR5) binding to HIV-1 gp120 are being considered as candidates for CD4-independent infection [27]. In addition, besides entering cells via an interaction between the virus envelope and cell surface receptors, HIV can infect cells by a phenomenon called antibody-dependent enhancement. This involves the binding of the Fab portion of non-neutralizing antibodies to the surface of the virion and transferring the virus into a cell through the complement or Fc receptor .

Does direct myocardial infection with HIV-1 play a role in the development of myocarditis and cardiac damage? The possibility that a primary cardiomyopathy may develop as a consequence of direct HIV-1 myocardial infection

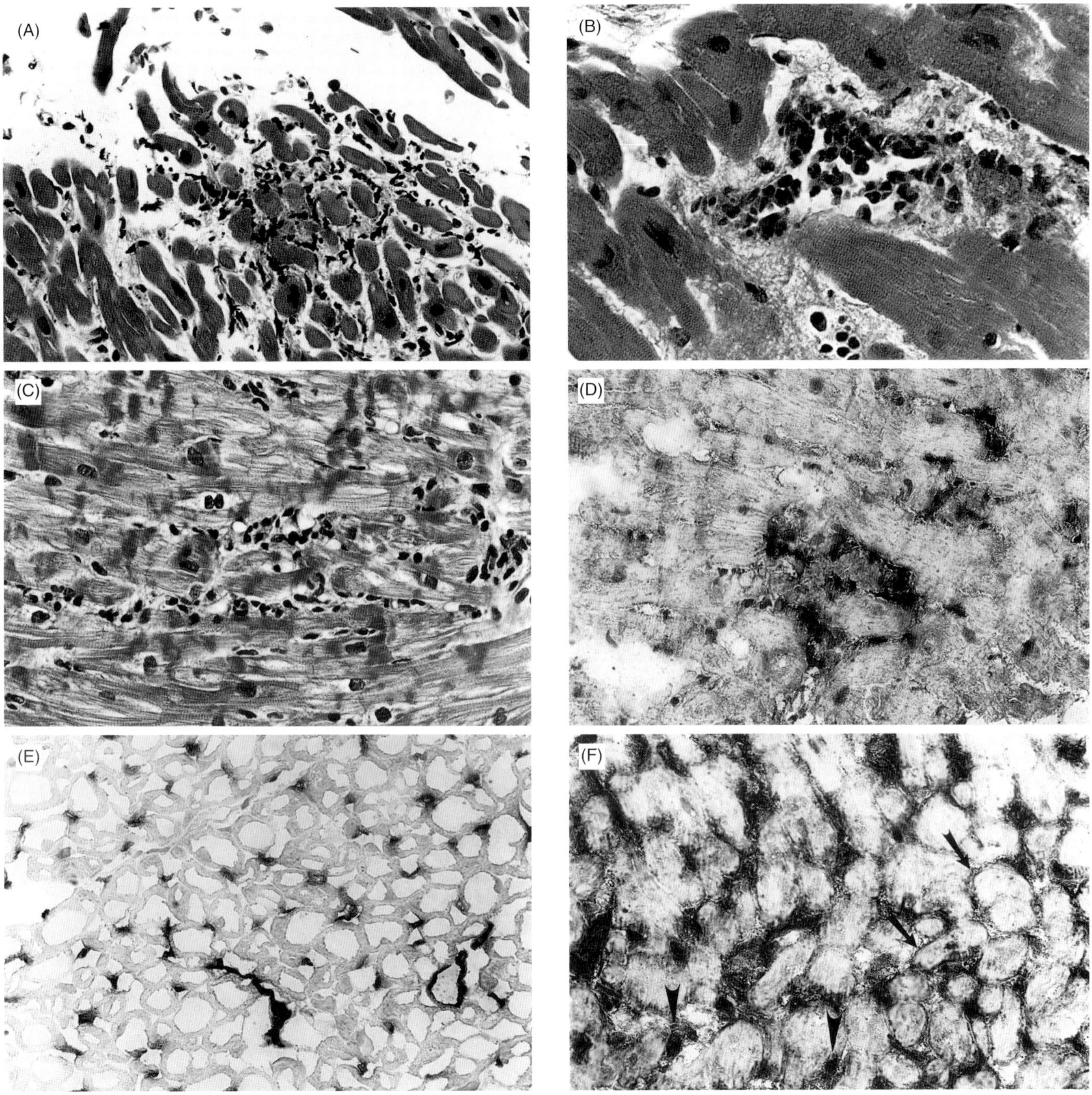


**Figure 26.1** *(A) Medium-powered photomicrograph taken from an endomyocardial biopsy specimen demonstrating active myocarditis. Note the interstitial collection of inflammatory cells surrounding a small group of necrotic myocytes. Haematoxylin and eosin (H & E) × 250. (B) Medium-powered photomicrograph taken from an endomyocardial biopsy specimen demonstrating eosinophilic myocarditis secondary to drug hypersensitivity. The patient presented with acute, rapid-onset congestive heart failure and was recently placed on penicillins. Note the cluster of perivascular eosinophils. H & E × 250. (C) Medium-powered photomicrograph taken from an endomyocardial biopsy specimen demonstrating bordeline myocarditis. Note the interstitial collection of inflammatory cells without evidence of myocyte necrosis. H & E × 400. (D) Immunoperoxidase staining of a frozen section with monoclonal antibody for CD8$^+$ lymphocytes in a sample showing histological evidence of borderline myocarditis. Clusters of CD8$^+$ lymphocytes stain within the myocardial intersititium (× 400). (E) Immunoperoxidase staining of a frozen section from a sample with no myocarditis with monoclonal antibody for human leucocyte antigen (HLA) ABC demonstrating baseline major histocompatibility complex (MHC) class I expression within myocardial microvascular endothelium (× 250). (F) Immunoperoxidase staining of a frozen section with monoclonal antibody for HLA ABC in a myocarditis sample demonstrating intense MHC class I expression throughout the myocardial interstitium. Note the intense staining within the microvascular endothelium (arrowheads), as well as discrete myocyte staining of MHC class I (arrows). This pattern of staining was routinely found in biopsy samples from both patients with readily diagnosed histological myocarditis and patients with only immunohistological evidence of increased myocardial inflammatory cells.*

is intriguing; however, the precise role of direct HIV-1 infection of myocytes in the development of cardiomyopathy remains poorly understood. One recent study by Rebolledo *et al.* [28] could not demonstrate foetal cardiac myocyte infection with wild-type HIV-1 virus. Several laboratories, however, have demonstrated the presence of HIV-1 gene transcripts within cardiac tissue from HIV-infected patients with myocarditis and cardiomyopathy, and photomicrographs of myocardial sections using *in situ* hybridization for HIV RNA have convincingly shown intense staining within myocytes [15, 17–19, 20] (Fig. 26.2). Grody *et al.* [19] detected HIV nucleic acids in 27% of patients who died of AIDS. The present anthors found positive hybridization signals for HIV-1 in five of 33 (15%) endomyocardial samples, while Barbaro *et al.* [15] detected HIV-1 nucleic acids in 58 of 76 (76%) endomyocardial samples. In all of these studies, only rare myocytes were infected with HIV-1 and these myocytes did not appear to elicit a localized inflammatory response. These findings are consistent with other studies of HIV-infected $CD4^-$ cells, which show low levels of infectivity (<1% of cells become infected), probably due to inefficient viral entry [25].

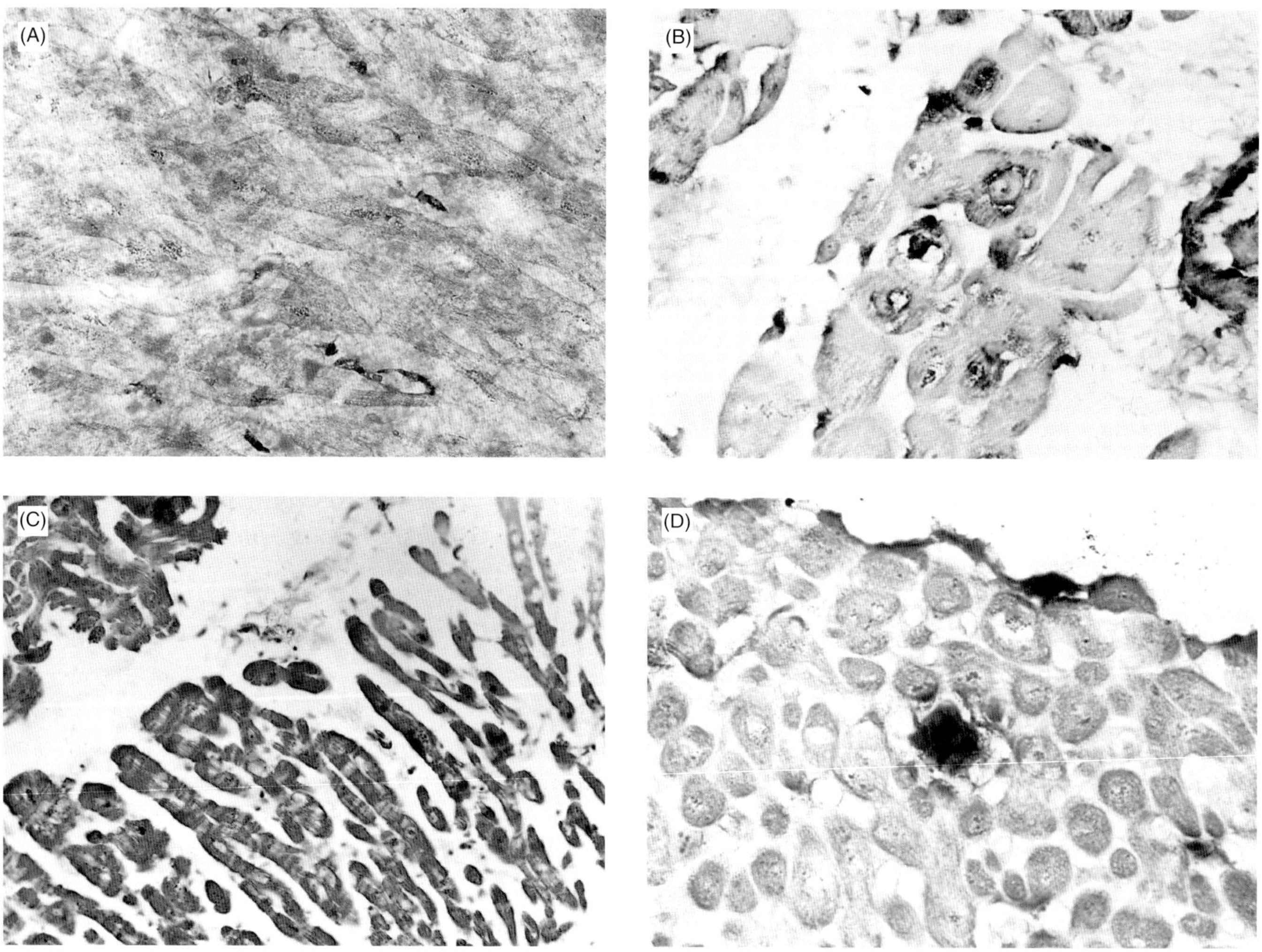


**Figure 26.2** *(A) In* situ *hybridization using the antisense riboprobe for cytomegalovirus (CMV) immediate-early (IE-2) genes in a control autopsy heart specimen from a patient with a history of CMV pneumonitis and encephalitis but no knwon cardiac disease during life. Note that the specific hybridization is limited focally to the microvascular endothelium. No specific myocyte hybridization is present (× 400). (B) In contrast, intense hybridization is present within the nuclear and perinuclear regions throughout the endomyocardial biopsy sample from an HIV-1-seropositive sample with active myocarditis (× 400). These findings suggest non-permissive (non-replicating) CMV infection which was consistent with the lack of histological evidence of myocytes nuclear inclusions typical of active CMV infection. (C) Same section as (B) treated with the control sense CMV IE riboprobe. Note the complete absence of positive hybridization within the microvascular endothelium or within myocytes (× 400). (D) In* situ *hybridization using the antisense riboprobe for HIV-1 genes demonstrating intense staining within a myocyte and several intersititial and endocardial cells (× 400).*

To address more specifically the issue of whether HIV-1 is cardiotropic *in vitro*, two studies sought to demonstrate HIV-1 infection of a human foetal cardiac myocyte cell line (termed W-1), useful as a surrogate to study the immunobiology of cardiac myocyte/lymphoid cell interactions [30, 31]. The results demonstrate that the W-1 cell line is capable of ingesting HIV-1 via the Fc receptor that is expressed by this cell line (Fig. 26.3). Only W-1 cells that were coincubated with HIV-1 antibody [immunoglobulin G (IgG)] and HIV-1 gave positive polymerase chain reaction (PCR) results. Controls consisted of W-1 myocytes with no HIV-1 antibody, W-1 cells with antibody and no virus, and W-1 cells alone. These results suggest that under certain conditions myocytes can indeed be infected by HIV-1, yet the possibility of HIV cardiotropism *in vitro* and the presence of HIV RNA within rare myocytes *in vivo* without an elicited immune response do not clearly indicate a direct role for the virus in the development of cardiac injury. The focal pattern of HIV gene expression seen in endomyocardial biospy specimens, and the lack of inflammation adjacent to myocytes positive for HIV RNA, may be more consistent with indirect HIV-mediated cardiac damage. In any case, with regard to the potential direct role of HIV-1 myocyte infection in the pathogenesis of HIV-related cardiomyopathy, studies are clearly needed to determine many remaining questions, including the following: (1) which myocardial cell types are susceptible to infection; (2) whether HIV-1 produces a latent or productive infection; (3) whether myocyte infection with HIV-1 induces MHC expression and becomes a target for immune-mediated injury; and (4) whether viral load is a variable in determining susceptibility to symptomatic heart disease.

It is, therefore, not known whether myocyte injury in HIV-related myocarditis can be explained by direct HIV-1 infection of myocytes, direct HIV-1 infection of other myocardial cells (e.g. interstitial dendritic cells and endothelial cells), other cardiotropic viruses (CMV, CVB, or EBV), cytotoxicity mediated by proinflammatory cytokines or viral proteins, or the initiation of cardiotropic virus-induced cardiac autoimmunity. Virus-induced myocyte antigen presentation in the setting of aberrant MHC expression is considered the stimulus for ongoing injury in most cases of human myocarditis [24, 32]. Overall, the results of histological and immunohistological studies in endomyocardial biopsy samples from patients with HIV-related cardiomyopathy strongly suggest that cardiotropic viral infection is likely to play some role in ongoing cardiac inflammation and injury. While the precise immunopathological mechanisms of myocardial injury need to be elucidated, the following may be involved: (1) viral infection of myocytes may irreversibly injure myocytes, directly eliciting a non-specific inflammatory response; (2) a $CD8^+$ T-cell response to virus-infected myocytes expressing endogenous viral peptides in association with MHC class I antigens results in myocyte lysis, possibly by apoptosis, and myocarditis; and (3) an aberrant autoimmune response is induced against autoantigenic peptides complexed to self-MHC molecules expressed on myocytes. This autoimmune response targets normal myocytes and produces myocarditis. Supportive evidence for all three possibilities, which probably act in concert *in vivo*, has been demonstrated in numerous experimental murine models of myocarditis.

## Potential role of cytokines and autoimmunity in HIV-related myocarditis and dilated cardiomyopathy

### Cytokines

The potential role of cytokines in HIV-related myocarditis and cardiomyopathy has been reviewed [20, 33] and is suggested by a variety of observations. (1) Patients with HIV-related cardiomyopathy may have significantly reduced systemic vascular resistance compared with patients without HIV infection who present with similarly depressed left ventricular function (Tables 26.5). This may be secondary to high circulating cytokine levels in HIV patients with cardiomyopathy, in particular those with severely depressed CD4 cell counts below 100/mm$^3$ [20]; (2) Matsumori *et al.* [34] demonstrated that approximately one-third of patients with idiopathic dilated cardiomyopathy and half with active myocarditis had elevated serum tumour necrosis factor-$\alpha$ (TNF-$\alpha$) levels. (3) Similarly, in experimental murine myocarditis, CVB3-infected mice demonstrate sustained elevations of serum levels of TNF-$\alpha$ and interleukin-1 (IL-1) throughout the acute myocarditic phase, as well as the chronic phase leading to cardiomyopathy [35].

### Autoimmunity

Many autoimmune-like serological abnormalities have been described in HIV-infected individuals, such as the presence of hypergammaglobulinaemia, circulating immune complexes, and anti-HILA class II antibodies [20, 36]. Also described are autoimmune processes such as idiopathic

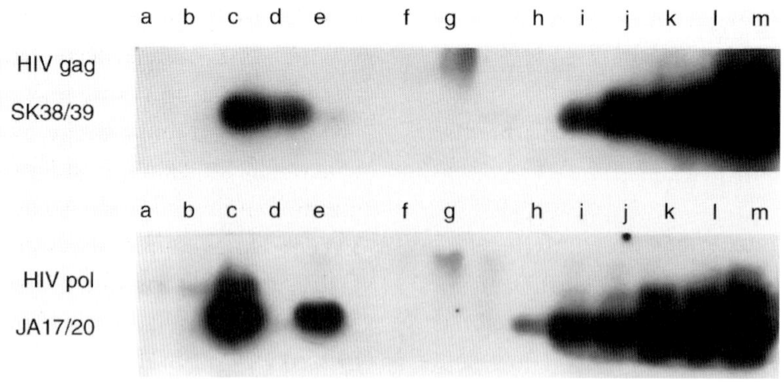


**Figure 26.3** *(a) Uninfected W-1 cells; and (b) 1 × 10*$^5$ *W-1 cells with 1 × 10*$^4$ *TCID50 of HIV-1, kvere kept overnight, washed, and then incubated for varying numbers of days. Data represent the results of day 3. However, results from day 7, 10, 14, and 21 were negative for both* gag *and* pol *primers. (c–f) W-1 cells (1 × 10*$^5$ *cells in each culture) were incubated with 10 mg/ml of a high-titred IgG isolated from a patient with HIV-1 (ELISA titer 1:100 000), and then 1 × 10*$^4$ *TCID50 of HIV-1 was added to each culture. Cultures were incubated for 24 h, washed, and then DNA-analysed for HIV-1 by PCR on day 3 (c),7 (d), 10 (e), and 14 (f). W-1 myocytes coincubated with HIV-1 and HIV-1 IgG became infected on days 3, 7, and 10. Cultures on days 21 and 28 were negative. (h–l) 8E5 cells stably infected with HIV-1. Varying concentrations of the 8E5 cell line were titrated with the uninfected H9 cell line at ratios of 1:10*$^3$ *(200 copies/sample), and 1:10*$^2$ *(2000 copies/sample), establishing that 1:10*$^6$ *infected cells can be detected. (m) Control CEM cell line infected with LAV. Supernatants at all time-points were assayed for reverse transcriptase (RT) and were negative. Negative RT in supernatants and the inability to culture HIV from infected W-1 cells after day 14 suggest that HIV infection of W-1 cells represents a non-replicating viral infection.*

thrombocytopenic purpura; rheumatological disorders such as Reiter's syndrome, Sjorgen's-like syndrome, and systemic lupus-like syndromes; bullous disease; and a variety of antibodies against non-T-lymphocytes. Longitudinal serological studies have also suggested that autoimmunity is already present in subgroups of patients and may be exacerbated by concurrent infection with HIV-1. Bona fide autoimmune phenomena such as autoimmune thrombocytopenia are frequently more prominent in patients with AIDS and low CD4 cell counts.

Evidence for cardiac-specific autoimmunity in patients with HIV-related cardiomyopathy has been found in studies in the present author's laboratory. Antiheart antibodies were identified using an enzyme-linked immunosorbent assay (ELISA) for three putative cardiac autoantigens previously described in patients with myocarditis and cardiomyopathy [32]: two mitochondrial proteins, adenine nucleotide translocator (ANT) and branched-chain ketoacid dehydrogenase (BCKD), and cardiac myosin. In positive non-HIV controls, elevated titres were found in 78% of patients with idiopathic dilated cardiomyopathy ($n = 78$) and 82% of patients with myocarditis ($n = 58$). In negative non-HIV controls, elevated titres were found in 11% of patients with ischaemic cardiomyopathy ($n = 58$), 4% of normal controls ($n = 100$), and less than 4% of patients with autoimmune diseases such as primary biliary cirrhosis ($n = 27$), rheumatoid arthritis ($n = 50$), and systemic lupus erythematosis ($n = 64$). In contrast, 52% of patients with HIV-related cardiomyopathy had elevated titres to one or more of the autoantigens tested. The presence of autoantibodies did not distinguish patients with CHF from their asymptomatic counterparts. However, sustained elevations over serial examinations were found in two-thirds of the patients who progressed to symptomatic cardiomyopathy, and in each instance, persistently elevated antiheart antibodies were present from 3 to 27 months before the development of CHF.

## Diagnostic cardiovascular evaluation in HIV infection

Recommendations for the diagnostic evaluation of HIV-related cardiomyopathy are summarized in Table 26.5. Clinically, the major goals are to establish the diagnosis of an

**Table 26.5** Diagnostic evaluation of cardiomyopathy in HIV infection

| | |
|---|---|
| **History and physical examination (attention to recent viral illness)** | |
| | Chest X-ray |
| | Echocardiogram |
| | Electrocardiogram |
| **Laboratory tests** | |
| | Complete blood count |
| | CPK MB |
| | Anti-nuclear antibody |
| | Serum selenium levels |
| | Urine VMA |
| | Thyroid function profile |
| | Serology (acute and convalescent) |
| | Coxsackievirus A and B |
| | Echovirus |
| | Influenza A and B |
| | Adenovirus |
| | Epstein–Barr virus |
| **Urinalysis** | |
| | Viral culture for enterovirus: pharynx, stool |
| | Toxicology screen |
| **Drug intervention** | |
| | Diuretic |
| | Inotropic agent |
| | Afterload reduction |
| | Consider drug respite for nucleoside analogues |
| | Rule out drug hypersensitivity |
| **Catheterization** | |
| | Endomyocardial biopsy (light microscopy, immunohistology staining) |
| | Right heart catheterization |
| **Possible additional studies** | |
| | Molecular probes for cardiotropic viruses |
| | Antiheart antibodies |

CPK MB = creatine phosphokinase microbiological assay; VMA = vanillylmandelic acid.

underlying heart muscle disease, determine whether it is reversible, and plan an appropriate treatment strategy [33]. It is important to try to date the onset of CHF symptoms. A rapid onset of symptoms suggests the presence of myocarditis. A history suggestive of coronary disease, alcohol abuse, or illicit drug use; a careful medication history with particular emphasis on new drugs, the duration of exposure to nucleoside analogues, and protease inhibitors; and history of non-cardiac toxicities to antiretroviral drugs should be sought.

Complete blood counts, antinuclear antibody evaluation, thyroid function tests, and urine for vanillylmandelic acid (VMA) excretion tests are obtained in patients with cardiomyopathy of unknown aetiology. A complete blood count serves to rule out peripheral eosinophilia (possible drug hypersensitivity) and to diagnose thrombocytopenia, which may indicate the patient's predisposition to autoimmune complications of HIV. Thyroid function tests and VMA tests rule out endocrinopathy, particularly hyperhyoidism and hypothyroidism, as well as phaeochromocytoma. Patients with advanced cardiomyopathy display signs and symptoms compatible with the presence of each of these disorders, and the distinguishing features may be obscured by the primary disease. Creatinine phosphokinase (CPK) elevations are infrequent in patients with myocarditis and usually suggest zidovudine-induced skeletal myositis. Acute and convalescent serological studies for evidence of exposure to cardiotropic viruses, and urine and stool viral cultures are listed in Table 26.5 but are not often useful in adult patients with suspected myocarditis.

The most useful diagnostic test is the echocardiogram, which allows for quantification of left ventricular function, size, valvular function, and concurrent pericardial abnormalities. A non-dilated, poorly contractile ventricle, particularly with a concurrent pericardial effusion, suggests the presence of acute myocarditis. Four-chamber dilatation, profound hypocontractile function, and thin ventricular walls suggest a more chronic condition. Patients with dilated cardiomyopathy often display electrocardiographic abnormalities owing to atrial enlargement, low voltage, and poor R-wave progression, often in pseudoinfarct pattern. Chest X-rays frequently show cardiomegaly with an increase in pulmonary vascularity, although patients with non-dilated cardiomyopathy have normal heart size and increased pulmonary vascularity. A large cardiac silhouette is more commonly noted in patients with large pericardial effusions than in those with dilated cardiomyopathy. Endomyocardial biopsy can be useful to diagnose myocarditis or to identify an opportunistic cardiac infection or cardiac malignancy.

## Therapy and management

Treatment of patients with HIV-related cardiomyopathy who present with CHF consists of the use of conventional treatment with digoxin, diuretics, vasodilators, and converting-enzyme inhibitors [37]. As mentioned above, patients with HIV-related cardiomyopathy may have significantly reduced systemic vascular resistance compared with patients without

**Table 26.6** Comparison of haemodynamic variables in patients with HIV-related and non-HIV-related myocarditis[a]

| | HIV-related ($n$ = 28) | Non-HIV-related ($n$ = 62) | $p$-Value |
|---|---|---|---|
| Heart rate (beats/min) | 103 | 99 | 0.51 |
| Cardiac index (l/m/m$^2$) | 3.1 | 2.4 | 0.02 |
| PCW (mean) (mmHg) | 13 | 16 | 0.16 |
| SVRI | 2453 | 3039 | 0.03 |
| LVSWI | 31.8 | 26.8 | 0.14 |

[a]Obtained during right-sided heart catheterization immediately after endomyocardial biopsy. PCW = pulmonary capillary wedge pressure; SVRI = systemic vascular resistance index; LVSWI = left ventricular stroke work index.

HIV infection who present with similarly depressed left ventricular function (Table 26.6). Therefore, afterload reduction may lead to hypotension in a subset of these patients and should be used judiciously.

Based on published results, patients with AIDS and severe left ventricular dysfunction with CHF appear to have a poor short-term prognosis, with approximately half dying of primary cardiac failure within 6–12 months of presentation [3, 5, 8–10, 13, 15]. Important exceptions to note are: (1) patients with cardiac dysfunction secondary to drug hypersensitivity (eosinophilic) myocarditis (e.g., secondary to penicillins and sulfa drugs) [17] or to drug cardiotoxicity (e.g., nucleoside analogues and pentamidine) [38, 39], in whom left ventricular function returns to normal following the discontinuation of the offending medication; (2) a small group of patients who present with HIV-related cardiomyopathy as a very early manifestation of HIV infection, in whom the cardiomyopathy resolves spontaneously within weeks of initiation of antiretroviral therapy; and (3) HIV-infected IVDUs who abuse cocaine and present with CHF that may resolve when the cocaine abuse is stopped.

Little is known about the role of antiviral therapy in HIV-related cardiomyopathy. Two patients with newly diagnosed HIV infection who presented with CHF responded dramatically to initiation of therapy with zidovudine, suggesting that a rapid reduction in viral load may have a dramatic effect on the myocardium. In contrast, patients with cardiomyopathy who are already taking antiretroviral therapy, particularly when there is a history of non-cardiac toxicity to antiretroviral therapy (e.g., skeletal myositis), may benefit from a brief respite from drugs and should be re-evaluated in 1 month [38]. If echocardiographic evidence of severe left ventricular dysfunction persists, endomyocardial biopsy should be considered to explore other causes of heart failure, as patients are unlikely to experience spontaneous remission at that point.

The recent development of highly active combination antiretroviral therapy has had a profound impact on the epidemiology of AIDS and on the lives of individual patients. Through combinations of antiretroviral drugs, especially protease inhibitors, viral suppression may be achieved. However, adherence to these complex medical regimens and drug interactions have been problems for many patients. In addition, the durability of viral suppression and clinical response are not yet well characterized. It is not clear how long viral suppression will last in individual patients. While the impact of newer combinations of antiretroviral therapies on the natural history of HIV-related cardiomyopathy needs to be studied, it is likely that patients with late-stage HIV infection will be at equivalent risk as the population on older regimens. In addition, newer antiretroviral agents have specific toxicities associated with thier use, which may create new cardiovascular syndromes.

Levy *et al.* [22] and Kaul *et al.* [40] each described one patient treated successfully with a combination of prednisone and azathiaprine. At The Johns Hopkins Hospital, all HIV-infected patients with severe left ventricular dysfunction and HYHA class III or IV CHF, myocarditis on biopsy, and circulating antiheart antibodies, were treated with conventional heart failure medications for 1 month. In a subgroup of 14 patients with persistent poor left ventricular function and S3 gallop on re-examination, immunosuppressive therapy was instituted with high-dose prednisone (1 mg/kg/day for 1 month followed by a gradual taper over 1 month). All patients had AIDS with median CD4 counts of 56/mm$^3$ (range 0–176) and did not have evidence of active viral infection. Of the 14 patients, eight had rapid marked improvement in left ventricular ejection fraction and early resolution of congestive symptoms. No patient experienced deterioration in cardiac function. Three required repeat therapy with prednisone after congestive symptoms and echocardiographic evidence of left ventricular dysfunction returned (Fig. 26.4). Of the 14 patients treated with immunosuppressive therapy, three were lost to follow-up at 5, 9, and 11 months after presentation with CHF. Of the remaining 11 patients, two were alive without

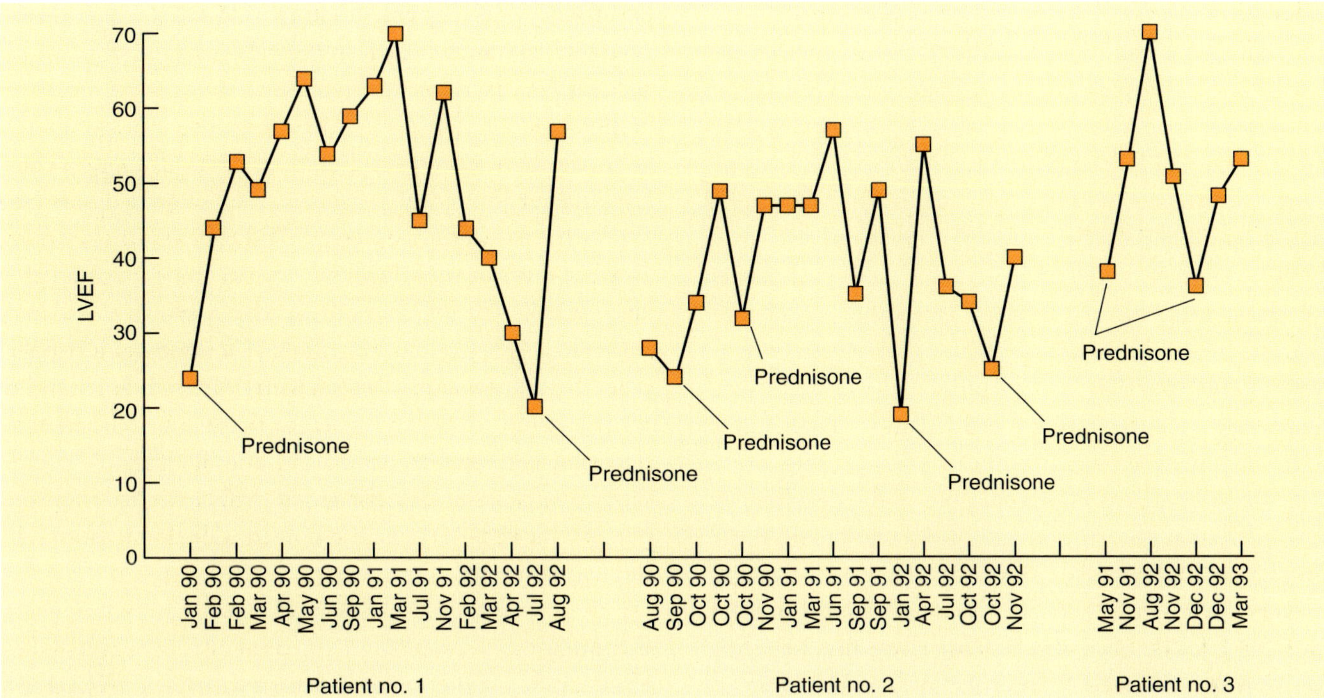


**Figure 26.4** *Left ventricular ejection fraction (LVEF) related to treatment with prednisone in three HIV-infected patients with myocarditis.*

cardiac dysfunction at 16 and 25 months. The remaining nine patients died between 3 and 35 months, although only three had primary cardiac deaths at 5, 9, and 10 months. Only one patient developed an opportunistic infection after a full course of immunosuppressive therapy.

It is clear that prospective studies are needed to define the potential role of immunosuppressive therapy in this disease, particularly in well-defined subsets of patients with HIV-related myocarditis and possible immune-mediated injury. In addition, a non-randomized study of a paediatric HIV infection recently suggested a possible role for intravenous immunoglobulin in HIV-related cardiomyopathy [41]. This immunomodulatory strategy will likewise require prospective clinical trials.

While the presence of asymptomatic HIV-related cardiac disease does not constitute a therapeutic challenge, proper identification of HIV-related cardiac disease, even occult disease, may have particular relevance in determining the feasibility of fluid replacement, as well as the antibiotic and tumour therapies commonly used in this population. For example, HIV-infected patients with occult cardiomyopathy may present clinically with acute pulmonary oedema after receiving intravenous hydration or blood products for dyspnoea of presumed pulmonary origin. Other forms of therapy such as intravenous trimethoprim–sulfamethoxasole require large volumes of fluid which must be used cautiously in patients with HIV-related cardiomyopathy. Lastly, anthracycline derivatives and interferon-$\alpha$ therapy, used as chemotherapeutic agents for Kaposi's sarcoma, may lead to further cardiac decompensation secondary to their independent cardiotoxicity.

## Potential effects of cocaine and alcohol on HIV-related cardiomyopathy

Although all forms of HIV-related heart disease have been described in each of the major HIV risk groups, HIV-seropositive IVDUs appear to be at increased risk for bacterial endocarditis and, possibly, the direct cardiotoxic manifestations of illicit drug use or alcohol. One key experience that points to a potential interaction between direct cardiotoxicity from illicit drug use and other toxins such as alcohol in HIV-infected IVDUs is that while left ventricular dysfunction occurs in most instances in patients with severely depressed circulating CD4 cell counts, HIV-infected IVDUs may develop severe cardiomyopathy and CHF when circulating CD4 cell counts are not markedly depressed.

## Cocaine

It is clear that cocaine is a cardiotoxic agent and may predispose to the development of cardiomyopathy. Other cardiovascular complications of cocaine abuse include chest pain, myocardial ischaemia and infarction, CHF, coronary spasm, cardiac arrhythmias, sudden death, myocarditis, dilated cardiomyopathy, infective endocarditis, aortic dissection, acute pulmonary oedema, and pathological alterations in blood vessels including accelerated atherosclerosis [42–45]. The precise pathogenic basis for these cardiovascular complications associated with cocaine use remains poorly understood and requires further study. In any case, the hypothesis that cocaine use in HIV-infected patients may predispose to the development of cardiomyopathy is critical from a public-health perspective. In the USA, 27% of all AIDS cases were diagnosed in IVDUs in 1994. In addition, over 5 million Americans use cocaine on a regular basis. The first issue that needs to be addressed is whether intravenous drug use alone plays an important causal role in the development of cardiomyopathy.

In a series of 534 consecutive endomyocardial biopsies performed at The Johns Hopkins Hospital between 1985 and 1990 [46], there were only six cases of cardiomyopathy in HIV-seronegative intravenous cocaine users, suggesting that cocaine-induced cardiomyopathy is rare in the non-HIV-infected population. In addition, global left ventricular hypokinesis was reported [16] in only one of 85 HIV-seronegative IVDUs (96% of whom were intravenous cocaine users), also supporting the hypothesis that in non-HIV-infected cohorts, intravenous drug use per se only explains a small proportion of cardiomyopathy cases. From a histological perspective, Virmani *et al.* [47] studied 40 medical examiner cases of cocaine-associated deaths and found evidence of myocarditis in 20%. Another study similarly found active myocarditis in 33% of autopsies from HIV-seronegative IVDUs with no clinical cardiac disease who experienced violent, trauma-related deaths [48]. These findings initially suggested that intravenous drug use may have contributed to the high prevalence of myocarditis in this population of HIV-infected patients. Examination of the frozen tissue from the HIV-seronegative group, however, failed to demonstrate increased myocyte expression of MHC class I, whereas 11 of 15 of the HIV-infected IVDUs with poor left ventricular function and myocarditis had abnormal myocyte expression of MHC class I. These findings strongly suggest that although histological myocarditis may be a non-specific findings in IVDUs, when associated with cardiomyopathy in the HIV-infected population, myocarditis is likely to represent a targeted immune response.

In the HIV-infected population, while it appears clear that intravenous cocaine users may develop cardiomyopathy with less severely depressed CD4 cell counts than non-IVDUs, it is not yet known whether cocaine use increases the overall risk for cardiomyopathy. Corallo *et al.* [11] reported a 41% prevalence of global left ventricular hypokinesis in predominantly IVDUs with AIDS, while Kinney *et al.* [7] found a lower prevalence of 10.5%. Further epidemiological studies comparing the incidence of cardiomyopathy in all HIV risk groups will be needed to define the specific role of cocaine use in the development of cardiomyopathy.

## Alcohol

Excessive consumption of alcohol is widely recognized as a common cause of dilated cardiomyopathy [49, 50]. The mechanisms responsible for alcohol-induced contractile dysfunction remain poorly characterized, yet there appears to be a direct correlation between alcohol consumption and depression of ejection fraction in populations of chronic alcoholics [51]. With regard to a potential synergism between alcohol use and cardiomyopathy in HIV-infected patients, several potential mechanisms may play a role. Alcohol may directly induce (1) myocyte injury. (2) Chronic alcohol use predisposing to exacerbation of viral myocarditis. Mice with experimental chronic alcoholism infected with *Trypanasoma cruzi* have a more severe myocarditis, higher levels of cardiac parasitaemia, and higher mortality rates [52]. Alcohol-induced immunosuppression may indeed predispose HIV-infected patients to higher cardiotropic virus titres which could induce more severe cardiac cellular injury; and (3) enhanced immune dysregulation induced by chronic alcohol abuse may predispose to exaggerated immune responses within the myocardium.

Whatever the pathogenic mechanisms that may play a role in the development of cardiomyopathy in HIV-infected patients abusing cocaine and/or alcohol, it is likely that multiple pathways converge to elicit cardiac injury. One such multiple pathway paradigm is described below when examining potential mechanisms responsible for the development of accelerated atherosclerosis in HIV-infected patients.

## Potential role of HIV infection and atherosclerosis

Recently, a lipodystrophy has been described in association with drug cocktails including protease inhibitors [53]. Fat wasting is seen from the arms, legs, and buttocks, while unusually large fat deposits in the abdomen and 'buffalo hump' fat pads on the back are seen. These anatomical findings have been associated with elevated serum cholesterol and triglyceride levels, which may predispose patients to severe premature coronary artery disease, angina, and heart attack [54–56]. While these preliminary findings do not warrant discontinuation of potential life-saving antiretroviral therapy in HIV-infected patients, they raise concerns regarding the cardiotoxicities that will be encountered during the next decade. Several types of arterial vascular lesion, including accelerated atherosclerosis and vasculitis, have already been described, even in children [57].

The association between HIV infection and an accelerated form of atherosclerosis has an appealing theoretical basis: (1) exposure to vasculotropic viruses such as CMV causing endothelial activation and injury; (2) the presence of activated macrophages triggered via enhanced production of cytokines by activated T-cells; (3) endothelial injury associated with HIV infection attributed to increased endothelial monocyte adherence resulting from upregulation of vascular endothelial adhesion molecules [58, 59]; (4) superimposed dyslipidaemia induced by newer antiretroviral regimens; (5) the atherogenic effects of cocaine with associated elevated circulating levels of catecholamines in the subpopulation of HIV-infected patients who abuse cocaine; and (6) the immunosuppression and immunodysregulation induced by cocaine and alcohol abuse increasing the potential for reactivation of latent CMV infection within myocardial endothelial cells, accelerating microvascular injury and leading to small-vessel disease and accelerated atherosclerosis in large epicardial vessels.

The present authors' anecdotal experience in three patients with acquired HIV infection following coronary artery bypass graft surgery is worrisome. These patients developed ischaemic dilated cardiomyopathy within months of the surgery and were found to have occluded grafts and progression of native coronary disease. It appears likely that as HIV-infected patients live longer and are exposed to pro-atherogenic drugs and cardiotropic viruses, the development of symptomatic atherosclerosis will require careful study.

## Conclusions

Since 1986, when HIV-related cardiomyopathy was first described clinically, numerous studies have found that HIV-infected patients are susceptible to a wide spectrum of cardiovascular abnormalities. To the clinician, the myriad of possible cardiac abnormalities in these patients poses unique diagnostic and therapeutic challenges. Any HIV-infected patient can develop symptomatic heart disease secondary to cardiomyopathy, cardiac tamponade, or endocarditis, although patients with severely depressed CD4 cell counts appear at particular risk. When patients present with new-onset CHF and are found to have depressed left ventricular function by echocardiography, the likelihood that an endomyocardial biopsy will demonstrate histological evidence of myocarditis is significantly higher than in the general population. Does the presence of myocarditis by histology and immunohistochemistry, along with the experimental evidence demonstrating that HIV-1 and a number of cardiotropic viruses (CVB, CMV, and EBV) are associated with HIV-related myocarditis, all strongly suggestive of a primary immune-mediated process within the myocardium, help clinicians in determining whether immunomodulative therapies should be considered? Today, the question remains as to whether immunosuppressive therapy has a role in the treatment of HIV-related cardiomyopathy and myocarditis. The Myocarditis Treatment Trial [60] failed to show a clinically significant benefit of prednisone therapy in (non-HIV) patients with histological evidence of active myocarditis. Similarly, while the presence of severe immunosuppression and immune dysregulation found in the HIV-infected population probably makes this patient group uniquely susceptible to cardiac inflammation, leading to progressive dysfunction, no specific immunosuppressive therapy has yet been shown to be effective. Randomized clinical trials in well-characterized patients are clearly needed to resolve these therapeutic issues.

Recent epidemiological trends indicate that the proportion of AIDS cases and new HIV infections are increasing among subpopulations that have been relatively under-represented in the USA. Increased proportions of HIV-infected women, African–Americans, and Hispanics, and infectious transmission through heterosexual transmission is likely to change the face of AIDS and AIDS-related syndromes, including heart disease. In addition, the clinical management of HIV infection and AIDS has become increasingly complex in recent years, and both newly approved and experimental therapeutic agents are constantly being used. The impact of these trends on the frequency of HIV-related cardiomyopathy, as well as the specific pathogenic mechanisms responsible for HIV-related cardiac dysfunction, will also need to be intensively studied and tracked.

## References


1. Horowitz HW, Telzak EE, Sepkowitz KA, Wormser GP. Human immunodeficiency virus infection, Part I. *Dis Mon* 1998; 44: 545–606.
2. Anderson DW, Virmani R. Emerging patterns of heart disease in human immunodeficiency virus infection. *Hum Pathol* 1990; 21: 253–7.
3. Cohen IS, Anderson DW, Virmani R *et al.* Congestive cardiomyopathy in association with the acquired immunodeficiency syndrome. *N Engl J Med* 1986; 315: 628–30.
4. Hsia J, Ross AM. Pericardial effusion and pericardiocentesis in human immunodeficiency virus infection. *Am J Cardiol* 1994; 74: 94–6.
5. Herskowitz A, Vlahov D, Willoughby S *et al.* Prevalence and incidence of left ventricular dysfunction in patients with human immunodeficiency virus infection. *Am J Cardiol* 1993; 71: 955–8.
6. Levy WS, Simon GL, Rios JC, Ross AM. Prevalence of cardiac abnormalities in human immunodeficiency virus infection. *Am J Cardiol* 1989; 63: 86–9.
7. Kinney EL, Brafman D, Wright RJ. Echocardiographic findings in patients with acquired immunodeficiency syndrome (AIDS) and AIDS-related complex (ARC). *Cathet Cardiovasc Diagn* 1989; 16: 182–5.
8. Monsuez JJ, Kinney EL, Vittecoq D *et al.* Comparison among acquired immune deficiency syndrome patients with and without clinical evidence of cardiac disease. *Am J Cardiol* 1988; 62: 1311–13.
9. Himelman RB, Chung WS, Chernoff DN *et al.* Cardiac manifestations of human immunodeficiency virus infection: a two-dimensional echocardiographic study. *J Am Coll Cardiol* 1989; 13: 1030–6.
10. Blanchard DG, Hagenhoff C, Chow LC *et al.* Reversibility of cardiac abnormalities in human immunodeficiency virus (HIV) infected individuals: a serial echocardiographic study. *J Am Coll Cardiol* 1991; 17: 1270–6.
11. Corallo S, Mutinelli MR, Moroni M *et al.* Echocardiography detects myocardial damage in AIDS: prospective study in 102 patients. *Eur Heart J* 1988; 9: 887–92.
12. Akhras F, Dubrey S, Gazzard B, Noble MIM. Emerging patterns of heart disease in HIV infected homosexual subjects with and without opportunistic infections; a prospective color flow Doppler echocardiographic study. *Eur Heart J* 1994; 15: 68–75.
13. Currie PF, Jacob AJ, Foreman AR *et al.* Heart muscle disease related to HIV infection: prognostic implications. *BMJ* 1994; 309: 1605–7.
14. De Castro S, d'Amati G, Gallo P *et al.* Frequency of development of acute global left ventricular dysfunction in human immunodeficiency virus infection. *J Am Coll Cardiol* 1994; 24: 1018–24.
15. Barbaro G, Di Lorenzo G, Grisorio B, Barbarini G. Incidence of dilated cardiomyopathy and detection of HIV in myocardial cells of HIV-positive patients. *N Engl J Med* 1998; 339: 1093–9.
16. Willoughby SB, Vlahov D, Herskowitz A. Frequency of left ventricular dysfunction and other echocardiographic abnormalities in human immunodeficiency virus seronegative intravenous drug users. *Am J Cardiol* 1993; 71: 446–7.
17. Herskowitz A, Wu T-C, Willoughby SB *et al.* Myocarditis and cardiotropic viral infection associated with severe left ventricular dysfunction in late stage infection with human immunodeficiency virus. *J Am Coll Cardiol* 1994; 24: 1025–32.
18. Wu TC, Pizzomo MC, Hayward GS *et al.* *In situ* detection of human cytomegalovirus immediate-early gene transcripts within cardiac myocytes of patients with HIV-associated cardiomyopathy. *AIDS* 1992; 6: 777–85.
19. Grody WW, Cheng L, Lewis W. Infection of the heart by the human immunodeficiency virus. *Am J Cardiol* 1990; 66: 203–6.
20. Herskowitz A, Willoughby S, Wu T-C *et al.* Immunopathogenesis of HIV-1 associated cardiomyopathy. *Clin Immunol Immunopathol* 1993; 68: 234–41.
21. Anderson DW, Virmani R, Reilly JM *et al.* Prevalent myocarditis at necropsy in the acquired immunodeficiency syndrome. *J Am Coll Cardiol* 1988; 12: 463–9.
22. Levy WS, Varghese PJ, Anderson DW *et al.* Myocarditis diagnosed by endomyocardial biopsy in human immunodeficiency infection with cardiac dysfunction. *Am J Cardiol* 1988; 62: 658–9.
23. Beschorner WE, Baughman KL, Turnicky RP *et al.* HIV associated myocarditis: pathology and immunopathology. *Am J Pathol* 1990; 137: 1365–71.
24. Herskowitz A, Ansari AA, Neumann DA *et al.* Induction of major histocompatibility complex (MHC) antigens within the myocardium of patients with active myocarditis: A nonhistologic marker of myocarditis. *J Am Coll Cardiol* 1990; 15: 624–32.
25. Levy JA. Pathogenesis of human immunodeficiency virus infection. *Microbiol Rev* 1993; 57: 183–9.
26. Ikeuchi K, Kim S, Byrn RA *et al.* Infection of nonlymphoid cells by human immunodeficiency virus Type 1 or Type 2. *J Virol* 1990; 64: 4226–31.
27. Hesselgesser J, Halks-Miller M, DelVecchio V *et al.* CD4-independent association between HIV-1 gp120 and CXCR4: functional chemokine receptors are expressed in human neurons. *Curr Biol* 1997; 7: 112–21.
28. Rebolledo MA, Krogstd P, Chen F *et al.* Infection of human fetal cardiac myocytes by a human immunodeficiency virus-1-dervied vector. *Circ Res* 1998; 83: 738–42.
29. Rodriguez ER, Nasim S, Hsia J *et al.* Cardiac myocytes and dendritic cells harbor human immunodeficiency virus (HIV) in infected patients with and without cardiac dysfunction: detection by multiplex, nested, polymerase chain reaction in individually microdissected cells from right ventricular endomyocardial biopsy tissue. *Am J Cardiol* 1991; 68: 1511–20.
30. Wang YC, Neckelmann N, Mayne A *et al.* Establishment of a human fetal cardiac myocyte cell line. *In Vitro Cell Dev Biol* 1991; 27A: 63–74.
31. Ansari AA, Kanter K, Wang YC *et al.* Major histocompatibility complex-expressing human cardiac myocytes are not the direct target of host cardiac-infiltrating cell: evidence for a prominent role of the indirect pathway in human cardiac allograft rejection. *Transplant Proc* 1993; 25: 89–93.

32. Ansari AA, Wang YC, Danner DJ *et al.* Abnormal expression of histocompatibility and mitochondrial antigens by cardiac tissue from patients with myocarditis and dilated cardiomyopathy. *Am J Pathol* 1991; 139: 59–67.
33. Herskowitz A, Baughman KL. Effect of HIV infection on the heart. In: ER Braunwald (ed.) *Heart disease, clinical update. Boston* 1994, 1–10.
34. Matsumori A, Yamada T, Suzuki H *et al.* Increased circulating cytokines in patients with myocarditis and cardiomyopathy. *Br Heart J* 1994; 72: 561–6.
35. Lane JR, Neumann DA, Lafond-Walker A *et al.* Interleukin 1 and tumor necrosis factor can promote coxsackievirus B-3-induced myocarditis in resistant B10.A mice. *J Exp Med* 1992; 175: 1123–9.
36. de Bracco MME, Borda E, Galassi N *et al.* Autoantibodies in HIV-infected patients that modulate the cholinergic activity of heart and gut tissue. *Autoimmunity* 1993; 14: 307–14.
37. Barbaro G, Barbarini G, Di Lorenzo G. Early impairment of systolic and diastolic function in asymptomatic HIV-positive patients: a multicenter echocardiographic and echo-Doppler study. *AIDS Res Hum Retroviruses* 1996; 12: 1559–63.
38. Herskowitz A, Willoughby SB, Baughman KL *et al.* Cardiomyopathy associated with anti-retroviral therapy in patients with human immunodeficiency virus infection: a report of six cases. *Ann Intern Med* 1992; 116: 311–13.
39. Domanski MJ, Sloas MM, Follmann DA *et al.* Effect of zidovudine and didanosine treatment on heart function in children infected with human immunodeficiency virus. *Pediatries* 1995; 127: 137–46.
40. Kaul S, Fishbein MC, Siegel RJ. Cardiac manifestations of acquired immune deficiency syndrome: a 1991 update. *Am Heart J* 1991; 122: 535–44.
41. Lipshultz SE, Orav EJ, Sanders SP, Colan SD. Immunoglobulins and left ventricular structure and function in pediatric HIV infection. *Circulation* 1995; 92: 2220–5.
42. Kloner RA, Hale S, Alker K, Rezkalla S. The effects of acute and chronic cocaine use on the heart. *Circulation* 1992; 85: 407–19.
43. Karch SB, Billingham ME. The pathology and etiology of cocaine-induced heart disease. *Arch Pathol Lab Med* 1988; 112: 225–30.
44. Mehta PM, Grainger TA, Lust RM *et al.* Effect of cocaine on left ventricular function: relation to increased wall stress and persistence after treatment. *Circulation* 1995; 91: 3002–9.
45. Pilati CF, Espinal AR, Pukys TF. Persistent left ventricular dysfunction after cocaine treatment in rabbits. *Proc Soc Exp Biol Med* 1993; 203: 100–7.
46. Herskowitz A, Campbell S, Deckers *et al.* Demographic features and prevalence of idiopathic myocarditis in patients undergoing endomyocardial biopsies at The Johns Hopkins Hospital. *Am J Cardiol* 1993; 71: 982–6.
47. Virmani R, Robinowitz M, Smialek JE, Smyth DF. Cardiovascular effects of cocaine: an autopsy study of 40 patients. *Am Heart J* 1988; 115: 1068–76.
48. Turnicky RP, Godin J, Smialek JE *et al.* Incidental myocarditis with intravenous drug abuse: the pathology, immunopathology, and potential implications for HIV associated myocarditis. *Hum Pathol* 1992; 23: 138–43.
49. Richardson PJ, Wodak AD. Alcohol-induced heart muscle disease. In: C Symons, T Evans, A Mitchell (eds) *Speficic heart muscle disease.* Bristol: G Wright PSG, 1983; 99–122.
50. Richardson PJ, Wodak AD, Atkinson L *et al.* Relation between alcohol intake, myocardial enzyme activity and myocardial function in dilated cardiomyopathy. *Br Heart J* 1986; 56: 165–70.
51. Urbano-Marquez A, Estruch R, Navarro-Lopez F *et al.* The effects of alcoholism on skeletal and cardiac muscle. *N Engl J Med* 1989; 320: 409–15.
52. Miller H, Abelmann WH. Effects of dietary ethanol upon experimental trypasosomal (*T. cruzi*) myocarditis. *Proc Soc Exp Biol Med* 1967; 126: 193–8.
53. SoRelle R. Vascular and lipid syndromes in selected HIV-infected patients. *Circulation* 1998; 98: 829–30.
54. Gallet B, Pulik M, Genet P *et al.* Lettor to the Editor. *Lancet* 1998; 351: 1958–9.
55. Henry K, Melroe H, Huebsch J *et al.* Severe premature coronary artery disease with protease inhibitors. *Lancet* 1998; 351: 1328.
56. Paton P, Tabib A, Loire R, Tete R. Coronary artery lesions and human immunodeficiency virus infection. *Res Virol* 1993; 144: 225–31.
57. Patel RC, Frishman WH. AIDS and the heart: clinicopathologic assessment. *Cardiovasc Pathol* 1995; 4: 173–83.
58. Zietz C, Hotz B, Sturzl M *et al.* Aortic endothelium in HIV-1 infection: chronic injury, activation and increased leucocyte adherence. *Am J Pathol* 1996; 149: 1887–98.
59. Dhawan S, Weeks BS, Soderland C *et al.* HIV-1 infection alters monocyte interaction with human microvascular endothelial cells. *J Immunol* 1995; 154: 422–32.
60. Mason JW, O'Connell JB, Herskowitz A *et al.* A clinical trial of immunosuppressive therapy for myocarditis. The Myocarditis Treatment Trial Investigators. *N Engl J Med* 1995; 333: 269–75.

# Cardiac involvement in systemic disorders

27

A. BURKE AND R. VIRMANI

## Introduction

Cardiac complications of non-cardiac diseases often result in significant morbidity and mortality. The effects of systemic diseases on the heart are usually complex and multifactorial, and often result in a dilated cardiomyopathy [1] (Table 27.1). These effects may be direct effects on the myocyte, with alterations in contractility or conduction or, more frequently, may be indirect. Indirect effects of systemic diseases on the heart include changes in vascular tone, metabolic changes that predispose to coronary disease, direct thrombotic or vasoactive effects on epicardial or intramural coronary arteries, changes in heart valve structure and function, and a combination of these factors. The eventual results on myocardial function may be due to ischaemia, interstitial diseases, hypertrophy, and inflammatory myocardial processes. The purpose of this chapter is to outline a few of the more common and important complications of systemic processes on the myocardium, with an emphasis on pathological alterations.

**Table 27.1** Secondary causes of dilated cardiomyopathy

| Condition | Frequency (%) |
|---|---|
| Primary cardiac causes[a] | 79 |
| Human immunodeficiency virus infection | 4.9 |
| Chronic alcoholism | 3.4 |
| Amyloidosis | 2.1 |
| Hypertension | 2.1 |
| Adriamycin toxicity | 1.3 |
| Cocaine abuse | 1.3 |
| Progressive systemic sclerosis | 1.0 |
| Systemic lupus erythematosus | 0.7 |
| Hyperthyroidism | 0.6 |
| Haemochromatosis | 0.4 |
| Sarcoidosis | 0.4 |
| Neuromuscular diseases | 0.4 |
| Hypothyroidism | 0.3 |
| Phaeochromocytoma | 0.15 |
| Polymyositis | 0.15 |
| Polyarteritis nodosa | 0.15 |
| Rheumatic carditis | 0.15 |
| Interleukin-2 toxicity | 0.15 |
| Prednisone toxicity | 0.15 |
| Histiocytosis X | 0.15 |
| Thrombotic thrombocytopenic purpura | 0.15 |
| Lithium toxicity | 0.15 |

(Adapted from ref. 1.)
[a]Including idiopathic dilated cardiomyopathy, myocarditis, coronary artery disease, peripartum cardiomyopathy, familiar cardiomyopathy, valvular myopathy, congenital heart disease, bypass surgery, atrial fibrillation.

## Cardiac complications of renal disease

### Left ventricular hypertrophy

Cardiac disease is the major cause of death in patients with end-stage renal disease (ESRD). Cross-sectional studies have shown that up to 80% of patients on dialysis have abnormal echocardiograms, with left ventricular hypertrophy being the most frequent finding (Fig. 27.1). The incidence of left ventricular hypertrophy in patients undergoing dialysis ranges from 50 to 90% [2–4]. In general, there is no difference in the frequency of left ventricular hypertrophy between patients treated by haemodialysis and those treated by chronic ambulatory peritoneal dialysis [5], although one study found a decreased prevalence in those treated with peritoneal dialysis [2]. Left ventricular hypertrophy is frequently noted in patients with moderate to severe chronic renal failure not requiring dialysis [6]. However, it is less frequently accompanied by left ventricular systolic dysfunction, compared with patients on peritoneal dialysis and haemodialysis [5]. The degree of left ventricular hypertrophy in patients with renal failure not requiring dialysis demonstrates a step-wise increase with decrease in renal function [4]. Left ventric-

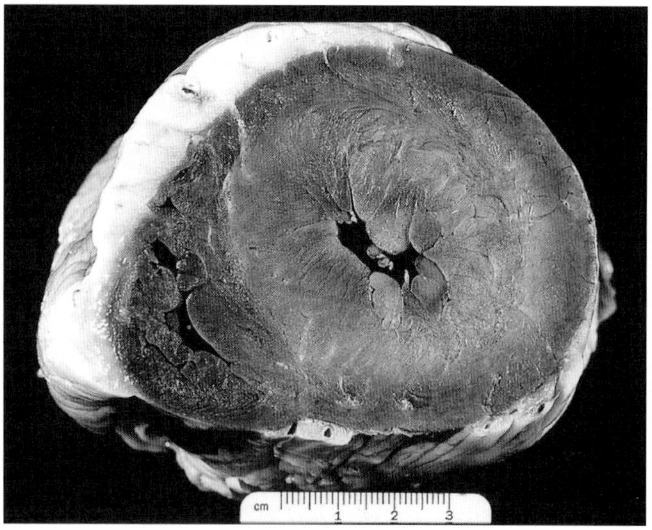


**Figure 27.1** *Concentric left ventricular hypertrophy, renal failure. Note the marked thickening of the left ventricular wall, approaching 2 cm, and the small chamber cavity. The patient was a 50-year-old male with a history of diabetes, end-stage renal failure, and left below-the-knee amputation, who was found unresponsive.*

ular hypertrophy as a complication of ESRD occurs in children as well as adults [7], and often affects the ventricular septum disproportionately [8]. In children, voltage criteria on the electrocardiogram (ECG) are of no value in detecting left ventricular hypertrophy, which must be evaluated by echocardiography [8].

The pathophysiology of left ventricular hypertrophy in renal failure patients is incompletely understood. Hypertension is an important contributor but is not the only stimulus, as normotensive patients with ESRD may show an increase in left ventricular mass over time [9]. Other factors include chronic flow overload, predominantly secondary to anaemia, and poorly understood neurohumoral alterations [10]. Factors that were independently related to left ventricular hypertrophy in some but not all studies are age, hypertension, high serum alkaline phosphatase level decreased haemoglobin level, increased endothelin level, and diabetes [2, 5, 11, 12]. Hyperparathyroidism has not been found to correlate with left ventricular mass [11]. In patients with moderately severe renal failure not requiring dialysis, age, hypertension, anaemia, and increased creatinine were independent predictors of left ventricular wall thickness [4]. In children, there is evidence that increased left ventricular mass occurs prior to the onset of anaemia or hypertension [7], and that anaemia has a more dominant influence on cardiovascular function than hypertension in end-stage renal failure [13].

Humoral factors that show an independent relationship with left ventricular hypertrophy in renal failure patients include increased plasma renin and endothelin levels. Because angiotensin II promotes growth in both fibroblasts and cardiac myocytes *in vitro*, a causal association with the development of left ventricular hypertrophy in chronic haemodialysis patients has been proposed [14]. The possible mechanism of endothelin-induced left ventricular hypertrophy remains speculative [15].

Diastolic function in renal failure-induced left ventricular hypertrophy is similar in degree to that seen in left ventricular hypertrophy without renal disease [16]. In patients on chronic ambulatory peritoneal dialysis diastolic dysfunction is most closely correlated with systolic blood pressure and creatinine levels, and not left ventricular mass [17].

The most serious complications of left ventricular hypertrophy in patients with renal disease are ventricular arrhythmias and sudden death [4]. Diastolic dysfunction associated with ventricular hypertrophy may cause unusual sensitivity to volume changes, such that hypotension, haemodynamic instability, supraventricular arrhythmias, and/or pulmonary oedema occur with small volume variations [10]. A syndrome of the hypertrophic, high cardiac output haemodialysis heart, characterized by a high cardiac output associated with left ventricular hypertrophy, right ventricular hypertrophy, and tricuspid insufficiency, has been described, and may require fistula revision and even a switch to peritoneal dialysis [18].

The treatment of left ventricular hypertrophy in patients with chronic renal failure includes control of hypertension, fluid overload, and uraemia [19]. The use of erythropoietin to treat anaemia has helped to reverse severe left ventricular hypertrophy, despite a small risk of exacerbating hypertension, perhaps mediated by endothelin and prostanoids [18, 20]. Antihypertensive monotherapy with the angiotensin-converting enzyme (ACE) inhibitors captopril and enalapril in patients with chronic renal failure results in regression of left ventricular mass index associated with a significant improvement in the diastolic function of the left ventricle without a demonstrable deterioration in left ventricular systolic performance [6].

Studies of animals with uraemia have shown several pathophysiological myocardial abnormalities related to left ventricular hypertrophy. These changes include interstitial myocardial fibrosis, for which parathyroid hormone is a permissive factor; reduced myocardial perfusion reserve, secondary to functional and structural changes of intramyocardial arteries and to reduced capillary density; and microvascular abnormalities resulting in reduce ischaemic tolerance. Also observed are diminished responsiveness to β-adrenergic stimulation, impaired maintenance of energy-rich nucleotide concentrations under conditions of ischaemia, abnormal control of intracellular calcium concentration, impaired insulin-mediated glucose uptake, and abnormalities of myocardial oxidative metabolism [21].

## Hypertrophic cardiomyopathy

Long-term haemodialysis has been reported to cause progression of left ventricular hypertrophy, with a tendency towards asymmetric septal hypertrophy that may be reversed by allotransplantation [22]. The frequency of septal asymmetry is low, however, and has been estimated at 3% [23]. A direct effect of increased plasma renin on increased septal thickness has been reported [14], as well as a high rate of septal asymmetry in children on dialysis [8].

## Cardiac failure

Heart failure is a common complication of ESRD, and may be the result of multiple factors, the most important being volume and pressure overload, and negative inotropic effects [24]. Volume overload develops from salt and fluid retention, chronic anaemia, and arteriovenous access fistulae. Pressure overload is largely the result of systemic hypertension, but may result in part from decreased aortic compliance [25]. Depressed cardiac function may occur as a result of hypoxaemia, elevated parathormone levels, metabolic and electrolyte abnormalities, and poorly defined uraemic toxins [24, 26]. Accelerated coronary artery disease and cardiac calcification frequently contribute to the pathogenesis of heart failure in patients with renal failure.

Although it is clear that hypertension is a determinant of left ventricular mass, the impaired diastolic function seen in uraemic patients appears to be independent of blood pressure, degree of hypertrophy, and metabolic changes, which suggests the existence of a specific cardiomyopathy [27]. The presence of interstitial fibrosis in pathological studies of uraemic heart disease supports the concept of a functional type of cardiomyopathy, which has led to the search for soluble 'cardiosuppressant' factors related to renal failure. Acetate ion (present in the dialysate) and secondary hyperparathyroidism do not appear to be clinically relevant myocardial depressant factors in patients with uraemia. The role of carnitine deficiency is not clarified, because most of the data are evaluated in poorly controlled study trials. Serum fractions and ultrafiltrates obtained from patients during dialysis suggest the existence of a water-soluble myocardial depressant of 10 000–30 000 mol. wt [28].

## Atherosclerosis

Coronary artery disease is the second most common cardiac finding in autopsies of patients dying of renal failure [29]. The high incidence of ischaemic heart disease may be a reflection of the high incidence of risk factors, such as hypertension and diabetes, in patients with renal disease. For unknown reasons, patients with chronic pyelonephritis or interstitial renal disease develop coronary artery disease more frequently than patients with other forms of chronic renal failure [30]. In addition to coronary risk factors, patients with renal disease have a higher incidence of lipid abnormalities [decreased high-density-lipoprotein, increased lipoprotein (a)], insulin resistance, and increased triglycerides. Other atherogenic factors in renal failure may include carnitine deficiency, increased parathormone levels, increased homocysteine, and enhanced fibrin and platelet deposition [30]. Elevated endothelin and homocysteine levels may participate in increased vascular stiffness [31]. Chronic ambulatory peritoneal dialysis may result in more lipid derangements than haemodialysis, and vessel calcification may play a role in atherosclerotic heart disease, but this is only an inference from several clinical observations [18].

## Calcification

An autopsy study in the early 1980s clearly established an association between cardiac calcification, especially of the mitral annulus, and chronic renal failure [32] (Fig. 27.2, 27.3). More recently, electron-beam computed tomographic studies have documented increased, rapidly progressing coronary artery calcification in patients in renal failure, compared with patients with coronary artery disease and normal renal function (Fig. 27.4). The coronary calcium score correlated with age, hypertension, and decreased bone mass, without an association with serum parathormone levels [33]. Mitral and aortic valve calcification is found in approximately 50% of patients [23, 33, 34]. Mitral valve calcification may progress to incompetence, which is a factor associated with decreased survival [35], whereas progression to mitral stenosis is uncommon

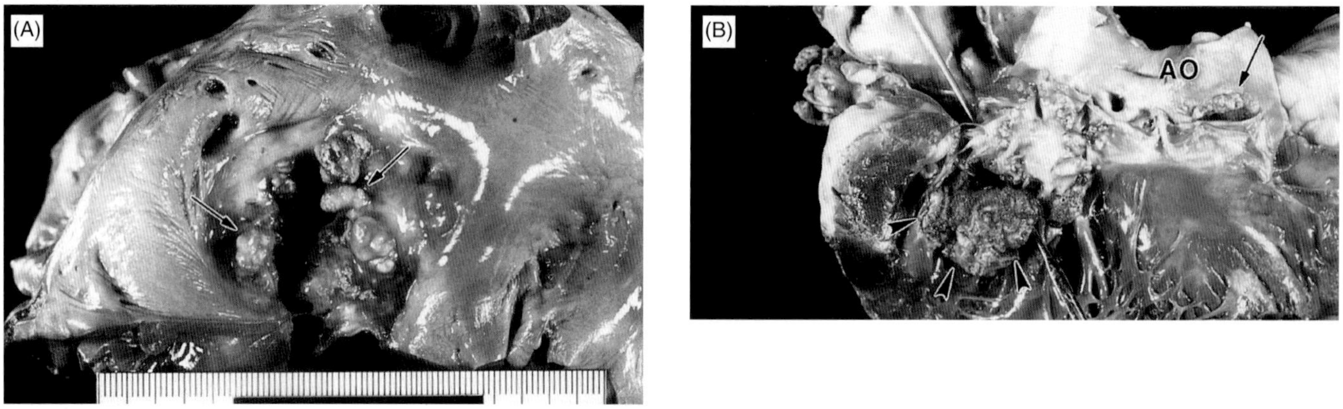


**Figure 27.2** *Mitral valve calcification, renal failure. (A) The mitral valve is viewed from the left atrium; note the left atrial appendage at the top of the photograph, and the atrial septum to the right. There is a large collection of calcified debris on the mitral valve* (arrows)*, resulting in severe stenosis. (B) The left ventricle is opened along the left ventricular outflow tact and a probe is placed in the mitral valve orifice. Note the large calcified nodule covering the mitral valve* (arrowheads)*. The aortic valve also shows focal calcific deposits at the sinotubular junction of the aorta (AO,* arrow*). The patient was a 56-year-old black male with end-stage renal disease on haemodialysis for 7 years and hypertension, who died from complications of sepsis and pneumonia.*

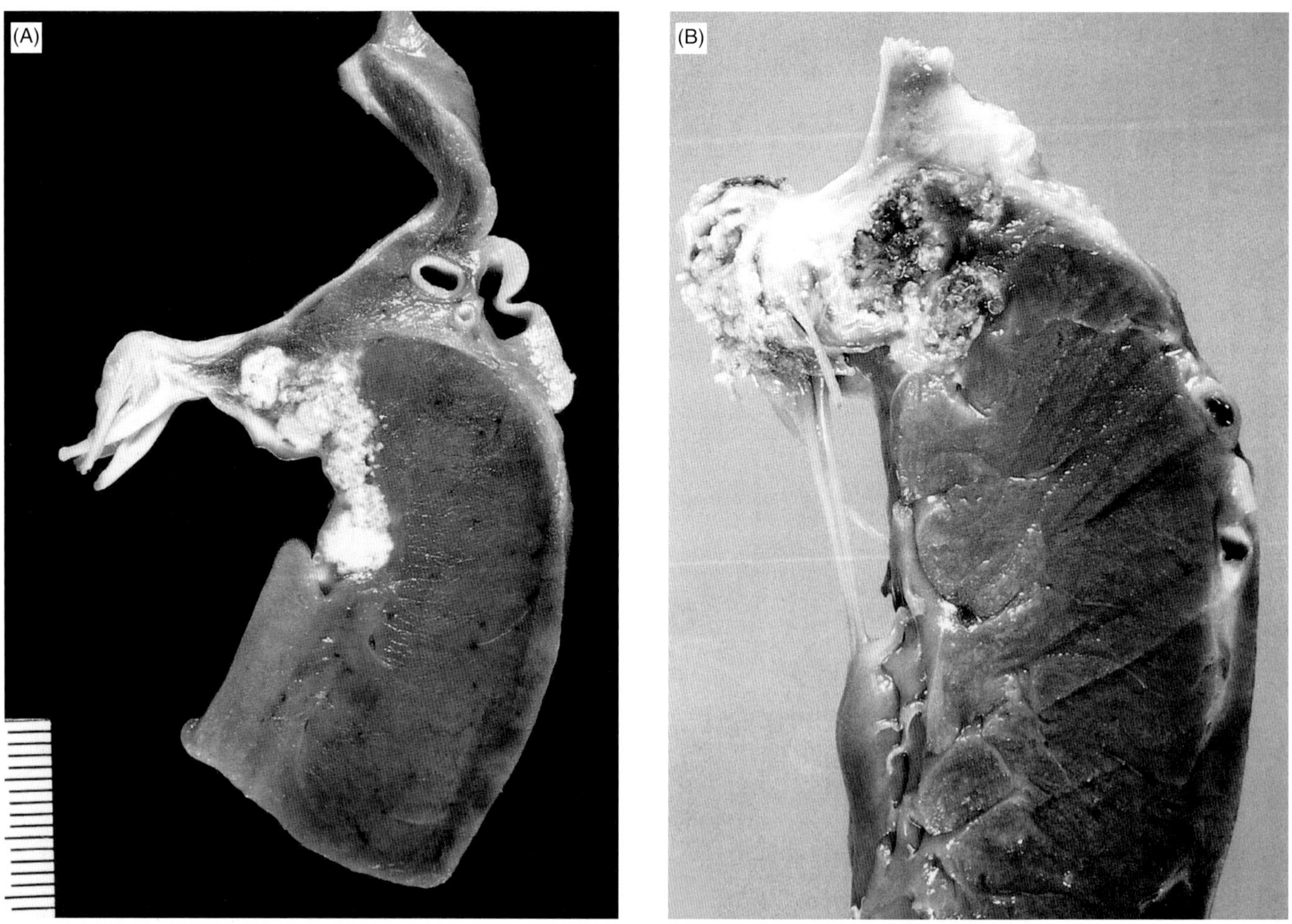


**Figure 27.3** *Mitral annular calcification, renal failure. The calcification is predominantly in the mitral annulus (compared with that shown in Fig. 27.2). These photographs show sections of the left ventricle and atrium including the mitral valve and mitral valve annulus. (A) The patient was a 40-year-old man with end-stage renal disease and a history of drug abuse, who was found unresponsive in a bath tub. (B) A 60-year-old patient who had a long history of dialysis-dependent renal failure (14.5 years). Moderate to severe mitral calcification was found at autopsy.*

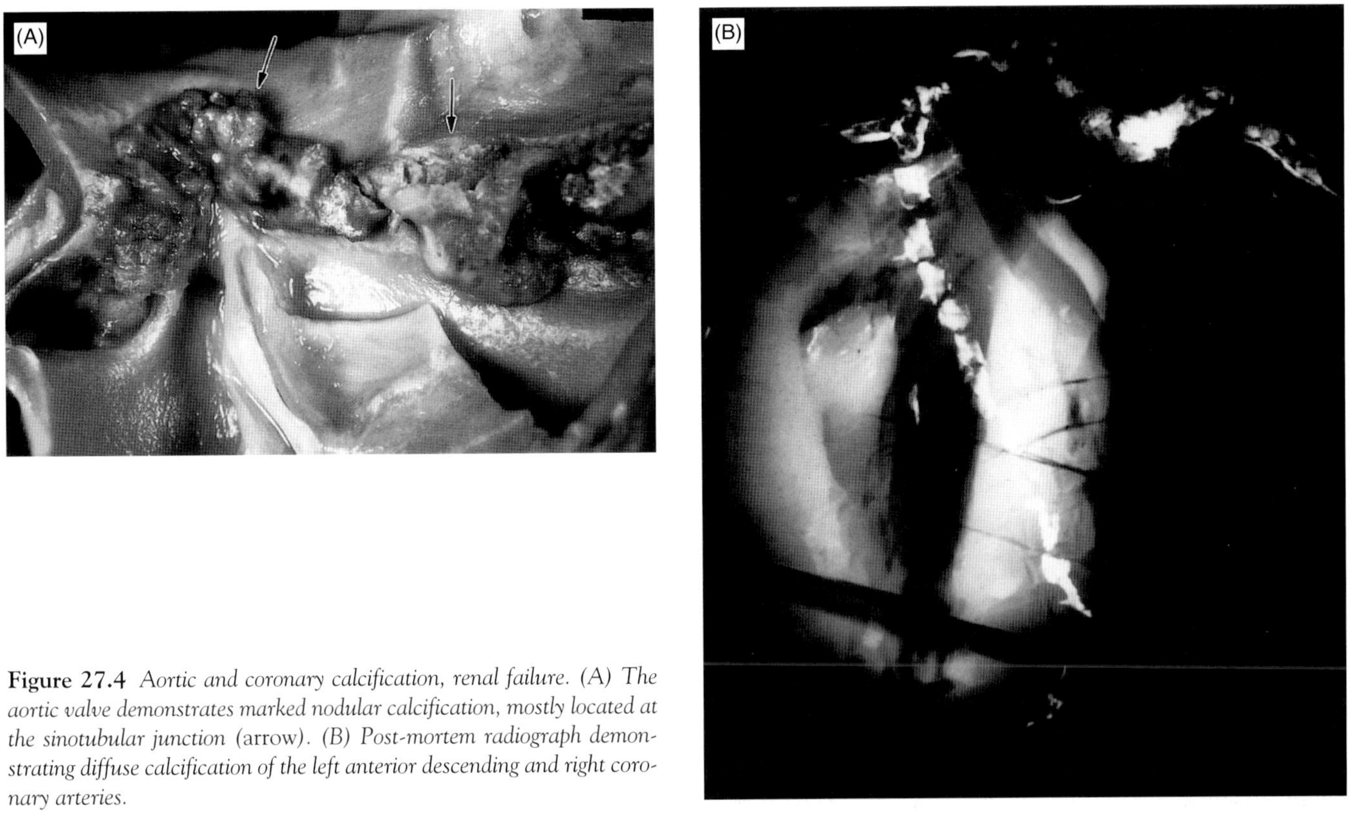


**Figure 27.4** *Aortic and coronary calcification, renal failure. (A) The aortic valve demonstrates marked nodular calcification, mostly located at the sinotubular junction* (arrow). *(B) Post-mortem radiograph demonstrating diffuse calcification of the left anterior descending and right coronary arteries.*

[36]. Mitral calcification in chronic renal failure is associated with hypertension [32, 37], underscoring the need for aggressive antihypertensive treatment in these patients. Occasionally, mitral valve replacement may be beneficial [38]. Calcification in renal failure patients may affect large portions of the vascular tree, resulting, rarely, in skin necrosis and calciphylaxis [39].

## Cardiac manifestations of systemic autoimmune disorders

### Rheumatoid arthritis

Cardiac involvement is commonly seen in patients with severe rheumatoid arthritis and, in clinical series, most frequently affects the pericardium and valves. Echocardiographic studies of patients with rheumatoid arthritis have demonstrated a high frequency of pericardial effusion, particularly posterior, aortic root dilatation and valvular thickening [40]. Patients without clinically overt heart disease may demonstrate left ventricular hypertrophy with filling impairment [41]. In contrast to progressive systemic sclerosis, left ventricular ejection fraction and wall thickness is only mildly affected [42].

Pericarditis is present in 11–50% of patients, and is confirmed by echocardiography, which shows a pericardial effusion. Occasionally, constrictive pericarditis may occur and result in congestive heart failure (CHF) [43]. Cardiac valve disease occurs in 10–25% of patients [44, 45], and consists of valve thickening, mitral prolapse and, uncommonly, valvular insufficiency, which rarely necessitates valve replacement. The order of frequency of valve involvement is that of rheumatic fever: mitral, aortic, tricuspid, and pulmonary. Histopathologically, rheumatoid nodules may be present at the base of the valves, with non-specific inflammation and fibrosis occurring on the valve leaflets. In autopsy series, approximately 50% of hearts from patients with rheumatoid cardiac disease demonstrate rheumatoid nodules, predominantly in the left ventricle free wall or mitral and aortic valves; in the remaining cases, there is non-specific scarring and inflammation [46]. Involvement of the coronary arteries by rheumatoid vasculitis is unusual, and generally restricted to smaller intramural vessels. Necrotizing fatal vasculitis, similar to polyarteritis nodosa, may involve the epicardial arteries and is the most common cause of myocardial infarction in patients with rheumatoid arthritis [46, 47]. Myocardial involvement by inflammation and rheumatoid nodules occurs in up to 20% of patients at autopsy, but rarely causes significant myocardial dysfunction [48]. In exceptional instances, rheumatoid nodules may embolize into the cerebral circulation or form pedunculated masses that are surgically excised [49, 50]. Heart block occurs in approximately 10% of patients with rheumatoid arthritis, and is usually first-degree atrioventricular block, uncommonly necessitating pacemaker placement. The pathological basis for heart block is usually the presence of rheumatoid nodules or scars in areas of the conduction system [51].

## Systemic lupus erythematosus

Cardiovascular manifestations develop in the majority of patients with systemic lupus erythematosus [52]. Echocardiographic studies of patients with lupus and cardiac symptoms demonstrate the most common structural abnormalities to be pericardial effusions (24%), ventricular enlargement (20%), mitral regurgitation (19%), and tricuspid regurgitation (14%). Although patients with lupus without cardiopulmonary symptoms do not have structural cardiac abnormalities, their ejection fractions and fractional shortenings are lower than those of control patients [53].

Severe coronary atherosclerosis resulting in angina pectoris and/or myocardial infarction may occur in young adults with lupus, particularly in those who developed risk factors such as hypertension and hyperlipidaemia while receiving prolonged corticosteroid therapy [52]. Coronary artery disease may also occur as a result of coronary vasculitis, which may be difficult to discern clinically from atherosclerosis [54]. However, the incidence of epicardial coronary vasculitis is very low compared with that seen in patients with rheumatoid arthritis.

In autopsy series, pericarditis has been found in 43–100% of patients [55]. Echocardiographically, effusions are present in 24–40% of patients [53, 56]. Cardiac tamponade and constrictive pericarditis are rare complications of lupus [52, 55, 57].

Endocarditis with superimposed non-bacterial verrucous vegetations (Libman–Sacks vegetations) is noted in more than 40% of hearts at autopsy, but is rarely diagnosed during life [55]. The most commonly affected valve is the mitral valve, followed by the aortic and tricuspid valves [58], and it is manifest echocardiographically by thickenings (50% of patients), vegetations (40%), insufficiency (30%), and stenoses (3–4%) [59]. Valve dysfunction, such as mitral and aortic insufficiency, occasionally manifest during life and occassionally necessitate surgery in the form of valve replacement [52, 60] or repair [61]. It has been hypothesized that steroid treatment of Libman–Sacks vegetations has resulted in an increased incidence of mitral insufficiency requiring surgery [60]. Inflammation of bioprosthetic valves has been reported as a complication of recurrent lupus valvulitis [62]. Mitral and aortic stenosis are rare complications of lupus [55]. Occasionally, valve replacement is necessary for severe mitral insufficiency [63] or because of infective endocarditis superimposed on Libman–Sacks vegetations [64]. Embolization of the vegetations may result in fatal coronary embolism [65]. The presence of valvular vegetations in patients with lupus erythematosus does not appear to be correlated with elevations of antiphospholipid antibodies [66, 67].

Myocarditis is clinically overt in 10% of patients with lupus erythematosus [55], and is found in 8–78% of autopsy series [55] (Fig. 27.5). An association has been reported between lupus myocarditis and skeletal myositis and antibodies to nuclear ribonucleoprotein [68]. Endomyocardial biopsy may be helpful in guiding immunosuppressive therapy [69]. Myocarditis may be associated with left ventricular dysfunction, and, in exceptional cases, aneurysm formation [70].

Neonatal heart block is a rare but well-known complication of newborns born to mothers with lupus erythematosus. It is currently not possible to identify those women whose fetuses will be affected, although immunogenetically, they appear to be more closely related to patients with

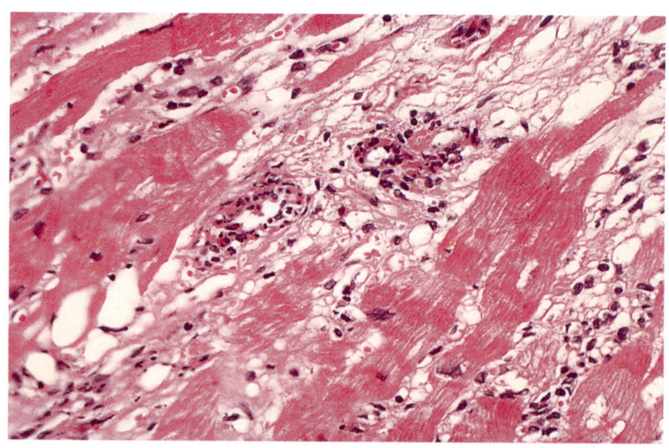

**Figure 27.5** *Myocarditis, lymphocytic, systemic lupus erythematosus. There is a small-vessel vasculitis in addition to interstitial inflammation and replacement fibrosis (endomyocardial biopsy). The patient was a 35-year-old woman with systemic lupus erythematosus who developed progressive exercise intolerance and congestive heart failure.*

Sjögren's syndrome than to those with classic lupus erythematosus. Bradycardia is generally identified between 16 and 24 weeks' gestation. Pathogenetically, it is believed that the maternal autoantibodies to 48 000 mol. wt SSB/La, 52 000 mol. wt SSA/Ro, and 60 000 mol. wt SSA/Ro ribonucleoproteins are involved in the disease [71]. Heart block is associated with an 80% infant survival rate at 3 years, and pacing is required in nearly two-thirds of affected children [71]. Although treatment of affected infants with dexamethasone has successfully diminished pericardial effusions, it has not reversed established third-degree block [72]. Recurrence of congenital heart block occurs in approximately 15% of subsequent pregnancies [71]. Significant structural abnormalities of the heart are not a component of neonatal lupus, but myocarditis and valvular lesions may complicate the heart block [73].

### Progressive systemic sclerosis (scleroderma)

Myocardial fibrosis is present at autopsy in 50% of patients with progressive systemic sclerosis. Scarring may involve the sinoatrial and atrioventricular nodes, and is often accompanied by pericardial inflammation [74]. Echocardiographic studies of patients with progressive systemic sclerosis demonstrate increased left ventricular mass and decreased ejection fraction, compared with control subjects and patients with other autoimmune diseases [42]; clinically significant left ventricular dysfunction is rare, however, as is dilated cardiomyopathy (Table 27.1). Symptomatic cardiac disease is most frequently manifest as pericarditis, which is present in 16% of patients with diffuse scleroderma and 30% of patients with limited scleroderma or CREST syndrome (calcinosis, Raynaud's disease, oesophageal dysfunction, sclerodactyly, and telangiectasia) [75]. Left ventricular function is generally normal in those with the CREST variant, in contrast to diffuse scleroderma [76]; right ventricular dysfunction may result from pulmonary hypertension in either disease. Ventricular conduction abnormalities are present in approximately 25% of patients; both left bundle branch block and right bundle branch block with left anterior fascicular block are associated with abnormal left ventricular function, whereas isolated right bundle branch block or left anterior fascicular block is associated with normal left ventricular function [77].

### Seronegative spondyloarthropathies

The seronegative spondyloarthropathies include ankylosing spondylitis, Reiter's syndrome, psoriatic arthritis, and arthritis associated with inflammatory bowel disease. Common features of these syndromes include a high prevalence of human leucocyte antigen (HLA) B27 major histocompatibility antigen, predominantly male involvement, putative association with prior infections such as with *Chlamydia* and *Klebsiella*, and sacroiliac arthritis. Cardiac manifestations are classically associated with ankylosing spondylitis [78], but have also been described in patients with Reiter's syndrome and, to a limited extent, in patients with psoriasiform arthritis [79, 80]. Cardiac disease in the seronegative spondyloarthropathies is generally limited to the aortic root, aortic valve, and conduction system, and generally manifests as aortic insufficiency or conduction disturbances [80].

In patients with ankylosing spondylitis and overt heart disease, 30% have evidence of aortic insufficiency on echocardiogram, and up to 10% develop clinically significant aortic insufficiency that may eventually necessitate valve replacement [79, 81]. Transoesophageal echocardiography demonstrates thickening of subaortic structures in the majority of patients with aortic insufficiency [81]. Patients with ankylosing spondylitis and cardiac abnormalities are older, have a longer disease duration, and have more peripheral joint disease than those without cardiac abnormalities [82]. Patients with Reiter's syndrome have a similar incidence of aortic insufficiency to those with ankylosing spondylitis [80]; coronary ostial stenosis has also been reported [83]. The incidence of heart block is approximately 33% in patients with ankylosing spondylitis [82], may be independently associated with the HLA-B27 antigen [84], and is more frequent in patients with aortic valve disease. Pathological studies of patients with Reiter's syndrome and ankylosing spondylitis have demonstrated aortic root inflammation [80, 85], and in those with ankylosing spondylitis a characteristic 'bump' is demonstrated on the anterior leaflet of the mitral valve [85].

### Vasculitic syndromes

Giant cell arteritis is a systemic vasculitis involving elastic and muscular arteries, with a propensity for cranial, especially temporal artery, involvement. The disease is rare in patients under the age of 50 years, and has a predilection for women of northern European descent. Polymyalgia rheumatica is a common overlap syndrome with giant cell arteritis, and occurs in 50% of patients. Aortic involvement occurs in 10 to 15% of patients, and manifests as aortic arch syndrome, aortic insufficiency [86], and aortic aneurysm

[87]. Patients with giant cell arteritis develop aortic aneurysms at a mean of 6 years after diagnosis, with a relative risk 17 times that of the normal population [88]. Aortic dissection and rupture are uncommon complications of giant cell aortitis [89], but are generally an underrecognized and potentially treatable cause of sudden death [87]. The aortic root and proximal ascending aorta are preferentially involved, and valve replacement with aortic root repair may be required [90–92]. Postoperative valve detachment is a recognized complication at the anastomotic site in patients with inflammatory aortic root disease [90]. Pathologically, the aortic wall demonstrates granulomatous destruction of the media, with fragmentation of the elastic lamellae, and giant cells are often numerous. In contrast with Takayasu's arteritis, there is relatively minimal intimal and adventitial scarring.

Polyarteritis nodosa and Wegener's granulomatosis may result in vasculitis of the epicardial and intramural myocardial arteries, but the coronary disease generally does not result in clinical symptoms [93, 94]. Occasionally, small-vessel disease may cause a dilated cardiomyopathy that becomes a presenting symptom of the illness (Table 27.1). Pathologically, there are necrotizing arteries similar to those seen in other organs. Churg–Strauss syndrome is a systemic vasculitis that is associated with tissue damage caused by eosinophilic infiltrates in the lungs, kidneys, skin, and other viscera. Cardiac manifestations overlap with eosinophilic endomyocardial fibrosis, or Loeffler's syndrome. Relapsing polychondritis is an inflammatory disease that characteristically involves cartilaginous tissues of the ear and trachea. Cardiovascular involvement is a fairly common complication and the second most frequent cause of mortality in this disease. Aortic root dilatation and mitral regurgitation may result in aortic and, less commonly, mitral valve replacement [95, 96]. Most patients are men, with a mean age of 39 years at the time of surgery. Complete heart block occurs rarely [97]. Pathologically, there is a non-specific aortitis, sometimes accompanied by a necrotizing vasculitis.

### Thrombotic autoimmune disorders

The antiphospholipid syndrome is characterized by thromboembolic events and recurrent spontaneous abortion [98]. The pathophysiological basis for the disease involves the formation of autoantibodies against phospholipids of either the lupus anticoagulant class or the anticardiolipin class. Approximately 50% of patients have clinically overt lupus erythematosus. Vascular manifestations of the disease include thrombosis and fibrointimal proliferation which lead to ischaemic infarction of the placenta or viscera [99]. Vascular inflammation is generally secondary to thrombosis, although a true vasculitis has been reported [100]. Cardiac manifestations of the antiphospholipid syndrome include Libman–Sacks valvar vegetations and atrial mural thrombi that have a tendency to calcify [101]. The laboratory diagnosis is based on abnormalities of phospholipid-dependent tests of coagulation, such as the activated partial thromboplastin time, in conjunction with solid-phase assay systems [radioimmunoassay or enzyme-linked immunosorbent assay (ELISA) for both anticardiolipin and lupus anticoagulants [98].

Thrombocytopenia occurs in approximately 1–3% of patients receiving intravenous heparin [102]. Immune-related thrombocytopenia (type II heparin-induced thrombocytopenia) is characterized by platelet counts dipping below $150 \times 10^9$/l (mean nadir $50 \times 10^9$/l), and is associated with a high risk of thromboembolic events [103]. Thromboembolic events that have been described in patients with type II heparin-induced thrombocytopenia include lower limb gangrene, stroke, acute myocardial infarction, deep venous thrombosis, and recurrent pulmonary embolism [104]. Patients with mural cardiac thrombi and thrombotic occlusion of coronary artery saphenous-vein bypass grafts have been described [105]. The treatment of heparin-induced thrombocytopenia includes immediate cessation of heparin, and substitution of other anticoagulants, such as danaparoid sodium and recombinant hirudin [103].

## Cardiac manifestations of haematological–oncological disorders

### Anaemia

In patients without heart disease, cardiac symptoms secondary to anaemia are uncommon. The resting cardiac output increases with haemoglobin values below 9 g/dl but, with gradual development of the anaemic state, patients have few adverse affects even with activity. Acute isovolaemic reduction of blood haemoglobin concentration to 5 g/dl in conscious, healthy, resting humans does not produce evidence of inadequate systemic oxygen delivery, as assessed by lack of change in oxygen consumption and plasma lactate concentration [106]. With haemoglobin levels lower than 4 g/dl CHF may ensue solely on the basis of the anaemia. However, in patients with coronary artery disease, angina may develop even in the presence of mild anaemia. Electrocardiographic changes of T-wave depression and inversion may occur in patients without heart disease when haemoglobin levels are below 7 g/dl [107].

Patients with chronic severe anaemia have a high output state due to low systemic vascular resistance. Enhanced activity of basal endothelium-derived relaxing factor makes an important contribution to the low systemic vascular resistance in chronic severe anaemia [108]. Echocardiography demonstrates eccentric hypertrophy with abnormal ratio of wall thickness to cavity diameter. Auscultation reveals a mid-systolic murmur due to increased velocity of blood flow across the semilunar valves. Diastolic murmurs due to increased flow across mitral and tricuspid valves may be similar to those of mitral or tricuspid stenosis, but they follow a third heart sound [107]. Correction of anaemia in patients with high-output heart failure should be accomplished with packed cells and diuretics, if necessary, to prevent worsening of CHF.

## Sickle cell disease

Echocardiograms of patients with sickle cell disease demonstrate increased left ventricular wall thickness and cavity diameter that correlate inversely with haemoglobin levels, especially as age advances [109]. Therefore, the cardiomyopathy of sickle cell disease is not significantly different from that of chronic anaemia of any cause. Left ventricular hypertrophy may be asymmetric, resulting in preferential septal hypertrophy [109]. Increases in wall thickness may be minimal compared with increases in left ventricular cavity diameter [110]. Ejection fractions are generally normal, but the velocity of circumferential fibre shortening is abnormally low [109]. The right ventricle may demonstrate significant dilatation and hypertrophy, resulting in tricuspid insufficiency and right heart failure, dependent on the degree of pulmonary hypertension resulting from thrombotic occlusion of pulmonary arteries. Sickle cell crises may result in acute myocardial infarction [111], transient atrioventricular block [112], and sudden death (Fig. 27.6). Sickle cell trait does not cause cardiac

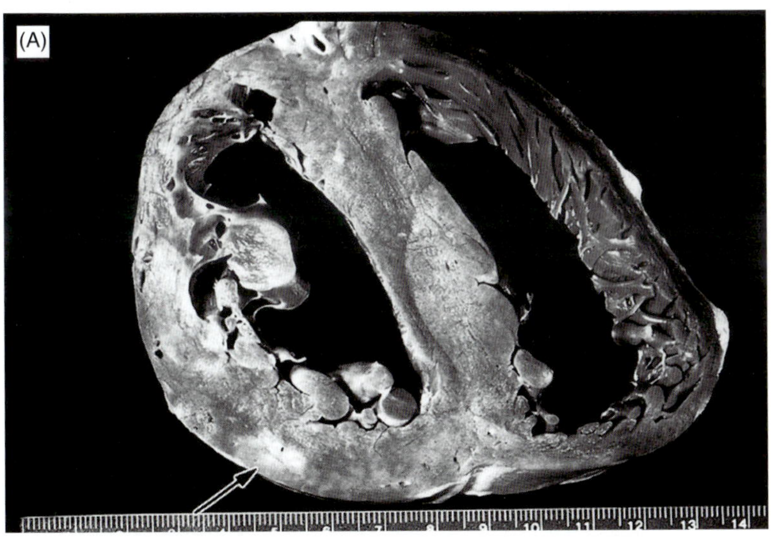


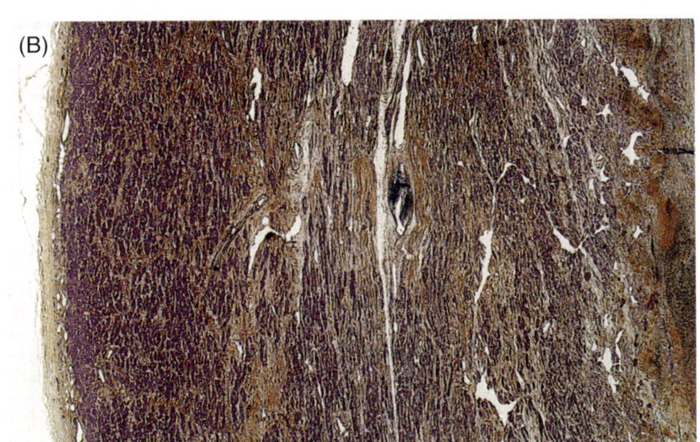


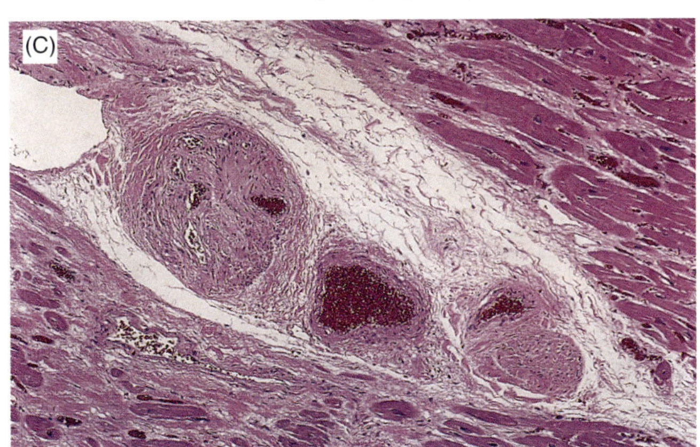


**Figure 27.6** *Cardiomyopathy of sickle cell disease. (A) Short-axis cut demonstrating marked biventricular dilatation and patchy left ventricular scars* (arrows). *(B) Histological preparation showing patchy fibrosis (yellow). Movat pentachrome. (C) Histological section demonstrating organizing thrombi within intramural coronary vessels* (arrow).

functional abnormalities. However, the trait may predispose to cardiac arrhythmias and sudden death in patients with heat stroke [113, 114].

### Thalassaemia

β-Thalassaemia major is associated with a high incidence of cardiac dysfunction. In contrast to sickle cell anaemia, in which myocardial damage is due primarily to high-output failure, pulmonary hypertension, and ischaemia, the cardiac abnormalities of β-thalassaemia are due largely to iron overload and cardiac inflammation [107]. In the early stages of the disease, diastolic abnormalities predominate, resulting in a mild restrictive cardiomyopathy [115]. Early mitral inflow velocity/peak late mitral inflow velocity, left atrial diameter, serum ferritin, and atrial natriuretic peptide levels are increased and are interrelated in the early stages of disease [116]. In later stages, after successive blood transfusions, approximately 6% of patients develop overt heart failure by the third decade [117]. Iron deposition within the myocardium may be demonstrated using ECG-gated spin echocardiography [118]. Myocarditis may be an important contributing factor to heart failure, in addition to the iron overload, and is diagnosed in up to 5% of these patients [119]. Pathologically, the myocardium demonstrates fibrosis, iron deposits, and myocyte hypertrophy [120]. The treatment of heart failure includes prevention by adequate chelation and ACE inhibitors, and administration of diuretics, vasodilators, inotropes, and antiarrhythmics [120].

### Haemochromatosis

Iron overload may adversely affect the heart regardless of the mechanisms, which include multiple transfusions in patients with anaemia, other forms of haemosiderosis, or primary haemochromatosis. The gene for hereditary haemochromatosis, an autosomal recessive disorder, is found in approximately 10% of Americans, most of whom are unaffected heterozygotes. Homozygotes represent 5 in 1000 white Americans. Symptoms of haemochromatosis include fatigue, palpitations, joint pains, and impotence. The diagnosis is made by high serum iron, high transferrin saturation, elevated serum ferritin, elevated transaminases, hyperglycaemia, and low values for thyroid-stimulating hormone (TSH) and gonadotropins. The most common cause of death is from cardiac failure and arrhythmias, followed by cirrhosis and hepatocellular carcinoma [121]. Occasionally, the presenting symptom of haemochromatosis may be dilated cardiomyopathy, diagnosed by endomyocardial biopsy (Table 27.1). The single laboratory test that correlates best with complications is the tissue iron concentration in liver biopsies [122]. Iron deposits within the heart may be identified by the used of computed tomography [123, 124]. CHF is treated with standard therapy, in conjunction with chelating agents for the prevention of progressive iron deposition. Ventricular tachycardias in patients with cardiac haemochromatosis may be successfully treated with amiodarone [125]. Pathologically, the heart in patients with haemochromatosis demonstrates intramyocyte iron, as demonstrated by Prussian blue stains, myocyte hypertrophy, and interstitial fibrosis (Fig. 27.7).

### Myeloproliferative syndromes

Hyperviscosity and thrombocytosis occur in patients with myeloproliferative syndromes, and may result in an increased incidence of ischaemic heart, peripheral, and

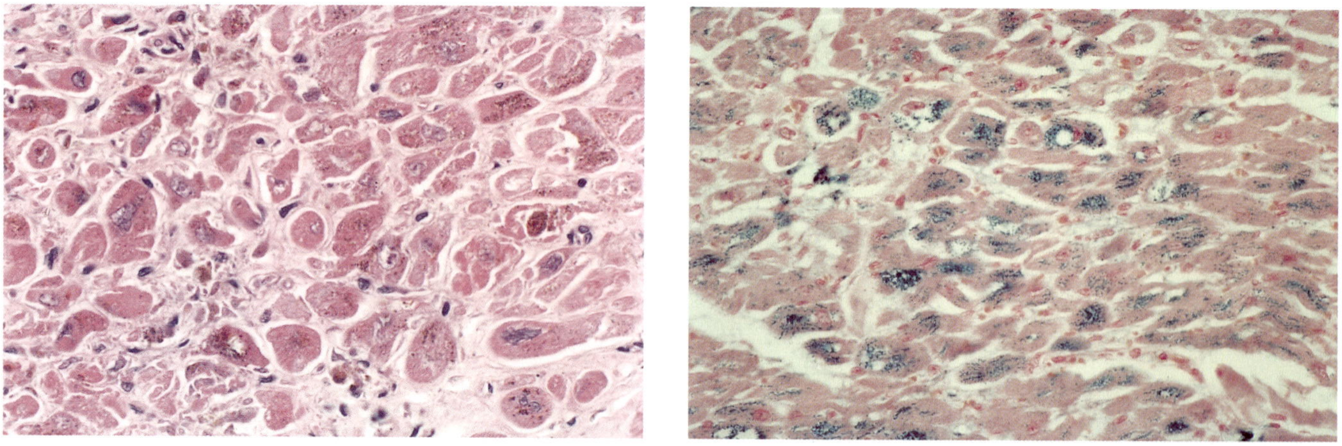

**Figure 27.7** *Haemochromatosis. (A) Histological section from the heart of a patient with haemochromatosis demonstrating increased brown iron pigment, myocyte size variation, and interstitial fibrosis. (B) Iron stain demonstrating increased iron (Prussian blue reagent) within myocytes.*

cerebrovascular disease [126]. Increased red blood cell mass may be a secondary phenomenon in patients with reduced oxygen transport or inappropriate erythropoietin secretion. Blood viscosity increases as the haematocrit rises above 50%, and CHF may ensue above levels of 60% as a result of hypervolaemia and augmented vascular resistance. Coronary thrombi may occur in patients with essential thrombocytosis in the absence of significant underlying coronary atherosclerosis [127]. The treatment of hyperviscosity and increased red blood cell mass includes phlebotomy and hydroxyurea.

## Thrombotic thrombocytopenic purpura

Thrombotic microangiopathy (thrombotic thrombocytopenic purpura/haemolytic uremic syndrome) is characterized by haemolytic anemia, red blood cell schistocytes on peripheral smear, and thrombocytopenia in the absence of activation of the clotting cascade [128]. In the haemolytic uraemic syndrome (HUS), renal symptoms dominate, whereas the central nervous system and to a lesser degree the heart are involved in thrombotic thrombocytopenic purpura (TTP). TTP is primarily seen in females, with a peak incidence in the fourth decade. The pathogenetic basis of TTP/HUS is unknown, but probably results from toxic endothelial damage following infections by verotoxin-producing *Escherichia coli* [129], viral infections including human immunodeficiency virus (HIV) [130], or autoimmune damage by circulating immune complexes. Predisposing conditions include pregnancy, systemic disease, malignant hypertension, HIV infection, cancer, systemic lupus erythematosus [131], sickle cell disease [132], and treatment with anticancer drugs. Endothelial damage results in release of von Willebrand factor multimers, and platelet activating factor. Clinically, heart failure may occur, and is occasionally rapidly progressive, resulting in death [133]. The initial presenting symptoms may be those of dilated cardiomyopathy (Table 27.1). At autopsy, thrombi are found (in decreasing order of frequency) in the brain, heart, lungs, kidneys, adrenals, spleen and liver. Characteristic cardiac findings include subepicardial haemorrhages, usually grossly evident, with microscopic platelet thrombus present within intramyocardial arterioles (Figure 27.8). Treatment includes plasma infusion and exchange, sometimes accompanied by antiplatelet drugs, prostacyclin analogs or steroids [128, 129, 134]. If instituted early in the disease course, treatment results in remission in the majority of patients.

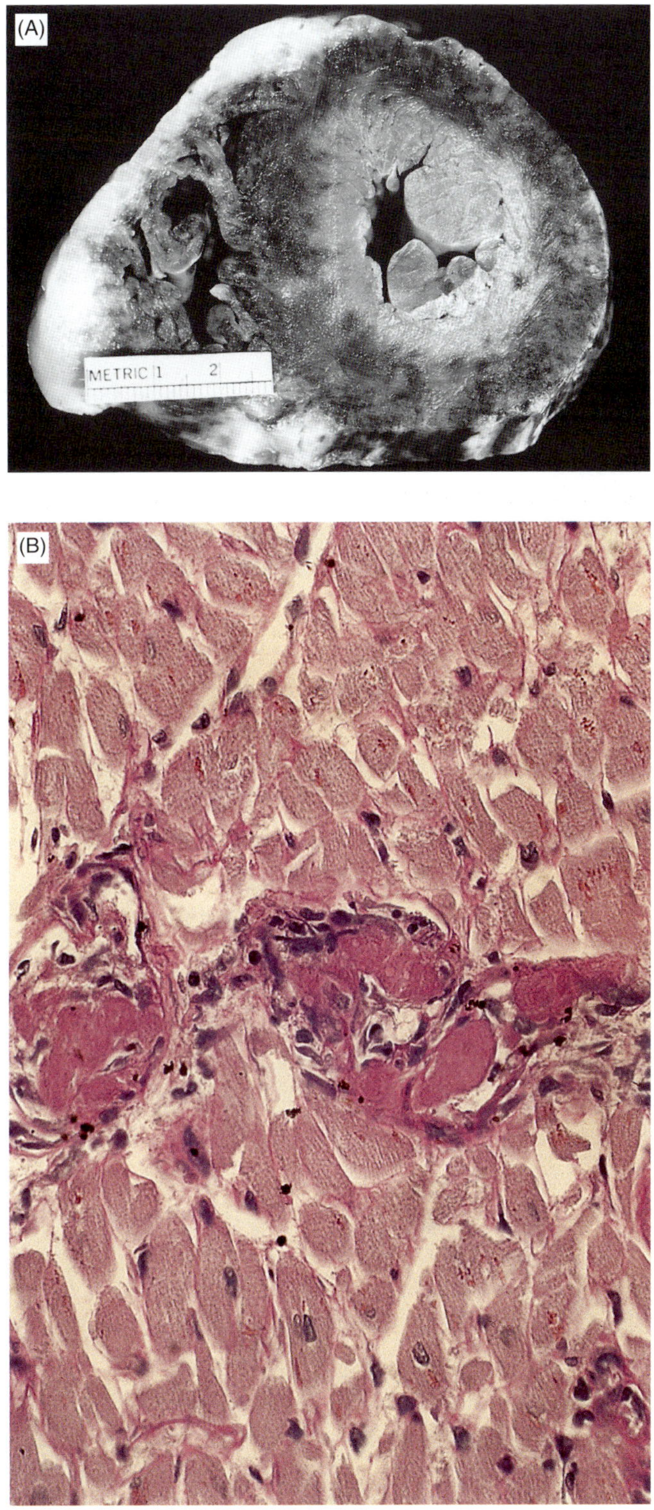


**Figure 27.8** *Thrombotic thrombocytopenic purpura. (A) Gross photograph of a heart from a patient dying soon after the diagnosis of microangiopathic haemolytic anaemia and severe thrombocytopenia demonstrating characteristic subepicardial haemorrhages. (B) Histological section demonstrating typical arteriolar thrombi distending the vessels and provoking an inflammatory reaction. Periodic acid–Schiff.*

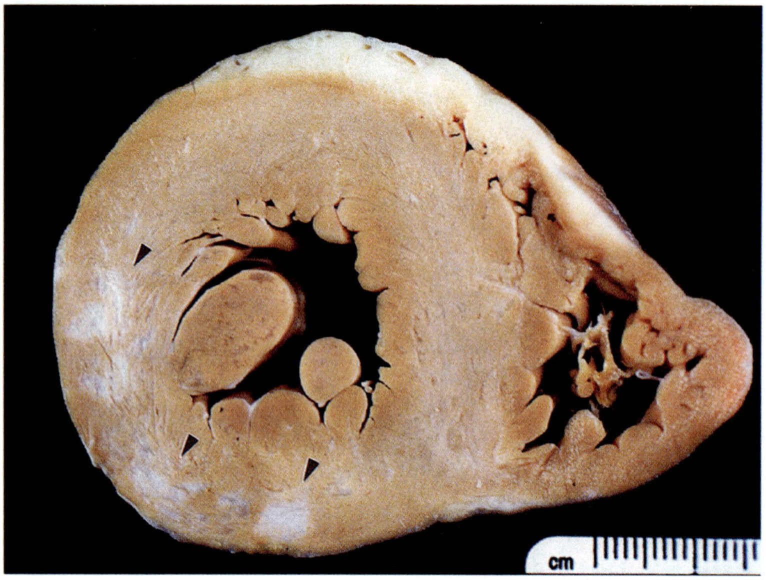


**Figure 27.9** *Duchenne's muscular dystrophy. Note scars in the posterolateral region of the left ventricle* (arrowheads). *The patient was a 12-year-old boy with a 9-year history of Duchenne's muscular dystrophy. He died several days after suffering a cardiac arrest hours after surgery for spinal fusion.*

### Metastatic tumours

Malignancies that involve the heart secondarily are, in order of frequency, carcinomas of the lung, lymphomas, carcinomas of the breast, leukaemia, malignant melanoma, hepatocellular carcinoma and carcinomas of the colon [135, 136]. The high incidence of cardiac metastases partly reflects the relatively high incidence of these tumours in the general population; relatively unusual tumours with a high propensity for cardiac spread include carcinomas of the thymus and thyroid, malignant melanoma, germ cell tumours, and renal cell carcinoma.

Malignancies spread to the heart by four paths: direct extension, usually from mediastinal tumour; haematogenous spread; lymphatic spread; and intracavitary extension from the inferior vena cava, or rarely the pulmonary veins. Although there are exceptions, epithelial malignancies typically spread to the heart by lymphatics. Melanoma, sarcomas, leukaemia and renal cell carcinoma metastasize to the heart by a haematogenous route, replacing large areas of myocardium not confined by vascular spaces. Lymphomas may involve the heart by most paths, including direct extension, haematogenous seeding or lymphatic spread. Melanomas, renal tumours, including Wilms' tumour and renal cell carcinoma, adrenal tumours, liver tumours, and uterine tumours are the most frequent intracavitary tumours. Renal cell and hepatocellular carcinomas may extend into the vena cava and the right atrium [137]. The treatment of metastatic cardiac tumours includes surgical removal, which may prolong life with minimal complications, especially for relatively slow-growing neoplasms [138–144].

## Neurological and neuromuscular disorders and cardiac disease

### Duchenne muscular dystrophy

Muscular dystrophies are genetic, inherent diseases of skeletal muscle marked by progressive muscle wasting. Duchenne (and the milder Becker) muscular dystrophies are caused by an X-linked mutation in the dystrophin gene, located at Xp21. The heart is commonly involved in Duchenne muscular dystrophy, resulting in degenerative changes in muscle fibers and fibrosis, most marked in the posterobasal region and adjacent lateral wall of the left ventricle [145] (Fig. 27.9). Ninety per cent of patients have loss of posteriorly directed electrical forces in the ECG, with tall right precordial R waves and deep Q waves in the left precordial and limb leads. Other abnormalities of conduction include sinus tachycardia, atrial ectopic beats, and ventricular premature complexes. Echocardiographically, hypokinesis of the posterobasal ventricular wall and changes indicative of decreased ventricular compliance are frequent [146]. In approximately 6% of men with idiopathic dilated cardiomyopathy, defects in the dystrophin gene may be identified, indicating that cardiac involvement may precede skeletal muscle involvement. Progressive cardiac dysfunction has also been reported in female carriers of the disease [147].

### Myotonic muscular dystrophy

Myotonic muscular dystrophy is a progressive, autosomal-recessive wasting disease primarily affecting facial, neck, and distal limb muscles. Cardiac involvement manifests most commonly as conduction defects, which may occur in the absence of severe skeletal disease [148]. First-degree heart block is the most common abnormality, and histological studies of the conduction system have demonstrated degeneration and fibrosis of the bundle of His and bundle branches [149]. Suggestions for clinical management include a careful cardiac history and a 12-lead ECG at least every year, with a low threshold for use of 24 h Holter monitoring [150]. The high frequency of cardiorespiratory complications during general anaesthesia is well known. A prolonged PR interval [151], as well as the size of the trinucleotide (cytosine-thymine-guanine) repeat expansion [148], are associated with an increased risk of cardiac events.

### Friedreich's ataxia

Approximately 20% of patients with Friedreich's ataxia, the most common form of hereditary spinocerebellar degenerative disease, develop a hypokinetic form of dilated cardiomyopathy. Cardiac deaths are common. Recently, Friedreich's ataxia has been associated with a mutation that consists of an unstable expansion of GAA trinucleotide repeat segments in the first intron of the gene on chromosome 9 encoding frataxin, a protein of unknown function highly expressed in the normal heart. Earlier phases of the cardiomyopathy are characterized by cardiac hypertrophy, which may be asymmetric or concentric [152], and cardiac abnormalities on echocardiography (up to 90% of patients) [153]. Wall motion abnormalities are often marked by the presence of Q waves on the ECG [154], and the severity of left ventricular hypertrophy is related to the number of GAA repeat segments [155] and early age at onset of disease [156]. Chest pain is only rarely a presenting symptom [153]. Pathologically, small-vessel disease of intramural coronary arteries has been described at autopsy.

### Desmin cardiomyopathy

Abnormal accumulations of desmin, a critical component of the cytoskeleton of cardiac myocytes, may result in cardiac and skeletal muscle disease. Desmin cardiomyopathy is characterized by progressive CHF, occurring usually in the second and third decades of life, and males and females are equally affected. The light microscopic features are nonspecific, but ultrastructurally there are degenerative alterations characterized by the accumulation of granular disordered filaments that stain for desmin by immunolabelling. Skeletal myopathy often accompanies the cardiomyopathy and periodic acid–Schiff (PAS) positive intracytoplasmic inclusions containing phosphorylated desmin may be seen in skeletal muscle. Abnormal collections of intermediate filaments have also been described in intestinal smooth muscle cells and the spinal cord. An association with mental retardation has been reported.

## Endocrine and nutritional diseases and the heart

### Acromegaly

Acromegaly is associated with increased cardiac morbidity and mortality. Echocardiographic studies on acromegalic patients show increased left ventricular mass and impaired diastolic filling [157], which may progress to intractable heart failure [158]. Coexistent diseases that frequently affect cardiac function in acromegalic patients include diabetes mellitus, hypertension, and coronary artery disease. Radionuclide angiography and echocardiography have shown that patients with acromegaly have impaired left ventricular diastolic filling at rest related to a greater index of left ventricular mass, even in the absence of systemic hypertension [159]. Pathologically, acromegalic cardiomyopathy is characterized by massive cardiac enlargement (Fig. 27.10), with myocardial hypertrophy, interstitial fibrosis, lymphomononuclear infiltration, and areas of monocyte necrosis [160]. Studies of patients with deficiency of growth hormones suggest that growth hormone plays a role in the control of cardiac wall stress and performance through a mechanism mediated by its effect on myocardial tissue growth [161]. Patients with childhood or adult-onset growth hormone deficiency have a reduced left ventricular mass and ejection fraction, and the indices of left ventricular systolic function remained markedly depressed during exercise [160]. Recombinant growth hormone increases myocardial mass and reduces left ventricular cavity size in patients with idiopathic dilated cardiomyopathy, resulting in improved haemodynamics, myocardial energy metabolism, and clinical status [162]. The treatment of acromegalic heart disease includes octreotide therapy, which improves cardiac structural and functional abnormalities, supporting the hypothesis of a

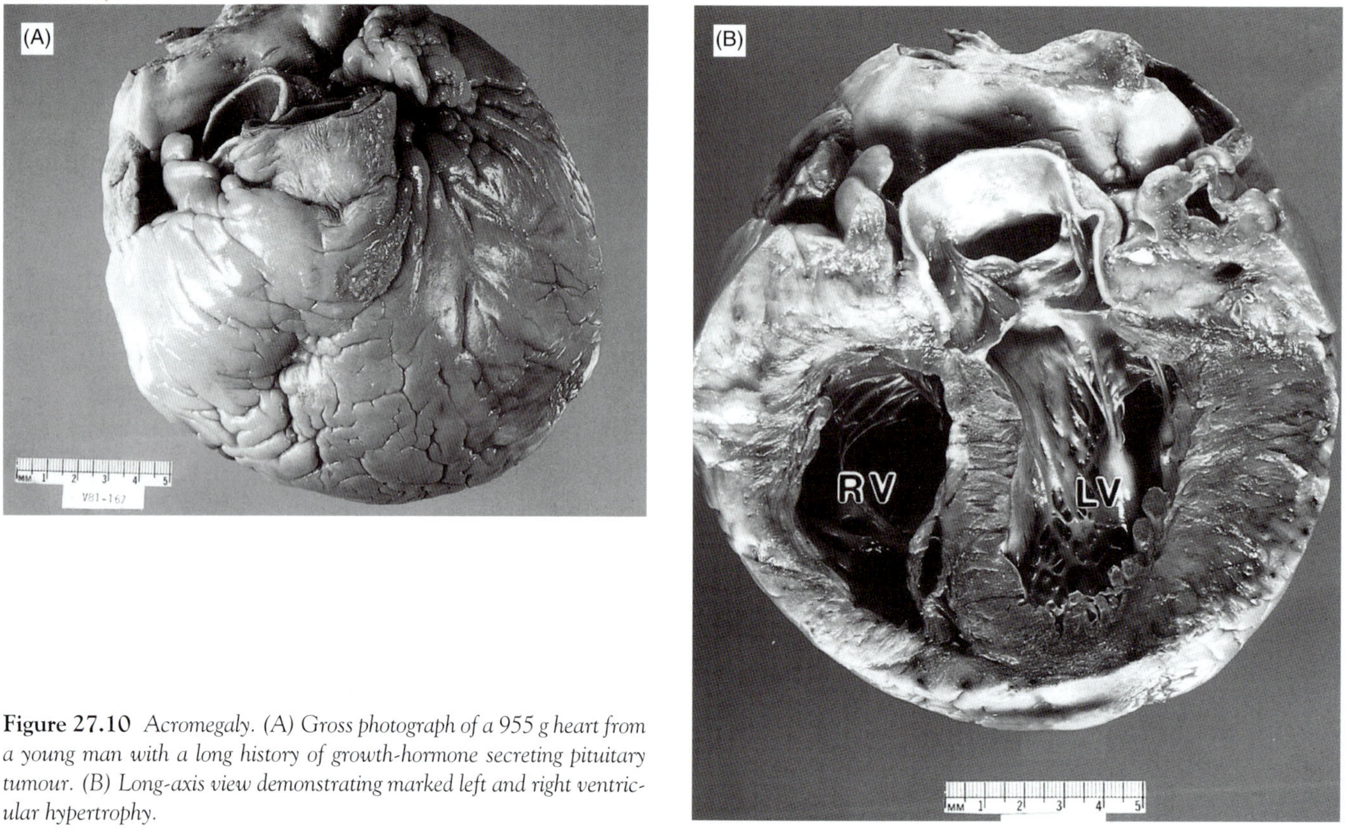


**Figure 27.10** *Acromegaly. (A) Gross photograph of a 955 g heart from a young man with a long history of growth-hormone secreting pituitary tumour. (B) Long-axis view demonstrating marked left and right ventricular hypertrophy.*

**Table 27.2** Clinical manifestation of hyperthyroidism

| Physical examination | Haemodynamic changes | Other |
|---|---|---|
| Hyperactive pericardium with resting tachycardia | ↑ Cardiac output | Atrial fibrillation |
| | ↑Systolic blood pressure | ST segment elevations |
| Accentuated first heart sound | Widened pulse pressure | ↓ QT interval |
| Possible third heart sound audible | ↓↓ Circulation time | ↑ PR interval |
| Systolic murmur | ↑ Cardiac index | Cardiac hypertrophy |
| Means–Lerman scratch | ↓ Arterial resistance | ↓ Contraction times |
| | ↑ Venous resistance | Wolff–Parkinson–White syndrome |
| | ↑ Systolic–diastolic function | |

(From ref. 165 with permission.)

specific heart disease secondary to high circulating growth hormone levels [163, 164].

## Thyroid disease

The cardiovascular symptoms of hyperthyroidism reflect increased cardiac output and, in some patients with chronic hyperthyroidism, CHF. These symptoms include palpitations, angina pectoris, dyspnoea on exertion, orthopnoea, and paroxysmal nocturnal dyspnoea (Table 27.2). Atrial fibrillation or CHF may be the only clinical manifestation of hyperthyroidism, especially in elderly patients with apathetic hyperthyroidism [166]. The CHF seen in patients with hyperthyroidism may be due in part to mitral insufficiency resulting from papillary muscle dysfunction [167]. Histologically, the cardiac findings are non-specific, and include myocyte necrosis, fibrosis, and round cell infiltration.

Thyrotoxicosis may exacerbate underlying heart disease, including heart failure of any cause, mitral valve prolapse, and angina. Occasionally, hyperthyroidism may result in

**Table 27.3** Clinical manifestations of hypothyroidism

| Physical examination | Hemodynamic changes | Other |
|---|---|---|
| Dyspnoea on exertion | ↓ Cardiac output | Pleural effusion |
| ↓ Exercise tolerance | ↓ Stroke volume | Ascites |
| Bradycardia; weak pulse | ↑ Circulation time | Non-pitting oedema |
| Hypertension | ↑ Peripheral vascular resistance | ↑ Conduction abnormalities |
| Faint heart sounds | | ↑ QT interval |
| Cardiac hypertrophy | | T-wave inversion |
| Congestive heart failure | | |

(From ref. 165 with permission.)

coronary spasm in the absence of coronary atherosclerosis [168]. Thyrotoxicosis-induced weakness of skeletal muscle may exacerbate dyspnoea in patients with or without heart failure.

Hypothyroidism, if longstanding, may result in a constellation of cardiac effects initially termed 'myxoedema heart' [169]. The pathophysiology of hypothyroid heart disease is generally considered to be the opposite of hyperthyroidism. The physiological effects on the circulation include decreased cardiac output, decreased stroke volume, and increased circulation time. There appears to be an increased risk of hypertension, owing to a persistent low renin state and increased peripheral vascular resistance (Table 27.3).

Therapy with (TSH) suppressive doses of $T_4$ has increased left ventricular contractility and induced mild myocardial hypertrophy. Whether $T_4$-treated patients under the age of 65 years have an increased risk of ischaemic heart is unclear [170]. Treating the hypothyroidism results in a lowering of cholesterol levels and an improved ratio of low-density lipoprotein (LDL) to high-density lipoprotein (HDL) cholesterol.

Thyroid hormone affects the cardiovascular system by three major mechanisms: cellular effects on the cardiac myocyte, interactions between thyroid hormone and the sympathoadrenal system, and peripheral haemodynamic changes that influence cardiac function [165]. The cellular effects of thyroid hormone on the cardiac myocyte are incompletely understood, but include nuclear as well as direct mechanisms. Extranuclear effects of thyroxin include increased activity of $Ca^{2+}$-adenosine triphosphatases (ATPases) of the myocardium, resulting in reduced sarcoplasmic calcium and improved myocardial relaxation and diastolic dysfunction [171]. Nuclear effects are delayed for 30 min to 1 h after administration of thyroid hormone, require ongoing protein synthesis, and are thought to result from the binding of thyroid hormone to two separate isoforms of the nuclear thyroid hormone receptor. This binding, which is specific to thyroid hormone response elements, affects transcription and translation of specific enzymes or contractile proteins [165], including myosin heavy chain-$\alpha$, $CA^{2+}$-ATPases, myosin heavy chain-$\beta$, and $Na^+/K^+$-ATPase. Hyperthyroidism may lead to increased $\beta$-sympathetic receptor expression on cardiac myocytes, and an increased metabolic state leading to elevated cardiac work and cardiac hypertrophy via an indirect mechanism.

## Adrenal disease

Cushing's syndrome results from increased levels of cortisol, and may occur from either oversecretion of adrenocorticotrophic hormone (ACTH) by the pituitary (sometimes referred to as Cushing's disease), primary tumours of the adrenal cortex, ectopic production of cortisol by non-adrenal tumours, or iatrogenic causes. The major cardiac complication of Cushing's syndrome, other than accelerated atherosclerosis, is concentric left ventricular hypertrophy. The aetiology of the ventricular remodelling in patients with Cushing's syndrome appears to occur regardless of the presence of coexistent hypertension [172]. The direct mechanism by which cortisol results in myocyte hypertrophy has not been elucidated. The mechanism of hypertension in patients with Cushing's syndrome is likely to be multifactorial, and is incompletely understood. Although sodium retention and volume expansion characterize cortisol-induced hypertension, the hypertension is largely independent of sodium and volume. Increased pressor responsiveness, particularly to catechols,

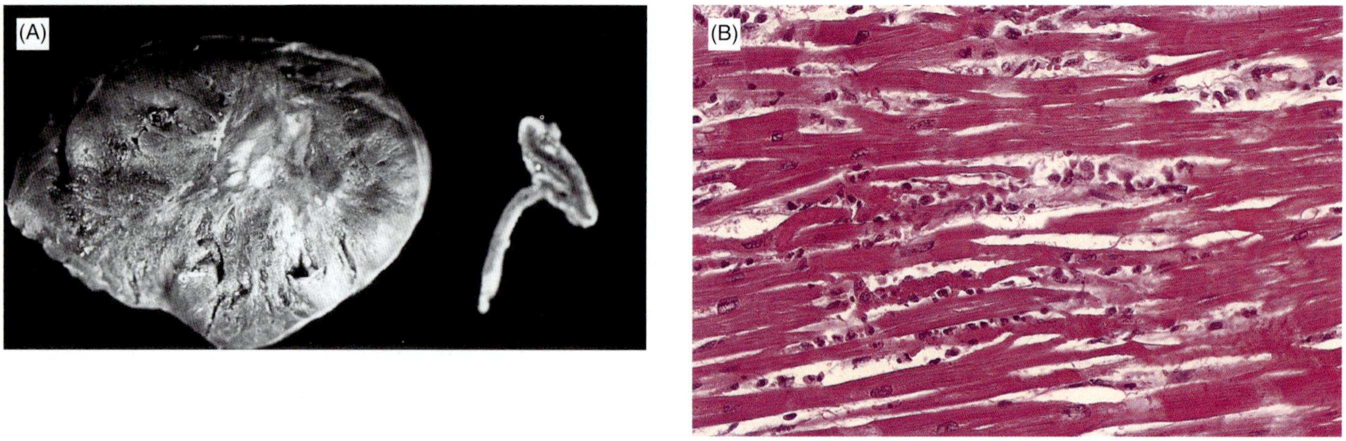


**Figure 27.11** *Phaeochromocytoma. (A) Note the large tumour replacing the adrenal gland on the left; the right adrenal gland is normal for comparison. (B) Catecholamine myocardial damage: there is multifocal myocyte damage with inflammatory infiltrates.*

is a prominent feature but whether these changes are sufficient to account for the hypertension remains unclear [173].

Low-renin hypertension caused by primary aldosteronism, or Conn's syndrome, is associated with a greater degree of left ventricular hypertrophy than essential hypertension, Cushing's disease, or phaeochromocytoma [174]. Other cardiac effects of primary aldosteronism are mediated by hypokalaemia and increased atrial pressure. Therefore, T-wave flattening or U-wave prominence on the ECG, and the presence of premature ventricular contractions, are often observed.

Adrenal insufficiency results in hypotension and may, when acute, result in hypovolaemic shock. In addition, a reversible dilated cardiomyopathy may occur [175].

## Phaeochromocytoma and catecholamine diseases

Increased catecholamine levels may result in chronic myocardial damage and CHF. Patients with phaeochromocytoma may present with a dilated cardiomyopathy that may be reversed by normalization of circulating catecholamines by medical or surgical means [176]. Other causes of increased catecholamine release, such as brain death or even severe emotional stress [177], may result in myocardial damage. Histologically, the major features of cardiomyopathy related to catecholamines are isolated cells or groups of myocytes showing contraction band necrosis (Fig. 27.11), with an associated inflammatory reaction composed of neutrophils and mononuclear cells. In cases of brain death, the degree of histological damage attributed to catecholamine toxicity has been related to the duration of the cerebral anoxia [178]. Catecholamine-mediated toxicity is believed to be the result of β-adrenoceptor-mediated cyclic adenosine monophosphate-dependent calcium overload of the cardiac myocyte [179, 180]. Rarely, phaeochromocytoma may be associated with a reversible form of apical hypertrophic cardiomyopathy, by mechanisms that are unexplained [181].

## Parathyroid disorders

As mentioned above, secondary hyperparathyroidism is involved in the pathogenesis of cardiac calcification in patients with renal failure. It is less clear, however, whether the cardiac hypertrophy seen in end-stage renal failure is mediated in part by hyperparathyroidism, or is due to other factors such as hypertension and anaemia. In primary hyperparathyroidism, there is an increased incidence of calcification of the mitral and aortic valves, an increased frequency of systemic hypertension, and impaired left ventricular filling during diastole [182]. Although parathyroidectomy successfully corrects the hypertension, there are few changes in other cardiac abnormalities. Concentric left ventricular hypertrophy has been reported.

Studies on cell cultures have demonstrated that cardiomyocytes and smooth muscle cells are target cells for parathyroid hormone and the structurally related peptide, parathyroid hormone-related peptide. Parathyroid hormone activates protein kinase C of cardiomyocytes, leading to hypertrophic growth and re-expression of foetal type proteins. Although this hypertrophic effect might theoretically contribute to left ventricular hypertrophy in haemodialysis patients with secondary hyperparathyroidism, such a relationship has yet to be demonstrated clinically on cardiac myocytes. Parathyroid hormone-related peptide activates protein kinase A via a N-terminal domain distinct from that identified on parathyroid hormone, and protein kinase C via a C-terminally located domain distinct from that found on parathyroid hormone. The precise clinical effects of these pathways are not clear [183]. Animal studies have shown that parathyroid hormone plays a permissive role in the development of cardiac fibrosis in uraemic rats [184].

## Diabetes mellitus

Diabetes mellitus has diverse affects on the cardiovascular system. These are mediated by changes in the lipid profile, direct effects of hyperglycaemia and hyperinsulinaemia, effects of diabetes on the autonomic system, and direct effects on the cardiac microcirculation and myocardium.

Diabetes often coexists with other risk factors for coronary artery disease, such as obesity and hypertension. Diabetics typically have increased plasma triglyceride levels and decreased HDL cholesterol, in conjunction with small, dense LDL particles. Insulin resistance may result in increases in circulating free fatty acids and triglyceride synthesis. Alteration of lipoprotein by glycation, especially LDL, may result in increased cholesterol ester accumulation in macrophages and the arterial wall, and there is evidence that oxidation of LDL may be increased in diabetics [185].

Increases in advanced glycation end-products have been demonstrated by immunolocalization techniques in the atherosclerotic plaques of experimental animals, and have been implicated in the pathogenesis of microvascular myocardial disease [186]. In conjunction with hyperlipidaemia, diabetes may increase circulating and tissue lipid peroxides, exacerbating the effect of hyperglycaemia alone. Glycation of apolipoprotein B may be associated with an increased risk of coronary events [187], and advanced glycation end-products may result in the upregulation of vascular adhesion molecules [188]. Findings in the extracellular matrix in experimental diabetic cardiomyopathy include distortion of myocardial capillaries, thickening of capillary walls, and disorganization of contractile fibres within cardiac myocytes. In humans, hyalinization of intramural arterioles has been demonstrated in endomyocardial biopsies of diabetic patients [189]. Decreased myocardial flow reserve, as demonstrated by positron emission tomography before and after dipyrimidole loading, has been documented in non-insulin-dependent diabetics, especially in males.

The clinical manifestations of cardiac disease among diabetics include acute myocardial infarction, CHF, cardiac autonomic dysfunction, and dilated cardiomyopathy in the absence of coronary artery disease. Pathological studies of coronary artery disease in patients dying suddenly show that diabetics are more likely to have extensive and distal disease, organized thrombi, and healed myocardial infarcts, and are less likely to have acute thrombi than normoglycaemics. Cardiac autonomic dysfunction is a correlate of peripheral somatic neuropathy, and is manifest by resting tachycardia, lack of beat-to-beat variability on the ECG, lack of heart rate change during the Valsalva manoeuvre, and increased heart rate with hypotension after standing [190]. The true risk of idiopathic dilated cardiomyopathy among diabetics is controversial, and has been estimated at 1.6 times that of the normal population [191]. Left ventricular dysfunction has been documented in patients with glucose intolerance and non-insulin-dependent diabetes mellitus, in the absence of coronary artery disease. Left ventricular end-systolic dimension, indexed to body surface area, has been shown to be greater in patients with non-insulin-dependent diabetes mellitus and in those with impaired glucose than in normoglycaemic persons, as is the ratio of the peak early diastolic velocity wave to the late diastolic wave [192].

## Obesity

Massive obesity is accompanied by an increase in blood volume and cardiac output, in proportion to the excess of body weight and the duration of obesity. Pedal oedema may occur as a consequence of elevated ventricular filling pressure, despite elevation of the cardiac output [193–195]. Circulatory congestive symptoms do not usually develop unless the degree of obesity is extreme and the body weight is greater than 135 kg [196]. Autopsy and echocardiographic studies have shown that heart mass is greater than expected in the massively obese (Fig. 27.12). Left ventricular dilatation and eccentric hypertrophy is commonly found and there is occasionally right ventricular hypertrophy [197]. Cardiac hypertrophy in obesity has been found to be different to the hypertrophy seen in hypertension: as opposed to concentric hypertrophy in hypertension, massive obesity appears to be associated with eccentric hypertrophy of the heart with chamber dilatation [198, 199]. The marked chronic increase in cardiac work caused

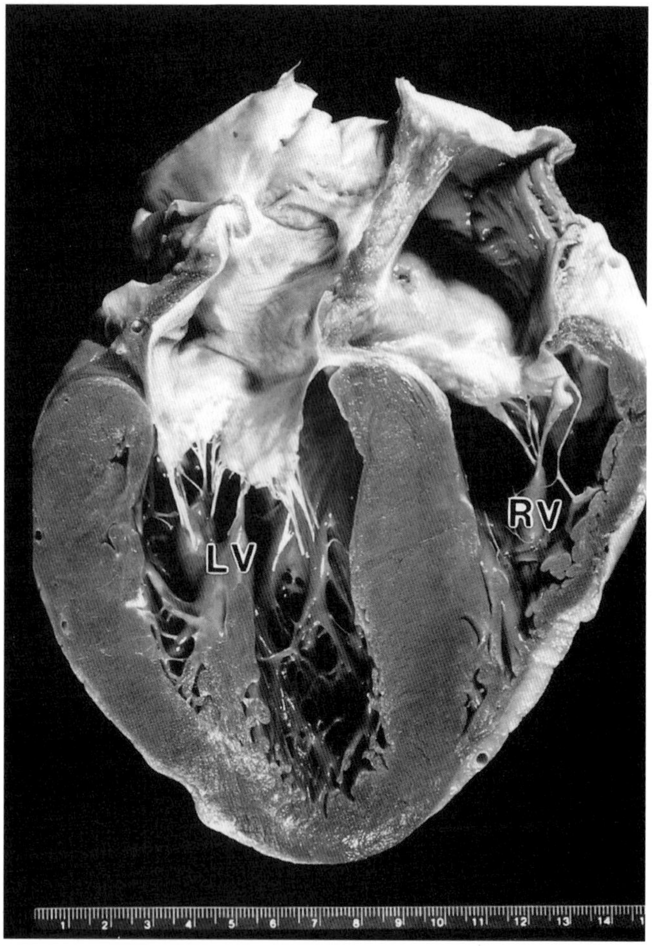


**Figure 27.12** *Obesity heart disease. The patient was a 156 kg male who died suddenly. At autopsy, the heart weighed 995 g, demonstrating left ventricular (LV) and right ventricular (RV) hypertrophy and dilatation.*

by increased cardiac output and peripheral resistance ultimately leads to heart failure and death. Somewhat surprisingly, the incidence of atherosclerosis has not been shown to be increased in morbid obesity [197]. A recent autopsy study of the morbidly obese has shown that heart weight remains constant as a percentage of body weight [200]. Obesity is characterized by increased ventricular and septal thickness, and left atrial and ventricular cavity size. These increases are mirrored by increased myocyte diameter and nuclear area. This study did not show a significant difference in the amount of atheroma or epicardial fat among groups of obese subjects and controls.

### Malnutrition and anorexia

The cardiac manifestations of severe malnutrition include autonomic dysfunction [201], long QT interval, valvular dysfunction, CHF, and sudden death. The prolonged QT interval may revert to normal after refeeding [202]; however, cardiac arrhythmias may also be associated with refeeding of anorectic patients, indicating that caloric prescription should be increased gradually and supplemental phosphorus commenced [203]. Reduced left ventricular mass may impair myocardial performance and result in CHF [204]. Echocardiographic studies of women with anorexia have shown that 62% have abnormalities of mitral valve motion, left ventricular chamber dimension and mass are decreased, cardiac index is reduced, and mid-wall shortening as a percentage of the values predicted from end-systolic stress is significantly impaired. This results in reduced left ventricular mass and filling associated with systolic dysfunction [205]. CHF may also occur in malnourished, severely ill elderly patients, and is associated with a significantly decreased survival [206]. Pathologically, heart weight may be decreased, myocytes are diminished in diameter with increased lipofuschin, and the epicardial fat undergoes brown fat change (Fig. 27.13). Morphometric analysis of electron micrographs of rat myocardium has shown an increase in capillary density, a decrease in capillary lumen cross-sectional area, and an increase in surface density of the myocytes during starvation, leading to a significant decrease in the diffusion distance for metabolites.

## Inherited metabolic disease and cardiomyopathy

A full discussion of the metabolic disorders and cardiac manifestations of inborn errors of metabolism is beyond the scope of this chapter. These disorders are typically expressed in infants and young children, and have little impact in the adult. Some relatively common metabolic disorders, however, may first present in adulthood, and are discussed below.

### Amino acid metabolism

Inherited errors of amino acid metabolism that affect the cardiovascular system include alkaptonuria (ochronosis), cystinosis, homocystinuria, and oxalosis (hyperoxaluria). Ochronosis (resulting from a deficiency of homogentisic acid oxidase) causes cardiovascular symptoms primarily by depositing brown–black pigment on the heart valves, arteries, veins, and capillaries. The major cardiovascular manifestations are aortic stenosis and accelerated atherosclerosis [207]. Homocystinuria is a rare inborn error of metabolism resulting in a high plasma homocysteine

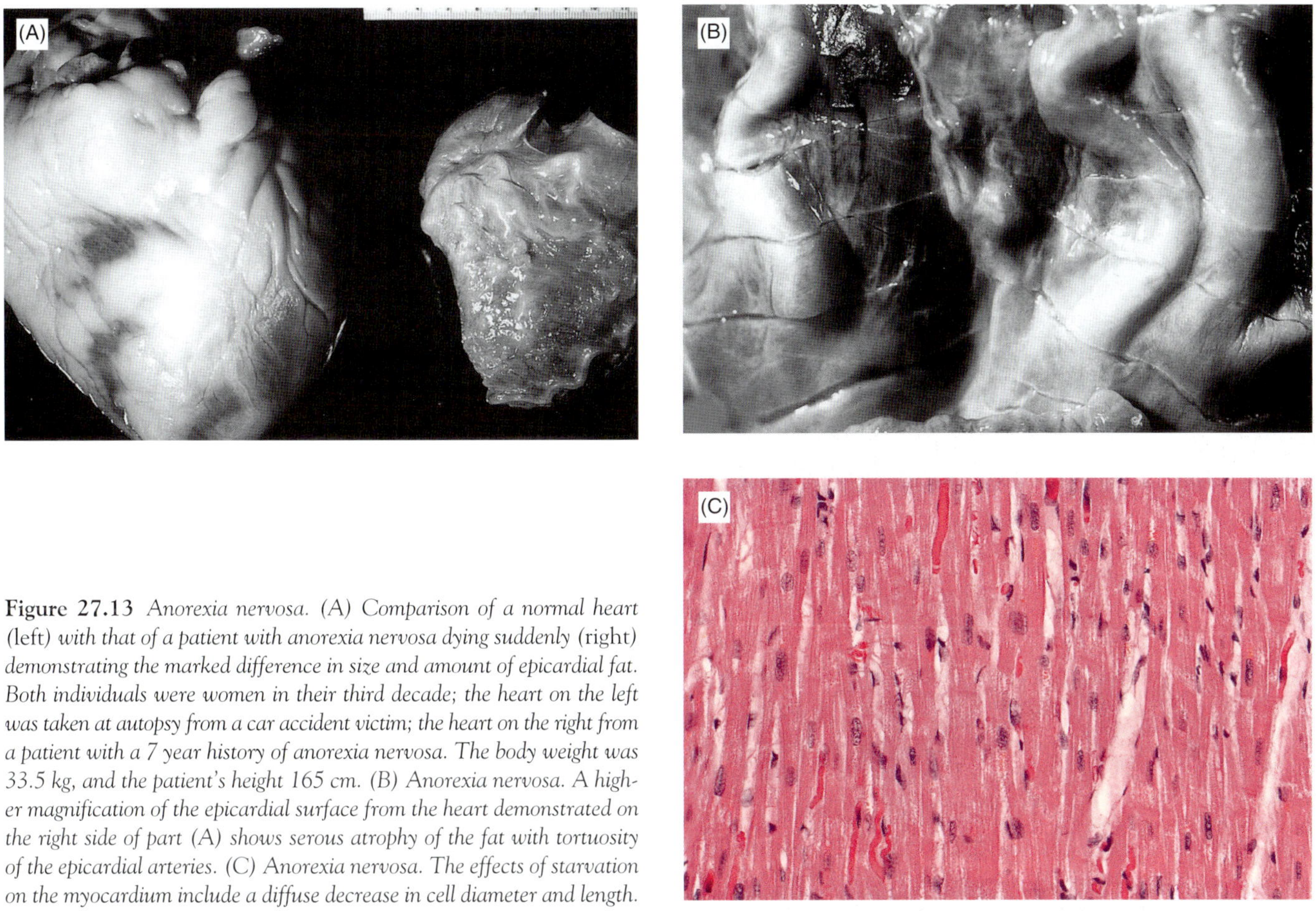


**Figure 27.13** *Anorexia nervosa. (A) Comparison of a normal heart (left) with that of a patient with anorexia nervosa dying suddenly (right) demonstrating the marked difference in size and amount of epicardial fat. Both individuals were women in their third decade; the heart on the left was taken at autopsy from a car accident victim; the heart on the right from a patient with a 7 year history of anorexia nervosa. The body weight was 33.5 kg, and the patient's height 165 cm. (B) Anorexia nervosa. A higher magnification of the epicardial surface from the heart demonstrated on the right side of part (A) shows serous atrophy of the fat with tortuosity of the epicardial arteries. (C) Anorexia nervosa. The effects of starvation on the myocardium include a diffuse decrease in cell diameter and length.*

(> 100 μmol/l) and premature mortality due to thromboembolic events [208]. The mechanism of the thrombosis is unclear, but may be related to an effect of homocysteine on coagulation, decreased resistance of the endothelium to thrombosis, and inhibition of nitric oxide-mediated vasodilation. Recently, several epidemiological studies have linked modest elevations of serum homocysteine with acute myocardial infarction, stroke, angina, vascular disease, and mortality in patients with known coronary artery disease [209–214]. Hyperoxaluria may result either from an inherited defect of alanine:glyoxylate aminotransferase or secondarily in patients with renal failure. Cardiac manifestations include conduction defects and dilated cardiomyopathy, which has been reported to reverse with normalization of serum oxalate levels [215].

## Carbohydrate metabolism

Of the glycogen storage diseases, types II–IV may cause cardiovascular dysfunction in infants and young children. Pompe's disease (infantile type II glycogen storage disease) is an autosomal-recessive condition caused by a deficiency of lysosomal α-1,4-glucosidase. Affected infants have profound cardiac dysfunction, with a large accumulation of glycogen in the myocytes. There is massive cardiomegaly and typically a dilated cardiomyopathy, which progresses to endocardial fibroelastosis and restrictive haemodynamic patterns. Adult-onset forms of glycogen storage disease II occur, but rarely result in cardiac dysfunction. Some forms of glycoproteinoses may result in cardiac hypertrophy, valve thickening, and conduction disturbances in infants and children; these include fucosidosis, mannosidosis, and mucolipidoses. Mucopolysaccharidoses are characterized by defects in the ability of lysosomes to catabolize proteoglycan and glycosaminoglycan, and result often in short stature, progressive coarsening of facial features, skeletal abnormalities, corneal clouding, mental retardation in most forms, and cardiovascular abnormalities. Children develop progressive cardiac symptoms due to cellular engorgement of the storage material within myocytes, coronary intima, and valve tissue.

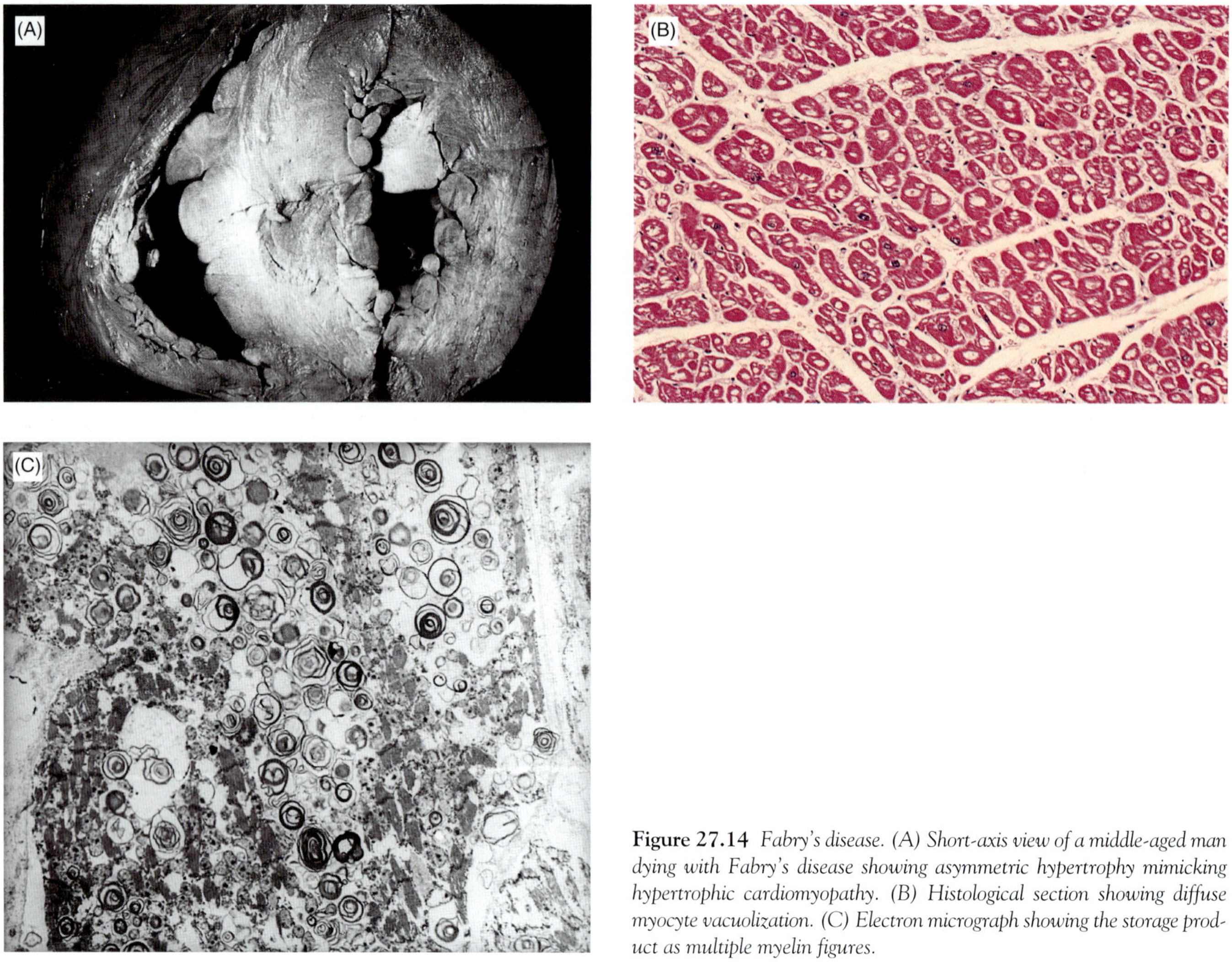


**Figure 27.14** *Fabry's disease. (A) Short-axis view of a middle-aged man dying with Fabry's disease showing asymmetric hypertrophy mimicking hypertrophic cardiomyopathy. (B) Histological section showing diffuse myocyte vacuolization. (C) Electron micrograph showing the storage product as multiple myelin figures.*

## Lipid disorders and Fabry's disease

Several lipid defects may cause cardiac dysfunction, but only one (Fabry's disease) typically presents in adulthood. The defects in fatty acid metabolism result in carnitine deficiency, and are most often caused by carnitine transport defects, medium-chain acyl-coenzyme A (CoA) dehydrogenase, or long-chain acyl-CoA dehydrogenase. Carnitine deficiency results in lipid accumulations in the myocardium and liver, and affected infants present with hypoglycaemia, coma, and CHF due to dilated cardiomyopathy. The sphingolipidoses with myocardial involvement include Fabry's disease ($\alpha$-galactosidase A deficiency), ceramidase deficiency (Farber's disease), and adult Gaucher's disease (glucocerebrosidase deficiency). Fabry's disease is an X-linked disorder that results in angiokeratomas, acroparesthaesias, hypohidrosis, and corneal opacities, as well as cardiomegaly secondary to accumulations of trihexosyl ceramide within myocytes. The left ventricular hypertrophy may be asymmetric, mimicking obstructive hypertrophic cardiomyopathy (Fig. 27.14). Recently, it has been suggested that approximately 3% of men with unexplained left ventricular hypertrophy have a heterozygous form of Fabry's disease [216]. Heterozygous females may develop cardiac disease similar to that of males.

## Connective tissue synthesis

Inherited disorders of connective tissue with cardiac manifestations include Marfan's disease, Ehlers–Danlos syndrome, cutis laxa, and pseudoxanthoma elasticum. Of these, only pseudoxanthoma elasticum typically causes myocardial dysfunction, generally due to intimal thickening and coronary artery obstruction [217].

## References


1. Kasper EK, Agema WR, Hutchins GM *et al.* The causes of dilated cardiomyopathy: a clinicopathologic review of 673 consecutive patients. *J Am Coll Cardiol* 1994; 23: 586–90.
2. Dai Y, He SJ, Yu Y *et al.* Correlative factors of left ventricular hypertrophy in end-stage renal disease. *J Tongji Med Univ* 1993; 13: 252–6.
3. Canziani ME, Cendoroglo Neto M, Saragoca MA *et al.* Hemodialysis versus continuous ambulatory peritoneal dialysis: effects on the heart. *Artif Organs* 1995; 19: 241–4.
4. Levin A, Singer J, Thompson CR *et al.* Prevalent left ventricular hypertrophy in the predialysis population: identifying opportunities for intervention. *Am J Kidney Dis* 1996; 27: 347–54.
5. Greaves SC, Gamble GD, Collins JF *et al.* Determinants of left ventricular hypertrophy and systolic dysfunction in chronic renal failure. *Am J Kidney Dis* 1994; 24: 768–76.
6. Dyadyk AI, Bagriy AE, Lebed IA *et al.* ACE inhibitors captopril and enalapril induce regression of left ventricular hypertrophy in hypertensive patients with chronic renal failure. *Nephrol Dial Transplant* 1997; 12. 945–51.
7. Johnstone LM, Jones CL, Grigg LE *et al.* Left ventricular abnormalities in children, adolescents and young adults with renal disease. *Kidney Int* 1996; 50: 998–1006.
8. Morris KP, Skinner JR, Wren C *et al.* Cardiac abnormalities in end stage renal failure and anaemia. *Arch Dis Child* 1993; 68: 637–43.
9. Rosansky SJ. Treatment of hypertension in renal failure patients: when do we overtreat? When do we undertreat? *Blood Purif* 1996; 14: 315–20.
10. London GM, Guerin AP, Marchais SJ. Pathophysiology of left ventricular hypertrophy in dialysis patients. *Blood Purif* 1994; 12: 277–83.
11. Harnett JD, Kent GM, Barre PE *et al.* Risk factors for the development of left ventricular hypertrophy in a prospectively followed cohort of dialysis patients. *J Am Soc Nephrol* 1994; 4: 1486–90.
12. Washio M, Okuda S, Mizoue T *et al.* Risk factors for left ventricular hypertrophy in chronic hemodialysis patients. *Clin Nephrol* 1997; 47: 362–6.
13. Morris KP, Skinner JR, Hunter S, Coulthard MG. Cardiovascular abnormalities in end stage renal failure: the effect of anaemia or uraemia? *Arch Dis Child* 1994; 71: 119–22.
14. Vlahakos DV, Hahalis G, Vassilakos P *et al.* Relationship between left ventricular hypertrophy and plasma renin activity in chronic hemodialysis patients. *J Am Soc Nephrol* 1997; 8: 1764–70.
15. Demuth K, Blacher J, Guerin AP *et al.* Endothelin and cardiovascular remodelling in end-stage renal disease. *Nephrol Dial Transplant* 1998; 13: 375–83.
16. Fujimoto S, Kagoshima T, Hashimoto T *et al.* Left ventricular diastolic function in patients on maintenance hemodialysis: comparison with hypertensive heart disease and hypertrophic cardiomyopathy. *Clin Nephrol* 1994; 42: 109–16.
17. Huting J, Alpert MA. Course of left ventricular diastolic dysfunction in end-stage renal disease on long-term continuous ambulatory peritoneal dialysis. *Clin Nephrol* 1993; 39: 81–7.
18. Prichard S, Sniderman A, Cianflone K, Marpole D. Cardiovascular disease in peritoneal dialysis. *Perit Dial Int* 1996; 16 (Suppl 1): S19–22.
19. Bech-Hanssen O, Wallentin I, Larsson O, Nyberg G. Reduced left ventricular hypertrophy in type 1 diabetic patients with end-stage renal failure. A comparison between groups investigated 1977–80 and 1991–93. *Nephrol Dial Transplant* 1996; 11: 1547–52.
20. Radermacher J, Koch KM. Treatment of renal anemia by erythropoietin substitution. The effects on the cardiovascular system. *Clin Nephrol* 1995; 44 (Suppl 1): S56–60.
21. Amann K, Ritz E. Cardiac disease in chronic uremia: pathophysiology. *Adv Ren Replace Ther* 1997; 4: 212–24.
22. De Lima JJ, Abensur H, da Fonseca JA *et al.* Comparison of echocardiographic changes associated with hemodialysis and renal transplantation. *Artif Organs* 1995; 19: 245–50.
23. Covic A, Goldsmith DJ, Georgescu G *et al.* Echocardiographic findings in long-term, long-hour hemodialysis patients. *Clin Nephrol* 1996; 45: 104–10.
24. Harnett JD, Foley RN, Kent GM *et al.* Congestive heart failure in dialysis patients: prevalence, incidence, prognosis and risk factors. *Kidney Int* 1995; 47: 884–90.
25. London GM, Pannier B, Guerin AP *et al.* Cardiac hypertrophy, aortic compliance, peripheral resistance, and wave reflection in end-stage renal disease. Comparative effects of ACE inhibition and calcium channel blockade. *Circulation* 1994; 90: 2786–96.
26. Blake P, Hasegawa Y, Khosla MC *et al.* Isolation of 'myocardial depressant factor(s)' from the ultrafiltrate of heart failure patients with acute renal failure. *Asaio J* 1996; 42: M911–15.
27. Facchin L, Vescovo G, Levedianos G *et al.* Left ventricular morphology and diastolic function in uraemia: echocardiographic evidence of a specific cardiomyopathy. *Br Heart J* 1995; 74: 174–9.
28. Horl WH, Riegel W. Cardiac depressant factors in renal disease. *Circulation* 1993; 87: IV77–82.
29. Ansari A, Kaupke CJ, Vaziri ND *et al.* Cardiac pathology in patients with end-stage renal disease maintained on hemodialysis. *Int J Artif Organs* 1993; 16: 31–6.
30. Leier CV, Boudoulas H. Renal disorders and heart disease. In: E Braunwald (ed.) *Heart disease: a textbook of cardiovascular medicine*. Philadelphia, PA: WB Saunders, 1997; 1914–38.
31. Blacher J, Demuth K, Guerin AP *et al.* Influence of biochemical alterations on arterial stiffness in patients with end-stage renal disease. *Arterioscler Thromb Vasc Biol* 1998; 18: 535–41.
32. Forman MB, Virmani R, Robertson RM, Stone WJ. Mitral annular calcification in chronic renal failure. *Chest* 1984; 85: 367–71.
33. Braun J, Oldendorf M, Moshage W *et al.* Electron beam computed tomography in the evaluation of cardiac calcification in chronic dialysis patients. *Am J Kidney Dis* 1996; 27: 394–401.
34. Mazzaferro S, Coen G, Bandini S *et al.* Role of aging, chronic renal failure and dialysis in the calcification of mitral annulus. *Nephrol Dial Transplant* 1993; 8: 335–40.
35. Huting J. Predictive value of mitral and aortic valve sclerosis for survival in end-stage renal disease on continuous ambulatory peritoneal dialysis. *Nephron* 1993; 64: 63–8.
36. D'Cruz IA, Madu EC. Progression to calcific mitral stenosis in end-stage renal disease. *Am J Kidney Dis* 1995; 26: 956–9.
37. Huting J. Mitral valve calcification as an index of left ventricular dysfunction in patients with end-stage renal disease on peritoneal dialysis. *Chest* 1994; 105: 383–8.
38. Toyoda Y, Shida T, Wakita N *et al.* Mitral valve replacement in a patient with an extensively calcified mitral annulus: report of a case. *Surg Today* 1998; 28: 427–9.
39. Rostaing L, el Feki S, Delisle MB *et al.* Calciphylaxis in a chronic hemodialysis patient with protein S deficiency. *Am J Nephrol* 1995; 15: 524–7.

40. Corrao S, Salli L, Arnone S *et al.* Cardiac involvement in rheumatoid arthritis: evidence of silent heart disease. *Eur Heart J* 1995; 16: 253–6.
41. Corrao S, Salli L, Arnone S *et al.* Echo-Doppler left ventricular filling abnormalities in patients with rheumatoid arthritis without clinically evident cardiovascular disease. *Eur J Clin Invest* 1996; 26: 293–7.
42. Toumanidis ST, Papamichael CM, Antoniades LG *et al.* Cardiac involvement in collagen diseases. *Eur Heart J* 1996; 16: 257–62.
43. McRorie ER, Wright RA, Errington ML, Luqmani RA. Rheumatoid constrictive pericarditis. *Br J Rheumatol* 1997; 36: 100–3.
44. Gabrielli F, Alcini E, Prima MA *et al.* Cardiac involvement in connective tissue diseases and primary antiphospholipid syndrome: echocardiographic assessment and correlation with antiphospholipid antibodies. *Acta Cardiol* 1996; 51: 425–39.
45. Mody G, Stevens JE, Meyers OL. The heart in rheumatoid arthritis: a clinical and echocardiographic study. *Q Med J* 1987; 247: 921–9.
46. Darcy TP, Virmani R. Coronary vasculitis. In: R Virmani, MB Forman (eds) *Nonatherosclerotic ischemic heart disease*. New York: Raven Press, 1989, 237–75.
47. Hidaka T, Suzuki K, Kawakami M *et al.* An autopsy case of malignant rheumatoid arthritis (MRA) which was difficult to distinguish from polyarteritis nodosa (PN). *Ryumachi* 1992; 32: 318–24.
48. Leibowitz WB. The heart in rheumatoid arthritis. *Ann Intern Med* 1963; 58: 102–24.
49. Mounet FS, Soula P, Concina P, Cerene A. A rare case of embolizing cardiac tumor: rheumatoid nodule of the mitral valve. *J Heart Valve Dis* 1997; 6: 77–8.
50. Webber MD, Selsky EJ, Roper PA. Identification of a mobile intracardiac rheumatoid nodule mimicking an atrial myxoma. *J Am Soc Echocardiogr* 1995; 8: 961–4.
51. Ahern M, Lever JV, Cosh J. Complete heart block in rheumatoid arthritis. *Ann Rheum Dis* 1983; 42: 389–95.
52. Ansari A, Larson PH, Bates HD. Cardiovascular manifestations of systemic lupus erythematosus: current perspective. *Prog Cardiovasc Dis* 1985; 27: 421–34.
53. Barton EN, Chung EE, Smikle MF *et al.* Asymptomatic cardiac involvement in systemic lupus erythematosus. *West Indian Med J* 1995; 44: 14–15.
54. Wilson VE, Eck SL, Bates ER. Evaluation and treatment of acute myocardial infarction complicating systemic lupus erythematosus. *Chest* 1992; 101: 420.
55. Doherty NE, Siegel RJ. Cardiovascular manifestations of systemic lupus erythematosus. *Am Heart J* 1985; 110: 1257–65.
56. Rantapaa-Dahlqvist S, Neumann-Andersen G, Backman C *et al.* Echocardiographic findings, lipids and lipoprotein(a) in patients with systemic lupus erythematosus. *Clin Rheumatol* 1997; 16: 140–8.
57. Lee IH, Yang SC, Kim TH *et al.* Cardiac tamponade as an initial manifestation of systemic lupus erythematosus — single case report. *J Korean Med Sci* 1997; 12: 75–7.
58. Morelli S, Perrone C, Valesini G. Tricuspid valve steno-insufficiency in systemic lupus erythematosus. *Lupus* 1995; 4: 318–20.
59. Roldan CA, Shively BK, Crawford MH. An echocardiographic study of valvular heart disease associated with systemic lupus erythematosus. *N Engl J Med* 1996; 335: 1424–30.
60. Morin AM, Boyer AS, Nataf P, Gandjbakhch I. Mitral insufficiency caused by systemic lupus erythematosus requiring valve replacement: three case reports and a review of the literature. *Thorac Cardiovasc Surg* 1996; 44: 313–16.
61. Kalangos A, Panos A, Sezerman O. Mitral valve repair in lupus valvulitis — report of a case and review of the literature. *J Heart Valve Dis* 1995; 4: 202–7.
62. Gordon RJ, Weilbaecher D, Davy SM *et al.* Valvulitis involving a bioprosthetic valve in a patient with systemic lupus erythematosus. *J Am Soc Echocardiogr* 1996; 9: 104–7.
63. Chauvaud SM, Kalangos A, Berrebi AJ *et al.* Systemic lupus erythematosus valvulitis: mitral valve replacement with a homograft. *Ann Thorac Surg* 1995; 60: 1803–5.
64. Demircin M, Dogan R, Peker O *et al.* Aortic insufficiency and enterococcal endocarditis complicating systemic lupus erythematosus. *Thorac Cardiovasc Surg* 1995; 43: 302–4.
65. Giri S, Parke AL, Mangion J *et al.* Lupus-related mitral valve disease: embolic coronary occlusion as a unique cause of myocardial infarction. *Can J Cardiol* 1997; 13: 859–63.
66. Gabrielli F, Alcini E, Di Prima MA *et al.* Cardiac valve involvement in systemic lupus erythematosus and primary antiphospholipid syndrome: lack of correlation with antiphospholipid antibodies. *Int J Cardiol* 1995; 51: 117–26.
67. Meyer O, Golstein M, Nicaise P *et al.* Heart valve disease in systemic lupus erythematosus. Role of antiphospholipid antibodies. *Clin Rev Allergy Immunol* 1995; 13: 49–56.
68. Borenstein DG, Fye WB, Arnett FC, Stevens MB. The myocarditis of systemic lupus erythematosus: association with myositis. *Ann Intern Med* 1978; 89: 619–24.
69. Fairfax MJ, Osborn TG, Williams GA *et al.* Endomyocardial biopsy in patients with systemic lupus erythematosus. *J Rheumatol* 1988; 15: 593–6.
70. Frustaci A, Gentiloni N, Caldarulo M. Acute myocarditis and left ventricular aneurysm as presentations of systemic lupus erythematosus. *Chest* 1996; 109: 282–4.
71. Buyon JP, Hiebert R, Copel J *et al.* Autoimmune-associated congenital heart block: demographics, mortality, morbidity and recurrence rates obtained from a national neonatal lupus registry. *J Am Coll Cardiol* 1998; 31: 1658–66.
72. Buyon JP. Neonatal lupus. *Curr Opin Rheumatol* 1996; 8: 485–90.
73. Ferrazzini G, Fasnacht M, Arbenz U *et al.* Neonatal lupus erythematosus with congenital heart block and severe heart failure due to myocarditis and endocardititis of the mitral valve. *Intensive Care Med* 1996; 22: 464–6.
74. Bulkley BH, Ridolfi RL, Salyer WR, Hutchins GM. Myocardial lesions of progressive systemic sclerosis. *Circulation* 1976; 53: 483–90.
75. Botstein GR, LeRoy EC. Primary heart disease in systemic sclerosis (scleroderma): advances in clinical and pathologic features, pathogenesis, and new therapeutic approaches. *Am Heart J* 1981; 102: 913–19.
76. Follansbee WP, Curtiss EI, Medsger TA Jr *et al.* Myocardial function and perfusion in the CREST syndrome variant of progressive systemic sclerosis. Exercise radionuclide evaluation and comparison with diffuse scleroderma. *Am J Med* 1984; 77: 489–96.
77. Follansbee WP, Curtiss EL, Rahko PS *et al.* The electrocardiogram in systemic sclerosis (scleroderma). Study of 102 consecutive cases with functional correlations and review of the literature. *Am J Med* 1985; 79: 183–92.
78. Ansell BM, Bywaters EGL, Doniach I. The aortic lesions of ankylosing spondylitis. *Br Heart J* 1958; 20: 507–15.
79. de Almeida FA, Albanesi Filho EM, de Albuquerque EM *et al.* Echocardiography in the evaluation of cardiac involvement in

seronegative spondylo-arthropathies. *Medicina (B Aires)* 1995; 55: 231–6.

80. Paulus HE, Pearson CM, Pitts W Jr. Aortic insufficiency in five patients with Reiter's syndrome. A detailed clinical and pathologic study. *Am J Med* 1972; 53: 464–72.
81. Arnason JA, Patel AK, Rahko PS, Sundstrom WR. Transthoracic and transesophageal echocardiographic evaluation of the aortic root and subvalvular structures in ankylosing spondylitis. *J Rheumatol* 1996; 23: 120–3.
82. O'Neill TW, King G, Graham IM *et al.* Echocardiographic abnormalities in ankylosing spondylitis. *Ann Rheum Dis* 1992; 51: 652–4.
83. Hoogland YT, Alexander EP, Patterson RH, Nashel DJ. Coronary artery stenosis in Reiter's syndrome: a complication of aortitis. *J Rheumatol* 1994; 21: 757–9.
84. Bergfeldt L. HLA-B27-associated cardiac disease. *Ann Intern Med* 1997; 127: 621–9.
85. Bulkley BH, Roberts WC. Ankylosing spondylitis and aortic regurgitation. Description of the characteristic cardiovascular lesion from study of eight necropsy patients. *Circulation* 1973; 48: 1014–27.
86. Costello JJ, Nicholson WJ. Severe aortic regurgitation as a late complication of temporal arteritis. *Chest* 1990; 98: 875–7.
87. Evans JM, Bowles CA, Bjornsson J *et al.* Thoracic aortic aneurysm and rupture in giant cell arteritis. A descriptive study of 41 cases. *Arthritis Rheum* 1994; 37: 1539–47.
88. Evans JO, Fallon WM, Hunder GG. Increased incidence of aortic aneurysm and dissection in giant cell (temporal) arteritis. A population-based study. *Ann Intern Med* 1995; 122: 502–7.
89. Ginsburg R. Aortic aneurysm and dissection in giant cell arteritis. *Ann Intern Med* 1996; 124: 615.
90. Eishi K, Nakajima S, Kitoh Y *et al.* Aortic root replacement with a cryopreserved aortic homograft in a patient with giant cell aortitis following two Bentall's type operations. *J Heart Valve Dis* 1995; 4: 509–12.
91. Richardson MP, Lever AM, Fink AM *et al.* Survival after aortic dissection in giant cell arteritis. *Ann Rheum Dis* 1996; 55: 332–3.
92. Lie JT. Aortic and extracranial large vessel giant cell arteritis: a review of 72 cases with histopathologic documentation. *Semin Arthritis Rheum* 1995; 24: 422–31.
93. Schrader ML, Hochman JS, Bulkley BH. The heart in polyarteritis nodosa: a clinicopathologic study. *Am Heart J* 1985; 109: 1313.
94. Morbini P, Dal Bello B, Arbustini E. Coronary artery inflammation and thrombosis in Wegener's granulomatosis–polyarteritis nodosa overlap syndrome. *G Ital Cardiol* 1998; 28: 377–82.
95. Lang-Lazdunski L, Pansard Y, Hvass U. Aortic valve replacement in relapsing polychondritis. *J Thorac Cardiovasc Surg* 1997; 114: 131–2.
96. Otasevic P, Pavlovski K, Popovic AD. Isolated mitral regurgitation complicating relapsing polychondritis. *Int J Cardiol* 1997; 60: 213–15.
97. Del Rosso A, Petix NR, Pratesi M, Bini A. Cardiovascular involvement in relapsing polychondritis. *Semin Arthritis Rheum* 1997; 26: 840–4.
98. Triplett DA. Protean clinical presentation of antiphospholipid-protein antibodies (APA). *Thromb Haemost* 1995; 74: 329–37.
99. Hughson MD, McCarty GA, Brumback RA. Spectrum of vascular pathology affecting patients with the antiphospholipid syndrome. *Hum Pathol* 1995; 26: 716–24.
100. Almeshari K, Alfurayh O, Akhtar M. Primary antiphospholipid syndrome and self-limited renal vasculitis during pregnancy: case report and review of the literature. *Am J Kidney Dis* 1994; 24: 505–8.
101. Gertner E, Leatherman J. Intracardiac mural thrombus mimicking atrial myxoma in the antiphospholipid syndrome. *J Rheumatol* 1992; 19: 1293–8.
102. Chong BH. Heparin-induced thrombocytopenia. *Br J Haematol* 1995; 89: 431–9.
103. Warkentin TE, Chong BH, Greinacher A. Heparin-induced thrombocytopenia: towards consensus. *Thromb Haemost* 1998; 79: 1–7.
104. Schmitt BP, Adelman B. Heparin-associated thrombocytopenia: a critical review and a pooled analysis. *Am J Med Sci* 1993; 305: 208–15.
105. Burke AP, Mezzetti T, Farb A *et al.* Multiple coronary artery graft occlusion in a fatal case of heparin-induced thrombocytopenia. *Chest* (in press).
106. Weiskopf RB, Viele MK, Feiner J *et al.* Human cardiovascular and metabolic response to actue, severe isovolemic anemia. *JAMA* 1998; 279: 217–21.
107. Shulman LN, Braunwald E, Rosenthal DS. Hematological–oncological disorders and heart disease. In: E Braunwald (ed.) *Heart disease: a textbook of cardiovascular medicine*. Philadelphia, PA: WB Saunders, 1997, 1786–808.
108. Anand IS, Chandrashekhar Y, Wander GS, Chawla LS. Endothelium-derived relaxing factor is important in mediating the high output state in chronic severe anemia. *J Am Coll Cardiol* 1995; 25: 1402–7.
109. Covitz W, Espeland M, Gallagher D *et al.* The heart in sickle cell anemia. The Cooperative Study of Sickle Cell Disease (CSSCD). *Chest* 1995; 108: 1214–19.
110. Braden DS, Covitz W, Milner PF. Cardiovascular function during rest and exercise in patients with sickle-cell anemia and coexisting alpha thalassemia-2. *Am J Hematol* 1996; 52: 96–102.
111. Martin CR, Johnson CS, Cobb C *et al.* Myocardial infarction in sickle cell disease. *J Natl Med Assoc* 1996; 88: 428–32.
112. Jaeggi E, Bolens M, Friedli B. Reversible second degree atrioventricular block after a severe sickle cell crisis. *Pediatr Cardiol* 1998; 19: 171–3.
113. Kark JA. Sickle-cell trait as an age-dependent risk factor for sudden death in physical training. *N Engl J Med* 1987; 317: 781–7.
114. Kark JA, Ward F. Exercise and hemoglobin S. *Semin Hematol* 1994; 31: 181–225.
115. Yaprak I, Aksit S, Ozturk C *et al.* Left ventricular diastolic abnormalities in children with beta-thalassemia major: a Doppler echocardiographic study. *Turk J Pediatr* 1998; 40: 201–9.
116. Brili SV, Tzonou AI, Castelanos SS *et al.* The effect of iron overload in the hearts of patients with beta-thalassemia. *Clin Cardiol* 1997; 20: 541–6.
117. Borgna-Pignatti C, Rugolotto S, De Stefano P *et al.* Survival and disease complications in thalassemia major. *Ann NY Acad Sci* 1998; 850: 227–31.
118. Mavrogeni SI, Maris T, Gouliamos A *et al.* Myocardial iron deposition in beta-thalassemia studied by magnetic resonance imaging. *Int J Card Imaging* 1998; 14: 117–22.
119. Kremastinos DT, Tiniakos G, Theodorakis GN *et al.* Myocarditis in beta-thalassemia major. A cause of heart failure. *Circulation* 1995; 91: 66–71.

120. Jessup M, Manno CS. Diagnosis and management of iron-induced heart disease in Cooley's anemia. *Ann NY Acad Sci* 1998; 850: 242–50.
121. Witte DL, Crosby WH, Edwards CQ *et al.* Practice guideline development task force of the College of American Pathologists. Hereditary hemochromatosis. *Clin Chim Acta* 1996; 245: 139–200.
122. Adams PC, Deugnier Y, Moirand R, Brissot P. The relationship between iron overload, clinical symptoms, and age in 410 patients with genetic hemochromatosis. *Hepatology* 1997; 25: 162–6.
123. Passen EL, Rodriguez ER, Neumann A *et al.* Images in cardiovascular medicine. Cardiac hemochromatosis. *Circulation* 1996; 94: 2302–3.
124. Niwano S, Yokoyama J, Niwano H, Aizawa Y. Images in cardiovascular medicine. Iron deposition in myocardium documented on standard computed tomography in cardiac hemochromatosis. *Circulation* 1998; 97: 2371.
125. Yalcinkaya S, Kumbasar SD, Semiz E *et al.* Sustained ventricular tachycardia in cardiac hemochromatosis treated with amiodarone. *J Electrocardiol* 1997; 30: 147–9.
126. Sagripanti A, Ferretti A, Nicolini A, Carpi A. Thrombotic and hemorrhagic complications in chronic myeloproliferative disorders. *Biomed Pharmacother* 1996; 50: 376–82.
127. Virmani R, Popovsky MA, Roberts WC. Thrombocytosis, coronary thrombosis and acute myocardial infarction. *Am J Med* 1979; 67: 498–506.
128. Bell WR. Thrombotic thrombocytopenic purpura/hemolytic uremic syndrome relapse: frequency, pathogenesis, and meaning. *Semin Hematol* 1997; 34: 134–9.
129. Ruggenenti P, Lutz J, Remuzzi G. Pathogenesis and treatment of thrombotic microangiopathy. *Kidney Int* 1997; 58 (Suppl): S97–101.
130. Ucar A, Fernandez HF, Byrnes JJ *et al.* Thrombotic microangiopathy and retroviral infections: a 13-year experience. *Am J Hematol* 1994; 45: 304–9.
131. Bray VJ, West SG, Kristo DA. Simultaneous presentation of thrombotic thrombocytopenic purpura and systemic lupus erythematosus. *South Med J* 1994; 87: 827–30.
132. Chinowsky MS. Thrombotic thrombocytopenic purpura associated with sickle cell-hemoglobin C disease. *South Med J* 1994; 87: 1168–71.
133. Khoo US, Dickens P, Cheung AN. Rapid death from thrombotic thrombocytopaenic purpura following caesarean section. *Forensic Sci Int* 1992; 54: 75–80.
134. Sagripanti A, Carpi A, Rosaia B *et al.* Iloprost in the treatment of thrombotic microangiopathy: report of thirteen cases. *Biomed Pharmacother* 1996; 50: 350–6.
135. Lam KY, Dickens P, Chan AC. Tumors of the heart. A 20-year experience with a review of 12,485 consecutive autopsies. *Arch Pathol Lab Med* 1993; 117: 1027–31.
136. Burke A, Virmani R. Tumors metastatic to the heart and pericardium. In: *Atlas of tumor pathology: tumors of the heart and great vessels*. Vol. 16. Washington, DC: Armed Forces Institute of Pathology, 1996, 195–210.
137. Tse HF, Lau CP, Lau YK, Lai CL. Transesophageal echocardiography in the detection of inferior vena cava and cardiac metastasis in hepatocellular carcinoma. *Clin Cardiol* 1996; 19: 211–13.
138. Abrams J, Talcott J, Corson JM. Pulmonary metastases in patients with low-grade endometrial stromal sarcoma. Clinicopathologic findings with immunohistochemical characterization. *Am J Surg Pathol* 1989; 13: 133–40.
139. Baba HA, Engers R, Heintzen MP. Right atrial metastasis as primary clinical manifestation of hepatocellular carcinoma. *Int J Cardiol* 1995; 47: 281–4.
140. Bartels P, O'Callaghan W, Peyton R. Metastatic liposarcoma of the right ventricle with outflow tract obstruction: restrictive pathophysiology predicts poor surgical outcome. *Am Heart J* 1988; 114: 696–8.
141. Bradley SM, Bolling SF. Late renal cell carcinoma metastasis to the left ventricular outflow tract. *Ann Thorac Surg* 1995; 60: 204–6.
142. Chen RH, Gaos CM, Frazier OH. Complete resection of a right atrial intracavitary metastatic melanoma. *Ann Thorac Surg* 1996; 61: 1255–7.
143. Patane J, Flum DR, McGinn JT Jr, Tyras DH. Surgical approach for renal cell carcinoma metastatic to the left atrium. *Ann Thorac Surg* 1996; 62: 891–2.
144. Riccioni L, Damiani S, Pasquinelli G, Scarani P. Solitary left ventricle metastasis by renal cell carcinoma with sarcomatoid features. *Tumori* 1996; 82: 266–9.
145. Ishikawa K. Cardiac involvement in progressive muscular dystrophy of the Duchenne type. *Jpn Heart J* 1997; 38: 163–80.
146. Brockmeier K, Schmitz L, von Moers A *et al.* X-chromosomal (p21) muscular dystrophy and left ventricular diastolic and systolic function. *Pediatr Cardiol* 1998; 19: 139–44.
147. Politano L, Nigro V, Nigro G *et al.* Development of cardiomyopathy in female carriers of Duchenne and Becker muscular dystrophies. *JAMA* 1996; 275: 1335–8.
148. Tokgozoglu LS, Ashizawa T, Pacifico A *et al.* Cardiac involvement in a large kindred with myotonic dystrophy. Quantitative assessment and relation to size of CTG repeat expansion. *JAMA* 1995; 274: 813–19.
149. Gharehbaghi-Schnell E, Finsterer J, Korschineck I *et al.* Myotonic dystrophy: molecular genetics and diagnosis. *Wien Klin Wochenschr* 1998; 110: 7–14.
150. Phillips MF, Harper PS. Cardiac disease in myotonic dystrophy. *Cardiovasc Res* 1997; 33: 13–22.
151. Colleran JA, Hawley RJ, Pinnow EE *et al.* Value of the electrocardiogram in determining cardiac events and mortality in myotonic dystrophy. *Am J Cardiol* 1997; 80: 1494–7.
152. Gunal N, Saraclar M, Ozkutlu S *et al.* Heart disease in Friedreich's ataxia: a clinical and echocardiographic study. *Acta Paediatr Jpn* 1996; 38: 308–11.
153. Ferres-Sanchez P, Subirana-Domenech M, Torner-Soler M. Chest pain during exercise as first manifestation of Friedreich's ataxia. *Br Heart J* 1995; 74: 464–7.
154. Casazza F, Morpurgo M. The varying evolution of Friedreich's ataxia cardiomyopathy. *Am J Cardiol* 1996; 77: 895–8.
155. Isnard R, Kalotka H, Durr A *et al.* Correlation between left ventricular hypertrophy and GAA trinucleotide repeat length in Friedreich's ataxia. *Circulation* 1997; 95: 2247–9.
156. Maione S, Giunta A, Filla A *et al.* May age onset be relevant in the occurrence of left ventricular hypertrophy in Friedreich's ataxia? *Clin Cardiol* 1997; 20: 141–5.
157. Giustina A, Boni E, Romanelli G *et al.* Cardiopulmonary performance during exercise in acromegaly, and the effects of acute sup-

pression of growth hormone hypersecretion with octreotide. *Am J Cardiol* 1995; 75: 1042–7.
158. Ohtsuka G, Aomi S, Koyanagi H *et al.* Heart valve operation in acromegaly. *Ann Thorac Surg* 1997; 64: 390–3.
159. Cuocolo A, Nicolai E, Fazio S *et al.* Impaired left ventricular diastolic filling in patients with acromegaly: assessment with radionuclide angiography. *J Nucl Med* 1995; 36: 196–201.
160. Lombardi G, Colao A, Cuocolo A *et al.* Cardiological aspects of growth hormone and insulin-like growth factor-I. *J Pediatr Endocrinol Metab* 1997; 10: 553–60.
161. Fazio S, Cittadini A, Sabatini D *et al.* Growth hormone and heart performance. A novel mechanism of cardiac wall stress regulation in humans. *Eur Heart J* 1997; 18: 340–7.
162. Lombardi G, Colao A, Marzullo P *et al.* Is growth hormone bad for your heart? Cardiovascular impact of GH deficiency and of acromegaly. *J Endocrinol* 1997; 155 (Suppl 1): S33–7, Discussion S39.
163. Merola B, Cittadini A, Colao A *et al.* Chronic treatment with the somatostatin analog octreotide improves cardiac abnormalities in acromegaly. *J Clin Endocrinol Metab* 1993; 77: 790–3.
164. Nishiki M, Murakami Y, Sohmiya M *et al.* Histopathological improvement of acromegalic cardiomyopathy by intermittent subcutaneous infusion of octreotide. *Endocr J* 1997; 44: 655–60.
165. Dillmann WH. Cardiac function in thyroid disease: clinical features and management considerations. *Ann Thorac Surg* 1993; 56: S9–14.
166. Aronow WS. The heart and thyroid disease. *Clin Geriatr Med* 1995; 11: 219–29.
167. Cavros NG, Old WD, Castro FD, Estep HL. Case report: reversible mitral regurgitation and congestive heart failure complicating thyrotoxicosis. *Am J Med Sci* 1996; 311: 142–4.
168. Masani ND, Northridge DB, Hall RJ. Severe coronary vasospasm associated with hyperthyroidism causing myocardial infarction. *Br Heart J* 1995; 74: 700–1.
169. Zondek H. Das myxoedemherz. *Muench Med Wochenschr* 1918; 65: 1180–1.
170. Bartalena L, Pinchera A. Effects of thyroxine excess on peripheral organs. *Acta Med Austriaca* 1994; 21: 60–5.
171. Davis PJ, Davis FB. Acute cellular actions of thyroid hormone and myocardial function. *Ann Thorac Surg* 1993; 56: S16–23.
172. Fallo F, Budano S, Sonino N *et al.* Left ventricular structural characteristics in Cushing's syndrome. *J Hum Hypertens* 1994; 8: 509–13.
173. Whitworth JA, Kelly JJ, Brown MA *et al.* Glucocorticoids and hypertension in man. *Clin Exp Hypertens* 1997; 19: 871–84.
174. Tanabe A, Naruse M, Naruse K *et al.* Left ventricular hypertrophy is more prominent in patients with primary aldosteronism than in patients with other types of secondary hypertension. *Hypertens Res* 1997; 20: 85–90.
175. Derish M, Eckert K, Chin C. Reversible cardiomyopathy in a child with Addison's disease. *Intensive Care Med* 1996; 22: 460–3.
176. Nanda AS, Feldman A, Liang CS. Acute reversal of pheochromocytoma-induced catecholamine cardiomyopathy. *Clin Cardiol* 1995; 18: 421–3.
177. Pavin D, Le Breton H, Daubert C. Human stress cardiomyopathy mimicking acute myocardial syndrome. *Heart* 1997; 78: 509–11.
178. Baroldi G, Di Pasquale G, Silver MD *et al.* Type and extent of myocardial injury related to brain damage and its significance in heart transplantation: a morphometric study. *J Heart Lung Transplant* 1997; 16: 994–1000.
179. Mann DL. Basic mechanisms of disease progression in the failing heart: the role of excessive adrenergic drive. *Prog Cardiovasc Dis* 1998; 48: 1–8.
180. Fenton RA, Galeckas KJ, Dobson JG Jr. Endogenous adenosine reduces depression of cardiac function induced by beta-adrenergic stimulation during low flow perfusion. *J Mol Cell Cardiol* 1995; 27: 2373–83.
181. Schuiki ER, Jenni R, Amann FW, Ziegler WH. A reversible form of apical left ventricular hypertrophy associated with pheochromocytoma. *J Am Soc Echocardiogr* 1993; 6: 327–31.
182. Dalberg K, Brodin LA, Juhlin-Dannfelt A, Farnebo LO. Cardiac function in primary hyperparathyroidism before and after operation. An echocardiographic study. *Eur J Surg* 1996; 162: 171–6.
183. Schluter KD, Piper HM. Cardiovascular actions of parathyroid hormone and parathyroid hormone-related peptide. *Cardiovasc Res* 1998; 37: 34–41.
184. Amann K, Ritz E, Wiest G *et al.* A role of parathyroid hormone for the activation of cardiac fibroblasts in uremia. *J Am Soc Nephrol* 1994; 4: 1814–19.
185. Williams GH, Lilly LS, Seely EW. The heart in endocrine and nutritional disorders. In: E Braunwald (ed.) *Heart disease: a textbook of cardiovascular medicine*. Philadelphia, PA: WB Saunders, 1997, 1887–913.
186. Sima A, Popov D, Starodub O *et al.* Pathobiology of the heart in experimental diabetes: immunolocalization of lipoproteins, immunoglobulin G, and advanced glycation endproducts proteins in diabetic and/or hyperlipidemic hamster. *Lab Invest* 1997; 77: 3–18.
187. Stitt AW, He C, Friedman S *et al.* Elevated AGE-modified ApoB in sera of euglycemic, normolipidemic patients with atherosclerosis: relationship to tissue AGEs. *Mol Med* 1997; 3: 617–27.
188. Vlassara H, Fuh H, Donnelly T, Cybulsky M. Advanced glycation endproducts promote adhesion molecule (VCAM-1, ICAM-1) expression and atheroma formation in normal rabbits. *Mol Med* 1995; 1: 447–56.
189. Sutherland CG, Fisher BM, Frier BM *et al.* Endomyocardial biopsy pathology in insulin-dependent diabetic patients with abnormal ventricular function. *Histopathology* 1989; 14: 593–602.
190. Spallone V, Menzinger G. Diagnosis of cardiovascular autonomic neuropathy in diabetes. *Diabetes* 1997; 46 (Suppl 2): S67–76.
191. Coughlin SS, Szklo M, Baughman K, Pearson TA. The epidemiology of idiopathic dilated cardiomyopathy in a biracial community. *Am J Epidemiol* 1990; 131: 48–56.
192. Celentano A, Vaccaro O, Tammaro P *et al.* Early abnormalities of cardiac function in non-insulin-dependent diabetes mellitus and impaired glucose tolerance. *Am J Cardiol* 1995; 76: 1173–6.
193. Nakajima T, Fujioka S, Tokunaga K *et al.* Correlation of intraabdominal fat accumulation and left ventricular performance in obesity. *Am J Cardiol* 1989; 64: 369–73.
194. Egan B, Fitzpatrick MA, Juni J *et al.* Importance of overweight in studies of left ventricular hypertrophy and diastolic function in mild systemic hypertension. *Am J Cardiol* 1989; 64: 752–5.

195. de Divitiis O, Fazio S, Petitto M *et al.* Obesity and cardiac function. *Circulation* 1981; 64: 477–82.
196. Alexander JK. The cardiomyopathy of obesity. *Prog Cardiovasc Dis* 1985; 27: 325–34.
197. Warnes CA, Roberts WC. The heart in massive (more than 300 pounds or 136 kilograms) obesity: analysis of 12 patients studied at necropsy. *Am J Cardiol* 1984; 54: 1087–91.
198. Messerli FH. Cardiovascular effects of obesity and hypertension. *Lancet* 1982; i: 1165–8.
199. Messerli FH, Ventura HO, Reisin ED *et al.* Obesity and essential hypertension. *Contrib Nephrol* 1982; 30: 116–23.
200. Duflou J, Virmani R, Rabin I *et al.* Sudden death as a result of heart disease in morbid obesity. *Am Heart J* 1995; 130: 306–13.
201. Rechlin T, Weis M, Ott C *et al.* Alterations of autonomic cardiac control in anorexia nervosa. *Biol Psychiatry* 1998; 43: 358–63.
202. Cooke RA, Chambers JB, Singh R *et al.* QT interval in anorexia nervosa. *Br Heart J* 1994; 72: 69–73.
203. Kohn MR, Golden NH, Shenker IR. Cardiac arrest and delirium: persentations of the refeeding syndrome in severely malnourished adolescents with anorexia nervosa. *J Adolesc Health* 1998; 22: 239–43.
204. Cooke RA, Chambers JB. Anorexia nervosa and the heart. *Br J Hosp Med* 1995; 54: 313–17.
205. de Simone G, Scalfi L, Galderisi M *et al.* Cardiac abnormalities in young women with anorexia nervosa. *Br Heart J* 1994; 71: 287–92.
206. Cederholm T, Jagren C, Hellstrom K. Outcome of protein-energy malnutrition in elderly medical patients. *Am J Med* 1995; 98: 67–74.
207. Kenny D, Ptacin MJ, Bamrah VS, Almagro U. Cardiovascular ochronosis: a case report and review of the medical literature. *Cardiology* 1990; 77: 477–83.
208. Mudd SH, Skovby F, Levy HL *et al.* The natural history of homocystinuria due to cystathionine beta-synthase deficiency. *Am J Hum Genet* 1985; 37: 1–31.
209. Arnesen E, Refsum H, Bonaa KH *et al.* Serum total homocysteine and coronary heart disease. *Int J Epidemiol* 1995; 24: 704–9.
210. Perry JJ. Serum total homocysteine concentration and risk of stroke. *Lancet* 1996; 348: 1526.
211. Verhoef P. Hennekens CH, Allen RH *et al.* Plasma total homocysteine and risk of angina pectoris with subsequent coronary artery bypass surgery. *Am J Cardiol* 1997; 79: 799–801.
212. Nygård O, Nordrehaug JE, Refsum H *et al.* Plasma homocysteine levels and mortality in patients with coronary artery disease. *N Engl J Med* 1997; 337: 230–6.
213. Robinson K, Arheart K, Refsum H *et al.* Low circulating folate and vitamin B6 concentrations: risk factors for stroke, peripheral vascular disease, and coronary artery disease. *Circulation* 1998; 97: 437–43.
214. Guba SC, Fink LM, Fonseca V. Hyperhomocysteinemia. An emerging and important risk factor for thromboembolic and cardiovascular disease. *Am J Clin Pathol* 1996; 106: 709–22.
215. Rodby RA, Tyszka TS, Williams. JW. Reversal of cardiac dysfunction secondary to type 1 primary hyperoxaluria after combined liver-kidney transplantation. *Am J Med* 1991; 90: 498–504.
216. Nakao S, Takenaka T, Maeda M *et al.* An atypical variant of Fabry's disease in men with left ventricular hypertrophy. *N Engl J Med* 1995; 333: 288–93.
217. Slade AK, John RM, Swanton RH. Pseudoxanthoma elasticum presenting with myocardial infarction. *Br Heart J* 1990; 63: 372–3.

# Iatrogenic diseases of the myocardium



I. CARRIÓ

## Introduction

A variety of drugs used for the treatment of non-cardiac ailments may result in myocardial damage. The damage may be acute or transient; sometimes it is associated with evidence of an inflammatory infiltrate with myocardial necrosis, whereas in other cases a hypersensitivity reaction may occur, without evidence of myocyte necrosis. Other substances that damage the myocardium produce chronic changes, with histological evidence of interstitial fibrosis and clinical symptoms of dilated cardiomyopathy. Most of these potentially cardiotoxic drugs are of proven efficacy for the treatment of various severe of life-threatening diseases and are unavoidable. Evaluation of the cardiotoxicity of these pharmacological agents is important since the residual cardiac damage determines the clinical outcome and quality of life after treatment, and may help in the development of potential cardioprotective strategies without the loss of therapeutic efficacy.

## Drugs known to result in myocardial abnormalities and common mechanisms of myocardial damage

Among the drugs known to cause myocardial abnormalities, antineoplastic drugs have been extensively studied, and a large body of data has accumulated demonstrating their dose-dependent cardiotoxicity. Anthracycline cardiotoxicity is caused by stimulated reactive oxygen metabolism. This augmented reactive oxygen flux causes free radical-mediated myocyte cell damage at specific sites. In addition, anthracyclines or their metabolites may trigger the release of endogenous substances such as histamine, arachidonic acid metabolites, platelet-activating factor, calcium, and other compounds potentially deleterious to the myocardium [1–4]. Other antineoplastic drugs have also been reported to result in myocardial damage and clinical symptoms of cardiotoxicity. High doses of cyclophosphamide are associated with electrocardiographic (ECG) changes, symptoms of congestive heart failure (CHF), and even death from haemorrhagic myocarditis [5]. The myocardial damage appears to results from direct endothelial damage produced by the drug and resultant fibrin microthrombi in the capillaries. 5-Fluorouracil is also associated with clinical signs of cardiotoxicity, manifested by chest pain, ECG changes, and arrhythmia. Swelling of myocardial fibres without an inflammatory infiltrate has been found at autopsy [6]. Newer antineoplastic drugs such as paclixatel also induce cardiotoxicity [7].

Interferon-$\alpha$ is often used to treat some malignancies and infections caused by human immunodeficiency virus (HIV). Up to 10% of patients treated with this leucocyte-derived protein may present with hypotension, tachycardia, and transient arrhythmias. Some of these patients develop clinical symptoms of CHF that may resolve with discontinuation of interferon administration [8]. The lymphokine interleukin-2, also used as an antineoplastic agent, produces cardiotoxicity in approximately 5% of patients, consisting of myocardial ischaemia, infarction, arrhythmias, and eosinophilic myocarditis [9].

Tricyclic antidepressants produce deleterious effects in patients with prior myocardial infarction or pre-existing ventricular arrhythmias, particularly when taken as an overdose [10]. Positive antimyosin uptake, indicating drug-induced myocardial damage, has been described in patients treated with tricyclic antidepressants [11]. The administration of phenothiazines has also been associated with ECG changes, atrial and ventricular arrhythmias and, rarely, sudden death [12]. Pathological alterations in the hearts of patients treated with these psychotropic drugs and who have had sudden death include the interstitial deposition of acid mucopolysaccharide, with myofibrillar degeneration, and endothelial proliferation in the small blood vessels [12]. Lithium carbonate, used occasionally in the treatment of patients with bipolar disorders, is frequently associated with electrocardiographic T-wave changes. Intoxication with lithium is associated with ventricular arrhythmias, atrioventricular conduction disturbances, and clinical symptoms of CHF. Myofibrillar degeneration associated with an interstitial lymphocytic infiltrate and fibrosis has been described in patients with signs of cardiotoxicity secondary to lithium therapy [13].

Emetine, which is used in the combined treatment of amoebiasis and schistosomiasis, often produces cardiovascular side-effects. Structural myocardial abnormalities at autopsy have included myofibrillar degeneration and necrosis, with an interstitial infiltrate of mononuclear cells and histiocytes [14]. Chloroquine is another cardiotoxic drug which is widely used to treat a variety of parasitic disorders. ECG changes have been reported after its administration, with conduction abnormalities and features of restrictive cardiomyopathy that may result in low cardiac output and death at toxic doses. Characteristic histological changes have also been observed by electron-microscopic examination [15].

High levels of circulating catecholamines are known to result in myocardial damage. Catecholamines may produce acute myocarditis, with focal myocardial necrosis, inflammation, epicardial haemorrhages, tachycardia, and arrhythmias [16]. A variety of pathogenetic mechanisms has been proposed [17], including a direct toxic effect, myocardial damage secondary to relative hypoxia due to persistently increased metabolic demands, or myocardial damage resulting from changes in autonomic nerve tone, calcium overload, free radicals, or increased membrane permeability [18].

Hypersensitivity myocarditis, characterized by peripheral eosinophilia and perivascular infiltration of the myocardium by lymphocytes, eosinophils, and histiocytes, with cell necrosis, may be occasionally caused by diverse drugs. Sudden death has been reported after serious adverse reactions to methyldopa, with histological findings characteristic of hypersensitivity myocarditis [19]. After severe allergic reactions to penicillin, sulfonamides and tetracycline, myocardial damage due to hypersensitivity myocarditis has also been occasionally reported [20]. Although most patients with hypersensitivity myocarditis are not critically ill, sudden death may occur, probably as consequence of a tachyarrhythmic episode.

The mechanisms of myocardial damage of anthracyclines have been extensively studied, since the number of cancer patients treated with anthracycline derivatives is enormous. Several biochemical alterations have been described that may lead to the pathogenesis of anthracycline-induced cardiomyopathy, including inhibition of nucleic acid and protein synthesis, release of vasoactive amine, alterations in adrenergic function, abnormalities in mitochondria, lysosomal changes, modifications of sarcolemmal calcium transport, attenuation of adenylate cyclase and adenosine triphosphatase (ATPase) activity, imbalance in myocardial electrolytes, formation of free radicals, lipid peroxidation, and depletion of non-protein tissue sulfhydryl groups [21, 22]. However, most of the studies support the view that an increase in oxidative stress, evidenced by an increase in free radicals and lipid peroxidation, as well as a decrease in antioxidants and sulfhydryl groups play predominant roles in the pathogenesis [21].

Increased oxidative stress produced by anthracyclines can be explained by their chemical structure, which is prone to the generation of free radicals. Adryamicin, for example, is a tetracyclic glycone to which an amino sugar is attached through a glycoside bond. The quinone ring, which is a part of the tetracycline moiety, undergoes redox cycling between quinone and semiquinone. During this process, the generated electrons are captured by oxidizing agents, including oxygen, which in turn initiates a chain reaction leading to the generation of free radical species. It is well known that an abundance of free oxygen radicals can lead to cardiomyocyte injury and cardiomyopathy [21]. Direct support for this concept of oxidative stress is provided by the detection of adriamycin-generated oxygen species by spin resonance spectroscopy of cytochrome P-450 reductase and xanthine oxidase have also been found to catalyse the reduction of the anthraquinone to a semiquinone free radical. Indirect support for the concept of oxidative stress is provided by studies that demonstrate an increase in tissue malondialdehyde, which is a product of lipid peroxidation [21]. Adriamycin has also been shown to counteract different antioxidant agents, thus contributing to net oxidative stress [21, 22].

## Clinical presentation and long-term sequelae of drug-induced myocardial damage

From a clinical standpoint, acute cardiotoxicity following

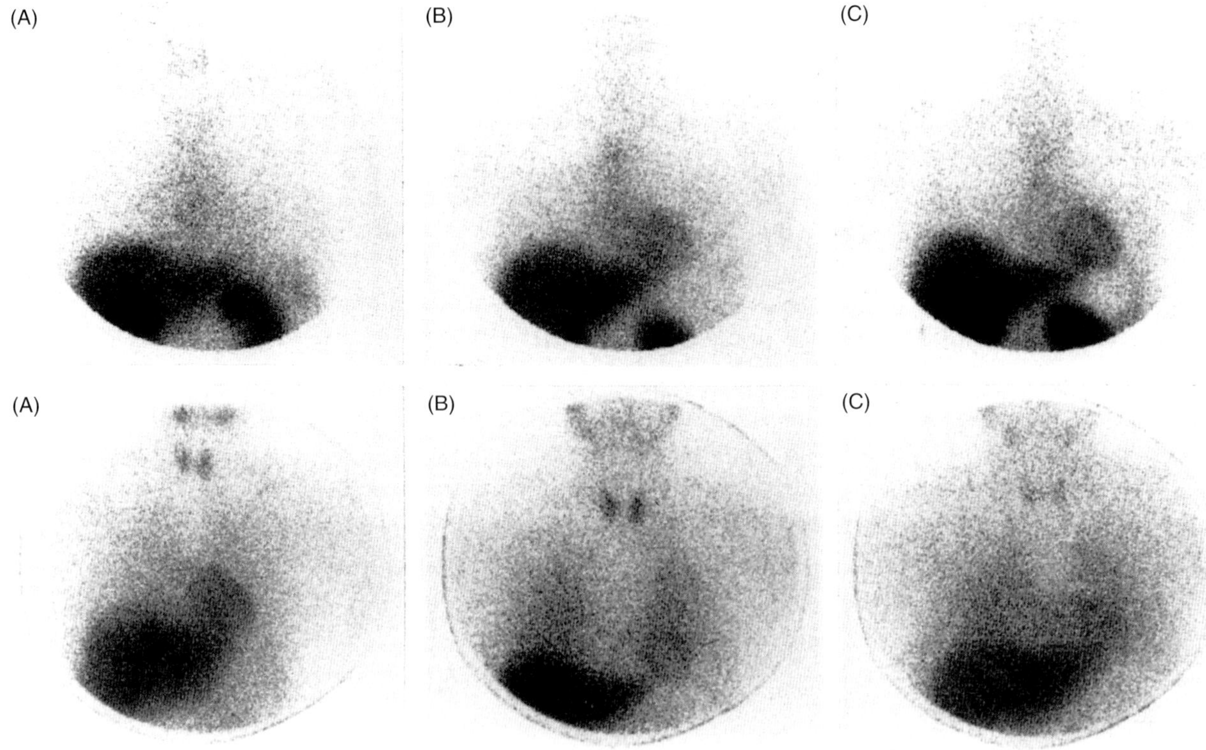


**Figure 28.1** *Serial images of a cancer patient treated with adriamycin, obtained at baseline (A), at intermediate cumulative doses (B), and at maximal doses of chemotherapy. Images obtained with antimyosin (top) show absent myocardial uptake at baseline with increasing uptake at intermediate and maximal doses, indicating progressive myocardial damage with cumulative adriamycin administration. Images obtained with MIBG (bottom) show normal uptake at baseline and a decrease in uptake at intermediate and maximal doses, indicating progressive adrenergic neuron function impairment with adryamicin administration. Using these radiotracers, abnormalities seen at intermediate doses usually precede functional deterioration.*

a single anthracycline dose appears distinctly different to the chronic cardiomyopathy that results from cumulative anthracycline dosage [23–25]. Acute toxicity is often subclinical, with acute and reversible electrocardiographic changes but without clinical evidence of myocardial dysfunction. This is observed in approximately 30% of patients within hours of adriamycin administration. In exceptional circumstances, acute cardiotoxicity develops after a single dose of adriamycin and presents as a pancarditis with overt biventricular failure. Important chronic anthracycline cardiotoxicity presents as congestive cardiomyopathy, which is characterized by a non-dilated, progressively low-output state that is unresponsive to cardiotonic agents.

Cardiotoxicity occurring well after chemotherapy had not been seriously considered until recent reports indicated an unexpectedly high incidence of late permanent cardiac functional abnormalities in cancer patients with prolonged survival [26, 27]. More than half of children with acute lymphoblastic leukaemia in whom complete clinical remission is induced by anthracycline chemotherapy have long-term abnormalities in contractility or ventricular wall thickness many years after completion of therapy [27]. Survivors of paediatric tumours constitute one of the largest new groups at risk for premature cardiovascular disease. The mechanisms of delayed anthracycline-associated cardiotoxicity are still unclear. Some reports suggest that anthracycline-induced inhibition of myocyte growth is the most likely aetiology. If this was the case, the myocardial insult should be age related, with maximal impact on very young patients. However, other studies have demonstrated a lack of correlation between age and late myocardial effects [27]. Furthermore, many patients who have late anthracycline-related myocardial dysfunction have more than one episode of CHF during follow-up, suggesting other mechanisms than the direct cardiac effect of the drug, such as additive myocardial damage of another origin or intercurrent viral illness. Prevention of late cardiotoxicity in long-term cancer survivors poses a new challenge to all medical professionals involved in the treatment of neoplastic diseases and its iatrogenic complications.

The traditionally accepted definition of anthracycline cardiotoxicity based on evolution of left ventricular systolic function has several drawbacks. Functional impairment is a consequence of myocardial cell damage caused by the administration of the cardiotoxic drug. Using an approach based on functional deterioration, cell damage below this threshold would not be considered as cardiotoxicity. In addition, alteration of various neurohumoral factors may also precede functional impairment and may constitute an important part of the spectrum of cardiotoxic effects of anthracycline administration [28]. Therefore, the definition of cardiotoxicity should be reviewed in the context of the natural history of the disease, and should relate to a better understanding of the myodegenerative and neurohumoral alterations that lead to the complex cardiomyopathy. Identification of the underlying pathogenetic tissular mechanisms at the subcellular level should lead to earlier diagnosis and facilitate prevention of the long-term deleterious effects of drug-induced cardiotoxicity. The most relevant clinical episodes of cardiotoxicity occur during antineoplastic treatment. Advances in chemotherapy prolong disease free intervals and overall survival, and contribute to improved cure rates. However, within the armamentarium of useful drug, in a continuously evolving field, anthracycline derivatives still play a major role. Despite advances in the search for less cardiotoxic analogues, cardiomyopathy remains the most serious toxic side-effect of anthracyclines, and limits their use in the treatment of lymphoma, leukaemia, and several solid tumours. Guidelines or recommendations for patient monitoring have been proposed with the hope of decreasing the incidence of acute and chronic cardiotoxicity. These guidelines should also result in a more meaningful evaluation of the cardiac effects of new chemotherapeutic agents and protocols. Continuing monitoring should facilitate earlier therapeutic intervention for cardiac decompensation, and therefore decrease the severity of clinical symptoms. Cardiac monitoring programmes should not, however, result in an excess of cancer-related deaths in an attempt to reduce cardiac deaths, i.e. cardiac risk reduction has to be weighed against a potential risk of inadequate antineoplastic effect.

Currently accepted guidelines [29] are as follows. Baseline left ventricular ejection fraction should be measured before administration of a dose of 100 mg/m$^2$ of adriamycin in all patients. Next, ejection fraction should be assessed at a dose of 300 mg/m$^2$ and again at 450 mg/m$^2$ if previous risk factors were present. A functional assessment should be undertaken before each subsequent dose. The chemotherapy should be discontinued if the ejection fraction decreases more than 10 points to an absolute value of less than 50%. Specific recommendations also exist for patients with abnormal baseline left ventricular ejection fraction, based on functional deterioration consequent to a high clinical likelihood of CHF.

Adherence to such surveillance regimens, based solely on functional assessment, has resulted in a significant reduction in the overall incidence of CHF [29]. In clinical practice, however, compliance with these guidelines is poor, mainly because unusual dedication is required on the part of the patient and referring physician. It is inconvenient and expensive for patients to undergo cardiac assessment and then chemotherapy at different hospitals and at different times. In consequence, many centres measure only a single left ventricular ejection fraction level at intermediate cumulative doses of chemotherapy to estimate the functional status and the patients ability to receive further chemotherapy.

From a clinical point of view, detection of the patients at risk of cardiomyopathy before ejection fraction deterioration is important, particularly since those patients could benefit from administration of alternative regimens that may avoid or delay functional impairment. Despite individual variability in terms of cardiac sensitivity to anthracyclines, patients with responding tumours could benefit from extending the anthracycline cumulative doses. Bearing this in mind, the question is, do available methods of screening adequately predict early or late cadiac outcomes? Left ventricular ejection fraction measurements do not seem to be sensitive enough to detect patients at risk of significant cardiotoxicity at an early stage of chemotherapy administration [30]. This is in keeping with the concept that a certain critical mass of cell damage is needed before functional impairment can be detected by existing conventional methods. Most studies take the prevention of CHF as the cardiac endpoint; however, taking into account the real incidence of CHF during chemotherapy with current protocols, this may not be a satisfactory endpoint. With increasing survival rates, late cardiotoxicity is becoming a more common clinical problem and it is important to find an endpoint that is more likely to predict the development of CHF at a later date [31–35]. Lipshultz *et al.* [31] showed that 65% of anthracycline-treated long-term survivors of childhood cancer have permanent functional cardiac abnormalities that may be progressive and result in late CHF. Late deterioration, probably due to myocyte degeneration with subsequent fibrosis, can be seen in patients with overt heart failure during chemotherapy but also in patients who had no cardiac symptoms acutely related to the chemotherapy. Prevention of these late effects may be crucial to improving the quality of life of long-term survivors.

Surveillance techniques should provide early identification of patients at risk of significant cardiotoxicity during chemotherapy, when changes in the schedule of administration can still be instituted or cardioprotective drugs be simultaneously administered. Such surveillance techniques should also help to reduce the incidence of long-term undersirable effects in patients with favourable outcomes.

## Assessment of drug-induced myocardial damage

Radionuclide ventriculography with serial resting left ventricular ejection fraction measurements is recognized as the best evaluated, most accurate, and most predictive method of assessing cardiac performance during chemotherapy. The strength of the method lies in its high reproducibility, since ejection fraction measurements can be performed with minimal intraobserver and interobserver variability. The weakness of the method is its limited sensitivity in detecting myocardial damage at an early stage. Assessment of diastolic function with radionuclide ventriculography, although advocated by some investigators as a more sensitive technique [36], has not gained general acceptance, mainly because of lesser reproducibility. The measurement of left ventricular ejection fraction during exercise [37] is not practical in cancer patients and may not be specific for cardiotoxicity. The measurements of resting left ventricular ejection fraction should be sufficiently later than the preceding drug dose to avoid transient effects of the drug as well as the false hypercontractility from the catecholamine release that follows acute administration of anthracyclines. Ejection fraction measurements should be scheduled 3 weeks after the last dose and 1 week before the next dose, with the patient normothermic and with a haemoglobin level at or above 9 g/dl.

Although left ventricular ejection fraction at rest is used by most oncologists to guide anthracycline therapy, several reports have shown that it may correlate poorly with endomyocardial biopsy grades, suggesting its limited sensitivity for assessing early myocardial damage [2, 3, 27]. All functional tests detect acute changes in ventricular function during chemotherapy; however, functional parameters depend on the loading state of the normal working ventricle and are affected by many factors including fever, peripheral vasodilation, reduced afterload, anaemia, sepsis, and renal failure [31]. With reduced afterload an abnormal ventricle can exhibit a normal ejection fraction, while with increased afterload even a normal ventricle may have low ejection fraction or impaired functional parameters. During intense chemotherapy, abnormal haemodynamics are common in cancer patients, limiting the sensitivity and specificity of functional assessment. Therefore, surveillance protocols should distinguish between these often confounding factor. For example, a progressive decrease in contractility over several consecutive tests would be more suggestive of cardiotoxicity, whereas a sudden change in one test from several stable normal values would be more likely to be due to other factors.

Serial echocardiography has been proposed as an alternative method for monitoring cardiotoxicity, especially in paediatric patients [38]. The technique is limited by variations in thoracic anatomy, such as emphysema, obesity, large breasts, tight intercostal spaces, and heavily calcified ribs, which may limit the availability of satisfactory acoustic windows. In addition, left ventricular ejection fractions measured by echocardiography are less reproducible than those obtained with radionuclide ventriculography. Although ultrasonic tissue characterization of anthracycline-induced myocardial damage is under active investigation, echocardiographic assessment of ventricular function through measurements of fractional shortening, isovolumetric relaxation time, and end-systolic wall stress is currently used to detect cardiomyopathy [39, 40]. As with radionuclide ventriculography, echocardiography cannot detect damage before haemodynamic deterioration, and frequent measurements must be obtained to identify consistent change in cardiac parameters anteceding clinically significant deterioration.

The ability of nuclear medicine to offer molecular insights may result in a better understanding of the pathophysiology of cardiotoxicity, improvement in early detection, and facilitation of better patient outcomes. For instance, $^{111}$In-antimyosin antibody studies allow *in vivo* non-invasive detection of myocardial damage. Binding of this antibody to intracellular myosin takes place only when sarcolemmal disruption occurs and the cell is irreversibly damaged. It has been shown that the morphological damage in the myocytes present in anthracycline cardiotoxicity can be detected by antimyosin scans, and that the intensity of the antibody uptake can be assessed by means of a heart-to-lung ratio [41]. In patients studied immediately after chemotherapy, antimyosin uptake is almost invariably seen, and is related to the severity of myocardial damage and the functional status of the patients after chemotherapy [41]. Sequential studies performed in individual patients demonstrate that antimyosin uptake relates to the cumulative dose of anthracyclines during chemotherapy [42]. Mild to moderate degrees of antibody uptake are seen at low or intermediate doses in patients who had normal baseline studies, while more intense antibody uptake is seen at higher cumulative doses. These studies also demonstrate that antimyosin uptake always precedes ejection fraction deterioration [41–43], and that those patients with intense antibody uptake at intermediate doses are those who are at risk of significant functional impairment at higher cumulative doses [43, 44]. Because of the higher sensitivity of antimyosin antibody studies, this technique has proven useful to compare cardiotoxicity of different anthracycline derivatives at therapeutic doses [42].

The sentitivity of antimyosin scans to detect myocardial cell damage and their ability to assess the time-course of such damage are well documented. It has been shown in several clinical conditions that the degree of antimyosin uptake relates to the extent and severity of myocyte damege, and that it can be reliably quantified in terms of the heart-to-lung ratio. The level of this ratio can be equated with the degree of myocardial damage, as shown in other types of diffuse myocardial disease such as heart transplant rejection or myocarditis, as well as anthracycline cardiotoxicity. The small dimensions of antimyosin Fab ($35 \times 65$ Å) allow it to enter the membrane gaps created by compliment membrane attack complexes or by inflammatory reactions [45]. This disruption of sarcolemmal continuity may subsequently result in myocyte necrosis [46]. Studies performed in patients without previous risk factors [41–44] have demonstrated conclusively that when a critical degree of myocardial cell damage is reached, as shown by a high heart-to-lung uptake ratio in antimyosin studies, a significant decrease in ejection fraction and symptoms of overt heart failure are more likely to occur with additional anthracycline administration.

Study of the uptake of radiolabelled Metaiodobenzylguanidine (MIBG) provides another useful method for assessing anthracycline cardiotoxicity. MIBG behaves similarly to noradrenaline and is taken up by myocardial sympathetic nerves. Several studies have shown that variations in myocardial MIBG uptake accurately reflect changes in myocardial adrenergic neuron integrity and function, and have been proposed to assess impairment of adrenergic innervation due to anthracycline cardiotoxicity. Decreased myocardial MIBG uptake has been observed in adriamycin-treated rats with limited morphological damage, such as vacuolar degeneration of the myocytes [47, 48]. In these animal studies, decreased myocardial MIBG uptake preceded ejection fraction deterioration. Valdés-Olmos *et al.* [49, 50] reported decreased myocardial MIBG uptake in patients with severely impaired ejection fraction after doxorubicin administration. Correlation with parameters derived from radionuclide angiocardiography suggested a global process of myocardial adrenergic derangement. Wakasugi *et al.* [48] demonstrated reduced myocardial tissue-bound noradrenaline and MIBG in adriamycin-treated rats. In that study, MIBG uptake revealed a dose-dependent decline which was probably due to either excessive compensatory byperadrenergic washout from the myocardium or direct adrenergic neuron damage. Hyperadrenergic washout seemed unlikely since myocardial noradrenaline did not decline as plasma noradrenaline levels increased with increasing dose, suggesting specific adrenergic neuron toxicity rather than a non-specific response to an impairment in ventricular function.

In a study comparing [$^{111}$In]antimyosin and MIBG in the assessment of anthracycline cardiotoxicity [51], some decrease in myocardial MIBG uptake was reported regardless of the functional status, suggesting a specific effect. Progressive myocyte necrosis during doxorubicin cardiotoxicity is associated with cardiac neuroadrenergic tissue necrosis. The clinical course of doxorubicin cardiotoxicity suggests altered neuroendocrine physiology [28]. This is supported by the observation of a decrease in β-adrenergic responsiveness and decreased myocardial cathecolamine stores with increased plasma catecholamines. In the same study [51], the decrease in myocardial MIBG accumulation paralleled the evolution of ejection fraction. At intermediate cumulative doses of

240–300 mg/m$^2$, 25% of patients presented with a mild reduction in MIBG uptake. At maximal cumulative doses, there was a significant decrease in MIBG uptake, consistent with impaired cardiac adrenergic activity. A direct relationship between a greater decrease in myocardial MIBG uptake and more severe functional impairment could not be obtained in this limited series of patients, although moderate to marked decreases in myocardial MIBG uptake at high cumulative doses were observed in all but one patient, with an absolute decrease in ejection fraction of more than 10%.

Perfusion agents have also been explored as potential tools for assessing anthracycline cardiotoxicity. Miyagawa *et al.* [52] showed decreased thallium washout rates from the myocardium of doxorubicin-treated rats. Piwnica-Worms *et al.* [53] observed altered mitochondrial energetics in cultured myocytes treated with adriamycin using *technetium-99m* ($^{99m}$*Tc)-Sestamibi*. These observations have not yet led to clinical studies. Takeishi *et al.* [54] used $^{123}$I-BMIPP for the identification of anthracycline cardiotoxicity. Metabolic changes in the myocardium as assessed by labelled fatty acids may also provide further insight into the mechanisms of cardiotoxicity. Particular attention should be paid in the future to the role of new drugs in combined chemotherapy; for example, it has been shown that paclitaxel may enhance the cardiotoxic effects of adriamycin by causing a significant delay in elimination [55].

It is difficult to anticipate how the early detection of cardiotoxicity with new non-invasive methods may influence management strategies in the future. The ideal test for monitoring drug cardiotoxicity should be non-injurious, inexpensive, and able to distinguish patients at risk of developing significant cardiotoxicity with higher doses from those at low risk. The test should not be too demanding in terms of hospital visits at different times to those for chemotherapy. Guidelines and recommendations to implement monitoring of cardiotoxicity should not be adopted as a mandatory format. Especially for new investigational agents, individual chemotherapy protocols will continue to redefine whether and how cardiac monitoring should be performed for that particular protocol. Mandatory guidelines that are demanding and difficult to follow add anxiety and cost to patients and their families. Although serial resting left ventricular ejection fraction measurements may remain the method of choice to monitor cardiotoxicity, it is possible that by using a more sensitive test, anthracycline administration could be individually tailored to meet specific clinical needs. A complementary approach of functional assessment, together with assessment of myocardial damage with antimyosin studies or of adrenergic innervation status with MIBG examinations, could be helpful for management of patients with previous risk factors or patients who are potential candidates for future repeat anthracycline administration. Early detection of cardiotoxicity in these circumstances could prompt changes in the schedule of administration or indicate the need for specific cardioprotection to prevent late undesirable cardiac effects of the chemotherapy.

There are no data on the value of assessing myocardial damage or myocardial innervation in other types of drug-induced cardiotoxicity, but it is reasonable to think that some of the concepts demonstrated in anthracycline cardiotoxicity can be similarly applied to other types of iatrogenic myocardial damage.

## Modulation of therapeutic regimens and cardioprotection for improvement of outcomes

If patients at risk of developing significant cardiotoxicity are detected at an early stage during drug administration, therapeutic regimens could be individually adjusted to prevent functional impairment. For example, anthracyclines are usually administered at 50–75 mg/m$^2$ with bolus injection at 3 week intervals, alone or combined with other chemotherapy. Using this approach, the incidence of clinically relevant cardiotoxicity is related to the cumulative dose: below a threshold of 550 mg/m$^2$ the incidence is less than 10%, while the incidence of CHF increases along a continuum above this dose threshold [29]. These observations led to the use of a maximum fixed dose of approximately 550 mg/m$^2$ in many protocols [56]. Alternative approaches include continuous infusion instead of bolus injection or the use of cardioprotective agents [57–60]. Since cardiotoxicity depends on peak plasma levels, continuous infusion may be less cardiotoxic than conventional bolus injection. Antimyosin studies performed in patients treated with continuous infusion techniques have shown less intense myocardial antimyosin uptake than patients treated with bolus administration, clearly indicating less severe cardiotoxicity [43]. In addition, continuous infusion regimens have demonstrated tumoricidal effects similar to those of bolus administration of anthracyclines [57]. However, the use of infusion pumps over 72 h is associated with problems at the site of injection, i.e., it may have the risk of infection, and cannot be used as the standard administration technique in all patients [58, 59]. Pharmacological cardioprotection with antioxidants or chelating agents also cannot be implemented as a routine and proper candidates should be carefully selected. The cost associated with these alternatives makes their widespread use impossible, indicating the need for proper selection of candidates.

The type of chemotherapeutic protocol is also important. In general, anthracyclines are given as adjuvant chemotherapy and as palliative chemotherapy for advanced disease. A total cumulative dose of doxorubicin over 360 mg/m$^2$ is seldom used in adjuvant chemotherapy [60]. A decrease in left ventricular ejection fraction by more than 10% with this cumulative dose is probably irrelevant. In this context, cardiotoxicity would be a major concern only if late undesirable effects can be caused by such limited doses. In the setting of palliative chemotherapy for advanced disease, higher doses of doxorubicin are administered, with an overall incidence of significant cardiotoxicity up to 20%. However, when dealing with a life-threatening disease with sometimes limited survival rates, cardiotoxicity may be of minor concern. In addition, if the reduction in anthracycline dose increases the death rate from cancer more than it decreases the morbidity and mortality from heart failure, more harm than good would be done by implementing such a reduction.

Cessation of the administration of anthracyclines at a fixed cumulative dose is a commonly practised approach that has important clinical implications which cannot be overlooked. Several studies have suggested that those patients in remission at doses of 450–550 mg/m$^2$ could have their remission time prolonged with additional administration of anthracyclines. Patients who can tolerate higher cumulative doses may benefit from additional anthracycline administration in terms of tumoricidal effect or duration of clinical response [56].

The use of cardioprotective drugs, such as antioxidants or chelating agents, has also been extensively investigated. One of the first antioxidants tested against adriamycin cardiomyopathy was vitamin E, with very encouraging initial findings. A bolus injection of vitamin E 24 h before adriamycin injection prevented the development of typical ultrastructural cardiomyopathic changes in mice [61]. However, in subsequent years, several conflicting reports appeared with respect to the efficacy of antioxidants, such as vitamin E, in mitigating the process of anthracycline cardiomyopathy. These differences may have been due to the experimental model as well as the type and dose of antioxidant used.

Subsequent studies suggested that vitamin E was cardioprotective only against the acute cardiotoxicity of adriamycin, whereas it offered limited protection against the development of chronic cardiomyopathy. The most attention has been aroused by the iron-chelating agent D-razoxane (ICRF-187). In an animal model, pretreatment with this compound significantly reduced the appearance of anthracycline cardiotoxicity, supporting the pathogenic role of oxidative stress in the development of cardiomyopathy [62]. This combination therapy was also introduced into clinical practice [63]. The mechanism by which the heart is protected by D-razoxane is not completely understood. It is possible that, being a strong iron chelator, this compound may prevent the generation of oxidative metabolites by the doxorubicin iron complex and may inhibit intracardiac peroxidative damage. Several prospective randomized, controlled clinical trials involving patients with cancer of the breast and lung, and paediatric soft-tissue sarcomas, have shown unequivocal evidence of substantial cardioprotection to several anthracyclines [64]. Adequate and effective cardioprotection is specially important in childhood malignancies where prevention of acute cardiac toxicity induced by anthracyclines should translate into prevention of chronic cardiac toxicity. A test capable of selecting patients ar risk of significant cardiotoxicity would help to pinpoint those who could most benefit from cardioprotection during anthracycline administration.

Probucol was introduced as a lipid-lowering drug. Its use subsequently declined because of an unfavourable effect on the plasma lipid profile, as demonstrated by a decrease in high-density lipoprotein levels. The chemical structure of probucol resembles vitamin E in that it has two phenolic groups, and very soon its strong antioxidant properties became evident. The beneficial effects of probucol against adriamycin-induced cardiomyopathy were tested in an animal model by Singal and co-workers [65]. When an optimal dose of probucol was used, adriamycin-induced cardiomyopathy was completly prevented. In addition, probucol did not affect the antitumour properties of adriamycin. Another important finding was that probucol alone as well as in combination with adriamycin caused an increase in endogenous antioxidant enzyme activities in the heart, making it an ideal agent for enhancing antioxidant defence in the membrane and cytosol compartment [65]. Clinical studies to assess the usefulness of probucol administered in conjunction with anthracycline chemotherapy should confirm these findings.

Most patients would accept some impairment of cardiac function if the potential for oncological cure would improve; minor functional abnormalities might represent an acceptable outcome, whereas disabling symptoms would not [18]. The potential cardiotoxicity that may detract from the future quality of life should be a concern in young patients with curable disease, while antitumoural effects might be the first priority in patients with advanced disease or aged patients under palliative therapy. Most patients wonder about the reversibility of undesirable effects. Eventual recovery of cardiac function in patients with anthracycline cardiotoxicity has been described [66]. The mechanism for eventual recovery is speculative but observations suggest the possibility of intrinsic healing of the damaged myocardium. Spontaneous reversal of myocardial dysfunction is also sometimes observed in myocarditis, peripartum cardiomyopathy, and alcoholic cardiomyopathy. Identification of variables predictive of spontaneous recovery and more favourable outcome, as well as determination of the role of intercurrent illness, would be clinically useful for the stratification and prognosis of the patients [67–70].

## Conclusions

The administration of a variety of drugs may result in myocardial damage. Among these, antineoplastic drugs used for management of non-cardiac diseases have been extensively studied. The most frequently observed mechanisms of myocardial damage induced by antineoplastic drugs are reactive oxygen flux and free radical-mediated cell damage. The clinical presentation of drug-induced myocardial damage involves a large spectrum of signs and symptoms, from acute, transient, and reversible changes, to chronic congestive cardiomyopathy or long-term functional subclinical abnormalities. The management of patients treated with potentially cardiotoxic drugs should include the prevention of acute toxic effects as well as undesirable long-term sequelae that adversely affect the quality of life. Functional tests used to monitor cardiotoxicity may not suffice for effective management. The lack of sensitivity of functional assessment in detecting early damage may be compensated by using tests to detect myocardial damage when changes in the administration regimens of the drug can still be implemented.

Early detection of cell damage or assessment of adrenergic neuron function may improve anthracine cardiotoxicity rather than by merely detecting and correcting haemodynamic abnormalities. The use of new agents to assess cardiotoxicity should provide a better understanding of the natural history of the disease, which could be followed by advances in the treatment of CHF and overall therapeutic success.

## References


1. Alexander J, Dainiak N, Berger HJ *et al.* Serial assessment of doxorubicin cardiotoxicity with quantitative radionuclide angiocardiography. *N Engl J Med* 1979; 300: 278–83.
2. Dardir MH, Ferrans VJ, Mikhael SY *et al.* Cardiac morphologic and functional changes induced by epirubicin chemotherapy. *J Clin Oncol* 1989; 7: 947–58.
3. Druck MM, Gulenchyn KY, Evans WK *et al.* Radionuclide angiography and endomyocardial biopsy in the assessment of doxorubicin cardiotoxicity. *Cancer* 1984; 53: 1667–74.
4. Rajagopalan S, Politi PM, Sinha BK, Myers CE. Adriamycin-induced free radical formation in the perfused rat heart: implications for cardiotoxicity.
5. Cazin B, Gorin NC, Laporte P *et al.* Cardiac complications after bone marrow transplantation. A report on a series of 63 consecutive transplantations. *Cancer* 1986; 57: 2061–5.
6. Martin M, Diaz Rubio E, Furio V *et al.* Lethal cardiac toxicity after cisplatin and 5-fluorouracil chemotherapy. Report of a case with a necropsy study. *Am J Clin Oncol* 1989; 12: 229–31.
7. Rowinsky EK, Eisenhauer EA, Chaudry V *et al.* Clinical toxicities encountered with paclixatel. *Sem Oncol* 1993; 20: 1–8. *Cancer Res* 1988; 48: 4766–9.
8. Deyton LR, Walker RE, Kovacs JA *et al.* Reversible cardiac dysfunction associated with interferon alfa therapy in AIDS patients with Kaposi's sarcoma. *N Engl J Med* 1989; 321: 1246–8.
9. Schutker LM, Hendricks CB, Holland KH *et al.* Eosinophilic myocarditis associated with high dose interleukin-2 therapy. *Am J Med* 1990; 88: 439–42.
10. Glassman AH, Roose SP, Bigger JT *et al.* The safety of tricyclic antidepressants in cardiac patients. *JAMA* 1993; 269: 2673–5.
11. Martí V, Ballester M, Udina C *et al.* Evaluation of myocardial cell damage by In-111-monoclonal antimyosin antibodies is patients under chronic tricyclic antidepressant drugs. *Circulation* 1995; 91: 1619–23.
12. Rael CL, Patel AK, LeRoy M. Drug induced torsade de pointes. *Clin Pharmac* 1985; 4: 675–80.
13. Brady HR, Horgan JH. Lithium and the heart: unanswered questions. *Chest* 1988; 93: 166–7.
14. Khan MI, Haider B, Thind IS. Emetine-induced cardiomyopathy in rabbits. *J Submicrosc Cytol Pathol* 1983; 8: 308–10.
15. Iglesias Cubero G, Rodriguez Reguero J, Royo Ortega JM. Restrictive cardiomyopathy caused by chloroquine. *Br Heart J* 1993; 69: 451–4.

16. Jiang JP, Downing SE. Catecholamine cardiomyopathy: review and analysis of pathogenetic mechanisms. *Yale J Biol Med* 1990; 581–6.
17. Raper R, Fischer M, Bihari D. Profound, reversible, myocardial depression in acute asthma treated with high dose catecholamines. *Crit Care Med* 1992; 20: 710–13.
18. Frustaci A, Loperfido F, Gentiloni N *et al.* Catecholamine induced cardiomyopathy in multiple endocrine neoplasia. *Chest* 1991; 99: 382–8.
19. Gravanis MB, Hertzler GL, Franch RH *et al.* Hypersensitivity myocarditis in heart transplant recipients. *J Heart Lung Transplant* 1991; 10: 688–90.
20. Burke AP, Saenger J, Mullik F, Virmani R. Hypersensitivity myocarditis. *Arch Pathol Lab Med* 1991; 115: 764–80.
21. Singal P, Iliskovic N, Li T, Kumar D. Adiamycin cardiomyopathy: pathophysiology and prevention. *FASEB J* 1997; 11: 931–6.
22. Monti E, Prosperi E, Supino R, Bottiroli G. Free radical-dependent DNA lesions are involved in the delayed cardiotoxicity induced by adriamycin in the rat. *Anticancer Res* 1995; 15: 193–7.
23. Lee BH, Goodenday LS, Muswick GJ *et al.* Alterations in left ventricular diastolic function with doxorubicin therapy. *J Am Coll Cardiol* 1987; 9: 184–8.
24. Mortensen SA, Olsen HS, Baandrup U. Chronic anthracycline cardiotoxicity: hemodynamic and histopathological manifestations suggesting a restrictive endomyocardial disease. *Br Heart J* 1986; 55: 274–82.
25. Severs NJ, Twist VW, Powell T. Acute effects of adriamycin on the macromolecular organization of the cardiac muscle cell plasma membrane. *Cardioscience* 1991; 2: 35–45.
26. Lipshultz SE, Colan SD, Gelber RD *et al.* Late cardiac effects of doxorubicin therapy for acute lymphoblastic leukaemia in childhood. *N Engl J Med* 1991; 324: 808–15.
27. Steinherz LJ, Steinherz PG, Tan C. Cardiac failure and dysrhythmias 6–19 years after anthracycline therapy: a series of 15 patients. *Med Pediatr Oncol* 1995; 24: 352–61.
28. Strashun A. Adriamycin, congestive cardiomyopathy, and metaiodobenzylguanidine (Editorial). *J Nucl Med* 1992; 33: 215–22.
29. Schwartz RG, Mckenzie MB, Alexander J *et al.* Congestive heart failure and left ventricular dysfunction complicating doxorubicin therapy. *Am J Med* 1987; 82: 1109–18.
30. Ewer MS, Ali MK, Mackey B *et al.* A comparison of cardiac biopsy grades and ejection fraction estimations in patients receiving adryamicin. *J Clin Oncol* 1984; 2: 112–17.
31. Lipshultz SE, Sanders SP, Goorin AM *et al.* Monitoring for anthracycline cardiotoxicity. *Pediatrics* 1994; 93: 433–7.
32. Blatt J, DeLaat C, Fricker FJ, Janosky JE. Pilot study of cardiac function after treatment of childhood Wilms' tumor with doxorubicin. *Pediatr Hematol Oncol* 1995; 12: 61–6.
33. Mameghan H, Fischer RJ, O'Gorman-Hughes D *et al.* Ewing's sarcoma: long term follow up in 49 patients treated from 1967 to 1989. *Int J Radiat Oncol Biol Phys* 1993; 25: 431–8.
34. Nakada S, Ogawa S, Hirayama T. Noninvasive evaluation of chronic cumulative and acute cardiotoxicity induced by anthracycline in children with acute leukemia. Assessment of mainly left ventricular contractile state by M mode echocardiography. *Nippon Ika Daigaku Zasshi* 1994; 61: 209–19.
35. Aviles A, Arevila N, Diaz Maqueo JC *et al.* Late cardiac toxicity of doxorubicin, epirubicin and mitoxantrone therapy for Hodgkin's disease in adults. *Leik Lymphoma* 1993; 11: 275–9.
36. Ganz WI, Sridar KS, Forness TJ. Detection of early anthracycline cardiotoxicity by monitoring the peak filling rate. *Am J Clin Oncol* 1993; 16: 109–12.
37. Palmeri ST, Bonow RO, Myers CE *et al.* Prospective evaluation of doxorubicin by rest and exercise radionuclide angiography. *Am J Cardiol* 1986; 58: 607–13.
38. Steinherz LJ, Graham T, Hurwitz R *et al.* Guidelines for cardiac monitoring of children during and after anthracycline therapy: report of the Cardiology Committee of the Children's Cancer Study Group. *Pediatrics* 1992; 89: 942–9.
39. Stoddard MF, Seeger J, Liddell NE *et al.* Prolongation of isovolumetric relaxation time as assessed by Doppler echocardiography predicts doxorubicin-induced systolic dysfunction in humans. *J Am Coll Cardiol* 1992; 20: 62–9.
40. Cittadini A, Fazio S, D'Ascia C *et al.* Subclinical cardiotoxicity by doxorubicin: a pulsed Doppler echocardiographic study. *Eur Heart J* 1991; 12: 1000–5.
41. Estorch M, Carrió I, Berná L *et al.* Indium-111-antimyosin scintigraphy after doxorubicin therapy in patients with advanced breast cancer. *J Nucl Med* 1990; 12: 1965–70.
42. Carrió I, Estorch M, Berná L *et al.* Assessment of anthracycline-induced myocardial damage by quantitative indium-111 myosin-specific monoclonal antibody studies. *Eur J Nucl Med* 1991; 18: 806–12.
43. Carrió I, Lopez-Pousa A, Estorch M *et al.* Detection of doxorubicin cardiotoxicity in patients with sarcomas by indium-111-antimyosin monoclonal antibody studies. *J Nucl Med* 1993; 34: 1503–7.
44. Valdés-Olmos R, Ten Bokkel Huinink WW, Ten Hoeve RF *et al.* Usefulness of indium-111 antimyosin scintigraphy in confirming myocardial injury in patients with anthracycline-associated left ventricular dysfunction. *Ann Oncol* 1994; 5: 617–27.
45. Narula J, Strauss HW, Khaw BA. Antimyosin positivity in doxorubicin cardiotoxicity: earlier than the conventional evidence. *J Nucl Med* 1993; 9: 1507–9.
46. Praet M, Ruysschaert JM. *In-vivo* and *in-vitro* mitochondrial membrane damages induced in mice by adriamycin and derivatives. *Biochim Biophys Acta* 1993; 1149: 79–85.
47. Wakasugi S, Wada A, Hasegawa Y *et al.* Detection of abnormal cardiac adrenergic neuron activity in adriamycin-induced cardiomyopathy with iodine-125-metaiodobenzylguanidine. *J Nucl Med* 1992; 33: 208–14.
48. Wakasugi S, Fischman AJ, Babich JW *et al.* Metaiodobenzylguanidine: evaluation of its potential as a tracer for monitoring doxorubicin cardiomyopathy. *J Nucl Med* 1993; 34: 1282–6.
49. Valdés-Olmos RA, ten Bokkel Huinink WW, Greve JC *et al.* I-123 MIBG and serial radionuclide angiocardiography in doxorubicin-related cardiotoxicity. *Clin Nucl Med* 1992; 17: 163–7.
50. Valdés Olmos RA, ten Bokkel Huinink WW, ten Hoeve RF *et al.* Assessment of anthracycline-related myocardial adrenetgic derangement by 123I-MIBG scintigraphy. *Eur J Cancer* 1995; 31A: 26–31.
51. Carrió I, Estorch M, Berná Ll *et al.* $^{111}$In-antimyosin and $^{123}$I-MIBG studies in the early assessment of doxorubicin cardiotoxicity. *J Nucl Med* 1995 (in press).
52. Miyagawa M, Tanada S, Hamamoto K. Scintigraphic evaluation of myocardial uptake of thallium 201 and technetium 99m pyrophosphate utilizing a rat model of chronic doxorubicin cardiotoxicity. *Eur J Nucl Med* 1991; 18: 332–8.
53. Piwnica-Worms D, Chiu ML, Kronauge JF. Detection of adriamycin-induced cardiotoxicity in cultured heart cells with technetium 99m-Sestamibi. *Cancer Chemother Pharmacol* 1993; 32: 385–91.

54. Takeishi Y, Sukekawa H, Sakurai T *et al.* Noninvasive identification of anthracycline cardiotoxicity: comparison of $^{123}$I-MIBG and $^{123}$I-BMIPP imaging. *Ann Nucl Med* 1994; 8: 177–82.
55. Gianni L, Munzone E, Capri G *et al.* Paclitaxel by 3-hour infusion in combination with bolus doxorubicin in women with untreated metastatic breast cancer. High antitumor efficacy and cardiac effects in a dose and sequence-finding study. *J Clin Oncol* 1995 (in press).
56. Van Hoff DD, Layard MW, Basa P *et al.* Risk factors for doxorubicin-induced congestive heart failure. *Ann Intern Med* 1979; 91: 710–17.
57. Speyer JL, Green MD, Kramer E *et al.* Protective effect of the bispiperazinedione ICRF-187 against doxorubicin induced cardiac toxicity in women with advanced breast cancer. *N Engl J Med* 1988; 319: 745–52.
58. Legha SS, Benjamin RS, Mackay B *et al.* Reduction of doxorubicin cardiotoxicity by prolonged continuous intravenous infusion. *Ann Intern Med* 1982; 96: 133–9.
59. Lokich J, Bothe A, Zipoli T *et al.* Constant infusion schedule for adryamicin: a phase I–II clinical trial of a 30 day schedule by ambulatory pump delivery system. *J Clin Oncol* 1983; 1: 24–8.
60. Bacci G, Picci P, Ferrari S *et al.* Influence of adriamycin dose in the outcome of patients with osteosarcoma treated with multidrug neoadjuvant chemotherapy: results of two sequential studies. *J Chemother* 1993; 5: 237–46.
61. Myers CE, McGuire WP, Liss RH *et al.* Adiamycin: the role of lipid peroxidation in cardiac toxicity and tumor response. *Science* 1977; 197: 165–7.
62. Nowak D, Pierscinski G, Drzewoski J. Ambroxol inhibits doxorubicin-induced lipid peroxidation in heart of mice. *Free Radical Biol Med* 1995; 19: 659–63.
63. Herman EH, Ferrans VJ. Reduction of chronic doxorubicin cardiotoxicity in dogs by pretreatment with (I)-1,2-bis(3,5-dioxopiperozinyl-1-yl) propane (ICRF-187). *Cancer Res* 1981; 41: 3436–40.
64. Hellmann K. Anthracycline cardiotoxicity prevention by dexrazoxane: breakthrough of a barrier — sharpens antitumor profile and therapeutic index. *J Clin Oncol* 1996; 2: 332–3.
65. Siveski-Iliskovic N, Hill M, Chow DA, Singal PK. Probucol protects against adriamycin cardiomyopathy without interfering with its antitumor effect. *Circulation* 1995; 91: 10–15.
66. Saini J, Rich MW, Lyss AP. Reversibility of severe left ventricular dysfunction due to doxorubicin cardiotoxicity. Report of three cases. *Ann Intern Med* 1987; 106: 814–16.
67. Gaudin PB, Hruban RH, Beschorner WE *et al.* Myocarditis associated with doxorubicin cardiotoxicity. *Am J Clin Pathol* 1993; 100: 158–63.
68. Ali MK, Ewer MS, Gibbs HR *et al.* Late doxorubicin-associated cardiotoxicity in children. The possible role of intercurrent viral infection. *Cancer* 1994; 74: 182–8.
69. Pihkala J, Saarinen UM, Lundstrom U *et al.* Effects of bone marrow transplantation on myocardial function in children. *Bone Marrow Transplant* 1994; 13: 149–55.
70. Nysom K, Holm K, Lipsitz R *et al.* Relationship between cumulative anthracycline dose and late cardiotoxicity in childhood acute lymphoblastic leukemia. *J Clin Oncol* 1998; 16: 545–50.

# SECTION IV

# Pathogenetic basis of management of cardiomyopathies

# Newer pharmacological options in myocardial diseases: reverse remodelling and retardation of inexorable decline in left ventricular function



E. J. EICHHORN

## Introduction

The concepts and paradigms of heart failure management have changed radically during the 1980s and 1990s. The treatment of chronic heart failure has shifted from pharmacological manipulation of haemodynamics to a strategy for protecting the heart from biological harm [1]. This shift in treatment has led to improvements in symptoms, function, and survival for these patients. However, despite medical advances for the treatment of congestive heart failure, including the use of angiotensin-converting enzyme (ACE) inhibitors, digitalis, and diuretics, the mortality for moderate to severe heart failure continues to be in excess of 20% per year for severely symptomatic patients and in excess of 10% per year for moderately symptomatic patients [2]. While cardiac transplantation provides a way to prolong the survival of patients in heart failure [3], the high cost, limited donor supply of hearts, and specialized and expensive follow-up care make this alternative possible for a very small minority of patients with heart failure. Thus, better prevention and improved medical care of patients with heart failure become critical.

Digitalis, diuretics, and ACE inhibitors play an important role in the long-term treatment of congestive heart failure. Aldosterone inhibitors have recently been shown to prolong survival in patients with advanced heart failure. β-Blockers clearly improve ventricular function and symptoms in patients with heart failure and prolong survival. Phosphodiesterase inhibitors and β-adrenergic agonists play a significant role in the acute treatment of heart failure, but may accelerate death if used chronically. On the horizon are newer agents which may benefit the biology of the myocyte and thus provide long-term benefit; however, clinical trials with these agents are lacking at this point in time.

## Pathophysiologic basis for pharmacological intervention in heart failure

In order to understand how best to treat chronic heart failure, it is imperative to understand the pathophysiology of the progression heart failure. Heart failure begins with an initial insult to ventricular function (Fig. 29.1) [1]. The most common aetiology for this is myocardial infarction or hypertension. Other causes include valvular heart disease, myocarditis, genetic causes, or an idiopathic aetiology. These insults result in left ventricular systolic and diastolic dysfunction leading to an increase in the load in the heart. An increase in preload results in atrial and ventricular stretch, activating several important neurohormonal systems [including angiotension II (AngII) [4, 5], cytokines [6], and atrial natriuretic factor [7]] which act in an autocrine/paracrine fashion. The reduced stroke volume resets baroreceptors, disinhibiting sympathetic discharge to the heart and peripheral tissues [8]. The renin–angiotensin system (RAS) and sympathetic nervous system (SNS) tend to cross-activate each other such that activation of one system tends to increase the activation of the other [9–11]. There may be concurrent activation of other potentially deleterious neurohormones such as endothelins [12, 13], vasopressin [14, 15], and cytokines, especially tumour necrosis factor (TNF)-α [6, 16].

In the short term, activation of the RAS and SNS provides inotropic and chronotropic support for the injured heart, and produces vasoconstriction and salt and water reabsorption [1, 17]. The vasoconstriction increases afterload and maintains blood pressure while the salt and water reabsorption results in an increase in preload, which increases the stroke volume by a Frank–Starling mechanism.

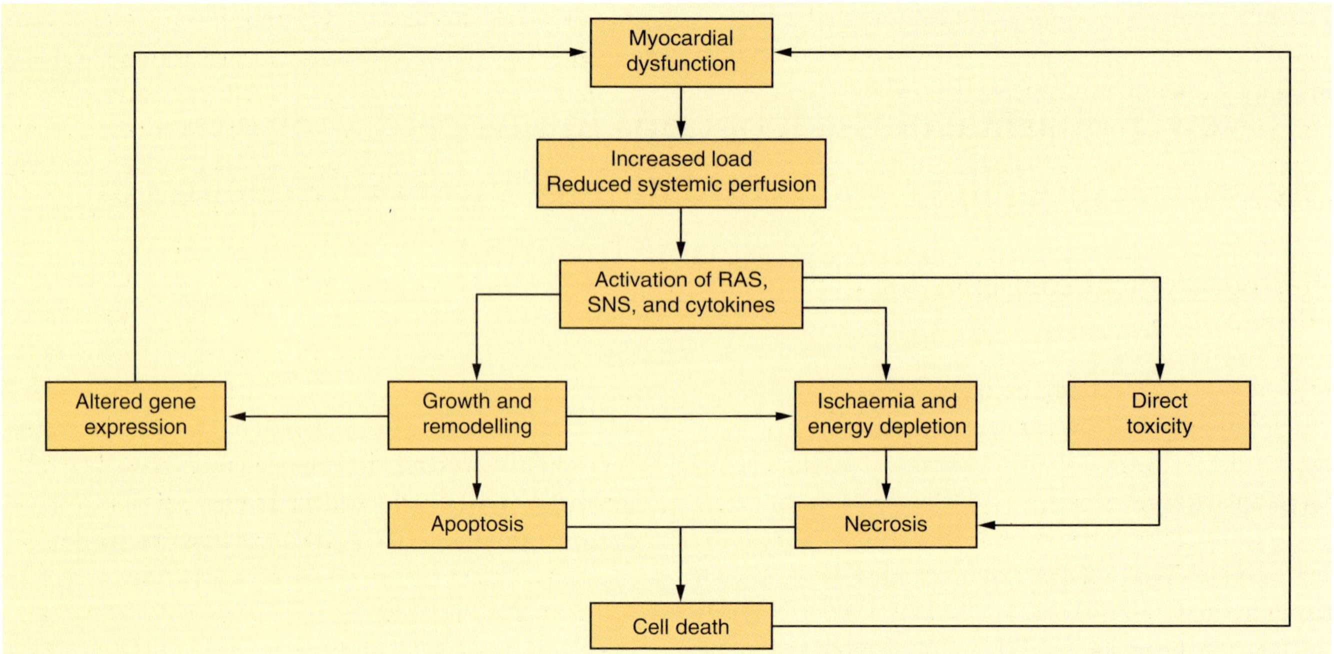


**Figure 29.1** *Pathophysiology of heart failure progression is depicted. Activation of neurohormones results in pathological growth of the ventricle leading to altered geometry and architecture, ischaemia and energy depletion, cell death by apoptosis and necrosis, and altered gene expression. This leads to a vicious cycle of more ventricular dysfunction and neurohormonal activation. Reprinted with permission of Americal Heart Association from reference 1.*

Over the long term, activation of these neurohormonal systems has a deleterious effect on the heart, invoking a pathological remodelling process that involves the myocytes as well as the interstitium [1, 18]. Noradrenaline [19, 20], angiotensin [4, 5 21], endothelins [22], and cytokines [23] are growth-promoting substances, both in myocytes and fibroblasts. Under the influence of these neurohormones, the heart, which is normally small and elliptical, becomes enlarged and spherical, with eccentric hypertrophy [24–26]. The shape changes because of myocyte elongation (as contractile units are laid down in series rather than in parallel) [27] and alterations in the interstitial network that maintains structural architecture [26, 28–30]. The enlarged ventricle is prone to increased (functional) mitral regurgitation [31] and elevated wall stress [24], which immediately lower ventricular performance. Subendocardial ischaemia may occur due to high wall stress and low coronary driving pressure (due to low stroke volume), leading to cell injury or stunning [32–34]. Cell injury leads to cell death and a vicious cycle of greater ventricular dysfunction is established (Fig. 29.1). These neurohormones may also be directly toxic to myocytes by causing calcium overload, increasing free radical formation, and energy depletion [35]. This leads to cell necrosis and further ventricular dysfunction. When these neurohormones activate growth pathways within the heart the adult myocyte is terminally differentiated and has limited ability to divide or form new myocytes [36], and will either grow pathologically or enter programmed cell death (apoptosis) [1, 37] Apoptosis leads to further ventricular dysfunction (Fig. 29.1). The pathological growth within the myocytes leads to a shift in isoforms, especially in contractile proteins such as myosin heavy chain [38]. The predominant isoform, $\alpha$-myosin heavy chain, is shifted to a less efficient, slower, more fetal-like $\beta$-isoform. This may lead to further contractile dysfunction. Thus, a vicious cycle is established leading to greater ventricular dysfunction and increased neurohormonal activation (Fig. 29.1).

Current strategies of the long-term treatment of heart failure are focused on antagonizing the neurohormonal and cytokine activation which lead to this progressive remodelling process. As the failing heart is haemodynamically dependent on neurohormonal activation to maintain circulation, neurohormonal antagonism requires slow withdrawal of this support to the heart. If these antagonists are administered too quickly, it can lead to haemodynamic deterioration in the form of hypotension, pulmonary oedema, and/or cardiogenic shock [39]. Indeed, this paradigm for the treatment of heart failure ignores short-term haemodynamic deterioration in favour of long-term biological improvement in chamber performance. This is in contrast with the view around the 1980s when drugs such as direct vasodilators or inotropic agents were used because they exhibited short-term haemodynamic improvement. At that time the long-term biological detrimental effects of these agents, which accelerated mortality in many cases, was not recognized.

## Pharmacological therapies for heart failure

### Angiotensin-converting enzyme inhibitors

ACE inhibitors work by antagonizing the conversion of angiotensin I to the vasoconstrictive and mitogenic AngII, and by inhibiting the breakdown of bradykinin, a substance which releases the growth inhibitory substance, nitric oxide. These effects result in vasodilatation and growth inhibition. As AngII produces a powerful growth signal in the heart [4, 5, 21], these agents inhibit the pathological growth process in myocytes and non-myocytes (fibroblasts) [28, 40–43]. ACE inhibitors retard pathological growth, which results in a slowing of ventricular dilatation and progressive increases in left ventricular mass in animal models [40–46] and humans who have chronic left ventricular dysfunction [47–49] or who have left ventricular dysfunction after myocardial infarction [50, 51].

#### *Effects on remodelling*

The Studies of Left Ventricular Dysfunction (SOLVD) study group examined the effects of enalapril on left ventricular volume and mass in patients with symptoms of mild to moderate heart failure and depressed left ventricular ejection fractions [47, 48]. Enalapril attenuated the progressive enlargement of end-diastolic and end-systolic volumes seen in the placebo group. Enalapril also attenuated the progressive increase in left ventricular mass, a surrogate marker of growth in the heart.

In both animal models of myocardial infarction and human clinical trials such as the Survival and Ventricular Enlargement (SAVE) trial, ACE inhibitors attenuated the progressive ventricular enlargement due to postmyocardial infarction remodelling [50–52]. Pfeffer, Mitchell, and associates [50, 53] showed that after an anterior wall myocardial infarction there is a progressive increase in end-diastolic and end-systolic volumes and an increase in the sphericity of the left ventricle between 3 weeks and 1 year. This change in geometry occurs at a time when infarct expansion has already occurred and thus represents ventricular remodelling. These late geometrical changes are prevented or retarded by ACE inhibitor therapy. In addition, those who receive an ACE inhibitor have reduced pulmonary capillary wedge pressure and better exercise tolerance. Sharpe *et al.* found a similar result in patients with inferior as well as anterior infarction [51].

The available data indicate that in patients with established dilated cardiomyopathies or with left ventricular (LV) dysfunction after myocardial infarction, administration of ACE inhibitors retards progression to increased LV mass and a more spherical shape, but do not actually regress hypertrophy or reverse the remodelling process [47–53]. Furthermore, there is no evidence from clinical investigations that ACE inhibitor therapy can lead to substantial improvement in intrinsic myocyte function. Although ACE inhibitors partially block the formation of AngII, thereby diminishing the effects of the RAS on the myocyte, and despite the fact that ACE inhibitors initially reduce adrenergic activity [10, 54], plasma noradrenaline increases over time and AngII escape (i.e. an increase in AngII formation via alternative pathways) increases [55–57]. These data suggest that progressive SNS and AngII activation occur even in the presence of ACE inhibitors and enforce the need for a concomitant, adjunctive, antineurohormonal strategy to block the long-term sequelae of noradrenaline and AngII on the heart. As the use of a β-blocking agent also results in further deactivation of the RAS, even in the presence of an ACE inhibitor [58], a combined strategy of ACE inhibitors and β-blockers makes intuitive sense.

#### *Clinical trials showing efficacy*

The short- and long-term effects of ACE inhibitors on haemodynamics were studied by the Captopril Multicenter Research Group [59]. Favourable acute haemodynamic effects included improved cardiac index, improved stroke work, reduction in systemic and pulmonary vascular resistance, and reductions in left and right heart filling pressures. After 8 weeks of therapy, repeat catheterization demonstrated sustained haemodynamic benefit based on the above parameters.

Both the Captopril–Digoxin Multicenter study [60] and the Captopril Multicenter Research Group [61] showed improvement in exercise tolerance and New York Heart Association (NYHA) functional class with ACE inhibitors compared to placebo. Thus, ACE inhibitors mildly improve the functional capacity of patients.

***Effect on survival***

In 1987, the CONSENSUS trial study group published their landmark trial of the effects of enalapril on mortality in 253 patients with severe heart failure (NYHA class IV) [62]. The addition of enalapril reduced mortality by 40% (from 44% to 26%) at 6 months.

In the National Institutes of Health (NIH)-sponsored SOLVD study, 6797 patients with an ejection fraction (EF) 0.35 were studied [63, 64]. During the 'treatment' trial, 2569 patients had mild to moderate symptoms of heart failure and were randomized to placebo ($n = 1284$) or enalapril ($n = 1285$) and followed for 41 months [63]. Enalapril treatment resulted in a 16% reduction in death [95% confidence interval (CI) = 5–26%, $p = 0.0036$], primarily due to a reduction in death from pump failure. In the 'prevention' trial, 4228 patients with no symptoms of heart failure but with an EF 0.35 were randomized to placebo ($n = 2117$) or enalapril ($n = 2111$) and followed for 37 months [64]. Despite a large number of cross-over patients from placebo to open-label ACE inhibitor (about 40%), enalapril resulted in a cardiovascular risk reduction of 12% (CI = −3 to 26%, $p = 0.12$) and a 20% reduction in hospitalization (95% CI = 9–30%, $p < 0.001$).

The recently completed ATLAS trial studied 3164 patients with NYHA class II–IV heart failure and LVEF ≤ 30% randomized to low dose (2.5–5.0 mg daily) or high dose (32.5–35.0 mg daily) lisinopril [65]. This study demonstrated an 8% reduction in the death rate which did not reach statistical significance ($p = 0.128$). However, the prespecified combination of death and hospitalization was reduced by 12% ($p = 0.002$). In addition, the high rate of open-label therapy and discontinuation of study drug may have precluded the study's ability to detect a mortality benefit from high-dose therapy. There is a some benefit from using higher doses of ACE inhibitors.

Echocardiographic and nuclear medicine substudies of the SOLVD patients examined the effect of enalapril on remodelling in the failing heart [47, 48]. Patients who received placebo had progressive enlargement of end-diastolic and end-systolic volumes and an increase in left ventricular mass. In contrast, patients who received enalapril had an attenuated effect on this remodelling process with no increase in volume or mass. These data suggest that ACE inhibitors prevent growth and progressive ventricular remodelling in patients with chronic heart failure, and this may translate into functional improvement and a mortality benefit.

In 1992, the SAVE investigators reported their findings of the effect of ACE inhibitors on mortality in 2231 post-myocardial infarction patients with an EF < 0.40 [52]. Patients were randomized 3–16 days after infarction to placebo ($n = 1116$) or captopril ($n = 1115$) and followed for 42 months. All-cause mortality was reduced in the captopril group by 19% (95% CI 3–32%, $p = 0.019$). In addition, captopril resulted in a 37% reduction in cardiovascular death ($p < 0.001$) and, as in the SOLVD trial, a 25% reduction in myocardial infarction ($p = 0.015$). Several other trials, similar to SAVE, using other ACE inhibitors, have been performed since then. These trials (AIRE [66], TRACE [67], and SMILE [68]) have all consistently shown a mortality reduction with ACE inhibitors. The data are overwhelming that patients with reduced LVEF should be placed on an ACE inhibitor.

***Adverse effects***

The most important side-effects of ACE inhibitors are: (1) hypotension on therapy initiation; (2) cough; (3) hyperkalaemia; (4) increased blood urea nitrogen (BUN) creatinine; and (5) angioedema [69]. The cough and angioedema appear to be mediated by the increase in bradykinin [69]. The increase in creatinine is due to the antagonism of efferent vasoconstriction in the glomerulus caused by inhibition of AngII formation (i.e. ACE inhibitors increase efferent vasodilation) [70, 71]. This causes a reduction in filtration pressure and leads to a decrease in filtration. This may be especially prominent in the presence of diuretics (which reduce preload, stroke volume, and renal perfusion) and non-steroidal anti-inflammatory drugs (NSAIDS, which promote afferent vasoconstriction in the glomerulus). In the presence of renal artery stenosis, this effect on BUN and creatinine may be especially prominent owing to poor renal perfusion. Angioedema is a rare side-effect of ACE inhibitors, but may be life-threatening if the ACE inhibitor is not stopped.

## Diuretics

Diuretics are the most commonly used drugs for the treatment of heart failure. They were first introduced into medical practice sometime after 1920 when the diuretic action of mercury was observed while treating patients with syphilis [72, 73]. Similar actions were noted with sulfonylureas, which led to the discovery of carbonic anhydrase inhibitors. In 1957, thiazide diuretics were discovered [74], and the loop diuretics came into being subsequently.

Diuretics act by preventing sodium reabsorption in the kidney and are defined by their site of action in the nephron [72]. The most common diuretics for use in heart failure are the loop diuretics (furosemide, bumetanide, torsemide, and ethacrynic acid). Other diuretics such as thiazide diuretics and potassium-sparing diuretics (spironolactone) are also used alone or in combination with loop diuretics. Diuretics are excellent at reducing preload, reducing fluid accumulation, and acutely improving dyspnoea [72].

*Clinical trials showing efficacy*

Since diuretics are so good at relieving symptoms of fluid overload, only one large placebo-controlled trial of diuretics has been conducted in patients with heart failure [75, 76]. Their efficacy has been readily apparent on an observational basis for years [72].

*Effects on survival*

One case-controlled study with thiazide diuretics in hypertensive patients suggests that at higher doses these agents may increase the risk of sudden death [77]. However, it is unclear whether these data will extend to the heart-failure population. Only one prospective survival trial of patients treated with diuretics has been performed to date. The recently completed RALES trial compared aldactone 25 mg daily and placebo on patients already treated with ACE inhibition and a loop diuretic [75, 76]. This dose of aldosterone is less than that necessary for effective diuresis, but is adequate for neurohormonal antagonism. The trial was stopped prematurely because of the mortality benefit (approximately 27% reduction in mortality) of aldactone. As aldosterone may have effects on chamber growth and remodelling (especially in terms of fibroblast effects) [26, 28], the inhibition of aldosterone (which is incomplete with just ACE inhibitors) may provide more complete protection from the pathological architectural changes which lead to progressive pump failure. In addition, the protection from hypokalaemia with aldactone may protect from sudden death, although the mechanism of this has yet to be confirmed. Despite the favourable effects of aldactone on survival of patients in heart failure, this result cannot be extrapolated to other diuretics which do not inhibit (and may in fact stimulate) the renin–angiotensin–aldosterone system.

*Adverse effects*

There are several important adverse effects of diuretics. The most important include: (1) electrolyte disturbance (hypokalaemia, hypomagnasaemia, hyponatraemia); (2) hypovolaemia and azotaemia (especially in combination with NSAIDs); (3) metabolic abnormalities [glucose intolerance, elevation of low-density and very-low density lipoproteins (LDLs and VLDLs), hyperuricaemia]; (4) activation of the RAS; and (5) arrhythmias [72, 78, 79].

Diuretics may result in total body and intracellular deficits of potassium and magnesium which may or may not be reflected by a measurable decrease in serum concentrations of these cations. Renal excretion of these cations is exacerbated by diuretic-induced hyperaldosteronism and metabolic alkalosis. The hypokalaemia cannot be corrected until the hypomagnesaemia has been corrected. Once corrected, hypokalaemia and hypomagnasaemia are best prevented by the use of: (1) potassium supplements; (2) potassium-sparing diuretics (which spare both potassium and magnesium); and (3) ACE inhibitors.

Prerenal azotaemia may be particularly marked if the patient has pre-existing renal or renal artery disease, is taking NSAIDs, or is using a concomitant ACE inhibitor [71]. NSAIDs interfere with the vasodilatory action of prostaglandins within the kidney. This may promote afferent vasoconstriction in the glomerulus, thereby reducing glomerular perfusion. ACE inhibitors promote efferent vasodilatation in the kidney, leading to reduced perfusion pressure. These actions increase the BUN.

Overuse of diuretics results in activation of the RAS, which may have long-term adverse effects on ventricular remodelling and patient survival [80, 81]. Diuretics should be used in combination with an ACE inhibitor and only to maintain a euvolaemic state. As aldactone has now been shown to increase survival in patients with heart failure [75, 76], it should be used in combination with an ACE inhibitor and a loop diuretic in patients with advanced heart failure and normal renal function.

## Digoxin

*Mechanism of action*

Digitalis preparations have been used for edema since the description in 1785 by Sir William Withering [82]. It has only been from the twentieth century that digitalis preparations have been considered useful in patients with heart failure and sinus rhythm [83–87], and only during the 1990s have the mechanisms been appreciated by which digoxin benefits the patient in heart failure.

Digitalis preparations work primarily by inhibiting Na/K-ATPase [88–92]. This leads to activation of the

Na/Ca exchanger in the sarcolemma and increased intracellular calcium concentration. This improves the contractile state. More recent data also suggest that the cardiac glycosides can alter ion selectivity of voltage-sensitive $Na^+$ channels in sarcolemmmal and T-tubular membranes, permitting $Ca^{2+}$ entry by a mechanism named 'slip mode conductance' [93]. However, digitalis also has two other important effects: (1) improvement in myocardial relaxation in patients with systolic dysfunction (a low ejection fraction) [94]; and (2) neurohormonal antagonism [95–102]. Digitalis may alter baroreflex desensitization in heart failure and reduce adrenergic activation [95–102]. Other beneficial neurohormonal effects include reductions in renin–angiotensin [97, 99] and TNF-$\alpha$ production [103], and an increase in counter-regulatory hormone (ANF and BNF) release [104]. Thus, digoxin may be a neurohormonal antagonist.

Digitalis also has electrophysiological effects. Digitalis preparations effect a slowing of sinus heart rate mediated through an increase in vagal tone [83, 97] and a reduction in sympathetic activity [95–102]. There is also an increase in refractoriness of the atrioventricular nodal tissues, which reduces ventricular response in patients with atrial fibrillation [83, 105, 106]. Since digoxin improves ventricular function in patients with heart failure [94, 100, 107–114], it is the drug of choice in patients with heart failure and atrial fibrillation who require immediate rate control [115].

### *Haemodynamic effects*

Digoxin does not alter central haemodynamics in normal controls, an effect which is most likely to be due to an increase in systemic vascular resistance (in normals) which offsets the increase in contractility [116–120]. However, in patients with chronic heart failure, it improves LVEF [60, 100, 121]. In addition to improving systolic performance in the failing heart, there appears to be at least an acute improvement in active relaxation with digitalis [94]. This effect is somewhat paradoxical as digitalis increases the concentration of intracellular calcium. However, the improvement in systolic performance may permit better elastic recoil of the ventricle, thereby improving relaxation. Resting and exercise haemodynamics are improved in part by reducing pulmonary capillary wedge pressure while increasing stroke work [113, 122, 123]. These improvements in haemodynamics are sustained during long-term therapy [113, 121, 124].

### *Clinical trials showing efficacy*

Digoxin has been shown to be efficacious at improving exercise tolerance and reducing the need for co-intervention (additional therapy for heart failure) [125]. Two withdrawal trials, the RADIANCE [126] and PROVED [127] studies, have shown the clinical benefit of digoxin therapy. In the RADIANCE study [126], 178 patients with moderate heart failure, EF $< 0.35$, and sinus rhythm were studied over 12 weeks in a double-blind, placebo-controlled fashion. Patients on ACE inhibitors and digoxin were randomized to continuing digoxin or switched from digoxin to placebo. Worsening heart failure developed in 23 placebo patients compared with four patients in the digoxin group ($p < 0.001$). All measures of functional capacity deteriorated in the patients receiving placebo compared with those continuing digoxin ($p = 0.033$ for maximal exercise tolerance, $p = 0.01$ for sub-maximal exercise endurance, and $p = 0.019$ for NYHA functional class). Patients switched to placebo also had decreased EF ($p = 0.001$) and increases in heart rate ($p = 0.001$). The PROVED trial was of similar design in 88 patients who were not taking ACE inhibitors [127]. This trial demonstrated worsened maximal exercise capacity ($p = 0.003$) and lower EF ($p = 0.016$) in those switched to placebo compared with those continuing digoxin.

The Digitalis Investigation Group (DIG) study was designed primarily as a mortality study of digoxin [128]. However, in this study, there was a significant reduction in hospitalizations for worsening heart failure in the digoxin treated group compared with the placebo group (910 versus 1180 patients hospitalized, $p < 0.001$), consistent with the findings of the PROVED and RADIANCE trials.

A recent study of heart-failure patients in sinus rhythm demonstrated that haemodynamic and autonomic improvement with digoxin was seen primarily at a low dose (0.125 mg daily; digoxin levels $0.8 \pm 0.5$ ng/ml) with no additional haemodynamic or autonomic benefit at higher doses (0.25 mg daily; digoxin levels $1.5 \pm 0.7$ ng/ml) [100].

### *Effect on survival*

The NIH-sponsored DIG trial studied 7788 patients in sinus rhythm and primarily moderate heart failure with a mean follow-up of 37 months [128]. Of these patients, 988 had a LVEF 45%. Approximately 70% of the patients in this study had coronary artery disease. The dose of digoxin was based on a normogram of the patient's size and weight. At the end of the study, there was no difference between treatment groups in all-cause mortality. However, there was a 14% reduction in pump failure death with a 12% increase in other cardiovascular (primarily sudden) deaths. There was also a significant reduction in the combination of death or hospitalization for congestive heart failure in patients on digoxin ($p < 0.001$). Thus, digoxin reduces hospitalization without an adverse effect on mortality.

A *post-hoc* analysis of the DIG study also found an association between the digoxin level and all-cause mortality. Above a digoxin level of 1.0 ng/ml, there was a marked increase in mortality. While this association is not cause-and-effect, when these data are combined with data showing that most of the benefit of digoxin is at a low dose for patients in sinus rhythm [100], one should consider using lower doses of digoxin for heart failure patients in sinus rhythm, keeping the level at approximately 0.8–1.0 ng/ml.

### *Adverse effects*

Digitalis toxicity is the most significant adverse effect of these preparations [129–131]. It should be remembered that quinidine, verapamil, and amiodarone have all been shown to decrease total body clearance of digoxin. In patients with renal insufficiency or prerenal azotaemia due to heart failure, digitalis levels and evidence of toxicity must be monitored closely. In the DIG trial, the incidence of hospitalization for suspected digoxin toxicity was 2% in patients taking digoxin compared with 0.9% in patients taking placebo [128]. The most common manifestations of digoxin intoxication were gastrointestinal and cardiac disturbances that included ventricular arrhythmias. One should distinguish between a digoxin effect (sagging of the ST segments), digoxin excess (atrioventricular block), digoxin intoxication (life-threatening arrhythmias), and digoxin overdose that in addition to arrhythmias is manifested by severe hyperkalaemia requiring dialysis. For severe, life-threatening arrhythmias, purified digoxin-specific Fab fragments are available [132, 133].

It is possible that a potassium-sparing diuretic such as aldactone may protect against digoxin-induced arrhythmias. Aldosterone has been shown to reduce serum and tissue potassium and magnesium levels [134, 135] and to cause the release of noradrenaline from the myocardium, potentiating digitalis-induced arrhythmias [136]. Aldosterone has also been shown to enhance the peripheral vasoconstrictor effects of digoxin and decrease atrial contractility. Thus, an aldosterone antagonist may be protective against the adverse effects of digoxin.

Digitalis intoxication may be potentiated by ischaemia for several reasons: (1) ischaemia by itself may inhibit Na/K-ATPase [137], thus enhancing the effect of digoxin on this targetor; (2) digitalis may mediate inappropriate coronary vasoconstriction in patients with ischaemia via an α-adrenergic mechanism [138–142]; and (3) digoxin may produce a sympathostimulatory effect in an ischaemic heart at the same dose at which it produces a sympathoinhibitory effect in the non-ischaemic situation [143]. Thus, the use of a concomitant β-adrenergic blocking agent may potentially reduce the ischaemia and arrhythmias caused by digoxin. While the beneficial effect of concomitant β-blocker therapy has been demonstrated in animal models, its effect in humans has yet to be established.

## β-Adrenergic blockers

### *Mechanism of action*

Despite the haemodynamic and survival benefits provided by ACE inhibitors, plasma noradrenaline continues to rise over time [55] and the mortality of patients treated with an ACE inhibitor remains high [62–64]. Blockade of the β-receptors in the heart results in an initial depression of LV function followed by late (after 1 month) paradoxical improvement in ventricular function over time [144], which is a biological effect [1, 145]. Multiple trials of β-adrenergic blockade have been performed to date and all have consistently shown two things: (1) β-adrenergic blockade when given carefully in a controlled fashion is safe; and (2) consistent improvement in LV function and functional class is demonstrated [146–161]. Only one β-blocker trial of greater than 1 month duration has failed to show an improvement in LV function [162]. In addition to improvement in LV performance and contractility, LV mechanical work increases with β-blockade, while myocardial oxygen consumption decreases [146]. This suggests improved myocardial efficiency. The improvement in LV function appears to be a dose-related phenomenon, with a greater dose of β-blocker producing greater improvement in ventricular function [148, 155]. This observation proves that the greater the protection from the deleterious effects of noradrenaline (cell death, alteration in phenotype), the greater the improvement in LV function. Indeed, β-blockers have been shown to increase message expression of adult α-myosin heavy chain and downregulate more fetal (and slower) β-myosin heavy chain in heart-failure patients treated for several months [38]. They have also reduce apoptosis in animal models of heart failure [163].

Thus, the antagonism of the growth stimulatory substances such as noradrenaline, AngII, aldosterone, endothelins, and cytokines provides a biological basis for improvement of LV function based on current paradigms of the progression of heart failure.

The patients who haemodynamically best respond to β-blocking agents are those with the most myocardial viability [164]. Thus, early treatment with β-blockers is critical. After 1 or more years of therapy with β-blockers, LV mass regresses and the ventricle reverse remodels to a more normal elliptical shape [144, 165]. This suggests that β-blockers, along with ACE inhibitors, not only stop the pathological growth process, but reverse it. This translates into improved clinical outcome.

### *Effects on survival*

The US Carvedilol Trials were a group of four studies examining exercise tolerance (moderate heart failure studies) and progression of disease (mild heart failure study) [155, 156, 166]. When the Data and Safety Monitoring Committee examined the data of all four trials together, there was a 65% reduction in all-cause mortality with carvedilol [risk ratio (RR) = 0.35, CI = 0.20–0.61, $p < 0.001$] [166]. While these studies suggested a mortality benefit of carvedilol, they were far from conclusive because of design problems (short follow-up, few events, study bias created by open-label run-in period).

The Cardiac Insufficiency Bisoprolol Study (CIBIS-1) trial randomized 641 patients with moderate heart failure to the $\beta_1$-selective agent bisoprolol or placebo [154]. While this trial was underpowered and only half of the patients were titrated to target dosage, there was a 20% reduction in mortality with bisoprolol (RR = 0.80, CI = 0.56–1.15), but this did not reach statistical significance ($p = 0.22$).

Two subsequent mortality trials, the second Cardiac Insufficiency Bisoprolol (CIBIS-2) [167] trial and the Metoprolol Randomized Intervention Trial in Heart Failure (MERIT-HF) [168, 169] were both powered and designed as mortality trials. Both of these trials were prematurely terminated by their respective Data and Safety Monitoring Committees because of the survival benefit of these agents. The CIBIS-2 trial recruited 2647 patients with NYHA class III–IV heart failure and an EF of 0.35 or less [167]. The patients were balanced in terms of demographics at baseline, and approximately 50% had ischaemic aetiology of heart failure. The $\beta_1$-selective agent, bisoprolol, reduced all-cause mortality by 34% ($p \leq 0.00006$) [167]. The placebo mortality in this trial was approximately 13% per year, which suggests that the heart failure population studied was not severely ill. Much of the reduction in mortality was due to a 44% reduction in sudden death ($p = 0.001$). While death due to pump failure was reduced by 26%, this did not reach statistical significance. The CIBIS-2 trial also demonstrated a 32% reduction in heart-failure hospitalizations with bisoprolol.

The MERIT-HF trial was also prematurely terminated because of benefit [169]. The 3991 patients in this study were predominantly NYHA class II-III with EF of 0.40 or less. Treatment with metoprolol CR/XL was associated with a 34% reduction in mortality ($p = 0.0062$ adjusted). Like the CIBIS-2 trial, the MERIT-HF study demonstrated a 41% reduction in sudden death ($p = 0.0002$), a 49% reduction in pump failure death ($p = 0.0023$), a 35% reduction in heart failure hospitalization ($p = 0.00001$), and an 18% reduction in all cause hospitalization ($p = 0.005$). The yearly mortality rate with placebo in this trial appears to be less than that of the CIBIS-2 trial (about 11% per year). Thus, the CIBIS-2 and MERIT-HF trials suggest that patients with mild to moderate heart failure have a survival benefit from bisoprolol or metoprolol CR/XL.

The CarvedilOl ProspEctive RaNdomIzed CUmulative Survival Trail (COPERNICUS) was a study of a non-selective β-blocking agent with α-blocking properties (carvedilol) in a low-ejection fraction, highly symptomatic population [170]. As compared to MERIT-HF [169] and CIBIS-2 [167] which excluded patients with ejection fractions of 0.40 and 0.35 or higher respectively, the COPERNICUS trial had a lower ejection fraction of 0.25 or below for entry. Entry into this study did not allow patients with significant peripheral or pulmonary oedema at the time of randomization, and thus was a somewhat selected population of patients with more advanced heart failure. Like the CIBIS-2 and MERIT-HF trials, this study demonstrated a 35% reduction in death (95% CI 19–48%, $p = 0.0014$ adjusted for interim analyses) with carvedilol. The annual placebo mortality in this trial was 18.5% which was higher than the 11.0% mortality in MERIT-HF and 13.2% in CIBIS-2 suggesting a more advanced heart failure population. A *post-hoc* analysis of the MERIT-HF study excluding patients with a left ventricular ejection fraction greater than 0.25 and NYHA functional class II demonstrated a similar result to COPERNICUS [171]. The annual placebo mortality was 19.1% in this analysis and there was a 39% reduction (95% CI 11–58% reduction, $p = 0.0086$) in mortality with metoprolol CR/XL. These data extend the spectrum of patients eligible to get β-blockade to patients with low ejection fraction and moderate to severe symptoms. However, these data do not establish the benefit of β-blockade for either Class IV patients who cannot reach compensation.

The β-blocker Evaluation of Survival Trial (BEST) also examined the effect of a non-selective β-blocking agent, bucindolol, on all cause mortality in patients with more advanced heart failure [172]. Patients in this study were NYHA functional class III or IV and had a left ventricular ejection fraction of 0.35 or less. This study also uniquely stratified patients in each site based on gender, ejection fraction ($>$ vs $\leq$ 0.20), presence or absence of coronary artery disease, and importantly race (black vs non-black). BEST was prematurely terminated by the Data and Safety Monitoring Committee based on 'the totality of evidence regarding the usefulness of β-blocker treatment derived from BEST and other studies'. The BEST study found a 10% reduction in mortality (95% CI −2 to 22% reduction, $p = 0.10$ unadjusted) with bucindolol. Bucindolol reduced cardiovascular mortality by 14% (95% CI = 1–26% reduction, $p = 0.04$) and reduced all cause hospitalization by 8% ($p = 0.08$). The lesser effect in BEST as compared to the other β-blocker mortality trials may be due to a different patient population studied, adverse sympatholytic effects of bucindolol, or chance. Bucindolol tended to have beneficial effects in less advanced heart failure patients and in non-black patients, while it had no benefit in NYHA class IV and in black patients. This most likely was due to greater sympatholytic effects of bucindolol in these two subgroups. As sympatholysis (as reflected by a drop in plasma norepinephrine) provides insurmountable loss of adrenergic support in hearts which are critically dependent on that support to maintain circulation in times of stress, an agent which removes that support may lead to an adverse outcome [173]. This may be especially a concern in the most advanced heart failure as seen in the NYHA class IV and black patients in BEST. As carvedilol, metoprolol CR/XL, and bisoprolol do not have the strong sympatholytic effects that bucindolol has, they may not produce adverse effects in very advanced heart failure as suggested by COPERNICUS [170] and the subgroup analysis of MERIT-HF [170].

There are theories that $\beta_1$-selective antagonists may not be as protective against sudden death as non-selective β-blockers [39, 174]. However, this has yet to be proven. The results of the CIBIS-II and MERIT-HF trials [167, 169] suggest that a $\beta_1$-selective agent will prolong survival and reduce sudden death. An ongoing trial, the Carvedilol or Metoprolol Trial (COMET) will examine the effects of carvedilol and metoprolol in a head-to-head comparison of mortality rates to determine whether there are advantages to a non-selective agent.

#### *Word of caution*

β-Adrenergic blocking agents are not rescue therapy for patients with the most advanced heart failure (i.e. patients on inotropic therapy in coronary care units or with decompensated heart failure). The initial effect of these agents is adrenergic withdrawal and sometimes worsening haemodynamics [39, 144]. Not every β-blocker can be used to treat heart failure as some are poorly tolerated, and the starting dose must be very low, with slow, weekly titration if the patient is stable. Guidelines for the initiation of β-blockers have been published [39]. There may be a subgroup of patients who do not benefit from this therapy and may worsen both haemodynamically and prognostically [175]. Future research will hopefully identify those patients who benefit and those who do not.

### Angiotensin receptor blockers

#### *Mechanism of action*

The recent Food and Drug Administration (FDA) approval of angiotensin receptor-blocking agents (ARBs) for hypertension has provided another agent to block the effects of Ang II. Most of the currently available ARBs (e.g. losartan, candasartan, irbesartan, valsartan) selectively block the AT1 receptor [176–178]. However, while these agents improve haemodynamics and exercise tolerance similarly to ACE inhibitors [179, 180], their mechanisms of action are different: (1) ARBs do not inhibit bradykinin breakdown like ACE inhibitors, which may result in nitrous oxide and prostacyclin release [181, 182]. These latter substances are growth inhibitors and may be beneficial in heart failure; (2) ARBs increase AngII levels locally by feedback mechanisms and the effect of AngII on the AT2 receptor (which is unblocked by selective AT1 blockade) is unknown (although some data suggest that the AT2 receptor may be a growth-inhibiting receptor that may mediate apoptosis in some conditions [183–185]); (3) differences may exist in the ability of ACE inhibitors and ARBs to reduce SNS activity [186]; and (4) ACE inhibitors decrease plasminogen activator inhibitor levels, but ARBs do not [187]. As these differences exist, and as

ACE inhibitors have been tried and tested in multiple clinical trials (while ARBs have not), ARBs cannot be freely substituted at this time for ACE inhibitors.

*Clinical trials showing efficacy*

The recent ELITE trials [188, 189] have suggested that these agents may be safe in patients with heart failure and conceivably could be slightly less beneficial as ACE inhibitors. In addition, the RAAS [190, 191], RESOLVD [192] and Val-HeFT [193] trials in humans as well as animal data [186, 194] suggest that there could be an additive benefit to an ACE inhibitor and an ARB working in concert. In the RESOLVD trial [192], a small study designed to look at exercise tolerance and LV function in patients on an ACE inhibitor, an ARB, or the combination, LV end-diastolic volumes at 43 weeks of therapy enlarged the least with combination therapy. This suggests that the least amount of pathological remodelling occurs with combination therapy. However, larger, better controlled studies are required to confirm this finding.

In the Val-HeFT study, 5010 heart failure patients taking an ACE inhibitor (or who were ACE intolerent) who had an EF $\leq$ 0.40 and were primarily NYHA class II–III were randomized to valasartan ($n = 2511$) or placebo ($n = 2499$) [193]. Valsartan did not reduce all cause mortality with a Risk ratio = 1.02 (95% CI = 0.90–1.15, $p$ = NS), but did reduce the prespecified combined endpoint of all cause mortality and morbidity (sudden death with resuscitation, heart failure hospitalization, need for IV inotrope or vasodilator for more than 4 hours), Risk ratio = 0.87 (95% CI = 0.79–0.96, $p = 0.009$). The reduction in morbidity was primarily due to a 28% reduction in hospitalization in the valsartan group ($p < 0.001$). However, subgroup analysis revealed that most of the benefit of valsartan was in patients who were not taking an ACE inhibitor. Furthermore, there was a trend to an increase in mortality and morbidity in patients taking β-blocker and ACE inhibitor who were randomized to valsartan. These data suggest that ARBs are slightly less effective than ACE inhibitors as monotherapy, and have little additional benefit as adjunctive therapy to ACE inhibitors. Based on Val-HeFT, they should not be added to the regimen of patients taking both a β-blocker and an ACE inhibitor. As β-blockers and ACE inhibitors are established therapy with proven mortality and morbidity benefits, ARBs should only be used when a patient is ACE inhibitor intolerent. The CHARM study is currently examining the effect of ARBs in ACE inhibitor intolerent patients, as adjunctive therapy of ACE inhibitors, and in patients with diastolic dysfunction.

*Adverse effects*

The most important side-effects are hypotension on therapy initiation, muscle cramps, and increased creatinine but, unlike ACE inhibitors, ARBs do not cause cough or angioedema because they do not inhibit bradykinin breakdown [188, 191, 195].

## Calcium channel blockers

*Mechanism of action*

These agents produce powerful vasodilator effects and variable negative inotropic effects by interfering with transmembrane calcium transients. Three generations of calcium antagonists currently exist (Table 29.1). The first-generation agents (verapamil, diltiazem, nifedipine) block the L-calcium channel and have direct negative inotropic effects on myocytes [196], while the second-generation agents (amlodipine, felodipine) are longer acting and much more vascular selective [197–200]. The third generation of agents (mibefradil) primarily block T-channels instead of the L-channels [201–204]. L-channels, or low voltage-gated calcium channels, are found in peripheral arteries, the ventricle, and the sinus node [205]. Blocking these channels results in the negative inotropic and chronotropic effects of the first-generation calcium blockers. The T-channels are found in the sinoartrial node, peripheral arteries, and neurohormonal cells of the kidney [205] and they may mediate a hypertrophic or growth response in myocytes [205–207]. T-channel blockade results in a reduction in heart rate and vasodilatation without reflex tachycardia or negative inotropic effects [203, 204]. In addition, as the T-channels may mediate a growth response [205–207], blockade may theoretically produce an anti-proliferative response [208].

While the short-term haemodynamic effects of first-generation agents appear to be beneficial due to vasodilatation [196, 209], long-term therapy results in no improvement in exercise tolerance [210], and even activation of deleterious neurohormones [209, 211, 212] that may cause ventricular enlargement [210]. The first-generation agents may worsen long-term outcome [213, 214] and are contraindicated in all patients with LV dysfunction.

By contrast, more recent studies with second-generation calcium antagonists are more promising. The PRAISE trials [215, 216] demonstrated no adverse effect of amlodipine on mortality in patients with heart failure as well as no benefit.

**Table 29.1** Calcium blocker effects in heart failure

| Agent | Half-life (h) | Effects in heart failure |
|---|---|---|
| *First generation* | | |
| Phenylalkylamine | | |
| Verapamil | 8 ± 6 | Negative inotrope |
| Benzothiazepine | | |
| Diltiazem | 4–6 | Negative inotrope; ↑ CHF exacerbation |
| 1,4-Dihydropyridine | | |
| Nifedipine | 5 | Negative inotrope; no exercise benefit; ↑ PRA; ↑ CHF exacerbation |
| Nicardipine | 1(IV) | Negative inotrope |
| *Second generation* | | |
| 1,4-Dihydropyridine | | |
| Felodipine | 15 ± 3 | No effect on mortality; no improvement in exercise or QOL |
| Amlodipine | 35–45 | Possible mild benefit in DCM; no change in PNE; may reduce cytokines |
| *Third generation* | | |
| Benzimidazolyl-substituted tetraline | | |
| Mibefradil | 10–15 | Adverse interaction with digoxin and antiarrhythmics |

↑ = increased; CHF = chronic heart failure; PRA = plasma renin activity; QOL = quality of life; DCM = dilated cardiomyopathy; PNE = plasma noradrenaline (norepinephrine).

A similar trial, V-HeFT III [217], using felodipine, found no effect of felodipine treatment on all-cause mortality. However, in patients with a more advanced NYHA class, there was a trend towards an adverse effect. The new third-generation agent mibefradil was recently tested in heart failure (MACH-1 trial) [218, 219]. This trial demonstrated an adverse interaction of mibefradil with several antiarrhythmic agents (including amiodarone) and digoxin, resulting in a trend towards increased mortality. Mibefradil was subsequently withdrawn from the market for use in hypertension. Based on these data, calcium blockers should not be given as front-line therapy for heart failure. They should be avoided in the presence of LV systolic dysfunction (i.e. a low LVEF) and only amlodipine should be used for refractory ischaemia or hypertension when other, more standard therapies (β-blockers, ACE inhibitors, nitrate).

## Inotropic agents

Most inotropic agents work by increasing cyclic adenosine monophosphate (cAMP), the intracellular messenger of the β-adrenergic system [220]. These agents improve haemodynamics, cardiac symptoms, and exercise tolerance [125, 221–227], but at moderate to high doses they may accelerate death [227–230]. This is best exemplified by the PROMISE trial [228], which examined the effect of high dose milrinone on survival in patients ($n$ = 1088) with moderate to severe heart failure who were receiving ACE inhibitors. After a median follow-up of 6.1 months, there was a 28% increase in cardiovascular mortality in the milrinone-treated group. The increase in mortality was greatest in the sickest patients (NYHA class IV), who most needed inotropic support. The cause of increased mortality was an increase in sudden death (arrhythmias), and there was no decrease in death from pump failure [231].

Use of intermittent dobutamine at moderate doses also improves exercise tolerance, but increases adverse events [227]. Thus, inotropic agents should only be used as short-term therapy for patients with decompensated heart failure or who are refractory to more standard therapies and need inotropic support to counteract fluid build-up. If used long term, inotropes should be at low dose and preferably in combination with β-blockade to prevent arrhythmic or ischaemic events [232]. The combination of low-dose inotropic therapy with β-blockade may have some long-term benefit [232], although this has yet to be proven. The inotropic drug used in combination with β-blockade should be one that does not work directly on the β-receptor (such as dobutamine) as these agents are less effective in the presence of a β-blocker and patients tend to develop tachyphylaxis. An agent that inhibits phosphodiesterase (such as milrinone or enoximone) is more effective in the presence of β-blockade since such agents are not dependent on agonist binding to the blocked receptor.

## New frontiers

### *Anticytokine therapy*

TNF-α is progressively activated as heart failure worsens [233, 234], much like the adrenergic nervous system and the RAS [81]. When expressed at sufficiently high concentrations, cytokines will mimic some aspects of the heart failure phenotype, including (but not limited to) progressive LV dysfunction, pulmonary oedema, LV remodelling, fetal gene expression, and cardiomyopathy [6, 235–237]. The most studied of these cytokines is TNF-α, a 17 000 mol.wt protein that acts through two distinct receptors, $TNFR_1$ and $TNFR_2$ [6]. TNF-α produces several powerful biological effects that include immunostimulation, mediation of host resistance to bacteria, activation of protein kinase C, and activation of the expression of a wide variety of genes involved in inflammation or cell growth [6, 238, 239]. TNF-α has been shown to be produced in the heart, and cardiac overexpression in transgenic animals results in myocarditis at high levels [235, 236] and the heart-failure phenotype at lower levels of expression [236, 237]. The heart-failure phenotype produced by overexpression of TNF-α includes replacement fibrosis similar to that found in dilated cardiomyopathy. This suggests that TNF-α may directly or indirectly activate fibroblasts and matrix metalloproteinases which play a key role in replacement fibrosis in dilated cardiomyopathy [240–243].

Recently, a recombinant dimer consisting of two p75-soluble TNF receptor molecules fused to the Fc fragment of human immunoglobulin $G_1$ ($IgG_1$) expressed in mammalian cells has been developed [244]. Data with recombinant TNF-α RII-soluble receptor-coupled antibodies have demonstrated short-term haemodynamic and functional improvement with this agent [244]. However, preliminary results of a clinical trial with this agent suggest a lack of effect on events. More anti-cytokine agents are being examined.

### *Endothelin antagonists*

Endothelin is the most powerful vasoconstrictor yet identified in the body [245, 246]. Endothelin-1 (ET-1) is elevated in patients with heart failure, and the plasma level of ET-1 correlates with pulmonary artery pressure and pulmonary vascular resistance [247, 248]. Endothelin acts on the endothelin A ($ET_A$) and B ($ET_B$) receptors on the myocyte [249, 250]. The endothelin receptors are linked to the activation of phospholipase C in a similar fashion to AngII [251, 252]. This pathway is known to stimulate proto-oncogenes such as c-*myc* and c-*fos* and promote cell growth and hypertrophy, and this has been shown for endothelin in an animal system [252–257]. In some animal systems, the endothelin pathway has been shown to activate tyrosine kinase, which leads to raf-MAP kinase activation and gene expression [258]. Thus, activation of the endothelin pathway may potentially result in abnormal growth patterns and pathological remodelling in the failing ventricle in a fashion similar to that in AngII.

The acute haemodynamic response to a non-selective $ET_A/ET_B$ antagonist, bosentan, is a reduction in mean arterial, pulmonary artery, and pulmonary capillary wedge pressures; a reduction in systemic and pulmonary vascular resistance; and an increase in stroke volume index [250]. Some animal data suggest that long-term use of an endothelin antagonist in animals with heart failure results in favourable effects on myocyte contractility, chamber remodelling, and mortality [259, 260]. While the acute haemodynamic profile appears favourable for this type of medication in heart-failure patients, the long-term effects on remodelling, haemodynamics, and survival are unknown. Several endothelin antagonists, both $ET_A$ selective and non-selective, are currently being evaluated in clinical trials. It is yet unclear whether $ET_A$ selective or $ET_A/ET_B$ non-selective blockade will provide more favourable outcomes.

### *Central sympatholytics*

Centrally acting agents such as clonidine, which reduce sympathetic discharge from the central nervous system, have been tested in small, short-term trials and shown to be of benefit [261–265]. Several newer agents are under development [266]. One of the main agents previously evaluated is moxonidine, which works by stimulating imidazoline receptors in the lateral reticular formation of the medulla and reducing sympathetic activation in a similar way to clonidine, but without the sedation, dry mouth, or impotence found with the latter (as there is much less stimulation of the $\alpha_2$-receptors in the pontomedullary region) [266, 267]. Moxonidine also activates renal imidazoline receptors, causing natriuresis. Centrally acting agents such as moxonidine reduce systemic vascular resistance, arterial pressure, and heart rate by reducing sympathetic discharge [267]. This unique combination of properties could make this type of agent better tolerated than many β-blockers in patients with heart failure, while reducing sympathetic activity. However, a large clinical trial with Moxonidine, the MOXCON study, was stopped prematurely for a greater than 50% increase in mortality as compared to placebo [173]. The reason for the increase in mortality may be similar to that seen in BEST. As sympatholysis provides insurmountable loss of adrenergic support in hearts which are critically dependent on that support to maintain circulation in times of stress, an agent which removes that support may lead to an adverse outcome. Thus, less potent sympatholytic agents may be tested in the future or this type of agent may have to be restricted to patients with less advanced heart failure. At the present time, these agents have no proven benefit and may be harmful.

### *Natriuretic factors*

Atrial and brain natriuretic factors (ANF and BNF) are peptides produced primarily in the atria and ventricles, respectively [7, 268–275]. Two other natruretic peptides, C-type natriuretic peptide (CNP) and urodilatin, have also been described [276, 277]. ANF is released in response to stretch or load [7, 274], while both pressure and volume overload have been implicated as stimuli for BNF release [278, 279]. These substances have significant natriuretic and vasodilatory properties which occur through activation of guanylate cyclase leading to increased cyclic guanine monophosphate (cGMP) [274, 275, 280–283]. Natriuretic peptides are cleared by the action of neutral endopeptidases [284, 285]. These natruretic peptides act as antagonists of the RAS and SNS [286–290] and, thus, act as growth inhibitors. While in some circumstances, ANF may increase myocyte apoptosis in some neonatal animal models [291], its effect in humans with heart failure is unknown.

ANF and BNF levels increase in heart failure [7, 292–298]. ANF levels appear to be a sensitive marker of filling pressures [7, 293] and, to a lesser degree, a marker of outcome [296, 297], while levels of BNF appear to be a stronger prognostic marker for overall outcome [299]. The stronger predictive value of BNF may be due to the fact that BNF is secreted primarily from the ventricle and has a much longer half-life, and so may better reflect the general diastolic function and heart-failure status of the patient over a period of time.

Infusion of ANF or BNF results in a drop in peripheral vascular resistance, arterial pressure, and pulmonary capillary wedge pressure, with little change or a mild increase in cardiac index [280, 286–288, 300–302]. Because BNF has a longer half-life than ANF, infusions of BNF may be beneficial for acute decompensation as well as chronic treatment of heart failure [303–307].

The administration of a neutral endopeptidase inhibitor to inhibit the metabolism of natriuretic peptides is another strategy for increasing the effect of the biological actions of these hormones [308–318]. The use of neutral endopeptidase inhibitors has been associated with an improvement in sodium excretion in heart-failure patients. Such agents may serve as an alternative to diuretics in the future and are under active investigation.

### *Dual metalloprotease inhibitors*

These agents may produce both antagonism of the RAS and neutral endopeptidase [319]. Thus, they may provide growth inhibition, vasodilatation, and natriuresis. The clinical results of this type of agent are still in very preliminary stages.

## Conclusions

A combination of myocyte hypertrophy, myocyte loss, and intrinsic cardiac myocytic dysfunction leads to ventricular remodelling and a decrease in systolic function and LVEF. Decreased LVEF is a powerful predictor of adverse outcome in patients with chronic heart failure [2, 320–323]. Thus, improved clinical outcome should result from strategies that reduce the biological signals responsible for myocyte growth dysfunction, and loss, and chamber remodelling. The use of combination therapy to antagonize multiple growth stimulatory signals (noradrenaline, AngII, aldosterone, endothelins, cytokines) appears to be the logical future of heart-failure therapy. Unfortunately, as new therapies develop, the patients suffer more from polypharmacy, the economic costs of numerous medications, and the side-effects of each agent. In addition, it becomes increasingly more difficult to prove the survival benefit of an individual agent since the benefits are additive among the approved agents that become 'standard of care' and are background therapy for clinical trials. More novel approaches in the future may therefore target common growth pathways within the myocyte (protein kinase C, calcineurin, etc.) which could be antagonized with single agents or with gene therapy.

It is clear that the paradigms for heart-failure progression have changed. No longer should the chronic treatment of heart failure be viewed in terms of haemodynamic goals achieved at the expense of a deleterious cell biology. Instead, the aim should be to improve the biology of the myocyte, even at the initial expense of haemodynamics. This paradigm is characterized by the beneficial effect on outcomes exemplified by β-adrenergic blockade. Future studies may better define newer adjunctive agents that will improve symptoms and outcome in heart-failure patients and may help to define the cellular pathways that can be altered to improve the biological properties of the myocyte.

## References


1. Eichhorn EJ, Bristow MR. Medical therapy can improve the biologic properties of the chronically failing heart: a new era in the treatment of heart failure. *Circulation* 1996; 94: 2285–96.
2. Eichhorn EJ. Prognosis determination in heart failure. *Am J Med* 2001; 110(2A): 14S–36S.
3. Hosenpud JD, Bennett LE, Keck BM *et al.* The registry of the International Society for Heart and Lung Transplantation: fourteenth official report — 1997. *J Heart Lung Transplant* 1997; 16: 691–712.
4. Sadoshima J, Izumo S. Signal transduction pathways of angiotensin II-induced c-*fos* gene expression in cardiac myocytes *in vitro*. Roles of phospholipid-derived second messengers. *Circ Res* 1993; 73: 424–38.
5. Sadoshima J, Xu Y, Slayter HS, Izumo S. Autocrine release of angiotensin II mediates stretch-induced hypertrophy of cardiac myocytes *in vitro*. *Cell* 1993; 75: 977–84.
6. Mann DL. The effect of tumour necrosis factor-alpha on cardiac structure and function: a tale of two cytokines. *J Cardiac Fail* 1996; 2 (Suppl): S165–72.
7. Edwards BS, Zimmerran RS, Schwab TR *et al.* Atrial stretch, not pressure, is the principal determinant controlling the acute release of atrial natriuretic factor. *Circ Res* 1988; 62: 191–5.
8. Leimbach WN, Wallin BG, Victor RG *et al.* Direct evidence from intraneural recordings for increased central sympathetic outflow in patients with heart failure. *Circulation* 1986; 73: 913–19.
9. McLeod AA, Brown JE, Kuhn C *et al.* Differentiation of hemodynamic, humoral and metabolic responses to $\beta_1$- and $\beta_2$-adrenergic stimulation in man using atenolol and propranolol. *Circulation* 1983; 67: 1076–84.
10. Bristow MR, Abraham WT. Anti-adrenergic effects of angiotensin converting enzyme inhibitors. *Eur Heart J* 1995; 16: 37–41.
11. Malik KU, Nasjletti A. Facilitation of adrenergic transmission by locally generated angiotensin II in rat mesenteric arteries. *Circ Res* 1976; 38: 26–30.
12. Cody RJ, Haas GJ, Binkley PF *et al.* Plasma endothelin correlates with the extent of pulmonary hypertension in patients with chronic congestive heart failure. *Circulation* 1992; 85: 504–9.
13. Rodeheffer RJ, Lerman A, Heublein DM, Burnett JCJ. Increased plasma concentrations of endothelin in congestive heart failure in humans. *Mayo Clin Proc* 1992; 67: 719–24.
14. Schrier RW, Bichet DG. Osmotic and nonosmotic control of vasopressin release and the pathogenesis of impaired water excretion in adrenal, thyroid, and edematous disorders. *J Lab Clin Med* 1981; 98: 1–15.
15. Bonjour JP, Malvin RL. Stimulation of ADH release by the renin–angiotensin system. *Am J Physiol* 1970; 218: 1555–9.
16. Torre-Amione G, Kapadia S, Benedict C *et al.* Proinflammatory cytokine levels in patients with depressed left ventricular ejection fraction: a report from the Studies of Left Ventricular Dysfunction (SOLVD). *J Am Coll Cardiol* 1996; 27: 1201–6.
17. Francis GS. The relationship of the sympathetic nervous system and the renin–angiotensin–aldosterone system in congestive heart failure. *Am Heart J* 1989; 118: 642–8.
18. Packer M, Lee WH, Kessler PD *et al.* Role of neurohormonal mechanisms in determining survival in patients with severe chronic heart failure. *Circulation* 1987; 75 (Suppl IV): IV-80–92.
19. Yamazaki T, Komuro I, Zou Y *et al.* Norepinephrine induces the raf-1 kinase/mitogen-activated protein kinase cascade through both $\alpha 1$- and $\beta$-adrenoceptors. *Circulation* 1997; 95: 1260–8.
20. Simpson P, McGrath A. Norepinephrine-stimulated hypertrophy of cultured rat myocardial cells is an alpha 1-adrenergic response. *J Clin Invest* 1983; 72: 732–7.
21. Sadoshima J, Qiu Z, Morgan JP, Izumo S. Angiotensin II and other hypertrophic stimuli mediated by G protein-coupled receptors activate tyrosine kinase, mitogen-activated protein kinase, and 90-kD S6 kinase in cardiac myocytes. The critical role of $Ca^{2+}$-dependent signaling. *Circ Res* 1995; 76: 1–15.
22. Shubeita HE, McDonough PM, Harris AN *et al.* Endothelin induction of inositol phospholipid hydrolysis, sarcomere assembly, and cardiac gene expression in ventricular myocytes: a paracrine mechanism for myocardial cell hypertrophy. *J Biol Chem* 1990; 265: 20 555–62.
23. Westwick JK, Weitzel C, Minden A *et al.* Tumor necrosis factor $\alpha$ stimulates AP-1 activity through prolonged activation of the c-Jun kinase. *J Biol Chem* 1994; 269: 26 396–401.
24. Grossman W, Jones D, McLaurin LP. Wall stress and patterns of hypertrophy in the human left ventricle. *J Clin Invest* 1975; 56: 56–64.
25. Sabbah HN, Goldstein S. Ventricular remodeling: consequences and therapy. *Eur Heart J* 1993; 14 (Suppl C): 24–9.
26. Weber KT, Anversa P, Armstrong PW *et al.* Remodeling and reparation of the cardiovascular system. *J Am Coll Cardiol* 1992; 20: 3–16.
27. Gerdes AM, Kellerman SE, Moore JA *et al.* Structural remodeling of cardiac myocytes in patients with ischemic cardiomyopathy. *Circulation* 1992; 86: 426–30.
28. Weber KT, Brilla CG. Pathological hypertrophy and cardiac interstitium. Fibrosis and renin–angiotensin–aldosterone system. *Circulation* 1991; 83: 1849–65.
29. Weber KT, Pick R, Janicki JS *et al.* Inadequate collagen tethers in dilated cardiomyopathy. *Am Heart J* 1988; 116: 1641–6.
30. Weber KT. Cardiac interstitium in health and disease: The fibrillar collagen matrix. *J Am Coll Cardiol* 1989; 13: 1637–52.
31. Kono T, Sabbah HN, Rosman H *et al.* Left ventricular shape is the primary determinant of functional mitral regurgitation in heart failure. *J Am Coll Cardiol* 1992; 20: 1594–8.
32. Sabbah HN, Sharov VG, Cook JM *et al.* Accumulation of collagen in the cardiac interstitium of dogs with chronic heart failure is associated with decreased capillary density and increased oxygen diffusion distance (Abstract). *J Am Coll Cardiol* 1995; 25: 222A.
33. Shimoyama H, Sabbh HN, Sharov VG *et al.* Accumulation of interstitial collagen in the failing left ventricular myocardium is associated with increased anaerobic metabolism among affected cardiomyocytes (Abstract). *J Am Coll Cardiol* 1994; 23: 98A.
34. Katz AM. Cellular mechanisms in congestive heart failure. *Am J Cardiol* 1988; 62: 3–8A.
35. Mann DL, Kent RL, Parsons B, Cooper G IV. Adrenergic effects on the biology of the adult mammalian cardiocyte. *Circulation* 1992; 85: 790–804.
36. Nadal-Ginard B. Commitment, fusion, and biochemical differentiation of a myogenic cell line in the absence of DNA synthesis. *Cell* 1978; 15: 855–64.
37. Thompson CB. Apoptosis in the pathogenesis and treatment of disease. *Science* 1995; 267: 1456–62.

38. Lowes BD, Minobe W, Abraham WT *et al.* Changes in gene expression in the intact human heart. Downregulation of α-myosin heavy chain in hypertrophied, failing ventricular myocardium. *J Clin Invest* 1997; 100: 2315–24.
39. Eichhorn EJ, Bristow MR. Practical guidelines for initiation of β-adrenergic blockade in patients with chronic heart failure. *Am J Cardiol* 1997; 79: 794–8.
40. Linz W, Scholkens BA, Ganten D. Converting enzyme inhibition specifically prevents the development and induces regression of cardiac hypertrophy in rats. *Clin Exp Hypertens* 1989; 11: 1325–50.
41. Baker KM, Chernin MI, Wixson SK, Aceto JF. Renin–angiotensin system involvement in pressure-overload cardiac hypertrophy in rats. *Am J Physiol* 1990; 259: H324–32.
42. Beinlich CJ, White GJ, Baker KM, Morgan HE. Angiotensin II and left ventricular growth in newborn pig heart. *J Mol Cell Cardiol* 1991; 23: 1031–8.
43. Brilla CG, Janicki JS, Weber KT. Cardioreparative effects of lisinopril in rats with genetic hypertension and left ventricular hypertrophy. *Circulation* 1991; 83: 1771–9.
44. Sabbah HN, Shimoyama H, Kono T *et al.* Effects of long-term monotherapy with enalapril, metoprolol, and digoxin on the progression of left ventricular dysfunction and dilation in dogs with reduced ejection fraction. *Criculation* 1994; 89: 2852–9.
45. McDonald KM, Rector T, Carlyle PF *et al.* Angiotensin-converting enzyme inhibition and beta-adrenoceptor blockade regress established ventricular remodeling in a canine model of discrete myocardial damage. *J Am Coll Cardiol* 1994; 24: 1762–8.
46. Pfeffer JM, Pfeffer MA, Braunwald E. Influence of chronic captopril therapy on the infarcted left ventricle of the rat. *Circ Res* 1985; 57: 84–95.
47. Konstam MA, Rousseau MF, Kronenberg MW *et al.* for the SOLVD Investigators. Effects of the angiotensin converting enzyme inhibitor enalapril on the long-term progression of left ventricular dysfunction in patients with heart failure. *Circulation* 1992; 86: 431–8.
48. Greenberg B, Quinones MA, Koilpillai C *et al.* for the SOLVD Investigators. Effects of long-term enalapril therapy on cardiac structure and function in patients with left ventricular dysfunction. Results of the SOLVD Echocardiography Substudy. *Circulation* 1995; 91: 2573–81.
49. Doherty NE, Seelos KC, Suzuki J-I *et al.* Application of cine nuclear magnetic resonance imaging for sequential evaluation of response to angiotensin-converting enzyme inhibitor therapy in dilated cardiomyopathy. *J Am Coll Cardiol* 1992; 19: 1294–302.
50. Mitchell GF, Lamas GA, Vaughan DE, Pfeffer MA. Left ventricular remodeling in the year after first anterior myocardial infarction: a quantitative analysis of contractile segment lengths and ventricular shape. *J Am Coll Cardiol* 1992; 19: 1136–44.
51. Sharpe N, Smith H, Murphy J *et al.* Early prevention of left ventricular dysfunction after myocardial infarction with angiotensin-converting-enzyme inhibition. *Lancet* 1991; 337: 872–6.
52. Pfeffer M, Braunwald E, Moye' L *et al.* on behalf of the SAVE Investigations. Effect of captopril on mortality and morbidity in patients with left ventricular, dysfunction after myocardial infarction. Results of survival and ventricular enlargement trial. *N Engl J Med* 1992; 327: 669–77.
53. Pfeffer MA, Lamas GA, Vaughan DE *et al.* Effect of captopril on progressive ventricular dilatation after anterior myocardial infarction. *N Engl J Med* 1988; 319: 80–6.
54. Gilbert EM, Sandoval A, Larrabee P *et al.* Lisinopril lowers cardiac adrenergic drive and increases β-receptor density in the failing human heart. *Circulation* 1993; 88: 472–80.
55. Francis GS, Cohn JN, Johnson G *et al.* for the V-HeFT VA Cooperative Studies Group. Plasma norepinephrine, plasma renin activity, and congestive heart failure. *Circulation* 1993; 87 (Suppl VI): VI-40–8.
56. van den Meiracker AH, Man in't Veld AJ, Admiraal PJ *et al.* Partial escape of angiotensin converting enzyme (ACE) inhibition during prolonged ACE inhibitor treatment: does it exist and does it affect antihypertensive response? *J Hypertens* 1992; 10: 803–12.
57. Hollenberg NK, Fisher ND, Price DA. Pathways for angiotensin II generation in intact human tissue: evidence from comparative pharmacological interruption of the renin system. *Hypertension* 1998; 32: 387–92.
58. Eichhorn EJ, McGhie AI, Bedotto JB *et al.* Effects of bucindolol on neurohormonal activation in congestive heart failure. *Am J Cardiol* 1991; 67: 67–73.
59. Captopril Multicenter Research Group. A cooperative multicenter study of captopril in congestive heart failure: hemodynamic effects and long-term response. *Am Heart J* 1985; 110: 439–47.
60. Captopril–Digoxin Multicenter Research Group. Comparative effects of therapy with captopril and digoxin in patients with mild to moderate heart failure. *JAMA* 1988; 259: 539–44.
61. Captopril Multicenter Research Group. A placebo-controlled trial of captopril in refractory chronic congestive heart failure. *J Am Coll Cardiol* 1983; 2: 755–63.
62. CONSENSUS Trial Study Group. Effects of enalapril on mortality in severe congestive heart failure: results of the Cooperative North Scandanavian Enalapril Survival Study (CONSENSUS). *N Engl J Med* 1987; 316: 1429–35.
63. SOLVD Investigators. Effect of enalapril on survival in patients with reduced left ventricular ejection fractions and congestive heart failure. *N Engl J Med* 1991; 325: 293–302.
64. SOLVD Investigators. Effect of enalapril on mortality and the development of heart failure in asymptomatic patients with reduced left ventricular ejection fractions. *N Engl J Med* 1992; 327: 685–91.
65. Packer M, Poole-Wilson PA, Armstrong PW, Cleland JGF, Horowitz JD, Massie BM, Ryden L, Thygesen K, Uretsky BF on behalf of the ATLAS Study Group. Comparative effects of low and high doses of the angiotensin-converting enzyme inhibitor, lisinopril, on morbidity and mortality in chronic heart failure. *Circulation* 1999; 100: 2312–18.
66. Acute Infarction Ramipril Efficacy (AIRE) Study Investigators. Effect of ramipril on mortality and morbidity of survivors of acute myocardial infarction with clinical evidence of heart failure. *Lancet* 1993; 342: 821–8.
67. Kober L, Torp-Pedersen C, Carlsen JE *et al.* A clinical trial of the angiotensin-converting-enzyme inhibitor trandolapril in patients with left ventricular dysfunction after myocardial infarction. Trandolapril Cardiac Evaluation (TRACE) Study Group. *N Engl J Med* 1995; 333: 1670–6.
68. Ambrosioni E, Borghi C, Magnani B for the Survival of Myocardial Infarction Long-Term Evaluation (SMILE) Study Investigators. The effect of the angiotensin-converting-enzyme inhibitor zofenopril on mortality and morbidity after anterior myocardial infarction. *N Engl J Med* 1995; 332: 80–5.
69. Held P, Swedberg K. ACE inhibitors in the treatment of heart failure. In: DB Barnett, H Pouleur, GS Francis (eds) *Congestive cardiac failure*. New York: Marcel Dekker, 1993, 169–83.
70. Abraham WT, Schrier RW. Renal salt and water handling in congestive heart failure. In: JD Hosenpud, BH Greenberg (eds) *Congestive heart failure*. New York: Springer, 1994; 161–73.

71. Dzau VJ, Packer M, Lilly LS *et al.* Prostaglandins in severe heart failure: relation to activation of the renin–angiotensin system and hyponatremia. *N Engl J Med* 1984; 310: 347–52.
72. Poole-Wilson PA. Diuretics for the treatment of heart failure. In: DB Barnett, H Pouleur, GS Francis (eds) *Congestive cardiac failure*. New York: Marcel Dekker, 1993, 103–17.
73. Pugh LGC, Wyndham CL. The circulatory effects of mercurial diuretics in congestive heart failure. *Clin Sci* 1949; 8: 11–19.
74. Novello FC, Sprague JM. Benzothiadiazine dioxides as novel diuretics. *J Am Chem Soc* 1957; 79: 2028–9.
75. Pitt B. ACE inhibitor co-therapy in patients with heart failure: rationale for the Randomized Aldactone Evaluation Study (RALES). *Eur Heart J* 1995; 16: 107–10.
76. Pitt B. RALES trial results presentation at the 71st Annual Scientific Session of the American Heart Association, 11 November 1998, Dallas, TX.
77. Siscovick DS, Raghunathan TE, Psaty BM *et al.* Diuretic therapy for hypertension and the risk of primary cardiac arrest. *N Engl J Med* 1994; 330: 1852–7.
78. Packer M, Gottlieb SS, Kessler PD. Hormone–electrolyte interactions in the pathogenesis of lethal cardiac arrhythmias in patients with congestive heart failure. *Am J Med* 1986; 80 (Suppl 4A): 23–9.
79. Singh BN, Hollenberg NK, Poole-Wilson PA, Robertson JIS. Diuretic-induced potassium and magnesium deficiency in relation to drug-induced QT prolongation, cardiac arrhythmias, and sudden death. *J Hypertens* 1992; 10: 301–16.
80. Bayliss J, Norell M, Canepa-Anson R *et al.* Untreated heart failure: clinical and neuroendocrine effects of introducing diuretics. *Br Heart J* 1987; 57: 17–22.
81. Francis GS, Benedict C, Johnstone DE *et al.* Comparison of neuroendocrine activation in patients with left ventricular dysfunction with and without congestive heart failure: a substudy of the studies of left ventricular dysfunction (SOLVD). *Circulation* 1990; 82: 1724–9.
82. Withering W. An account of the foxglove and some of its medical uses, with practical remarks on dropsy, and other diseases. In: FA Willins, TE Keys (eds) *Classics of cardiology*. Volume I. New York: Henry Schuman, Dover Publications, 1941, 231–52.
83. Gheorghiade M. Digoxin. *Cardiology Clinics: Annual of Drug Therapy* 1997; 1: 81–103.
84. Yusuf S. Clinical experience in protecting the failing heart. *Clin Cardiol* 1993; 16: II-27–9.
85. Christian HA. Digitalis effects in chronic cardiac cases with regular rhythm in contrast to auricular fibrillation. *Med Clin North Am* 1922; 5: 1173–90.
86. Luten D. Clinical studies of digitalis: effects produced by administration of massive dosage to patients with normal mechanism. *Arch Intern Med* 1924; 33: 251–78.
87. Marvin HM. Digitalis and diuretics in heart failure with regular rhythm, with special reference to importance of etiologic classification of heart disease. *J Clin Invest* 1927; 3: 521–39.
88. Godraind T. Stimulation and inhibition of the $Na^+$, $K^+$ pump by cardiac glycosides. In: K Greef (ed.) *Cardiac glycosides: Part I. Experimental pharmacology*. New York: Springer, 1981, 381–406.
89. Packer M. End of the oldest controversy in medicine. Are we ready to conclude the debate on digitalis? *N Engl J Med* 1997; 336: 575–6.
90. Kelly RA, Smith TW. Pharmacological treatment of heart failure. In: JG Hardman, LE Limbird, PB Molinoff *et al.* (eds) *Goodman and Gilman's Pharmacological basis of therapeutics*. 9th edition. New York: McGraw-Hill, 1996, 809–38.
91. Little WC, Rossi Jr, Freeman GL. Comparison of effects of dobutamine and ouabain on left ventricular contraction and relaxation in closed-chest dogs. *J Clin Invest* 1987; 80: 613–20.
92. Pw L, Cs H, Swaminathan R. The chronic effects of long-term digoxin administration on $Na^+/K^+$-ATPase activity in rat tissues. *Int J Cardiol* 1993; 40: 95–100.
93. Santana LF, Gomez AM, Lederer MJ. $Ca^{2+}$ flux through promiscuous cardiac $Na^+$ channels: slip mode conductance. *Science* 1998; 279: 1027–33.
94. Eichhorn EJ, Willard JE, Alvarez L *et al.* Are contraction and relaxation coupled in patients with and without congestive heart failure? *Circulation* 1992; 85: 2132–9.
95. van Veldhuisen DJ, Man in't Veld AJ, Dunselman PHJM *et al.* on behalf of the DIMT Study Group. Double-blind placebo-controlled study of ibopamine and digoxin in patients with mild to moderate heart failure: results of the Dutch Ibopamine Multicenter trial (DIMT). *J Am Coll Cardiol* 1993; 22: 1564–73.
96. Ferguson DW, Berg WJ, Sanders JS *et al.* Sympathoinhibitory responses to digitalis glycosides in heart failure patients. Direct evidence from sympathetic neural recordings. *Circulation* 1989; 80: 65–77.
97. Krum H, Bigger JT, Goldsmith RL, Packer M. Effect of long-term digoxin therapy on autonomic function in patients with chronic heart failure. *J Am Coll Cardiol* 1995; 25: 289–94.
98. Gheorghiade M, Ferguson D. Digoxin: a neurohormonal modulator in heart failure? *Circulation* 1991; 84: 2181–6.
99. Ribner HS, Plucinski DA, Hsieh AM *et al.* Acute effects of digoxin on total systemic vascular resistance in congestive heart failure due to dilated cardiomyopathy: a hemodynamic–hormonal study. *Am J Cardiol* 1985; 56: 896–904.
100. Slatton ML, Irani WN, Hall SA *et al.* Does digoxin provide additional hemodynamic and autonomic benefit at higher doses in patients with mild to moderate heart failure and normal sinus rhythm? *J Am Coll Cardiol* 1997; 29: 1206–13.
101. Gheorghiade M, Hall V, Fenn NM, Goldstein S. Chronic effects of digoxin withdrawal on neurohormones in patients with stable heart failure treated with converting enzyme inhibitors (Abstract). *Eur Heart J* 1993; 14 (Suppl): 131.
102. Newton GE, Tong JH, Schofield AM *et al.* Digoxin reduces cardiac sympathetic activity in severe congestive heart failure. *J Am Coll Cardiol* 1996; 28: 155–61.
103. Matsumori A, Ono K, Nishio R *et al.* Modulation of cytokine production and protection against lethal endotoxemia by the cardiac glycoside ouabain. *Circulation* 1997; 96: 1501–6.
104. Tsutamoto T, Wada A, Maeda K *et al.* Digitalis increases brain natriuretic peptide in patients with severe congestive heart failure. *Am Heart J* 1997; 134: 910–16.
105. Gold H, Cattell M, Greiner T *et al.* Clinical pharmacology of digoxin. *J Pharmacol Exp Ther* 1953; 109: 45–57.
106. Redfors A. The effect of different digoxin doses on subjective symptoms and physical working capacity in patients with atrial fibrillation. *Acta Med Scand* 1971; 190: 307–20.
107. Cattell M, Gold H. The influence of digitalis glycosides on the force of contraction of mammalian cardiac muscle. *J Pharmacol Exp Ther* 1938; 62: 116–25.
108. Bloomfield RA, Rapaport B, Milnor JP *et al.* The effects of the cardiac glycosides upon the dynamics of the circulation in congestive heart failure: I. Ouabain. *J Clin Invest* 1948; 27: 588–99.
109. McMichael J, Sharpey-Schafer EP. The action of intravenous digoxin in man. *Q J Med* 1944; 13: 123–35.

110. Selzer A, Kelly J. Action of digitalis upon the non-failing heart: a critical review. *Prog Cardiovasc Dis* 1964; 3: 273–83.
111. Selzer A, Malmborg R. Hemodynamic effect of digoxin in latent cardiac failure. *Circulation* 1962; 25: 695–702.
112. Stead EA, Warren JV, Brannon ES. Effect of lanatoside C on the circulation of patients with congestive heart failure: a study using catheterization of the right side of the heart. *Arch Intern Med* 1948; 81: 282–91.
113. Arnold SB, Byrd RC, Meister W *et al.* Long-term digitalis therapy improves left ventricular function in heart failure. *N Engl J Med* 1980; 303: 1443–8.
114. Hasenfuss G, Mulieri LA, Allen PD *et al.* Influence of isoproterenol and ouabain on excitation–contraction coupling, cross-bridge function and energetics in failing human myocardium. *Circulation* 1996; 94: 3155–60.
115. Sarter BH, Marchlinski FE. Redefining the role of digoxin in the treatment of atrial fibrillation. *Am J Cardiol* 1992; 69: 71–81G.
116. Braunwald E. Effects of digitalis on the normal and the failing heart. *J Am Coll Cardiol* 1985; 5: 51–9A.
117. Braunwald E, Bloodwell RD, Goldberg LI, Morrow AG. Studies on digitalis: IV. Observations in man on the effects of digitalis preparations on the contractility of the nonfailing heart and on total vascular resistance. *J Clin Invest* 1961; 40: 52–9.
118. Mason DT, Braunwald E. Studies on digitalis: IX. Effects of ouabain on the non-failing heart. *J Clin Invest* 1963; 42: 1105–11.
119. Mason DT, Braunwald E. Studies on digitalis: IX. Effects of ouabain on forearm vascular resistance and venous tone in normal subjects and in patients with heart failure. *J Clin Invest* 1964; 43: 532–43.
120. Rudman T, Gorcyzca CA, Pastor BH. The effect of digitalis on the cardiac output of the normal heart at rest and during exercise. *Ann Intern Med* 1961; 55: 620–31.
121. Gheorghiade M, Hall VB, Jacobsen G *et al.* Effects of increasing maintenance dose of digoxin on left ventricular function and neurohormones in patients with chronic heart failure treated with diuretics and angiotensin-converting enzyme inhibitors. *Circulation* 1995; 92: 1801–7.
122. Gheorghiade M, Hall V, Lakier J, Goldstein S. Comparative hemodynamic and neurohormonal effects of intravenous captopril and digoxin and their combinations in patients with severe heart failure. *J Am Coll Cardiol* 1989; 13: 134–42.
123. Tisdale JE, Gheorghiade M. Acute hemodynamic effects of digoxin alone or in combination with other vasoactive agents in patients with congestive heart failure. *Am J Cardiol* 1992; 69: 34–47G.
124. Guyatt GH, Sullivan MJ, Fallen EL *et al.* A controlled trial of digoxin in congestive heart failure. *Am J Cardiol* 1988; 61: 371–5.
125. Dibianco R, Shabetai R, Kostuk W *et al.* A comparison of oral milrinone, digoxin, and their combination in the treatment of patients with chronic heart failure. *N Engl J Med* 1989; 320: 677–83.
126. Packer M, Gheorghiade M, Young JB *et al.* for the RADIANCE Study. Withdrawal of digoxin from patients with chronic heart failure treated with angiotensin-converting-enzyme inhibitors. *N Engl J Med* 1993; 329: 1–7.
127. Uretsky BF, Young JB, Shahidi FE *et al.* on behalf of the PROVED Investigative Group. Randomized study assessing the effect of digoxin withdrawal in patients with mild to moderate congestive heart failure. Results of the PROVED trial. *J Am Coll Cardiol* 1993; 22: 955–62.
128. Digitalis Investigation Group. The effect of digoxin on mortality and morbidity in patients with heart failure. *N Engl J Med* 1997; 336: 525–33.
129. Smith TW, Antman EM, Friedman PL *et al.* Digitalis glycosides: mechanisms and manifestations of toxicity. *Prog Cardiovasc Dis* 1984; 26: 413–58, 495–540.
130. Smith TW, Haber E. Digoxin intoxication: the relationship of clinical presentation to serum digoxin concentration. *J Clin Invest* 1970; 49: 2377–86.
131. Beller GA, Smith TW, Abelmann WH *et al.* Digitalis intoxication: a prospective clinical study with serum level correlations. *N Engl J Med* 1971; 284: 989–97.
132. Antman EM, Wenger TL, Butler VP Jr *et al.* Treatment of 150 cases of life-threatening digitalis intoxication with digoxin-specific Fab antibody fragments: final report of a multicenter study. *Circulation* 1990; 81: 1744–52.
133. Hickey AR, Wenger TL, Carpenter VP *et al.* Digoxin immune Fab therapy in the management of digitalis intoxication: safety and efficacy results of an observational surveillance study. *J Am Coll Cardiol* 1991; 17: 590–8.
134. Schohn DC, Jahn HA, Pelletier BC. Dose-related cardiovascular effects of spironolatone. *Am J Cardiol* 1993; 71: 40–5A.
135. Mironneau J. Calcium channel antagonist effect of spironolactone on aldosterone antagonist. *Am J Cardiol* 1995; 65: 7–8K.
136. Brilla CG, Matsubara LS, Weber KT. Antifibrotic effects of spironolactone in preventing myocardial fibrosis in systemic arterial hypertension. *Am J Cardiol* 1993; 71: 12–16A.
137. Beller GA, Conroy J, Smith TW. Ischemia-induced alterations in myocardial ($Na^+$–$K^+$)-ATPase and cardiac glycoside bindings. *J Clin Invest* 1976; 57: 341–50.
138. Tanz RD. Possible contribution of digitalis-induced coronary constriction to toxicity. *Am Heart J* 1986; 111: 812–17.
139. Watanabe AM. Digitalis and the autonomic nervous system. *J Am Coll Cardiol* 1985; 5: 35–42A.
140. Sagar KB, Hanson EC, Powell WJ. Neurogenic coronary vasoconstrictor effects of digitalis during acute global ischemia in dogs. *J Clin Invest* 1977; 60: 1248–57.
141. Vatner SF, Higgins CB, Franklin D, Braunwald E. Effects of a digitalis glycoside on coronary and systemic dynamics in conscious dogs. *Circ Res* 1971; 28: 470–9.
142. Cooke IP, Shepherd JT, Vanhyoutte PM. Vasoconstriction induced by ouabain in the canine coronary artery: contribution of adrenergic and nonadrenergic responses. *Cardiovasc Drugs Ther* 1988; 2: 255–63.
143. Hewett KW, Rosen MR. Alpha and beta adrenergic interactions with ouabain-induced delayed afterdepolarizations. *J Pharmacol Exp Ther* 1984; 229: 188–92.
144. Hall SA, Cigarroa CG, Marcoux L *et al.* Time Course of improvement in left ventricular function, mass, and geometry in patients with congestive heart failure treated with β-adrenergic blockade. *J Am Coll Cardiol* 1995; 25: 1154–61.
145. Bristow MR, Gilbert EM. Improvement in cardiac myocyte function by biological effects of medical therapy: a new concept in the treatment of heart failure. *Eur Heart J* 1995; 16 (Suppl F): 20–31.
146. Eichhorn EJ, Heesch CM, Barnett JH *et al.* Effect of metoprolol on myocardial function and energetics in patients with nonischemic dilated cardiomyopathy: a randomized, double-blind, placebo-controlled study. *J Am Coll Cardiol* 1994; 24: 1310–20.
147. Waagstein F, Bristow MR, Swedberg *et al.* for the Metoprolol in Dilated Cardiomyopathy (MDC) Trial Study Group. Beneficial effects of metoprolol in idiopathic dilated cardiomyopathy. *Lancet* 1993; 342: 1441–6.

148. Bristow MR, O'Connell JB, Gilbert EM *et al.* for the Bucindolol Investigators. Dose–response of chronic β-blocker treatment in heart failure from either idiopathic dilated or ischemic cardiomyopathy. *Circulation* 1994; 89: 1632–42.
149. Australia–New Zealand Heart Failure Research Collaborative Group. Effects of carvedilol, a vasodilator-β-blocker, in patients with congestive heart failure due to ischemic heart disease. *Circulation* 1995; 92: 212–18.
150. Gilbert EM, Anderson JL, Deitchman D *et al.* Chronic β-blocker–vasodilator therapy improves cardiac function in idiopathic dilated cardiomyopathy: a double-blind, randomized study of bucindolol versus placebo. *Am J Med* 1990; 88: 223–9.
151. Woodley SL, Gilbert EM, Anderson JL *et al.* β-Blockade with bucindolol in heart failure due to ischemic vs idiopathic dilated cardiomyopathy. *Circulation* 1991; 84: 2426–41.
152. Olsen SL, Gilbert EM, Renlund DG *et al.* Carvedilol improves left ventricular function and symptoms in chronic heart failure: a double-blind randomized study. *J Am Coll Cardiol* 1995; 25: 1225–31.
153. Wisenbaugh T, Katz I, Davis J *et al.* Long-term (3 month) effects of a new beta-blocker (nebivolol) on cardiac performance in dilated cardiomyopathy. *J Am Coll Cardiol* 1993; 21: 1094–100.
154. CIBIS Investigators and Committees. A randomized trial of beta-blockade in heart failure: the Cardiac Insufficiency Bisoprolol Study (CIBIS). *Circulation* 1994; 90: 1765–73.
155. Bristow MR, Gilbert EM, Abraham WT *et al.* for the MOCHA Investigators. Carvedilol produces dose-related improvements in left ventricular function and survival in subjects with chronic heart failure. *Circulation* 1996; 94: 2807–16.
156. Packer M, Colucci WS, Sackner-Bernstein JD *et al.* for the PRECISE Study Group. Double-blind, placebo-controlled study of the effects of carvedilol in patients with moderate to severe heart failure. The PRECISE trial. *Circulation* 1996; 94: 2793–9.
157. Engelmeier RS, O'Connell JB, Walsh R *et al.* Improvement in symptoms and exercise tolerance by metoprolol in patients with dilated cardiomyopathy: a double-blind, randomized, placebo-controlled trial. *Circulation* 1985; 72: 536–46.
158. Pollock SG, Lytash J, Tedesco C *et al.* Usefulness of bucindolol in congestive heart failure. *Am J Cardiol* 1990; 66: 603–7.
159. Paolisso G, Gambardella A, Marrazzo G *et al.* Metabolic and cardiovascular benefits deriving from β-adrenergic blockade in chronic congestive heart failure. *Am Heart J* 1992; 123: 103–10.
160. Krum H, Sackner-Bernstein J, Goldsmith RL *et al.* Double-blind, placebo-controlled study of the long-term efficacy of carvedilol in patients with severe chronic heart failure. *Circulation* 1995; 92: 1499–506.
161. Fisher ML, Gottlieb SS, Plotnick GD *et al.* Beneficial effects of metoprolol in heart failure associated with coronary artery disease: a randomized trial. *J Am Coll Cardiol* 1994; 23: 943–50.
162. Dubach P, Bonetti P, Schertler Th *et al.* Beta blockade in CHF: not a class effect? Influence of bisoprolol on left ventricular size and function (Abstract). *Circulation* 1998; 98 (Suppl I): I-365.
163. Sabbah HN, Sharov VG, Gupta RC, Todor A, Singh V, Goldstein S. Chronic therapy with metoprolol attenuates cardiomyocyte apoptosis in dogs with heart failure. *J Am Coll Cardiol* 2000; 36: 1698–1705.
164. Eichhorn EJ, Grayburn PA, Mayer S *et al.* for The BEST Investigators. Myocardial viability by dobutamine stress echocardiography predicts improvement in ejection fraction with β-blockade in patients with heart failure: The BEST Trial. *J Am Coll Cardiol* 2001; 37: 179A.
165. Lowes BD, Gill EA, Abraham WT, Larrain JR, Robertson AD, Bristow MR, Gilbert EM. Effects of carvedilol on left ventricular mass, chamber geometry, and mitral regurgitation in chronic heart failure. *Am J Cardiol* 1999; 83: 1201–5.
166. Packer M, Bristow MR, Cohn JN *et al.* for the US Carvedilol Heart Failure Study Group. Effect of carvedilol on morbidity and mortality in chronic heart failure. *N Engl J Med* 1996; 334: 1349–55.
167. CIBIS-II Investigators and Committees. The Cardiac Insufficiency Bisoprolol Study II (CIBIS-II): a randomised trial. *Lancet* 1999; 353: 9–13.
168. International Steering Committee on Behalf of the MERIT-HF Study Group. Rationale, design, and organization of the Metoprolol CR/XL randomized intervention trial in heart failure (MERIT-HF). *Am J Cardiol* 1997; 80 (9B): 54–8J.
169. MERIT-HF Study Group. Effect of metoprolol CR/XL in chronic heart failure: Metoprolol CR/XL Randomised Interventions Trial in Congestive Heart Failure (MERIT-HF). *Lancet* 1999; 353: 2001–7.
170. Packer M, Coats AJS, Fowler MB *et al.* Effect of carvedilol on survival in severe chronic heart failure. *N Engl J Med* 2001; 344: 1651–8.
171. Goldstein S, Waagstein F, Hjalmarson A. The effect of metoprolol CR/XL in patients with severe heart failure in MERIT-HF. *J Am Coll Cardiol* 2001; 37 (Suppl A): 183A (abstr).
172. Eichhorn EJ, Domanski MJ, Krause-Steinrauf H, Bristow MR, Lavori PW for The BEST Investigators. A trial of the beta-adrenergic blocker bucindolol in patients with advanced chronic heart failure. *N Engl J Med* 2001; 344: 1659–67.
173. Cohn JN, Coats AJ. Heart failure 99 – the MOXCON story. *Int J Cardiol* 1999; 71(2): 109–11.
174. Eichhorn EJ, Hjalmarson Å. β-Blocker treatment for chronic heart failure: the frog prince. *Circulation* 1994; 90: 2153–6.
175. Lechat P, Escolano S, Golmard JL *et al.* on behalf of the CIBIS Investigators. Prognostic value of bisoprolol-induced hemodynamic effects in heart failure during the Cardiac Insufficiency Bisoprolol Study (CIBIS). *Circulation* 1997; 96: 2197–205.
176. Eberhardt RT, Kevak RM, Kang PM, Frishman WH. Angiotensin II receptor blockade: an innovative approach to cardiovascular pharmacotherapy. *J Clin Pharmacol* 1993; 33: 1023–38.
177. Wong PC, Price WA, Chiu AT *et al.* Nonpeptide angiotensin II receptor antagonists. VIII. Characterization of functional antagonism displayed by DuP 753, an orally active antihypertensive agent. *J Pharmacol Exp Ther* 1990; 252: 719–25.
178. Cazaubon C, Gougat J, Bousquet F *et al.* Pharmacological characterization of SR 47436, a new nonpeptide AT1 subtype angiotensin II receptor antagonist. *J Pharmacol Exp Ther* 1993; 265: 826–34.
179. Dickstein K, Chang P, Willenheimer R *et al.* Comparison of the effects of losartan and enalapril on clinical status and exercise performance in patients with moderate or severe chronic heart failure. *J Am Coll Cardiol* 1995; 26: 438–45.
180. Crozier I, Ikram H, Awan N *et al.* for the Losartan Hemodynamic Study Group. Losartan in heart failure. Hemodynamic effects and tolerability. *Circulation* 1995; 91: 691–7.
181. Hirsch H, Bijou R, Yuen J *et al.* Enalaprilat-mediated vasodilation is attenuated by indomethacin in congestive heart failure and completely abolished in normal subjects (Abstract). *Circulation* 1993; 88 (Suppl I): I-293.
182. Nakamura M, Funakoshi T, Arakawa N *et al.* Effect of angiotensin-converting enzyme inhibitors on endothelium-dependent peripheral

vasodilation in patients with chronic heart failure. *J Am Coll Cardiol* 1994; 24: 1321–7.
183. Booz GW, Baker KM. Role of type 1 and type 2 angiotensin receptors in angiotensin II-induced cardiomyocyte hypertrophy. *Hypertension* 1996; 28: 635–40.
184. Dzau VJ, Horiuchi M. Differential expression of angiotensin receptor subtypes in the myocardium: a hypothesis. *Eur Heart J* 1996; 17: 978–80.
185. Tanaka M, Ohnishi J, Ozawa Y *et al.* Characterization of angiotensin II receptor type 2 during differentiation and apoptosis of rat ovarian cultured granulosa cells. *Biochem Biophys Res Commun* 1995; 207: 593–8.
186. Spinale FG, de Gasparo M, Whitebread S *et al.* Modulation of the renin–angiotensin pathway through enzyme inhibition and specific receptor blockade in pacing-induced heart failure. I. Effects on left ventricular performance and neurohormonal systems. *Circulation* 1997; 96: 2385–96.
187. Ridker PM, Gaboury CL, Conlin PR *et al.* Stimulation of plasminogen activator inhibitor *in vivo* by infusion of angiotensin II: evidence of a potential interaction between the renin– angiotensin system and fibrinolytic function. *Circulation* 1993; 87: 1969–73.
188. Pitt B, Segal R, Martinez FA *et al.* on behalf of ELITE Study Investigators. Randomised trial of losartan versus captopril in patients over 65 with heart failure (Evaluation of Losartan in the Elderly Study, ELITE). *Lancet* 1997; 349: 747–52.
189. Pitt B, Poole-Wilson P, Segal R *et al.* on behalf of the ELITE II Investigators. Effect of losartan compared with captopril on mortality in patients with symptomatic heart failure: randomised trial – the Losartan Heart Failure Survival Study ELITE II. *Lancet* 2000; 355: 1582–7.
190. Pitt B, Dickstein K, Benedict CR *et al.* for the RAAS Investigators. The Randomized Angiotensin Receptor Antagonist–ACE Inhibitor Study (RAAS) — Pilot Study (Abstract). *Circulation* 1996; 94 (Suppl I): I-428.
191. Pitt B, Chang P, Grossman W *et al.* Rationale, background, and design of the Randomized Angiotensin Receptor Antagonist–Angiotensin–Converting Enzyme Inhibitor Study (RAAS). *Am J Cardiol* 1996; 78: 1129–31.
192. McKelvie RS, Yusuf S, Pericak D *et al.* Comparison of candesartan, enalapril, and their combination in congestive heart failure. Randomized Evaluation of Strategies for Left Ventricular Dysfunction (RESOLVD) Pilot Study. *Circulation* 1999; 100: 1056–64.
193. Cohn JN. Presentation at American Heart Association Scientific Sessions, Nov. 15, 2000, New Orleans, LA.
194. Shen Y-T, Lynch JJ, Wiedmann RT *et al.* Angiotensin II receptor antagonist enhances the effects of angiotensin converting enzyme inhibitor in conscious pigs with congestive heart failure (Abstract). *J Am Coll Cardiol* 1997; 29 (Suppl A): 244A.
195. Pylypchuk GB. ACE inhibitor-versus angiotensin II blocker-induced cough and angioedema. *Ann Pharmacother* 1998; 32: 1060–6.
196. Aroney CN, Semigran MJ, Dec GW *et al.* Inotropic effect of nicardipine in patients with heart failure: assessment by left ventricular end-systolic pressure-volume analysis. *J Am Coll Cardiol* 1989; 14: 1331–8.
197. Reid JL, Meredith PA, Donnelly R, Elliott HL. Pharmacokinetics of calcium antagonists. *J Cardiovasc Pharmacol* 1988; 12 (Suppl 7): S55–9.
198. Burges RA, Dodd MG, Gardiner DG. Pharmacologic profile of amlodipine. *Am J Cardiol* 1989; 64: 10–20I.
199. Fleckenstein A, Frey M, Zorn J, Fleckenstein-Grun G. Amlodipine, a new 1,4-dihydropyridine calcium antagonist with a particularly strong antihypertensive profile. *Am J Cardiol* 1989; 64: 21–34I.
200. Gradman AH. Hemodynamic effects of the vascular selective calcium antagonist felodipine in patients with impaired left ventricular function. *Am Heart J* 1992; 123: 273–8.
201. Massie BM. Mibefradil: a selective T-type calcium antagonist. *Am J Cardiol* 1997; 80: 23–32I.
202. Abernethy DR. Pharmacologic and pharmacokinetic profile of mibefradil, a T- and L-type calcium channel antagonist. *Am J Cardiol* 1997; 80: 4–11C.
203. Clozel JP, Veniant M, Osterrieder W. The structurally novel $Ca^{2+}$ channel blocker Ro 40-5967, which binds to the [$^3$H]desmethoxyverapamil receptor, is devoid of the negative inotropic effects of verapamil in normal and failing rat hearts. *Cardiovasc Drugs Ther* 1990; 4: 731–6.
204. Veniant M, Clozel JP, Wolfgang R. Ro 40-5967, in contrast to diltiazem does not reduce left ventricular contractility in rats with chronic myocardial infarction. *J Cardiovasc Pharmacol* 1991; 17: 272–84.
205. Katz AM. Calcium channel diversity in the cardiovascular system. *J Am Coll Cardiol* 1996; 28: 522–9.
206. Nuss HB, Houser SR. T-type $Ca^{2+}$ current is expressed in hypertrophied adult feline left ventricular myocytes. *Circ Res* 1993; 73: 777–82.
207. Sen L, Smith TW. T-type $Ca^{2+}$ channels are abnormal in genetically determined cardiomyopathic hamster hearts. *Circ Res* 1994; 75: 149–55.
208. Schmitt R, Clozel J-P, Iberg N, Buhler FR. Mibefradil prevents neointima formation after vascular injury in rasts. Possible role of the blockade of the T-type voltage-operated calcium channel. *Arterioscler Thromb Vasc Biol* 1995; 15: 1161–5.
209. Fifer MA, Colucci WS, Lorell BH *et al.* Inotropic, vascular and neuroendocrine effects of nifedipine in heart failure: comparison with nitroprusside. *J Am Coll Cardiol* 1985; 5: 731–7.
210. Agostoni PG, DeCesare N, Doria E *et al.* Afterload reduction: a comparison of captopril and nifedipine in dilated cardiomyopathy. *Br Heart J* 1986; 55: 391–9.
211. Elkayam U, Roth A, Hsueh W *et al.* Neurohormonal consequences of vasodilator therapy with hydralazine and nifedipine in severe congestive heart failure. *Am Heart J* 1986; 111: 1130–8.
212. Prida XE, Kubo SH, Laragh JH, Cody RJ. Evaluation of calcium-mediated vasoconstriction in chronic congestive heart failure. *Am J Med* 1983; 75: 795–800.
213. Elkayam U, Amin J, Mehra A *et al.* A prospective, randomized, double-blind, crossover study to compare the efficacy and safety of chronic nifedipine therapy with that of isosorbide dinitrate and their combination in the treatment of chronic congestive heart failure. *Circulation* 1990; 82: 1954–61.
214. Goldstein RE, Boccuzzi SJ, Cruess D, Nattel S, the Adverse Experience Committee and the Multicenter Diltiazem Postinfarction Research Group. Diltiazem increases late-onset congestive heart failure in postinfarction patients with early reduction in ejection fraction. *Circulation* 1991; 83: 52–60.
215. Packer M, O'Connor CM, Ghali JK *et al.* for the Prospective Randomized Amlodipine Survival Evaluation Study Group. Effect of amlodipine on morbidity and mortality in severe chronic heart failure. *N Engl J Med* 1996; 335: 1107–14.
216. Packer M. Presentation at the American College of Cardiology Scientific Sessions, March 15, 2000, Anaheim, CA.

217. Cohn JN, Ziesche S, Smith R *et al.* for the Vasodilator-heart Failure Trial (V-HeFT) Study Group. Effect of the calcium antagonist felodipine as supplementary vasodilator therapy in patients with chronic heart failure treated with enalapril. V-HeFT III. *Circulation* 1997; 96: 856–63.
218. Levine TB for the MACH-1 Investigators. The design of the mortality assessment in congestive heart failure trial (MACH-1, Mibefradil). *Clin Cardiol* 1997; 20: 320–6.
219. Elkayam U. MACH-1 presentation at the European Society of Cardiology Scientific Sessions, 23 August 1998, Vienna, Austria.
220. Colucci WS, Wright RF, Braunwald E. New positive inotropic agents in the treatment of congestive heart failure. *N Engl J Med* 1986; 314: 290–9.
221. Massie BM, Berk MR, Brozena SC *et al.* for the FACET Investigators. Can further benefit be achieved by adding flosequinan to patients with congestive heart failure who remain symptomatic on diuretic, digoxin, and an angiotensin converting enzyme inhibitor? *Circulation* 1993; 88: 492–501.
222. Packer M, Narahara KA, Elkayam U *et al.* and the Principal Investigators of the REFLECT Study. Double-blind, placebo-controlled study of the efficacy of flosequinan in patients with chronic heart failure. *J Am Coll Cardiol* 1993; 22: 65–72.
223. German and Austrian Xamoterol Group. Double-blind placebo-controlled comparison of digoxin and xamoterol in chronic heart failure. *Lancet* 1988; i: 489–93.
224. Uretsky BF, Generalovick T, Reddy PS *et al.* The acute hemodynamic effects of a new agent, MDL 17,043, in the treatment of congestive heart failure. *Circulation* 1983; 67: 823–8.
225. Monrad ES, Baim DS, Smith HS, Lanoue AS. Milrinone, dobutamine, and nitroprusside: comparative effects on hemodynamics and myocardial energetics in patients with severe congestive heart failure. *Circulation* 1986; 73 (Suppl III): III-168–74.
226. Gottlieb SS, Kukin ML, Penn J *et al.* Sustained hemodynamic response to flosequinan in patients with heart failure receiving angiotensin-converting enzyme inhibitors. *J Am Coll Cardiol* 1993; 22: 963–7.
227. Dies F, Krell MJ, Whitlow P *et al.* Intermittent dobutamine in ambulatory outpatients with chronic cardiac failure (Abstract). *Circulation* 1986; 74 (Suppl II): II-38.
228. Packer M, Carver JR, Chesebro JH *et al.* and the PROMISE investigators. Effect of milrinone on mortality in severe chronic heart failure. The prospective randomized milrinone survival evaluation (PROMISE). *N Engl J Med* 1991; 325: 1468–75.
229. Packer M, Rouleau J, Swedberg K and the PROFILE Investigators & Coordinators. Effect of flosequinan on survival in chronic heart failure: preliminary results of the PROFILE study (Abstract). *Circulation* 1993; 88 (Suppl I): I-301.
230. Xamoterol in Severe Heart Failure Study Group. Xamoterol in severe heart failure. *Lancet* 1990; 336: 1–6.
231. Packer M, Francis GS, Abrams J *et al.* Oral milrinone increases the risk of sudden death in severe chronic heart failure: the PROMISE trial (Abstract). *Circulation* 1991; 84: II-310.
232. Shakar SF, Abraham WT, Gilbert EM *et al.* Combined oral positive inotropic and beta-blocker therapy for treatment of refractory class IV heart failure. *J Am Coll Cardiol* 1998; 31: 1336–40.
233. Torre-Amione G, Kapadia S, Benedict C *et al.* Proinflammatory cytokine levels in patients with depressed left ventricular ejection fraction: a report from the Studies of Left Ventricular Dysfunction (SOLVD). *J Am Coll Cardiol* 1996; 27: 1201–6.
234. Levine B, Kalman J, Mayer L *et al.* Elevated circulating levels of tumor necrosis factor in severe chronic heart failure. *N Engl J Med* 1990; 323: 236–41.
235. Kubota T, McTiernan CF, Frye CS *et al.* Cardiac-specific overexpression of tumor necrosis factor-alpha causes lethal myocarditis in transgenic mice. *J Card Fail* 1997; 3: 117–24.
236. Bryant D, Becker L, Richardson J *et al.* Cardiac failure in transgenic mice with myocardial expression of tumor necrosis factor-$\alpha$. *Circulation* 1998; 97: 1375–81.
237. Kubota T, McTiernan CF, Frye CS *et al.* Dilated cardiomyopathy in transgenic mice with cardiac-specific overexpression of tumor necrosis factor-$\alpha$. *Circ Res* 1997; 81: 627–35.
238. Bristow MR. Tumor necrosis factor-$\alpha$ and cardiomyopathy. *Circulation* 1998; 97: 1375–81.
239. Vileek J, Lee TH. Tumor necrosis factor. *J Biol Chem* 1991; 266: 7313–16.
240. Cleutjens JPM. The role of metalloproteinases in heart disease. *Cardiovasc Res* 1996; 32: 816–21.
241. Mann DL, Spinale FG. Activation of matrix metalloproteinases in the failing human heart. Breaking the tie that binds. *Circulation* 1998; 98: 1699–702.
242. Bozkurt B, Kribbs SB, Clubb FJ *et al.* Pathophysiologically relevant concentrations of tumor necrosis factor-$\alpha$ promote progressive left ventricular dysfunction and remodeling in rats. *Circulation* 1998; 97: 1382–91.
243. Stetler-Stevenson W. Dynamics of matrix turnover during pathologic remodeling of the extracellular matrix. *Am J Pathol* 1996; 148: 1345–50.
244. Deswal A, Bozhurt B, Seta Y, Parilti-Eiswirth S, Hayes FA, Blosch C, Mann DL. Safety and efficacy of a soluble p75 tumor necrosis factor receptor (Enbrel, Etanercept) in patients with advanced heart failure. *Circulation* 1999; 99: 3224–6.
245. Yanagisawa M, Kurihara H, Kimura S *et al.* A novel potent vasoconstrictor peptide produced by vascular endothelial cells. *Nature* 1988; 332: 411–15.
246. Stevenson LW, Fonarow GC. Endothelin and the vascular choir in heart failure. *J Am Coll Cardiol* 1992; 20: 854–7.
247. Cody RJ, Haas GJ, Binkley PF *et al.* Plasma endothelin correlates with the extent of pulmonary hypertension in patients with chronic congestive heart failure. *Circulation* 1992; 85: 504–9.
248. Tsutamoto T, Wada A, Maeda Y *et al.* Relation between endothelin-1 spillover in the lungs and pulmonary vascular resistance in patients with chronic heart failure. *J Am Coll Cardiol* 1994; 23: 1427–33.
249. Sakurai T, Yanagisawa M, Takuwa Y *et al.* Cloning a cDNA encoding non-isopeptide-selective subtype of the endothelin receptor. *Nature* 1990; 348: 732–5.
250. Kiowski W, Sutsch G, Hunziker P *et al.* Evidence for endothelin-1-mediated vasoconstriction in severe chronic heart failure. *Lancet* 1995; 346: 732–6.
251. Shubeita HE, McDonough PM, Harris AN *et al.* Endothelin induction of inositol phospholipid hydrolysis, sarcomere assembly, and cardiac gene expression in ventricular myocytes. *J Biol Chem* 1990; 265: 20 555–62.
252. Lamers JMJ, Eskildsen-Helmond YEG, Resink AM *et al.* Endothelin-1 induced phopholipase C-$\beta$ and D and protein kinase C isoenzyme signaling leading to hypertrophy in rat cardiomyocytes. *J Cardiovasc Pharmacol* 1995; 26 (Suppl 3): S100–3.
253. Simonson MS, Wann S, Mene P *et al.* Endothelin stimulates phospholipase C, $Na^+/H^+$ exchange, c-*fos* expression, and mitogenesis in rat mesangial cells. *J Clin Invest* 1989; 83: 708–12.

254. Ito H, Hirata Y, Hiroe M *et al.* Endothelin-1 induces hypertrophy with enhanced expression of muscle-specific genes in cultured neonatal rat cardiomyocytes. *Circ Res* 1991; 69: 209–15.
255. Shichiri M, Hirata Y, Nakajima T *et al.* Endothelin-1 is an autocrine/paracrine growth factor for human cancer cell lines. *J Clin Invest* 1991; 87: 1867–71.
256. Sakai S, Yorikane R, Miyauchi T *et al.* Altered production of endothelin-1 in the hypertrophied rat heart. *J Cardiovasc Pharmacol* 1995; 26 (Suppl 3): S452–5.
257. Simonson MS, Wann S, Mene P *et al.* Endothelin stimulates phospholipase C $Na^+/H^+$ exchange, c-fos expression, and mitogenesis in rat mesangial cells. *J Clin Invest* 1989; 83: 708–12.
258. Haneda M, Kikkawa R, Koya D *et al.* Endothelin-1 stimulates tyrosine phosphorylation of p125 focal adhesion kinase in mesangial cells. *J Am Soc Nephrol* 1995; 6: 1504–10.
259. Mulder P, Richard V, Derumeaux G *et al.* Role of endogenous endothelin in chronic heart failure. Effect of long-term treatment with an endothelin antagonist on survival, hemodynamics, and cardiac remodeling. *Circulation* 1997; 96: 1976–82.
260. Spinale FG, Walker JD, Mukherjee R *et al.* Concomitant endothelin receptor subtype-A blockade during the progression of pacing-induced congestive heart failure in rabbits. Beneficial effects on left ventricular and myocyte function. *Circulation* 1997; 95: 1918–29.
261. Giles TD, Iteld BJ, Mautner RK *et al.* Short-term effects of intravenous clonidine in congestive heart failure. *Clin Pharmacol Ther* 1981; 30: 724–8.
262. Giles TD, Thomas MG, Sander GE, Quiroz AC. Central alpha-adrenergic agonists in chronic heart failure and ischemic heart disease. *J Cardiovasc Pharmacol* 1985; 7 (Suppl 8): S51–5.
263. Giles TD, Sander GE, Thomas MG, Quiroz AC. Alpha-adrenergic mechanisms in the pathophysiology of left ventricular heart failure an analysis of their role in systolic and diastolic dysfunction. *J Mol Cell Cardiol* 1986; 18 (Suppl 5): 33–43.
264. Giles TD, Thomas MG, Quiroz AC *et al.* Acute and short-term effects of clonidine in heart failure. *Angiology* 1987; 38: 537–48.
265. Manmontri A, MacLeod SM. Centrally acting sympatholytic agents in the treatment of congestive heart failure. A review of the literature. *Drugs* 1990; 40: 169–75.
266. van Zwieten PA. Central imidazoline ($I_1$) receptors as targets of centrally acting antihypertensives: moxonidine and rilmenidine. *J Hypertens* 1997; 15: 117–25.
267. Dickstein K, Kopp U, Manhenke C *et al.* The hemodynamic and neurohormonal effects of moxonidine, a sympathetic inhibitor, in congestive heart failure (Abstract). *J Am Coll Cardiol* 1997; 29 (Suppl): 170A.
268. Kangawa D, Matsuo H. Purification and complete amino acid sequence of alpha human atrial natriuretic polypeptide (a-hANP). *Biochem Biophys Res Commun* 1984; 118: 131–9.
269. Genest J, Cantin M. Atrial natriuretic factor. *Circulation* 1987; 75 (Suppl I): I-118–24.
270. Hamid Q, Wharton J, Terenghi G *et al.* Localization of atrial natriuretic peptide mRNA and immunoreactivity in the rat heart and human atrial appendage. *Proc Natl Acad Sci USA* 1987; 84: 6760–4.
271. Sudoh T, Maekawa K, Kojima M *et al.* Cloning and sequence analysis of cDNA encoding a predursor for human brain natriuretic peptide. *Biochem Biophys Res Commun* 1989; 159: 1427–34.
272. Nakao K, Mukoyama M, Hosoda K *et al.* Biosynthesis, secretion, and receptor selectivity of human brain natriuretic peptide. *Can J Physiol Pharmacol* 1991; 69: 1500–6.
273. Tateyama H, Hino J, Minamino N *et al.* Characterization of immunoreactive brain natriuretic peptide in human cardiac atrium. *Biochem Biophys Res Commun* 1990; 166: 1080–7.
274. Bonow RO. New insights into the cardiac natriuretic peptides. *Circulation* 1996; 93: 1946–50.
275. Boland DG, Abraham WT. Natriuretic peptides in heart failure. *Congest Heart Fail* 1998; March/April: 23–33.
276. Sudoh T, Minamino N, Kangawa K, Matsuo H. C-type natriuretic peptide (CNP): a new member of natriuretic peptide family identified in porcine brain. *Biochem Biophys Res Commun* 1990; 168: 863–70.
277. Feller SM, Gagelmann M, Forssmann WG. Urodilatin: a newly described member of the ANP family. *Trends Pharmacol Sci* 1989; 10: 93–4.
278. Yoshimura M, Yasue H, Okumura K *et al.* Different secretion patterns of atrial natriuretic peptide and brain natriuretic peptide in patients with congestive heart faliure. *Circulation* 1993; 87: 464–9.
279. Yoshibaysahi M, Kamiya T, Saito Y, Matsuo H. Increased plasma levels of brain natriuretic peptide in hypertrophic cardiomyopathy. *N Eng J Med* 1993; 329: 433–4.
280. Weidmann P, Hasler L, Gnadinger MP *et al.* Blood levels and renal effects of atrial netriuretic peptide in normal man. *J Clin Invest* 1986; 77: 734–42.
281. Zeidel ML. Hormonal regulation of inner medullary collecting duct sodium transport. *Am J Physiol* 1991; 265: F159–73.
282. Kleinert HD, Maack T, Atlas SA *et al.* Atrial natriuretic factor inhibits angiotensin-, norepinephrine-, and postassium-induced vascular contractility. *Hypertension* 1984; 6 (Suppl I): I-143–7.
283. Geller DM, Currie MG, Wakitani K *et al.* Atriopeptins: a family of potent biologically active peptides derived from mammalian atria. *Biochem Biophys Res Commun* 1984; 120: 333–8.
284. Stephenson SL, Kenny AJ. The hydrolysis of alpha-human atrial natriuretic peptide by pig kidney microvillar membranes is initiated by endopeptidase-24.11. *Biochem J* 1987; 243: 183–7.
285. Olins GM, Spear KL, Siegel NR *et al.* Atrial peptide inactivation by rabbit-kidney brush-border membranes. *Eur J Biochem* 1987; 170: 431–4.
286. Saito Y, Nakao K, Nishimura K *et al.* Clinical application of atrial natriuretic polypeptide in patients with congestive heart failure: beneficial effects on left ventricular function. *Circulation* 1987; 76: 115–24.
287. Molina CR, Fowler MB, McCrory S *et al.* Hemodynamic, renal, and endocrine effects of atrial natriuretic peptide infusion in severe heart failure. *J Am Coll Cardiol* 1988; 12: 175–86.
288. Cody RJ, Atlas SA, Laragh JH *et al.* Atrial natriuretic factor in normal subjects and heart failure patients: plasma levels and renal, hormonal, and hemodynamic responses to peptide infusion. *J Clin Invest* 1986; 78: 1362–74.
289. Richards AM, McDonald D, Fitzpatrick MA *et al.* Atrial natriuretic hormone has biological effects in man at physiological plasma concentrations. *J Clin Endocrinol Metab* 1988; 67: 1134–9.
290. Floras JS. Sympathoinhibitory effects of atrial natriuretic factor in normal humans. *Circulation* 1990; 81: 1860–73.
291. Wu C-F, Bishopric NH, Pratt RE. Atrial natriuretic peptide induces apoptosis in neonatal rat cardiac myocytes. *J Biol Chem* 1997; 272: 14 860–6.
292. Shenker Y, Sider RS, Ostafin EA, Grekin RJ. Plasma levels of immunoreactive atrial natriuretic factor in healthy subjects and in patients with edema. *J Clin Invest* 1985; 76: 1684–7.
293. Raine AEG, Erne P, Burgisser E *et al.* Atrial natriuretic peptide and atrial pressure in patients with congestive heart failure. *N Engl J Med* 1986; 315: 533–7.

294. Burnett JC Jr, Kao PC, Hu DC *et al.* Atrial natriuretic peptide elevation in congestive heart failure in the human. *Science* 1986; 231: 1145–7.
295. Wei CM, Heutlein DM, Perrella MA *et al.* Natriuretic peptide system in human heart failure. *Circulation* 1993; 88: 1004–9.
296. Gottlieb SS, Kukin ML, Ahern D, Packer M. Prognostic importance of atrial natriuretic peptide in patients with chronic heart failure. *J Am Coll Cardiol* 1989; 13: 1334–9.
297. Swedberg K, Eneroth P, Kjekshus J, Wilhelmsen L for the CONSENSUS Trial Study Group. Hormones regulating cardiovascular function in patients with severe congestive heart failure and their relation to mortality. *Circulation* 1990; 82: 1730–6.
298. Yasue H, Yoshimura M, Sumida H *et al.* Localization and mechanism of secretion of B-type natriuretic peptide in comparison with those of A-type natriuretic peptide in normal subjects and patients with heart failure. *Circulation* 1994; 90: 195–203.
299. Tsutamoto T, Wada A, Maeda K *et al.* Attenuation of compensation of endogenous cardiac natriuretic peptide system in chronic heart failure. Prognostic role of plasma brain natriuretic peptide concentration in patients with chronic symptomatic left ventricular dysfunction. *Circulation* 1997; 96: 509–16.
300. Hermann HC, Rosenthal AD, Davis CA. Cardiovascular effects of intracoronary atrial natriuretic peptide administration in man. *Am Heart J* 1990; 120: 308–15.
301. Anand IS, Kalra GS, Ferrari R *et al.* Hemodynamic hormonal, and renal effects of atrial natriuretic peptide in untreated congestive cardiac failure. *Am Heart J* 1989; 118: 500–5.
302. Crozier IG, Nicholls MG, Ikram H *et al.* Haemodynamic effects of atrial natriuretic peptide infusion in heart failure. *Lancet* 1986; ii: 1242–5.
303. Yoshimura M, Yasue H, Morita E *et al.* Hemodynamic, renal, and hormonal responses to brain natriuretic peptide infusion in patients with congestive heart failure. *Circulation* 1991; 84: 1581–8.
304. Hobbs RE, Miller LW, Bott-Silverman C *et al.* Hemodynamic effects of a single intravenous injection of synthetic human brain natriuretic peptide in patients with heart failure secondary to ischemic or idiopathic dilated cardiomyopathy. *Am J Cardiol* 1996; 78: 896–901.
305. Marcus LS, Hart D, Packer M *et al.* Hemodynamic and renal excretory effects of human brain natriuretic peptide infusion in patients with congestive heart failure. *Circulation* 1996; 94: 3184–9.
306. Gomes MPV, Hobbs RE. B-type (brain) natriuretic peptide: a new therapeutic agent for the treatment of heart failure. *Congest Heart Fail* 1998; 4: 15–21.
307. Abraham WT, Lowes BD, Ferguson DA *et al.* Systemic hemodynamic, neurohormonal, and renal effects of a steady-state infusion of human brain natriuretic peptide in patients with hemodynamically decompensated heart failure. *J Card Fail* 1998; 4: 37–44.
308. Roques BP, Noble F, Dauge V, Fournie-Zaluski MC. Neutral endopeptidase 24.11: structure, inhibition, and experimental and clinical pharmacology. *Pharmacol Rev* 1993; 45: 87–146.
309. Richards M, Espiner E, Frampton C *et al.* Inhibition of endopeptidase EC 24.11 in humans: renal and endocrine effects. *Hypertension* 1990; 16: 269–76.
310. Margulies KB, Cavero PG, Seymour AA *et al.* Neutral endopeptidase inhibition potentiates the renal actions of atrial natriuretic factor. *Kidney Int* 1990; 38: 67–72.
311. Jardine A, McConnell J, Dilly SG *et al.* Pharmacologic elevation of endogenous ANF in man using the atriopeptidase inhibitor (UK 69578) (Abstract). *J Am Coll Cardiol* 1989; 13: 76A.
312. Rademaker MT, Charles CJ, Espiner EA *et al.* Neutral endopeptidase inhibition: augmented atrial and brain natriuretic peptide, haemodynamic and natriuretic responses in ovine heart failure. *Clin Sci* 1996; 91: 283–91.
313. Wegner M, Hirth-Dietrich C, Stasch JP. Role of neutral endopeptidase 24.11 in AV fistular rat model of heart failure. *Cardiovasc Res* 1996; 31: 891–8.
314. Cleland JG, Swedberg K. Lack of efficacy of neutral endopeptidase inhibitor ecadotril in heart failure. The International Ecadotril Multi-centre Dose-ranging Study Investigators (Letter). *Lancet* 1998; 351: 1657–8.
315. Norcini G, Morazzoni G, Pocchiari F *et al.* Phosphonamide inhibitors of neutral endopeptidase (EC 3.4.24.11). *J Enzyme Inhib* 1997; 12: 71–7.
316. Kentsch M, Otter W, Drummer C *et al.* Neutral endopeptidase 24.11 inhibition may not exhibit beneficial haemodynamic effects in patients with congestive heart failure. *Eur J Clin Pharmacol* 1996; 51: 269–72.
317. Rademaker MT, Fitzpatrick MA, Charles CJ *et al.* Comparison of chronic neutral endopeptidase inhibition and furosemide in an ovine model of heart failure. *J Cardiovasc Pharmacol* 1996; 27: 439–46.
318. Kimmelstiel CD, Perrone R, Kilcoyne L *et al.* Effects of renal neutral endopeptidase inhibition on sodium excretion, renal hemodynamics and neurohormonal activation in patients with congestive heart failure. *Cardiology* 1996; 87: 46–53.
319. Robl JA, Sun CQ, Stevenson J *et al.* Dual metalloprotease inhibitors: mercaptoacetyl-based fused heterocyclic dipeptide mimetics as inhibitors of angiotensin-converting enzyme and neutral endopeptidase. *J Med Chem* 1997; 40: 1570–7.
320. Cohn JN, Johnson GR, Shabetai R *et al.* for the V-HeFT VA Cooperative Studies Group. Ejection fraction, peak exercise oxygen consumption, cardiothoracic ratio, ventricular arrhythmias, and plasma norepinephrine as determinants of prognosis in heart failure. *Circulation* 1993; 87 (Suppl VI): VI-5–16.
321. Cohn JN, Rector TS. Prognosis of congestive heart failure and predictors of mortality. *Am J Cardiol* 1988; 62: 25–30A.
322. Glover DR, Littler WA. Factors influencing survival and mode of death in severe chronic ischaemic cardiac failure. *Br Heart J* 1987; 57: 125–32.
323. Unverferth DV, Magorien RD, Moeschberger ML *et al.* Factors influencing the one-year mortality of dilated cardiomyopathy. *Am J Cardiol* 1984; 54: 147–52.

# Targeting genes and modulating signal transduction in cardiomyopathies

30

R. J. HAJJAR, T. L. FORCE AND A. ROSENZWEIG

## Introduction

Targeting genes to the heart through somatic gene transfer has the potential to alter the approach to patients with cardiomyopathy in two distinct, yet related, ways. First, the ability to manipulate signal transduction pathways in relevant *in vitro* and *in vivo* models of cardiovascular disease allows the role of these pathways in disease pathogenesis to be tested. In this way, disease mechanisms and causal relationships can be elucidated and potential targets for therapeutic intervention can be identified. Moreover, gene transfer allows rapid integration into clinically relevant models of the latest developments in molecular and cell biology. Once a target has been identified, the full spectrum of therapeutic avenues is available for consideration. These include traditional pharmacological agents, targeted synthesis of small molecule agonists or antagonists, or delivery of biological agents (cells, antibodies, genetic material). Gene transfer allows hypotheses about the mechanisms of disease to be tested and, it is hoped, therapy to be tailored accordingly. Secondly, investigators learn valuable lessons about local modulation of these pathways through somatic gene transfer. Ultimately, gene transfer, which serves initially as an experimental tool, may provide a novel therapeutic approach.

Signal transduction encompasses a broad range of molecular mechanisms linking external stimuli to intracellular responses. Stimuli may include soluble factors such as growth factors, hormones, or cytokines, as well as mechanical forces, or signals transmitted directly from one cell to another. Whatever the source, these signals initiate a carefully orchestrated cascade of molecular interactions that ultimately determine the cell's response or phenotype. In the myopathic heart, a several important stimuli have been delineated, but unequivocally identifying the mechanisms by which these stimuli contribute to the observed pathology is frequently confounded by simultaneous alterations in multiple signalling pathways in the complex milieu of the failing heart. Gene transfer allows one to overexpress either a normal (wild-type) form of a specific signalling molecule or a mutant that has either no activity (null mutant) or actually blocks the endogenous activity of this molecule (dominant negative mutant). By perturbing a specific signalling pathway in this manner, the functional relevance of this pathway to the pathogenesis of the cardiomyopathy can be assessed.

To understand efforts at targeting genes to modulate the pathogenesis of cardiomyopathies, an understanding of both the technology of gene transfer and the biology of signal transduction as it relates to cardiomyopathies is required. Dramatic advances have been made in both areas in recent years, some of which will be highlighted here. First, cardiovascular somatic gene transfer is considered and both the vectors employed and current approaches to *in vivo* delivery of these vectors to the heart are reviewed. Secondly, specific targets relevant to cardiomyopathy that are currently being investigated in experimental models are considered. Phenotypes to be considered include abnormalities of contractile function, cardiac hypertrophy, and cardiomyocyte apoptosis. In each section, the primary signalling pathways thought to contribute these pathological phenotypes are discussed.

## Targeting genes to the heart

### Overview

A brief review of essential genetic principles and a few definitions will be useful to the clinical reader.

The inheritable blueprint for mammalian cells is stored primarily in the form of deoxyribonucleic acid (DNA) packaged into chromosomes located in the cell's nucleus. This DNA serves as a template for the transcription of messenger ribonucleic acid (mRNA). mRNA moves to the cytoplasm where it, in turn, serves as a template for the synthesis of the proteins that fulfil the structural and functional missions of the cell. The DNA ultimately responsible for the production of a particular protein is referred to as a gene. Each gene includes not only the DNA sequence (coding sequence) that directs which amino acids are assembled into the protein, but also other sequences that are not ultimately translated into protein. These non-coding regions include the gene's promoter, which controls the transcription of mRNA from the gene and frequently other sequences, called introns, interspaced throughout the coding sequence. During the generation of mRNA these introns are removed.

In the laboratory, DNA is more stable and easier to manipulate than RNA. For this reason, a mRNA sequence is frequently used to generate a complementary DNA molecule (cDNA) that can then be more conveniently handled in the laboratory. The cDNA contains the full coding sequence for a specific protein, but it must be combined with other sequences for expression in mammalian cells. Of particular importance is a mammalian promoter which can direct the production of mRNA from the cDNA template. The promoter, cDNA, and other sequences incorporated to facilitate expression comprise a unit referred to as a mammalian expression cassette. Delivery of a competent mammalian expression cassette to the cell nucleus results in the production of mRNA, which moves to the cytoplasm and serves as a template for the ribosomal production of the encoded protein. The amount of protein produced is critically dependent not only on elements of the incorporated sequence (e.g. the promoter), but also on a complex array of ancillary issues that affect the ability of the cDNA to reach the nucleus and be transcribed.

## Somatic gene transfer

Introduction of genetic material into the cells and tissues of the body is termed somatic gene transfer, in contradistinction to genetic manipulation of the germline, as in a transgenic mouse model. Despite the nomenclature, the material being transferred is most commonly not the gene but rather cDNA in a mammalian expression cassette. The cDNA may be delivered in its pure form (naked DNA) or packaged in association with a variety of vehicles or vectors designed to enhance gene transfer. Available vectors are conceptually divided into non-viral vectors employing physical–chemical gene delivery and recombinant viral vectors in which the cDNA of interest has been incorporated into a virus, which is then used to infect the target cell and in the process conveys the exogenous cDNA.

Expression of the transferred gene (or transgene) can be quantified in two fundamental ways: the efficiency and level of expression. Efficiency refers to the number of cells expressing the transgene divided by total number of cells in the population, and is usually denoted as a percentage. The level of expression indicates the total amount of exogenous protein expressed. While these parameters are conceptually distinct, they are often related in practical terms. For example, the determined efficiency of gene transfer depends critically on the sensitivity of the assay used to detect gene expression. Using a more sensitive assay, expression may be detectable in a higher percentage of the cell population even though the intrinsic efficiency of gene transfer has not changed. In addition, an increase in the level of expression, perhaps through the use of a stronger promoter, usually improves the calculated efficiency since transgene expression now exceeds the threshold necessary for detection in more cells.

As systems for cardiovascular gene transfer are developed, reporter genes encoding proteins that are easily identified and/or quantitated are frequently used. In general, these proteins have either enzymatic activity (e.g. β-galactosidase, luciferase) or intrinsic fluorescent properties (e.g. green fluorescent protein). While reporter constructs have proven extremely useful in establishing and characterizing gene transfer models, it is important to realize that they are an imperfect model for the ultimate goal of such studies. First, the expressed reporter protein may have effects that confound experimental results: β-Galactosidase, for example, evokes a significant host immune response which can be difficult to distinguish from the response to the vector itself [1]. Secondly, the level of expression detectable for a particular reporter gene depends on the sensitivity of the assay system and probably bears no relationship to a biologically relevant functional endpoint. The level of expression required of the relevant transgene to mediate a specific effect varies tremendously with the specific application and may be either grossly overestimated or underestimated by the use of a reporter construct. Therefore, the appropriate tools (vector, construct, delivery system) also differ with the specific application. To test the ability of a particular gene transfer approach to modulate a particular biological pathway, it is ultimately necessary to do just that without interposing a surrogate marker.

While an exhaustive review of vector systems is beyond the scope of this chapter, certain general principles can be identified. Non-viral vectors have thus far had unacceptably low transfection efficiencies for *in vivo* applications that require transduction of a large proportion of myocytes. However, applications that require only a low level of expression in a small percentage of cells may well be suitable for such approaches. The use of viral vectors significantly heightens biosafety concerns about possible contamination with replication-competent virus and the transgene-independent host response to the vector itself. Among viral vectors, retroviruses have been the most extensively studied and used clinically. However, retroviral vectors require an actively dividing host cell and are therefore not generally suitable for cardiac gene transfer. Recombinant adenoviral vectors, in contrast, can infect and transduce non-replicating cells. Many investigators have now demonstrated the feasibility of both *in vitro* and *in vivo* cardiac gene transfer and these vectors will be considered in more detail.

## Adenoviral vectors

Adenoviruses are a family of double-stranded DNA viruses that cause a variety of clinical diseases including acute upper respiratory illnesses, conjunctivitis, and gastroenteritis [2]. In a normal host, these illnesses are self-limited and terminated by the host's immune response to the virus. Viral replication and expression of most viral gene products are critically dependent on a family of transcription factors encoded in the *E1* locus of the virus. Substitution of an engineered mammalian expression cassette for *E1* results in a 'first-generation' recombinant adenoviral vector that can infect many mammalian cells but can replicate effectively only in a helper cell line that has been engineered to provide the products of *E1*. In a normal mammalian cell, the recombinant adenovirus is internalized and its DNA is efficiently transported to the cell nucleus. In the absence of *E1* products, the endogenous viral promoters are relatively quiescent, while the mammalian expression cassette has been engineered to yield high-level transgene expression. In this way, highly evolved viral mechanisms are exploited to facilitate delivery and expression of the transgene.

Recombinant adenoviral vectors offer several significant advantages. The viruses can be prepared at extremely high titre, infect non-replicating cells, and allow incorporation of relatively large or even multiple cDNAs. Recombinant adenoviral vectors offer the opportunity to investigate the role of local signal transduction pathways in both *in vitro* and *in vivo* model systems. These vectors confer high-efficiency and high-level transduction of cardiomyocytes *in vitro* [3, 4]. Numerous investigators have also achieved *in vivo* cardiac gene transfer using recombinant adenoviral vectors carrying reporter genes [5–9]. In addition, using an *in vivo* perfusion approach (Fig. 30.1), the feasibility of modulating ventricular funcion through direct *in vivo* adenoviral gene transfer has been demonstrated [9]. In this approach, the viral solution is injected above the aortic valve while the aorta and pulmonary artery are transiently cross-clamped. The virus is thereby forced down the coronaries, resulting in relatively diffuse transduction of the myocardium. Alternative approaches, such as direct myocardial injection and selective coronary cannulation, are also being actively pursued, but result in focal transgene expression and may be more applicable to focal diseases such as ischaemic heart disease rather than cardiomyopathies which often affect the heart more globally. Nevertheless, these early animal studies establish that *in vivo* adenoviral gene transfer can not only achieve transgene expression in the myocardium, but also modulate intrinsic functional properties of the intact heart. While expression and functional effects need to be assessed for each application individually, these data encouragingly suggest that recombinant adenoviral vectors with this transduction technique produce functionally important expression in a substantial proportion of the myocardium. Moreover, neither the *in vivo* gene transfer protocol nor control viruses (carrying reporter genes alone) affect left ventricular function [9].

The effectiveness of the normal host immune response to adenovirus accounts for the self-limited nature of infections caused by wild-type genes and contributes to the favourable biosafety profile of recombinant adenoviral vectors. However, it also results in the major disadvantages of adenoviral gene transfer: transience of expression and a potentially deleterious host immune/inflammatory response to the vectors themselves. Gene transfer to adult myocardium *in vivo* has generally been found to mediate hgih-level expression for 1–2 weeks [5–8, 10, 11]. Four days after transduction, a significant mononuclear leucocyte infiltrate becomes evident and is probably the predominant mechanism limiting the duration of expression [12]. By

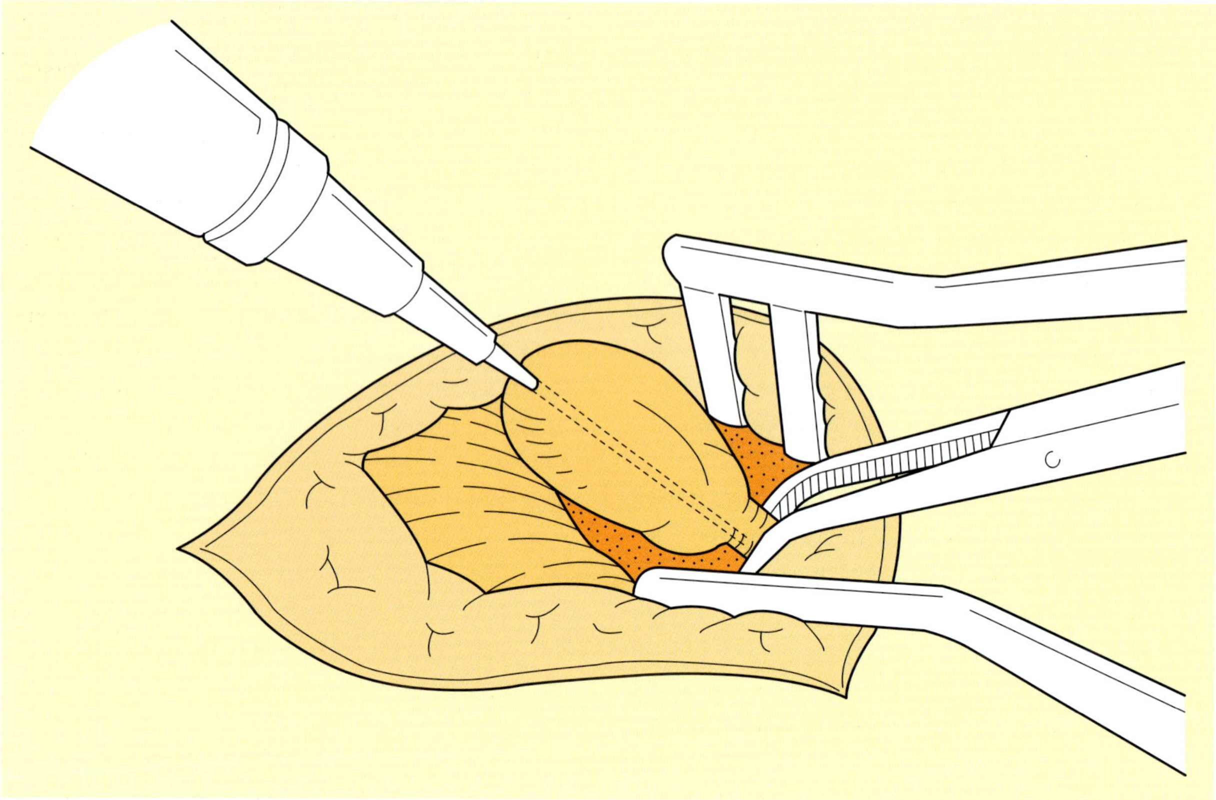

**Figure 30.1** *Cardiac delivery of recombinant adenoviral vectors to whole heart* in vivo. *To achieve generalized cardiac gene transfer, viral solution is injection above the aortic valve while the aorta and pulmonary artery are transiently cross-clamped. Animals tolerate the procedure well and injection of control virus has no significant physiological effects on ventricular function. In contrast, this method achieves expression of functionally relevant transgenes in a proportion of the myocardium sufficient to modulate overall left ventricular function [9].*

2–4 weeks after infection, transgene expression has usually either declined dramatically or been extinguished completely. The decrease in transgene expression can also be associated with local scarring and disruption of normal architectural features around the site of injection by 3–4 months after injection, which may also be exacerbated by the mechanical trauma of direct myocardial injection [12].

## Improved vectors

The initial working hypothesis that adenoviral replication and gene expression require *E1* translates into a reasonable but imperfect model. Either because the requirement for *E1* products is incomplete or because other transcription factors in the host cell can genetically complement the *E1* deletion, expression of other viral gene products can occur after infection with *E1*-deleted adenoviral vectors [13]. Moreover, *in vivo* the host immune response appears to be directed, at least in part, to viral antigens expressed after infection [1, 13]. Therefore, recent efforts have been focused on improving the initial first-generation adenoviral vectors by further crippling critical viral genes. In this way, additional barriers to viral gene expression and replication will exist, and even complementation of the *E1* deletion (by host transcription factors or another viral infection) will not restore viral functions. The consequent reduction in viral antigen production would then be predicted to attenuate the host immune response and prolong the duration of transgene expression.

Proof for this concept was first provided by second-generation adenovirus vectors which contain a single-base substitution in the *E2a*-encoded DNA-binding protein, part of the adenovirus-specific DNA polymerase [13]. Gene transfer to mouse liver *in vivo* with these second-generation vectors lasted for over 70 days (compared with 14 days with first-generation constructs) and invoked much less leucocyte infiltration [13]. Although this work first established the validity of this approach to improving adenoviral vectors, the temperature-sensitive mutation resulted in slower growth and lower yields, substantially increasing the associated labour and expense.

Adenoviral vectors are currently being developed that either delete additional essential viral genes, such as E4 [14–17], or use a 'helper virus' strategy to generate a 'gutted' virus virtually devoid of all viral genes [18, 19]. These approaches need to be empirically tested. Moreover, gene transfer results often differ for different species and different target organs. Subsequent viral vectors need to be rigorously compared for cardiovascular gene transfer in realistic, preclinical models before the potential of vectors already available in basic laboratories can be assessed fully. Nevertheless, it seems reasonable to anticipate that significant advances in the available gene transfer vectors will occur in coming years that will open a wider array of clinical problems to this approach. In the meantime, vectors that are currently in use provide a powerful experimental tool to help in the understanding of the pathophysiology of cardiomyopathies and thus to identify targets for intervention. Clinical use of current vector systems is likely to prove effective only in the minority of specific situations where the clinical and biological goals are suited to current technological limitations.

## Specific targets: contractile function

The intrinsic contractile function of the heart depends on a number of subcellular mechanisms which include: (1) neurohormonal receptors that can significantly modulate cardiac function; (2) various processes responsible for excitation–contraction coupling; and (3) contractile proteins [20]. In the setting of heart failure, alterations occur in all three subcellular mechanisms [20–24]. Although a number of abnormalities has been identified in failing hearts, it is not clear whether these changes are adaptive or pathogenic. Targeting these mechanisms by gene transfer allows investigators to test the role of these mechanisms in the pathogenesis of heart failure and cardiomyopathy, and in developing strategies for gene therapy.

### Neurohormonal receptors

The autonomic nervous system, through adrenergic and cholinergic stimulation of sarcolemmal receptors, profoundly affects the function of the heart. As shown in Figure 30.2, these receptors are coupled to G proteins, which elicit a spectrum of biochemical activities.

#### *β-Adrenergic receptors and G proteins*

Cardiac β-adrenergic receptors are mainly of the $\beta_1$-receptor type, although about 20% are of the $\beta_2$-subtype [25]; both β-receptors are coupled to heterotrimeric G proteins. Occupancy of the β-adrenergic receptor by G proteins leads to activation of adenylyl cyclase and the formation of cyclic adenosine monophosphate (cAMP), an important second messenger in myocardial cells [25]. G proteins consist of α, β, and γ subunits, and are further subdivided depending on the subunit into $G_s$, $G_i$, $G_q$, or $G_{12/13}$. Upon receptor stimulation, the heterotrimer splits into the guanosine triphosphate (GTP) bound and activated α-subunit and the β/γ subunits. The GTP-bound $Gs_\alpha$ subunit stimulates adenylyl cyclase activity, generating cAMP. Human ventricular myocardium also contains a third β-receptor, the $\beta_3$ subtype [26], which couples to $G_i$, resulting in the inhibition of adenylyl cyclase activity. Stimulation of $\beta_3$-receptors has a negative inotropic effect, but the mechanisms underlying this effect are not clear. Upon occupancy, $\beta_1$- and $\beta_2$-receptors are phosphorylated by a family of β-adrenergic receptor kinases (βARK), which cause desensitization of the receptors [27, 28].

#### *Cyclic AMP*

cAMP is an important modulator of cardiac cellular function. Most of the effects of cAMP are mediated by cAMP-dependent protein kinases that phosphorylate a number of intracellular enzymes. Phosphorylation of L-type calcium ($Ca^{2+}$) channels increases the entry of $Ca^{2+}$ through the channel; phosphorylation of phospholamban removes the inhibition of phospholamban on the sarcoplasmic reticulum $Ca^{2+}$-ATPase (SERCA), allowing the $Ca^{2+}$ pump of the sarcoplasmic reticulum (SR) to lower intracellular $Ca^{2+}$ at a faster rate during relaxation; and phosphorylation of troponin I decreases the sensitivity of the myofilaments to $Ca^{2+}$, allowing faster release of $Ca^{2+}$ during relaxation. The turnover of cAMP is rapid, with a balance between its formation by adenylyl cyclase and its breakdown by phosphodiesterase [29–35].

#### *$\alpha_1$-Receptors, angiotensin II type 1 and endothelin*

Agonists that bind these receptors are potent inducers of cardiac hypertrophy. These receptors share the property of activating phospholipase Cβ (PLCβ) through a G protein, $G_q$. Activated PLCβ hydrolyses membrane-bound phosphatidylinositol biphosphate ($PIP_2$), releasing inositol triphosphate ($IP_3$) and 1,2-diacylglycerol (DAG). $IP_3$ releases $Ca^{2+}$ from the (SR), while DAG activates protein kinase C (PKC). Both increased cytosolic [$Ca^{2+}$] and PKC regulate the growth and hypertrophy of myocardial cells [36, 37].

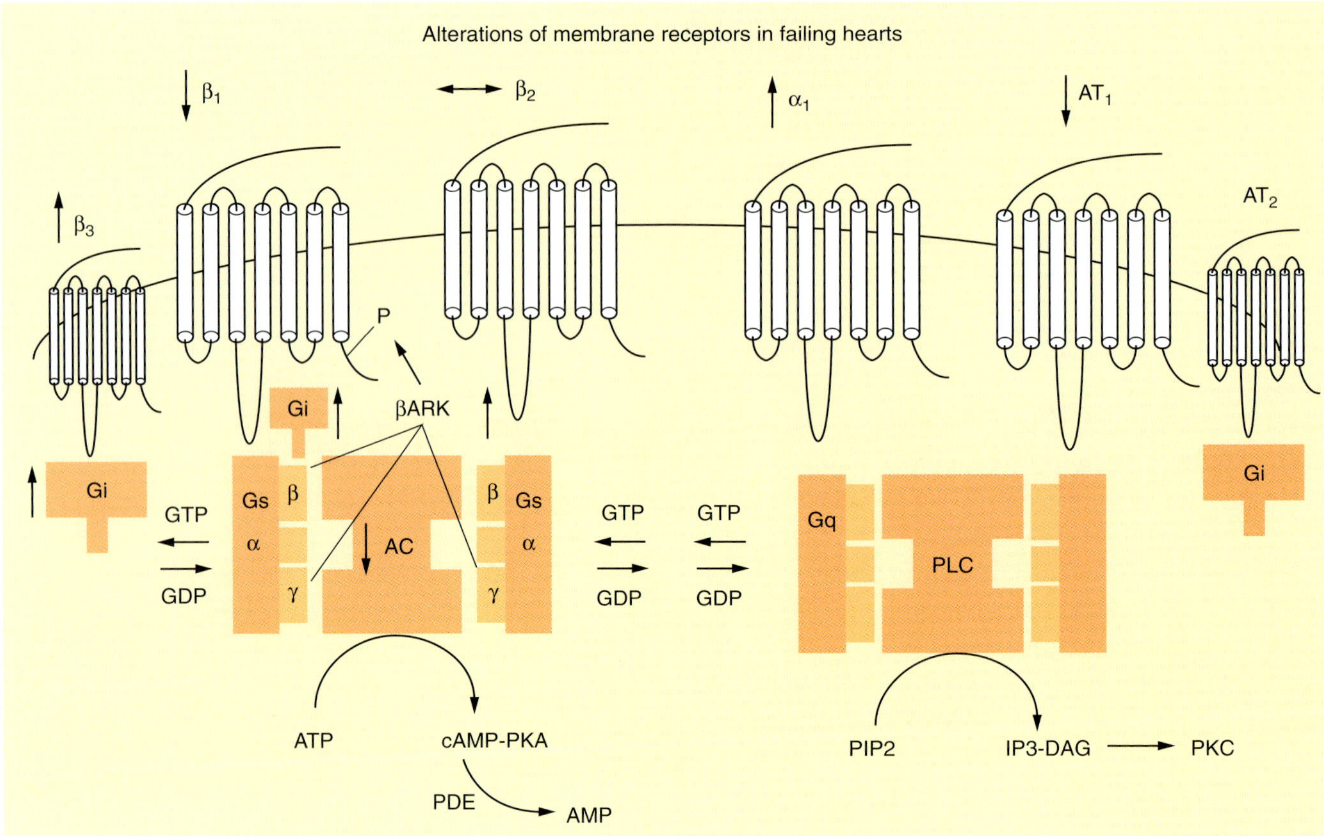


**Figure 30.2** *Alterations in the major components of β-adrenergic signal transduction and the angiotensin receptor signalling pathways in failing human hearts.* $\beta_1$, $\beta_2$, $\beta_3$ = *β-adrenergic receptors;* $\alpha_1$ = *α-adrenergic receptors; β-ARK = β-adrenergic receptor kinase; AT1, AT2 = angiotensin receptors; AC = adenylyl cyclase; Gs (α, β, γ) = subunits of the stimulatory G protein; Gi = inhibitory G protein; PLC = phospholipase C; PKA = protein kinase A; PDE = phosphodiesterase;* $PIP_2$ = *phosphatidyl inositol biphosphate;* $IP_3$ = *inositol triphosphate; DAG = diacyl glycerol; PKC = protein kinase C; ATP = adenosine triphosphate; cAMP = cyclic adenosine monophosphate.*

Heart failure is accompanied by multiple changes in the β-receptor adenylyl cyclase pathways [25, 29, 31, 35, 36, 38, 39]. The density of the $\beta_1$-receptors is reduced and the extent of this reduction correlates with the severity of ventricular dysfunction. This is the most consistently observed abnormality of the β-adrenergic pathway. The second β-adrenergic abnormality in failing myocardium is an uncoupling of the $\beta_1$- and $\beta_2$-receptors from $G_s$. The third abnormality is an upregulation of β-adrenergic receptor kinase [25, 29, 31, 35, 36, 38, 39]. With β-receptor occupancy, βARK binds to G protein β and γ subunits, uncoupling the β-receptors. Another signal transduction abnormality in the failing heart is an increase in the functional activity of $G_i$ in the face of normal levels of $G_s$. This upregulation of $G_i$ induces an uncoupling of the β-receptors from adenylyl cyclase, and a reduction in cAMP levels. The abundance of $\alpha_1$-receptors increases modestly during heart failure, which may lead to a greater stimulus to hypertrophy. However, the correlation between the density of $\alpha_1$-receptors and the rate of progression of hypertrophy remains unclear. In contrast, the density of activated T-cell-1 (AT1) receptors, which are coupled to many of the same effector enzyme systems as $\alpha_1$-receptors, decrease in failing hearts. Since a balance exists between AT1 with its growth-promoting activity and AT2 with its putative proapoptotic activity, a relative increase in AT2 receptors may lead to an increase in apoptosis (37).

## Excitation–contraction coupling

The understanding of excitation–contraction coupling in mammalian myocytes continues to evolve [23, 40]. Traditionally, the process of excitation leading to contraction and relaxation has been thought to occur through a series of co-

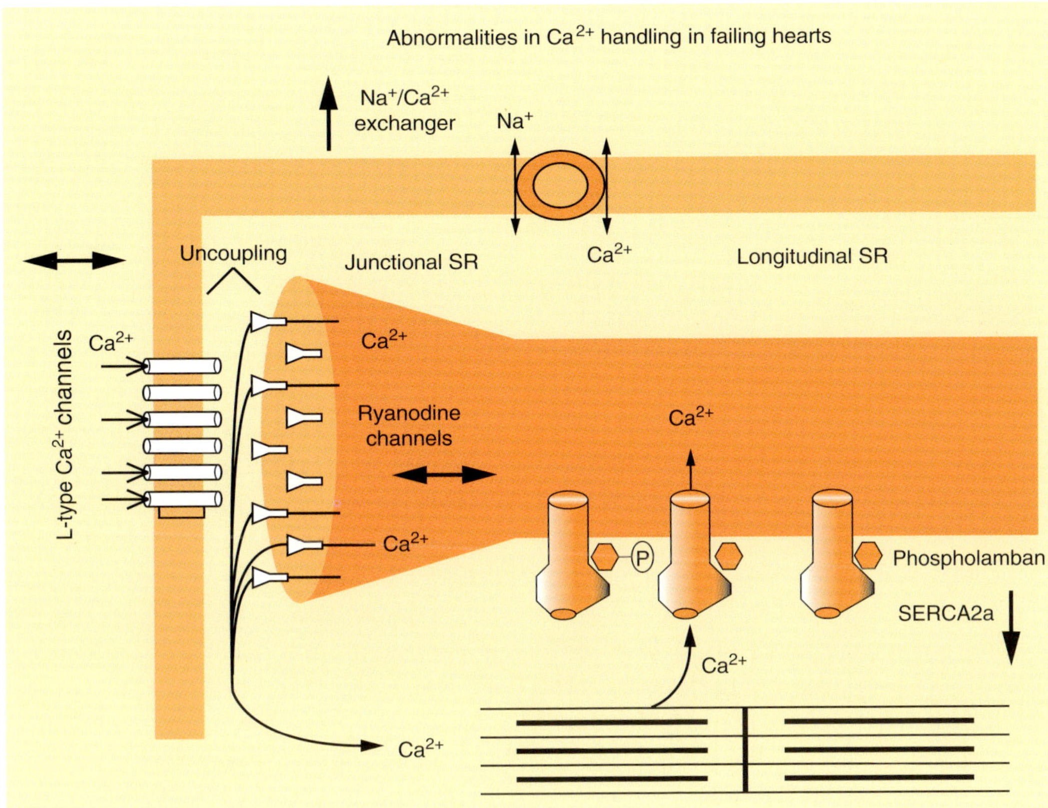


**Figure 30.3** *Abnormalities of channels and transporters responsible for $Ca^{2+}$ handling in failing human hearts. SR = sarcoplasmic reticulum; SERCA2a = cardiac sarcoplasmic reticulum $Ca^{2+}$-ATPase pump.*

ordinated steps. Electrical excitation across the sarcolemma leads to the opening of voltage-gated $Ca^{2+}$ channels, allowing the entry of a small amount of $Ca^{2+}$, which triggers the release of a larger amount of $Ca^{2+}$ from the SR through the ryanodine receptors [20]. This increase in $Ca^{2+}$ activates the myofilaments, resulting in contraction. Relaxation occurs when $Ca^{2+}$ is released from the myofilaments and is taken up by the SR $Ca^{2+}$-(ATPase) (SERCA2a) pump into the SR and extruded from the cell by the Na/Ca exchanger. The calcium pumping activity of SERCA2a is influenced by phospholamban. In the unphosphorylated state, phospholamban inhibits $Ca^{2+}$-ATPase, whereas phosphorylation of phospholamban by cAMP-dependent protein kinase and by $Ca^{2+}$-calmodulin-dependent protein kinase reverses this inhibition [41]. This mechanism has been refined by recent data using confocal microscopy which showed the presence of intracellular calcium sparks, arising from a cluster of ryanodine receptors in close proximity to a voltage-dependent calcium channel. With this mechanism, labelled local control, the coupling of a calcium channel with a cluster of ryanodine receptors allows $Ca^{2+}$ influx through a single $Ca^{2+}$ channel to increase the local concentration of $Ca^{2+}$ in the vicinity of the ryanodine receptors, producing a $Ca^{2+}$ spark [23, 40, 42]. When a large number of $Ca^{2+}$ channels is activated, multiple $Ca^{2+}$ sparks combine to increase cytosolic $Ca^{2+}$, which leads to myofilament activation.

### *Abnormal calcium handling in failing hearts*

Calcium transients recorded from failing human myocardial cells or trabeculae are significantly prolonged, with an elevated end-diastolic intracellular $Ca^{2+}$ concentration [43, 44]. At higher levels of stimulation, the amount of $Ca^{2+}$ released from the SR has also been found to be decreased in failing human hearts. Since calcium handling is regulated by the voltage-dependent $Ca^{2+}$ channel, the SR $Ca^{2+}$ release channels, the SERCA2a/phospholamban complex, and the Na/Ca exchanger, several studies have focused on the relative changes in these proteins in myopathic and normal hearts (Fig. 30.3).

The activities of both the L-type $Ca^{2+}$ channels and the ryanodine release channels in patients with dilated cardiomyopathy, recorded under voltage-clamp conditions, are essentially the same as those in normal subjects [45]. The mRNA levels of the ryanodine release channels are also not significantly different in hearts with dilated cardiomyopathy and normal hearts [45]. However, even though the L-type $Ca^{2+}$ channels and the ryanodine release channels may be expressed in normal amounts, their ability to function may be abnormal in failing hearts. It has recently been shown that in failing myocardial cells, L-type $Ca^{2+}$ channels have a reduced ability to activate the adjacent ryanodine receptors [45]. This points towards impaired coupling between L-type $Ca^{2+}$ channels and adjacent ryanodine receptors. It is still unclear whether all forms of heart failure have this type of coupling abnormality but it would seem that this defect in the microenvironment of adjacent channels may be the basis for disease states in the heart.

The steady-state levels of SERCA2a mRNA are markedly reduced in both failing human hearts and experimental models of heart failure [21, 34, 36, 46]. Associated with a decrease in mRNA, there is a decrease in SR $Ca^{2+}$-ATPase activity and SR $Ca^{2+}$ uptake from SR vesicles and membranes isolated from failing human hearts. In some studies, the protein levels of SR $Ca^{2+}$-ATPase in failing human hearts have been shown to be significantly reduced, while other studies have failed to show significant changes between protein levels of SR $Ca^{2+}$-ATPase in non-failing and failing human myocardium [21].

There is an increase in both mRNA and protein levels of the Na/Ca exchanger from the myocardium of failing human hearts [47, 48]. The enhanced expression of the exchanger has been hypothesized to be of functional relevance since the Na/Ca exchanger brings $Ca^{2+}$ into the cell or extrudes it from the cell. A transfer of $Ca^{2+}$ removal from SR to $Na^+$-mediated extrusion would have consequences for $Na^+$ homoeostasis within the cell. Several observations are consistent with a change in $Na^+$ control in failing human myocardium. In muscle strips from failing human hearts, there is an increase in sensitivity to compounds that produce positive inotropic effects through raised intacellular $Na^+$, either by inhibiting Na/K-ATPase or by opening $Na^+$ channels. It has been suggested that the relaxation abnormalities produced by the loss of SERCA2a activity could be, at least partially, compensated by the increase in Na/Ca exchanger activity [47, 48].

## Contractile proteins

Several abnormalities occur at the level of the contractile proteins in failing myocardium (Fig. 30.4) [49]. There is a decrease in α-major histocompatability complex (MHC) with an increase in β-MHC. There is also a decrease in myosin light chain kinase [50]. Overall, there is a 20–30% decrease in myofibrillar protein content. In non-failing myocardium, there is one single predominant isoform for troponin T, referred to as troponin $T_1$ [36]. A second isoform (troponin $T_2$) increases substantially in the ventricular myocardium of patients with heart failure [36]. The shifts and changes in the contractile proteins have direct consequences on the functional properties of muscle contraction. An increase in β-MHC results in a decrease in the cross-bridge cycling rate [51] and an increase in energy conservation, since fewer ATP molecules are split. It also leads to slower contraction and relaxation phases, which are characteristic of failing myocardium. An increase in troponin $T_2$ leads to a decrease in the sensitivity of the myofilaments to $Ca^{2+}$ and an abnormal response to agents targeting the filaments [52].

## Targeting specific pathways

### *β-Adrenergic pathway*

The feasibility of restoring the β-adrenergic signalling deficiencies that are characteristic of heart failure has been tested in cultured adult ventricular myocytes using adenoviral vectors encoding the $\beta_2$-adrenergic receptors and a βARK1 inhibitor, consisting of the carboxyl-terminus of βARK1 [53]. Both transgenes were shown to increase significantly isoproterenol-stimulated cAMP in normal isolated ventricular myocytes. Overexpression of these transgenes has been tested in failing cardiomyocytes. In isolated ventricular myocytes from rabbits that have been chronically paced to produce haemodynamic failure, β-adrenergic signalling defects include downregulation of myocardial β-adrenergic receptors, functional β-receptor uncoupling, and upregulation of the β-adrenergic receptor kinase [53, 54]. Adenoviral-mediated gene transfer of the human $\beta_2$-adrenergic receptor or an inhibitor of βARK1 to these failing myocytes led to the restoration of β-receptor signalling [54]. These results demonstrated that defects present in this critical myocardial signalling pathway can be corrected *in vitro* using genetic modification, raising the possibility of novel inotropic therapies for heart failure including the inhibition of βARK1 activity in the heart.

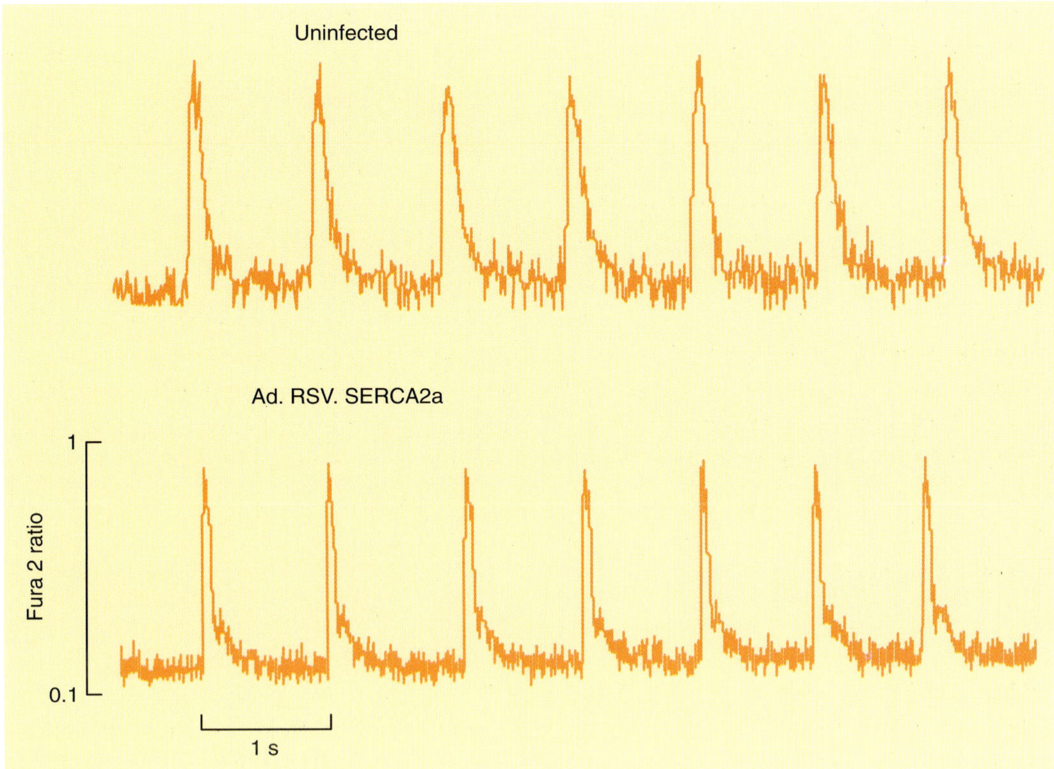


**Figure 30.4** *Abnormalities in contractile proteins in failing human hearts. MLCK = myosin light chain kinase; MHC = myosin heavy chain; TnT = troponin T; TnC = troponin C; TnI = troponin I.*

### *Sarcoplasmic reticulum $Ca^{2+}$-ATPase pump/phospholamban*

The relative ratio of phospholamban/SERCA2a is an important determinant of SR function in cardiac mycocytes [41]. Using adenoviral gene transfer, it was shown that increasing SERCA2a levels leads to an increase SR $Ca^{2+}$-ATPase activity, a faster relaxation phase, an increase in the amount of $Ca^{2+}$ released, and a decrease in diastolic $Ca^{2+}$ (Fig. 30.5) [4]. An increased ratio of phospholamban to SERCA2a is an important characteristic of both human and experimental heart failure [41]: both are characterized by prolonged $Ca^{2+}$ transient and impaired relaxation. Using adenoviral vectors, increasing levels of phospholamban relative to SERCA2a in isolated cardiac myocytes significantly altered intracellular $Ca^{2+}$ handling in isolated cardiomyocytes by prolonging the relaxation phase of the $Ca^{2+}$ transient, decreasing $Ca^{2+}$ release, and increasing resting $Ca^{2+}$ [3, 4]. These results support the hypothesis that altering the relative ratio of phospholamban to SERCA2a accounts for the abnormalities in $Ca^{2+}$ handling observed in failing ventricular myocardium [3, 4]. In earlier studies, it was shown that overexpressing SERCA2a can largely 'rescue' the phenotype created by increasing the phospholamban to SERCA2a ratio [3, 4]. This rescue effect by SERCA2a is especially encouraging since it suggests that restoring the normal phospholamban/SERCA2a ratio through somatic gene transfer could correct the abnormalities of $Ca^{2+}$ handling and contraction seen in failing hearts. Adenovirus-mediated expression of a SERCA2 transgene in cultured neonatal myocytes treated with phorbol-12-myristate-13-acetate (PMA), a compound that decreases endogenous SERCA2 espression and results in prolongation of $Ca^{2+}$ transients, can reconstitute depressed endogenous SERCA2 levels, shorten prolonged $Ca^{2+}$ transients, and augment SR $Ca^{2+}$ uptake [55]. It is conceivable that such an approach might be used *in vivo* to normalize altered $Ca^{2+}$ regulation in human heart failure. It is also conceivable that by decreasing levels of phospholamban using antisense

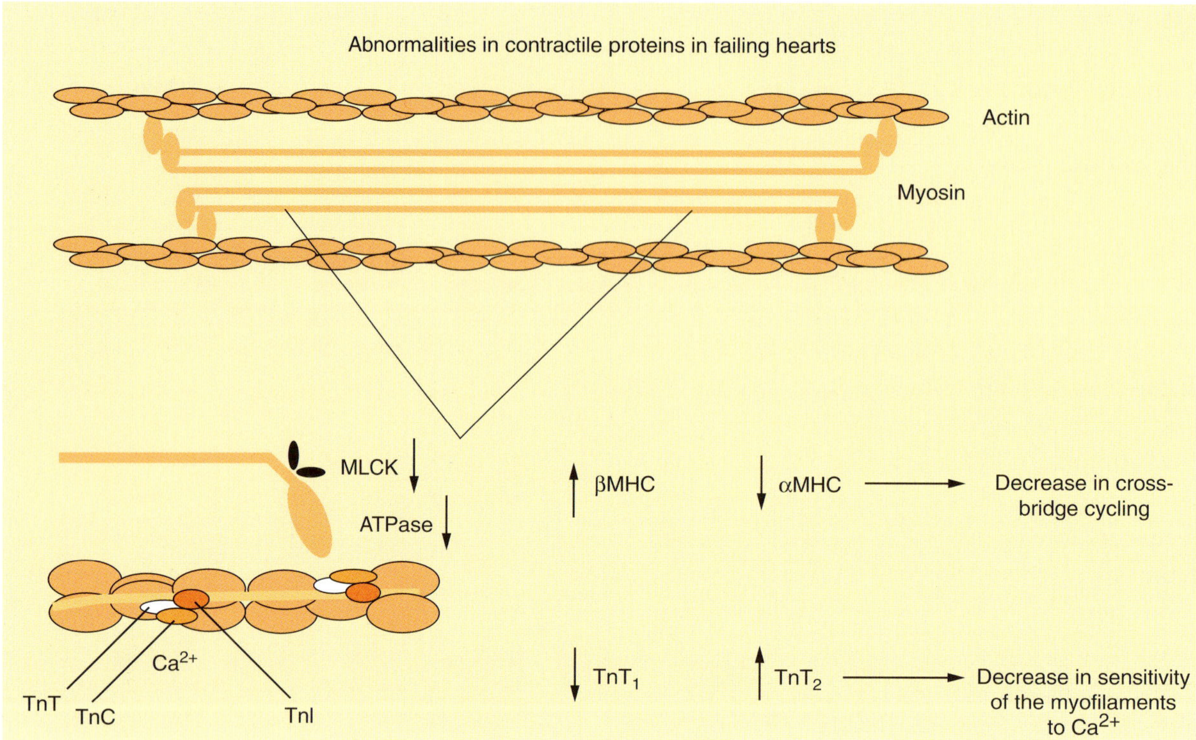


**Figure 30.5** *Effects of SERCA2a overexpression on calcium transients in cardiomyocytes. Intracellular calcium, measured by the fluorescent protein FURA-2, in an uninfected cardiomyocyte, and a cardiomyocyte infected for 48 h with an adenovirus carrying the SERCA2a gene under the control of the RSV promoter, stimulated at 1 Hz. Note the faster relaxation in the cardiomyocyte overexpression SERCA2a.*

strategies, the SERCA2a/phospholamban ratio can be normalized.

*In vivo*, using the methods of adenoviral gene transfer described earlier, overexpression of phospholamban was shown to decrease developed pressure, increase the time-course for relaxation, and significantly decrease-dP/dt [4]. These features reconstitute characteristic abnormalities of failing hearts in experimental models. Preliminary results have shown that overexpression of SERCA2a in a rat model of pressure-overload hypertrophy improves left ventricular systolic and diastolic function. Further work is needed in different animal models to verify that overexpression of SERCA2a or alterations in the phospholamban/SERCA2a ratio will yield beneficial contractile effects in failing hearts.

### *Troponin complex*

Adenoviral-mediated genetic modification of the highly regulated myofilaments has been successfully achieved in cardiac myocytes. Unlike the expression of membrane-bound receptors and transporters which can be rapidly integrated into the cell membranes and become functional, integration of specific contractile proteins requires the replacement of endogenous myofibrillar proteins [56, 57]. For this reason, adenovirus-mediated gene transfer of contractile proteins has been shown to take effect over 7 days. The effects of adenovirus-mediated slow skeletal troponin I (ssTnI) gene transfer on myofilament structure and function in adult cardiac myocytes in primary culture have been examined recently [56, 57]. In functional studies on permeabilized single cardiac myocytes, the threshold for $Ca^{2+}$-activated contraction was significantly lowered in adult cardiac myocytes expressing ssTnI relative to control values [56, 57]. Furthermore, $Ca^{2+}$-activated tension development was enhanced in cardiac myocytes expressing ssTnI compared with control values under conditions mimicking the acidosis found during myocardial ischaemia. These results demonstrated the utility of adenovirus vectors for efficient genetic modification of the cardiac myofilament for structure–function studies in cardiac myocytes and highlighted the possibility of their use in disease states.

## Hypertrophy

### Stress-activated protein kinase/p38 and cyclosporin/NFAT3 pathways

***Identifying candidate targets***

Based on a number of studies using expression of constitutively active or dominant inhibitory mutants of various signalling molecules in transgenic animals, several cytosolic signalling pathways have been implicated in the hypertrophic response of the heart. Many of these molecules are not ideal targets for inhibition since they occupy very proximal positions in signalling cascades and would be likely to have far-reaching effects in the intact animal. For example, one of the first signalling molecules expressed in the heart of transgenic animals and associated with cardiac hypertrophy is the small G protein, Ras. Ras regulates a multitude of cellular pathways including activation of the extracellular signal regulated kinases (Erk-1 and Erk-2), a subfamily of the mitogen-activated protein kinase (MARK) superfamily (reviewed in refs. 58 and 59). Ras also regulates two families of stress-response protein kinases, the stress-activated protein kinases (SAPKs, also known as c-Jun N-terminal kinases or JNKs), and the p38 family, kinases that are also part of the MAPK superfamily. Ras also regulates, in part, the activation of phosphoinositide 3 kinase which, in turn, plays a role in regulating the protein kinases Akt/PKB and the p70 ribosomal S6 kinase. Biological functions regulated by Ras include such basic processes as cellular proliferation, cellular differentiation, and apoptosis. Consequently, strategies designed to block the hypertrophic response by inhibiting Ras activity would be likely to produce many untoward effects.

Another problem with identifying signalling molecules that are candidate targets for modulation with gene transfer is that some molecules are not integral to the hypertrophic response but, when inhibited, block the response. These proteins serve permissive functions which are essential for basic cellular processes. For example, inhibition of the p70 ribosomal S6 kinase was shown to block the hypertrophic response to angiotensin II (AngII) but it is unlikely that the kinase directly regulates major components of the hypertrophic response [60]. Rather, the kinase plays a critical role in the translational control of several mRNAs which encode key elements of the translational apparatus and, therefore, are essential for any response that requires enhanced protein synthesis, including not only hypertrophy but also the mitogenic response [61].

**Stress-response protein kinases as targets**

MAP kinase cascades consist of a three-tiered module in which a MAP kinase kinase kinase (MAPKKK) activates the downstream MEK (MAPK/ERK kinase) which, in turn, activates the MAPK by phosphorylating it on threonine and tyrosine residues within the catalytic domain (reviewed in refs. 58 and 62). When activated, the MAPKs translocate to the nucleus where many of their primary targets, transcription factors, are located [63]. It is these transcription factors that regulate the induction of sets of genes which largely determine the ultimate biological response of the cell.

SAPKs and p38s are activated in response to a variety of cellular stresses including inflammatory cytokines [tumour necrosis factor (TNF) and interleukin-1 (IL-1)], ischaemia– reperfusion, and a number of environmental stresses including heat, osmolar stress, oxidant stress, ionizing radiation, and ultraviolet irradiation. Recent studies of cardiomyocytes *in vitro* have suggested that the SAPKs and the p38s are also activated by a variety of hypertrophic stimuli, including cell stretch and several neurohormonal agents such as endothelin-1 (ET-1), AngII, and phenylephrine. These studies suggest that the SAPKs and p38s transduce critical signals governing the hypertrophic response and might be appropriate targets for inhibition. Two groups have demonstrated that constitutive activation of p38, induced by expression of activated mutants of MKK6 or MKK3, MEKs that are the immediate upstream activators of p38, increased cell size, enhanced the expression of atrial natriuretic factor (ANF), and enhanced sarcomeric organization [64, 65]. Overexpression of wild-type or constitutively active MKK7 (a MEK which is upstream of the SAPKs) also increased cell size, and enhanced ANF expression and sarcomere organization [66].

These studies [64–66] confirmed that the sustained activation of either the p38 or SAPK pathways is sufficient to induce cardiomyocyte hypertrophy. However, studies such as these force constitutive activation of signalling pathways by overexpressing activated mutants or wild-type components of these cascades in cardiomyocytes *in vitro* or in the hearts of transgenic animals. This results in supranormal and prolonged activation of normal downstream targets and, in some cases, activation of other signalling pathways that are not activated under physiological conditions. This makes it difficult to ascribe any effects to one specific pathway unless one can also demonstrate that the pathway is necessary for the hypertrophic response to physiologically relevant stimuli (discussed in ref. 67).

One strategy employed to prove that a pathway is necessary for a hypertrophic response is to express inactive mutants of the MEK immediately upstream of the MAPK postulated to play a role in the response. These inactive mutants function as dominant inhibitors of activation of the relevant MAPKs. There are two types of these mutants. In the first, the critical lysine in the ATP-binding site of the kinase is mutated (often to arginine, methionine, or alanine). Consequently, ATP cannot bind to the kinase and, therefore, the mutant cannot phosphorylate or activate the MAPK. In the second type of inactivating mutation, the two residues of the MEK that are phosphorylated by the upstream MAPKKK are mutated to residues that cannot be phosphorylated. Both types of dominant inhibitory mutant function by sequestering either upstream MAPKKKs and/or the MAPK, and have been shown to block activation of the SAPKs or p38s in response to a variety of agonists and to suppress such cellular responses as apoptosis in response to several stimuli in a number of cell types [68, 69].

One study used adenovirus-mediated gene transfer to express SEK-1(KR), a kinase inactive mutant of SEK-1, in neonatal rat cardiomyocytes [70]. SEK-1, like MKK7, is a MEK in the SAPK pathway. This approach takes advantage of the relative specificity of the MEKs for the MAPKs. That is, at the level of the MEKs there is relatively little cross-talk between the various MAPK pathways. Similar selectivity exists for the kinase-inactive mutants of the MEKs which, unless grossly overexpressed, do not block activation of the other MAPK pathways. Thus, expression of SEK-1(KR) could be titrated to inhibit completely agonist-induced SAPK activation without inhibiting activation of the ERKs or p38s. Expression of SEK-1(KR) in neonatal rat cardiomyocytes abrogated the hypertrophic response to ET-1 as determined by protein synthesis, ANF expression, and sarcomere organization. In contrast, PD98059, a specific inhibitor of MEK-1, a MEK upstream of the ERKs, and SB203580, an inhibitor of p38s, failed to block ET-1-induced cardiomyocyte hypertrophy [70].

This type of intervention appears to be feasible in the intact animal using the method of adenoviral gene transfer *in vivo*. The critical determinant of whether a specific pathway can be blocked with this approach is the level of expression of the dominant inhibitory mutant. Based on studies in cultured cells and, more recently, gene transfer *in vivo*, it appears that the dominant inhibitory transgene must be expressed at levels at least as great as the native, wild-type kinase to inhibit significantly signal transduction down the pathway. These levels of expression of SEK-1(KR) have been achieved [70]. Since the SAPKs are markedly activated in the heart by pressure overload, the role of the SAPK pathway in the development of pressure overload hypertrophy is currently being evaluated.

Many stimuli, including cellular stretch [71], peptide growth factors [e.g. fibroblast growth factor (FGF) and platelet-derived growth factor (PDGF)], transforming growth factor-β (TGF-β), some cytokines (cardiotrophin-1 and leukaemia inhibitory factor), and neurohormonal agents (AngII, ET-1, and α-adrenergic agents such as phenylephrine) can cause myocyte hypertrophy *in vitro* [72–75]. Which of these play important roles *in vivo* are not clear, but the neurohormonal agents are excellent candidates. These agents interact with serpentine receptors coupled to heterotrimeric G proteins of the $G_q$ family [74, 76, 77]. Recently, studies that blocked signalling from $G_q$-linked receptors by overexpressing the carboxy-terminal tail of the αq subunit in the hearts of transgenic mice inhibited the development of pressure overload hypertrophy, suggesting that signalling from $G_q$-linked receptors may play a critical role *in vivo* [78]. Since inhibition of Et-1- and AngII-induced activation of the SAPKs blocks myocyte hypertrophy *in vitro*, the SAPKs may be ideal targets for blocking the hypertrophic response *in vivo*.

Several studies also support a role for the p38s in the hypertrophic response of cardiomyocytes [64, 65, 79]. This is not surprising since the SAPKs and p38s are activated by many, although not all, of the same stimuli and they share some common substrates (e.g. the transcription factors Elk-1 and ATF-2). Most studies which have explored the role of the p38s in hypertrophy have employed chemical inhibitors of the pyridinyl imidazole class (SB203580 and SB202190). While these studies suggest a role for the p38s in cardiomyocyte hypertrophy in response to ET-1 and phenylephrine, sole reliance on the inhibitors is problematic since the drugs do not inhibit two isoforms of p38 (p38γ and p38δ) and, more importantly, inhibit several SAPK isoforms at concentrations commonly employed in published studies [80]. Thus, while it is likely that the SAPKs and p38s may serve redundant functions in at least some components of the hypertrophic response, it is critical to employ concentrations of a drug that specifically inhibits p38s in the system being studied. Alternatively, adenovirus-mediated gene transfer of dominant inhibitory MEKs upstream of p38s, MKK3 and MKK6, should allow one to dissect the role of p38s in hypertrophy.

## Calcineurin and hypertrophy

A second cytosolic signalling pathway that appears to be an important modulator of the hypertrophic response is controlled by the calcium- and calmodulin-dependent protein serine/threonine phosphatase, calcineurin or protein phosphatase 2B [81, 82]. Molkentin *et al.* [82] demonstrated that expression of activated calcineurin was sufficient to induce hypertrophy in transgenic mice, a response that was blocked by treatment with an inhibitor of calcineurin, cyclosporin A (CsA). Furthermore, CsA and FK506, another calcineurin inhibitor, blocked AngII- and phenylephrine-induced hypertrophy in cardiomyocytes in culture.

In cardiomyocytes, calcineurin, activated by calmodulin binding in the presence of elevated cytosolic free $Ca^{2+}$, dephosphorylates the transcription factor, nuclear factor of activated T-cells-3 (NF-AT3). NF-AT3 then translocates to the nucleus where it binds to GGAAAT sequences in the promoters of various genes and activates transcription from those genes. Although calcineurin has many effects on cells in addition to activation of NF-ATs, including modulation of the activity of the ryanodine and inositol trisphosphate receptors, activation of nitric oxide synthase, and regulation of $Na^+$–$K^+$-ATPase, Molkentin *et al.* were able to induce hypertrophy in transgenic mice by expressing activated NF-AT3. These data strongly suggested that the calcineurin effect was mediated via activation of NF-AT3 and not via another of calcineurin's many effects.

Can the data suggesting that the SAPKs are necessary for the hypertrophic response be reconciled with the data suggesting that the calcineurin/NF-AT pathway is necessary? In T-cells, the full response to activation of the T-cell receptor requires co-operative interactions between NF-ATs and another transcription factor, activator protein-1 (AP-1). Alone, NF-AT and AP-1 bind weakly to composite NF-AT/AP-1 sites in the promoters of several immune response genes. When both factors are present, however, binding is co-operative and gene expression is maximal [83].

### *SAPKs and p38 regulate the activity of AP-1*

AP-1 is composed of a heterodimer of c-Jun and c-Fos. The SAPKs phosphorylate two serine residues in the amino-terminal region of c-Jun, thereby increasing its transcriptional activating activity (Fig. 30.6) [84, 85]. In addition, the SAPKs or p38 can phosphorylate and activate the ternary complex factor (TCF) Elk-1, which controls induction of c-fos. This may enhance transcription from the NF-AT/AP-1 composite sites by inducing an increase in c-Fos levels. p38, via activation of the transcription factor MEF-2c, can induce increases in c-Jun levels and, thereby, increase AP-1 activity. Finally, p38 also phosphorylates and activates another protein kinase, mitogen-activated protein kinase activated protein kinase-2 (MAPKAP-K2), which phosphorylates and activates the transcription factor cAMP response element binding protein (CREB) [86]. Since CREB also regulates induction of c-Fos in response to cellular stresses, p38 may regulate c-Fos levels via activation of CREB (Fig. 30.6).

It has been postulated [70, 82] that the costimulatory pathway of T-cells, which requires both calcineurin/NF-ATs and activated SAPKs/AP-1, may be operative in the hypertrophic response of cardiomyocytes. Data identifying calcineurin/NF-AT3 [70] and the SAPKs [82] as necessary for the hypertrophic response strongly suggest that this is the case. If so, both pathways would probably be necessary for the full expression of the hypertrophic response to physiological stimuli, although if either is markedly constitutively activated, that may be sufficient by itself to induce hypertrophy. The current consensus is that the SAPK and calcineurin pathways are parallel and their signals are integrated at the promoters of relevant genes by co-operative interaction of NF-AT and AP-1. However, cyclosporin A (CsA) has been shown to inhibit SAPK activation in some cells, raising the possibility that calcineurin could be upstream of the SAPKs in a linear pathway signalling hypertrophy [87, 88].

Although chemical inhibitors of calcineurin are available, the many targets of calcineurin and the toxicity resulting from that inhibition make the phosphatase a poor candidate for the design of inhibitors. Similarly, inhibitors of NF-AT3 would need to be targeted to the less well-conserved regions of the molecule or the inhibitor would be likely to interact with all NF-ATs, leading to immune compromise. Another approach would be to target the protein kinase which phosphorylates NF-AT3, leading to its export from the nucleus and termination of the signal. Two kinases appear to be involved in this process: an as yet unidentified priming kinase and glycogen synthase kinase-3 (GSK-3) [89]. GSK-3 is active in the unstimulated cell, and

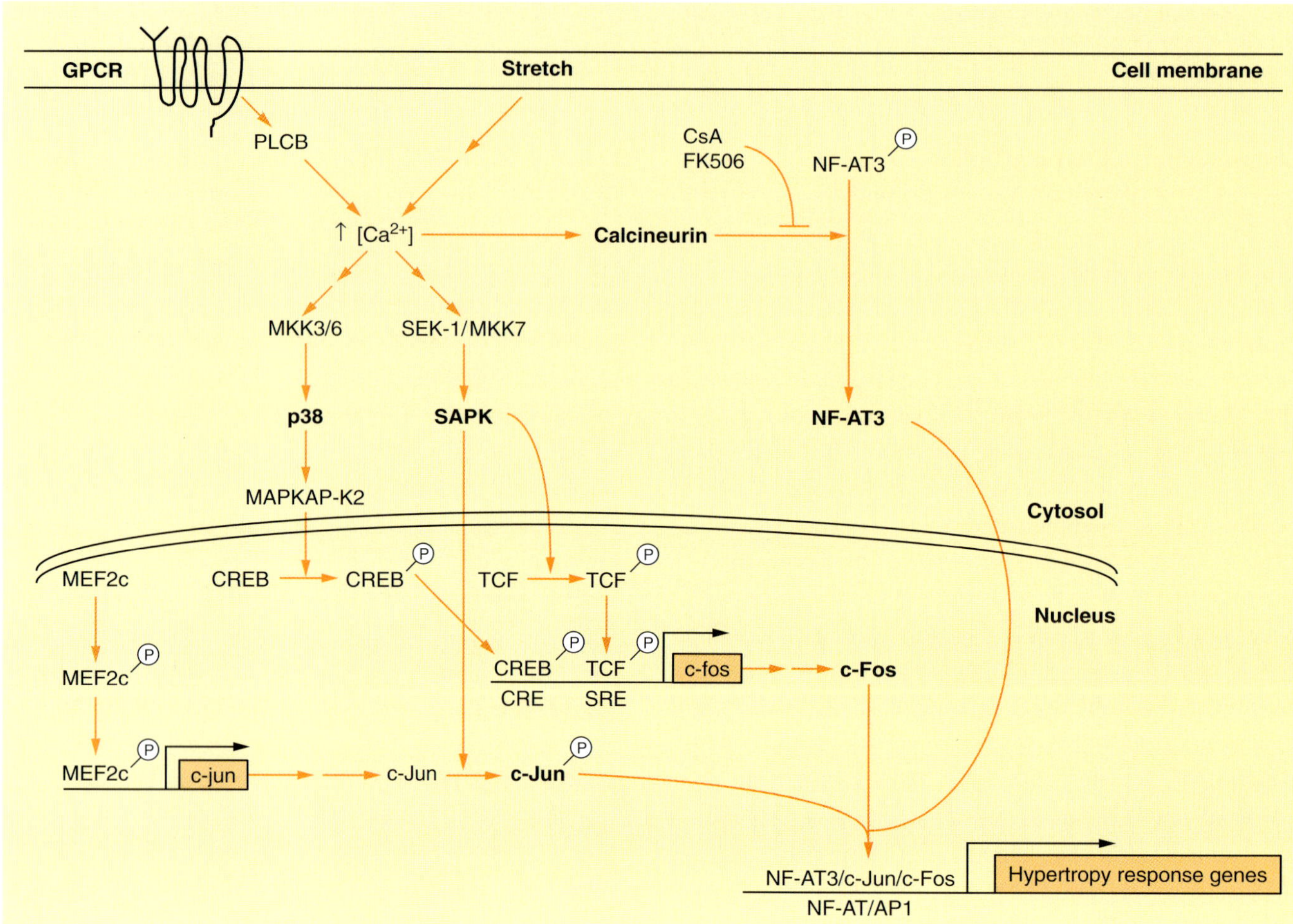


**Figure 30.6** *Postulated role and mechanisms of activation of the costimulatory pathway in cardiomyocytes. Exposure of cells to stretch or agonists with G protein-coupled receptors (GPCR) induces an increase in cytosolic free [$Ca^{2+}$]. This triggers activation of the SAPK/p38 pathways and calcineurin. SAPK targets include the transcription factor c-Jun (increases transcriptional activating activity) and the ternary complex factor (TCF) Elk-1 (increases transcriptional activating activity and DNA binding activity directed at serum response elements, contained in many genes including the c-fos gene). p38 targets include the transcription factors MEF2c and, via activation of MAPKAP-K2, CREB, which, in part, which induce expression of c-jun and c-fos genes, respectively. Calcineurin dephosphorylates NF-AT3, allowing it to translocate to the nucleus. c-Jun, c-Fos, and NF-AT3 demonstrate co-operative binding at composite NF-AT/AP-1 sites which are postulaed to be in the promoters of various genes that are critical to the hypertrophic response.*

is inactivated by phosphorylation at Ser-9 by Akt/PKB and other mitogen-activated kinases. GSK-3 activity reappears as cytosolic free $Ca^{2+}$ returns towards the resting level. As opposed to the strategies outlined above for blocking the activation of a pathway by gene transfer of a dominant inhibitory mutant, inhibition of calcineurin/ NF-AT3 signalling in the adult heart might better be accomplished by gene transfer of a GSK-3 mutant which cannot be inactivated (e.g. Ser-9 mutated to Ala).

## Non-specificity remains a problem

Not surprisingly, many of the cytosolic signalling pathways which appear to regulate expression of the hypertrophic phenotype are pathways that are highly conserved throughout evolution, a fact that attests to their central role in development and differentiation. The potential problems associated with inhibiting (or activating) signalling molecules that are very proximal in signalling pathways were discussed above, but even when one considers signalling molecules that are relatively far downstream in a pathway, the risk of untoward effects is great. For example, in addition to their putative roles in hypertrophy, both the SAPKs and GSK-3 are downstream components of Wnt signalling pathways that are essential for normal development in

*Drosophila* and mammals. The identification of targets which, when persistently inhibited or activated, block hypertrophy but do not produce unwanted effects will be difficult. The hope is that, for example, specific SAPK or p38 isoforms will govern specific responses in the heart and that by targeting those specific isoforms, the undesired effects of across-the-board inhibition of all SAPKs, p38s, or other signalling molecules will be minimized [64].

## Apoptosis

### Apoptosis in cardiovascular disease

Death of heart muscle results in an irreversible decrease in cardiac function which correlates with overall morbidity and mortality in many different clinical settings. Since adult cardiomyocytes are postmitotic, damaged heart muscle cannot generally be regenerated through cell division. Therefore, cardiomyocyte loss (as well as the consequent deterioration in cardiac function) is cumulative over the lifetime of an individual. This may contribute to the observation that heart failure currently accounts for a large proportion of admission diagnoses, particularly among the elderly [90, 91]. For these reasons, understanding how cardiomyocyte death is controlled and identifying possible opportunities for intervention have significant clinical implications.

It has recently been recognized that, in response to specific stimuli, cells can activate intrinsic suicide pathways and undergo programmed cell death or apoptosis. During this process, cell membranes bleb and the cell nucleus undergoes the characteristic morphological changes associated with fragmentation of chromosomal DNA [92]. The development of these changes is highly conserved, thus allowing identification of useful morphological and biochemical markers of apoptosis [92, 93].

Using these markers, apoptosis has been identified in a wide variety of conditions. There is evidence of progressive cell loss and fibrosis with chronic pressure overload in a variety of heart-failure models [94]. Recent studies have documented apoptosis in experimental heart failure [95–97] and in human cardiomyopathy [98]. Markers of programmed cell death are also apparent in right ventricular dysplasia [99], transplanted cardiac allografts [100], and during normal cardiomyocyte development [101]. Cardiomyocyte apoptosis is particularly prominent in models of ischaemia–reperfusion injury [102], affecting a significant proportion of cardiomyocytes in the affected area. Apoptosis has recently been documented in acute human myocardial infarction associated with patent infarct-related arteries [103]. In this setting it is significantly more common in the border zones adjacent to infarction [103].

However, two critical questions remain unanswered in this context. First, what is the functional contribution of apoptosis to the pathogenesis of these disorders? Secondly, what are the intracellular pathways that determine whether cardiomyocytes undergo apoptosis? It is possible that cardiomyocyte apoptosis is an epiphenomenon that reflects rather than causes the progression of these conditions. Moreover, programmed cell death could even play a protective role in some settings, such as myocarditis. The functional relevance of apoptosis is extremely difficult to assess in clinical studies, but data are beginning to emerge from animal studies that cardiomyocyte apoptosis contributes significantly to disease pathogenesis in some settings [104]. Such studies highlight the general area of programmed cell death as a potential target for therapy in cardiomyopathies; however, little is known about the intracellular pathways that determine whether cardiomyocytes undergo this process.

Fortunately, in this context, one may learn from recent progress studying apoptosis in simpler biological systems. Major advances in the understanding of the molecular basis of programmed cell death have resulted from studies of development in the nematode *C. elegans* and extrapolation from these studies to vertebrate systems [105]. A search for mammalian homologues of the *C. elegans* death genes (ced-3 and ced-4) led to the identification of the interleukin-1β-converting enzyme (ICE) family of proteases and their role in apoptosis [105]. More than ten homologues of human origin have been described which share substrate structural preferences and are proteolytically activated [106]. The nomenclature of this family has recently been standardized to caspases (for **c**ysteine **as**partic acid-specific prote**ases**), followed by an Arabic numeral indicating the order of discovery (Table 30.1) [106]. Recent reports have noted altered expression of apoptosis-related genes after myocardial infarction [107] or hypoxia [108]. In general, however, modulation of cell death pathways occurs not through altered expression of these genes but rather through the proteolytic activation of existing proenzymes [109], permitting the activated form of these enzymes to be identified by immunoblotting. The viral protein crmA appears to be a specific and powerful inhibitor of caspase family members and blocks programmed cell death in a

**Table 30.1** Nomenclature of interleukin-1β-converting enzyme (ICE) family proteases or caspases

| Caspase member | Caspase-1 | Caspase-2 | Caspase-3 | Caspase-4 | Caspase-5 | Caspase-6 | Caspase-7 | Caspase-8 | Caspase-9 | Caspase-10 |
|---|---|---|---|---|---|---|---|---|---|---|
| Previous name(s) | ICE | ICH-1 | CPP32, Yama, apopain | TX, ICH-2, $ICE_{rel}$-II | $ICE_{rel}$-III, TY | Mch2 | Mch3, ICE-LAP3, CMH-1 | MACH, FLICE, Mch5 | ICE-LAP6, Mch6 | Mch 4 |

variety of settings [110–115]. Even non-viral overexpression of crmA is sufficient to block apoptosis in response to pharmacological doses of TNF-α and cycloheximide [116]. Thus, somatic gene transfer of crmA or similar inhibitors to the heart in models of cardiac disease provides a way to simultaneous assess the contribution of crmA-sensitive pathways to cardiac apoptosis as well as their functional importance.

Despite identification of many molecular participants in this process (Table 30.1), a coherent and comprehensive model has not yet been assembled. Most current models place caspase-3 downstream of caspases-1, -8, and -10 [117, 118]. Therefore, several different upstream pathways may independently lead to caspase-3 activation and apoptosis [117]. Similarly, many downstream substrates have been identified [119]. It remains unclear which of the identified substrates are critical participants and which merely markers of apoptosis [119]. However, caspase activation results in cleavage of poly(ADP-ribose) polymerase (PARP) to a characteristic fragment that correlates well with caspase activity and apoptosis [119, 120], and thus serves as a useful general index of caspase-mediated apoptosis.

## *In vivo* inhibition of cardiac apoptosis by caspase inhibitor

The specific inhibitor of caspase proteases, benzyloxycarbonyl-Val-Ala-Asp fluoromethylketone (zVAD-FMK), has recently been demonstrated to reduce cardiomyocyte apoptosis *in vivo* in a rat model of ischaemia–reperfusion injury [104]. Importantly, this reduction in apoptosis resulted in both a reduction in infarct size and an improvement in left ventricular haemodynamic measurements. These results provide important evidence of the functional relevance of apoptosis in a model of cardiovascular disease. However, the reduction in infarct size was modest and it is likely that the specific functional contribution of these pathways will differ substantially in different cardiovascular conditions. Moreover, using this approach it is impossible to correlate precisely the effects of the intervention with phenotype and the possibility of systemic effects of this reagent have not been fully explored.

## Insulin-like growth factor-I in apoptosis

In addition to the caspases described above, a number of viability factors has been identified that can play an important role in modulation of apoptosis. These include growth factors such as insulin-like growth factor-I (IGF-I), which blocks apoptosis in many settings [121–123], including models of cardiac ischaemia–reperfusion injury [124]. In general, this IGF-I rescue effect appears to be mediated through IGF-I receptor-dependent suppression of caspase-mediated cell death [125].

## Insulin-like growth factor-I-mediated signalling pathways

The IGF-I receptor (IGF-IR) is a tyrosine kinase consisting of two 135 000 mol.wt α-subunits and two 95 000 mol.wt β-subunits. IGF-I binds the α-subunits which activates the tyrosine kinase activity of the β-subunits. Binding of IGF-I to IGF-IR initiates signalling through two distinct pathways: (1) phosphorylation of insulin receptor substrate-1 (IRS-1) with activation of phosphatidylinositol (PI)-3 kinase; and (2) the Ras/MAPK pathway (see Fig. 30.7) [126]. The phosphorylation of IRS-1/activation of PI-3 kinase pathway appears critical to the ability of IGF-I to block programmed cell death [127–129]. The activation of Ras/MAP kinase is necessary for malignant transformation, may contribute to cardiac hypertrophy [130], and may also be antiapoptotic [131].

Several independent lines of evidence support the concept that IGF-IR downstream signalling pathways are distinct and can be differentially activated. First, a constitutively active IGF-IR mutant activates PI-3 kinase but not MAPK [132]. Secondly, Chinese hamster ovary

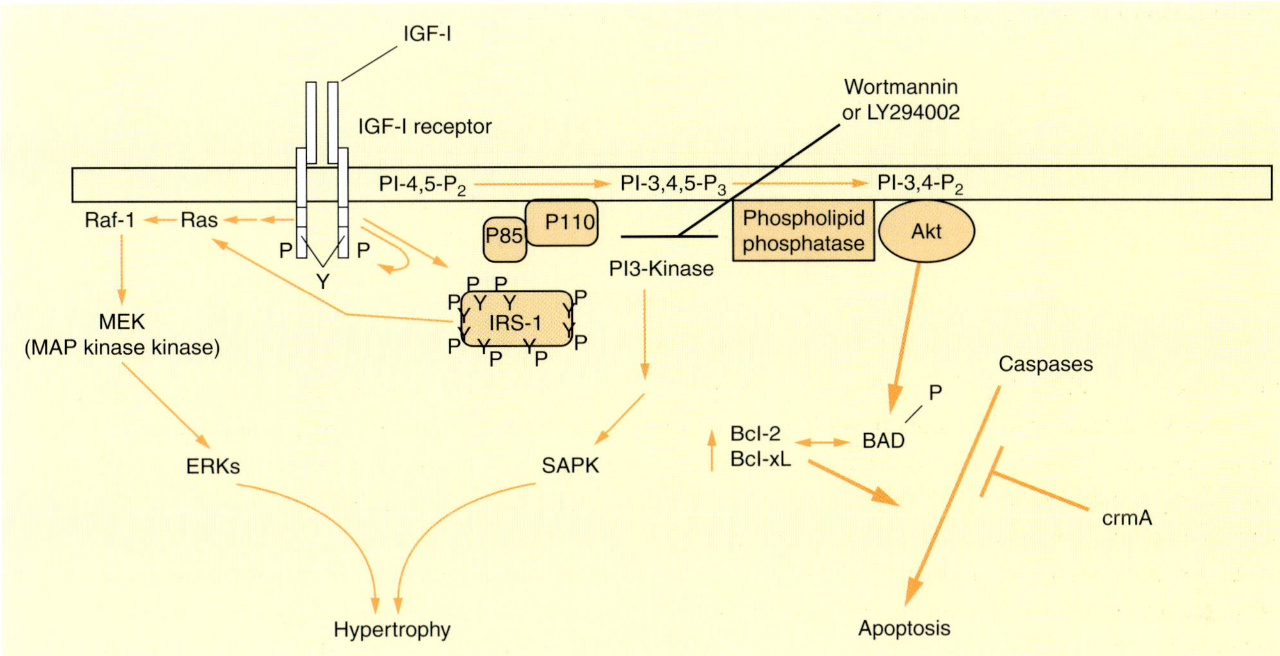


**Figure 30.7** *Insulin-like growth factor-I (IGF-I) receptor-mediated signalling pathways. After IGF-I binds to the IGF-I receptor (IGF-IR), the receptor phosphorylates and activates IRS-1 and PI3-kinase (among other SH domain-containing proteins). Activation of IGF-IR also results in phosphorylation of Shc which forms complexes with Grb2 in association with the guanine nucleotide exchange factor Sos, which activates Ras. Ras activation leads to MAP kinase activation through a series of intermediaries depicted schematically. Wortmannin and LY294002 act as specific pharmacological inhibitors of PI3-kinase.*

(CHO) cells that express a dominant negative adapter subunit of PI-3 kinase inhibit its activation but not that of Ras/MAPK [133]. Thirdly, the constitutively active PI-3 kinase BD110 [134] has been shown not to activate MAP kinase pathways [134]. Fourthly, pharmacological blockade of PI-3 kinase with wortmannin inhibits its activation but has no effect on the activation of Ras/MAPK [132]. Finally, inhibitors or Ras activation have been identified that do not inhibit PI-3 kinase activation [135].

Although the receptor-mediated effects of IGF-I represent a complex array of downstream signalling pathways (Fig. 30.7), the ability of IGF-I to block apoptosis directly is generally dependent on activation of PI-3 kinase [136]. PI-3 kinase, in turn, activates the serine–threonine kinase, Akt [137]. Recent studies have demonstrated that Akt is the downstream target of PI-3 kinase that is both necessary and sufficient to mediate inhibition of apoptosis in several cell types [138–142]. In some cell types, Akt appears to work through phosphorylation of BAD, releasing Bcl-2 family members which ultimately inhibit caspase-mediated cell death [143]. Therefore, PI-3 kinase appears to be a critical component in a signal transduction pathway mechanistically linking viability factors, such as IGF-I, to caspases through activation of the serine–threonine kinase, Akt, in many other cellular systems. However, it is important to emphasize that critical roles for these molecules have not been established in cardiomyocytes. Adenoviral vectors carrying previously described wild-type, constitutively active, or dominant negative forms of PI-3 kinase and Akt provide a nearly unique tool for testing the relevance of these pathways in *in vitro* and *in vivo* models of cardiac disease.

## Insulin-like growth factor-I in the cardiovascular system

In the heart, acute infarction is associated with an increase in both IGF-I and IGF-IR [144]. IGF-I enhances ventricular function during the onset of heart failure in rats with myocardial infarction [145, 146]. In addition, IGF-I has been shown to stimulate the synthesis of cardiac contractile proteins [147], and also has systemic effects which could impact cardiovascular conditions such as an increase in endothelial nitric oxide release [148]. Therefore, to understand the cardiovascular effects of IGF-I, it is important to differentiate between local and systemic actions, and to assess the independently effects on apoptosis and on cardiocyte function.

Treatment with growth hormone (GH), which has been shown to lead to beneficial remodelling in heart failure [149], increases the content of IGF-I in myocytes and induces the expression of mRNA for IGF-I in heart and skeletal muscle [150]. For these reasons, IGF-I has been postulated to mediate locally many of the beneficial effects of GH. Cardiac overexpression of IGF-I in transgenic mice leads to cardiomegaly through an increase in the number of cardiocytes, without cellular hypertrophy [151]. However, this finding may well reflect the effect of increased IGF-I throughout development and would be expected to differ from the effect on postmitotic adult cardiocytes. Systemic administration of either GH or IGF-I for 4 weeks in rats resulted in cellular and gross hypertrophy [152], which was accompanied by an increase in cardiac index and a decrease in systemic vascular resistance [152]. All parameters of cardiac function improved, both *in vivo* and in isolated perfused Langendorff preparations.

In animal models, both systemic IGf-I [124] and cardiac [153] IGF-I overexpression can reduce cardiocyte apoptosis. In an *in vivo* rat model of ischaemia–reperfusion, pretreatment with a single intraperitoneal injection of IGF-I reduced cardiocyte apoptosis by approximately 50% in the area of injury [124]. More recently, transgenic mice overexpressing IGF-I were found to have less myocyte apoptosis and improved cardiac function in an infarction model [153]. While it is tempting to speculate that these beneficial effects were mediated by local activation of downstream IGF-I signalling pathways, the systemic effects of IGF-I could also affect these results. IGF-I-mediated increases in nitric oxide [148] could affect two critical determinants of postischaemic injury, namely leucocyte infiltration [154–156] and vascular tone [157, 158]. Results in transgenic mice are further confounded by the developmental effects of constitutive IGF-I overexpression, such as cardiocyte hyperplasia [153]. Somatic gene transfer offers an alternative strategy to investigate the effects of local IGF-I signalling pathways without the developmental confounders inherent in transgenic systems.

Given the beneficial cardiac effects of IGF-I, an alternative strategy might be systemic treatment with this growth factor. However, chronic systemic administration of IGF-I poses several theoretical problems. First, its efficacy may be undermined by IGF serum binding proteins. Secondly, systemic IGF-I may inadvertently amplify distant occult malignancies through activation of MAPK pathways. Thirdly, exposure to chronic IGF-I leads to cardiac hypertrophy in a number of animal models [145, 152], which is also thought to correlate with MAPK activation. Although there is some indication that IGF-I-induced hypertrophy may be beneficial in some settings [152], induction of hypertrophy raises concern because, in clinical studies, cardiac hypertrophy virtually always correlates with significant cardiac morbidity and mortality [159]. Local and specific modulation of IGF-I downstream signalling pathways would avoid these disadvantages of systemic IGF-I administration. Once the critical pathways have been identified, somatic gene transfer also offers a potential therapeutic avenue by specifically activating beneficial pathways. However, it is also possible that pharmacological approaches such as screening for or chemical synthesis of specific small molecule modulators of these pathways could be exploited.

## Models of cardiomyocyte apoptosis

Cardiomyocyte apoptosis can be assessed in a variety of *in vitro* and *in vivo* models to permit evaluation of the role of specific signalling pathways. Cultured neonatal rat cardiomyocytes undergo apoptosis in response to a variety of traditional apoptotic stimuli [160]. These include TNF-$\alpha$ and cycloheximide, either individually or in combination, as well as pathophysiologically relevant stimuli such as hypoxia [160].

Apoptosis may be analysed through a variety of complementary techniques designed to identify the characteristic histological or biochemical hallmarks of programmed cell death. These include nuclear morphology (Hoechst staining), DNA laddering, TUNEL assay, flow cytometry using propidium iodide or fluorescein isothiocyanate conjugated annexin V to detect the presence of surface phosphatidylserine [161, 162], and commercially available enzyme-linked immunosorbent assay (ELISA) kits designed to detect histone associated DNA fragments. It is important to realize that many of these assays measure different indicators and that while the overall results are generally consistent between assays, the specific numbers may vary with the assay. The TUNEL assay allows one to identify the apoptotic cells by colocalizing a lineage-specific marker, but may be difficult to quantitate. Flow cytometry and ELISA for histone-associated DNA are inherently quantitative but more applicable to cultured cells than tissue culture sections. DNA laddering is the biochemical hallmark of apoptosis and provides a highly specific marker that can be applied to cultured cells or tissues. While not inherently quantitative, the intensity of laddering is usually a reasonably accurate reflection of the amount of apoptosis. However, these biochemical assays do not identify the nature of the apoptotic cells, and it is important to remember that other cell types may contribute to such findings in *in vivo* and even *in vitro*.

### Insulin-like growth factor-I blocks apoptosis of cardiomyocytes *in vitro*

As noted above, IGF-I is a potent viability factor in many systems. IGF-I also has beneficial effects on cardiomyocyte function in a variety of experimental models. Moreover, growth hormone, which in this context may act primarily by elevating IGF-I levels [150], has recently been demonstrated to have clinical benefits in heart failure [149]. The mechanisms underlying all of these benefits have not yet been fully elucidated.

IGF-I also has a direct beneficial effect in blocking apoptosis of cultured cardiomyocytes [160, 163]. For example, transient hypoxia increases cardiomyocyte apoptosis, which is significantly attenuated by prior treatment with IGF-I [163]. Moreover, this benefit is attenuated by simultaneous treatment with PI-3 kinase inhibitors such as wortmannin or LY294002 [163]. While it is tempting to speculate that the *in vivo* benefits of IGF-I may reflect activation of these signalling pathways, many other direct and indirect effects may play important roles not evident in simple *in vitro* models. At present, these signalling pathways represent logical candidates for a role in the control of cardiomyocyte apoptosis. Somatic gene transfer provides a way to manipulate these pathways *in vitro* and *in vivo* and thus to test whether these candidates are appropriate targets for future efforts at intervention. Modulation of these pathways in relevant *in vivo* models allows one not only to test the role of a particular molecule but simultaneously to assess its functional relevance in disease pathogenesis.

## Future directions

While it is tempting to become impatient with delays in the clinical application of the approaches described above, it is important to remember that researchers are still very much in the early phases of a newly developing field. Although substantial progress has been made, before gene therapy can become a practical reality for cardiovascular disease in general and cardiomyopathies in particular, many hurdles need to be overcome. Newer vectors that provide prolonged, high-level, preferably cardiac-specific transgene expression, need to be developed. Extensive *in vivo* testing of these is necessary to clarify their effectiveness and safety. Although early human trials will be likely to rely on direct cardiac injection of vectors, minimally invasive delivery systems for either perfusion or injection need to be developed to realize fully the potential of this therapeutic approach. However, the technological promise is empty if it is not founded on a solid understanding of disease pathogenesis and this may represent the most challenging hurdle to gene therapy. Furtunately, it is also one of the most interesting aspects and even the currently available gene transfer vectors can help in this regard. By using somatic gene transfer as an experimental tool, researchers can help to elucidate the pathophysiology of cardiovascular diseases and explore the functional impact of modulating specific targets. Simultaneously, an appreciation of the power and limitations of specific vectors and delivery systems develops, along with an understanding of how they interact with the host. All of these elements are necessary for somatic gene targeting to become a practical reality in cardiomyopathy.

## References


1. Yang Y, Jooss KU, Su Q *et al*. Immune responses to viral antigens versus transgene product in the elimination of recombinant adenovirus-infected hepatocytes *in vivo*. *Gene Therapy* 1996; 3: 137–44.
2. Horwitz MS. Adenoviridae and their replication. In: Fields BN, Knipe DM, Chanock RM *et al*. (eds) *Fundamental virology*. Vol. 1. New York: Raven Press, 771–816.
3. Hajjar RJ, Schmidt U, Kang JX *et al*. Adenoviral gene transfer of phospholamban in isolated rat cardiomyocytes. Rescue effects by concomitant gene transfer of sarcoplasmic reticulum Ca(2+)-ATPase. *Circ Res* 1997; 81: 145–53.
4. Hajjar RJ, Kang JX, Gwathmey JK, Rosenzweig A. Physiological effects of adenoviral gene transfer of sarcoplasmic reticulum calcium ATPase in isolated rat myocytes. *Circulation* 1997; 95: 423–9.
5. Guzman RJ, Lemarchand P, Crystal RG, Epstein SE, Finkel T. Efficient gene transfer into myocardium by direct injection of adenovirus vectors. *Circ Res* 1993; 73: 1202–7.
6. Magovern CJ, Mack CA, Zhang J *et al*. Direct *in vivo* gene transfer to canine myocardium using a replication-deficient adenovirus vector. *Ann Thorac Surg* 1996; 62: 425–33.
7. Lee J, Laks H, Drinkwater DC *et al*. Cardiac gene transfer by intracoronary infusion of adenovirus vector-mediated reporter gene in the transplanted mouse heart. *J Thorac Cardiovasc Surg* 1996; 111: 246–52.

8. Kass-Eisler A, Falck-Pedersen AE, Alvira M *et al.* Quantitative determination of adenovirus-mediated gene delivery to rat cardiac myocytes *in vitro* and *in vivo*. *Proc Natl Acad Sci USA* 1993; 90: 11 498–502.
9. Hajjar R, Schmidt U, Matsui T *et al.* Modulation of ventricular function through gene transfer *in vivo*. *Proc Natl Acad Sci USA* 1998; 95: 5251–6.
10. French BA, Mazur W, Geske RS, Bolli R. Direct *in vivo* gene transfer into porcine myocardium using replication-deficient adenoviral vectors. *Circulation* 1994; 90: 2414–24.
11. Barr E, Carroll J, Kalynych AM, Tripathy SK *et al.* Efficient catheter-mediated gene transfer into the heart using replication-defective adenovirus. *Gene Ther* 1994; 1: 51–8.
12. Quinones M, Leor J, Kloner R *et al.* Avoidance of immune response prolongs expression of genes delivered to the adult rat myocardium by replication-defective adenovirus. *Circulation* 1996; 94: 1394–401.
13. Engelhardt JF, Ye X, Doranz B, Wilson JM. Ablation of E2A in recombinant adenoviruses improves transgene persistence and decreases inflammatory response in mouse liver. *Proc Natl Acad Sci USA* 1994; 91: 6196–200.
14. Krougliak V, Graham FL. Development of cell lines capable of complementing E1, E4, and protein IX defective adenovirus type 5 mutants. *Hum Gene Therapy* 1995; 6: 1575–86.
15. Yeh P, Dedieu JF, Orsini C *et al.* Efficient dual transcomplementation of adenovirus E1 and E4 regions from a 293-derived cell line expressiong a minimal E4 functional unit. *J Virol* 1996; 70: 559–65.
16. Brough DE, Lizonova A, Hsu C *et al.* A gene transfer vector-cell line system for complete functional complementation of adenovirus early regions E1 and E4. *J Virol* 1996; 70: 6497–501.
17. Gao GP, Yang Y, Wilson JM. Biology of adenovirus vectors with E1 and E4 deletions for liver-directed gene therapy. *J Virol* 1996; 70: 8934–43.
18. Fisher KJ, Choi H, Burda J *et al.* Recombinant adenovirus deleted of all viral genes for gene therapy of cystic fibrosis. *Virology* 1996; 217: 11–22.
19. Kochanek S, Clemens PR, Mitani K *et al.* A new adenoviral vector: replacement of all viral coding sequences with 28 kb of DNA independently expressing both full-length dystrophin and beta-galactosidase. *Proc Natl Acd Sci USA* 1996; 93: 5731–6.
20. Barry WH, Bridge JHB. Intracellular calcium homeostasis in cardiac myocytes. *Circulation* 1993; 87: 1806–15.
21. Arai M, Matsui H, Periasamy M. Sarcoplasmic reticulum gene expression in cardiac hypertrophy and heart failure. *Circ Res* 1994; 74: 555–64.
22. Aviv A. Recent advances in cellular $Ca^{2+}$ homeostasis: implications to altered regulations of cellular $Ca^{2+}$ and $Na^{(+)}$–$H^{+}$ exchange in essential hypertension. *Curr Opin Cardiol* 1996; 11: 477–82.
23. Balke CW, Gold MR. Excitation–contraction–relaxation coupling in the normal and failing heart. *Heart Dis Stroke* 1993; 2: 150–5.
24. Liao R, Helm PA, Hajjar RJ *et al.* $[Ca^{2+}]_i$ in human heart failure: a review and discussion of current areas of controversy. *Yale J Biol Med* 1994; 67: 247–64.
25. Bristow MR. Mechanism of action of beta-blocking agents in heart failure. *Am J Cardiol* 1997; 80: 26–40L.
26. Gauthier C, Tavernier G, Charpentier F *et al.* Functional β3 adrenoreceptor in the human heart. *J Clin Invest* 1996; 98: 556–62.
27. Lefkowitz RJ. G proteins in medicine. *N Engl J Med* 1995; 332: 186–7.
28. Lefkowitz RJ, Pitcher J, Krueger K, Daaka Y. Mechanisms of beta-adrenergic receptor desensitization and resensitization. *Adv Pharmacol* 1998; 42: 416–20.
29. Bohm M, Flesch M, Schnabel P. Beta-adrenergic signal transduction in the failing and hypertrophied myocardium. *J Mol Med* 1997; 75: 842–8.
30. Muller FU, Boknik P, Knapp J *et al.* Quantification of the cAMP response element binding protein in ventricular nuclear protein from failing and nonfailing human hearts. *Biochem Biophys Res Commun* 1997; 236: 351–4.
31. Bohm M, Flesch M, Schnabel P. Role of G-proteins in altered beta-adrenergic responsiveness in the failing and hypertrophied myocardium. *Basic Res Cardiol* 1996; 91: 47–51.
32. Lohse MJ, Engelhardt S, Danner S, Bohm M. Mechanisms of beta-adrenergic receptor desensitization: from molecular biology to heart failure. *Basic Res Cardiol* 1996; 91: 29–34.
33. Flesch M, Erdmann E, Bohm M. Changes in beta-adrenoceptors and G-proteins during the transition from cardiac hypertrophy to heart failure. *J Card Fail* 1996; 2: S35–43.
34. Flesch M, Schwinger RH, Schnabel P *et al.* Sarcoplasmic reticulum $Ca^{2+}$-ATPase and phospholamban mRNA and protein levels in end-stage heart failure due to ischemic or dilated cardiomyopathy. *J Mol Med* 1996; 74: 321–32.
35. Bohm M. Alterations of beta-adrenoceptor-G-protein-regulated adenylyl cyclase in heart failure. *Mol Cell Biochem* 1995; 147: 147–60.
36. Colucci WS. Molecular and cellular mechanisms of myocardial failure. *Am J Cardiol* 1997; 80: 15–25L.
37. Asano K, Dutcher DL, Port JD *et al.* Selective downregulation of the angiotensin II AT1-receptor subtype in failing human ventricular myocardium. *Circulation* 1997; 95: 1193–200.
38. Rockman HA, Choi DJ, Rahman NU *et al.* Receptor-specific *in vivo* desensitization by the G protein-coupled receptor kinase-5 in transgenic mice. *Proc Natl Acad Sci USA* 1996; 93: 9954–9.
39. Rockman HA, Koch WJ, Milano CA, Lefkowitz RJ. Myocardial beta-adrenergic receptor signaling *in vivo*: insights from transgenic mice. *J Mol Med* 1996; 74: 489–95.
40. Balke CW, Egan TM, Wier WG. Processes that remove calcium from the cytoplasm during excitation–contraction coupling in intact rat heart cells. *J Physiol* 1994; 474: 447–62.
41. Koss KL, Kranias EG. Phospholamban: a prominent regulator of myocardial contractility. *Circ Res* 1996; 79: 1059–63.
42. Wier WG, Lopez-Lopez JR, Shacklock PS, Balke CW. Calcium signalling in cardiac muscle cells. *Ciba Found Symp* 1995; 188: 146–60.
43. Gwathmey JK, Bentivegna LA, Ransil BJ *et al.* Relationship of abnormal intracellular calcium mobilisation to myocyte hypertrophy in human ventricular myocardium. *Cardiovasc Res* 1993; 27: 199–203.
44. Gwathmey JK, Morgan JP. Sarcoplasmic reticulum calcium mobilization in right ventricular pressure-overload hypertrophy in the ferret: relationships to diastolic dysfunction and a negative treppe. *Pflugers Arch Eur J Physiol* 1993; 422: 599–608.
45. Gomez AM, Valdivia HH, Cheng H *et al.* Defective excitation–contraction coupling in experimental cardiac hypertrophy and heart failure. *Science* 1997; 276: 800–6.
46. Schwartz K, Mercadier JJ. Molecular and cellular biology of heart failure. *Curr Opin Cardiol* 1996; 11: 227–36.
47. Flesch M, Putz F, Schwinger RH, Bohm M. Functional relevance of an enhanced expression of the $Na^{(+)}$–$Ca^{2+}$ exchanger in the failing human heart. *Ann NY Acad Sci* 1996; 779: 539–42.
48. Flesch M, Schwinger RH, Schiffer F *et al.* Evidence for functional relevance of an enhanced expression of the $Na^{(+)}$–$Ca^{2+}$ exchanger in failing human myocardium. *Circulation* 1996; 94: 992–1002.
49. Katz AM. The cardiomyopathy of overload: an unnatural growth response. *Eur Heart J* 1995; 16: 110–14.

50. Nakao K, Minobe W, Roden R *et al.* Myosin heavy chain gene expression in human heart failure. *J Clin Invest* 1997; 100: 2362–70.
51. Hajjar RJ, Gwathmey JK. Cross-bridge dynamics in human ventricular myocardium. Regulation of contractility in the failing heart. *Circulation* 1992; 86: 1819–26.
52. Hajjar RJ, Gwathmey JK, Briggs GM, Morgan JP. Differential effect of DPI 201–106 on the sensitivity of the myofilaments to $Ca^{2+}$ in intact and skinned trabeculae from control and myopathic human hearts. *J Clin Invest* 1988; 82: 1578–84.
53. Drazner MH, Peppel KC, Dyer S *et al.* Potentiation of beta-adrenergic signaling by adenoviral-mediated gene transfer in adult rabbit ventricular myocytes. *J Clin Invest* 1997; 99: 288–96.
54. Akhter SA, Skaer CA, Kypson AP *et al.* Restoration of beta-adrenergic signaling in failing cardiac ventricular myocytes via denoviral-mediated gene transfer. *Proc Natl Acad Sci USA* 1997; 94: 12 100–5.
55. Giordano FJ, He H, McDonough P *et al.* Adenovirus-mediated gene transfer reconstitutes depressed sarcoplasmic reticulum $Ca^{2+}$-ATPase levels and shortens prolonged cardiac myocyte $Ca^{2+}$ transients. *Circulation* 1997; 96: 400–3.
56. Westfall MV, Rust EM, Metzger JM. Slow skeletal troponin I gene transfer, expression, and myofilament incorporation enhances adult cardiac myocyte contractile function. *Proc Natl Acad Sci USA* 1997; 94: 5444–9.
57. Westfall MV, Rust EM, Albayya F, Metzger JM. Adenovirus-mediated myofilament gene transfer into adult cardiac myocytes. *Methods Cell Biol* 1997; 52: 307–22.
58. Force T, Pombo CM, Avruch JA, Bonventre JV, Kyriakis JM. Stress-activated protein kinases in cardiovascular disease. *Circ Res* 1996; 78: 947–53.
59. Kyriakis JM, Avruch J. Protein kinase cascades activated by stress and inflammatory cytokines. *BioEssays* 1996; 18: 567–77.
60. Sadoshima J, Izumo S. Rapamycin selectively inhibits angiotensin II-induced increase in protein synthesis in cardiac myocytes *in vitro*. *Circ Res* 1995; 77: 1040–52.
61. Pullen N, Dennis PB, Andjelkovic M *et al.* Phosphorylation and activation of p70S6K by PDK1. *Science* 1998; 279: 707–10.
62. Kyriakis JM, Avruch J. Sounding the alarm: protein kinase cascades activated by stress and inflammation. *J Biol Chem* 1996; 271: 24 313–16.
63. Lenormand P, Sardet C, Pages G *et al.* Growth factors induce nuclear translocation of MAP kinases (p42 and p44) but not of their activator MAP kinase kinase (p45) in fibroblasts. *J Cell Biol* 1993; 122: 1079–88.
64. Wang Y, Huang S, Sah VP, Ross J *et al.* Cardiac muscle cell hypertrophy and apoptosis induced by distinct members of the p38 mitogen-activated protein kinase family. *J Biol Chem* 1998; 273: 2161–8.
65. Zechner D, Thuerauf DJ, Hanford DS *et al.* A role for the p38 mitogen-activated protein kinase pathway in myocardial cell growth, sarcomeric organization, and cardiac-specific gene expression. *J Cell Biol* 1997; 139: 115–27.
66. Wang Y, Su B, Sah VP *et al.* Cardiac hypertrophy induced by mitogen-activated protein kinase kinase 7, a specific activator for c-Jun $NH_2$-terminal kinase in ventricular muscle cells. *J Biol Chem* 1998; 273: 5423–6.
67. Cohen P. The search for physiological substrates of mitogen- and stress-activated protein kinases in mammalian cells. *Trends Cell Biol* 1997; 7: 353–61.
68. Verheij M, Bose R, Hua Lin X *et al.* Requirement for ceramide-initiated SAPK/JNK signalling in stress-induced apoptosis. *Nature* 1996; 380: 75–9.
69. Zanke BW, Boudreau K, Rubie E *et al.* The stress-activated protein kinase pathway mediates cell death following injury induced by cis-platinum, UV irradiation or heat. *Curr Biol* 1996; 6: 606–13.
70. Choukroun G, Hajjar R, Bonventre JV *et al.* Role of the stress-activated protein kinases in endothelin-induced cardiomyocyte hypertrophy. *J Clin Invest* 1998; 102: 1311–20.
71. Komuro I, Yazaki Y. Control of cardiac gene expression by mechanical stress. *Annu Rev Physiol* 1993; 55: 55–75.
72. Pennica D, Shaw KJ, Swanson TA *et al.* Cardiotrophin-1. Biological activities and binding to the leukemia inhibitory factor receptor/gp130 complex. *J Biol Chem* 1995; 270: 10 915–22.
73. Parker TG, Schneider MD. Peptide growth factor can provoke 'fetal' contractile protein gene expression in rat cardiac myocytes. *J Clin Invest* 1990; 85: 507–14.
74. Yamazaki T, Yazaki Y. Is there a major involvement of the renin–angiotensin system in cardiac hypertrophy. *Circ Res* 1997; 81: 639–42.
75. Sakai S, Miyauchi T, Kobayashi M *et al.* Inhibition of myocardial endothelin pathway improves long-term survival in heart failure. *Nature* 1996; 385: 353–5.
76. Shubita HE, McDonough PM, Harris AN *et al.* Endothelin induction of inositol phospholipid hydrolysis, sarcomere assembly, and cardiac gene expression in ventricular myocytes. *J Biol Chem* 1990; 265: 20 555–62.
77. Sadoshima J, Xu Y, Slayter HS, Izumo S. Autocrine release of angiotensin II mediates stretch-induced hypertrophy of cardiac myocytes *in vitro*. *Cell* 1993; 75: 977–84.
78. Akhter SA, Luttrell LM, Rockman HA *et al.* Targeting the receptor-Gq interface to inhibit *in vivo* pressure overload myocardial hypertrophy. *Science* 1998; 280: 574–7.
79. Nemoto S, Zelin S, Lin A. Opposing effects of Jun kinase and p38 mitogen-activated protein kinases on cardiomyocyte hypertrophy. *Mol Cell Biol* 1998; 18: 3518–26.
80. Whitmarsh AJ, Yang S-H, Su M-S *et al.* Role of p38 and JNK mitogen-activated protein kinases in activation of ternary complex factors. *Mol Cell Biol* 1997; 17: 2360–71.
81. Klee CB, Ren H, Wang X. Regulation of the calmodulin-stimulated protein phosphatase, calcineurin. *J Biol Chem* 1998; 273: 13 367–70.
82. Molkentin JD, Lu JR, Antos CL *et al.* A calcineurin-dependent transcriptional pathway for cardiac hypertrophy. *Cell* 1998; 93: 215–28.
83. Chen L, Glover JNM, Hogan PG *et al.* Structure of the DNA-binding domains from NFAT, Fos, and Jun bound specifically to DNA. *Nature* 1998; 392: 42–8.
84. Pulverer B, Kyriakis JM, Avruch J *et al.* Phophorylation of *c-jun* mediated by MAP kinases. *Nature* 1991; 353: 670–4.
85. Karin M. The regulation of AP-1 activity by mitogen-activated protein kinases. *J Biol Chem* 1995; 270: 16 483–6.
86. Tan Y, Rouse J, Zhang A *et al.* FGF and stress regulate CREB and ATF-1 via a pathway involving p38 MAP kinase and MAPKAP kinase-2. *EMBO J* 1996; 15: 4629–42.
87. Matsuda S, Moriguchi T, Koyasu S, Nishida E. T lymphocyte activation signals for interleukin-2 production involve activation of MKK6-p38 and MKK7-SAPK/JNK signaling pathways sensitive to cyclosporin A. *J Biol Chem* 1998; 273: 12 378–82.

88. Su B, Jacinot E, Masahiko H *et al.* JNK is involved in signal integration during costimulation of T lymphocytes. *Cell* 1994; 77: 727–36.
89. Beals CR, Sheridan CM, Turck CW *et al.* Nuclear export of NF-ATc enhanced by glycogen synthase kinase-3. *Science* 1997; 275: 1930–4.
90. Taffet GE, Teasdale TA, Bleyer AJ *et al.* Survival of elderly men with congestive heart failure. *Age Ageing* 1992; 21: 49–55.
91. Duncan AK, Vittone J, Fleming KC, Smith HC. Cardiovascular disease in elderly patients. *Mayo Clin Proc* 1996; 71: 184–96.
92. Sgonc R, Wick G. Methods for the detection of apoptosis. *Int Arch Allergy Immunol* 1994; 105: 327–32.
93. Compton MM. A biochemical hallmark of apoptosis: internucleosomal degradation of the genome. *Cancer Metastasis Rev* 1992; 11: 105–19.
94. Capasso JM, Palackal T, Olivetti G, Anversa P. Left ventricular failure induced by long-term hypertension in rats. *Circ Res* 1990; 66: 1400–12.
95. Cheng W, Li B, Kajstura J *et al.* Stretch-induced programmed myocyte cell death. *J Clin Invest* 1995; 96: 2247–59.
96. Liu Y, Cigola E, Cheng W *et al.* Myocyte nuclear mitotic division and programmed myocyte cell death characterize the cardiac myopathy induced by rapid ventricular pacing in dogs. *Lab Invest* 1995; 73: 771–87.
97. Sharov VG, Sabbah HN, Shimoyama H *et al.* Evidence of cardiocyte apoptosis in myocardium of dogs with chronic heart failure. *Am J Pathol* 1996; 148: 141–9.
98. Narula J, Haider N, Virmani R *et al.* Apoptosis in myocytes in end-stage heart failure. *N Engl J Med* 1996; 335: 1182–9.
99. Mallat Z, Tedgui A, Fontaliran F *et al.* Evidence of apoptosis in arrhythmogenic right ventricular dysplasia. *N Engl J Med* 1996; 335: 1190–6.
100. Szabolcs M, Michler RE, Yang X *et al.* Apoptosis of cardiac myocytes during cardiac allograft rejection: relation to induction of nitric oxide synthase. *Circulation* 1996; 94: 1665–73.
101. Fernandez E, Garry DJ, Epstein JA *et al.* Programmed cell death in mouse cardiac and skeletal muscle development. *Circulation* 1996; 94: I-281.
102. Gottlieb RA, Burleson KO, Kloner RA *et al.* Reperfusion injury induces apoptosis in rabbit cardiomyocytes. *J Clin Invest* 1994; 94: 1621–8.
103. Saraste A, Pulkki K, Kallajoki M *et al.* Apoptosis in human acute myocardial infarction. *Circulation* 1997; 95: 320–3.
104. Yaoita H, Ogawa K, Maehara K, Maruyama Y. Attenuation of ischemia/reperfusion injury in rats by a caspase inhibitor. *Circulation* 1998; 97: 276–81.
105. Yuan J. Evolutionary conservation of a genetic pathway of programmed cell death. *J Cell Biochem* 1996; 60: 4–11.
106. Alnemri E, Livingston D, Nicholson D *et al.* Human ICE/CED-3 protease nomenclature. *Cell* 1996; 87: 171–2.
107. Misao J, Hayakawa Y, Ohno M *et al.* Expression of bcl-2 protein, an inhibitor of apoptosis, and bax, an accelerator of apoptosis in ventricular myocytes of human hearts with myocardial infarction. *Circulation* 1996; 94: 1506–12.
108. Tanaka M, Ito H, Adachi S *et al.* Hypoxia induces apoptosis with enhanced expression of Fas antigen messenger RNA in cultured neonatal rat cardiomyocytes. *Circ Res* 1994; 75: 426–33.
109. Vaux DL, Strasser A. The molecular biology of apoptosis. *Proc Natl Acad Sci USA* 1996; 93: 2239–44.
110. Gagliardini V, Fernandez PA, Lee RK *et al.* Prevention of vertebrate neuronal death by the crmA gene. *Science* 1994; 263: 826–8.
111. Komiyama T, Ray CA, Pickup DJ *et al.* Inhibition of interleukin-1 beta converting enzyme by the cowpox virus serpin CrmA. An example of cross-class inhibition. *J Biol Chem* 1994; 269: 19 331–7.
112. Los M, Van de Craen M, Penning LC *et al.* Requirement of an ICE/CED-3 protease for Fas/APO-1-mediated apoptosis. *Nature* 1995; 375: 81–3.
113. Tewari M, Dixit VM. Fas- and tumor necrosis factor-induced apoptosis is inhibited by the poxvirus crmA gene product. *J Biol Chem* 1995; 270: 3255–60.
114. Tewari M, Telford WG, Miller RA, Dixit VM. CrmA, a poxvirus-encoded serpin, inhibits cytotoxic T-lymphocyte-mediated apoptosis. *J Biol Chem* 1995; 270: 22 705–8.
115. Tewari M, Quan LT, O'Rourke K *et al.* Yama/CPP32 beta, a mammalian homolog of CED-3, is a CrmA-inhibitable protease that cleaves the death substrate poly(ADP-ribose) polymerase. *Cell* 1995; 81: 801–9.
116. Miura M, Friedlander RM, Yuan J. Tumor necrosis factor-induced apoptosis is mediated by a CrmA-sensitive cell death pathway. *Proc Natl Acad Sci USA* 1995; 92: 8318–22.
117. Nicholson DW, Ali A, Thornberry NA *et al.* Identification and inhibition of the ICE/CED-3 protease necessary for mammalian apoptosis. *Nature* 1995; 376: 37–43.
118. Fernandes-Alnemri T, Armstrong RC, Krebs J *et al. In vitro* activation of CPP32 and Mch3 by Mch4, a novel human apoptotic cysteine protease containing two FADD-like domains. *Proc Natl Acad Sci USA* 1996; 93: 7464–9.
119. Patel T, Gores G, Kaufman S. The role of proteases during apoptosis. *FASEB J* 1996; 10: 587–97.
120. Kaufmann SH, Desnoyers S, Ottaviano Y *et al.* Specific proteolytic cleavage of poly(ADP-ribose) polymerase: an early marker of chemotherapy-induced apoptosis. *Cancer Res* 1993; 53: 3976–85.
121. Rodriguez-Tarduchy G, Collins MK, Garcia I, Lopez-Rivas A. Insulin-like growth factor-I inhibits apoptosis in IL-3-dependent hemopoietic cells. *J Immunol* 1992; 149: 535–40.
122. Stewart CE, Rotwein P. Insulin-like growth factor-II is an autocrine survival factor for differentiating myoblasts. *J Biol Chem* 1996; 271: 11 330–8.
123. Gluckman P, Klempt N, Guan J *et al.* A role for IGF-1 in the rescue of CNS neurons following hypoxic–ischemic injury. *Biochem Biophys Res Commun* 1992; 182: 593–9.
124. Buerke M, Murohara T, Skurk C *et al.* Cardioprotective effect of insulin-like growth factor I in myocardial ischemia followed by reperfusion. *Proc Natl Acad Sci USA* 1995; 92: 8031–5.
125. Jung Y, Miura M, Yuan J. Suppression of interleukin-1 beta-converting enzyme-mediated cell death by insulin-like growth factor. *J Biol Chem* 1996; 271: 5112–17.
126. LeRoith D, Werner H, Beitner-Johnson B, Roberts C. Molecular and cellular aspects of the insulin-like growth factor I receptor. *Endocr Rev* 1995; 16: 143–63.
127. Yao R, Cooper GM. Requirement for phosphatidylinositol-3 kinase in the prevention of apoptosis by nerve growth factor. *Science* 1995; 267: 2003–6.
128. Minshall C, Arkins S, Freund GG, Kelley KW. Requirement for phosphatidylinositol 3′-kinase to protect hemopoietic progenitors against apoptosis depends upon the extracellular survival factor. *J Immunol* 1996; 156: 939–47.
129. Scheid MP, Lauener RW, Duronio V. Role of phosphatidylinositol 3-OH-kinase activity in the inhibition of apoptosis in haemopoietic cells: phosphatidylinositol 3-OH-kinase inhibitors reveal a

difference in signalling between interleukin-3 and granulocyte-macrophage colony stimulating factor. *Biochem J* 1995; 312: 159–62.
130. Yamazaki T, Komuro I, Kudoh S *et al.* Mechanical stress activates protein kinase cascade of phosphorylation in neonatal rat cardiac myocytes. *J Clin Invest* 1995; 96: 438–46.
131. Xia Z, Dickens M, Raingeaud J *et al.* Opposing effects of ERK and JNK-p38 MAP kinases on apoptosis. *Science* 1995; 270: 1326–31.
132. Takahashi K, Yonezawa K, Nishimoto I. Insulin-like growth factor I receptor activated by a transmembrane mutaion. *J Biol Chem* 1995; 270: 19 041–5.
133. Hara K, Yonezawa K, Sakaue H, Ando A *et al.* 1-Phosphatidylinositol 3-kinase activity is required for insulin-stimulated glucose transport but not for RAS activation in CHO cells. *Proc Natl Acad Sci USA* 1994; 91: 7415–19.
134. Kobayashi M, Nagata S, Kita Y *et al.* Expression of a constitutively active phosphatidylinositol 3-kinase induces process formation in rat PC12 cells. Use of Cre/loxP recombination system. *J Biol Chem* 1997; 272: 16 089–92.
135. Sakaue M, Bowtell D, Kasuga M. A dominant-negative mutant of mSOS1 inhibits insulin-induced Ras activation and reveals Ras-dependnet and -independent insulin signaling pathways. *Mol Cell Biol* 1995; 15: 379–88.
136. Yao R, Cooper GM. Growth factor-dependent survival of rodent fibroblasts requires phosphatidylinositol 3-kinase but is independent of pp70S6K activity. *Oncogene* 1996; 13: 343–51.
137. Datta K, Bellacosa A, Chan TO, Tsichlis PN. Akt is a direct target of the phosphatidylinositol 3-kinase. Activation by growth factors, v-src and v-Ha-ras, in Sf9 and mammalian cells. *J Biol Chem* 1996; 271: 30 835–9.
138. Dudek H, Datta SR, Franke TF *et al.* Regulation of neuronal survival by the serine–threonine protein kinase Akt. *Science* 1997; 275: 661–5.
139. Kauffmann-Zeh A, Rodriguez-Viciana P, Ulrich E *et al.* Suppression of c-Myc-induced apoptosis by Ras signalling through PI(3)K and PKB. *Nature* 1997; 385: 544–8.
140. Franke TF, Kaplan DR, Cantley LC, Toker A. Direct regulation of the Akt proto-oncogene product by phosphatidylinositol-3,4-bisphosphate. *Science* 1997; 275: 665–8.
141. Franke TF, Kaplan DR, Cantley LC. PI3K: downstream AKTion blocks apoptosis. *Cell* 1997; 88: 435–7.
142. Kulik G, Klippel A, Weber MJ. Antiapoptotic signalling by the insulin-like growth factor I receptor, phosphatidylinositol 3-kinase, and Akt. *Mol Cell Biol* 1997; 17: 1595–606.
143. Datta SR, Dudek H, Tao X *et al.* Akt phosphorylation of BAD couples survival signals to the cell-intrinsic death machinery. *Cell* 1997; 91: 231–41.
144. Reiss K, Kajstura J, Zhang X *et al.* Acute myocardial infarction leads to upregulation of the IGF-1 autocrine system, DNA replication, and nuclear mitotic division in the remaining viable cardiac myocytes. *Exp Cell Res* 1994; 213: 463–72.
145. Duerr RL, Huang S, Miraliakbar HR *et al.* Insulin-like growth factor-1 enhances ventricular hypertrophy and function during the onset of experimental cardiac failure. *J Clin Invest* 1995; 95: 619–27.
146. Cheng W, Reiss K, Li P *et al.* Aging does not affect the activation of the myocyte insulin-like growth factor-1 autocrine system after infarction and ventricular failure in Fischer 344 rats. *Circ Res* 1996; 78: 536–46.
147. Young LH, Hu X, Yin R *et al.* IGF-1 increases heart myosin heavy chain and actin synthesis in the awake rat. *Circulation* 1996; 94: 1–67.
148. Tsukahara H, Gordienko DV, Tonshoff B *et al.* Direct demonstration of insulin-like growth factor-I-induced nitric oxide production by endothelial cells. *Kidney Int* 1994; 45: 598–604.
149. Fazio S, Sabatini D, Capaldo B *et al.* A preliminary study of growth hormone in the treatment of dilated cardiomyopathy. *N Engl J Med* 1996; 334: 809–14.
150. Isgaard J, Nilsson A, Vikman K, Isaksson OG. Growth hormone regulates the level of insulin-like growth factor-I mRNA in rat skeletal muscle. *J Endocr* 1989; 120: 107–12.
151. Reiss K, Cheng W, Ferber A *et al.* Overexpression of insulin-like growth factor-1 in the heart is coupled with myocyte proliferation in transgenic mice. *Proc Natl Acad Sci USA* 1996; 93: 8630–5.
152. Cittadini A, Stromer H, Katz SE *et al.* Differential cardiac effects of growth hormone and insulin-like growth factor-1 in the rat. A combined *in vivo* and *in vitro* evaluation. *Circulation* 1996; 93: 800–9.
153. Li Q, Li B, Wang X *et al.* Overexpression of insulin-like growth factor-1 in mice protects from myocyte death after infarction, attenuating ventricular dilation, wall stress, and cardiac hypertrophy. *J Clin Invest* 1997; 100: 1991–9.
154. Khan BV, Harrison DG, Olbrych MT *et al.* Nitric oxide regulates vascular cell adhesion molecule 1 gene expression and redox-sensitive transcriptional events in human vascular endothelial cells. *Proc Natl Acad Sci USA* 1996; 93: 9114–19.
155. Kubes P, Kurose I, Granger DN. NO donors prevent integrin-induced leukocyte adhesion but not P-selectin-dependent rolling in postischemic venules. *Am J Physiol* 1994; 267: H931–7.
156. Provost P, Lam JY, Lacoste L *et al.* Endothelium-derived nitric oxide attenuates neutrophil adhesion to endothelium under arterial flow conditions. *Arterioscler Thromb* 1994; 14: 331–5.
157. Huang PL, Huang Z, Mashimo H *et al.* Hypertension in mice lacking the gene for endothelial nitric oxide synthase. *Nature* 1995; 377: 239–42.
158. Harrison DG, Kurz MA, Quillen JE *et al.* Normal and pathophysiologic considerations of endothelial regulation of vascular tone and their relevance to nitrate therapy. *Am J Cardiol* 1992; 70: 11–17B.
159. Krumholz HM, Larson M, Levy D. Prognosis of left ventricular geometric patterns in the Framingham Heart Study. *J Am Coll Cardiol* 1995; 25: 879–84.
160. Umansky S, Cuenco G, Khutzian S *et al.* Post-ischemic apoptotic death of rat neonatal cardiomyocytes. *Cell Death differentiation* 1995; 2: 235–241.
161. Koopman G, Reutelingsperger CP, Kuijten GA *et al.* Annexin V for flow cytometric detection of phosphatidylserine expression on B cells undergoing apoptosis. *Blood* 1994; 84: 1415–20.
162. Vermes I, Haanen C, Steffens-Nakken H, Reutelinsperger C. A novel assay for apoptosis. Flow cytometric detection of phosphatidylserine expression on early apoptotic cells using fluorescein labelled Annexin V. *J Immunol Methods* 1995; 184: 39–51.
163. Matsui T, Li L, del Monte F *et al.* Adenoviral gene transfer of activated phosphatidylinositol 3′-kinase and Akt inhibits apoptosis of hypoxic cardiomyocytes *in vitro*. *Circulation* 1999; 100: 2373–9.

# Congestive heart failure: contemporary medical therapy 31

R. M. DELGADO III AND J. T. WILLERSON

## Introduction

Heart failure is the end result of various heart diseases that damage the myocardium. Previous chapters in this book have described the myriad ways in which myocardial damage may occur. If this damage occurs beyond a threshold amount, clinical congestive heart failure (CHF) will result. This sets into motion the frequently described vicious cycle of CHF in which lowered systemic perfusion leads to activation of systemic mechanisms that may contribute to progressive myocardial dysfunction (Figure 31.1). This model is oversimplified in that there is now evidence that many other systemic and myocardial systems are also upregulated by the altered haemodynamics of heart failure. A common theme to be found in this chapter is that the medical interventions that interrupt this vicious cycle of progression seem to have the greatest effect in slowing the progression of the disease.

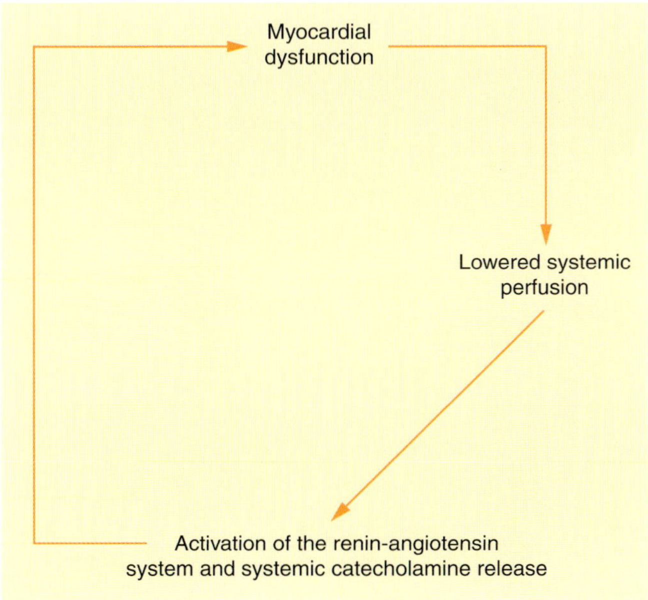


**Figure 31.1** *The vicious cycle of heart failure. Myocardial dysfunction leads to impaired hemodynamics which then causes activation of the renin–angiotensin system and systemic catecholamine release. This, in turn, leads to further myocardial dysfunction.*

As we have improved our methods of treating once fatal conditions, such as acute coronary syndromes, the incidence and prevalence of heart failure has risen. Heart failure now, directly or indirectly, contributes to the death of approximately 250 000 individuals per year and causes substantial morbidity with over 3 million hospitalizations per year [1–3]. As the population ages, there is a projected two- to three-fold increase in prevalence in the next decade [4]. Thus, it is very important to develop improved therapies based on the understanding of mechanisms involved in the development and progression of heart failure.

During 1999 and 2000, guidelines have been developed by the Heart Failure Society of America and the American Heart Association and American College of Cardiology [5–6]. These guidelines are based on the synthesis of data from large clinical studies in chronic heart failure by experts in the field. These guidelines form the basis for treatment and recommendations made in this chapter. The major classes of drugs used to treat heart failure are described, along with their proposed mechanisms of action and the data to support their use. Finally, current areas of investigation and speculation on the future of medical management of heart failure are presented.

## Angiotensin-converting enzyme inhibitors

Angiotensin-converting enzyme (ACE) inhibitors are the best studied class of drugs for the treatment of CHF. There is definitive evidence that ACE inhibitors reduce mortality and morbidity in patients with heart failure (Table 31.1). A strong statement can now be made that all patients with

**Table 31.1** Large pharmaceutical studies on heart failure and their clinical outcomes

| Trial name | NYHA class | Number of patients | Follow-up (months) | Primary endpoint | Therapy | Findings |
|---|---|---|---|---|---|---|
| CONSENSUS | IV | 253 | 6 | Mortality | Enalapril vs placebo | Enalapril > placebo |
| SOLVD (treatment) | II–IV | 2569 | N/A | Mortality | Enalapril vs placebo | Enalapril > placebo |
| DIG | N/A | 7788 | 37 | Mortality | Digoxin | No difference |
| MDC | | 383 | 18 | Mortality | Metoprolol vs placebo | Metoprolol > placebo |
| GESICA | II–IV | 516 | 24 | Mortality | Amiodarone vs placebo | Amiodarone > placebo in subgroups |
| CHF-STAT | II–IV | 674 | 24 | Mortality | Amiodarone vs placebo | No difference |
| ELITE | II–IV | 722 | 11 | Mortality | Losartan vs captopril | Losartan > captopril |
| ELITE II | II–IV | 3152 | 24 | Mortality | Losartan vs captopril | No difference |
| RESOLVD | II–IV | 768 | 10 | Symptoms and LV remodelling | Candesartan vs enalapril vs both | Combination prevents LV remodelling |
| MERIT-HF | II–IV | 3991 | 12 | Mortality | Metoprolol vs placebo | Metoprolol > placebo |
| US CARVEDILOL (four studies) | II–IV | 1094 | 7–8 | Exercise tolerance and quality of life | Carvedilol vs placebo | Carvedilol > placebo |
| CIBIS I | III–IV | 641 | 21 | Mortality | Bisoprolol vs placebo | No difference |
| CIBIS II | II–IV | 2647 | 16 | Mortality | Bisoprolol vs placebo | Bisoprolol > placebo |
| BEST | III–IV | 2708 | N/A | Mortality | Bucindolol vs placebo | No difference |
| RALES | IV | 1663 | 24 | Mortality | Spironolactone vs placebo | Spironolactone > placebo |
| COPERNICUS | IIIB–IV | 1800 | Early termination | Mortality | Carvedilol vs placebo | Carvedilol > placebo |

heart failure due to left ventricular (LV) systolic dysfunction should receive an ACE inhibitor, unless they are intolerant to the drug [5–9].

ACE inhibitors work by inhibiting the renin–angiotensin system (RAS) through the blockade of ACE [a key catalytic protein in the generation of angiotensin (AngII)], the breakdown of bradykinin, and the formation of aldosterone. Inhibiting this system reduces sodium and water retention and causes arterial vasodilatation and venodilatation, thereby unloading the heart through its influence in reducing venous return to the right heart and decreasing resistance to ejection by the left heart. By these mechanisms, ACE inhibitors break the vicious cycle of heart failure (Fig. 31.1). ACE inhibitors play a role in tissue remodelling at the myocyte level and in vascular remodelling in the systemic vasculature.

The SOLVD trial established that these drugs provide symptomatic relief and favourably affect the risk of morbidity and mortality in patients with symptomatic heart failure [10]. The SOLVD trial showed that ACE inhibitors were also beneficial in patients with asymptomatic LV systolic dysfunction by decreasing the likelihood of hospitalization for heart failure [11] (Table 31.1). The CONSENSUS study showed that ACE inhibitors favourably affect mortality in patients with severe heart failure [New York Heart-Association (NYHA) class IV] [12] (Table 31.1). A more recent analysis of trials conducted with various ACE inhibitors in patients with CHF shows that the beneficial effects of these drugs seem to be a class effect without a significant benefit of one drug over another. This does not exclude the possibility, however, that an ACE inhibitor with relatively greater vascular or tissue effect might not have a greater effect in vascular or myocyte protection [13].

There are contraindications to the use of these drugs, such as hypotension, relative hyperkalaemia, and the deterioration of renal function. For these reasons, it is recommended that initial doses be small with careful up titration over a period of weeks, until the target dose is achieved. Worsening renal insufficiency appears to occur mostly in patients with renal vascular disease, although it may also occur in patients with severe heart failure.

Hyperkalaemia develops in some patients with concomitant renal disease and in some who are treated with potassium-sparing diuretics. In these cases, patients should be closely monitored in the first few days and weeks after initiation of the ACE inhibitor. Cough occurs in 15–30% of treated patients and is the most common reason for discontinuation of these drugs [14, 15]. In patients in whom the cough is persistent and troublesome, therapy with angiotensin II receptor blockers (ARBs) or the combination of hydralazine and isosorbide dinitrate may be used. Angio-oedema occurs in less than 1% of patients receiving an ACE inhibitor, although this may be a life-threatening side-effect (15).

It is important to realize that even though some side-effects may occur early in treatment, they do not generally prevent long-term use of ACE inhibitors. In addition, symptomatic improvement may not be seen until patients have received treatment for several weeks or months. Furthermore, ACE inhibitors may reduce the risk of disease progression, even if symptoms have not responded favourably to treatment. Selected ACE inhibitor trials are listed in Table 31.1.

## Angiotensin II receptor blockers

ARBs act by inhibiting this receptor for AngII on the cell membrane. The clinical effects of these drugs are similar to ACE inhibitors, although it is unclear whether they have the same tissue effects, such as the vascular remodelling effects of ACE inhibitors. They are capable of substantial reduction in blood pressure in patients with systemic arterial hypertension, and they lower systemic vascular resistance in patients with heart failure [16].

The ELITE study compared losartan (an ARB) with captopril (an ACE inhibitor) and showed a small mortality benefit for losartan over captopril in elderly patients with CHF [17] (Table 31.1). However, a follow-up study, ELITE II, a much larger study with more than 3000 patients, showed no mortality benefit of losartan over captopril [18]. The dose of losartan used in this study was 50 mg/day, which is a relatively low dose, and it is possible that a higher dose of the ARB might be more effective. It was found in this study that the ARB was better tolerated than the SCE inhibitor, primarily because of the coughing associated with ACE inhibitors.

Studies with other ARBs, such as the RESOLVD trial, which evaluated candesartan and enalapril, showed no benefit of the ARB over the ACE inhibitor [19]. Prior to the emergence of ARBs, the combination of hydralazine and isosorbide dinitrate was used in patients who were intolerant to ACE inhibitors. Early studies show that this combination was better than placebo, but not as good as ACE inhibitors in the treatment of heart failure [20].

The current recommendation is that patients should be treated with an ACE inhibitor, and only if truly intolerant should then be treated with the combination of hydralazine and isosorbide dinitrate or an ARB. Patients who develop worsening renal function, ACE inhibitor, hypotension or hyperkalaemia with an ACE inhibitor often have the same effects with an ARB. Thus, care must be used in these patients to try to avoid and certainly to detect these side-effects. Studies are underway presently to determine whether or not the conbination of ACE inhibitors and ARBs is better than ACE inhibitors alone in the treatment of heart failure.

## Diuretic therapy

The goal of diuretic therapy is to improve symptoms related to congestion. Dietary sodium restriction is important in patients who have intravascular volume overload, as this may decrease their need for diuretic therapy and may mitigate metabolic abnormalities associated with diuretic therapy. Thiazide diuretics may be effective in treating some patients with mild fluid overload and relatively normal renal function. Most patients, however, require loop diuretics to reduce filling pressure and intravascular volume. Patients with severe heart failure and compromised renal function may require the use of two or more diuretics with different mechanisms of action. Most patients with symptomatic CHF require maintenance doses of a diuretic. These patients should be educated to look for signs of volume overload and instructed to record their weights daily, at the same time of day, after voiding. Patients can be given a range for weight gain or loss, after which they should contact their physician.

Non-steroidal anti-inflammatory drugs should be used carefully in patients on diuretics, as they may increase the tendency of diuretics to cause azotaemia [21–23]. These anti-inflammatory drugs may also decrease the effects of ACE inhibitors, thereby leading to haemodynamic decompensation in an otherwise stable patient. The newer cyclooxygenase II specific anti-inflammatory drugs (COX-2 inhibitors) appear to have a lower incidence of this problem. The most important adverse effect of diuretics in this patient population is electrolyte depletion, particularly hypokalaemia. Depletion of potassium and magnesium may produce serious arrhythmias [24]. This risk is particularly high when diuretics that do not spare potassium are used at the same time. Potassium-sparing diuretics, such as spironolactone, which will be discussed in a subsequent section, may help to prevent potassium depletion, as does the careful administration of exogenous potassium.

Diuetics are known to increase activation of the RAS and perhaps other neurohormonal systems [25]. This may exacerbate electrolyte depletion and promote progression of heart failure over the long term. Volume depletion with excessive use of diuretics may lead to azotaemia and hypotension, placing the patient in a vicious cycle of hyperkalaemia and digitalis toxicity. This is also seen when patients have conditions that lead to volume depletion, such as vomiting, diarrhoea, or a febrile illness. In these circumstances, patients should be taken off their diuretics and monitored closely with volume repletion, if necessary. Finally, an ACE inhibitor and or ARB therapy may decrease the need for diuretics and prevent the need for potassium supplementation in some patients receiving diuretic therapy.

## Digoxin

Digoxin has been used for more than 200 years in the treatment of heart failure and atrial arrhythmias. Nevertheless, there is some controversy as to whether digoxin should be used in patients with CHF in normal sinus rhythm. It is clear that digoxin is beneficial in patients with symptomatic heart failure and associated atrial fibrillation. Currently, the US Food and Drug Administration has given approval for digoxin use for the treatment of mild to moderate heart failure in patients with or without atrial fibrillation [26].

Digoxin is currently the only oral drug with positive inotropic effects approved for long-term management of CHF. Digoxin's weak positive inotropic effect is due to inhibition of sodium-potassium-adenosine triphosphatase (Na/K-ATPase), which results in an increase in intracelluar calcium. Digoxin also has an important neurohormonal-modulating effect with a sympathoinhibitory effect, which is independent of its inotropic action [27, 28].

The DIG trial was a placebo-controlled, double-blind, randomized study of more than 7000 patients that included a 3 year follow-up and showed a neutral effect of digoxin on mortality [29]. However, fewer patients in the digoxin-treated group were hospitalized for worsening of their heart failure, and a smaller number of patients required additional interventions to treat worsening heart failure.

The PROVED and RADIANCE trials show that patients who are on digoxin, diuretics, and ACE inhibitor therapy were less likely to have worsening of their heart failure than patients treated with a diuretic, an ACE inhibitor or a diuretic with digoxin [30]. A subgroup analysis of the DIG trial indicated that patients with severe NYHA class IV heart failure also benefit from digoxin. A retrospective analysis of the PROVED and RADIANCE data showed that patients with mild heart failure withdrawn from digoxin had an increased risk of worsening of their heart failure. Thus, patients with LV systolic dysfunction and mild symptoms of heart failure probably benefit clinically and symptomatically from digoxin therapy [31].

Recent data suggest that the dose of digoxin should be 0.125 or 0.25 mg once per day based on body weight and renal function, and that higher doses are not necessary to derive neurohormonal and functional benefits [32, 33]. In patients who have CHF and atrial fibrillation with a rapid ventricular response, it is not recommended that doses greater than 0.25 mg/day be used for heart-rate control, but rather that a β-blocker or amiodarone be added to help to control heart rate, if needed [5]. If amiodarone is used for this purpose, it is important to reduce the dose of digoxin or monitor its levels closely, since amiodarone reduces renal and non-renal clearance of digoxin, thereby increasing serum concentrations.

## β-Blockers

β-Blockers have been studied in patients with heart failure since the 1970s, and they have slowly gained favour in its treatment [34]. Small, early studies showed that β-blockers were safe, when initiated at low doses and titrated up slowly under observation [35]. In studies that followed patients for more than 3 months, improvements left ventricular in ejection fraction (LVEF) and symptoms were often shown [36]. These studies led to other large-scale studies, and clinical trials using β-blockers in patients with CHF that now include more than 10 000 patients [37, 38].

It is now clear that β-blockers represent a significant advance in the treatment of heart failure, although difficulty in initiation and the early need for gradual upward titration in dose have led to slow initial usage. Current recommendations by the Heart Failure Society of America are that β-blockers should be routinely administered in clinically stable patients with LV systolic dysfunction (LVEF ≤

40%) and mild to moderate symptoms of heart failure (NYHA class II–III), and that these patients should already be on standard therapy with an ACE inhibitor, diuretics, and digoxin [5].

It is important to consider specific β-blockers, because although $\beta_1$-selective and non-selective β-blockers appear to have similar efficacy in heart failure, β-blockers with intrinsic sympathomimetic activity may have a negative impact on mortality, and thus should not be used.

Metoprolol has been studied in two trials and found to be of benefit. In the Metoprolol in Dilated Cardiomyopathy (MDC) study, 383 patients with non-ischaemic heart failure and classs II–III symptoms were evaluated [36]. The results showed a 34% reduction in risk of need for cardiac transplantation listing, although the absolute reduction in deaths was not statistically significant [36]. The MERIT-HF trial used metoprolol CR-XL and included 3999 patients with NYHA class II–IV heart failure [39]. The patients were initiated on a low dose of 12.5–25 mg/day and up-titrated to a target dose of 200 mg/day during an 8 week period. Premature discontinuation of the drug was similar between treated and placebo groups. The metoprolol-treated group showed a 34% reduction in mortality ($p$ = 0.0062) [40].

The effect of bisoprolol was evaluated in the CIBIS studies. In the CIBIS I study, 641 patients with NYHA class III–IV heart failure were evaluated [41]. An initial dose of 1.25 mg/day was up-titrated to a maximum of 5 mg/day. This study found no significant difference in all-cause mortality. However, the risk of hospitalization was reduced by 34%. These findings led to the larger CIBIS II study which investigated 2647 patients over 1.3 years [42]. Most patients received ACE inhibitors, diuretics, and digoxin and more than 80% had NYHA class III heart failure. The target dose range of bisoprolol was increased to 10 mg/day. This study showed an annual reduction in mortality of 34% and a 32% decrease in hospitalization.

Metoprolol and bisoprolol are $\beta_1$-selective β-blockers. In contrast, carvedilol is a non-selective $\beta_1$- and $\beta_2$-blocker with additional α-adrenergic blocker and free radical scavenging properties. It has been studied in multiple trials and shown to be beneficial in the treatment of heart failure. The US Carvedilol studies comprised four different study populations and included a total of 1094 patients [43–45]. Doses of carvedilol ranged from 3.125 mg twice a day to 50 mg twice a day, and patients were up-titrated as in other studies. The treated patients had a LVEF of <35% and were in NYHA classes II–IV. The studies were terminated early because of a reduced mortality associated with the use of carvedilol across the four combined trials. In addition, the mortality risk was 65% lower in the treated group, and the combined risk of hospitalization or death was reduced by 38% compared with placebo.

Some have questioned the validity of the survival analysis in the US Carvedilol trials because mortality was not the primary endpoint, and only one of the four trials achieved a significant result when mortality was analysed as a primary endpoint. Despite this, the overall survival benefit and reduction in hospitalization have been accepted as significant. Analysis of individual studies shows that there seems to be a greater benefit in patients who have more severe heart failure, and that higher doses, 25 mg twice a day, are better than lower doses [45]. Current recommendations are to attempt to achieve 25 mg twice a day and 50 mg twice a day in patients weighing more than 80 kg.

The Australian/New Zealand Carvedilol study included 415 patients with ischaemic cardiomyopathy, NYHA class I–III symptoms, and a LVEF < 45% [46]. This study of patients with less severe heart failure showed a decrease in the combined risk of all-cause mortality and hospitalization of 26% in the carvedilol-treated patients. The recent COPERNICUS trial, designed to assess the use of carvedilol in patients with severe heart failure (NYHA class III–IV), has recently been completed. Preliminary results demonstrate positive benefits with carvedilol therapy in this population with more severe heart failure.

Based on these studies, it is believed that β-blockers not only have significant mortality and symptomatic benefit in the short to medium term, but also seem to slow the progression of heart failure and attenuate LV remodelling. For example, the LV diastolic dimension may be significantly reduced in β-blocker-treated patients. In addition, β-blockers are often able to improve LVEF in some patients, especially those with concomitant hypertension; in some cases, it has been possible to remove patients from the transplant waiting list.

It is clear from prior studies that β-blockers are beneficial in patients after myocardial infarction and following coronary revascularization. In addition, β-blockers are capable of decreasing LV hypertrophy. Given these findings and the belief that β-blockers slow progression of LV dysfunction (both systolic and diastolic dysfunction), it has now been recommended that β-blockers be considered for use in patients with an LVEF <40%, even when they are asymptomatic (NYHA class I) [5]. In this circumstance, ACE inhibitors should also be used, based on data from the SOLVD prevention study [11]. A study comparing metoprolol and carvedilol is currently underway to determine whether one has benefit over the other.

Initiation of β-blocker therapy is often difficult and requires frequent follow-up and close monitoring. Patients should be clinically stable on standard therapy, including an ACE inhibitor and digoxin, for at least 2–3 weeks before initiating the β-blocker. However, it is widely believed that patients can be initiated on the lowest doses of β-blockers during hospitalization for an acute exacerbation, if they are monitored closely. An upcoming study will assess whether the positive inotropic agent milrinone may be used to facilitate initiation of β-blockers in patients with recent decompensation of their heart failure.

β-Blockers should be initiated at their lowest recommended doses and up-titrated very slowly, generally every 2 weeks over a period of 2 months. Patients should be evaluated by a physician or physician extender during each titration period. In many patients, the up-titration must occur over prolonged periods, and it is not always possible to achieve maximal doses in all patients. However, even moderate doses have shown clinical benefits and should be achieved, if at all possible.

If patients are experiencing worsening symptoms or side-effects due to a β-blocker, the up-titration should not be performed. It may be necessary to adjust other medications during the up-titration periods, such as lowering the diuretic dose in patients who have orthostatic symptoms, which is the most common side-effect of carvedilol. Patients should be reassured that orthostatic symptoms may occur in the first few days after up-titration but usually improve. Worsening of congestive symptoms is uncommon during initiation, but when they occur they can often be easily managed with titration of diuretics. Symptomatic bradycardia may develop in patients who are also receiving digoxin and amiodarone. In these patients, slow withdrawal of the amiodarone or digoxin and monitoring of serum digoxin levels often will achieve clinical stability [5].

The non-selective β-blockers may be more prone to causing bronchospasm. In patients who experience this side-effect, $\beta_1$-selective β-blockers should be preferentially used. In patients who develop severe bronchospasm, the β-blocker will need to be discontinued. It is not advisable to give these agents to patients with a history of severe asthma or with wheezing on examination. Abrupt discontinuation of the β-blocker is not recommended. There are reports of sudden cardiac death after abrupt discontinuation of β-blockers, especially in patients with coronary artery disease [47, 48]. Finally, when using β-blockers in patients with heart failure, patient education is very important. As such, heart failure educational programmes are becoming more available and are especially useful for this purpose [49].

## Spironolactone

The recent RALES trial demonstrated the benefit of low-dose spironolactone in survival of patients with severe NYHA class IV heart failure [50] (Table 31.1). This study was developed as a result of emerging evidence that aldosterone appears to play an important role in the pathophysiology of CHF. Aldosterone has been shown to increase sympathetic activation and parasympathetic inhibition and to promote cardiac and vascular structural remodelling through collagen synthesis [51–53]. In addition, aldosterone enhances sodium retention and potassium and magnesium loss in patients with heart failure [54].

Early studies of ACE inhibitors in patients with heart failure showed a divergence of mortality curves soon after initiation of the ACE inhibitor, but the mortality curves then appear to run parallel over the long term. It has been postulated that this effect may be due to a transient decrease in aldosterone secretion caused by the ACE inhibition. Despite continuation of the ACE inhibitor, there is a return of serum aldosterone levels similar to that prior to initiation of the ACE inhibition [55]. This may help to explain the benefit provided by aldosterone inhibition in patients with heart failure.

The RALES trial, which had an endpoint of all-cause mortality, included 1663 patients with severe heart failure and LVEF of <35%. There was a 46% mortality rate in the placebo group compared with 35% in the spironolactone-treated group ($p < 0.001$) [50] (Table 31.1). Both sudden death and death from progressive heart failure were reduced. In addition, the frequency of hospitalization for patients with heart failure was 35% lower in the aldosterone-treated group ($p < 0.001$), and there was a greater improvement in NYHA class in the treated group. Since this was a selected group of patients, transferring these data to clinical practice must be done with care.

Current recommendations for use of spironolactone in patients with heart failure limit it to use in patients who have NYHA class IV symptoms. Spironolactone should be initiated at a dose of 12.5 or 25 mg/day and maximized at 25 mg/day. It should not be used in patients with a serum potassium of ≥ 5.0 mmol/l or a serum creatinine of ≥ 2.5 mg/dl. Potassium supplements should be decreased or stopped, and serum potassium should be monitored closely. Spironolactone should be used carefully in patients with low cardiac output and/or with recent fluctuations in renal function. Hyperkalaemia is the most important side-effect, but gynaecomastia sometimes with breast pain may also occur with chronic use.

Aldosterone antagonism represents yet another modality of therapy in patients with heart failure, which targets a specific hormone known to be deranged in this disease state. Future studies will demonstrate whether or not this multitargeted approach results in long-term slowing or some reversal of the disease process.

## Anticoagulation and antiplatelet therapy

Warfarin has been studied in patients with heart failure and found to be effective in preventing thromboembolic complications in patients with intermittent atrial fibrillation and in patients with prior thromboembolic events. These findings have led to its recommendation for use in heart-failure patients with these complications [7, 8]. There are no data to support using warfarin in patients without atrial fibrillation or prior thromboembolic events, and expert opinions vary. Some have advocated its use in patients with a LV diastolic dimension of greater than 6 cm or patients with spontaneous echo contrast noted on echocardiogram. It does seem clear, however, that patients with evidence of a mural thrombus should receive warfarin anticoagulation, but there is also no clear recommendation as to the appropriate dose. Current practice seems to favour an International Normalized Ratio (INR) range from 2.0 to 3.0. Future studies will address these issues and compare warfarin with aspirin and other antiplatelet agents.

Aspirin has important effects in patients with coronary artery disease and atherosclerosis [56]. A retrospective analysis of studies with ACE inhibitors in patients with heart failure and postmyocardial infarction has shown that there may be a drug interaction between aspirin and ACE inhibitors [57, 58]. Despite this, there is no conclusive evidence from a study designed to examine the question of whether or not aspirin and ACE inhibitors together abrogate the expected beneficial effect in patients with heart failure. Aspirin appears to diminish the haemodynamic effects of ACE inhibitors, but this may be counterbalanced by the positive effect of aspirin in reducing ischaemic events through its antithrombotic effect [59]. The mechanism of action of aspirin appears to be due its inhibition of thromboxane $A_2$ synthesis. Newer antagonists of adenosine diphosphate, such as ticlopidine and clopidogrel, do not exhibit this effect [60]. Clopidogrel has been compared with aspirin in a large study (CAPRIE trial) and shown to prevent vascular events in patients with atherosclerotic disease slightly but statistically significantly better than aspirin [61]. Further studies are needed to determine the role of adenosine diphosphate antagonists in preventing thrombosis in patients with heart failure.

## Antiarrhythmic therapy

Sudden death continues to be a common cause of death in heart-failure patients. The most important initiating cause of sudden death is remains unclear, but could be bradyarrhythmia, tachyarrhythmia or haemodynamic causes. Therefore, it is difficult to assess the benefit of antiarrhythmic therapy without performing large clinical trials. It appears that class III antiarrhythmic drugs may hold the greatest promise for prevention of sudden death in patients with heart failure. Studies involving D-sotalol and dofetilide have not shown an improvement in mortality [62, 63]. However, in selected studies, amiodarone has shown an improvement in mortality.

The GESICA trial studied 516 patients with severe CHF with NYHA class III–IV symptoms and a mean LVEF of 20%. This study showed a 28% reduction in all-cause mortality, which was the primary endpoint, and the trial was terminated prematurely. An analysis of the data revealed that sudden cardiac death and death due to progressive heart failure were both reduced by comparable amounts. In addition, the beneficial effects were seen mainly in patients with a resting heart rate of 90 beats/min [64].

The CHF-STAT study involved 674 patients with a greater proportion of ischaemic cardiomyopathy patients than the GESICA study and with slightly less severe CHF. It showed a trend towards improved survival with amiodarone in patients with non-ischemic heart failure but no significant improvement in patients with coronary heart disease ($p = 0.07$) [65]. In addition, the amiodarone-treated patients showed improved LVEF, but in patients with a symptomatic non-sustained ventricular tachycardia there was no benefit. These seemingly conflicting results may have been due to differences in the population of patients studied. Based on this, amiodarone cannot be generally recommended for the prevention of arrhythmias and sudden cardiac death in heart-failure patients. However, it can be recommended as the drug of choice for treatment of supraventricular tachycardia not controlled by digoxin or β-blockers in patients with heart failure [5].

There have been several studies on the use of implantable cardiac defibrillators in the treatment of life-threatening arrhythmias in patients with heart failure. However, these studies have not specifically been performed on heart-failure patients [66–68]. Studies are underway with defibrillators as well as a combination device, which includes a multisite pacemaker and defibrillator, in patients with CHF. Presently, the recommendations for use of defibrillators in heart-failure patients mirror those in patients without heart failure, i.e. they should be used in patients who have been resuscitated from an arrhythmic sudden cardiac death and in those with haemodynamically destabilizing or sustained or repetitive ventricular tachycardia.

## Medical management of decompensated heart failure

There is controversy concerning the use of inotropic therapy in decompensated and chronic advanced heart failure. It is clear that in the acutely decompensated state, inotropes may be used to preserve end-organ function and to stabilize an unstable patient. Controversy exists, however, over the role of inotropic agents in the long-term management of patients with severe CHF despite optimal oral medical therapy.

The most commonly used inotropic agents in the management of decompensated advanced heart failure include dobutamine, milrinone, and dopamine. Dobutamine is a β-antagonist, which increases myocardial contractility and causes peripheral vasodilatation by stimulation of β-receptors. It is effective in increasing stroke volume but must be combined with a vasodilator, such as nitroprusside, or a diuretic to reduce filling pressures [69, 70]. Dobutamine increases myocardial oxygen consumption and may cause tachycardia and increased arrhythmogenicity [69, 71, 72]. Dopamine acts on peripheral dopaminergic receptors, promotes vasodilatation of some vascular beds at low doses, and improves renal blood flow. At low doses, dopamine may facilitate diuresis in patients with severe refractory heart failure and renal insufficiency, and exerts no important efffect on myocardial oxygen consumption. It is often useful in combination with other vasodilators, such as nitroprusside or milrinone.

Phosphodiesterase inhibitors (PDEIs), such as milrinone and amrinone, offer some advantages over β-agonists, particularly in chronic heart-failure patients [69, 73–76]. These drugs reduce right ventricular afterload better than dobutamine and lower pulmonary capillary wedge pressure with less of an increase in myocardial oxygen consumption [73–76]. As they are not dependent on β-receptors for their action, these agents seem to cause less tachycardia and can be used in combination with β-blockers [77]. Lower doses of PDEIs should be used in patients at high risk for arrhythmias, as these agents have arrhythmogenic potential. Care must be used in treating patients with renal insufficiency, because drug toxicity can occur in renally impaired patients, leading to proarrhythmia effects. The half-life of milrinone is approximately 2.5 h. Thus, its onset of action after initiation and loss of effect after discontinuation take longer than with β-agonists. Because of its theoretical benefits over dobutamine and its ability to be used with β-blockers, milrinone is now finding an important role in the management of severe heart failure. In patients considered for cardiac transplantation or in those listed for transplantation and being bridged to transplant, milrinone offers the advantage of lowering pulmonary vascular resistance and thus the chance of developing donor right heart failure after transplant. The long-term outpatient use of milrinone is controversial in that it may increase mortality. Studies to examine this question are difficult to perform owing to the severity of illness of the patients; therefore, the decision to use inotropes must take into account benefit in symptoms versus the possibility of increased mortality risk.

## Future medical management of heart failure

Medical interventions in heart failure are designed to interrupt deranged counterregulatory systems. As new physiological derangements are found, new classes of drugs are being studied for heart-failure treatment; for example, inhibitors of endothelin receptors are being studied, as are agents that block the metabolism of atrial naturetic peptide. The future may see a complicated and expanding array of drugs used to block deranged systems in heart failure.

There is an alternative area of investigation in which agents are used to try to slow or reverse the progression of heart failure by inhibiting adverse remodelling at a basic level. These agents may be able to halt the disease process before systemic counterregulatory consequences occur. Inflammation of the myocardium may play a role in this process and inhibitors of inflammation and agents that modulate the remodelling process, such as inhibitors of tumour necrosis factor-α and matrix metalloproteinases, may play a role in the future in stabilizing or reversing the course of heart failure.

## References


1. Massie BM, Shah NB. Evolving trends in the epidemiologic factors of heart failure: rationale for preventive strategies and comprehensive disease management. *Am Heart J* 1997; 133: 703–12.
2. Graves EJ. National hospital discharge survey: annual summary, 1993. *Vital and Heatlh Statistics*, Volume 121, Series 13: data from National Health Survey. Washington DC: US Government Printing Office, 1995, 1–63.
3. Centers for Disease Control and Prevention. Cerebrovascular disease mortality and Medicare hospitalization — United States, 1980–1990. MMWR 1992; 41: 447–80.
4. Eriksson H. Heart failure: a growing public health problem. *J Intern Med* 1995; 237: 135–41.
5. HFSA Guidelines for Management of patients with Heart Failure Caused by Left Ventricular Systolic Dysfunction — Pharmacological Approaches. *J Card Fail* 1999; 5: 357–82.
6. Packer M, Cohn JN on behalf of the Steering Committee and Membership of the Advisory Council to Improve Outcomes Nationwide in Heart Failure. Consensus recommendations for the management of chronic heart failure. *Am J Cardiol* 1999; 83 (Suppl): 1–38A.
7. Konstam MA, Dracup K, Baker D *et al.* Heart failure: evaluation and care of patients with left ventricular systolic dysfunction. Rockville, MD: Agency for Health Care Policy and Research, US Department of Health and Human Services, 1994.
8. ACC/AHA Task Force on Practice Guidelines. Guidelines for the evaluation and management of heart failure. *Circulation* 1995; 92: 2764–84.
9. Task Force of the Working Group for Heart Failure and the European Society of Cardiology. The treatment of heart failure. *Eur Heart J* 1997; 18: 736–53.
10. SOLVD Investigators. Effect of enalapril on survival in patients with reduced left ventricular ejection fractions and congestive heart failure. *N Engl J Med* 1991; 22: 1411–17.
11. SOLVD Investigators. Effect of enalapril on mortality and the development on heart failure in asymptomatic patients with reduced left ventricular ejection fractions. *N Engl J Med* 1992; 327: 375–80.
12. CONSENSUS Trial Study Group. Effects of enalapril on mortality in severe congestive heart failure: results of the Cooperative North Scandinavian Enalapril Survival Study (CONSENSUS). *N Engl J Med* 1987; 316: 1429–35.
13. Yusuf S, Sleight P, Pogue J *et al.* Effects of an angiotensin-converting-enzyme inhibitor, ramipril, on cardiovascular events in high-risk patients. The Heart Outcomes Prevention Evaluation Study Investigators. *N Engl J Med* 2000; 342: 145–53.
14. Packer M, Kessler PD, Gottilieb SS. Adverse effects of converting-enzyme inhibition in patients with severe congestive heart failure: pathophysiology and management. *Postgrad Med J* 1986; 62 (Suppl 1): 179–82.
15. Israili ZH, Hall WD. Cough and angioneurotic edema associated with angiotesin-converting enzyme inhibitor therapy: a review of the literature and pathophysiology. *Ann Intern Med* 1992; 117: 234–42.
16. Crozier I, Ikram H, Awan N *et al.* for the Losartan Hemodynamic Study Group. Losartan in heart failure: hemodynamic effects and tolerability. *Circulation* 1995; 91: 691–7.
17. Pitt B, Segal R, Martinez FA *et al.* Randomized trial of losartan versus captopril in patients over 65 with heart failure (ELITE). *Lancet* 1997; 349: 747–51.
18. Pitt B, Poole-Wilson P, Segal R *et al.* Effects of losartan versus captopril on mortality in patients with symptomatic heart failure: rationale, design, and baseline characteristics of the patients in the Losartan Heart Failure Survival Study (ELITE II). *J Card Fail* 1999; 5: 146–54.
19. Yusuf A, Maggioni AP, Held P *et al.* Effects of candesartan, enalapril or their combinations on exercise capacity, ventricular function, clinical deterioration, and quality of life in heart failure: Randomized Evaluation of Strategies for Left Ventricular Dysfunction (RESOLVD) (Abstract). *Circulation* 1997; 96: I-452.
20. Cohn JN, Johnson G, Ziesche S *et al.* A comparison of enalapril with hydralazine-isosorbide dinitrate in the treatment of chronic congestive heart failure. *N Engl J Med* 1991; 325: 303–10.
21. Herchuelz A, Derenne F, Deger F *et al.* Interaction between nonsteroidal anti-inflammatory drugs and loop diuretics: modulation by sodium balance. *J Pharmacol Exp Ther* 1989; 248: 1175–81.
22. Dzau VJ, Packer M, Lilly LS *et al.* Prostaglandins in severe heart failure: relation to activation of the renin–angiotensin system and hyponatermia. *N Engl J Med* 1984; 310: 347–52.
23. Gottlieb SS, Robinson S, Krichten CM *et al.* Renal response to indomethacin in congestive heart failure secondary to ischemic or idiopathic dilated cardiomyopathy. *Am J Cardiol* 1992; 70: 890–3.
24. Steiness E. Olesen KH. Cardiac arrhythmias induced by hypokalemia and potassium loss during maintenance digoxin therapy. *Br Heart J* 1976; 38: 167–72.
25. Francis GS, Benedict C, Johnston DE *et al.* Comparison of neuroendocrine activation in patients with left ventricular dysfunction with and without congestive heart failure: a substudy of the Studies of Left Ventricular Dysfunction (SOLVD). *Circulation* 1990; 82: 1724–9.
26. Lanoxin Package Insert. GlaxoWellcome, 1997.
27. Gheorghiade M, Ferguson D. Digoxin: a neurohormonal modulator in heart failure? *Circulation* 1991; 84: 2181–6.
28. Ferguson DW, Berg WJ, Sander JS *et al.* Sympathoinhibitory responses to digitalis glycosides in heart failure patients: direct evidence from sympathetic neural recordings. *Circulation* 1989; 80: 65–77.
29. Digitalis Investigation Group. The effect of digoxin on mortality and morbidity in patients with heart failure. *N Engl J Med* 1997; 336: 525–33.
30. Young JB, Gheorghiade M, Uretsky BF *et al.* Superiority of 'triple' drug therapy in heart failure: insights from the PROVED and RADIANCE trials. *J Am Coll Cardiol* 1998; 32: 686–92.

31. Adams KF, Gheorghiade M, Uretsky BF *et al.* Patients with mild heart failure worsen during withdrawal from digoxin therapy. *J Am Coll Cardiol* 1997; 30: 42–8.
32. Gheorghiade M, Hall VB, Jacobsen G *et al.* Effects of increasing maintenance dose of digoxin on left ventricular function and neurohormones in patients with chronic heart failure treated with diuretics and angiotensin-converting enzyme inhibitors. *Circulation* 1995; 92: 1801–17.
33. Slatton ML, Irani WN, Hall SA *et al.* Does digoxin provide additional hemodynamic and autonomic benefit at higher doses in patients with mild to moderate heart failure and normal sinus rhythm? *J Am Coll Cardiol* 1997; 29: 1206–13.
34. Swedberg K, Hjalmarson A, Waagstein F *et al.* Prolongation of survival in congestive cardiomyopathy by beta-receptor blockade. Beneficial effects of metoprolol in idiopathic dilated cardiomyopathy. *Lancet* 1979; i: 374–6.
35. Bristow MR. O'Connell JB, Gilbert EM *et al.* Dose–response of chronic β-blocker treatment in heart failure from either idiopathic dilated or ischemic cardiomyopathy. *Circulation* 1994; 89: 1632–42.
36. Waagstein F, Bristow MR, Swedberg K *et al.* Beneficial effects of metoprolol in idiopathic dilated cardiomyopathy: Metoprolol in Dilated Cardiomyopathy (MDC) Trial Study Group. *Lancet* 1993; 342: 1441–6.
37. Heidenreich PA, Lee TT, Massie BM. Effect of beta-blockade on mortality in patients with heart failure: a meta-analysis of randomized clinical trials. *J Am Coll Cardiol* 1997; 30: 27–34.
38. Lechat P, Packer M, Chalon S *et al.* Clinical effects of beta-adrenergic blockade in chronic heart failure: a meta-analysis of double-blind, placebo-controlled, randomized trials. *Circulation* 1998; 98: 1184–91.
39. International Steering Committee. Rationale, design, and organization of the Metoprolol CR/XL Randomized Intervention Trial in Heart Failure (MERIT-HF). *Am J Cardiol* 1997; 80 (Suppl): 54–8J.
40. MERIT-HF Study Group. Effect of metoprolol CR/XL in chronic heart failure: metoprolol CR/XL randomized intervention trial in congestive heart failure (MERIT-HF). *Lancet* 1999; 353: 2001–7.
41. CIBIS Investigators and Committees. A randomized trial of beta-blockade in heart failure: the Cardiac Insufficiency Bisoprolol Study (CIBIS). *Circulation* 1994; 90: 1765–73.
42. CIBIS Investigators and Committees. The Cardiac Insufficiency Bisoprolol Study II (CIBIS-II). A randomized trial of beta-blockade in heart failure. *Lancet* 1999; 353: 9–13.
43. Packer M, Bristow MR, Cohn JN *et al.* The effect of carvedilol on morbidity and mortality in patients with chronic heart failure. *N Engl J Med* 1996; 334: 1349–55.
44. Goldsmith SR, Dick C. Differentiating systolic from diastolic heart failure: pathophysiologic and therapeutic considerations. *Am J Med* 1993; 95: 645–55.
45. Cohn JN, Archibald DG, Ziesche S *et al.* Effect of vasodilator therapy on mortality in chronic congestive heart failure: results of a Veterans Administration Cooperative Study. *N Engl J Med* 1986; 314: 1547–52.
46. Cohn JN, Johnson G, Ziesche S *et al.* A comparison of enalapril with hydralazine–isosorbide dinitrate in the treatment of chronic congestive heart failure. *N Engl J Med* 1991; 325: 303–10.
47. Waagstein F, Caidahl K, Wallentin I *et al.* Long-term beta-blockade in dilated cardiomyopathy: effects of short-term and long-term metoptolol followed by withdrawal and readministration of metoprolol. *Circulation* 1989; 80: 551–63.
48. Morimoto S, Shimizu K, Yamada K *et al.* Can beta-blocker therapy be withdrawn from patients with dilated cardiomyopathy? *Am Heart J* 1999; 137: 456–9.
49. Uretsky BF, Pina I, Quigg RJ *et al.* Beyond drug therapy: nonpharmacologic care of the patient with advanced heart failure. *Am Heart J* 1998; 135: S264–84.
50. Pitt B, Zannad F, Remme WJ *et al.* The effect of spironolactone on morbidity and mortality in patients with severe heart failure. *N Engl J Med* 1999; 341: 709–17.
51. Wang W. Chronic administration of aldosterone depresses baroreceptor reflex function in the dog. *Hypertension* 1994; 24: 571–5.
52. Weber KT, Brilla CG. Pathological hypertrophy and cardiac interstitium: fibrosis and renin–angiotensin–aldosterone system. *Circulation* 1991; 83: 1849–65.
53. Duprez DA, De Buyzere ML, Rietzchel ER *et al.* Inverse relationship between aldosterone and large artery compliance in chronically treated heart failure patients. *Eur Heart J* 1998; 19: 1371–6.
54. Dzau VJ, Colucci WS, Hollenberg NK *et al.* Relation of the renin–angiotensin–aldosterone system to clinical state in congestive heart failure. *Circulation* 1981; 63: 645–51.
55. Struthers AD. Aldosterone escape during angiotensin-converting enzyme inhibitor therapy in chronic heart failure. *J Card Fail* 1996; 2: 47–54.
56. Antiplatelet Trialist's Collaboration. Collaborative overview of randomized trials of antiplatelet therapy-I. Prevention of death, myocardial infarction and stroke by prolonged antiplatelet therapy in various categories of patients. *BMJ* 1994; 308: 81–106.
57. Nguyen KN, Aursnes I, Kjekshus J. Interaction between enalapril and aspirin on mortality after acute myocardial infarction: subgroup analysis of the Cooperative New Scandinavian Enalapril Survival Study II (CONSENSUS II). *Am J Cardiol* 1997; 79: 115–19.
58. Peterson JG, Lauer MS, Young JB *et al.* Evidence for an adverse interaction between ACE inhibitors and aspirin following a myocardial infarction: the GUSTO-1 Trial (Abstract). *J Am Coll Cardiol* 1998; 31: 96A.
59. Oosterga M, Anthonio RL, de Kam PJ *et al.* Effects of aspirin on angiotensin-converting enzyme inhibition and left ventricular dilation one year after acute myocardial infarction. *Am J Card* 1998; 82: 1178–81.
60. Sharis PJ, Cannon CP, Loscalzo J. The antiplatelet effects of ticlopidine and clopidogrel. *Ann Intern Med* 1998; 129: 394–405.
61. CAPRIE: Steering Committee. A randomized, blinded trial of clopidogrel versus aspirin in patients at risk of ischemic events. *Lancet* 1996; 348: 1329–39.
62. Waldo AL, Camm AJ, deRuyter H *et al.* Effect of D-sotalol on morality in patients with left ventricular dysfunction after recent and remote myocardial infarction. *Lancet* 1996; 348: 7–12.
63. Bloch-Thompsen PE for the DIAMOND-MI Investigators. Danish investigation of arrhythmia and mortality on dofetilide (Abstract). Presented at the 70th Scientific Sessions of the American Heart Association. *Clin Cardiol* 1998; 21: 52–4.
64. Doval HC, Nul DR, Grencelli HO *et al.* for the GESICA Investigators. Randomized trial of low-dose amiodarone in severe congestive heart failure. *Lancet* 1994; 33: 77–82.
65. Sullican MJ, Higginbotham MB, Cobb FR. Exercise training in patients with severe left ventricular dysfunction: hemodynamic and metabolic effects. *Circulation* 1988; 78: 506–15.
66. Moss AJ, Hall WJ, Cannon DS *et al.* for the MADIT Investigators. Improved survival with an implanted defibrillator in patients with

coronary disease at high risk for ventricular arrhythmia. *N Engl J Med* 1996; 335: 1933–40.
67. AVID Investigators. A comparison of antiarrhythmic drug therapy or implantable defibrillators in patients resuscitated from near-fatal ventricular arrhythmias. *N Engl J Med* 1997; 337: 1576–83.
68. Cappato R. Secondary prevention of sudden death: the Dutch Study, the Antiarrhythmic Versus Implantable Defibrillator Trial, the Cardiac Arrest Study Hamburg, and the Canadian Implantable Defibrillator Study. *Am J Cardiol* 1999; 83 (Suppl): 68–73D.
69. Monrad ES, Baim DS, Smith HS *et al.* Milrinone, dobutamine, and nitroprusside: comparative effects on hemodynamics and myocardial energetics in patients with severe congestive heart failure. *Circulation* 1986; 73 (Suppl III): III-168–74.
70. Leier CV, Heban PT, Huss P. Comparative systemic and regional hemodynamic effects of dopamine and dobutamine in patients with cardiomyopathic heart failure. *Circulation* 1978; 58: 466–75.
71. Unverferth DA, Blanford M, Kates *et al.* Tolerance to dobutamine after a 72 hour continuous infusion. *Am J Med* 1980; 69: 262–6.
72. Takaoka H, Takeuchi M, Hata K *et al.* Beneficial effects of a $Ca^{2+}$ sensitizer, MCI-154, on the myocardial oxygen consumption–cardiac output relation in patients with left ventricular dysfunction after myocardial infarction: comparison with dobutamine and phosphodiesterase inhibitor. *Am Heart J* 1997; 133: 283–9.
73. Karlsberg RP, DeWood MA, DeMaria AN *et al.* for the Milrinone–Dobutamine Study Group. Comparative efficacy of short-term intravenous infusions of milrinone and dobutamine in acute congestive heart failure following acute myocardial infarction. *Clin Cardiol* 1996; 19: 21–30.
74. Colucci WS, Wright RF, Jaski BE *et al.* Milrinone and dobutamine in severe heart failure: differing hemodynamic effects and individual patient responsiveness. *Circulation* 1984; 73 (Suppl 3): III-175–83.
75. Eichhorn EJ, Konstam MA, Weiland DS *et al.* Differential effects of milrinone and dobutamine on right ventricular preload, afterload and systolic performance in congestive heart failure secondary to ischemic or idiopathic dilated cardiomyopathy. *Am J Cardiol* 1987; 60: 1329–33.
76. Jaski BE, Fifer MA, Wright RF *et al.* Positive inotropic and vasodilator actions of milrinone in patients with severe congestive heart failure. Dose–response relationships and comparison to nitroprusside. *J Clin Invest* 1985; 75: 643–9.
77. Tsvetkova TO, Farber DJ, Abraham WT *et al.* Comparative hemodynamic effects of milrinone and dobutamine in heart failure patients treated chronically with carvedilol (Abstract). *J Card Fail* 1998; 4 (3 Suppl 1): 36.

# SECTION V

# Pathogenetic basis of surgical management in end-stage heart failure

# Exploiting the understanding of pathogenic mechanisms in developing surgical interventions



M. ARGENZIANO AND E. A. ROSE

## Introduction

The different forms of cardiomyopathy vary widely in aetiology, pathophysiology, and natural history. Accordingly, multiple therapeutic modalities are utilized in the management of these disorders, and include pharmacological and medical approaches as well as surgical interventions. In this chapter, the surgical treatments of heart failure and its causes are discussed, with particular attention being paid to the development of procedures based on specific pathogenetic mechanisms. Although the discussion that follows is by no means comprehensive, it is intended to provide examples of operations that either halt or reverse the pathological processes responsible for heart failure, and to explore the pathophysiological basis for the efficacy of these procedures.

## Surgical approaches to the treatment of heart failure

Many surgical procedures have been conceived and used in the prevention and treatment of heart failure, with varying indications, degrees of efficacy, and associated risks. For the purposes of this chapter, the major surgical approaches to heart failure management are categorized according to their principal mode of therapeutic benefit: (1) repair of structural defects causing pressure and volume overload; (2) anatomical remodelling of the ventricle; (3) revascularization of ischaemic myocardium; and (4) ventricular assistance or replacement.

### Correction of conditions resulting in ventricular pressure and volume overload

Perhaps the most straightforward approach to the surgical management of heart failure is represented by operations that aim to correct structural abnormalities responsible for myocardial dysfunction, such as aortic stenosis (AS), aortic insufficiency (AI), mitral regurgitation (MR), and hypertrophic cardiomyopathy (HCM). The aetiology and pathological basis of myocardial dysfunction in these disorders may be quite variable, and while causing minimal symptomatic cardiac dysfunction in early stages, may lead to progressive heart failure. If irreversible, as is often the case in its later stages, heart failure may complicate surgical correction of the original pathological process. For these reasons, and because operations for valvular disorders and HCM are performed on a spectrum of patients ranging from the healthy to the severely ill, numerous options exist in the surgical management of these entities. In this section, the variable pathological manifestations and corresponding surgical treatments of this category of myocardial disorders are examined.

#### *Operations for hypertrophic cardiomyopathy*

HCM, also known as idiopathic hypertrophic subaortic stenosis (IHSS), is a complex familial cardiac disease with unique pathophysiological characteristics and heterogeneous expression, resulting in a diversity of morphological, functional, and clinical features [1, 2]. Caused by a mutation in one of four genes that encode for cardiac sarcomeric proteins [3, 4], HCM is inherited as an autosomal dominant trait and has an estimated prevalence of about 1 in 500 [5]. Although asymmetric hypertrophy of the anterior ventricular septum is the most common morphological characteristic of this disease, other patterns of involvement, including diffuse left ventricular (LV) hypertrophy and minimal localized ventricular thickening, are common. At the microscopic level, a characteristically disorganized cellular architecture is seen in most cases, with chaotic myocyte arrangements and interconnections [6]. It is thought that

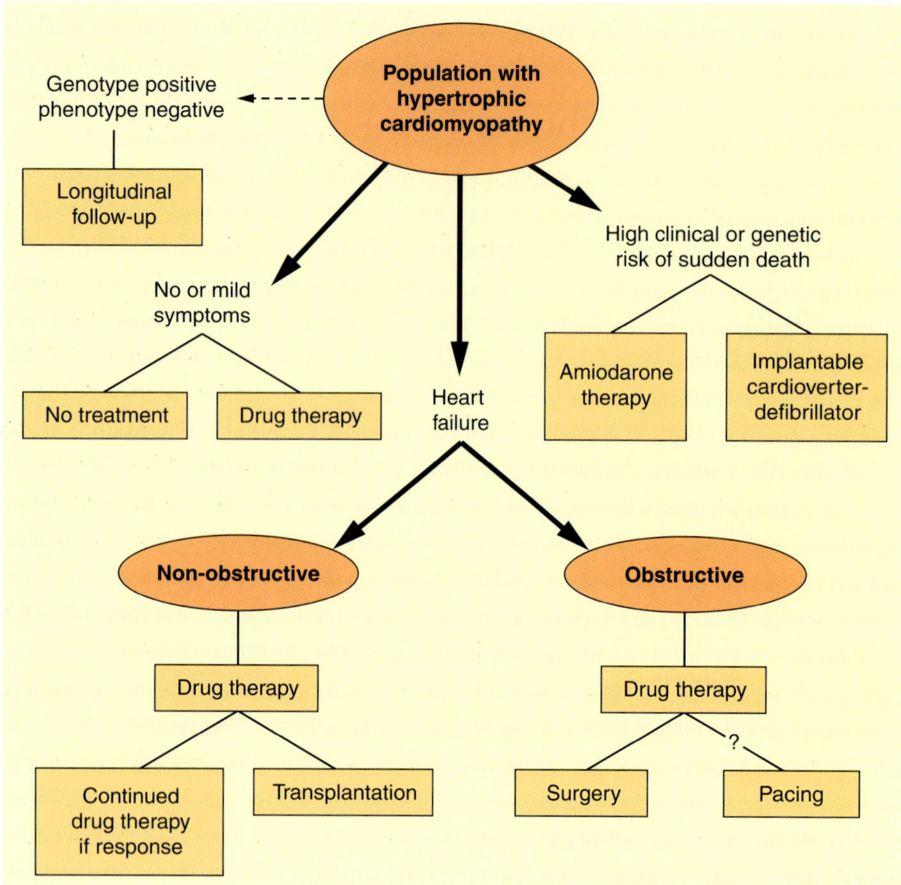


**Figure 32.1** *The principal clinical presentations of hypertrophic cardiomyopathy and corresponding treatment strategies. The size of the arrows indicates the approximate proportion of patients with hypertrophic cardiomyopathy in each subgroup. The dashed arrow indicates the present uncertainties regarding the size of this subgroup, and the question mark indicates the uncertainties regarding the therapeutic efficacy of pacing. The drugs are specified in the text.*

this cellular disorganization may impair normal electrophysiological impulses, thereby serving as an arrhythmogenic substrate. Other abnormalities are also frequently encountered, including malformations of the mitral valve apparatus [7], anomalous papillary muscle insertion directly into the anterior mitral leaflet [8], and collagen deposition throughout the LV wall. This abnormal distribution of collagen is thought to induce a sort of vascular remodelling, resulting in increased ventricular stiffness [9] and abnormal intramural coronary arteries with thickened walls and narrowed lumens [10].

The clinical course of HCM varies widely, ranging from patients who remain asymptomatic with normal life expectancy to those with progressive heart failure, disabling angina, or sudden death. The pathophysiological processes responsible for these clinical sequelae are multiple, and include diastolic dysfunction resulting from impaired relaxation of the non-compliant left ventricle [11], dynamic obstruction of the LV outflow tract by septal hypertrophy or mitral valve systolic anterior motion [12], myocardial ischaemia due to impaired coronary vasodilator reserve [10], and supraventricular and ventricular arrhythmias [11]. Therefore, management of patients with HCM depends not only on the constellation of clinical manifestations encountered, but also on the presumed underlying pathological process (Fig. 32.1).

When arrhythmias are the main source of symptomatology, in the form of either atrial fibrillation (which occurs in 25% of HCM patients) or syncopal episodes (which are likely to be due to ventricular tachyarrhythmias and are a risk factor for subsequent sudden death), medical therapy with amiodarone and other agents is the mainstay of treatment. In patients deemed at high risk of sudden death, insertion of an implantable cardioverter–defibrillator (ICD) is the most definitive therapeutic option.

In cases where heart failure is the predominant clinical manifestation, initial therapy is pharmacological, including calcium channel-blocking and β-blocking agents, which decrease contractility and systolic ventricular pressures. If symptoms do not subside, further management is dictated by the presence or absence of LV outflow obstruction. For patients with refractory symptoms of heart failure and subaortic pressure gradients greater than 50 mmHg, the standard option is ventricular septal myectomy (the Morrow procedure), in which a small amount of muscle is resected from the proximal ventricular septum [11]. By eliminating the outflow obstruction, this operation normalizes ventricular pressures in 90% of patients and results in symptomatic improvement in 70% [13]. Unfortunately, only 5% of HCM patients are candidates for the Morrow procedure, since in most cases a significant subaortic gradient is not demonstrable. Because ventricular hypertrophy is not always localized in the basal septum, and since abnormalities of the mitral valve and subvalvular apparatus have been implicated in the pathophysiology of HCM, some authors have advocated mitral valve replacement [14], mitral valve plication [15], or partial papillary muscle excision [16] alone or in combination with septal myectomy. Although theoretically reasonable options, these procedures are likely to be associated with higher rates of morbidity than simple myotomy–myectomy, and must be applied in carefully selected cases.

Finally, the observed clinical improvement and reduction of subaortic gradients in several HCM patients undergoing dual-chamber pacing for conduction defects has prompted the suggestion that DDD pacing may benefit patients with symptomatic HCM (Fig. 32.2). Postulated mechanisms by which synchronous atrioventricular pacing might ameliorate the pathophysiological derangements of HCM include inhibition of detrimental septal motion by ventricular pre-excitation [17], reduction of the outflow gradient by depression of systolic function [18], reduction of mitral valve anterior systolic motion and subsequent regurgitation [19], and improved diastolic filling [20]. Despite these theoretical considerations, early reports of pacing-induced regression of ventricular hypertrophy [21] have not been substantiated, and the role of pacing in the treatment of this disorder remains highly controversial.

Thus, in the management of HCM, an understanding of the pathological processes responsible for the clinical manifestations is critical, since only a small percentage of patients (i.e. those with heart failure and LV outflow obstruction) are candidates for septal myectomy, and another small group may benefit from implantable defibrillator or permanent pacemaker insertion.

### *Operative treatment of aortic stenosis*

Aortic valvular stenosis is characterized by an increased resistance to LV ejection, resulting in pressure overload and progressive LV hypertrophy and dilatation. Patients with AS are often asymptomatic, and those with mild to moderate disease may not have perceptible symptoms. In fact, several studies have documented a relatively benign long-term course for patients with mild AS. In one longitudinal study of such patients, aortic valve replacement was required in only 8% after 10 years and 22% after 20 years of follow-up [22]. However, some authors have documented more rapid progression of mild to moderate AS in some patients, with a mean rate of increase in aortic gradient of 7.2 mmHg per year [23], especially in patients with aortic valve calcification or concomitant coronary artery disease. Consequently, although patients with mild or moderate AS are at low risk for mortality, close follow-up is warranted in order to identify patients with rapid progression to significant stenosis.

Compared with mild or moderate AS, significant AS, characterized by a valve area of less than 0.7 $cm^2$, is associated with a more malignant course. In studies of patients with haemodynamically significant AS who refused surgery, 5-year mortality rates of 64–75% have been observed [24, 25]. Although cardiac mortality from AS is uncommon in the absence of symptoms, significant AS is known to result in the onset of angina, syncope, or heart failure in 40% of patients within 2 years of diagnosis [26]. With the onset of symptoms, the risk of mortality increases significantly. Average survival in patients with significant AS is 4–5 years after the onset of angina, 2–3 years after the onset of syncope, and 1–2 years after the onset of heart failure [27]. This underscores the importance of close clinical follow-up in patients with AS and the advisability of aortic valve replacement soon after the appearance of symptoms.

Since the onset of angina or syncope usually precedes the development of overt heart failure in patients who develop symptomitic AS, most patients undergoing aortic valve replacement have normal or only mildly impaired LV function. Even in cases of significant ventricular dysfunction due to longstanding AS, the relief of pressure overload afforded by valve replacement usually results in substantial improvement, if not normalization, of ventricular performance. However, despite early symptomatic improvement in these patients, late ventricular dysfunction and overt heart failure are observed in a significant proportion. In fact, almost two-thirds of all deaths occurring more than 12 years after aortic valve replacement are caused by congestive heart failure [24]. Patients at risk for this late

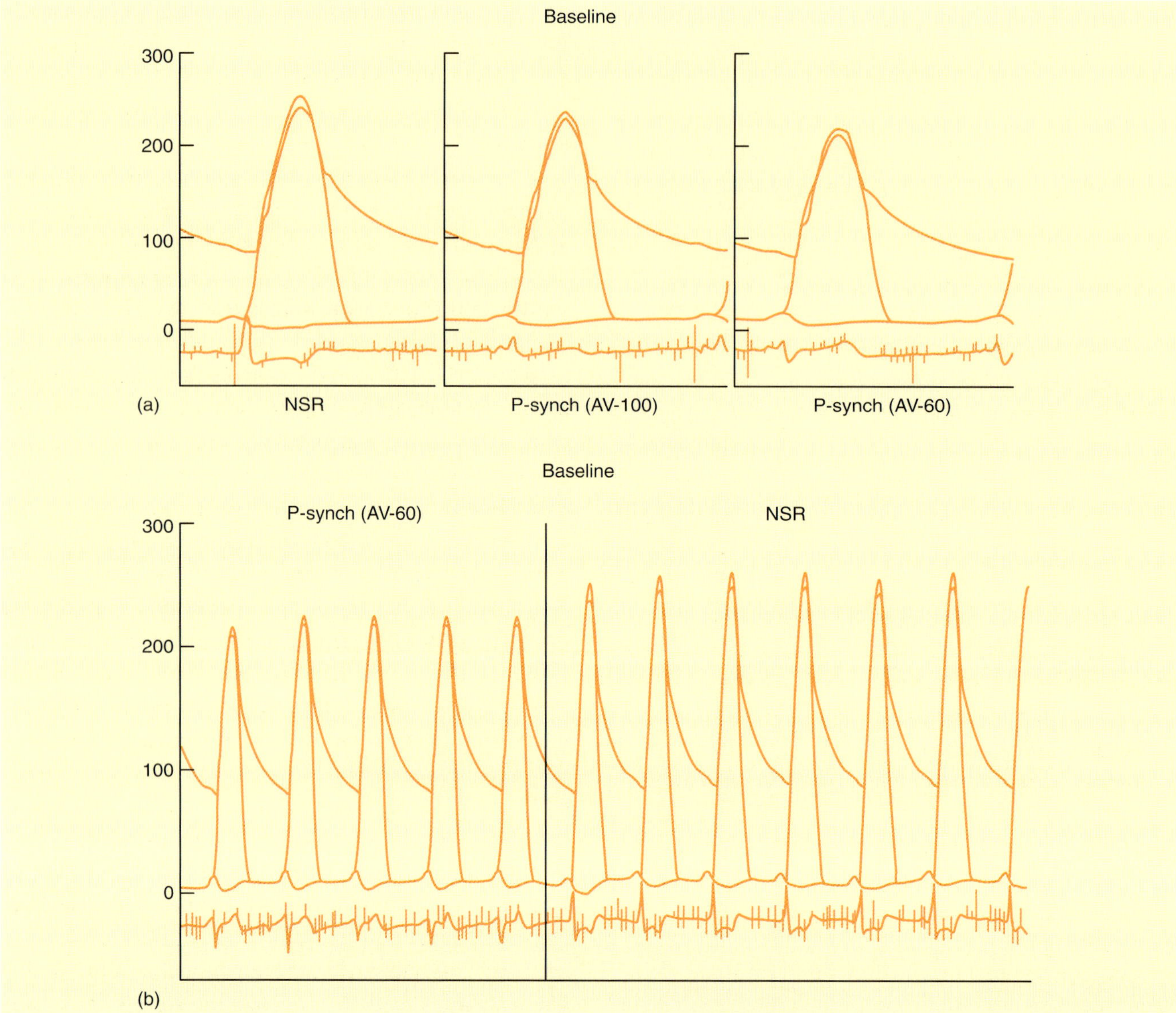


**Figure 32.2** *High-fidelity pressure recordings from left ventricle, ascending aorta, and left atrium obtained from 74-year-old woman with hypertrophic cardiomyopathy and labile outflow tract gradient. Doppler echocardiography performed 10 days before hemodynamic catheterization study revealed minimal outflow obstruction in resting state, but gradient >80 mmHg after amyl nitrate inhalation. (a) In baseline state without outflow tract gradient, dual-chamber pacing a successively shorter AV intervals (P-synch) results in progression lengthening of the QRS duration (i.e. complete capture or pacemaker preexcitation) and reduction of intraventricular pressures. This is most likely a result of dyssynchronous ventricular activation and consequent dyssynergic ventricular contraction. Left atrial contraction with short AV delay pacing occurs closer to onset of ventricular contraction, but does not compromise contribution to left ventricular filling. (b) Sudden termination of ventricular pacing with resumption of sinus rhythm (NSR) results in immediate return of baseline left ventricular and aortic pressures.*

complication are those with preoperative evidence of advanced disease, including ventricular dysfunction, high peak-to-peak systolic gradient, abnormal cardiothoracic index, and ventricular ectopic beats.

Notwithstanding the beneficial effects of pressure unloading on the hypertrophied ventricle in cases of pure AS, it is more difficult to predict the surgical outcome of patients with LV dysfunction and AS in the setting of significant coronary artery disease. In these cases, the relative contributions of ischaemia and pressure overload on ventricular dysfunction may be unclear, and in the absence of concomitant successful revascularization of viable myocardium, isolated aortic valve replacement may not improve ventricular function. In a study of 14 patients with critical AS (valve area ≤ 0.4 $cm^2$) and severe ventricular dysfunction, depressed intrinsic contractility, manifested as a mean systolic aortic valve gradient of less than 30 mmHg, was predictive of a poor clinical outcome [28]. Thus, while patients with AS and ventricular dysfunction due to irreversible processes such as dilated cardiomyopathy, transmural infarction, or non-revascularizable coronary disease often report significant resolution of symptoms after valve replacement, there may not be significant improvement in objective indices of ventricular performance. Furthermore, even patients with progressive ventricular dysfunction due solely to AS eventually reach a point where valve replacement may no longer produce clinical improvement.

In summary, the natural history of severe or symptomatic AS is fairly malignant, since most patients with significant stenosis eventually become symptomatic, and most patients with symptoms die prematurely without aortic valve replacement. Although ventricular dysfunction and clinical heart failure are risk factors for death in patients with significant AS, these processes are usually reversible if aortic valve replacement is undertaken before permanent ventricular damage ensues and in combination with myocardial revascularization in cases of concomitant ischaemic disease. Although patients with longstanding high-grade AS and significant ventricular hypertrophy usually enjoy early symptomatic improvement after surgery, they may be at risk for increased operative mortality, less certain postoperative improvement, and development of late congestive heart failure.

### *Operative treatment of aortic insufficiency*

Aortic regurgitation results in a volume overload of the left ventricle, leading to eccentric ventricular hypertrophy. Because the ventricle thickens as it dilates, the ratio of wall thickness to chamber size remains stable, and a normal ejection fraction is maintained despite increases in end-diastolic volume. Consequently, patients with AI may remain well-compensated and asymptomatic until late in their course. In several studies of the natural history of AI, the clinical course has been shown to be indolent and relatively benign. In one report [29], only 25% of asymptomatic patients with severe (3+ to 4+) aortic regurgitation required aortic valve replacement after 7 years of follow-up, and in a more recent study [30] which followed asymptomatic patients for over 11 years, surgery was prompted by the onset of symptoms or ventricular dysfunction in less than 5% of the patients per year. While these observations may suggest that the majority of patients with severe but asymptomatic AI will never develop symptoms or ventricular failure, longstanding disease eventually leads to decreases in ejection fraction and cardiac output associated with increases in end-diastolic volume. Although the mechanisms of this functional deterioration are not precisely defined, afterload mismatch and inadequate hypertrophy have been implicated. Once ventricular function declines and symptoms of dyspnoea, syncope, or angina supervene, mean survival is only 3–5 years.

Because AI, if allowed to progress indefinitely, eventually leads to ventricular decompensation, clinical heart failure, and death, many patients have aortic valve replacement (AVR). However, for a number of reasons, the decision to proceed with surgery and the appropriate timing of this intervention may not be straightforward. Although many patients tolerate longstanding severe AI without significant clinical manifestations, patients undergoing AVR after the onset of symptoms or ventricular dysfunction are less likely to improve postoperatively and are at increased risk for the development of advanced heart failure [24]. Furthermore, progressive and irreversible ventricular dysfunction may develop in the absence of symptoms. For these reasons, patients with significant AI should be followed closely, and surgery recommended while patients are still asymptomatic or minimally symptomatic and at the first sign of ventricular dysfunction on routine testing. Several authors have attempted to identify preoperative predictors of outcome after AVR for AI, and in two echocardiographic studies [31], preoperative left ventricular end-systolic dimension of more than 55 mm and fractional shortening of less than 25% were associated with an increased risk of postoperative and late death from congestive heart failure. These and other studies have confirmed the importance of surgical intervention prior to the onset of impaired systolic function, ventricular enlargement, or increased systolic wall stress.

The echocardiographic variables cited above have also been found to predict the eventual need for surgery in asymptomatic patients with AI. In one study [32], asymptomatic patients with an end-systolic dimension less than 40 mm required surgery at a rate of only 5% per year with no mortality, while in another [29], 19% of patients with an end-systolic dimension greater than 50 mm developed symptoms, ventricular dysfunction, or sudden death. Finally, several studies have documented the importance of exercise tolerance in the determination of prognosis after

AVR for chronic AI, with preserved exercise tolerance predictive of improved survival and increased reversibility of ventricular dysfunction after surgery. In addition, evaluation of ventricular function during exercise may help to identify patients with early ventricular dysfunction that is masked clinically by a reduction in physical activity.

In summary, patients with significant AI and symptoms of heart failure, angina, or syncope are a high risk for mortality without AVR Asymptomatic patients with severe AI should be followed closely, with regular evaluation of ventricular function at rest and during exercise. AVR is offered to these patients if ventricular function deteriorates, as manifested by a reduced ejection fraction, increased end-systolic dimension, or decreased percentage of fractional shortening. Importantly, the presence of symptoms is associated with decreased postoperative survival and reversibility of ventricular dysfunction, underscoring the need for surgical intervention while patients are still asymptomatic.

### *Mitral valve repair and replacement*

In Western countries, the major cause of MR is degenerative valve disease that results in ruptured chordae and flail mitral leaflets [33]. Although patients with MR may be asymptomatic for many years, the LV volume overload caused by increasing MR leads to progressive ventricular dilatation and dysfunction. As will be discussed in this section, a variety of factors may conceal the severity of myocardial compromise until significant irreversible damage has occurred. Although it is recognized that operative intervention is indicated in patients with severe MR (in which 10-year surgery-free survival is only 10%) [33], the timing and choice of operation are associated with some controversy.

Heart failure is the leading cause of mortality in patients with MR, even after surgical correction of the volume overload [34]. In fact, up to 30% of patients experience postoperative LV dysfunction [35], often without preoperative evidence of heart failure or decreased ejection fraction. This postoperative decrement in LV function may be attributed to a number of factors. The preoperative ejection fraction and systolic function are often overestimated in patients with MR, since the low-pressure atrium decreases effective afterload. When this low-pressure decompression is eliminated, afterload increases and preload decreases, with resultant depression of the ejection fraction. Also, in the case of traditional mitral valve replacement

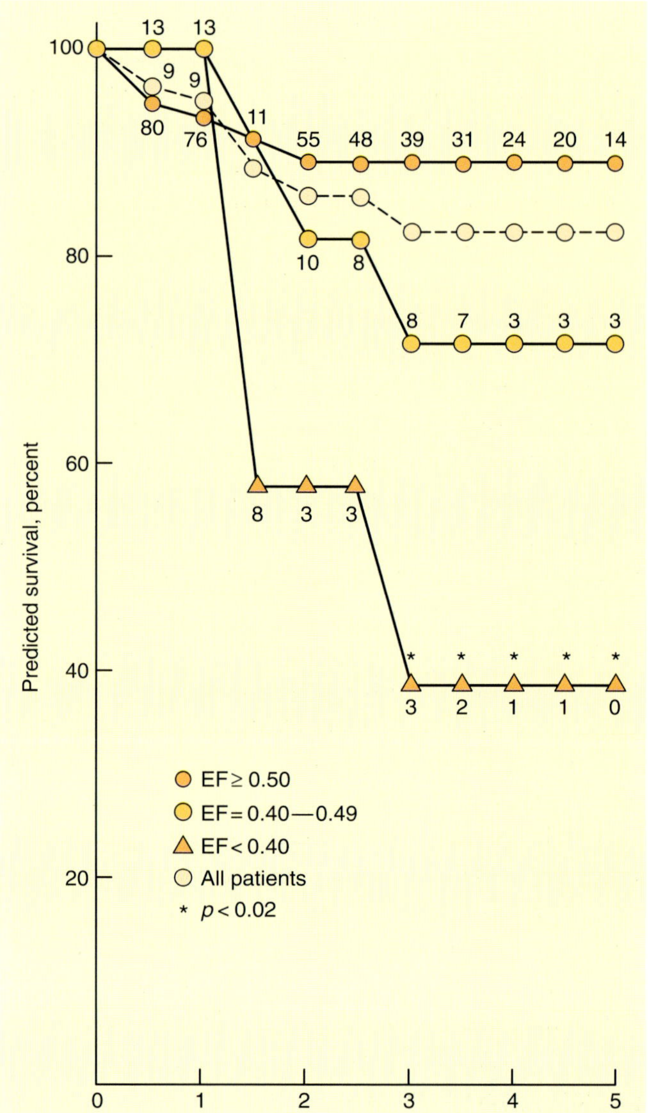


**Figure 32.3** *Life-table survival curves showing predicted survival of the overall study population and the study population stratified accordingly to left ventricular ejection fraction (EF). The overall 5-year survival was 82%, but survival even at 3 years in patients with an ejection fraction below 0.40 was only 38%.*

(MVR), resection of the anterior and posterior valve leaflets disrupts the subvalvular apparatus, which is important in maintaining LV volume, geometry, and systolic performance [36, 37].

Notwithstanding the relative unpredictability of postoperative function, the most important determinant of postoperative survival is the preoperative ejection fraction. In one study [37], 5-year survival after MVR was 90% for patients with a preoperative ejection fraction greater than 0.50 but only 38% for those with an ejection fraction less than 0.40 (Fig. 32.3). Thus, surgery is generally recommended for patients with significant MR while the ejection fraction is still above 0.60 in adults and 0.50 in children [34]. In addition, the observation that patients with longstanding MR have clinical outcomes inferior to those with short-lived disease has led to the recommendation that early surgery be offered to patients who are expected eventually to require operation [39].

As mentioned above, the pathophysiological basis of myocardial dysfunction in MR due to degenerative valve disease is chronic volume overload resulting in ventricular dilatation. However, in ischaemic mitral insufficiency, myocardial ischaemia or infarction may be the dominant causative mechanism. In this entity, papillary muscle dysfunction results in mitral valve prolapse and clinically significant MR. Although loss of papillary contractile function due to ischaemia or infarction is necessary for the development of ischaemic MR, ventricular dilatation or widening of the mitral annulus are also thought to be critical in this process [40]. In the early stages of ischaemic MR, myocardial revascularization may be sufficient to reverse the pathological process, but if permanent ventricular damage has been sustained or irreversible ventricular or annular dilatation has ensued, MVR or repair may be necessary as well.

Although surgical intervention is recommended and highly successful in patients with MR and preserved systolic function, a more challenging cohort of potential surgical candidates comprises patients with clinical signs of heart failure or evidence of depressed systolic function. In these patients, MVR can be expected to depress myocardial performance further, and as cited above, is associated with a high perioperative mortality rate and poor long-term survival. Thus, compared with patients with AI, who generally benefit from valve replacement regardless of severity of ventricular dysfunction (albeit with increased operative mortality), patients with severe heart failure due to MR have a significantly poorer prognosis. For these reasons, alternatives to MVR have been developed, with the intention of avoiding or minimizing the pathological processes responsible for postoperative deterioration in systolic performance.

As described above, an important pathogenetic determinant of ventricular dysfunction after conventional MVR is elimination of valvular–ventricular interactions induced by disruption of the subvalvular apparatus [37]. The specific mechanisms by which papillary–ventricular attachments enhance systolic function include preload enhancement of midwall LV fibres (via inhibition of LV sphericalization) [41] and reduction of regional midwall afterload (via provision of structural support) [42]. Thus, techniques of mitral valve repair and replacement with chordal preservation have been developed. Specific techniques include prosthetic ring annuloplasty; anterior leaflet fixation to secondary chordae; chordal transposition, replacement, or elongation; and papillary muscle plication or resection [43].

Several experimental and clinical studies have compared the effects of conventional MVR and chordal-preserving procedures on ventricular function. In most clinical studies [44–48], MVR resulted in decreased cardiac output, increased LV end-diastolic pressure, and decreased ejection fraction (due to decreased end-diastolic volume, with no change in end-systolic volume), while chordal-sparing procedures resulted in preserved cardiac output and ejection fraction associated with reductions in both end-diastolic and -systolic volumes (Fig. 32.4). In a recent comparison of conventional MVR to chordal-preserving procedures [59], these findings were confirmed, with the additional observation that chordal sparing was associated with superior preservation of ventricular geometry. These and other studies confirm the clinical importance of preserving the subvalvular apparatus when feasible. A representation of the differential effects of mitral valve repair and replacement on postoperative ejection fraction is depicted in Figure 32.5. Clinical reports have demonstrated a significant reduction in operative mortality and improvement in long-term survival in patients undergoing chordal-sparing procedures [50–52]. The decreased morbidity and mortality noted after mitral valve repair procedures is probably due to improved preservation of ventricular function as well as to decreased operative time and technical complexity. The importance of the latter factor is illustrated by the experience with acute ischaemic mitral regurgitation, in which high mortality rates have been significantly reduced by the choice of mitral valve repair over replacement [53].

In summary, the modern surgical management of MR is based on a continually evolving understanding of pathological determinants of valvular and ventricular dysfunction. Major advances that have been achieved utilizing this knowledge include an awareness of the importance of preoperative ventricular function on outcome and an appreciation of the positive clinical impact of procedures that preserve the subvalvular apparatus.

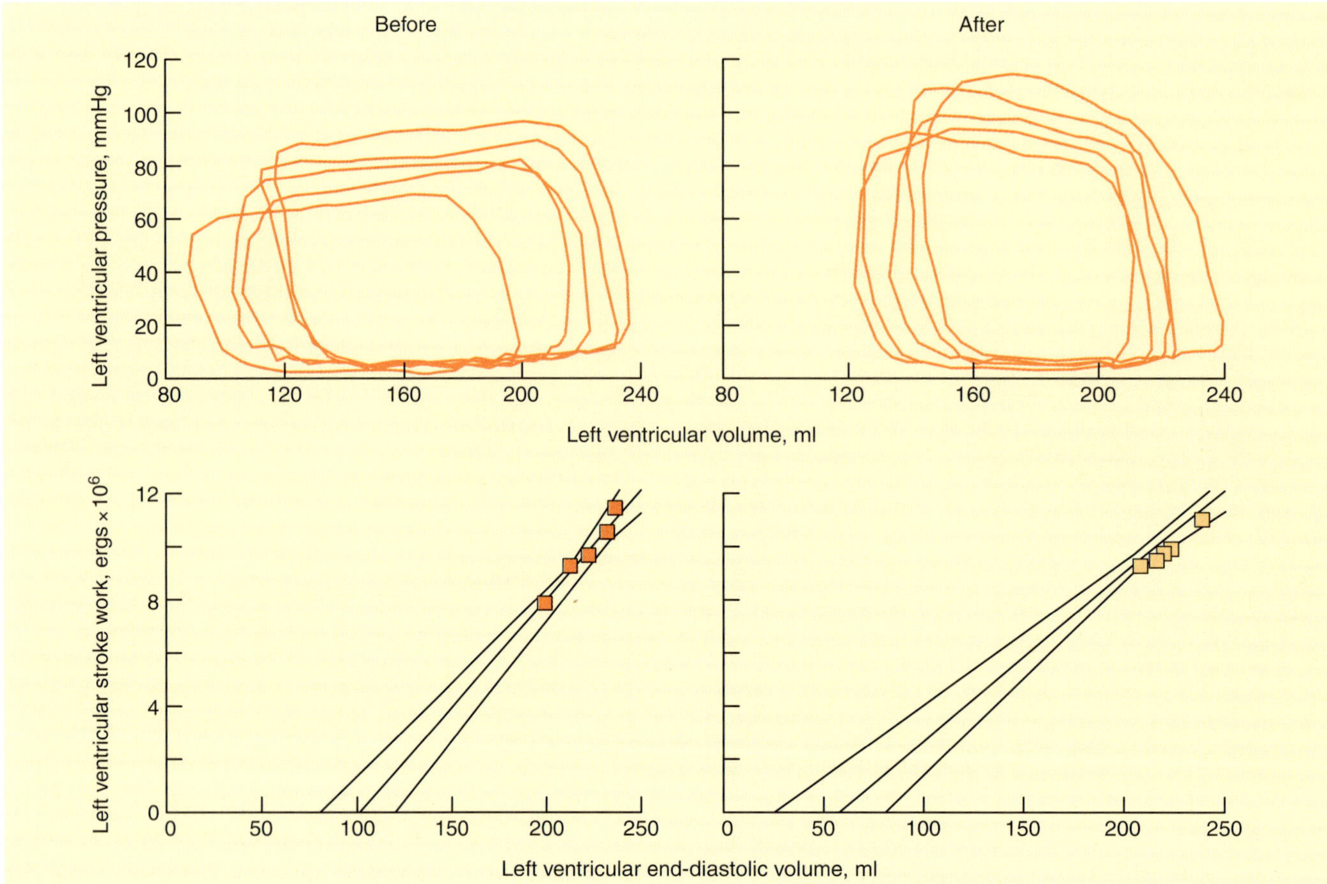


**Figure 32.4** *Left ventricular pressure-volume loops (top) and stroke work/end-diastolic volume relationships (bottom) in a patient with mitral regurgitation before (left) and immediately after (right) standard mitral valve replacement resecting the mitral leaflets. Left ventricular pressure was measured with a micromanometer and volume with RNA techniques at multiple steady-state preloads produced by infusion or withdrawal from the aortic cannula. While systolic left ventricular pressure increased and total ejection fraction decreased after valve replacement, global ventricular pump function (lower panels) did not significantly change after resection of the mitral apparatus either in this typical patient.*

## Anatomic remodelling of the ventricle

As illustrated in the previous section, discrete anatomical abnormalities may impart significant strains on the ventricle, eventually leading to progressive heart failure. In these cases, the benefits of operative management are largely based on the removal of specific pathogenetic influences on ventricular function. In other cases, however, ventricular failure ensues from irreversible processes, such as idiopathic dilated cardiomyopathy or myocardial infarction complicated by development of a ventricular aneurysm. In this section, pathological entities and procedures designed to reconstruct physically the failing, dilated ventricle will be examined.

### *Ventricular aneurysmectomy*

Left ventricular aneurysms (LVAs) are characterized anatomically by thinning of the ventricle wall in an area of scar due to a transmural myocardial infarction [54], and functionally by paradoxical motion of the aneurysmal segment with distortion of ventricular geometry. Although most ventricular aneurysms are considered chronic, developing over time after the initial myocardial injury, they may develop immediately after acute myocardial infarction. Acute LVA is usually not managed surgically, but is rather allowed to 'mature' while haemodynamic stability is established by pharmacological agents, mechanical support, or myocardial revascularization.

Because of recent improvements in the medical management of acute myocardial infarction, congestive heart failure, and ventricular arrhythmias, the number of patients requiring surgical treatment of chronic ventricular aneurysms has decreased. However, the primary indications for surgical intervention have not changed, and

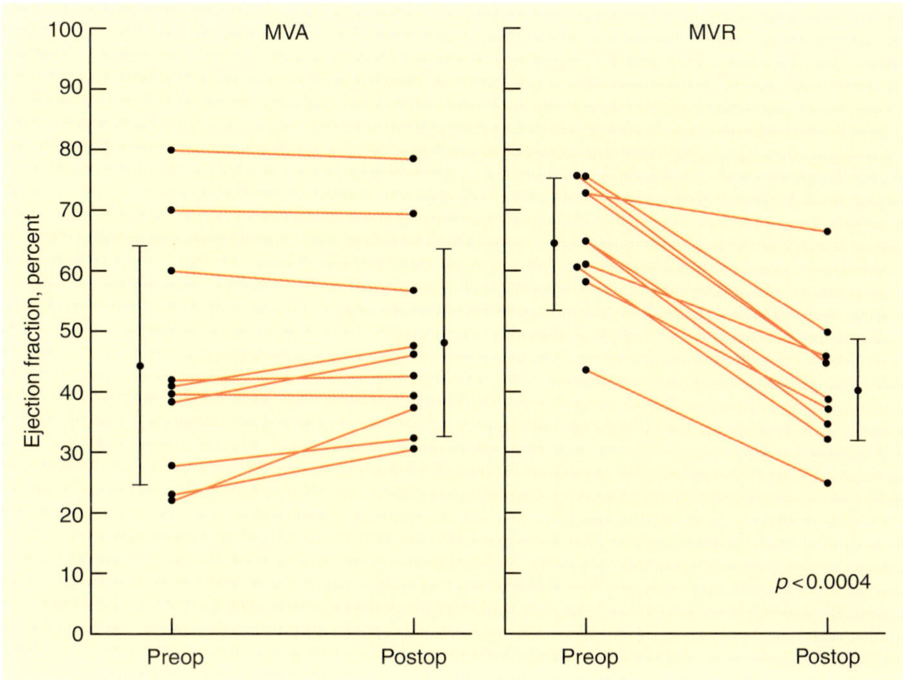


**Figure 32.5** *Levels of ventricular dysfunction in patients with mitral valve repair (left) compared with patients with mitral valve replacement (right).*

include medically refractory heart failure, angina pectoris, ventricular tachyarrhythmias, and thromboembolism. While patients with these manifestations are known to have a poor long-term survival without surgical intervention, asymptomatic patients have a reported 90% 5-year survival with medical therapy alone [55]. Although this might suggest that surgical intervention should be reserved for symptomatic patients only, it has been observed that asymptomatic patients are at risk for rapidly progressive heart failure due to decompensation of a chronically volume-overloaded and dilated left ventricle, resulting in global (and inoperable) ventricular dysfunction. For this reason, surgical management is offered to asymptomatic patients with chronic LVA who manifest evidence of progressive ventricular dilatation or dysfunction, increasing MR, or aneurysmal enlargement [54].

The pathophysiological effects of an LVA on ventricular function are mediated by two major mechanisms. First, paradoxical motion of the aneurysmal free wall and septum results in volume overload and dilatation of the remaining functional myocardium, since the stroke volume must be increased to fill the aneurysm while maintaining forward cardiac output. Pathologically, this paradoxical motion is caused not only by stretching of the aneurysmal scar, but also of the border zones of viable myocardium that surround the aneurysm [56]. This may explain the observation that patients undergoing standard aneurysmal resection, in which a peripheral strip of aneurymal tissue is left behind and closed linearly (avoiding the border zone), often do not enjoy significant improvements in ventricular function [57]. The second mechanism responsible for progressive deterioration of ventricular function involves distortion of normal ventricular geometry. As the base of an enlarging ventricular aneurysm dilates, it carries the adjacent normal free wall away from the septum, disturbing the normal parallel relationship of the septum and lateral free wall. This and other distortions of ventricular geometry may significantly decrease contractile efficiency even when local myocardial contractility is normal [57, 58].

Early attempts at surgical treatment of LVAs were based on the assumption that simple resection was the optimal way to relieve volume overload of the remaining ventricular myocardium, and open aneurysm resection with linear closure of the ventriculotomy, introduced by Cooley in 1958 [59], remained the standard technique for over 25 years. However, the frequent inability to document improvement in ventricular performance and the continued high mortality of this approach led to modifications based on an improved understanding of the underlying pathological basis of ventricular dysfunction. As mentioned above, simple resection and closure of the aneurysmal segment removes the actual aneurysm as a source of effective 'regurgitant volume', but does not eliminate the paradoxical motions of the border zone or septal myocardium, which remain as continued sources of volume strain on the ventricle postoperatively. Furthermore, distortions of ventricular geometry are not effectively restored with simple linear closure, which may actually induce further abnormalities in ventricular morphology, especially in large aneurysms.

The Jatene [60] and Dor [61] techniques of ventricular aneurysmorrhaphy were conceived to correct the constellation of pathophysiological defects described above. Although individually distinct techniques with significant differences, they share the common objective of improving ventricular function by eliminating paradoxical motion of the free wall and septum, and restoring global ventricular geometry. In the Jatene technique, after the actual aneurysm is resected, the aneurysmal portion of the septum is imbricated, which stabilizes it against the surrounding contracting ventricle and restores the normal conical shape of the distal deptum. Next, the base of the resected aneurysm is approximated with a circumferential pursestring suture, which draws the ventricular free wall back towards the septum, restoring the more oblique, conical relationship of these structures. Finally, the remaining ventricular defect is closed, either primarily or with a bovine pericardial patch. In the Dor endoventricular circular patch plasty, the aneurysmal free wall is resected, and the defect bridged with an endocardial patch. In this operation, the aneurysmal septum is not imbricated, but is instead excluded from the ventricular cavity by fixation of the endocardial patch to the junction of the septal endocardial scar and normal septal myocardium. After placement of a pursestring suture around the base of the defect (in this case proximal to the excluded septal segment), the endocardial patch is sewn circumferentially to the edges of remaining myocardium. While restoring ventricular geometry, this manoeuvre also prevents paradoxical motion of the diseased septum and border zone by excluding these areas from the forces of ventricular contraction.

The theoretical advantages of the Jatene and Dor techniques of ventricular aneurysmorrhaphy over traditional simple closure have been supported by encouraging clinical results. In a report describing the Jatene experience, surgical mortality was 5.8% and both early and late postoperative testing revealed improved ventricular function [58]. In Dor's experience, surgical mortality has been less than 7%, and postoperative evaluation has confirmed improvement in ejection fraction and control of ventricular arrhythmias in the majority of patients [62]. Nonetheless, attempts to compare the results of these techniques with new modifications of the linear closure technique [63] have thus far been inconclusive because of a lack of randomization and failure to control for variables such as infarct size and the effect of concomitant revascularization on ventricular function.

As in the case of the chordal-preserving mitral valve operations discussed in the previous section, the surgical management of ventricular aneurysms has undergone significant evolution as an improved understanding of underlying pathogenetic processes has been achieved. In this respect, the Jatene and Dor techniques represent examples of surgical interventions designed specifically to address complex and multifactorial pathological processes that had been previously unappreciated or ignored.

### *Partial left ventriculectomy (Batista procedure)*

No cardiac surgical procedure has received more recent attention (and been the subject of more controversy) than the partial left ventriculectomy (PLV) introduced by Batista [64] a few years ago. In this operation, significant portions of left ventricular myocardium are resected in an attempt to restore normal geometry to ventricles rendered dysfunctional by cardiomyopathic dilatation. Either alone or in combination with valve replacement or repair, proponents of this operation [65, 66] believe that these geometrical changes lead to normalization of cardiovascular physiology and improved pump function. As with the treatment of ventricular aneurysms, this surgical approach to idiopathic dilated cardiomyopathy seeks to reverse myocardial dysfunction by correcting pathological ventricular geometry.

The pathophysiological mechanisms responsible for the development of dilated cardiomyopathy are complex and not fully understood. By a variety of processes, myocyte loss and dysfunction (a detailed consideration of which is beyond the scope of this chapter) leads to compensatory LV dilatation, which acts to preserve cardiac output as contractility declines [67, 68]. However, progressive LV dilatation results in increased wall stress (as predicted by the law of LaPlace), resulting in increased energy expenditure and decreased pump efficiency [68]. Distortion of ventricular geometry by continued dilatation results in further derangements in ventricular function, which may be compounded by papillary dysfunction and MR.

In turn, mitral insufficiency leads to volume overload of the ventricle, which induces further compensatory dilatation [69]. Haemodynamically, these pathological changes result in increased LV filling pressure and decreased myocardial contractility, ejection fraction, and cardiac index.

Early experience with PLV in patients with end-stage dilated cardiomyopathy has yielded mixed results. Few clinical reports (and no randomized studies) exist in the published literature, and the majority describes small numbers of patients undergoing multiple variations of PLV either alone or in combination with other procedures. Furthermore, the variable degree to which haemodynamic, echocardiographic, and physiological data are collected, as well as the limited length of follow-up, allow for only cursory judgements to be made regarding the physiological effects and clinical efficacy of this novel operation. In three recent articles [65, 66, 70] by authors with reasonably large PLV experience, several important observations were made. Postoperatively, all investigators noted increases in LV ejection fraction attributable to decreased end-diastolic volume in the face of unchanged end-systolic volume. However, more detailed evaluation of ventricular function revealed conflicting results. In one study [66], increases in ejection fraction were not accompanied by improvements in load-independent measures of contractility, such as end-systolic elastance, and were in fact associated with decreases in diastolic compliance which were judged to be detrimental to overall ventricular function. Similarly, an article by surgeons who combined PLV with mitral valve repair and annuloplasty [70] observed that increased ejection fraction did not translate into improved cardiac index despite significant reductions in mitral regurgitation. In this group's experience, 15% of patients suffered immediate haemodynamic collapse requiring the support of left ventricular assist devices (LVADs). Conversely, a third group [65] reported improvements in cardiac index, stroke index, and stroke-work index after PLV, coupled with reductions in diastolic stiffness, myocardial wall stress, and severity of clinical heart failure.

In response to the relative paucity of physiological data available from clinical series and the current absence of adequate animal models of dilated cardiomyopathy, a theoretical analysis has been published of pressure–volume and stress–strain relationships resulting from PLV with varying amounts of muscle resection [71]. This analysis revealed, as did one clinical report [66], that improvements in systolic function induced by reduction of ventricular mass and diameter were accompanied by decreases in diastolic compliance (Fig. 32.6), resulting in depression of overall pump function. Furthermore, it was concluded that increases in ejection fraction and elastance may be difficult to interpret in the setting of decreased end-diastolic volume and altered ventricular geometry, and may not necessarily correlate with improved ventricular performance. Nonetheless, this analysis also predicted a decrease in myocardial wall stress,

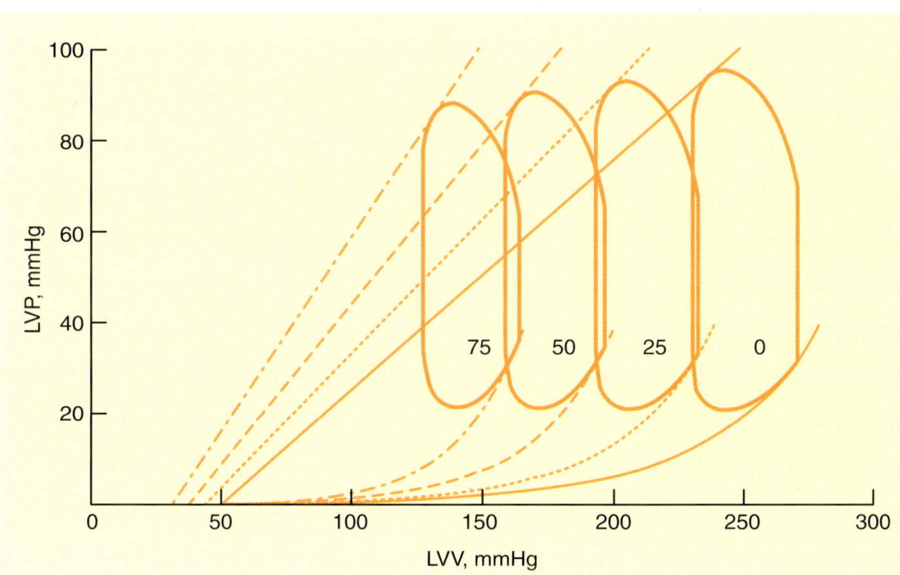


**Figure 32.6** *Left ventricular pressure-volume loops (LVP and LVV) are shown at each of the four levels of mass reduction (0, 25, 50, and 75 g of tissue removed). The pressure-volume loops shift to the left in response to mass reduction. Also shown on this graph are the ESPVRs (straight lines that intersect the end-systolic point of the respective pressure-volume loop) and the EDPVRs (curvilinear relations that intersect the end diastolic point of the respective pressure-volume loop). A mass is reduced from 0 to 75 g (solid line, dotted line, dashed line dotted/dashed line), the ESPVR slope increases, and the curvature of the EDPVR increases, both relations tend to move in a parallel fashion.*

an important mechanism by which PLV might improve cardiac function and clinical status. Current evidence suggests that reduction of ventricular wall stress may induce regression of myocyte hypertrophy ('reverse remodelling') and diminution of contractile dysfunction mediated by subendocardial ischaemia [72, 73].

Notwithstanding these and other postulated haemodynamic and physiological effects of PLV, clinical successes have been reported by several authors, with significant prolongation of life expectancy in many patients with end-stage heart failure [70, 71, 74]. Unfortunately, the clinical efficacy of PLV has varied widely within most series, with at least as many clinical failures as successes. For this reason, current efforts are being directed at identifying clinical and physiological predictors of haemodynamic improvement and long-term survival after PLV. In one study of the effect of myocardial histology on functional outcome [66], postoperative improvement in ventricular function was found to be correlated with the degree of myocyte hypertrophy and inversely proportional to the degree of myocardial fibrosis. Similarly, McCarthy *et al.* [70] noted poorer results in patients with myocardial fibrosis, myocarditis, and ischaemic cardiomyopathy, and superior outcomes in those sensitive to inotropic agents. These findings suggest that the extent of clinical improvement after PLV may depend on the ability of diseased myocytes to regain normal functional morphology. Thus, the reversibility of pathological ventricular remodelling, as assessed by myocardial histology or other means, may represent a preoperative predictor of success after PLV.

The early experience with PLV raises many more questions than it answers. Although the operation induces physiological and structural changes that would be expected to improve cardiac function, these improvements are not always observed or do not always result in clinically measurable success. Nonetheless, a significant proportion of patients undergoing PLV enjoys at least short-term improvement in clinical status. In the face of an increasing worldwide prevalence of end-stage heart failure and the limited options for treatment of this disorder, further study of this potentially beneficial operation is warranted, and will at the very least lead to a better understanding of the pathogenetic basis of heart failure.

## Operations for ischaemic cardiomyopathy

Ischaemic cardiomyopathy is diagnosed in 300 000 Americans each year, and 80 000 deaths are attributed to this condition annually [75]. The majority of patients with coronary artery disease and severe LV dysfunction will receive medical management, which often results in poor long-term survival. Because heart transplantation is only available to approximately 2000 patients per year owing to a limited donor organ supply, the only recourse for most patients who are unresponsive to medical therapy is surgical revascularization. Since it is difficult to predict which patients will show improvements in ventricular function postoperatively, and because of the high mortality in patients who do not benefit from revascularization, many such patients are not offered coronary artery bypass grafts (CABG). Nonetheless, several studies have documented the feasibility of surgical revascularization in patients with severe ventricular dysfunction. In one study [76], 83 patients with a mean ejection fraction of 24% underwent CABG at one institution and 39 patients with a mean ejection fraction of 18% were surgically revascularized at another. In both series, patients experienced improvements in ventricular function and subjective symptoms with a low perioperative mortality rate and a 3-year survival rate of over 80%. In another study, 42 patients with an ejection fraction less than 20% underwent CABG with improved postoperative ventricular function, operative mortality rate of 4.8%, and 1-year survival rate of 88% [77]. Finally, in a retrospective review of patients undergoing either medical therapy or surgical revascularization while awaiting heart transplantation [78], those undergoing CABG had a 5-year survival rate of 80%, compared with only 28% in medically managed patients. The operative mortality rate in this series was 20%, illustrating the high risk of surgery in this patient population.

Because of the unpredictability of functional improvement after high-risk surgical revascularization, several studies have attempted to identify preoperative factors associated with improved outcome. Currently, resurrection of ischaemic but viable ('hibernating') myocardium is thought to be the main mechanism by which ventricular function may improve after surgical revascularization, and this concept is supported by the historical observation that patients with heart failure and angina fare better after revascularization than those without angina. In one study of 57 patients with a mean ejection rate of 28% [79], the only clinical variable found to predict a favourable outcome was the presence of significant areas of hibernating myocardium, manifested as a large reversible defect on preoperative thallium-201 scanning. Because the presence of revascularizable ischaemic myocardium is highly correlated with the presence of angina or previous myocardial infarction [80], these factors are considered as positive predictors of outcome after high-risk CABG. Finally, the current ability to identify areas of viable myocardium by thallium-201 scintigraphy, single-photon emission computed tomography (SPECT), and positron emission tomography (PET) has allowed the more precise identification of patients who are likely to benefit from surgical revascularization. In this regard, the accuracy and clinical value of dobutamine stress echocardiography have been recently validated [81].

Despite the positive prognostic significance of the presence of hibernating myocardium, other preoperative variables have been shown to influence surgical results in patients with ischaemic cardiomyopathy. In a retrospective study of patients undergoing CABG with an ejection fraction of less than 20% [76], predictors of poor outcome included advanced age, female gender, increased severity of coronary artery disease, and the presence of ventricular arrhythmias. In another study [82], peripheral vascular disease, hypertension, and increased LV filling pressures were associated with decreased postoperative survival. Thus, although the presence of ischaemic but viable myocardium should weigh heavily in the decision to proceed with surgical revascularization in patients with ventricular dysfunction, a number of other factors must also be taken into consideration that may predict a significant risk of failure.

Several other factors may influence outcome after high-risk myocardial revascularization. Just as for any coronary bypass operation, success depends on optimal myocardial protection. Both the use of retrograde cardioplegia, which induces more uniform and complete myocardial cooling in the presence of severe coronary artery disease, and blood cardioplegia, which enhances myocardial protection during aortic cross-clamping, have been shown to decrease postoperative mortality in patients undergoing high-risk CABG. In addition, the quality of the distal coronary vasculature is critically important prognostically, since effective revascularization cannot be attained in the absence of suitable target vessels. In one study of high-risk CABG patients [83], the only two predictors of increased mortality were advanced age and poor vessel quality, leading the authors to suggest that older patients with poor target vessels be refused surgery regardless of the potential for rescuscitation of viable myocardium.

Patients with end-stage heart failure due to ischaemic heart disease present a significant therapeutic challenge. Despite the recent development of pharmacological agents that may prolong life expectancy in these patients, surgical revascularization represents a potentially life-saving option in the absence of the availability of heart transplantation. Advanced diagnostic techniques may aid in the identification of patients with hibernating myocardium, who generally benefit functionally from revascularization. However, significant comorbid conditions, the severity of heart failure, and the quality of the distal coronary vasculature are important determinants of functional recovery and survival that should not be ignored. A representative diagnostic and management algorithm for the management of ischaemic cardiomyopathy is reproduced in Figure 32.7.

## Ventricular assistance and replacement

In the spectrum of procedures performed for the treatment of heart failure, by far the most dramatic interventions are those designed directly to replace or augment ventricular pump function. Two examples of this form of therapy are dynamic cardiomyoplasty and LVADs. Although these modalities were conceived purely as forms of mechanical ventricular assistance, experience has revealed more subtle effects on ventricular function, with potential influences on ventricular remodelling and functional recovery. Although fraught with limitations, each of these technologies provides a unique opportunity to study the impact of significant mechanical unloading on the natural history of pathological ventricular remodelling and dilatation.

### *Dynamic cardiomyoplasty*

Dynamic cardiomyoplasty (DCM) is a surgical treatment of dilated cardiomyopathy in which the latissimus dorsi muscle is mobilized and wrapped circumferentially around the heart and then stimulated synchronously with the cardiac cycle. Effectively, the muscle wrap acts as an autologous external compression device, augmenting synchronized systolic pressure. Initially conceived in the early 1970s, this technique of myocardial assistance has undergone phase I and II clinical trials, and a phase III prospective trial is currently underway [84]. At medium-term follow-up, the majority of patients undergoing DCM will enjoy substantial improvements in functional status, even though objective haemodynamic improvements are often not demonstrable [85]. Although DCM was originally

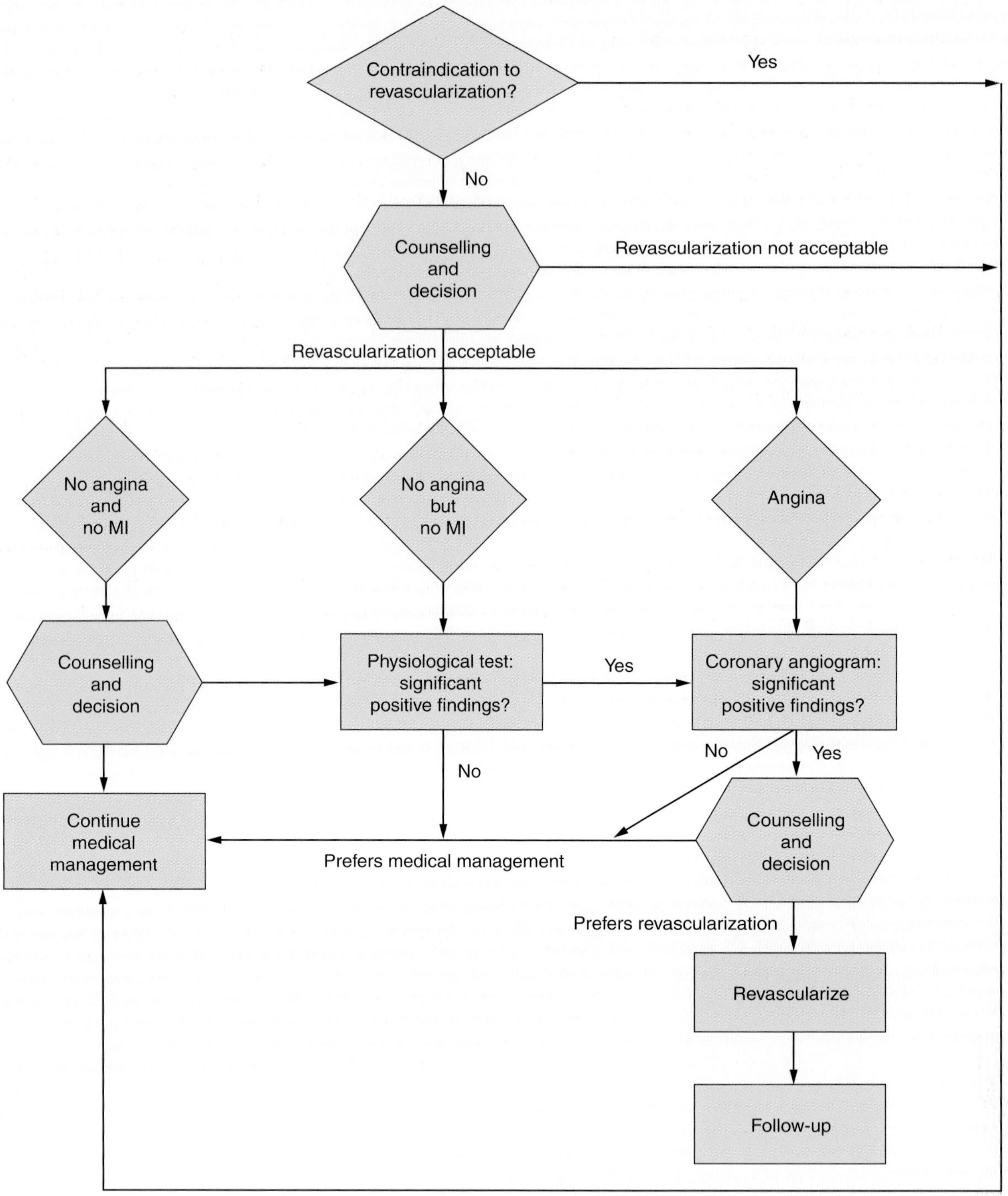


**Figure 32.7** *Evaluation and treatment of coronary artery disease in patients with heart failure.*

thought to improve cardiac function simply by providing systolic 'squeeze' to the failing ventricle, subsequent experimental and clinical studies suggest that the mechanisms by which DCM influences myocardial function may be considerably more complex, and may include stabilization of ventricular volumes by the girdling effect of the muscle wrap [86]. However, because of discordant results on the effects of DCM on myocardial performance [87, 88], no consensus has been reached regarding actual mechanisms of action.

There are several reasons for the often conflicting results reported in studies of DCM. The systolic effects of dynamic cardiomyoplasty are critically dependent on the conditioning of the latissimus muscle and proper synchronization of contraction with the systolic cycle. Because significant phenotypic changes are induced in skeletal muscle during conditioning by continuous electrical stimulation [87], results from studies using unconditioned muscle wraps underestimate the degree to which a properly conditioned muscle may augment systolic function. Conversely, although studies performed in optimally synchronized muscle wraps have demonstrated improvements in many indices of systolic function, including stroke volume, end-systolic elastance, and peak –d*P*/dt, none of these benefits has been demonstrated at clinically achievable levels of synchronization.

In recent well-controlled experimental [89] and clinical [90] studies, DCM has been shown to increase ejection fraction and peak ejection rate while decreasing end-diastolic volume, end-systolic volume, and end-diastolic pressure (Fig. 32.8). Although this reduction in ventricular volume and pressure had no effect on cardiac index, it enhanced effective contractility and reduced myocardial wall stress. The latter finding supports previous studies which have reported beneficial effects of DCM on myocardial stress–strain relationships [91, 92]. An additional finding was a reduction in wall motion asynchrony, a common characteristic of failing ventricles. It has been postulated that by contracting at the appropriate point in mid-to-late systole, the muscle wrap could improve ejection dynamics by acting as a 'time-varying afterload reducer', lowering ventricular volumes and pressures near the end of the systolic contraction phase [92, 93].

Although the above studies have confirmed the capacity of DCM to augment systolic function under certain conditions, the facts that significant clinical improvement has been demonstrated in patients without evidence of improved contractility suggests that other mechanisms are also operative. Significant evidence points to the existence of at least two other mechanisms by which DCM

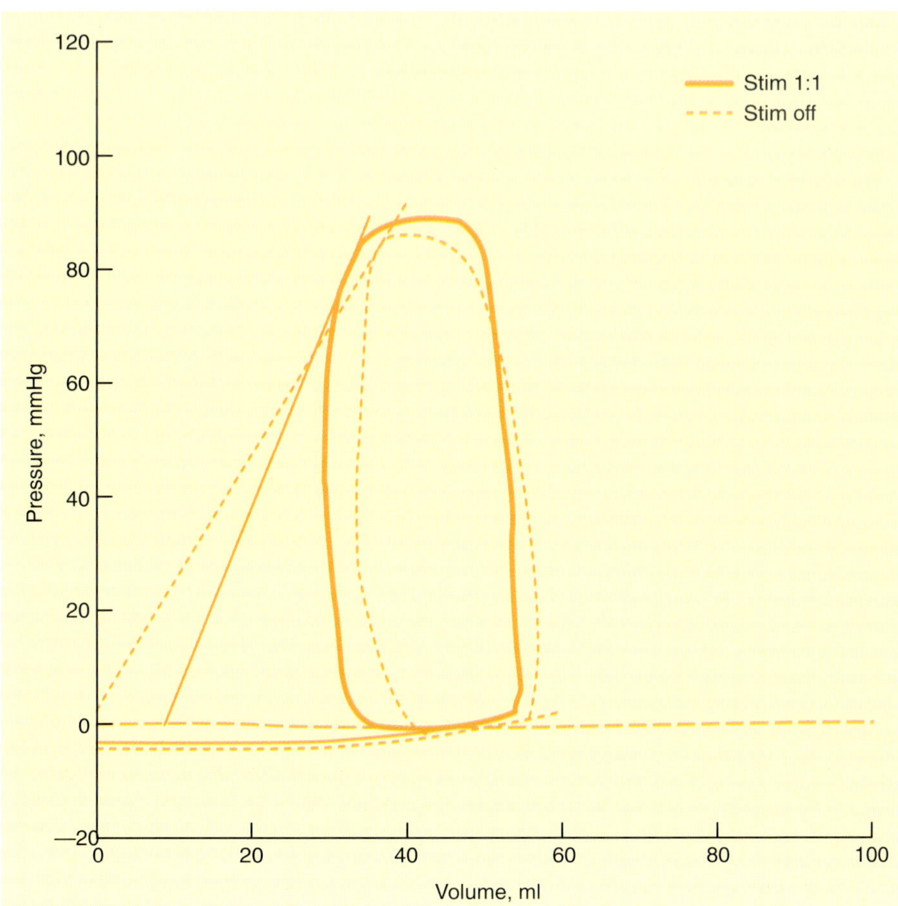


**Figure 32.8** *Improvement in end-systolic pressure–volume relationships during active stimulation in a dynamic cardiomyoplasty model.*

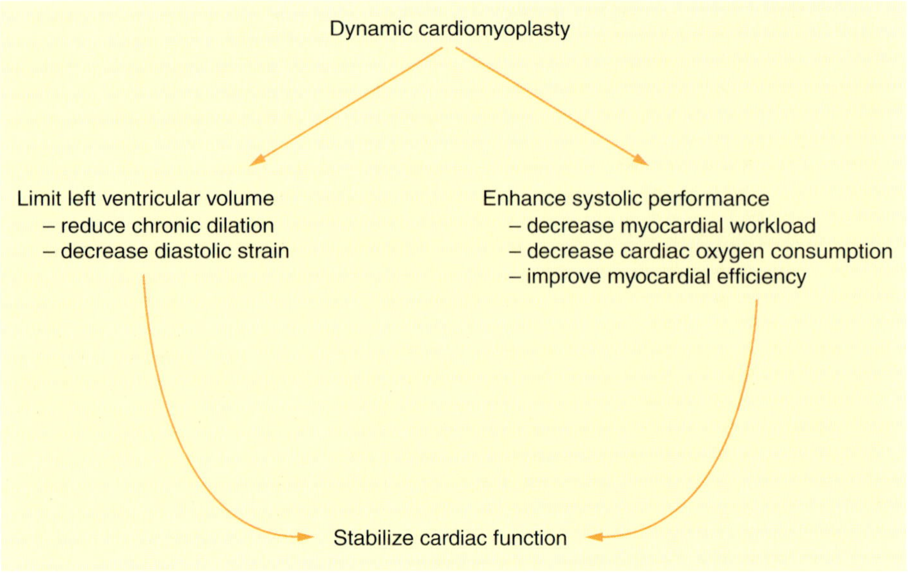


**Figure 32.9** *Proposed mechanisms of cardiomyoplasty. Dynamic cardiomyoplasty acts by at least two mechanisms. Girding effects on the left ventricle limit the chronic dilation associated with heart failure and thus decrease diastolic strain. Enhancement of effective contractility with skeletal muscle assistance decreases myocardial workload and thus decreases cardiac oxygen consumption and increases myocardial efficiency. Both of these presumably act to stabilize cardiac function over time.*

ameliorates the severity of clinical heart failure (Fig. 32.9): (1) the passive constraint or 'girdling effect' of the muscle wrap, whether stimulated or not, restrains the ventricle from further dilatation and prevents continuing increases in myocardial tension by stabilizing cavitary radius [94]; (2) the aforementioned reduction in wall stress effected by dynamic systolic compression may serve to reduce the stimulation of pathological myocyte hypertrophy and remodelling. Thus, by limiting ventricular dilatation and decreasing wall stress, DCM may stem or even reverse pathological ventricular remodelling [95].

### *Ventricular assist devices*

LVADs have emerged as a promising option in the treatment of end-stage heart failure, and are currently used both for temporary support in acute postcardiotomy shock and as a bridge to transplantation in chronic heart failure. The success of these devices in restoring haemodynamic stability and maintaining organ perfusion for extended periods has led to the suggestion that they be implanted in patients as an alternative to transplantation, and a randomized trial investigating this possibility is currently underway [96]. In addition to the beneficial haemodynamic effects imparted by these devices, several reports have suggested that prolonged LVAD support might allow recovery of native cardiac function, allowing device explantation without transplantation [97–99].

Ventricular remodelling is the term used to describe modifications in biochemical composition of the ventricular wall, orientation of cardiac myocytes, and chamber geometry that are responsible for the initially compensatory and later maladaptive changes characteristics of dilated cardiomyopathy [97]. It is hypothesized that these changes are mediated by physical stresses as well as an abnormal neurohormonal milieu [100]. Both angiotensin-converting enzyme inhibitors and nitrates have been shown to attenuate ventricular enlargement after myocardial infarction, suggesting that reduction in wall stress may be an important factor in the reversal of pathological remodelling [101, 102]. In addition, in patients with chronic heart failure, β-blocker therapy has been shown to reduce ventricular mass and normalize ventricular shape [103]. However, because the unloading effects of these agents are necessarily limited by systemic hypotension and organ hypoperfusion, the extent to which significant reverse remodelling can be induced pharmacologically is unclear.

Compared with medical afterload reduction, LVAD support can achieve more complete ventricular unloading, dramatically reducing ventricular pressures and volumes [97]. It has therefore been suggested that mechanical unloading might induce significant reversal of ventricular remodelling, and this concept is supported by reports detailing reductions in ventricular size [97, 104], evidence of spontaneous ventricular ejection and improved cardiac function [99, 105], and the histological demonstration of improved myocardial architecture [106] in patients supported by LVAD. In one study [97], LVAD support was shown to reverse ventricular dilatation and restore the end-diastolic

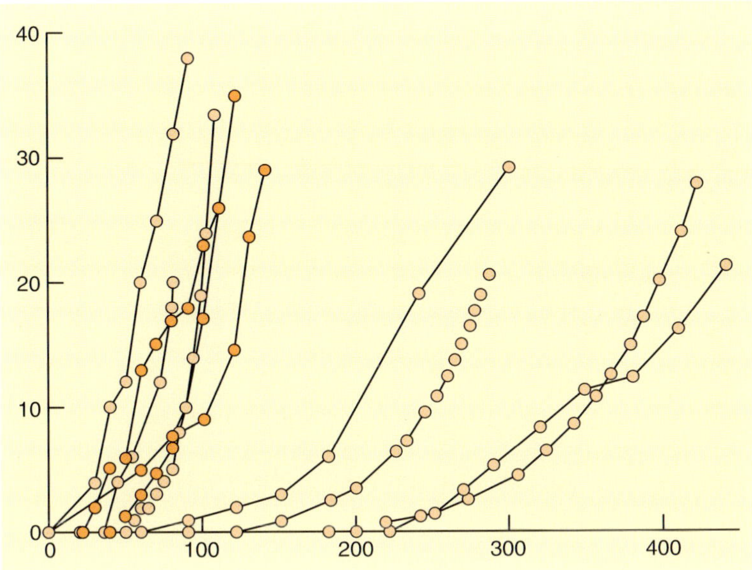


**Figure 32.10** *Graph showing end-diastolic pressure-volume relation (PVR) of hearts from four medically treated patients with end-stage idiopathic cardiomyopathy (●), three heart failure patients after prolonged left ventricular assist device (LVAD) support (●), and three normal subjects (●). Whereas EDPVRs of hearts from medically treated patients were shifted far to the right of the normal hearts, EDPVRs from the LVAD groups were close to normal. The x-axis shows volume in milliliters; y-axis, pressure in mmHg.*

pressure–volume relationship towards normal (Fig. 32.10), and in another [107], two patients were reported to recover sufficient cardiac function to allow device explantation without transplantation. However, in a recent investigation [108], early reductions in ventricular size induced by LVAD support were not accompanied by later decreases in chamber volume or improvements in LV fractional shortening. In addition, although this study demonstrated improvements in histological markers for myocyte damage, with reduced contraction band necrosis and wavy fibres, it also documented an increase in ventricular fibrosis. Finally, it should be noted that in one of the two cases of LVAD explantation cited above, recurrent ventricular dilatation and clinical heart failure ensued, illustrating the potentially temporary effects of LVAD unloading on myocardial architecture.

The mechanisms by which LVAD support improves ventricular geometry and induces at least temporary remodelling are not fully understood, but two major processes are likely to be involved. First, decreases in LV volume and pressure result in reduction of myocardial wall stress, a known contributor to the progression of pathological remodelling. These decreases in oxygen demand are accompanied by an improved nutrient supply, resulting from increased systolic pressure and decreased diastolic transmural pressure. Secondly, it has been shown that the plasma concentration of several neurohormones which regulate myocardial growth (such as aldosterone, renin, and catecholamines) normalize during LVAD support [109]. Since the abnormal elaboration of these and other factors is thought to contribute to the maladaptive neurohumoral milieu of heart failure, the potential role of LVAD support in reducing this pathological stimulus cannot be ignored. Nonetheless, in a recent study [111], improvements in ventricular volume and diastolic pressure–volume relationships induced by LVAD support were significantly diminished by device inflow valve regurgitation, suggesting that effective pressure–volume unloading is the major stimulus for reverse remodelling (Fig. 32.11).

In summary, LVAD support provides immediate ventricular unloading and improves haemodynamics, leading to normalization of ventricular volume, diastolic pressure–volume relationships, and some elements of myocardial histology. However, these effects may only be temporary, since device removal invariably exposes the heart to previously pathological neurohumoral, genetic, and mechanical influences. In combination with medical or genetic manipulations aimed at correction of underlying pathogenetic mechanisms, LVAD support may play a role in the initiation and maintenance of reverse remodelling of the failing ventricle. At present, however, it is more likely that LVAD explantation will result in sustained myocardial recovery in patients with reversible disease processes, such as myocarditis or postcardiotomy failure due to reversible ischaemia or myocardial stunning.

### *Heart transplantation*

Heart failure affects over 400 000 people in the USA each

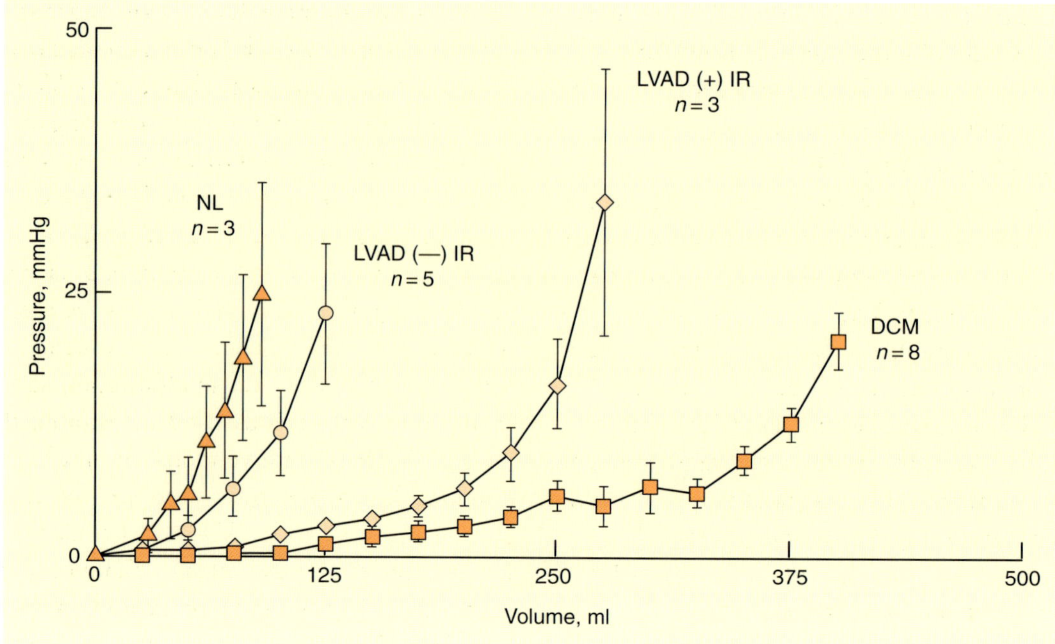


**Figure 32.11** *End-diatolic pressure-volume relationship determined at time of cardiac transplantation. Values are reported as mean ± standard deviation. (DCM = dialated cardiomyopathy; IR = inflow regurgitation; LVAD = left ventricular assist device; NL = normal.)*

year, and despite the administration of ever-improving pharmacological agents and the application of surgical techniques described in this chapter, results in the death of 250 000 patients each year. When maximal medical therapy is insufficient to stabilize myocardial function and surgical options fail or do not exist, heart transplantation is the final recourse. Because a limited pool of donor organs exists, with only 2000 heart transplants performed annually, priority is given to patients with limited life expectancy and no medical or surgical alternatives.

Current eligibility criteria for cardiac transplantation include end-stage heart failure with a life expectancy of less than 1 year, inoperable coronary artery disease with intractable anginal symptoms, or malignant ventricular arrhythmias unresponsive to medical or surgical therapy. In addition, patients with NYHA class III or IV heart failure refractory to maximal medical therapy are considered eligible if LV ejection rate is less than 20% and functional capacity is severely impaired, as assessed by determination of maximum oxygen consumption ($VO_{2\,max}$). Studies have demonstrated the utility of this latter measure in the selection of appropriately disabled candidates, predicting a survival benefit in patients with a pretransplant $VO_{2\,max} \leq$ 14 ml/kg per minute [111]. Although an infrequent indication, the successful transplantation of patients with cardiac tumours has also been reported [112]. Given current advances in the medical management of heart failure, haemodynamic support by mechanical ventricular assistance and dynamic cardiomyoplasty, and myocardial revascularization techniques, it is clear that the definitions of medically and surgically refractory end-stage heart failure have evolved and will continue to do so.

Exclusionary criteria have been formulated in an attempt to identify patients in whom the risk of death from transplant failure or from comorbid conditions does not justify the use of a scarce and valuable organ. Significant end-organ dysfunction, evidenced by reductions in creatinine clearance, elevations in serum creatinine and total bilirubin, or significant coagulopathy, is considered a contraindication to transplantation, as are active infection; recent pulmonary infarction; excessive obesity; evidence of drug, tobacco, or alcohol abuse; and active mental illness or psychosocial instability. Based on the well-established association of severe pulmonary hypertension with post-transplant right heart failure and death [113, 114], demonstration of pharmacological reversibility of pulmonary hypertension is considered an absolute requirement. Finally, because of rigorous immunosuppressive regimens and the potential need for intensification of this therapy during episodes of acute rejection, transplantation is not considered an option for patients with active or recent malignancy or the presence of antibodies to the human immunodeficiency virus (HIV).

Survival rates for cardiac transplantation at the present authors' institution have improved during the cyclosporine era, with a current actuarial survival of 85% at 1 year and approaching 70% at 5 years. These rates compare favourably with worldwide data of the Registry of the International Society for Heart and Lung Transplantation, which indicate 1- and 5-year survival estimates of 78% and 67%, respectively [107]. As in other series, the most frequent causes of death within the first year of cardiac transplantation are acute rejection and infection, while graft coronary artery disease (CAD) or allograft vasculopathy is the leading cause of death after the first year.

Episodes of acute rejection, diagnosed by routine endomyocardial biopsy and/or the new onset of clinical symptoms or alterations in cardiac function, are a common occurrence in the first year after transplantation [115]. Although the prevalence of rejection has declined in the era of immunosuppressive triple therapy, a recent analysis of the authors' experience [116] revealed an actuarial freedom from rejection rate of 45% at 1 year, with nearly 80% of first year rejections occurring within the first 3 months after transplantation. There were no significant differences in rejection frequency and actuarial freedom from rejection between primary transplant and retransplanted patients. An algorithm for treatment of rejection has been published previously [117]. In brief, low-grade (I or II) and clinically asymptomatic grade III rejection is treated with oral steroid boost therapy, which is followed by weekly endomyocardial biopsy until histological resolution is confirmed. In cases of persistent rejection, a second steroid boost is given intravenously. Patients not responding to a second steroid dose and all patients manifesting haemodynamic instability receive intravenous OKT3 or antithymocyte globulin (if hypersensitive to OKT3). In the authors' reported experience, 52% and 36% of rejection episodes have responded to oral and intravenous steroid therapy, respectively, with the remainder being treated with specific anti-T-cell or anti-B cell modalities.

Accelerated graft CAD remains a major complication and is the leading cause of late death after cardiac transplantation [118]. Angiographic evidence of graft CAD has been reported in as many as 45% of cardiac transplant patients surviving more than 3 years, and is associated with a five-fold increased risk of other cardiac events, such as myocardial infarction, heart failure, or sudden death [119]. Although the exact pathogenic basis of graft CAD is not known, both immunological and non-immunological mechanisms have been proposed for the development of the diffuse concentric myointimal proliferation characteristic of this process [120]. Current approaches in the prevention of graft CAD include aggressive therapy of acute rejection episodes as well as risk-factor modification through weight loss and lipid-lowering strategies, even though no objective data exist demonstrating the beneficial impact of these interventions on graft vasculopathy. Pharmacological therapies proposed for the prevention and treatment of graft CAD have included platelet-modifying agents [121] and calcium channel blockers [122]. Although early enthusiasm for the use of aspirin and dipyridamole has been tempered by equivocal long-term results, short-term studies using quantitative angiography and intravascular ultrasound have confirmed the ability of diltiazem to prevent and even induce regression of graft CAD. Finally, percutaneous coronary atherectomy and angioplasty have been successfully performed for discrete proximal stenoses in cardiac transplant patients [123], but it is presently unclear whether these techniques will have a significant impact in the treatment of graft CAD, which is usually diffuse and involves both proximal and distal coronary vessels.

## Conclusions

This review has surveyed the current landscape of available surgical treatments for heart failure and its causes, from the straightforward and efficacious mitral valve repair for early mitral regurgitation to the complex and highly controversial 'Batista' procedure for end-stage dilated cardiomyopathy. While some procedures aim to correct specific abnormalities responsible for the deterioration of ventricular function, others more ambitiously attempt to reverse this deterioration either by physically reconstructing the ventricle or by providing direct mechanical assistance. While the surgical options for the treatment of heart failure are almost as diverse as the pathological processes that they seek to address, they share a common goal: restoration of function through correction of specific pathogenetic mechanisms. The development of mechanism-specific interventions such as these requires a high degree of flexibility, allowing for the evolution of new or modified techniques as pathological processes are elucidated and more completely understood. As the development of surgical interventions for heart failure and other cardiac disorders proceeds into the twenty-first century, this flexibility must be maintained. As the understanding of pathological cardiac processes reaches the previously unforeseeable degree of detail made possible by recent advances in molecular biology and genetic engineering, the development of surgical and medical therapies for heart failure will necessarily require the modification of previous notions and the introduction of new concepts and technologies.

## References


1. Spirito P, Seidman CE, McKenna WJ, Maron BJ. The management of hypertrophic cardiomyopathy. *N Engl J Med* 1997; 336: 775–85.
2. Maron BJ. Hypertrophic cardiomyopathy. *Lancet* 1997; 350: 127–33.
3. Watkins H, Rosenzweig A, Hwang D-S *et al.* Characteristics and prognostic implications of myosin missense mutations in familial hypertrophic cardiomyopathy. *N Engl J Med* 1992; 326: 1108–14.
4. Thierfelder L, Watkins H, MacRae C *et al.* Alpha-tropomyosin and cardiac troponin T mutations cause familial hypertropjic cardiomyopathy: a disease of the sarcomere. *Cell* 1994; 77: 701–12.
5. Maron BJ, Gardin JM, Flack JM *et al.* Assessment of the prevalence of hypertrophic cardiomyopathy in a general population of young adults: echocardiographic analysis of 4111 subjects in the CARDIA study. *Circulation* 1995; 92: 785–9.
6. Maron BJ, Roberts WC. Quantitative analysis of cardiac muscle cell disorganisation in the ventricular septum of patients with hypertrophic cardiomyopathy. *Circulation* 1979; 59: 689–706.
7. Klues HG, Maron BJ, Dollar AL, Roberts WC. Diversity of structural mitral valve alterations in hypertrophic cardiomyopathy. *Circulation* 1992; 85: 1651–60.
8. Klues HG, Roberts WC, Maron BJ. Anomalous insertion of papillary muscle directly into anterior mitral valve leaflet in hypertrophic cardiomyopathy: significance in producing left ventricular outflow obstruction. *Circulation* 1991; 84: 1188–97.
9. Nihoyannopoulos P, Karatasakis G, Frenneaux M *et al.* Diastolic function in hypertrophic cardiomyopathy: relation to exercise capacity. *J Am Coll Cardiol* 1992; 19: 536–40.
10. Maron BJ, Wolfson JK, Epstein SE, Roberts WC. Intramural ('small vessel') coronary artery disease in hypertrophic cardiomyopathy. *J Am Coll Cardiol* 1986; 8: 545–57.
11. Wigle ED, Sasson Z, Henderson MA *et al.* Hypertrophic cardiomyopathy: the importance of the site and extent of hypertrophy. *Prog Cardiovasc Dis* 1985; 28: 1–83.
12. Maron BJ, Bonow RO, Cannon RO *et al.* Hypertrophic cardiomyopathy: interrelation of clinical manifestations, pathophysiology, and therapy. *N Engl J Med* 1987; 316: 780–9, 844–52.
13. Wigle ED, Rakowski H, Kimball BP, Williams WG. Hypertrophic cardiomyopathy: clinical spectrum and treatment. *Circulation* 1995; 92: 1680–92.
14. Cooley DA, Leachman RD, Hallman GL. Idopathic hypertrophic subaortic stenosis: surgical treatment including mitral valve replacement. *Arch Surg* 1971; 103: 606–12.
15. McIntosh CL, Maron BJ, Cannon RO, Klues HG. Initial results of combined anterior mitral leaflet plication and ventricular septal myotomy–myectomy for relief of left ventricular outflow tract obstruction in patients with hypertrophic cardiomyopathy. *Circulation* 1992; 86 (Suppl II): II-60–7.
16. Schoedube FA, Klues HG, Reith S *et al.* Long-term clinical and echocardiographic follow-up after surgical correction of hypertrophic obstructive cardiomyopathy with extended myectomy and reconstruction of the subvalvular mitral apparatus. *Circulation* 1995; 92 (Suppl II): II-122–7.
17. Duport G, Valeix B, Lefevre J *et al.* Interet de la stimulation ventriculaire droite permanente dans la cardiomyopathie obstructive. *Nouv Presse Med* 1978; 138: 2868–9.
18. Bedotto JB, Grayburn PA, Black WH *et al.* Alterations in left ventricular relaxation during atrioventricular pacing in humans. *J Am Coll Cardiol* 1990; 15: 658–64.
19. Gras D, Mabo P, DePlace C *et al.* Outcome of mitral regurgitation in obstructive hypertrophic cardiomyopathy treated by DDD pacing. *Circulation* 1994; 90 (Suppl): I-443.
20. Erwin J, McWilliams E, Gearty G *et al.* Hemodynamic assessment of dual chamber pacing in hypertrophic obstructive cardiomyopathy using radionuclide ventriculography. *Br Heart J* 1986; 55: 507.
21. Fananapazir L, Epstein ND, Curiel RV *et al.* Long-term results of dual-chamber DDD pacing in obstructive hypertrophic cardiomyopathy: evidence for progressive symptomatic and hemodynamic improvement and reduction of left ventricular hypertrophy. *Circulation* 1994; 90: 2731–42.
22. Horstkotte D, Loogen F. The natural history of aortic valve stenosis. *Eur Heart J* 1988; 9 (Suppl E): 57–64.
23. Peter M, Hoffmann A, Parker C *et al.* Progression of aortic stenosis. Role of age and concomitant coronary artery disease. *Chest* 1993; 103: 1715–19.
24. Chizner MA, Pearle DL, deLeon AC Jr. The natural history of aortic stenosis in adults. *Am Heart J* 1980; 99: 419–24.
25. O'Keefe JH Jr, Vliestra RE, Bailey KR, Holmes DR Jr. Natural history of candidates for balloon aortic valvuloplasty. *Mayo Clin Proc* 1987; 62: 986–91.
26. Pagani FD, Bolling SF. Valve surgery in patients with severe left ventricular dysfunction. In: EA Rose, LW Stevenson (eds) *Management of end-stage heart disease*. Philadelphia PA: Lippincott-Raven, 1998, 165–74.
27. Ross J Jr, Braunwald E. Aortic stenosis. *Circulation* 1968; 38 (Suppl 5): V61+.
28. Carabello BA, Green LH, Grossman W *et al.* Hemodynamic determinanants of prognosis of aortic valve replacement in critical aortic stenosis and advanced congestive heart failure. *Circulation* 1980; 62: 42–8.
29. Bonow RO, Rosing DR, McIntosh CI *et al.* The natural history of asymptomatic patients with aortic regurgitation and normal left ventricular function. *Circulation* 1983; 68: 509–17.
30. Bonow RO, Lakatos E, Maron BJ, Epstein SE. Serial long-term assessment of the natural history of asymptomatic patients with

chronic aortic regurgitation and normal left ventricular function. *Circulation* 1991; 84: 1625–35.
31. Henry WL, Bonow RO, Borer JS *et al*. Observations on the optimum time for operative intervention for aortic regurgitation: I. Evaluation of the results of aortic valve replacement in symptomatic patients. *Circulation* 1980; 61: 471–83.
33. Henry WL, Bonow RO, Rosing DR, Epstein SE. Observations on the optimum time for operative intervention for aortic regurgitation: II. Serial echocardiographic evaluation of asymptomatic patients. *Circulation* 1980; 61: 484–92.
33. Enriquez-Sarano M, Tajik A, Schaff H *et al*. Echocardiographic prediction of survival after surgical correction of organic mitral regurgitation. *Circulation* 1994; 90: 830–7.
34. Wisenbaugh T, Skudicky D, Sareli P. Prediction of outcome after valve replacement for rheumatic mitral regurgitation in the era of chordal preservation. *Circulation* 1994; 89: 191–7.
35. Enriquez-Sarano M, Tajik A, Schaff H *et al*. Echocardiographic prediction of left ventricular function after correction of mitral regurgitation: results and clinical implications. *J Am Coll Cardiol* 1994; 24: 1536–43.
36. Lillehei CW, Levy MJ, Bonnabeau RC. Mitral valve replacement with preservation of papillary muscles and chordae tendinae. *J Thorac Cardiovasc Surg* 1964; 47: 532–43.
37. Sarris GE, Miller DC. Role of the mitral subvalvular apparatus in left ventricular systolic mechanics. *Semin Thorac Cardiovasc Surg* 1989; 1: 133–42.
38. Phillips HR, Levine FH, Carter JE *et al*. Mitral valve replacement for isolated mitral regurgitation: analysis of clinical course and late postoperative left ventricular ejection fraction. *Am J Cardiol* 1981; 48: 647–54.
39. Enriquez-Sarano M, Schaff H, Frye R. Early surgery for mitral regurgitation: the advantages of youth. *Circulation* 1997; 96: 4121–23.
40. Fishbein MC. Mitral insufficiency in coronary artery disease. *Semin Thorac Cardiovasc Surg* 1989; 1: 129–32.
41. Spence PA, Peniston CM, David TE *et al*. Toward a better understanding of the etiology of left ventricular dysfunction after mitral valve replacement: an experimental study with possible clinical implications. *Ann Thorac Surg* 1986; 41: 363–71.
42. March RJ, Waters KA, Talbot T *et al*. Influence of native mitral apparatus on three-dimensional left ventricular geometry following mitral valve replacement. *Surg Forum* 1986; 17: 306–8.
43. McBride LR, Carpentier A. Surgical anatomy of cardiac valves and techniques of valve reconstruction. In: AE Baue *et al*. (eds) *Glenn's Thoracic and cardiovascular surgery*. Volume II. 6th edition. Norwalk, CT: Appleton & Lange, 1967–71.
44. Rastelli GC, Kirklin JW. Hemodynamic state early after prosthetic replacement of the mitral valve. *Circulation* 1966; 34: 448–61.
45. Boucher CA, Bingham JB, Osbakken MD *et al*. Early changes in left ventricular size and function after correction of left ventricular volume overload. *Am J Cardiol* 1981; 47: 991–1004.
46. Rouleau CA, Frye RL, Ellis FH Jr. Hemodynamic state early after open mitral valve replacement and reconstruction. *J Thorac Cardiovasc Surg* 1969; 58: 870–8.
47. Kennedy JW, Doces JG, Stewart DK. Left ventricular function before and following treatment of mitral valve disease. *Am Heart J* 1979; 97: 592–8.
48. Morton MJ, Bohnsted SW, Pantley GA *et al*. Effect of successful mitral valve replacement on left ventricular function. *Circulation* 1980; 62: III-208.
49. Ren J-F, Aksut S, Lighty GW Jr *et al*. Mitral valve repair is superior to valve replacement for the early preservation of cardiac function: relation of ventricular geometry to function. *Am Heart J* 1996; 131: 974–81.
50. Galloway AC, Colvin SB, Baumann FG *et al*. A comparison of mitral valve reconstruction with mitral valve replacement: intermediate-term results. *Ann Thorac Surg* 1989; 47: 655–62.
51. Sand ME, Naftel DC, Blackstone EH *et al*. A comparison of repair and replacement for mitral valve incompetence. *J Thorac Cardiovasc Surg* 1987; 94: 208–19.
52. Perier P, Deloche A, Chauvaud S *et al*. Comparative evaluation of mitral valve repair and replacement with Starr, Bjork, and porcine valve prostheses. *Circulation* 1984; 70 (Suppl I): I-187.
53. Rankin JS, Livesey SA, Smith R *et al*. Trends in the surgical treatment of ischemic mitral regurgitation: effects of mitral valve repair on hospital mortality. *Semin Thorac Cardiovasc Surg* 1989; 1: 149–63.
54. Cox JL. Left ventricular aneurysms: pathophysiologic observations and standard resection. *Semin Thorac Cardiovasc Surg* 1997; 9: 113–22.
55. Grondin P, Kretz JG, Bical O *et al*. Natural history of succular aneurysms of the left ventricle. *J Thorac Cardiovasc Surg* 1979; 77: 57–62.
56. Moulton MJ, Downing SW, Creswell LI *et al*. Mechanical dysfunction in the border zone of an ovine model of left ventricular aneurysm. *Ann Thorac Surg* 1995; 60: 986–8.
57. Cox JL. Surgical management of left ventricular aneurysms: a clarification of the similarities and differences between the Jetene and Dor techniques. *Semin Thorac Cardiovasc Surg* 1997; 9: 131–8.
58. Jatene AD. Surgical treatment of left ventricular aneurysm. In: AE Baue *et al*. (eds) *Glenn's Thoracic and cardiovascular surgery*. Volume II. 5th edition. Norwalk, CT: Appleton P Lange, 1829.
59. Cooley DA, Collins HA, Morris GC, Chapman DW. Ventricular aneurysm after myocardial infarction. Surgical excision with use of temporary cardiopulmonary bypass. *JAMA* 1958; 167: 557.
60. Jatene AD. Left ventricular aneurysmectomy: resection or reconstruction. *J Thorac Cardiovasc Surg* 1985; 89: 321–8.
61. Dor V, Saab M, Coste P *et al*. Left ventricular aneurysm. A new surgical approach. *Thorac Cardiovasc Surg* 1989; 37: 11–19.
62. Dor V, Sabatier M, Di Donato M *et al*. Late hemodynamic results after left ventricular patch repair associated with coronary grafting in patients with post-infarction akinetic or dyskinetic aneurysm of the left ventricle. *J Thorac Cardiovasc Surg* 1995; 110: 1291–301.
63. Mickleborough LL. Ventricular aneurysmectomy and surgical ablative approaches for malignant arrhythmias. In: EA Rose, LW Stevenson (eds) *Management of end-stage heart disease*. Philadelphia PA: Lippincott-Raven, 1998; 155–64.
64. Batista RJV, Dantos JLV, Takeshita N *et al*. Partial left ventriculectomy to improve left ventricular function in end-stage heart disease. *J Card Surg* 1996; 11: 96–7.
65. Moreira LEP, Stolf NAG, Bocchi EA *et al*. Partial left ventriculectomy with mitral valve preservation in the treatment of patients with dilated cardiomyopathy. *J Thorac Cardiovasc Surg* 1998; 115: 800–7.
66. Gorcsan J III, Feldman AM, Kormos RL *et al*. Heterogeneous immediate effects of partial left ventriculectomy on cardiac performance. *Circulation* 1998; 97: 839–42.
67. Cohn JN. Structural basis for heart failure: ventricular remodeling and its pharmacological inhibition. *Circulation* 1995; 91: 2504–7.

68. Packer M. Pathophysiology of chronic heart failure. *Lancet* 1992; 340: 88–92.
69. Blondheim DS, Jacobs LE, Kotler MN *et al.* Dilated cardiomyopathy with mitral regurgitation: decreased survival despite a low frequency of left ventricular thrombus. *Am Heart J* 1991; 122: 763–71.
70. McCarthy PM, Starling RC, Wong J *et al.* Early results with partial left ventriculectomy. *J Thorac Cardiovasc Surg* 1997; 114: 755–65.
71. Dickstein ML, Spotnitz HM, Rose EA, Burkhoff D. Heart reduction surgery: an analysis of the impact on cardiac function. *J Thorac Cardiovasc Surg* 1997; 113: 1032–40.
72. Rubin SA, Fishbein MC, Swan HJ. Compensatory hypertrophy in the heart after myocardial infarction in the rat. *J Am Coll Cardiol* 1983; 1: 435–41.
73. Strobeck EJ, Sonnenblick EH. Pathophysiology of heart failure. In: HJ Levine *et al.* (eds) *The ventricle: basic and clinical aspects*. Boston, MA: Martinus Nijhoff, 1985, 209–24.
74. Batista RJ, Verde J, Nery P *et al.* Partial left ventriculectomy to treat end-stage heart disease. *Ann Thorac Surg* 1997; 64: 634–8.
75. Kern JA, Kron IL. High-risk myocardial revascularization. In: EA Rose, LW Stevenson (eds) *Management of end-stage heart disease*. Philadelphia, PA: Lippincott-Raven, 1998, 149–53.
76. Elefteriades JA, Kron IL. CABG in advanced left ventricular dysfunction. *Cardiol Clin* 1995; 1: 35–42.
77. Lansman SL, Cohen M, Galla JD *et al.* Coronary bypass with ejection fraction of 0.20 or less using centigrade cardioplegia: long-term followup. *Ann Thorac Surg* 1993; 56: 480–5.
78. Luciani GB, Faggian G, Razzolini R. Severe ischemic left ventricular failure: coronary operation of heart transplantation. *Ann Thorac Surg* 1993; 55: 719–23.
79. Chan RKM, Raman J, Lee KG *et al.* Prediction of outcome after revascularization in patients with poor left ventricular function. *Ann Thorac Surg* 1996; 61: 1428–34.
80. Konstam M, Dracup K, Baker D *et al.* Heart failure: evaluation and care of patients with left-ventricular systolic dysfunction. Clinical practice guideline No. 11. AHCPR Publication No. 94-0612. Rockville, MD: Agency for Health Care Policy and Research, Public Health Service, US Department of Health and Human Services, June 1994, 67–77.
81. Hennessy TG, Codd MB, McCarthy C *et al.* Dobutamine stress echocardiography in the detection of coronary artery disease in the clinical practice setting. *Int J Cardiol* 1997; 62: 55–62.
82. Milano CA, White WD, Smith LR *et al.* Coronary artery bypass in patients with severely depressed ventricular function. *Ann Thorac Surg* 1993; 56: 487–93.
83. Langenburg SE, Buchanan SA, Blackbourne LH *et al.* Predicting survival after coronary revascularization for ischemic cardiomyopathy. *Ann Thorac Surg* 1995; 60: 1193–7.
84. Chiu RC-J. Dynamic cardiomyoplasty for heart failure. *Br Heart J* 1995; 73: 1–3.
85. Furnary AP, Jessup M, Moreira LEP. Multicenter trial of dynamic cardiomyoplasty for chronic heart failure. The American cardiomyoplasty group. *J Am Coll Cardiol* 1995; 28: 1175–80.
86. Hagege AA, Desnos M, Fernandez F *et al.* Clinical study of the effects of latissimus dorsi muscle flap stimulation after cardiomyoplasty. *Circulation* 1995; 92 (Suppl): II-210–15.
87. Lee KF, Wechsler AS. Dynamic cardiomyoplasty. *Adv Card Surg* 1993; 4: 207–36.
88. Jatene AD, Moreira LFP, Stolf NAG *et al.* Left ventricular function changes after cardiomyoplasty in patients with dilated cardiomyopathy. *J Thorac Cardiovasc Surg* 1991; 102: 132–9.
89. Patel HJ, Lankford EB, Polidori DJ *et al.* Dynamic cardiomyoplasty: its chronic and acute effects on the failing heart. *J Thorac Cardiovasc Surg* 1997; 114: 169–78.
90. Schreuder JJ, van der Veen FH, van der Velde ET *et al.* Left ventricular pressure–volume relationships before and after cardiomyoplasty in patients with heart failure. *Circulation* 1997; 96: 2978–86.
91. Lee KL, Dignan RJ, Dyke CM *et al.* Effects of dynamic cardiomyoplasty on left ventricular performance and myocardial mechanics in dilated cardiomyopathy. *J Thorac Cardiovasc Surg* 1991; 102: 124–31.
92. Bellotti G, Moraes A, Bocchi E *et al.* Late effects of cardiomyoplasty on left ventricular mechanics and diastolic filling. *Circulation* 1993; 88: 304–8.
93. Brutsaert DL, Sys SU. Relaxation and diastole of the heart. *Physiol Rev* 1989; 69: 1228–315.
94. Capouya ER, Gerber RS, Drinkwater DC Jr *et al.* Girdling effect of nonstimulated cardiomyoplasty on left ventricular function. *Ann Thorac Surg* 1993; 56: 867–71.
95. Mott BD, Oh JH, Misawa Y *et al.* Mechanisms of cardiomyoplasty: comparative effects of adynamic versus dynamic cardiomyoplasty. *Ann Thorac Surg* 1998; 65: 1039–45.
96. Rose EA, Goldstein DJ. Wearable long-term mechanical support for patients with end-stage heart disease: a tenable goal. *Ann Thorac Surg* 1996; 61: 399–402.
97. Levin HR, Oz MC, Chen JM *et al.* Reversal of chronic ventricular dilation in patients with end-stage cardiomyopathy by prolonged mechanical unloading. *Circulation* 1995; 91: 2717–20.
98. Mandarino WA, Gorscan TA, Pham S *et al.* Estimation of left ventricular function in patients with left ventricular assist devices. *ASAIO J* 1995; 41: M544–7.
99. Frazier OH. First use of an untethered, vented electric device for long-term support. *Circulation* 1994; 89: 2908–14.
100. Pfeffer MA, Brauwald E. Ventricular remodeling after myocardial infarction: experimental observations and clinical implications. *Circulation* 1994; 81: 1161–72.
101. Jugdutt BL, Warnica JW. Intravenous nitroglycerin therapy to limit myocardial infarct size, expansion and complications: effect of timing, dosage and infarct location. *Circulation* 1988; 78: 906–19.
102. Pfeffer MA, Lamas G, Vaughan D *et al.* Effect of captopril on progressive ventricular dilation after anterior myocardial infarction. *N Engl J Med* 1988; 319: 80–6.
103. Hall S, Cigarroa C, Marcouz L *et al.* Regression of hypertrophy and alteration in left ventricular geometry in patients with congestive heart failure treated with beta-adrenergic blockade. *Circulation* 1994; 90 (Suppl I): I-543.
104. Burnett CM, Duncan M, Frazier OH *et al.* Improved multiorgan function after prolonged univentricular support. *Ann Thorac Surg* 1993; 55: 65–71.
105. McCarthy PM, Sabik JF. Implantable circulatory support devices as a bridge to heart transplantation. *Semin Thorac Surg* 1994; 6: 174–80.
106. Sceinin SA, Capek P, Radovancevic B. The effect of prolonged left ventricular support on myocardial histopathology in patients with end-stage cardiomyopathy. *ASAIO J* 1992; 38: M271–4.
107. Oz MC, Argenziano M, Catanese KA *et al.* Bridge experience with long-term implantable left ventricular assist devices: are they an alternative to transplantation? *Circulation* 1997; 95: 1844–52.

108. McCarthy PM, Nakatani S, Vargo R *et al.* Structural and left ventricular histologic changes after implantable LVAD insertion. *Ann Thorac Surg* 1995; 59: 609–13.
109. Levin HR, Chen JM, Oz MC *et al.* Potential for left ventricular assist devices as outpatient therapy while awaiting transplantation. *Ann Thorac Surg* 1994; 58: 1515–20.
110. Moazami N, Argenziano M, Kohomoto T *et al.* Inflow valve regurgitation during left ventricular assist device support may interfere with reverse ventricular remodeling. *Ann Thorac Surg* 1998; 65: 628–31.
111. Mancini DM, Eisen H, Kussmaul W *et al.* Value of peak exercise oxygen consumption for optimal timing of cardiac transplantation in ambulatory patients with heart failure. *Circulation* 1991; 83: 778–86.
112. Goldstein DJ, Oz MC, Rose EA *et al.* Experience with heart transplantation for cardiac tumors. *J Heart Lung Transplant* 1995; 14: 382–6.
113. Sarris GE, Moore KA, Schroeder JS *et al.* Cardiac transplantation: the Stanford experience in the cyclosporine era. *J Thorac Cardiovasc Surg* 1994; 108: 240–52.
114. Semigran MJ, Cockrill BA, Kacmarek R *et al.* Hemodynamic effects of inhaled nitric oxide in heart failure. *J Am Coll Cardiol* 1994; 24: 982–8.
115. Sarris GE, Moore KA, Schroeder JS *et al.* Cardiac transplantation: the Stanford experience in the cyclosporine era. *J Thorac Cardiovasc Surg* 1994; 108: 240–52.
116. Michler RE, Chen JM, Mancini DM *et al.* Sixteen years of cardiac transplantation: the Columbia–Presbyterian Medical Center Experience 1977 to 1993. In: *Clinical transplants*, Los Angles, 1993, 109–18.
117. Caves PL, Stinson EB, Billingham ME *et al.* Diagnosis of human cardiac allograft rejection by serial cardiac biopsy. *J Thorac Cardiovasc Surg* 1973; 66: 461–6.
120. Gao SZ, Schroeder JS, Alderman EL *et al.* Prevalence of accelerated coronary artery disease in heart transplant survivors: comparison of cyclosporine and azathioprine regimens. *Circulation* 1989; 80 (Suppl): III-100–5.
121. Uretsky BF, Murali S, Reddy PS *et al.* Development of coronary artery disease in cardiac transplant recipients receiving immunosuppressive therapy with cyclosporine and prednisone. *Circulation* 1987; 76: 827–34.
122. Billingham ME. Histopathology of graft coronary disease. *J Heart Lung Transplant* 1992; 3: 538–44.
123. Griepp RB, Stinson EB, Bieber CD *et al.* Control of graft atherosclerosis in human heart transplant recipients. *Surgery* 1977; 81: 262–9.
124. Schroeder JS, Gao SZ, Alderman EL *et al.* A preliminary study of diltiazem in the prevention of coronary artery disease in heart transplant recipients. *N Engl J Med* 1993; 328: 164–70.
125. Votapka TV, Swartz MT, Reedy JE *et al.* Heart transplantation charges: status 1 versus status 2 patients. *J Heart Lung Transplant* 1995; 14: 366–72.

# Revascularization as an alternative to transplantation 33

S. WESTABY, K. SAATVEDT AND O. H. FRAZIER

Improvements in the treatment of acute myocardial infarction have decreased early mortality, but generated large numbers of patients with chronic heart failure [1] (Fig. 33.1). Severely symptomatic heart failure derives only limited benefit from medical treatment alone. Up to one-third of patients gain no symptomatic relief from angiotensin converting enzyme (ACE) inhibitors, and episodes of decompensation through cardiac dysrhythmia or pulmonary oedema necessitate repeated hospital admissions. Despite the advances in medical therapy the degree of left ventricular dysfunction remains a strong predictor of mortality with an annual rate of 16% from cardiogenic shock and 8% from dysrhythmia [2]. Five-year mortality from heart failure exceeds that of most malignant tumours. Meanwhile cardiac transplantation is restricted to a highly selected younger age group without significant co-morbidity.

It is now apparent that transplant-listed patients with ischaemic heart disease who do not receive a donor organ may have a 3–4-year survival that equates with those successfully transplanted [3]. In fact, many patients with markedly reduced left ventricular ejection fraction (LVEF) can survive for years with good functional capacity. Consequently it is extremely difficult to decide when to schedule transplantation unless the patient is already committed to a left ventricular assist device for cardiogenic shock. In relation to LVEF the Parsonnet scoring system consistently predicts higher than actual risk (observed/expected $<1$) for conventional surgical procedures [4]. The situation now merits a detailed re-evaluation of potential surgical alternatives for so-called 'end-stage' heart failure patients.

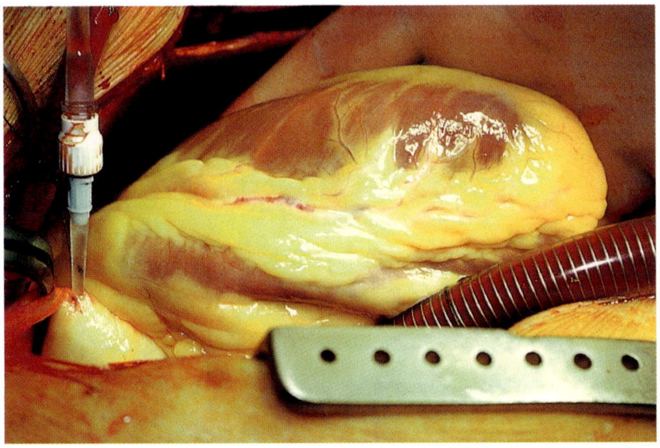

**Figure 33.1** *Urgent revascularization of an occluded left anterior descending coronary artery following attempted PTCA. There is an evolving acute infarction throughout the anterolateral myocardium.*

## The pathophysiology of myocardial ischaemia

Acute coronary occlusion causes irreversible cell necrosis and myocardial infarction within minutes. There is only sufficient oxygen in the myocardium to supply energy for two to three beats. The high energy phosphates, ATP and creatine phosphate may provide energy for a further six to ten beats, but are broken down to xanthine and hypoxanthine which are then lost from the myocardium. The fall in ATP accelerates glycolysis and increases the level of protons (since there is no washout) thereby causing impairment of mechanical function (Fig. 33.2). Oxygen free radicals are generated whilst the cellular enzyme systems which protect again free radicals are depressed. Although the total tissue ATP level does not fall for several minutes, creatine phosphate (the myocardial energy reserve system) has decreased by 80% in 3 minutes. At the same time ischaemia impairs the deacylation–reacylation cycle of the membrane phospholipids through the decrease in ATP and an increase in AMP (and therefore a decrease in the activity of acyl-COA synthetase). This results in accumulation of the fatty acids and lysophospholipids which cause derangement of cell membranes directly or through

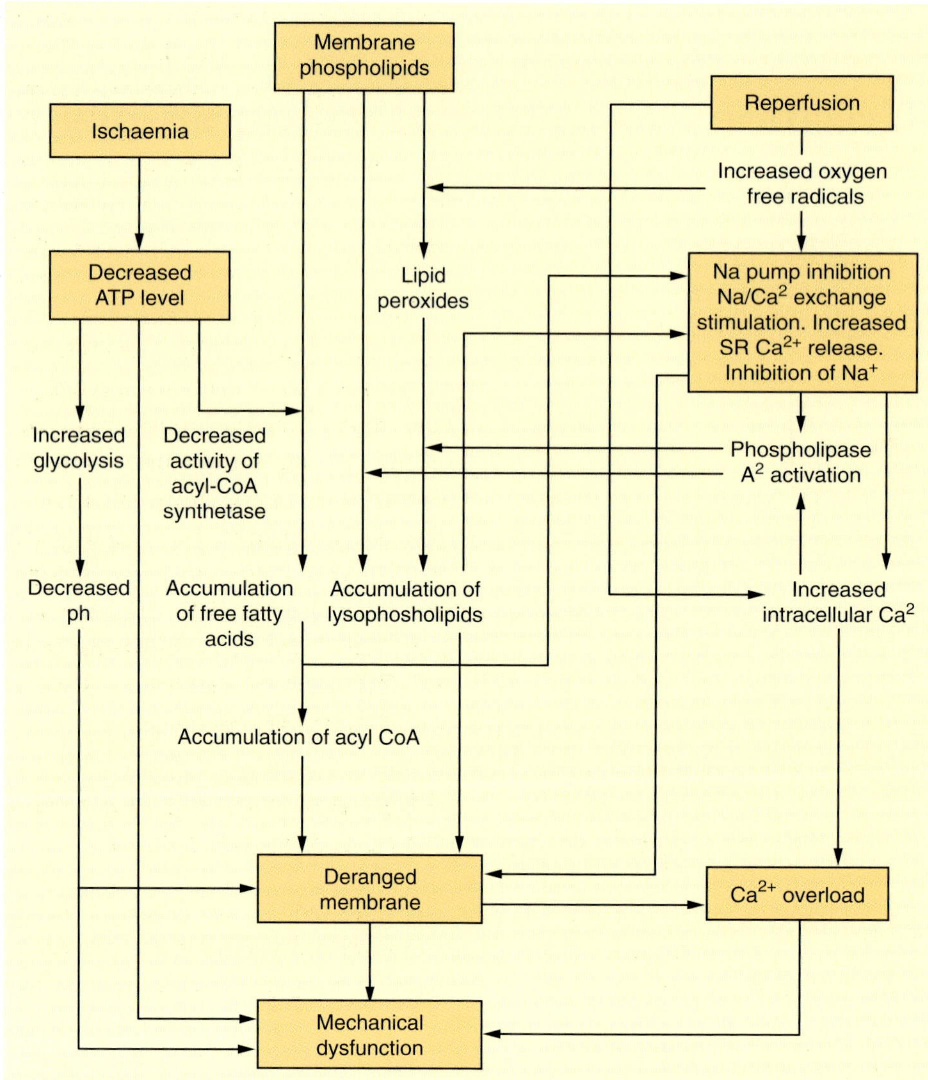


**Figure 33.2** *Flow diagram illustrating the molecular biology of acute myocardial ischaemia (from Yasushi Abito MD, Asastrikawa Medical College, Japan).*

accumulation of acyl-COA and acyl carnitine. This leads to mechanical dysfunction.

After reperfusion, the normal energy state is not restored for up to 1 week when high energy phosphates are re-synthesized [5]. Whilst the level of ATP rises oxygen free radicals inhibit the sodium pump, stimulate sodium/calcium exchange, increase calcium release from the sarcoplasmic reticulum and inhibit an inactivation process of the sodium channel. All these changes increase the intracellular calcium, which increases the activity of phospholipases (accelerating breakdown of membrane phospholipids) and produces calcium overload and hence mechanical dysfunction. Oxygen free radicals also produce peroxidation of membrane phospholipids, which are easily cleaved by phospholipase $A_2$. Therefore, mechanical function cannot recover immediately after reperfusion (Fig. 33.3).

Changes in the electrocardiogram appear in 3 seconds and pain at about 1 minute. The ischaemic muscle has reduced tension during systole and becomes stretched by intraventricular pressure. The fall in systolic tension occurs through intracellular acidosis, lack of energy substrate and accumulation of phosphates and magnesium. Contraction is prolonged more than normal leading to an uncoordinated contraction/relaxation pattern. Beta-adrenoceptor antagonists and calcium channel blockers attenuate the mechanical dysfunction induced by ischaemia-reperfusion by decreasing cardiac function. They can also inhibit peroxidation of phospholipids by mechanisms other than their

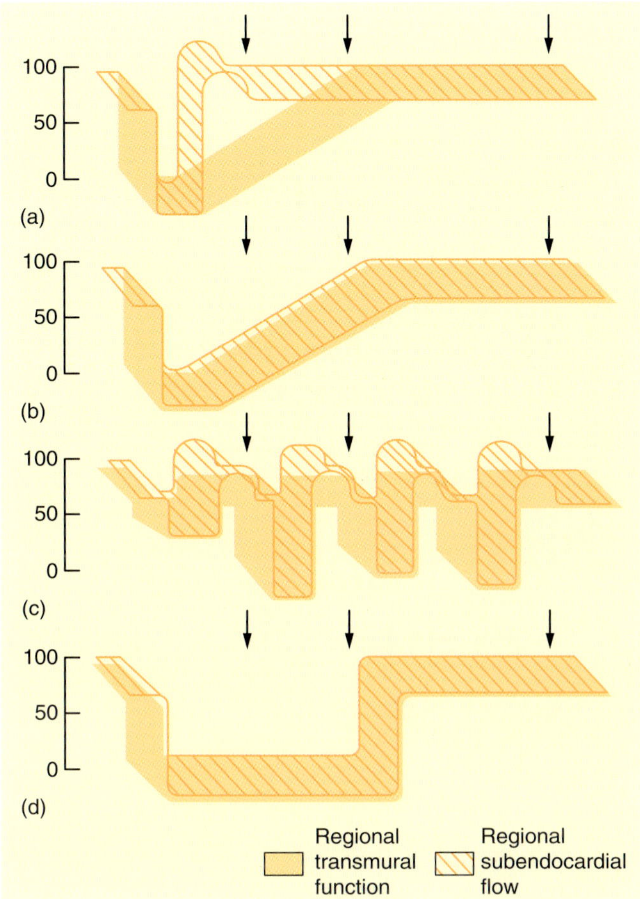


**Figure 33.3** *Differential diagnosis of reversible wall motion abnormalities which may occur in a patient with critical coronary stenoses (from Roberto Bolli MD, Baylor College of Medicine, Houston). (a) Brief episode of ischaemia followed by rapid restoration of flow and by stunning (reperfusion–contraction mismatch). (b) Brief episode of ischaemia followed by gradual restoration of subendocardial flow due to slow lysis of thrombus and/or slow release of vasoconstriction. There is no stunning because flow and function are 'matched'. (c) Recurrent brief episodes of silent ischaemia. In this case there is no stunning since flow and function are matched. (d) Myocardial hibernation/low coronary flow with appropriately matched function. If function is measured at the points marked by the arrows, the situations depicted in panels b, c and d could be mistaken for stunning unless flow is measured at the same time as function. The differential diagnosis of a reversible wall motion abnormality consequently requires simultaneous measurement of flow and function in order to distinguish stunning from silent isibenia or hibernation.*

energy-sparing effects though overdosage causes mechanical dysfunction. Drugs that inhibit the sodium channel (such as lidocaine) also protect the myocardium from ischaemia-reperfusion mechanical dysfunction.

Repeated episodes of ischaemia are associated with impaired ionic flux in the calcium and potassium channels of the sarcoplasmic reticulum. Potassium loss during short periods of ischaemia is not restored for up to 30 minutes. Repeated ischaemia leads to cumulative loss of ions and impaired function (stunning) [6]. The contractile function of stunned myocardium can be restored by inotropes or an increase in extracellular calcium suggesting that the abnormality is unrelated to the contractile proteins. Even after short periods of myocardial ischaemia contractile function and many metabolic changes may not recover for several weeks. Although short periods of ischaemia are followed by a hyperaemic vasodilatory response, areas of ischaemia with evolving necrosis have reduced blood flow by the no/reflow phenomenon. In this case there is vascular smooth muscle contraction, oedema around the necrotic tissue, contracture of myocytes and plugging of arterioles through endothelial oedema. If coronary flow is repeatedly inadequate (for instance, during repeated exercise in the presence of a fixed high-grade coronary stenosis), then myocardial function may remain impaired continuously with a chronic reduction in contractile reserve [7]. This is the hibernation which may be reversed by revascularization (Fig. 33.3).

## The impact of reperfusion during acute myocardial infarction

Reperfusion by thrombolysis or acute PTCA during the narrow time frame when the myocyte is in a state of critical ischaemia (but remains viable) has been shown to reduce cell death, limit infarct size and increase survival [8]. In the event of incomplete or delayed reperfusion, oxidative stress has been shown to induce apoptosis over and above that induced by ischaemia alone [9] (Fig. 33.4). Incomplete myocardial infarction leaves viable, but ischaemic myocardium within the involved segments. In the absence of revascularization this flow metabolism mismatch results in an unstable substrate for postinfarction dysrhythmic events and mortality independent of age or LVEF (event rate 43% versus 8% for scar) [10].

It is now apparent that aggressive early treatment of myocardial infarction with cardiogenic shock can modify clinical outcome. From the Shock Trial Registry, which enrolled 1090 patients with cardiogenic shock from 36 centres, the impact of surgery or thrombolysis, intra-aortic balloon pump counter-pulsation (IABP), and the combinations were compared with medical treatment [11]. Individually, patients treated with thrombolysis had lower in-hospital mortality than those who were not (54% versus 64%, $p = 0.005$). Those selected for IABP insertion also

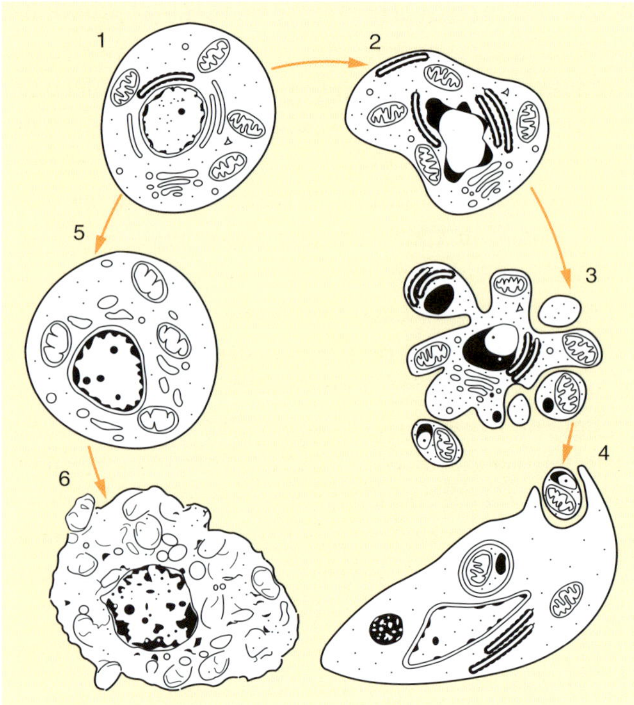


**Figure 33.4** *The difference between apoptosis and necrosis. The normal cell is shown at (1). The ultrastructural changes in apoptosis are shown to the right and those of necrosis to the left. Apoptosis begins with compaction and segregation of chromatin into sharply delineated masses, which lie against the nuclear and cellular outlines. Rapid progression of the process over a few minutes results in nuclear fragmentation and convolution of the cell surface with development of pedunculated protruberances (3). These then detach to produce membrane bound apoptotic bodies, which are phagocytosed and destroyed by adjacent cells (4). In contrast necrosis of an irreversible injured cell begins with clumping of chromatin into ill-defined masses, gross swelling of organalles and the appearance of floculent densities in the matrix of mitochondria. The membranes then break down and the cell disintegrates promoting an inflammatory response in the interstitium (6).*

had a lower in-hospital mortality than those who were not (50% versus 72%, $p < 0.0001$). A combination of thrombolysis with IABP provided the lowest mortality (47%). Those who received neither had a mortality of 77%, those with IABP alone 52%, and those with thrombolysis alone 63% ($p < 0.0001$). Coronary revascularization (CABG) rates differed amongst the groups. Only 18% of patients who received neither thrombolysis nor IABP underwent revascularization. The figure was similar for thrombolysis alone (20%), whereas those who received an IABP with or without thrombolysis had a 70% incidence of revascularization ($p < 0.0001$). Notably the deployment of urgent revascularization significantly reduced in-hospital death for cardiogenic shock patients (revascularization 3% mortality versus no revascularization 78%, $p < 0.0001$). These findings show that during cardogenic shock the combination of thrombolysis, IABP, and urgent revascularization (PTCA or CABG) greatly reduced hospital mortality in comparison with medical management alone.

## The pathological spectrum of myocardial dysfunction

Thrombolysis and acute PTCA frequently cause incomplete or delayed reperfusion which may preserve myocardial viability, but result in akinesia or dyskinesia of involved segments. Consequently impaired left ventricular function may be due to a number of different pathological entities:

- **Permanent myocyte loss due to infarction with scar formation.** The development of a Q-wave on the electrocardiogram is generally accepted as confirmatory evidence of a myocardial infarction (Fig. 33.5), but the presence of a Q-wave is a poor index of the extent of infarction. Infarct size can be reduced by prompt thrombolysis, PTCA or surgical revascularization, but some degree of necrosis is inevitable even if clinically silent. Full thickness infarction heals by scar formation with the potential to develop a left ventricular aneurysm.
- **Chronic dysfunction in viable myocardium subtended by stenosed coronary arteries.** This is myocardium (as opposed to scar) where the ischaemic insult is insufficient to cause necrosis but the tissue remains jeopardized and prone to repeated episodes of ischaemia. Areas of necrosis and fibrosis may eventually develop in the ischaemic area.
- **Changes in the remote myocardium.** Adverse remodelling occurs in normal myocardium through increased

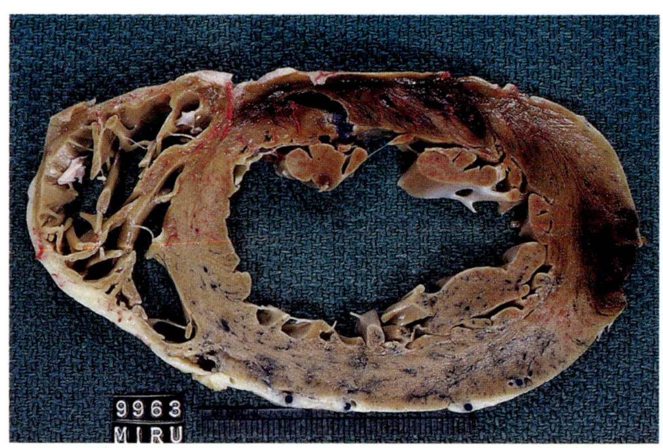


**Figure 33.5** *Section through the left ventricular wall after full thickness acute myocardial infarction. There is extensive necrosis and haemorrhage into the site of the infarction.*

wall stress, metabolic, genetic and neurohormonal changes (Fig. 33.6). Revascularization and surgical reverse remodelling can be used to attenuate the deterioration in remote myocardial function.

## Stunning and hibernation

'Stunning' is defined as myocardium with impaired contractility after transient coronary occlusion salvaged by re-perfusion, but exhibiting prolonged postischaemic dysfunction. This may last hours to weeks. In myocardial stunning there is a flow/contraction mismatch, but well preserved myocardial ultra-structure. Stunned myocardium (global or regional) often occurs after acute myocardial infarction, as well as after cardioplegic arrest during heart operations.

The effects of stunning were outlined by Topol *et al.* [13]. This group evaluated myocardial functional recovery in 20 consecutive myocardial infarction patients who received thrombolysis and in some cases PTCA. After restoration of blood flow to areas of evolving infarction, there was no immediate (or 24 hours) improvement in left ventricular wall motion, but 10 days later 23 of 28 reperfused infarct segments demonstrated improved wall motion compared with only six of 20 non-reperfused segments.

With repeated episodes of ischaemia the myocardium remains jeopardized and exhibits markedly reduced contraction. The concept of chronic flow/contraction mismatch but reversible ischaemic left ventricular dysfunction was introduced in the mid-1980s by Rahimtoolah to account for the improvement in LVEF seen after CABG in heart failure patients [14] (Fig. 33.7). Rahimtoolah first reported the case of a patient with an occluded left anterior descending coronary artery, an akinetic anteroapical wall, and a global ejection fraction of 37%. After CABG, function of the anteroapical region returned to normal and the LVEF increased to 76%. It is now apparent that up to 40% of left ventricular segments with Q-waves or dyskinesia following myocardial infarction are not irreversibly damaged [15]. This information was obtained essentially because surgeons were determined to bypass coronary arteries whether or not the cardiologist predicted benefit.

Hibernating myocardium is usually defined as a state of persistently impaired left ventricular function at rest caused by reduced coronary blood flow (Fig. 33.8) that can be partially or completely restored to normal if the myocardial oxygen/demand relationship is favourably altered. Improvement may occur either through restoration of blood flow or reduced oxygen demand. Inotropic support can produce

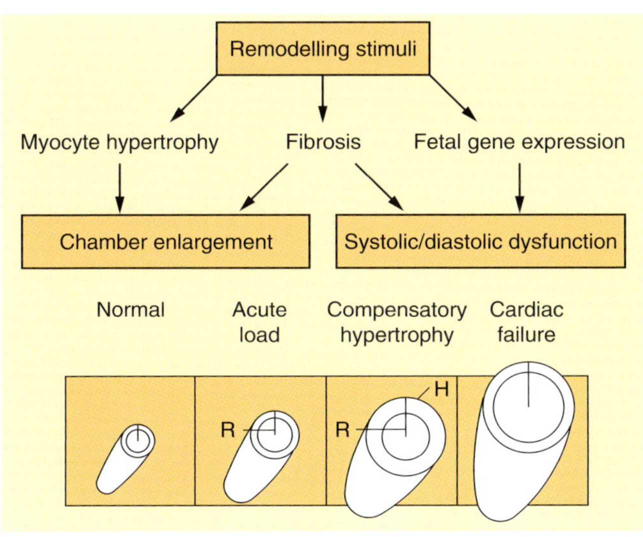


**Figure 33.6** *Remodelling stimuli, progressively affect the shape and function of the left ventricle (R = radius, H = hypertrophy).*

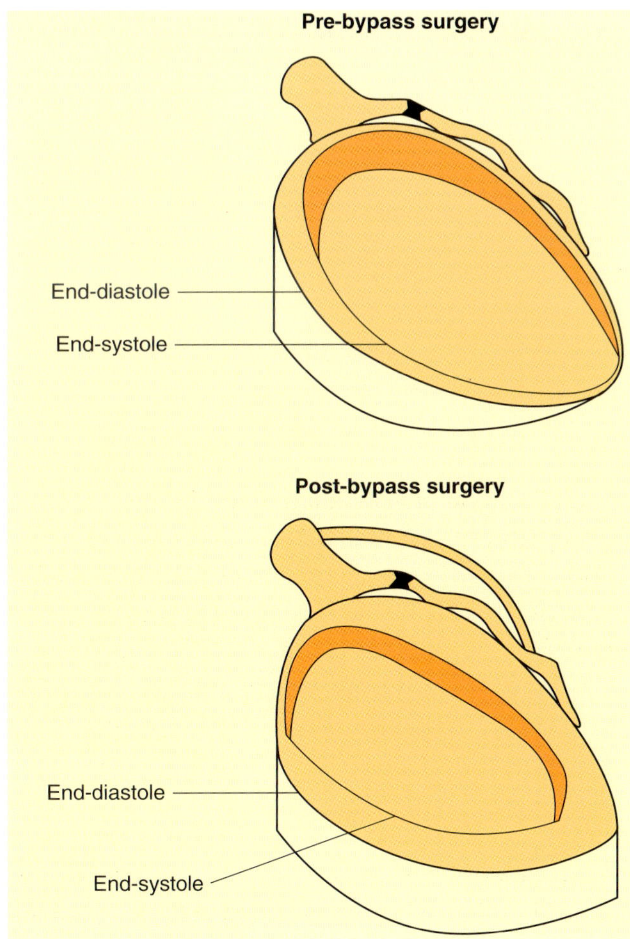


**Figure 33.7** *The influence of surgical revascularization on hibernating myocardium as described by Rahimtoola. Restoration of blood flow restores myocardial function.*

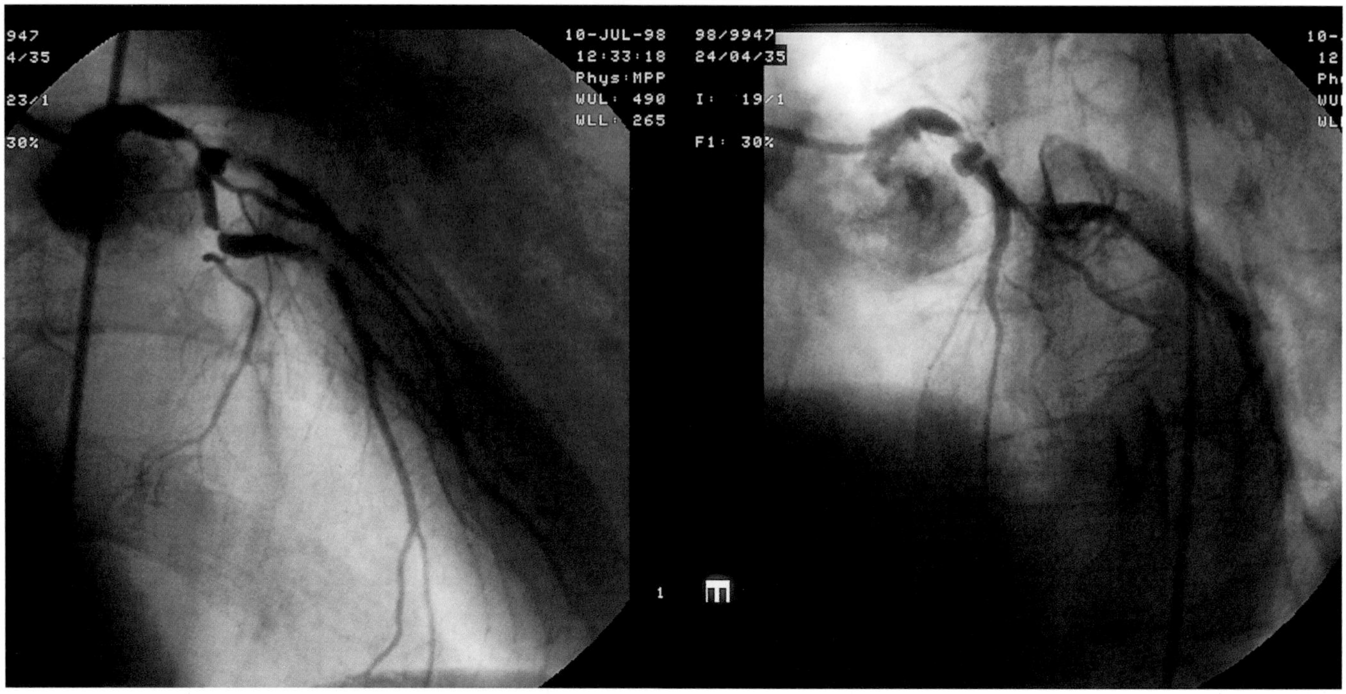


**Figure 33.8** *High grade lesions in the proximal left coronary left artery, which caused repetitive stunning and then hibernation. Akinesia existed throughout the anterolateral surface, but without Q-waves or history of myocardial infarction.*

temporary improvement in contraction. However, recent data suggest that blood flow in hibernating myocardial segments is not always decreased to the same extent that would account for the degree of cardiac dysfunction [16]. Some consider that hibernating myocardium is actually a manifestation of repeated myocardial stunning, perhaps the result of impairment in coronary flow reserve. Ross has described hibernation as perfusion/contraction matching in ischaemic areas with a high degree of interstitial fibrosis, myocytolysis or loss of sarcomeres [17]. Hearst has defined hibernation as exquisitely regulated tissue successfully adapting its activity to the prevailing circumstances [18]. The sustained balance between reduced regional myocardial blood flow and decreased contractile function is associated with a recovery of metabolic parameters during chronic ischaemia. However, in contrast with the normal myocardial architecture in stunning, hibernation is associated with loss of myofilaments, disorganization of the cyto-skeleton, degeneration of the sarcoplasmic reticulum and atrophy or apoptosis in areas of persistent low flow ischaemia. Recently Rinaldi *et al.* have shown that in patients with coronary artery disease and stable exertional angina repetitive episodes of ischaemia lead to profound and persistent postischaemic dysfunction [19]. A number of investigations using PET have shown that transmural blood flow in hibernating myocardial segments is generally within the range of values seen in healthy volunteers with echocardiographically normal LV function [20]. A reduction of about 20% can be found in other cases. However, a loss of systolic wall thickening or presence of scar (wall thinning) may account for the 20% under estimation of regional radioactivity counts, thereby explaining an apparent hypo-perfusion in some dysfunctional segments.

## Impaired coronary flow reserve: a link between stunning and hibernation?

Coronary flow reserve (the ratio of myocardial blood flow during pharmacologically induced hyperaemia to baseline flow), decreases as coronary stenosis severity increases and the impairment is more severe in those regions with resting myocardial dysfunction. In patients with coronary stenoses Uren *et al.* demonstrated that flow reserve decreases in proportion to the degree of obstruction and is abolished altogether for stenoses >80% of the luminal diameter [21] (Fig. 33.9a, b). Under these circumstances an increase in cardiac workload above baseline cannot be met by an increase in myocardial blood flow thereby leading to ischaemia. Therefore, in patients with severe coronary disease the limited flow reserve causes myocardial ischaemia,

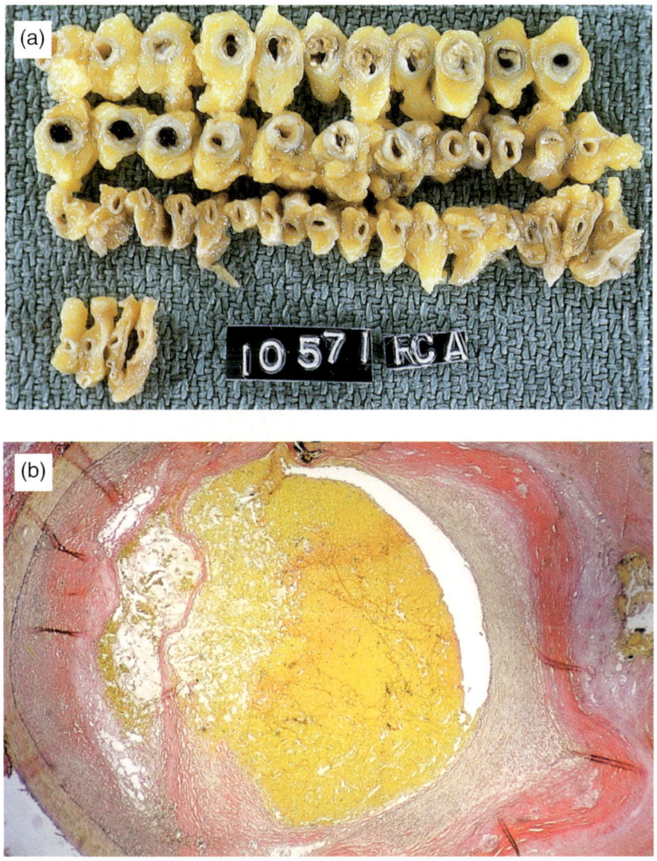


**Figure 33.9** *(a) Multiple sections through a diffusely diseased right coronary artery. (b) Ninety per cent occlusion of the vessel lumen.*

(often asymptomatic) even for small increases of oxygen demand associated with ordinary daily activities. Regardless of blood flow under basal conditions, marked ischaemia occurs when oxygen demand is increased. Thus, intermittent episodes of ischaemia (and postischaemic stunning) might play a role in the development of chronically reversible left ventricular dysfunction (Fig. 33.3). Under these conditions CABG has the potential to eliminate the chronic ischaemic dysfunction by restoring flow reserve.

In summary, the original hypothesis that a prolonged reduction in resting myocardial blood flow is responsible for hibernation in humans with chronic postischaemic ventricular dysfunction is inaccurate. The concept that stunning and hibernation are causally related by a constraint in flow reserve is supported by recent experimental studies [22, 23]. These indicate that flow beyond the stenosed coronary artery subtending the region of chronic dysfunction falls after a period of chronic stunning and that severe reduction in coronary flow reserve is present in areas of akinesia or dyskinesia. It is likely that repeated episodes of ischaemia and reperfusion may eventually lead to sustained changes in the function of the coronary micro-circulation [24]. This suggestion is supported by the finding that ventricular function may be slow to improve (over months) after revascularization [25].

## The relationship between stunning, hibernation and heart failure

The relationship between myocardial stunning or hibernation and heart failure remains complex. Some patients with coronary disease do not stun, others suffer repeated but clinically silent episodes of stunning after normal daily activities [26]. If such episodes are frequent with incomplete recovery of contractile function before the next insult, chronic ventricular dysfunction may ensue. This repetitive stunning may trigger the development of myocardial hibernation, which is associated with changes in myocyte metabolism and structure [27]. Structural changes depend on the time that the blood supply to the myocardium remains jeopardized during demand ischaemia. Thus, myocardium may progress from a phase of functional hibernation (without changes in the contractile protein apparatus) to a phase of 'structural hibernation' with morphological abnormalities within the myocyte (loss of myofibrillar material and accumulation of glycogen) [28]. In structural hibernation, functional recovery after revascularization is more prolonged and dependent on new protein synthesis and myocyte repair. In the absence of revascularization, repetitive ischaemia may progress to myocyte necrosis or apoptosis, which indicates that hibernating myocardium is not fully adapted to chronic under-perfusion [29]. Cellular degeneration and myocyte loss are accompanied by reparative fibrosis. They combine to cause degeneration in the structural and functional integrity of the left ventricle. Consequently if revascularization is to succeed it should be applied early before functional hibernation progresses to structural hibernation.

## Changes in the remote myocardium after infarction

The components of postinfarction ventricular remodelling include infarct expansion, neurohormonal activation, myocardial hypertrophy and global left ventricular dilatation (Fig. 33.10) [30]. Myocardial necrosis triggers an inflammatory reaction with neutrophil infiltration and release of proteolytic enzymes. Collagen breakdown predominates up to 14 days following infarction when serum

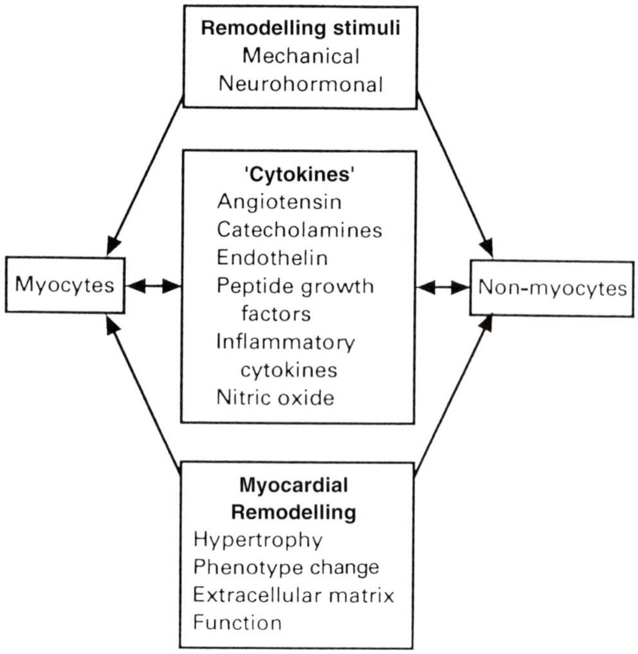


**Figure 33.10** *Mechanical and neurohormonal remodelling stimuli which act on myocytes and non-myocytes.*

levels of matrix metalloproteinases (zinc-dependent collagenase) are raised [31]. Subsequently endogenous tissue inhibitors of matrix metalloproteinase prevail and the activity shifts from collagen degradation and infarct expansion to fibroblast infiltration, collagen deposition and scar formation. The left ventricle progressively dilates and assumes a more spherical as opposed to elliptical contour (Fig. 33.11).

The workload of the myocardium remote from the infarction is increased both by loss of contraction in the scar, and dysfunctional changes. Increased wall stress results in lengthening and thinning of the left ventricular wall through lateral slippage of myocardial planes [32]. During the lytic phase the surface area occupied by the infarcted region increases and may lead to free wall or septal rupture. In the early stages ventricular dilatation serves to maintain stroke volume through the Starling curve. The changes in ventricular geometry, local wall strain and filling pressures combine to increase the metabolic requirements of the remote myocardium, which plays the crucial role in main-

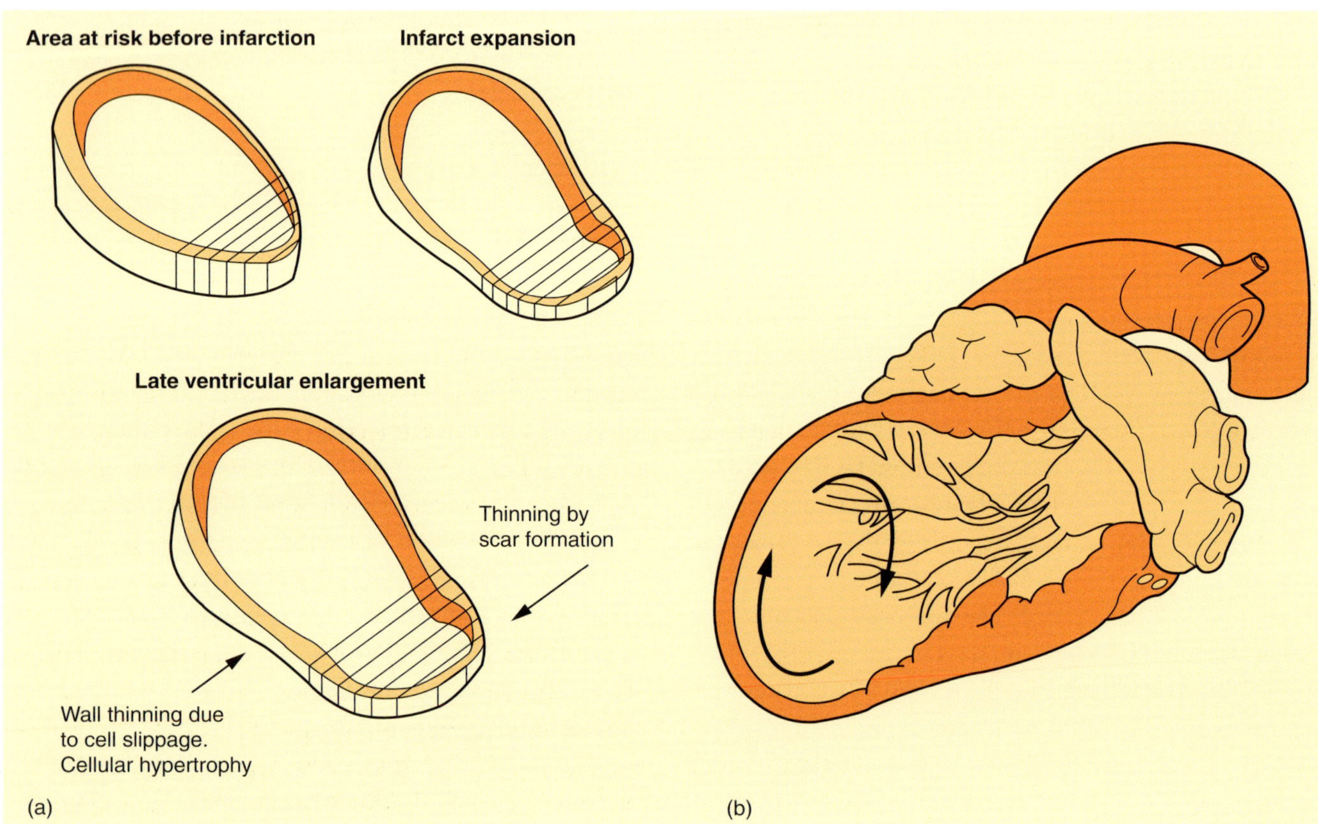


**Figure 33.11** *(a) Increased sphericity of the left ventricle following anterolateral myocardial infarction. (b) The changes in ventricular geometry, end-diastolic pressure and local wall strain combine to increase the metabolic requirements of the normal myocardium, which undergoes compensatory hypertrophy.*

taining cardiac output. These working segments undergo compensatory hypertrophy [33]. Increased sympathetic drive maintains cardiac output through inotropic and chronotropic actions, but aggravates infarct expansion and promotes ventricular remodelling. Elevated plasma neurohormonal levels are closely related to infarct size and the degree of left ventricular dysfunction [34].

In the long term, sympathetic activation contributes to the re-expression of a fetal gene programme (Table 33.2) and left ventricular hypertrophy, which may ultimately exacerbate ventricular dilatation [34]. The hypertrophic stimuli consist of neurohormonal agents (noradrenalin, angiotensin 2 and endothelin), local growth promoting peptides (insulin growth factor 1, cardiotrophin 1, fibroblast growth factor) and physical factors causing myocyte stretch (increased preload and afterload, increased wall tension). These stimuli act on specific cell surface receptors which activate a cascade of intracellular signalling pathways. Re-expression of the fetal gene programme induces myocyte hypertrophy by stimulating deposition of sarcoplasmic elements (Fig. 33.12) [35]. This results in elongation of the myocyte and a pattern of hypertrophy which causes global left ventricular dilatation and wall thinning. These myocytes may also have impaired contractility. As a result the greater left ventricular mass to cavity volume ratio may lead to endocardial ischaemia as the capillary network fails to keep pace with tissue growth. Eventually the adaptive mechanisms are unable to compensate adequately leading to persistent abnormal loading conditions.

When the infarcted region occupies more than 10% of the total myocardial mass (40% of all transmural myocardial infarctions), the left ventricle progressively enlarges with the onset of symptomatic heart failure. When more

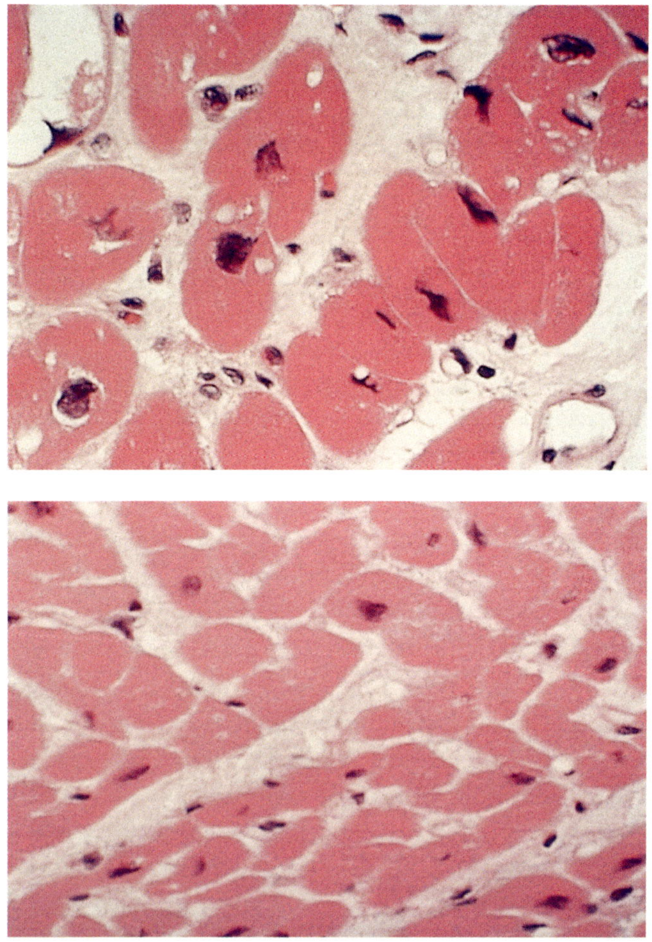

**Figure 33.12** *Section through hypertrophied myocytes in heart failure (above) compared with normal myocardial architecture (below). Re-expression of the fetal gene programme in heart failure induces myocyte hypertrophy by stimulating the production of sarcoplasmic elements.*

than 50% of the myocardium is impaired increased wall tension causes sub-endocardial ischaemia in the remote myocardium. This triggers left ventricular failure.

The relationship between the extent of myocardial infarction, the degree of left ventricular dysfunction and late mortality was well defined by Yoshida and Gould (Table 33.2) [36]. These investigators showed that a myocardial infarction of >23% of the left ventricular circumference caused impaired LVEF (<43%) and a 3-year mortality of 43%. This contrasted with myocardial infarction of less extent, which carried 3-year mortality of only 5%. In those patients with LVEF <43%, the 3-year mortality was 38% in contrast to only 6% when LVEF >43%. However, LVEF alone was a poor predictor of late mortality in patients with hibernating myocardium. The presence of viable myocardium (as determined by positron emission tomography)

**Table 33.1** Myocardial phenotype in adult, fetal and hypertrophic hearts

| Phenotype | Adult | Fetal | Hypertrophy/ failure |
|---|---|---|---|
| Cardiac actin | +++ | + | + |
| Skeletal actin | + | +++ | +++ |
| Smooth muscle actin | + | +++ | +++ |
| $\alpha$ Myosin heavy chain | +++ | + | + |
| $\beta$ Myosin heavy chain | + | +++ | +++ |
| SR $Ca^{2+}$ ATPase | +++ | + | + |

**Table 33.2** Relation between infarct size and mortality

| | Three-year mortality (%) | $p$ value |
|---|---|---|
| Myocardial infarction or scar ≥ 23% | 43 | 0.014 |
| Myocardial infarction or scar <23% | 5 | |
| EF<43% | 38 | 0.029 |
| EF>43% | 6 | |
| EF≤ 43% without viable myocardium | 63 | 0.059 |
| EF≤ 43% with viable myocardium* | 13 | |

*For all patients with viable myocardium the 3-year mortality rate was 8% (80% had CABG). For patients with only fixed scar >23% mortality rate was 50% ($p$ = 0.018, only 40% had CABG). EF, ejection fraction. (Adapted from Yoshida and Gould, 1993.)

is an independent predictor of survival as well as identifying those with impaired LVEF who are most likely to benefit from revascularization [37]. Three-year mortality in patients with LVEF <43% and no viable myocardium was 63% in contrast to 13% for those with viable myocardium submitted for revascularization [36]. For patients with only fixed scar in the territory at risk from coronary occlusion, the mortality rate of 50% at 3 years was no different with or without revascularization, thereby suggesting no benefit of CABG in this subgroup.

### Selection of heart failure patients for revascularization

Currently, PTCA or CABG are applied predominantly on the basis of symptoms and angiographic findings. In the presence of poor left ventricular function without angina or knowledge of myocardial viability, it is unlikely that more than 50% of patients will achieve benefit [38]. Revascularization does not improve the function of scar tissue and it is difficult or impossible on the basis of the ECG, coronary angiography or ventriculogram to determine which areas of the myocardium might benefit from enhanced perfusion. From the now historic CASS Registry, 5-year survival for medically treated patients with LVEF < 25%, was only 41% as compared to 62% of those treated by CABG [39]. For many of these patients fatigue and breathlessness are the predominant symptoms (New York Heart Association (NYHA) class III or IV) and prognosis is poor despite medical therapy. Absence of angina and a results-orientated environment mitigate against CABG for many, but in an increasingly aged population there are hundred of thousands of these patients and transplant donor availability is falling. Only around 10% of potential candidates will eventually receive an organ and in an attempt to lower waiting-list mortality, many transplant centres now select out more patients for high-risk coronary bypass. In turn, increasingly reliable methods have evolved to identify reversible wall motion abnormalities in an attempt to improve the safety and efficacy of CABG.

## Myocardial viability assessment

The goal of myocardial viability assessment is to prospectively identify potentially reversible left ventricular dysfunction in patients whose prognosis may be favourably altered by CABG (Fig. 33.13).

Differentiation between reversible ischaemia and scar can sometimes be made on clinical grounds, for instance in the presence of angina which responds to sublingual nitrate therapy. In the absence of anginal symptoms more objective evidence is required to differentiate between those who will or will not derive benefit from improved myocardial blood flow.

Strategies that have emerged to differentiate between viable and non-viable myocardium include the evaluation of regional perfusion, cell membrane integrity, and metabolism with nuclear techniques; assessment of contractile reserve using dobutamine echocardiography or magnetic resonance imaging; and assessment of microvascular integrity using contrast echocardiograpy. Most of these techniques are reasonably accurate in predicting functional recovery after CABG, but some points regarding their application are worth stressing. First, the patients should have documented coronary artery disease with left ventricular dysfunction, and be potential candidates for CABG. Second, the methods utilized for viability assessment have consid-

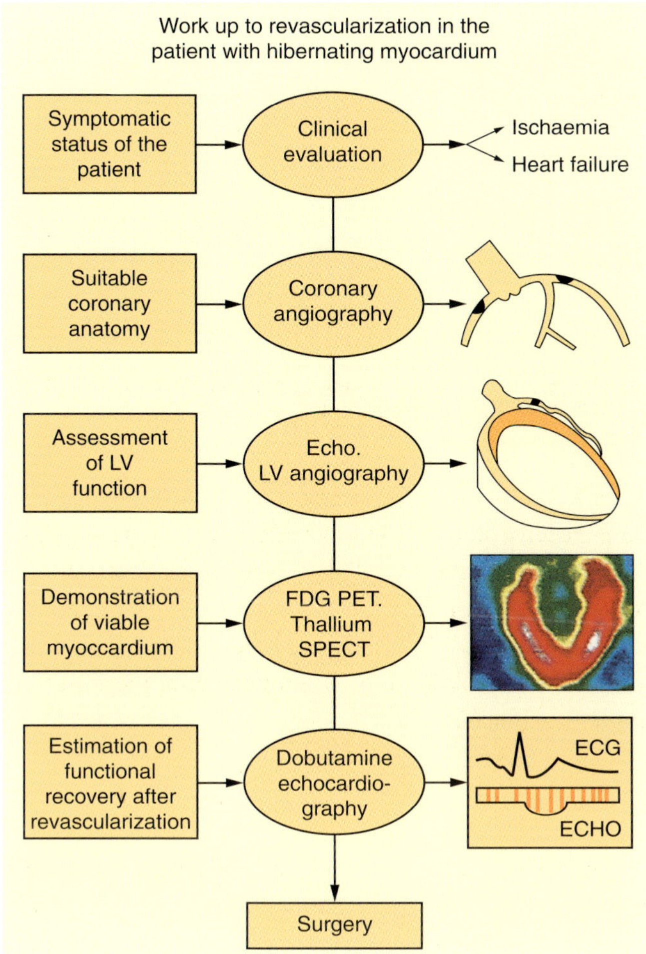


**Figure 33.13** *Scheme for assessment of hibernating myocardium and suitability for surgical revascularization in patients with coronary artery disease and impaired left ventricular function.*

erable overlap with the techniques employed for diagnostic or prognostic evaluation of patients with coronary artery disease, such as the stress-redistribution thallium study. Often, a reasonable assessment of myocardial viability can be obtained with relatively minor modifications of existing protocols, such as reinjection of thallium to demonstrate fixed thallium defects on conventional stress-redistribution images [40]. For patients in whom the question of myocardial viability is primary, however, it is important to decide upon the tracer, the technique, and the technology that can best address the clinical query. Third, the presence of myocardial viability is not an all-or-none phenomenon. In abnormally contracting myocardium, there may be a mixture of scar and viable myocytes. The utility of viability assessment rests on the assumption that without a certain critical proportion of viable myocytes in asynergic segments, CABG will not have therapeutic benefit.

### Stress echocardiography

Patients with poor LVEF, but reversible ischaemia, retain a significant degree of inotropic reserve in the areas of dyskinesia [41]. This is the basis of prediction of recovery using dobutamine stress echocardiography. This involves peripheral venous infusion of low dose (5 and 10 μg/kg/minute) dobutamine during continuing ECG and echocardiographic monitoring. These parameters are recorded at the beginning of the study and every 3 minutes thereafter until completion of the 3-minute dose increment. Beta-blockers are withdrawn at least 24 hours before investigation. A normal segmental response to dobutamine is defined as a progressive enhancement in contractility during stress. Ischaemia is identified by stress-induced wall motion abnormality. Akinetic myocardium at baseline is considered as responsive to dobutamine if wall motion improves by at least one full grade, or as non-responsive if regional wall motion does not change. A global wall motion score is calculated at baseline and at all stages of dobutamine stress. Left ventricular volumes and LVEF are calculated in each patient at rest and at 10 μg/kg/minute of dobutamine. Left ventricular volumes are computed echocardiographically at end-diastole and end-systole for comparison of baseline with stress.

Reversal of regional asynergy during inotropic stimulation predicts functional recovery after revascularization. A greater than 20% improvement of the systolic wall thickening score during dobutamine infusion has a sensitivity of 82% and specificity of 86% for recovery at postsurgical follow-up. Van Overscheld *et al.* showed an improvement of the regional wall motion score by an average of $6.1 \pm 2.4$ grades during low-dose dobutamine in patients with reversible dysfunction, compared with only $1.8 \pm 4.2$ grades in patients with persisting postoperative dysfunction [42]. Enhanced regional wall motion occurred almost exclusively in previously hypokinetic segments. In those who showed improvement in LVEF and end-systolic volume (LVESV) after surgery, enhanced contractility involved both akinetic and hypokinetic segments. The cut-off value which best differentiated between reversible and non-reversible left ventricular dysfunction during dobutamine infusion was an improved regional wall motion score of at least four full grades.

La Canna *et al.* have shown that the basic echocardiographic parameter 'preserved diastolic thickness' invariably correlates with successful surgical revascularization [43] (Fig. 33.14). Myocardial wall thickening on echocardiography also correlates well with histological findings at intra-operative biopsy obtained from hibernating myocardial segments. Nevertheless the apparent maintenance of myocardial thickness and myocyte function, either metabolic or pharmacologically induced, may still not ultimately and conclusively depict the degree of reversibility of structural abnormalities. At present functional tests (dobutamine or other inotrope related echocardiography) reliably indicate potential for early left ventricular recovery after CABG, whereas metabolic investigations (e.g. rest-redistribution radionuclide tests or PET) are better prognosticators of long-term outcome. The major limits of dobutamine echocardiography are:

- the occurrence of ischaemia caused by inotrope stimulation in the presence of a severe reduction in coronary flow, and
- the reduction in beta-receptor density in heart failure, which limits the response of the myocardium to dobutamine infuction.

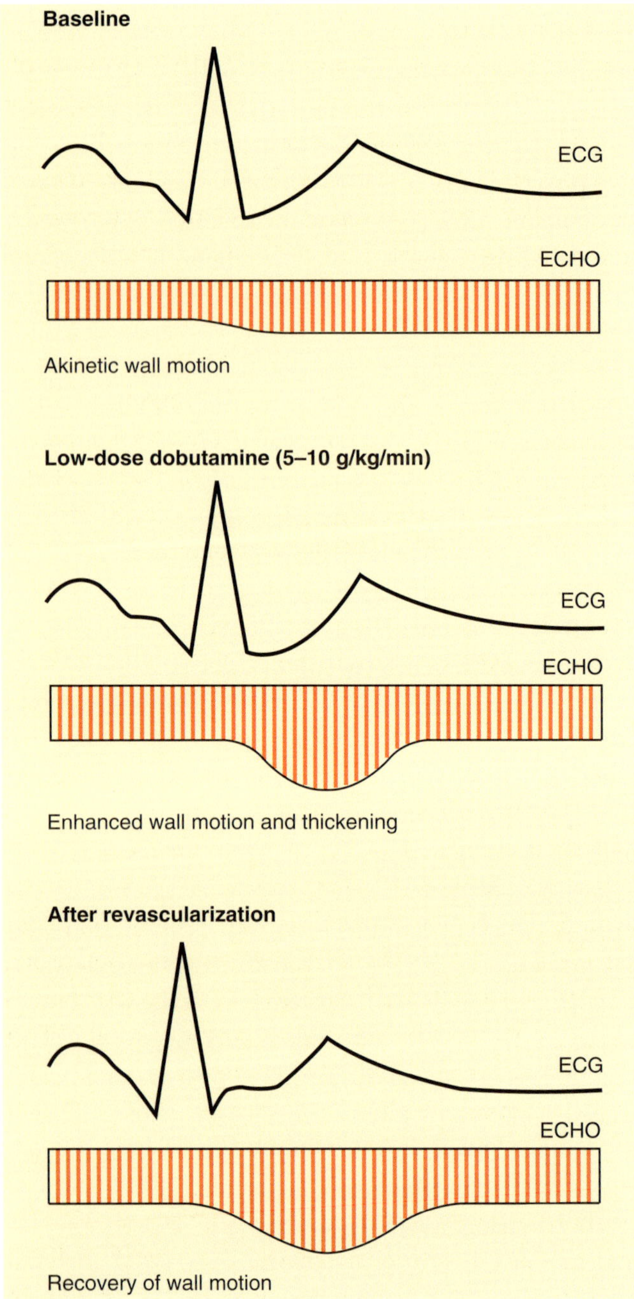


**Figure 33.14** *Diagram illustrating the influence of dobutamine infusion on myocardial contractility and wall thickening in patients with hibernation and potentially reversible wall motion abnormalities (from Giovanni La Canna, Brescia, Italy).*

One criticism of dobutamine echocardiography is that it frequently overestimates wall motion improvement after revascularization and provides only moderate inter-institutional agreement (about 70%) [44]. As an alternative Rocci *et al.*, assessed LVEF response at rest, low-dose dobutamine infusion and peak stress using the bi-plane disc method [45]. They found that improvement in global LVEF predicted postrevascularization recovery significantly better than segmental wall motion changes (72% versus 53%, $p = 0.003$). A biphasic LVEF response with greater than 20% improvement at low doses, then subsequent worsening at peak stress had the highest predictive value (80%) for late functional recovery.

## Positron emission tomography

The use of metabolic radiotracers with positron emission tomography (PET) is generally considered the non-invasive 'gold-standard' for viability assessment [46]. The principle underlying the use of a metabolic tracer is that viable myocytes are metabolically active, while scarred tissue is metabolically inert.

Ischaemia produces a number of alterations in myocardial metabolism. The tricarboxylic acid cycle, the primary source of high-energy phosphates in oxidative metabolism, is compromised in the setting of reduced perfusion and oxygen supply. The loss of oxidative potential results in a compensatory shift towards increased glucose utilization brought about by glycogen breakdown and increased glucose uptake. Whilst fatty acid and acetate tracers have been used to track oxidative metabolism experimentally, the tracer that has gained most clinical use is $^{18}$F-fluorodeoxyglucose (FDG). FDG is a metabolic marker that competes for hexokinase and tracks transmembrane exchange of glucose [47]. In ischaemic myocardium glucose utilization is increased, and thus FDG is concentrated in areas of ischaemic left ventricular dysfunction.

In the PET scan the combined evaluation of regional myocardial blood flow and glucose metabolism provides specific metabolic patterns to differentiate between ischaemic, but viable myocardium as opposed to scar. Increased glucose uptake in segments with reduced blood flow (flow/metabolism mismatch) provides evidence of viable myocardium whilst a segmental concordant reduction in glucose utilization and perfusion demonstrates scar tissue. The overall accuracy of FDG PET for predicting functional recovery after CABG is 80–90%. There is a well-documented correlation between the extent of preoperative mismatch with PET and improvement in LVEF after CABG. Tillisch showed that when more than two segments (out of a potential eight) were revascularized then the LVEF increased from a mean of 30 ± 11% to 45 ± 14% [48]. When less than two segments were involved, there was no improvement in LVEF. DiCarli and colleagues showed that the preoperative extent of flow/metabolism mismatch is correlated linearly with the magnitude of improvement in heart failure symptoms with CABG [49]. Using the Specific Activity Scale, patients with large mismatches (>18%) particularly in the left anterior descending territory had greatest benefit improving their functional state by 107%. Before CABG many of these patients were unable to shower, whereas afterwards they walked 4 mph on level ground without limitation. For patients without mismatch or areas <18% the improvement in functional status was limited to 32% and 42%, respectively. The investigators concluded that the degree of improvement in heart failure symptoms after CABG for ischaemic cardiomyopathy was directly related to the extent of myocardial viability determined preoperatively by PET. Surprisingly patients with angina did not have larger areas of hibernation. On the contrary the hibernating areas were frequently larger in the absence of angina.

Pagano and colleagues compared the predictive value of dobutamine echocardiography with PET in coronary patients with overt heart failure [50]. Assessment 6 months after CABG showed 57% of dysfunctional left ventricular segments to have improved with an overall increase in LVEF from 23& to 32% ($p < 0.0001$). Whilst dobutamine echocardiography and PET had similar predictive values (68% and 66%) in the identification of hibernating myocardium, dobutamine echocardiography had a significantly lower negative predictive value than PET (54% versus 96%, $p = 0.0001$). A significant linear correlation was found between the number of PET viable segments and the changes in LVEF after CABG ($R = 0.65, p = 0.0001$). Haas and colleagues retrospectively compared patients with advanced coronary disease and LVEF <35% who were chosen for CABG either on the basis of clinical presentation and angiographic findings or after assessment of hibernating myocardium using PET [51]. These investigators found the PET assessed group to have substantially less hospital mortality (11.4% versus 0, $p = 0.04$) and better 12-month survival (97% versus 79%, $p = 0.01$). Those assessed for hibernating myocardium required lower doses of inotropes and were significantly less likely to develop low output syndrome. The authors concluded that viability studies improve selection of heart failure patients for CABG and resulted in lower risk of mortality or perioperative complications.

### Viability assessment with SPECT imaging

Though radiotracers used for single photon emission computed tomography (SPECT) display different cellular kinetics, their uptake by the myocardium reflects both perfusion and cell membrane (sarcolemmal or mitochondrial) integrity, and therefore, viability [52]. With quantitative techniques, much information can be gained from a single scan.

*Thallium imaging.* The initial distribution of thallium is primarily a function of blood flow (first-pass extraction in the range of 85%), whilst the later redistribution (over 3–4 hours) is a function of regional blood volume and is unrelated to flow. Distribution of thallium begins within 10–15 minutes after injection and is delayed in regions of poor perfusion. The rate of thallium clearance from areas of myocardium depends on the concentration gradient between the myocytes and the blood. The reversibility of a myocardial defect (from the initial to delayed redistribution images over time) denotes tissue viability. Stress testing (exercise or pharmacology) is used to induce ischaemia with this technique and provides important diagnostic and prognostic information about inducible ischaemia and viability (Fig. 33.15). However, in some patients, stress-redistribution imaging may underestimate the amount of hibernating myocardium. Though late (24 hours), thallium redistribution imaging improves detection, up to 37% of territories that remain irreversible on both 3–4-hour and 24-hour studies (suggesting scar formation) may show recovery of function after CABG [53].

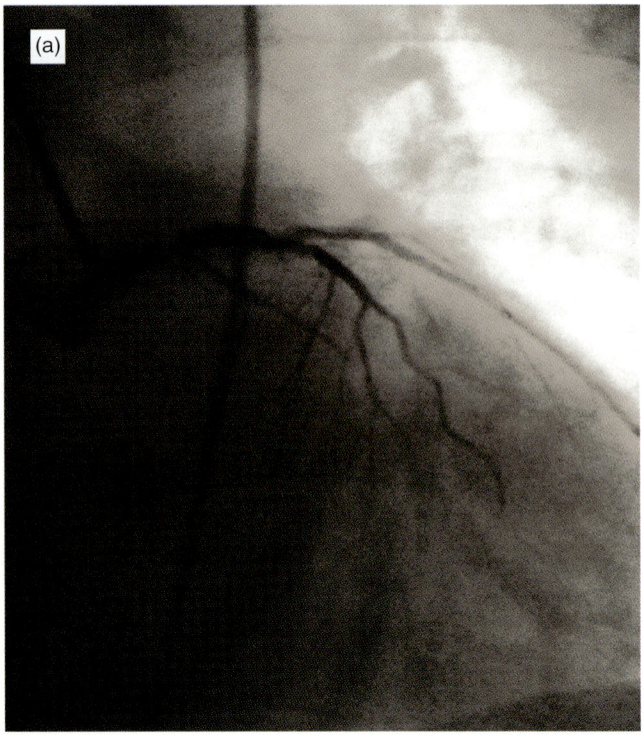


Reinjection of thallium at rest following stress-redistribution imaging improves the identification of hibernating myocardium in up to 49% of the apparently irreversible 3–4-hour defects similarly for 39% of irreversible defects on 24-hour redistribution images [54]. Consequently stress-redistribution-reinjection thallium imaging yields good positive and negative predictive accuracy (80–90% range) for recovery of myocardial function after CABG. Similarly, the correlation between stress-redistribution-reinjection thallium and FDG PET imaging is excellent (up to 88%) when quantitative image analysis is employed [55].

Rest-redistribution thallium imaging is an alternative to reinjection imaging after stress in heart failure patients in whom exercise testing is contraindicated. If the clinical question addresses the presence of viable myocardium within akinetic segments (and not inducible ischaemia), it is reasonable to perform a rest-redistribution thallium SPECT. As for reinjection imaging, rest-redistribution imaging is reliable in predicting improvement in systolic function after CABG.

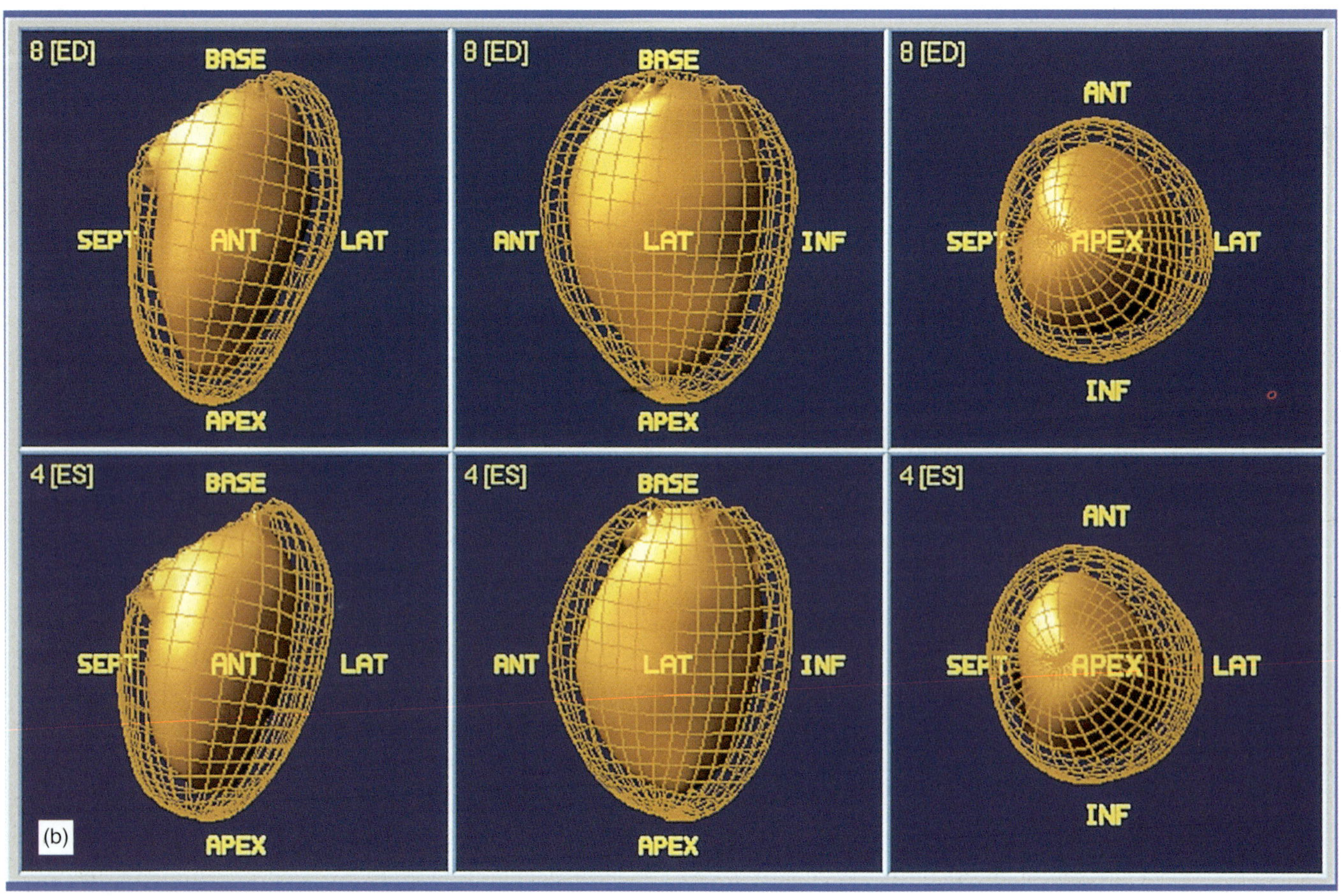


**Figure 33.15** *Viability assessment with SPECT imaging (a). Severe atheroma throughout the left coronary artery (b).*

*Technetium-99m labelled perfusion tracers.* Clinical studies have shown that the accuracy of sestamibi, teboroxime, and tetrofosmin (three technetium-99m labelled tracers with US Food and Drug Administration approval) is similar to that of thallium for detecting coronary artery disease [56]. Whether they provide similar information to thallium with regards to myocardial perfusion defect size, defect reversibility, and viability is uncertain.

Most information about myocardial viability assessment comes from studies with sestamibi. Sestamibi is a lipophilic cationic complex which is taken up passively by myocyte sarcolemmal and mitochondrial membranes. At equilibrium, it is retained within the mitochondria by a large negative transmembrane potential, and thus reflects cellular viability. Early initial experience with quantitative sestamibi uptake performed at rest, resulted in favourable positive (80%) and negative (96%) predictive values for functional recovery after CABG [57]. However, other investigations suggest that sestamibi may underestimate myocardial viability particularly in patients with severe left ventricular dysfunction [58]. The experience with tetrofosmin, teboroxime and newer technetium-based agents for viability assessment is limited.

## Relationship of perfusion, inducible ischaemia, and flow reserve to viability

The relationship between perfusion and viability is complex. Particularly since ischaemic myocardial dysfunction frequently involves a combination of chronic hypoperfusion and/or repetitive episodes of ischaemia (i.e. the coexistence of classic models of hibernation and stunning). The concept that perfusion imaging may be used as a marker of myocardial viability is supported by two lines of investigation:

- that a threshold of flow exists below which viability is not sustainable and
- that intact coronary flow reserve translates into sustainable viability.

In adequately perfused segments retention of vasodilator capacity (i.e. intact coronary flow reserve), appears also to be a marker of myocardial viability. Areas of abnormal coronary flow reserve with PET usually correspond to reversible defects with SPECT imaging [59]. Evidence suggest that reversibility of a perfusion defect (inducible ischaemia) on stress-redistribution-reinjection thallium imaging is a strong predictor of functional recovery after CABG [53].

Promising new techniques such as functional magnetic resonance imaging, assessment of microvascular integrity with echocardiography, and new technetium-99m radiotracers are currently under investigation. Refinement of existing methods by attenuation and scatter correction and gating of perfusion images, may further improve the prediction of recovery of hibernating myocardium and global left ventricular function in the surgical candidate.

## Prognostic implications of myocardial viability assessment

Despite the preponderance of literature using change in ventricular function as an endpoint, the real purpose of CABG is to improve patient outcome, as determined by symptoms and mortality. While assessment of ventricular function seems to be a fair surrogate for studies of outcome, (given the relationship between impaired ventricular function and mortality), this relationship may not persist after CABG [60]. The prognostic significance of viability assessment has been addressed in a number of clinical trials. The importance of perfusion-metabolism mismatch on PET imaging has been confirmed in several studies with an average follow-up of at least 1 year. Despite non-randomization of therapy, the findings have been remarkably consistent. Patients with perfusion-metabolism mismatch have very high mortality if medically managed, and much lower mortality if revascularized. Patients with matched defects, indicating scar, manifest no such difference in outcome between medical and surgical treatment [61]. Recent studies with thallium imaging also indicate the potential prognostic significance of viability assessment using SPECT, although the number of patients remains small.

## Conduct of CABG for the heart failure patient

Patients are selected for CABG with two or more segments of hibernating myocardium, adequate target vessels, a pulmonary artery pressure <60 mmHg and well-preserved right ventricular function. The ethos for CABG in the failing ventricle can be summarized as simplicity, safety and speed. An intra-aortic balloon pump is usually employed preoperatively. Only good target vessels to reversibly ischaemic myocardium are grafted to keep the cross-clamp (myocardial ischaemia) time short. All patients should receive a left internal thoracic artery graft to the most important branch of the left coronary (Fig. 33.16).

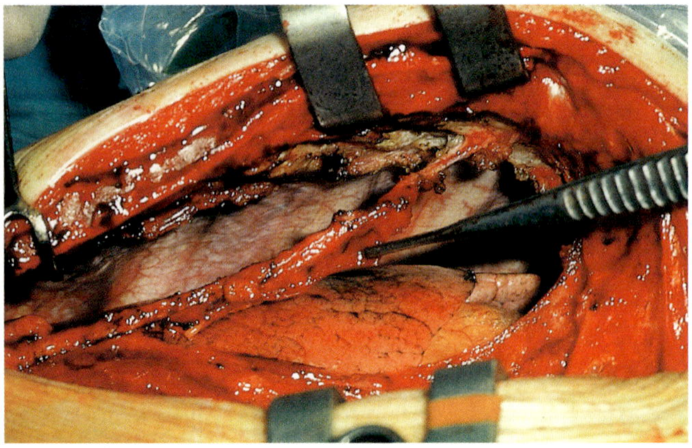

**Figure 33.16** *Harvesting of the left internal thoracic artery.*

Predicting the need for postoperative inotropic support, vein grafts may prove more reliable than radial artery grafts (Fig. 33.17a, b) which exhibit spasm with some inotropes. Jegaden and co-authors reported problems with the use of arterial grafts, compared with the left internal thoracic artery plus vein grafts, in patients with poor left ventricular function [62]. Arterial graft patients had more perioperative events and no survival benefit. Others have reported similar lack of benefit, though recently the problem of spasm has been addressed successfully by pretreatment of radial arterial grafts with the long acting agent phenoxybenzamine instead of papaverine. This policy may improve survival benefit for multiple arterial graft operations as has been suggested for non-heart failure patients.

Myocardial protection is at the discretion of the surgeon but satisfactory results have been reported with retrograde warm blood cardioplegia (which avoids maldistribution through high-grade coronary stenoses) or with temperature guided antegrade cardioplegia [63]. With this technique myocardial segments which failed to cool appropriately with antegrade cardioplegia are grafted first and then repeat cardioplegia delivered via the grafts. In view of the need to minimize myocardial ischaemia the decision to correct moderate mitral regurgitation or to perform left ventricular restoration surgery must be taken carefully. However, correction of moderate and severe mitral regurgitation improves cardiac output and reduces volume overload in the already dilated ventricle [64].

There are a number of situations where mitral valve repair with CABG improves the outlook for the heart failure patient [64]. These are:

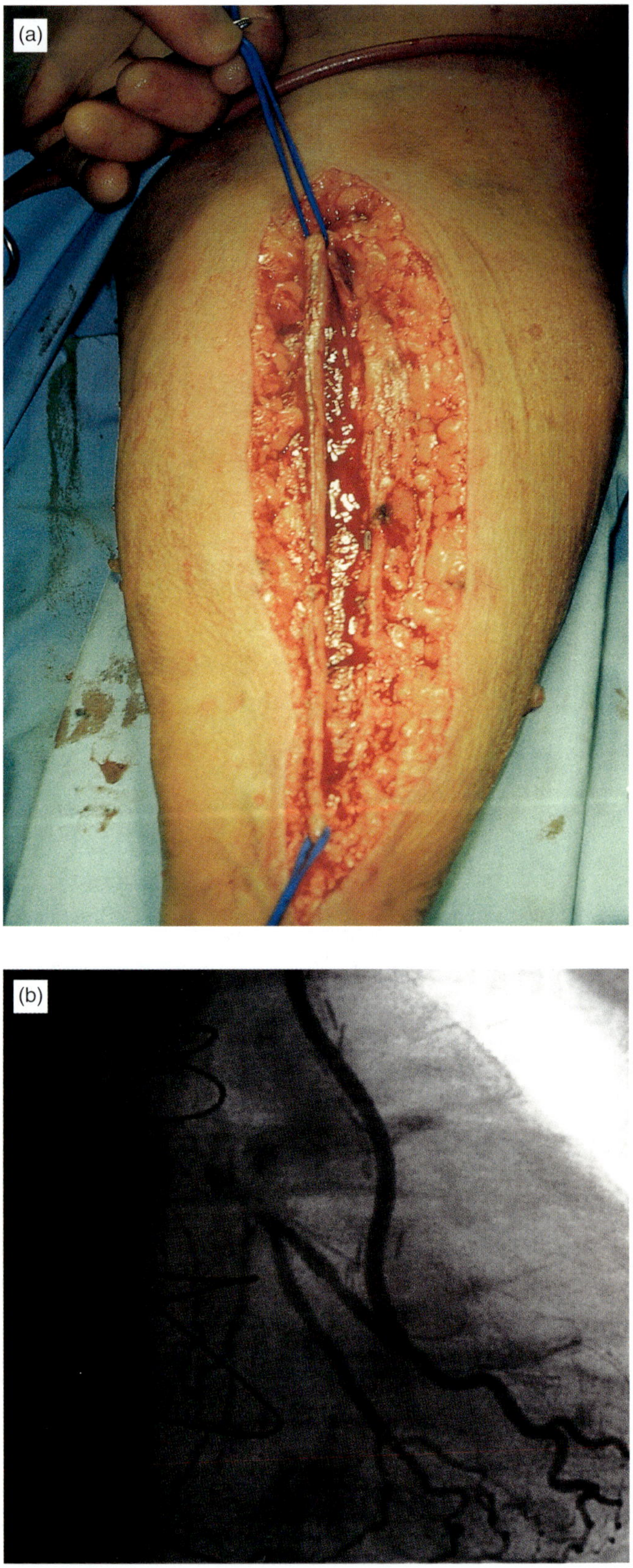


**Figure 33.17** *(a) Harvesting of the radial artery in an obese female patient with poor long saphenous veins. (b) Postoperative angiographic study of a radial artery graft to the disconnected circumflex coronary system (courtesy of David Taggart, Oxford Heart Centre, UK).*

- Chronic progressive dyspnoea (NYHA III or IV) associated with previous myocardial infarction, an enlarged dysfunctional left ventricle and varying degrees of pulmonary hypertension. This comprises the largest group.
- Ischaemia manifest by angina and variable mitral regurgitation which becomes significantly worse during an acute ischaemic episode, causing dyspnoea at rest or left ventricular failure with pulmonary oedema.
- Acute myocardial ischaemia or infarction located infero-basally (right coronary or dominant circumflex distribution), which causes sudden posteromedial papillary muscle dysfunction and mitral regurgitation.
- Acute catastrophic pulmonary oedema which may occur suddenly after myocardial infarction due to papillary muscle rupture.

Guidelines for mitral repair in ischaemic regurgitation are a left ventricular end systolic volume index >80 ml/m$^2$ or a calculated regurgitant fraction >50% of the forward LVEF [65]. Patients with angina, good target vessels, mild to moderate regurgitation and reversible ischaemia posterolaterally on the PET scan, can be treated by CABG alone.

The Alfieri stitch is a very simple and effective manoeuvre for ischaemic patients [66] (Fig. 33.18). The alternative is mitral annuloplasty with significant under sizing of the valve ring which increases leaflet coaptation [67]. Systolic anterior motion is avoided because of widening of the aorta-mitral angle and increased left ventricular size.

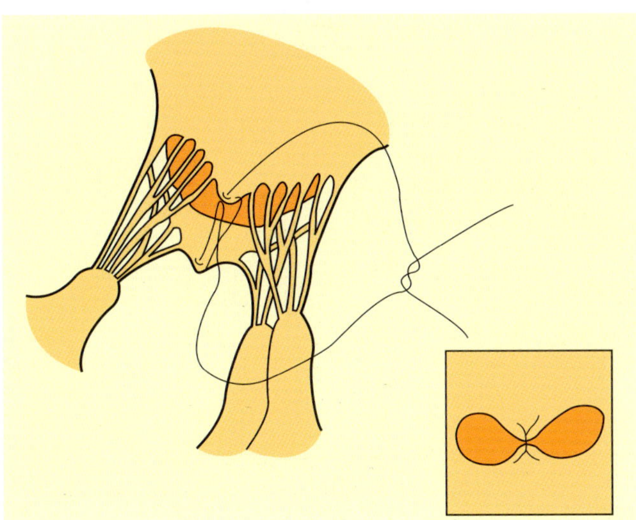

**Figure 33.18** *The simple Alfieri mitral valve repair to reduce or eliminate ischaemic mitral regurgitation. The central portions of the anterior and posterior leaflet are sewn together to produce a double channel mitral orifice.*

The undersized ring remodels the base of the myopathic heart helping to re-establish an elliptical shape to the ventricle. Should valve replacement prove necessary as much of the sub-valvar apparatus as possible should be conserved to maintain left ventricular geometry and function. The application of left ventricular restoration surgery is consider in the next chapter. Suffice it to say here that without intervention a left ventricular end systolic volume index (LVESVI) > 60 ml/m$^2$ predicts 33% 1-year mortality.

## Outcome following revascularization of the poor left ventricle

In any coronary population the survival benefit after CABG is greatest for those with severe angina, three-vessel disease and advanced left ventricular dysfunction [68]. These are the patients at greatest risk from continued medical therapy [69]. For patients with ischaemic or acutely injured myocardium, CABG prolongs life, improves functional status, and diminishes the prevalence of sudden cardiac death caused by arrhythmias. In the past perioperative mortality has been reported to be between 10–37%, though recently much lower mortality has been attributed to advances in myocardial protection [70]. In addition to parameters of left ventricular dysfunction, unfavourable patient characteristics including advanced age, female gender, severity of coronary artery disease, presence of preoperative dysrhythmia or renal failure have been shown to contribute to mortality [71].

In a series of patients referred for cardiac transplantation Hausmann and colleagues compared 225 who underwent CABG with 231 others who remained on the transplant list [72]. The important differences between the groups were the longer duration of symptoms, the presence of right heart failure and a greater incidence of previous CABG in the heart transplant recipients (Table 33.3). Operative risk in the CABG group was significantly higher for those with a greatly increased left ventricular end diastolic pressure (LVEDP >24 mmHg), a low preoperative cardiac output (<2.0 l/min/m$^2$), and for patients in NYHA class IV. Hospital mortality (30 day) was 7.1% for the CABG patients versus 18.2% in the transplant group. There was no significant difference in CABG mortality in patients with LVEF between 10–20% versus those between 20–30%. Hospital mortality for those with unstable angina or acute myocardial infarction was 16.7% as compared to those with stable angina or no angina, which was 5.3%. In patients that had suffered two or more previous myocardial infarctions

**Table 33.3** Guidelines for coronary bypass versus transplantation in end-stage coronary artery disease

| CABG | Transplant |
|---|---|
| Prevailing hibernation | Prevailing scar |
| Short duration of heart failure | Prolonged heart failure |
| Low dose diuretics | High dose diuretics |
| No right ventricular failure | Chronic right ventricular failure |
| Stable cardiac output | Progressively lower output |
| Cardiac index > 2.0 l/min/m$^2$ | Cardiac index < 2.0 l/min/m$^2$ |
| LVEDP < 24 mmHg | LVEDP > 24 mmHg |
| Good target vessels | Poor vessels |
| First operation | Previous revascularization |

LVEDP, left ventricular end diastolic pressure.

hospital mortality was 11.3% versus 5.8% for those with only one previous event. Use of the left internal thoracic artery provided lower (5.2%) operative mortality than for vein grafts alone (7.8%). Survival for the CABG group was 78.9% after 6 years versus 68.9% in the transplant group. Late investigation of CABG patients showed a significant decrease in mean pulmonary artery and pulmonary capillary wedge pressures. Left ventricular ejection fraction improved from a mean of 0.23% to 0.39% ($p < 0.0001$).

In a similar study Tjan and colleagues compared the outcome in 51 potential transplant candidates (LVEF < 20%), who underwent CABG instead with 163 transplant patients with ischaemic cardiomyopathy [73]. The survival analysis was performed on the basis of intention to treat, independent of subsequent transplantation. Groups were comparable with regard to left ventricular function, pulmonary capillary wedge pressure and serum creatinine. Patients in the CABG group were older (63 ± 8) ($p = 0.001$) and included a higher percentage of women. One-year survival was similar in both groups (CABG 71.9% versus transplantation 66.3%). Of the CABG patients perioperative survival was 88.2% with preoperative serum creatinine and the non-usage of the internal thoracic artery predicting adverse outcome. The authors concluded that following evaluation for cardiac transplantation up to 50% of patients could be referred for CABG, after assessing myocardial viability and general risk factors such as age, peripheral vascular disease, and history of hypertension. Selection according to preoperative LVEF was not useful, whilst the degree of viable myocardium was predictive of outcome. The authors recommend preoperative use of the intra-aortic balloon pump and left ventricular assist device standby during the procedure. With worsening donor availability others support the policy of revascularization as an alternative to transplantation [74–76].

Kaul and colleagues identified risk factors for hospital mortality in patients with LVEF <20%, reversible ischaemia, and operable target vessels [74]. Primary indications for surgery were unstable angina (35%), return of symptoms after previous CABG (20%), congestive heart failure with reversible ischaemia (26%) and recurrent ventricular arrhythmia's (20%). Overall actuarial survival was 82%, 79% and 73% at 1, 2 and 5 years, respectively. Patients who did not receive retrograde cardioplegia, older patients, and those with preoperative ventricular dysrhythmias or renal failure had an increased risk of hospital mortality. Patients with congestive symptoms and those requiring extensive or redo CABG were at increased risk of death throughout the follow-up period. Hospital mortality increased as the number of distal anastomosis performed increased thereby emphasizing the need for short cross-clamp times.

At present the long-term outcome after CABG is poorly defined. Only structurally preserved and perfused myocytes show substantial postrevascularization recovery and improvement in left ventricular mechanics overall is neither uniform nor stable with time. Myocardial ultrastructure is an important determinant of recovery, which is limited as mycardial fibrosis progresses [78]. The presence of a well developed coronary collateral circulation is a positive predictor of functional improvement. Patients with worse preoperative function have limited perioperative recovery and may manifest a rapid decline in LVEF over time with early recurrence of heart failure symptoms. The supposition is that these patients with less than optimal outcome despite assessment of viability have major structural derangement within the hypocontractile zones with gradual loss of recovered myocardial function through progressive myocyte degeneration (i.e. unrelenting ischaemic cardiomyopathy). The time limited benefits of CABG in advanced left ventricular function were demonstrated by Luciani who showed only 47% of patients to be free of heart failure symptoms 5 years post-CABG despite 75% survival at this time [74]. However, CABG appeared to influence the mode of death. Most late deaths occurred through left ventricular failure and not arrhythmia which otherwise accounts for more than 60% of deaths in unoperated patients with ischaemic cardiomyopathy.

**Table 33.4** Decision making in the surgery of end stage ischaemic heart disease

| Condition | Intervention |
|---|---|
| Reversible ischemia LVESVI < 60 ml/m$^2$ | CABG alone |
| Full thickness scar and left ventricular aneurysm | Linear resection ± CABG |
| Akinetic/dyskinetic left ventricle<br>LVESVI > 60 ml/m$^2$ with reversible ischaemia | CABG + LV restoration surgery |
| Class III/IV mitral regurgitation | Mitral repair ± CABG |
| No reversible ischaemia LVESVI > 100 ml/m$^2$<br>Pulmonary hypertension (PAP > 70 mmHg)<br>Right ventricular failure | Left ventricular assist device or transplantation (no conservative option) |

LVESVI, left ventricular end systolic volume index (normal is < 30 ml/m$^2$); CABG, coronary artery bypass grafting; PAP, pulmonary artery pressure. (Adapted from Hausmann *et al.*, 1997.)

In summary, up to 50% of ischaemic patients submitted for transplantation (and many more deemed unsuitable) have hibernating myocardium and may respond favourably to CABG. PET and dobutamine stress echocardiography are currently the best predictors of functional recovery in hibernating myocardium. Those without viable muscle derive limited or no benefit from CABG at high operative risk. Long-term outlook for those with initial improvement after CABG is uncertain, but limited by myocardial fibrosis in non-ischaemic segments following ventricular remodelling.

However, medium-term outcome is considerably better than the prospect of a transplant waiting list. Consequently, a more aggressive approach to investigation and treatment is warranted for patients with advanced ischaemic heart disease and poor left ventricular function. Guidelines for surgical decision making in end stage ischaemic heart disease are summarized in Table 33.4.

## References


1. Théroux P, Willerson JT, Armstrong PW (2000) Progress in the treatment of acute coronary syndromes. A 50 year perspective (1950–2000). *Circulation* **10**: IV-2–IV-13.
2. Di Carli MF, Maddhai J, Rockhsar S *et al.* (1998) Long term survival of patients with coronary artery disease and left ventricular dysfunction: implications for the role of myocardial viability assessment in management decisions. *J Thorac Cardiovasc Surg* **11**: 997–1004.
3. Louie HW, Laks A, Milgalter E *et al.* (1991) Ischemic cardiomyopathy: criteria for coronary revascularization and cardiac transplantation. *Circulation* **84**(suppl) III: 290–5.
4. Wechsler AS (1996) Editorial on Coronary artery bypass grafting in patients with an ejection fraction of twenty percent or less. *J Thorac Cardiovasc Surg* **III**: 998–1000.
5. Braunwald E, Klorer RA (1992) The stunned myocardium: prolonged, postischemic ventricular dysfunction. *Circulation* **86**: 1146–9.
6. Bolli R (1992) Myocardial 'stunning' in man. *Circulation* **86**: 1671–91.
7. Marban E (1991) Myocardial stunning and hibernation. The physiology behind the colloquialisms. *Circulation* **83**: 681–8.
8. Bagmir F and Fast Revascularization During Instability in Coronary Artery Disease Investigators (1999) Invasive compared with noninvasive treatment in unstable coronary artery disease: FRISC II prospective randomised multicentre study. *Lancet* **354**: 708–15.
9. Sabbah HN (2000) Apoptotic cell death in heart failure. *Cardiovasc Res* **45**: 704–12.
10. Laek. S, Marwick TH, Cook SA *et al.* (1994) Prognosis of patients with left ventricular dysfunction with and without viable myocardium after myocardial infarction. Relative efficacy of medical therapy and revascularization. *Circulation* **90**: 2687–94.
11. Sanborn TA, Sleeper LA, Bates ER *et al.* (2000) Impact of thrombolysis, intra-aortic balloon counterpulsation and their combination in cardiogenic shock complicating acute myocardial infarction: a report from the SHOCK Trial Registry. Should we emergently revascularise occluded coronaries for cardiogenic shock? *J Am Coll Cardiol* **36**(suppl A): 1123–9.
12. Braunwald E (1990) The stunned myocardium: newer insights into mechanisms and clinical implications. *J Thorac Cardiovasc Surg* 100: 310–11.
13. Topol EJ, Weiss JL, Guzman PA *et al.* (1984) Immediate improvement of dysfunctional myocardial segments after coronary revascularization: detection by intraoperative transoesophageal echocardiography. *J Am Coll Cardiol* **4**: 1123–9.
14. Rahimtoola SH (1989) The hibernating myocardium. *Am Heart J* **117**: 211–21.
15. Arnese M, Cornel JH, Salustri A *et al.* (1995) Prediction of improvement of regional left ventricular function after surgical revascularization. A comparison of low-dose dobutamine echocardiography with 201TI single-photon emission computed tomography. *Circulation* **91**: 2748–52.
16. Camici PG, Rimoldi O (1997) Resting myocardial blood flow in patients with hibernating myocardium quantified by positron emission tomography. *Basic Res Cardiol* **92**: 6–8.

17. Ross J Jr (1991) Myocardial perfusion-contraction matching. Implications for coronary heart disease and hibernation. *Circulation* **83**: 1076–83.
18. Hearse DJ, Bolli R (1992) Reperfusion induced injury: manifestations, mechanism and clinical relevance. *Cardiovasc Res* **26**: 101–8.
19. Rinaldi CA, Masani ND, Linka AZ, Hall RJ (1999) Effect of repetitive episodes of exercise induced myocardial ischemia on left ventricular function in patients with chronic stable angina: evidence for cumulative stunning or ischemic preconditioning? *Heart* **81**: 404–11.
20. Gerber BLJL, Vanoverschelde A, Bol *et al.* (1994) Myocardial blood flow, glucose uptake and recruitment of inotropic reserve in chronic left ventricular ischemic dysfunction. Implications for the pathophysiology of chronic myocardial hibernation. *Circulation* 651–9.
21. Uren NGJA Melin B, De Bruyne W *et al.* (1994) Myocardial blood flow as a function of coronary stenosis severity in man. *New Engl J Med* **330**: 1782–8.
22. Fallavollita JA, Perry BJ, Canty JM, Jr. (1995) $^{18}$F-2-deoxyglucose deposition and regional flow in pigs with chronically dysfunctional myocardium. Evidence for transmural variations in chronic hibernating myocardium. *Circulation* 1900–9.
23. Lim HJA, Fallavollita, Hard R, Kerr CW *et al.* (1999) Profound apoptosis-mediated regional myocyte loss and compensatory hypertrophy in pigs with hibernating myocardium. *Circulation* **100**: 2380–6.
24. Bolli RJF, Triana, Jeroudi MO (1990) Prolonged impairment of coronary vasodilation after reversible ischemia. Evidence of microvascular stunning. *Circulation* **67**: 332–43.
25. Spyrou N, Khan MA, Rosen SD *et al.* (2000) Persistent but reversible coronary microvascular dysfunction after bypass grafting. *Am J Physiol* (in press).
26. Ambrosio GS, Betocchi L, Pace MA, Losi *et al.* (1996) Prolonged impairment of regional contractile function after resolution of exercise-induced angina. Evidence of myocardial stunning in patients with coronary artery disease. *Circulation* **94**: 2455–64.
27. Camici PG, Wijns WM, Borgers R *et al.* (1997) Pathophysiological mechanisms of chronic reversible left ventricular dysfunction due to coronary artery disease (hibernating myocardium). *Circulation* **96**: 3205–14.
28. Schwarz ER, Schaper J, von Dahl C *et al.* (1996) Myocyte degeneration and cell death in hibernating human myocardium. *J Am Coll Cardiol* **27**: 1577–85.
29. Elsasser AM, Schelpper WP, Klovekorn WJ *et al.* (1997) Hibernating myocardium: an incomplete adaptation to ischemia. *Circulation* **96**: 2920–31.
30. Braunwald E, Bristow MR (2000) Congestive heart failure: fifty years of progress. *Circulation* **102**(suppl IV): IV-14–IV-23.
31. Wessner JF Jr (1991) Matrix metalloproteinases and their inhibitors in connective tissue remodelling. *FASEB J* **5**: 2145–54.
32. Olivetti G, Capasso JM, Sonneblick EH *et al.* (1990) Side to side slippage of myocytes participates in ventricular remodeling acutely myocardial infarction in rats. *Circ Res* **67**: 23–34.
33. Pfeffer MA (1995) Left ventricular remodelling after acute myocardial infarction. *Annu Rev Med* **46**: 455–66.
34. Cohn JN, Johnson GR, Shabetai R *et al.* (1993) Ejection fraction, peak exercise oxygen consumption, cardiothoracic ratio, ventricular arrhythmias and plasma nor-epinephrine as determinants of prognosis in heart failure. *Circulation* **87**(suppl VI): VI-5–VI-16.
35. Lorell BH, Carbello BA (2000) Left ventricular hypertrophy. Pathogenesis, detection and prognosis. *Circulation* **102**: 470–79.
36. Yoshida F, Gould KL (1993) Quantitative relation of myocardial infarct size and myocardial viability by positron emission tomography to left ventricular ejection fraction and 3 year mortality with and without revascularization. *J Am Coll Cardiol* **22**: 984–97.
37. Lee KS, Marwick TH, Cook SA *et al.* (1994) Prognosis of patients with left ventricular dysfunction, with and without viable myocardium after myocardial infarction. Relative efficacy of medical therapy and revascularization. *Circulation* **90**: 2687–94.
38. Marwick T, MacIntyre WJ, Lafont A *et al.* (1992) Metabolic response of hibernating and infarcted myocardium to revascularization: a follow up study of perfusion, function and metabolism. *Circulation* **85**: 1347–53.
39. Emond M, Mock MB, Davis KB *et al.* (1994) Long term survival of medically treated patients in the coronary artery surgery study (CASS). *Circulation* **90**: 2645–57.
40. Kiat H, Berman DS, Maddahi J *et al.* (1988) Late reversibility of tomographic myocardial TI-201 defects: an accurate marker of myocardial viability. *J Am Coll Cardiol* **12**: 955–62.
41. Williams MJ, Odabashiar J, Lauer MS *et al.* (1996) Prognostic value of dobutamine echocardiography in patients with left ventricular dysfunction. *J Am Coll Cardiol* **27**: 132–9.
42. Vanoverschelde J-LJ, Berger BL, D'Handt A-M *et al.* (1995) Preoperative selection of patients with severely impaired left ventricular function for coronary revascularization. Role of low dose dobutamine echocardiography and exercise redistribution – reinjection thallium SPECT. *Circulation* **92**(suppl II): II.37–II.44.
43. La Canna G, Alfieri O, Giubbini R *et al.* (1994) Echocardiography during infusion of dobutamine for identification of reversible dysfunction in patients with chronic coronary artery disease. *J Am Coll Cardiol* **23**: 617–26.
44. La Canna G, Rahimtoola SH, Visioli O *et al.* (2000) Sensitivity, specificity and predictive accuracies of noninvasive tests, singly and in combination, for diagnosis of hibernating myocardium. *Eur Heart J* **21**: 1358–67.
45. Roccli G, Poldermass D, Bax JJ *et al.* (2000) Usefulness of the ejection fraction response to dobutamine infusion in predicting functional recovery after coronary artery bypass grafting in patients with left ventricular dysfunction. *Am J Cardiol* **85**: 1440–4.
46. Camici P, Ferrannini E, Opie LH (1986) Myocardial metabolism in ischemic heart disease: basic principles and application to imaging by positron emission tomography. *Circulation* **74**: 81–8.
47. Camicio P, Araujo LI, Spinks T *et al.* (1986) Increased uptake of $^{18}$F-fluorodeoxyglucose in postischemic myocardium of patients with exercise induced angina. *Circulation* **74**: 81–8.
48. Tillisch J, Brunken R, Marshall R *et al.* (1986) Reversibility of cardiac wall motion abnormalities predicted by positron tomography. *N Engl J Med* **314**: 884–8.
49. DiCarli MF, Davidson M, Little R *et al.* (1994) Value of metabolic imaging with positron emission tomography for evaluating prognosis in patients with coronary artery disease and left ventricular dysfunction. *Am J Cardiol* **73**: 527–33.
50. Pagano D, Lewis DME, Townend JN *et al.* (1999) Revascularization for postischemic heart failure: how myocardial viability affects survival. *Heart* **82**: 684–8.
51. Haas F, Haehnel CJ, Picker W *et al.* (1997) Preoperative positron emission tomographic viability assessment and perioperative and postoperative risk in patients with advanced ischemic heart disease. *J Am Coll Cardiol* 1693–700.

52. Beller GA, Ragosta M, Watson DD, Gimple LW (1992) Myocardial thallium-201, scintigraphy for assessment of viability in patients with severe left ventricular dysfunction. *Am J Cardiol* **70**: 18E–22E.
53. Ragosta M, Beller GA, Watson DD *et al.* (1993) Quantitative planar rest redistribution TI-201 imaging in detection of myocardial viability and prediction of improvement in left ventricular function after coronary bypass surgery in patients with severely depressed left ventricular function. *Circulation* **87**: 1630–41.
54. Dilsizian V, Rocco TP, Freedman NM *et al.* (1990) Enhanced detection of ischemic, but viable myocardium by the reinjection of thallium after stress redistribution imaging. *N Engl J Med* **323**: 141–6.
55. Bonow RO, Dilsizian V, Cuocolo A, Bacharach SL (1991) Identification of viable myocardium in patients with coronary artery disease and left ventricular dysfunction: comparison of thallium scintigraphy with reinjection and PET imaging with 18-F-fluorodeoxy glucose. *Circulation* **83**: 26–37.
56. Willerson JT (1990) Technetium-99m MIBI as a myocardial perfusion agent. *Circulation* **82**: 1067–9.
57. Bisi G, Sciagra R, Sartoso GM *et al.* (1993) Nitrate sestamibi perfusion imaging: predictive value for the outcome of coronary revascularization. *Circulation* **88**: 1058–64.
58. Soufer R, Dey HM, Markey J *et al.* (1993) Inferior wall myocardial viability is underestimated on sestamibi SPECT: comparison to FDG positron emission tomography. *Circulation* **88**: 1059–66.
59. Altehoefer C, von Dahl J, Biedermann M *et al.* (1994) Significance of defect severity in technetium-99m MIBI SPECT at rest to assess myocardial viability: comparison with fluoride-18-FDG PET. *J Nucl Med* **35**: 569–74.
60. Samady H, Elefteriades JA, Abbot BG *et al.* (1999) Failure to improve left ventricular function after coronary revascularization for ischemic cardiomyopathy is not associated with worse outcome. *Circulation* **100**: 1298–304.
61. Lee K, Marwick TH, Cook SA *et al.* (1994) Prognosis of patients with left ventricular dysfunction with and without viable myocardium after myocardial infarction. Relative efficacy of medical therapy and revascularization. *Circulation* **90**: 2687–94.
62. Jegaden O, Bontemps L, DeGevigney A *et al.* (1998) Does the extended use of arterial grafts compromise myocardial recovery after coronary artery bypass grafting in left ventricular dysfunction? *Eur J Cardiothorac Surg* **14**: 353–9.
63. Mickleborough LL, Maruyama H, Yasushi T *et al.* (1995) Results of revascularization in patients with severe left ventricular dysfunction. *Circulation* (suppl 2): 73–9.
64. David T.E. (1994) Techniques and results of mitral valve repair for ischemic mitral regurgitation. *J Cardiac Surg* **9**(suppl): 274–7.
65. Yamaguchi A, Ino T, Adachi H *et al.* (1998) Left ventricular volume predicts postoperative course in patients with ischemic cardiomyopathy. *Ann Thorac Surg* **65**: 434–8.
66. Maisano F, Redaelli A, Pennati G *et al.* (1999) The haemodynamic effects of double orifice valve repair for mitral regurgitation: a 3D computative model. *Eur J Cardiothorac Surg* **15**: 419–25.
67. Bach DS, Boling SF (1995) Early improvement in congestive heart failure after correction of secondary mitral regurgitation in end stage cardiomyopathy. *Am Heart J* **129**: 1165–70.
68. Pigott JD, Kouchoukos NT, Oberman A *et al.* (1985) Late results of surgical and medical therapy for patients with coronary artery disease and depressed myocardial function. *J Am Coll Cardiol* **5**: 1036–45.
69. Emond M, Mock MB, Davis KB *et al.* (1994) Long term survival of medically treated patients in the coronary artery surgery study (CASS). *Circulation* **90**: 2645–57.
70. Lansman SL, Cohen M, Galla JD *et al.* (1993) Coronary bypass with ejection fraction of 0.20 or less using centigrade cardioplegia: long term follow up. *Ann Thorac Surg* **56**: 480–6.
71. Blitz A, Laks H. (1996) The role of coronary revascularization in the management of heart failure: identification of candidates and review of results. *Curr Op Cardiol* **11**: 276–90.
72. Hausmann H, Warnecke H, Ennker J *et al.* (1993) Survival predictors in patients with a left ventricular ejection fraction of 10–30% receiving a coronary bypass analysis of preoperative variables. *Cardiovasc Surg* **1**: 558–62.
73. Tjan TDT, Kondruweit M, Scheld HH *et al.* (2000) The bad ventricle – revascularization versus transplantation. *J Thorac Cardiovasc Surg* **48**: 9–14.
74. Luciani GB, Faggani G, Razzaloni R *et al.* (1993) Severe ischemic left ventricular failure: coronary operation or heart transplantation? *Ann Thorac Surg* **55**: 719–23.
75. Blakeman BM, Pifasse R, Sullivan H *et al.* (1990) High-risk heart surgery in the heart transplant candidate. *J Heart Transplant* **9**: 468–72.
76. Louie HW, Laks H, Milgater *et al.* (1991) Ischemic cardiomyopathy: criteria for coronary revascularization and cardiac transplantation. *Circulation* **84**(suppl III): III-290–III-295.
77. Kaul TK, Agnihotri AK, Fields BL *et al.* (1996) Coronary artery bypass grafting in patients with an ejection fraction of twenty percent or less. *J Thorac Cardiovasc Surg* **111**: 1001–12.
78. Flameng W, Suy R, Schwarz F *et al.* (1981) Ultrastructural correlates of left ventricular contraction abnormalities in patients with chronic ischemic heart disease: determinants of reversible segmental asynergy post revascularization surgery. *Am Heart J* **102**: 846–57.

# Surgical restoration of the failing left ventricle 

S. WESTABY, T. KATSUMATA AND O. H. FRAZIER

As the incidence of symptomatic heart failure rises in an increasingly elderly population there is a substantial need for improved surgical options. Whilst the survival benefits of medical treatment are limited combinations of conventional surgical operations with improved medical management are providing clinical outcomes which surpass those of cardiac transplantation [1]. In the presence of extensive ischaemic damage surgical revascularization alone will only improve outlook in patients with hibernating myocardium [2]. Others with partial or full thickness scar can nevertheless be improved by surgical reversal of the remodelling process. The common basis for heart failure in ischaemic and idiopathic dilated cardiomyopathy is conversion of the normal elliptical ventricle into a spherical shape (Fig. 34.1). Increased sphericity and the presence of mitral regurgitation are markers of worse prognosis (1-year mortality 54–70%) [3]. In the failing heart mitral regurgitation occurs secondary to annular dilatation, and altered left ventricular geometry with or without papillary muscle dysfunction [4]. Volume overload causes progressive left ventricular and annular dilatation, worsened mitral regurgitation and decreased survival.

The following account of current and emerging surgical strategies for heart failure concentrates on those patients with left ventricular ejection fraction (LVEF) $< 30\%$, mean pulmonary artery pressure $> 25$ mmHg, left ventricular circumferential akinesia or dyskinesia $>60\%$ and left ventricular end-diastolic volume (LVEDV) $>250$ ml (LVEDV index $>140$ ml). Most of these patients are New York Heart Association (NYHA) functional class III or IV with medical treatment. Early conventional surgical operations can improve symptoms or may prevent further deterioration, but ineffective treatment allows progressive decline.

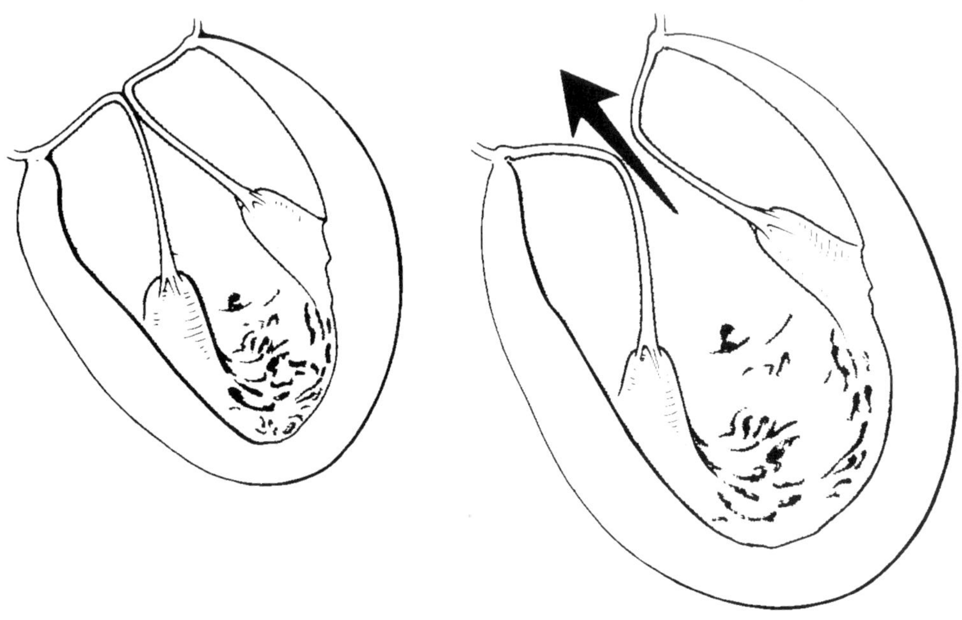

**Figure 36.1** *In heart failure the normal elliptical left ventricular shape progressively becomes spherical with hypertrophy of functioning myocardium to compensate for increased wall stress. Dilatation of the ventricle results in enlargement of the mitral annulus and restrictive motion of the leaflets, secondary to distraction of the papillary muscles. Mitral regurgitation is progressive and a marker of worse prognosis.*

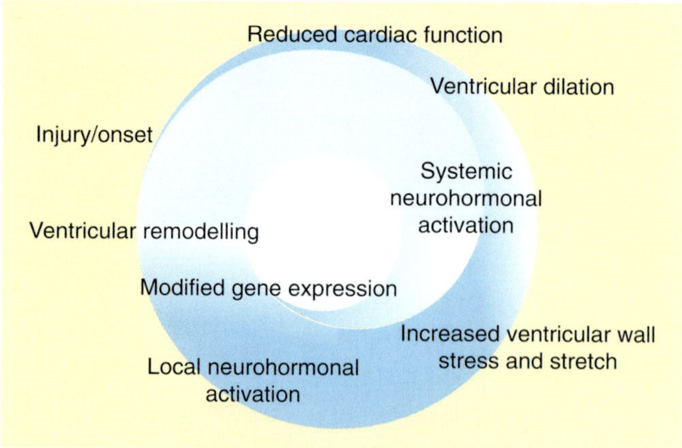


**Figure 34.2** *Diagram to illustrate those factors which contribute to progression of ventricular remodelling in heart failure.*

As the heart dilates both systolic and diastolic wall stress increase through their physical relationship with diameter and intra-cavity pressure (Fig. 34.2). Compensatory hypertrophy occurs when the heart thickens in an attempt to normalize wall stress, but in the vast majority of patients with systolic dysfunction, myocyte hypertrophy does not prevent further deterioration. The left ventricle continues to dilate, diastolic filling pressures rise, after load increases due to vasoconstriction and wall stress becomes exceptionally high. With cellular hypertrophy there are changes in myocyte genetic expression to foetal type with down regulation of those genes functional in the adult heart [5]. Cardiac fibroblasts begin to produce large amounts of extracellular matrix causing interstitial fibrosis within the myocardium (Fig. 34.3). The progression of morphological changes (dilatation) and reduction in ejection fraction are closely linked. The dilated ventricle suffers elevated wall tension because myocardial thickness does not increase to compensate for the greater radius. An increase in myocardial oxygen demand coincides with impairment of subendocardial blood flow through high filling pressures.

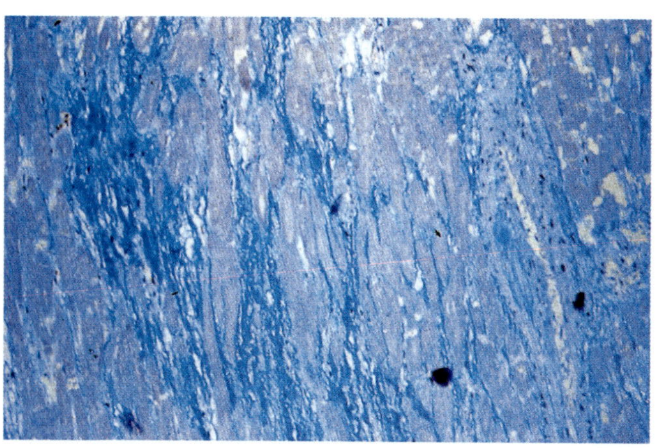

**Figure 34.3** *Diffuse interstitial fibrosis in the heart failure myocardium.*

Exercise capacity has a poor relationship with left ventricular function, although LVEF is an important determinant of survival. Patients with an LVEF >40% have modest annual mortality rate (<10%), whilst those with LVEF <30% have annual mortality rates exceeding 25% [6]. For patients with LVEF 15–40% there is an almost linear relationship between LVEF and annual mortality rate. The condition of the left ventricle is therefore an important determinant of survival independent of the severity of symptoms. A low EF (<30%) indicates that the ventricle has remodelled, but a dilated chamber with low LVEF can eject the same stroke volume as a normal ventricle with an LVEF of 60%. As LVEF decreases it does not necessarily reflect an impairment of contraction, but rather a remodelling of the ventricle. Consequently an important goal of both medical and surgical therapy for congestive heart failure is to prevent progression of the remodelling process. Neurohormonal agents including angiotensin, norepinephrine, endothelin, aldosterone and cyclic guanosine monophosphate (GMP) influence the remodelling process. In particular the relationship between plasma norepinephrine and mortality is clearly defined [7]. Patients with a plasma norepinephrine <600 pg/ml have the lowest cumulative mortality rate compared with those whose plasma norepinephrine levels exceed 900 pg/ml who have a short life expectancy. Activation of the sympathetic nervous system is therefore an important contributor to mortality.

New surgical treatments for heart failure now focus on preventing progressive left ventricular dysfunction and promoting symptomatic relief. Currently moderation of left ventricular remodelling in coronary disease, dilated cardiomyopathy, long-standing valvular disease, or hypertension is first attempted with ACE inhibitors, nitrates, calcium channel blockers or beta-blockers. When these measures fail to control symptoms (or progressive cardiac enlargement) surgical methods should now be considered. As in valvular heart disease surgery to improve ventricular function should occur before remodelling is rendered irreversible by myocardial fibrosis. For instance the 'Cor bovinum' of chronic aortic regurgitation has an inordinately high risk of surgical mortality and little functional rehabilitation in survivors.

## Ventricular restoration in ischaemic heart disease

Coronary artery disease produces a spectrum of myocardial pathology which ranges from functional hibernation to transmural fibrous scar after full thickness myocardial infarction (Fig. 34.4). Between these extremes is a range of ischaemic change modified over time by thrombolytic therapy, acute PTCA, or treatment of hypertension and risk factors.

Most ventricular aneurysms are apical in location. They occur after acute occlusion of the left anterior descending coronary artery in the absence of collateral circulation. Some aneurysms extend beyond the apex depending on the distribution of the vessel. The diagonal branch and the anterior papillary muscle are displaced laterally secondary to infarct expansion and thinning. Posterior aneurysms may occur after occlusion of the posterior descending artery and involve the posterior papillary muscle. In both anterior and posterior aneurysms the inter-ventricular septum may be involved in the scarring and thinning process. Occasionally an aneurysm may occur in the distribution of the obtuse marginal or diagonal branches (Fig. 34.5).

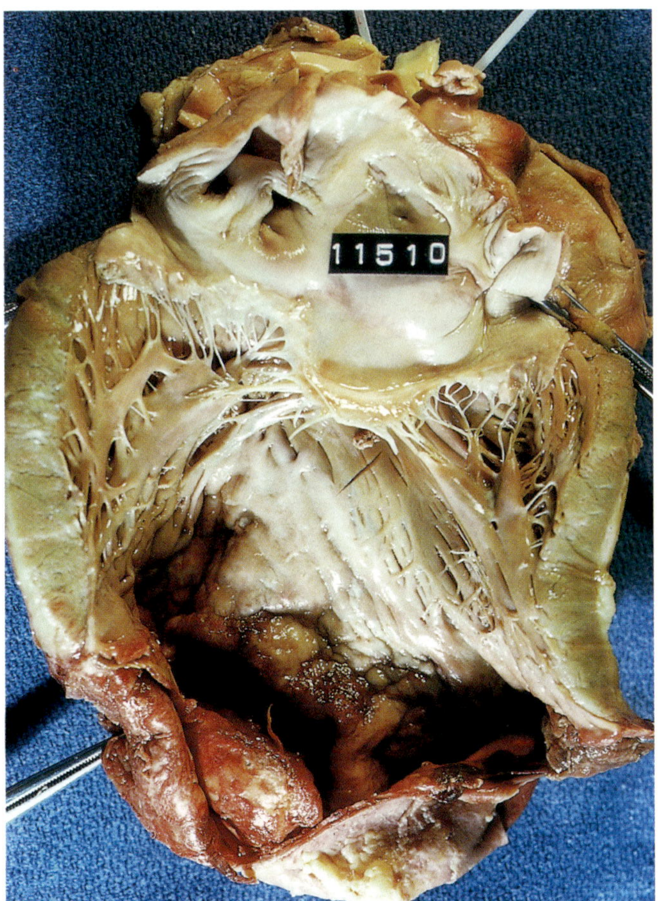


**Figure 34.4** *Full thickness myocardial scar and left ventricular aneurysm, which caused death from heart failure.*

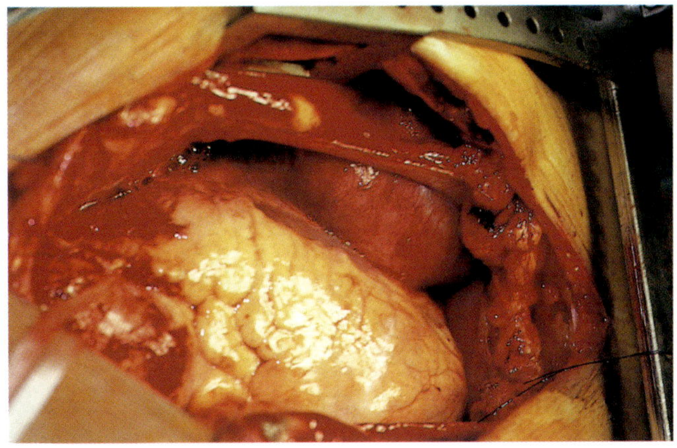

**Figure 34.5** *Unusual sacular left ventricular aneurysm following occlusion of a large circumflex marginal artery.*

The wall of a mature aneurysm is a thin white fibrous scar visible externally. There is a smooth non-trabeculated endocardial surface (Fig. 34.6) clearly demarcated from viable myocardium. More than 50% of classic left ventricular aneurysms contain mural thrombus attached to the endocardial surface. A total of 10–15% have extensive calcification within the scar. This calcification is primarily subendocardial and mid-myocardial in distribution and the over-lying pericardium is densely adherent to the epicardial surface (Fig. 34.7a, b).

Classic left ventricular aneurysms are uncommon in the era of thrombolytic re-cannalization of the occluded artery. Thrombolysis limits myocardial necrosis to the subendocardial area by preserving perfusion to the subepicardial zone. The epicardial appearance may be of diffuse scattered punctate scars interspersed with viable myocardium of

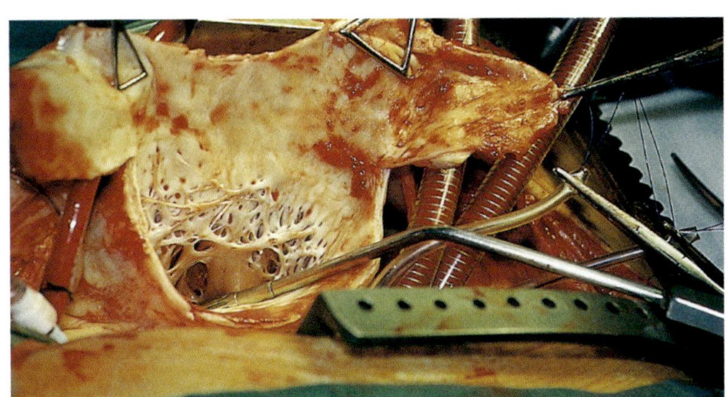

**Figure 34.6** *Anterolateral left ventricular scar showing the smooth non-trabeculated endocardial surface of a left ventricular aneurysm.*

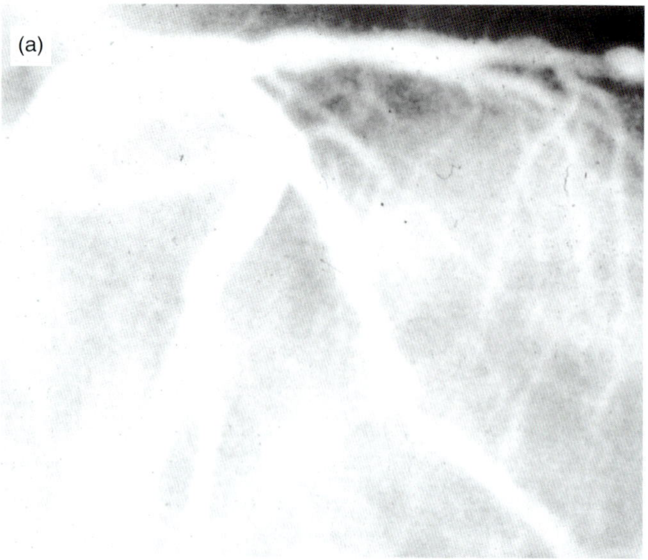


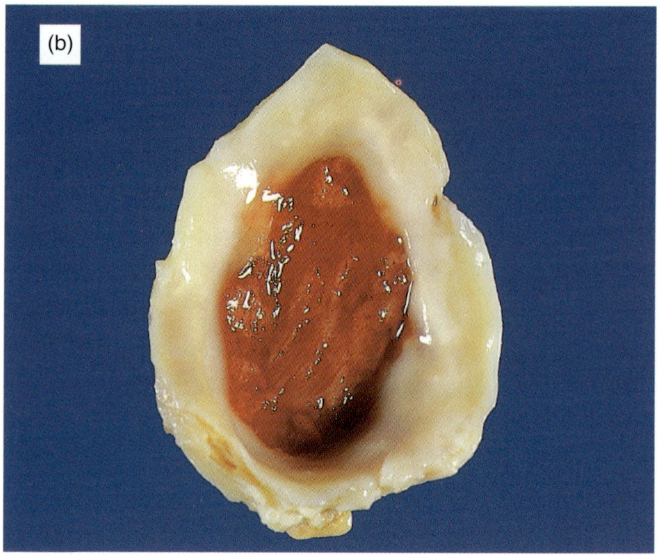


**Figure 34.7** *(a) Diffuse left coronary artery disease with previous occlusion of left anterior descending branch. This resulted in an extensive calcified anterolateral infarction and left ventricular dilatation. (b) This solid calcific endocardial plaque containing thrombus was excised during the Dor operation.*

normal thickness. The endocardium beneath retains its trabeculations and the patchy scarring is not clearly demarcated from the rest of the wall. Mural thrombi are not usually present and the pericardium is not adherent. Salvage of the epicardial surface prevents dyskinesia so that the involved segments manifest local parietal akinesia rather than paradoxical movement. At operation the akinetic area may be hidden under a deceptively normal epicardial muscle layer. The degree of thinning is not apparent on direct vision and akinetic areas seen on ventriculography may correspond with a thick myocardial wall mixed with scar.

The non-aneurysmal part of the left ventricular wall is subject to increased systolic wall stress as the cavity size increases through bulging of the dyskinetic portion. Inactivation (by akinesis or dyskinesis) of 20% of the left ventricular circumference is required before ventricular dilatation occurs, but the larger the akinetic segment the greater the enlargement. The progressive hypertrophy and systolic wall stress as ventricular size increases account for the worsening symptoms in these patients. Stroke volume and global ejection fraction gradually decline as myocardial ischaemia develops in the non-aneurysmal portion.

Paradoxical wall motion reduces the efficiency of the ventricle because systolic work is wasted on expansion of the aneurysm. In small aneurysms (usually without heart failure symptoms) survival is determined primarily by the severity of the coronary disease. Prognosis is worse with dyskinesia than akinesia (where the fibrous area remains

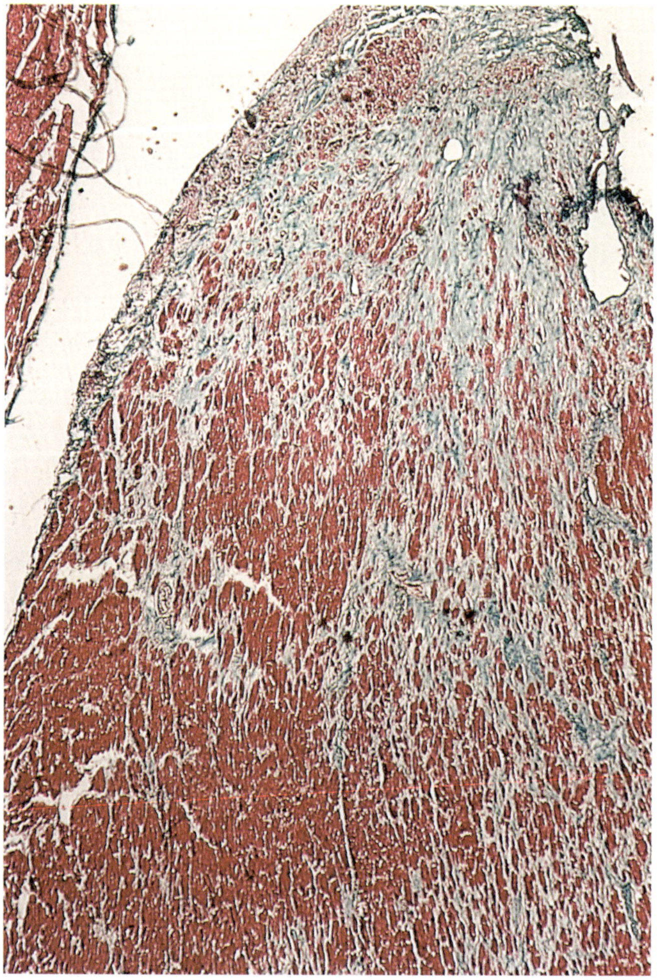

**Figure 34.8** *Ischaemic fibrosis of the anterolateral papillary muscle in a heart failure patient with mitral regurgitation.*

immobile during systole). Functional characteristics of the remainder of the ventricle are also determinants of outcome. When the papillary muscles are ischaemic (Fig. 34.8) or if changes in ventricular geometry interfere with the subvalvar apparatus, mitral regurgitation compromises survival.

### Indications for surgery

Worsening prognosis is associated with greater aneurysm size, decreased global LVEF and more extensive coronary disease [8]. Modern medical therapy is often effective in controlling symptoms and the patient may survive for many years before haemodynamic decompensation. However, once decompensation begins (Fig. 34.9), functional deterioration may occur rapidly and increase the risk of surgical mortality. For this reason, ventricular restoration surgery should be considered in asymptomatic patients with critical coronary stenoses, but bypassable vessels. Surgery is also indicated for asymptomatic patients when there is deteriorating left ventricular function on non-invasive testing (increasing diastolic dimensions, decreasing ejection fraction or increasing mitral regurgitation). Functional deterioration is heralded by angina of increased severity, congestive heart failure or the occurrence of ventricular arrhythmias or embolic events. Dor recommends surgery when heart failure symptoms predominate over angina, when the patient reaches NYHA III or IV, when LVEF is <30%, LVAP >15 mmHg and when the percentage of asynergic left ventricular circumference exceeds 60% [9]. As enthusiasm for left ventricular restoration increases some proponents now suggest that all patients with myocardial infarction should be followed by coronary angiography, echocardiography and electrophysiological assessment. If a wall motion abnormality >20% of the left ventricular circumference is found, surgical restoration should be considered to prevent deterioration in healthy myocardium.

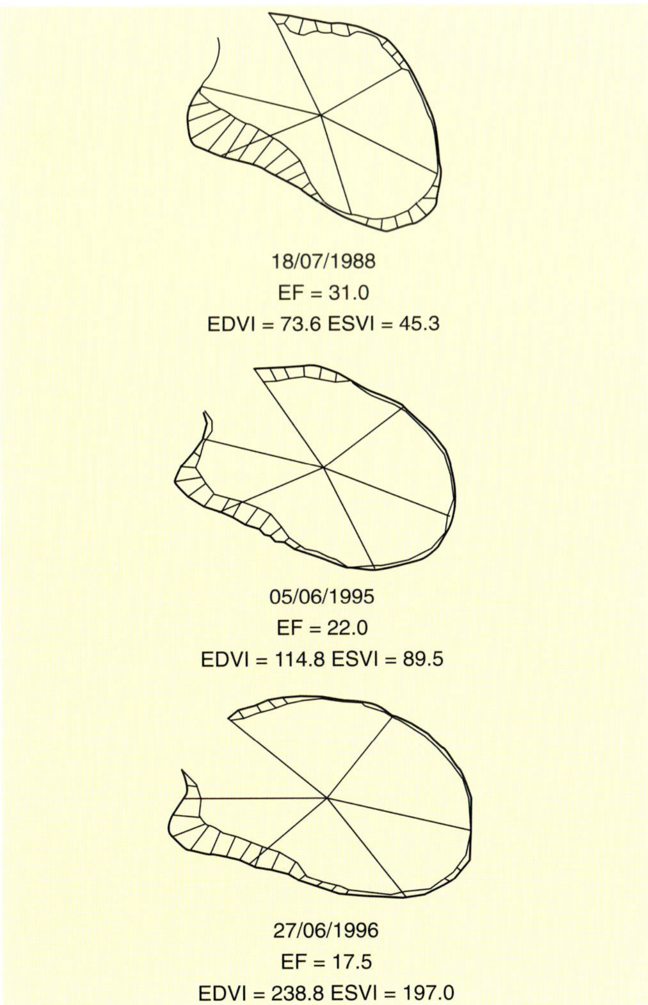


**Figure 34.9** *Progression of left ventricular remodelling over time after anterolateral infarction (courtesy of Dr Vincent Dor). (EF – ejection fraction, EDVI – end diastolic volume index, ESVI – end systolic volume index.)*

## The surgical approach

Echocardiographically or angiocardiographically, an aneurysm is defined as an area of left ventricle, which is demarcated from surrounding chamber by hypokinesis, akinesis or dyskinesis (Fig. 34.10). Pathologically the area of abnormal wall motion may consist of thin scar or a variable thickness of scar mixed with viable myocardium.

The surgery of left ventricular aneurysm began in 1944 when Beck reinforced a dyskinetic lesion with fascia lata in an attempt to prevent paradoxical motion. Bailey (1955) used a side-biting clamp to plicate the aneurysmal segment in the precardiopulmonary bypass era. With the availability of cardiopulmonary bypass Cooley performed the first successful open excision of a left ventricular aneurysm (1958) [10]. In classic descriptions of the operation the thinned area is excised leaving behind a rim of scar to facilitate linear closure (Fig. 34.11a, b). Achievable with relatively low mortality, this simple approach can eliminate congestive heart failure, angina or thromboembolic complications. However, over-enthusiastic resection may produce a small poorly compliant ventricle with perioperative mortality or failure to improve symptoms (Fig. 34.12). In order to avoid this complication more complex repair techniques have evolved to restore the ventricle from its globular to an elliptical shape.

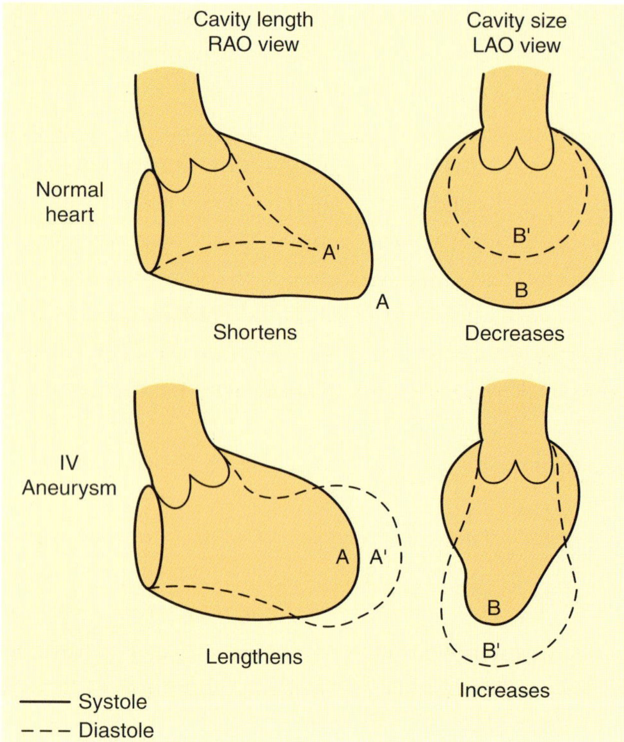


**Figure 34.10** *Normal left ventricular wall motion (above) and paradoxical motion in a left ventricular aneurysm.*

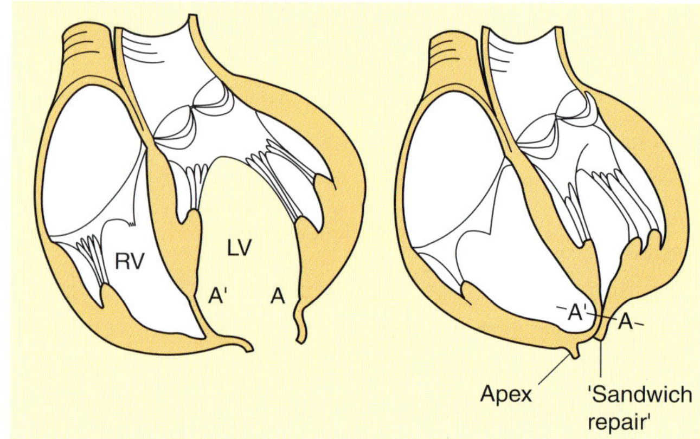


**Figure 34.12** *Diagram illustrating excision of the left ventricular aneurysm sac followed by linear repair. This may result in too small a left ventricular cavity with impaired diastolic function.*

On simple ventriculography it is impossible to determine whether an aneurysmal segment would benefit from revascularization (to recruite hibernating myocardium) or resection. Preoperative assessment by dobutamine echocardiography, PET or radio-isotope perfusion scans are used to distinguish scar from hibernating myocardium. In many patients the decision between revascularization or resection is made only at the time of surgery with the left ventricle decompressed but beating during cardiopulmonary bypass. Thinned paradoxically distending transmural scar is easily recognized and resected. Should the epicardium of an akinetic segment appear normal, the degree of thinning is assessed by needle aspiration [11]. When the territory consists of thick myocardium interspersed with scar, then revascularization is performed.

When myocardial thinning is demonstrated (or in the event of uncertainty) a 3.0 cm ventriculotomy is performed through the akinetic area about 2.0 cm parallel to the distal left anterior descending coronary. Inspection and palpation of the contracting muscle will determine the transition zone between vigorously contracting and non-contracting muscle. The morphological appearance ranges from:

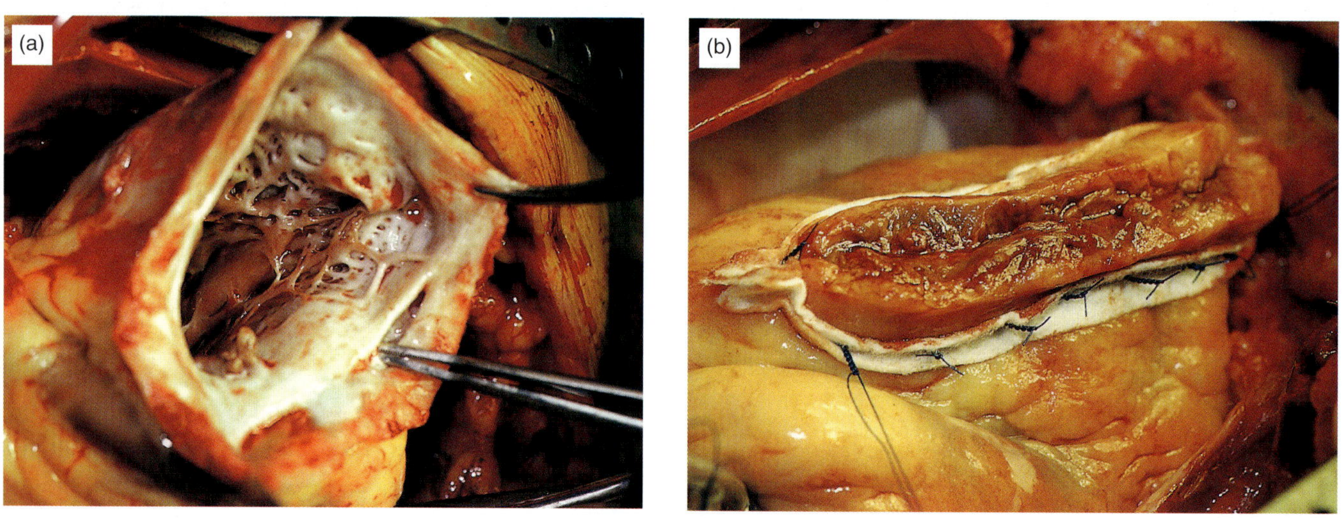


**Figure 34.11** *(a) Large anterolateral left ventricular aneurysm during surgical repair. The aneurysm sac has been excised leaving a 1cm fibrous margin to facilitate closure. (b) Linear closure of the left ventricular wall after aneurysm resection.*

- full thickness scar (now uncommon)
- trabecular scar with no clear circumferential transition to normal muscle or
- predominantly normal muscle that is non-contractile (most common).

In the absence of full thickness scar with paradoxical motion, the Dor procedure is undertaken to restore left ventricular geometry from the poorly defined spherical apex to the normal elliptical shape (surgical anterior ventricular restoration) [12] (Fig. 34.13). This is a more reproducible procedure than linear aneurysmectomy for patient in whom chamber geometry and residual cavity size are unpredictable. Linear closure is performed only when the residual chamber can be of relatively normal size and shape without distortion of the papillary muscle or septal anatomy. In the presence of extensive endocardial calcification the epicardium over the plaque is incised and the calcified tissue removed *en bloc* by carefully dissecting this layer from the surrounding tissues (Fig. 34.7b). Calcification often extends over the endocardial surface well beyond the planned area of resection.

### The Dor procedure

Palpation of the open beating ventricle defines the transition zone between contracting and non-contracting muscle and guides extension of the incision from base to apex for full exposure. Thombus is removed and the extent of the endocardial scar assessed. If there is a history of ventricular tachycardia the endocardial scar is excised and cryotherapy applied to the edges of the resection. The aim is then to provide an elliptical shape to the remaining ventricular cavity by excluding non-contractile septal, posterior or lateral areas. The transition zone between contracting muscle and the akinetic area is used to define the site of the circumferential 'Fontan' suture employed to create a surgical neck between the ventricular cavity and excluded akinetic ventricular wall. The 2/0 monofilament suture is passed through fibrous myocardium just distal to the transition zone towards the edge of the heart. The suture is then tightened to leave a defect in the left ventricular wall of about 2.5 cm in diameter. The patch should be made about 3 cm in diameter to compensate for the space taken by the suture line. The outer rim of the Dacron is used to anchor extra haemostatic sutures (Fig. 34.14). After de-airing the redundant excluded ventricular wall is used to cover the patch and eliminate bleeding. Coronary bypass is applied to stenosed arteries including the proximal part of an occluded left anterior descending coronary so that septal branches are revascularized. The past 10–15 years has witnessed substantial improvement in myocardial protection resulting in a fall of mortality to <5% in patients with or without concomitant coronary artery bypass grafting. There are relatively few contra-indications for left ventricular restoration surgery in symptomatic patients, but operative mortality is significantly increased (>10%) and functional benefit decreases in those who present with severe heart failure or cardiogenic shock without angina [13].

## Results of surgery

There are no prospective randomized studies to compare survival after surgical versus medical treatment in asymptomatic patients. Surgery in this category remains an individual judgment based upon the location and extent of the coronary artery disease, age, results of viability studies and co-morbid conditions.

For left ventricular aneurysm resection the most important variable to determine surgical risk and late mortality is the preoperative left ventricular function. Hospital mortality is <3% for patients with an ejection fraction of >30%. In contrast a patient with three vessel disease operated after prolonged congestive heart failure has an 80–100% risk of hospital mortality. Mickelborough reported a consecutive series of 92 patients in whom the operative mortality was 3% despite diffuse coronary artery disease, advanced left ventricular dysfunction and ventricular arrhythmias [11]. Eighteen per cent of these patients required intra-aortic balloon pump support postoperatively. The average increase in ejection fraction was only 7% though postoperative echocardiographic data demonstrated a significant decrease in left ventricular dimensions and mitral regurgitation. Actuarial survival, including hospital deaths, was 88% at 1 year, 86% at 2 years and 80% at 5 years. There was no difference in survival in patients with preoperative LVEF >20% and those with LVEF <20%. Global LVEF was a poor predictor of operative risk, though assessment of contractility of the non-aneurysmal segments was an important determinant of outcome. The outcome varies in different series, but in general, 3 day, 1-, 3- and 5-year survival has been in the order of 90%, 85%, 75% and 65%. This survival is better than from non-surgical treatment, but does not take into account the influence of concomitant myocardial revascularization. Long-term

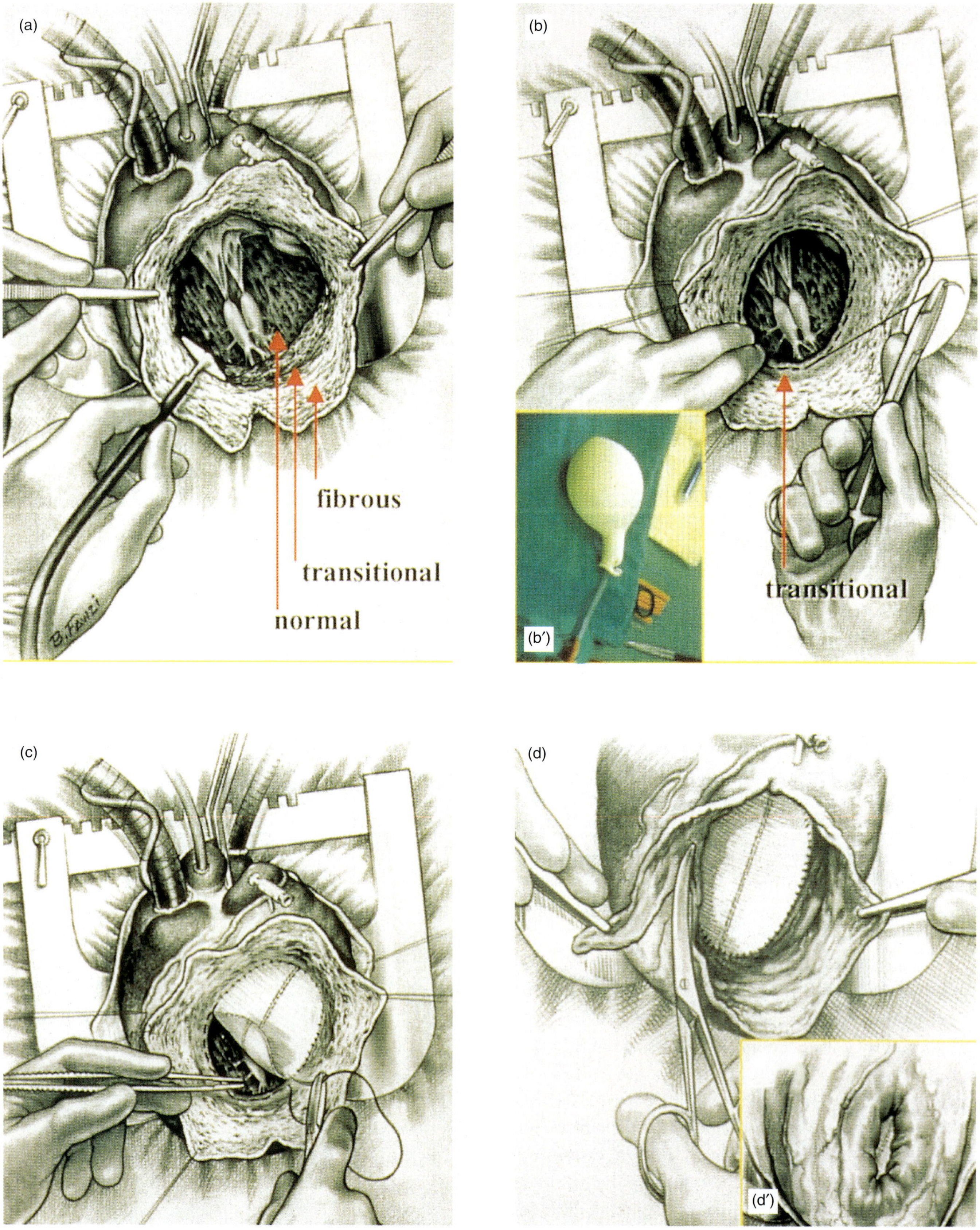


**Figure 34.13** *The Dor procedure to surgically remodel the left ventricular cavities from a spherical to elliptical shape. An inflatable balloon can be used to ensure adequate residual left ventricular volume as the Fontan suture is tightened (courtesy of Dr Vincent Dor).*

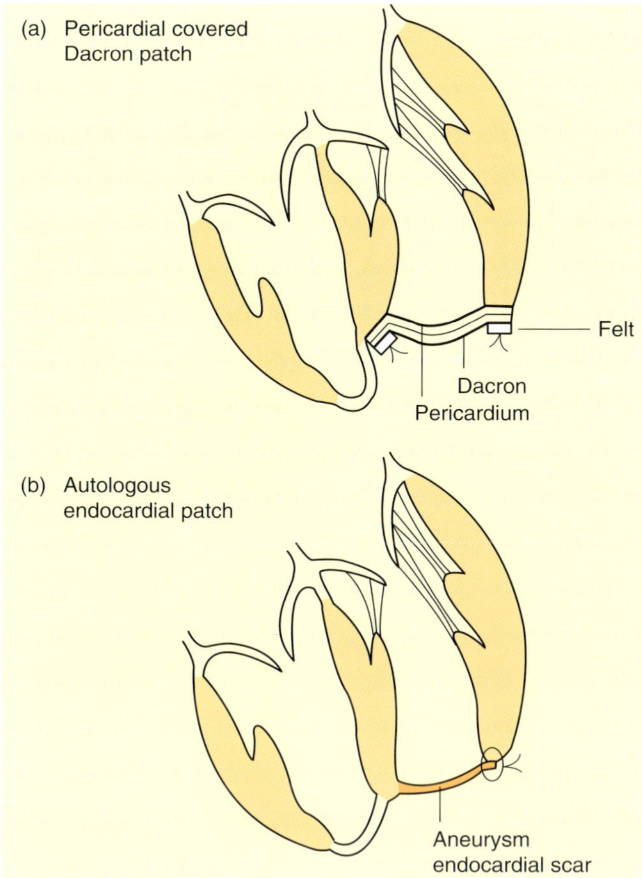


**Figure 34.14** *Diagrammatic illustration of the Dor operation using (a) pericardial covered Dacron patch and (b) autogenous endocardium from septal scar.*

survival is better for patients presenting with angina rather than congestive heart failure, in those with single- or two-vessel disease rather than diffuse three vessel disease, and when myocardial revascularization is complete. Five-year survival in this group of patients approaches 85%. For asymptomatic patients the 5-year survival exceeds 90%.

Dor studied a cohort of 781 ventricular restoration patients (age 59± 7 years) with mean ejection fraction 17 ± 3%. All patients were NYHA class III or IV and were followed on average of 2 years [14]. Many of the operations included subtotal endocardiectomy and cryotherapy for spontaneous or inducible ventricular tachycardia. Hospital mortality was 19.3%. Ejection fraction improved from 17 ± 3% to 37 ± 10% ($p < 0.0001$) (Fig. 34.15). On multivariate analysis factors which influenced early mortality were the presence of critical narrowing in the circumflex artery and the duration of cardiopulmonary bypass. At 1-year follow-up a significant improvement in NYHA class was observed with no patient remaining in NYHA IV. The improvement in LVEF was maintained (39 ± 11%) as well as the reduction in inducible and spontaneous ventricular tachycardia. Late mortality was 10% at 5 years.

Buckberg and colleagues applied a modified Dor procedure to a group of elderly patients (mean age 77 years), all in NYHA class IV [15]. These patients had multiple admissions for congestive heart failure, some with cardiac cachexia. Left ventricular volumes and LVEF were calculated pre- and postoperatively from biplane cineangiography. (Table 34.1) Preoperatively, the mean LVEF was 20% (±8.5%), end-diastolic volume was 311 ± 105 ml, and end-systolic volume was 243 ± 81 (LVEDV index 169 ± 55 ml/m$^2$; LVESV index 132 ± 41 ml/m$^2$). Postoperative LVEF increased from 20 to 35%. The average diastolic volume (LVEDV) was reduced by 80 ml (312–225 ml) an average of 28%. The left ventricular end systolic volume

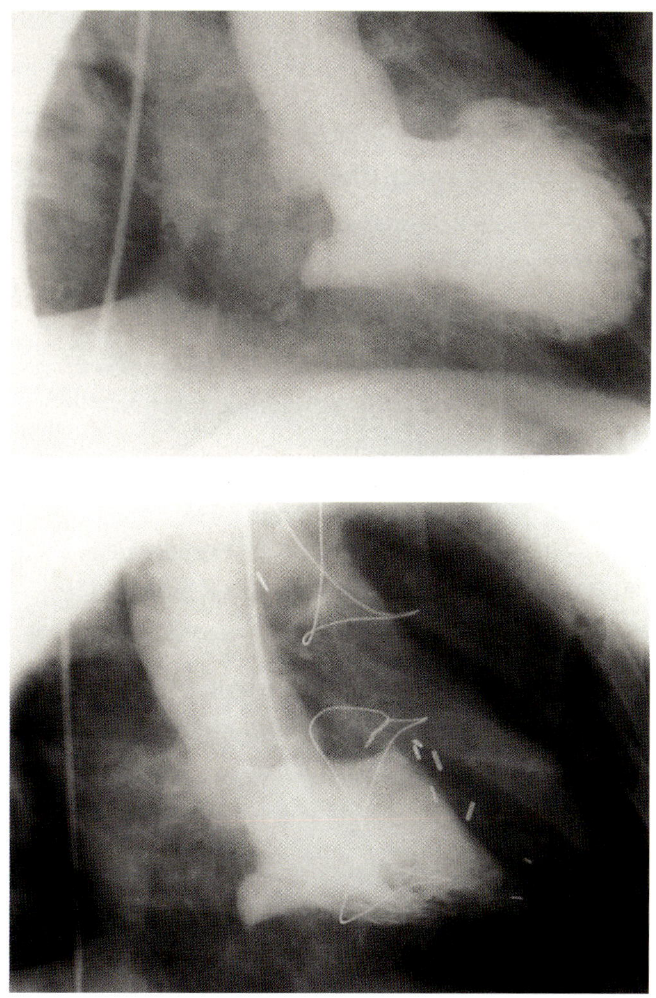

**Figure 34.15** *Pre- and postoperative ventriculography illustrating the outcome after the Dor operation. Dyskinetic anterolateral left ventricular wall is excluded. The remodelled ventricle is restored to an elliptical shape.*

**Table 34.1** Left ventricular volume indices

| | Normal | Restoration surgery indicated | Severe heart failure |
|---|---|---|---|
| LVEDVI[a] | 75 ml/m$^2$ | >180 ml/m$^2$ | >300 ml/m$^2$ |
| LVESVI[b] | 25 ml/m$^2$ | >60 ml/m$^2$ | >100 ml/m$^2$ |

[a]Left ventricular end diastolic volume index. [b]Left ventricular end systolic volume index. CABG for hibernating myocardium improves LVEF only if LVESVI<100 ml/m$^2$.

(LVESV) was reduced from 243 to 149 ml; an average of 49%. The left ventricular end-diastolic volume index was reduced by 48 ml/m$^2$ (170–121 ml/m$^2$). The left ventricular end-systolic volume index (LVESVI) was reduced 45 ml/m$^2$ (132–81 ml/m$^2$). These elderly patients had gross left ventricular enlargement. The substantial improvement following left ventricular restoration surgery contrasts with the changes manifest by patients undergoing coronary revascularization alone. For coronary patients with LVEF averaging 25% postrevascularization LVEF increases to around 30% as long as preoperative LVESVI was <100 ml/m$^2$, but does not change if preoperative LVESVI exceeds 100 ml/m$^2$ [16]. Absence of improvement in large ventricles following CABG alone is consistent with the findings of Yamaguchi who documented higher mortality and congestive heart failure in patients with LVESVI >100 ml/m$^2$ [16].

Buckberg and colleagues documented improved contractility of remote muscle after restoration to an elliptical shape and attributes improvement to the change in myocardial morphology. Spotnitz has described transmural shearing planes on cross-sections of the myocardium [17]. Contractile fibres run perpendicular to these planes and thickening of contracting heart muscle is produced by torsion or deformation of these fibres. This change in myocardial thickening is responsible for left ventricular ejection and is evident during magnetic resonance imaging of the left ventricular wall. The torsion is related to the angle of fibre orientation with a conical formation towards the apex. The Dor procedure restores apical fibre orientation and improves wall thickening during ventricular contraction. Restoration produces a more normal orientation of sinobulbar and circular muscle around the ventricle and re-establishes an ellipsoid form to improve systolic twisting compression. Energy demands are diminished simultaneously since oxygen requirements are related to wall stress.

The immediate improvement in ventricular function contrasts with delayed recovery after revascularization of hibernating myocardium. Surgical restoration excludes the akinetic anterior segment providing improved contractility from shape alteration [18].

## Left ventricular volume reduction in idiopathic dilated cardiomyopathy

Ventricular aneurysm operations and the Dor procedure in part improve remote ventricular muscle function secondary to the physical principle of Laplace (wall tension = intraventricular pressure × left ventricular radius + 2 × wall thickness).

In dilated cardiomyopathy the left ventricular cavity dimensions enlarge, wall tension increases and contractility is further impaired leading to a downward spiral of worsening left ventricular function. Wall stress is one of the major determinants of myocardial oxygen requirement so that a reduction in wall stress may retard deterioration in left ventricular function, particularly in ischaemic patients.

Partial left ventriculectomy (PLV) was introduced by Batista in Brazil to reduce left ventricular volume, improve LVEF and relieve symptoms in congestive heart failure patients without access to transplantation [19] (Fig. 34.16a, b). The underlying concept is that a reduction of left ventricular diameter and wall stress with a relative increase in left ventricular wall thickness can reset the parameters of the Laplace principle and improve cardiac output. Batista's convincing presentations using bovine and snake hearts led to widespread adoption of the operation in the absence of outcome data. Only now is information available to define both early mortality and the effect on intermediate term survival. In turn, experimental data were obtained, which address the mechanisms of symptomatic improvement.

### Indications for partial left ventriculectomy

There are no clear guidelines for PLV in patients with left ventricular global dysfunction. There are no convincing data on long-term survival, functional status, cardiac performance, or sustainability of volume reduction. Prohibitive short-term mortality has been reported, but without definition of preoperative risk factors [20]. In early reports virtually all NYHA class III or IV adult patients, with end-diastolic dimension (LVEDD) >7 cm were candidates for this procedure (Table 34.2) [21–23]. Suggested inclusion

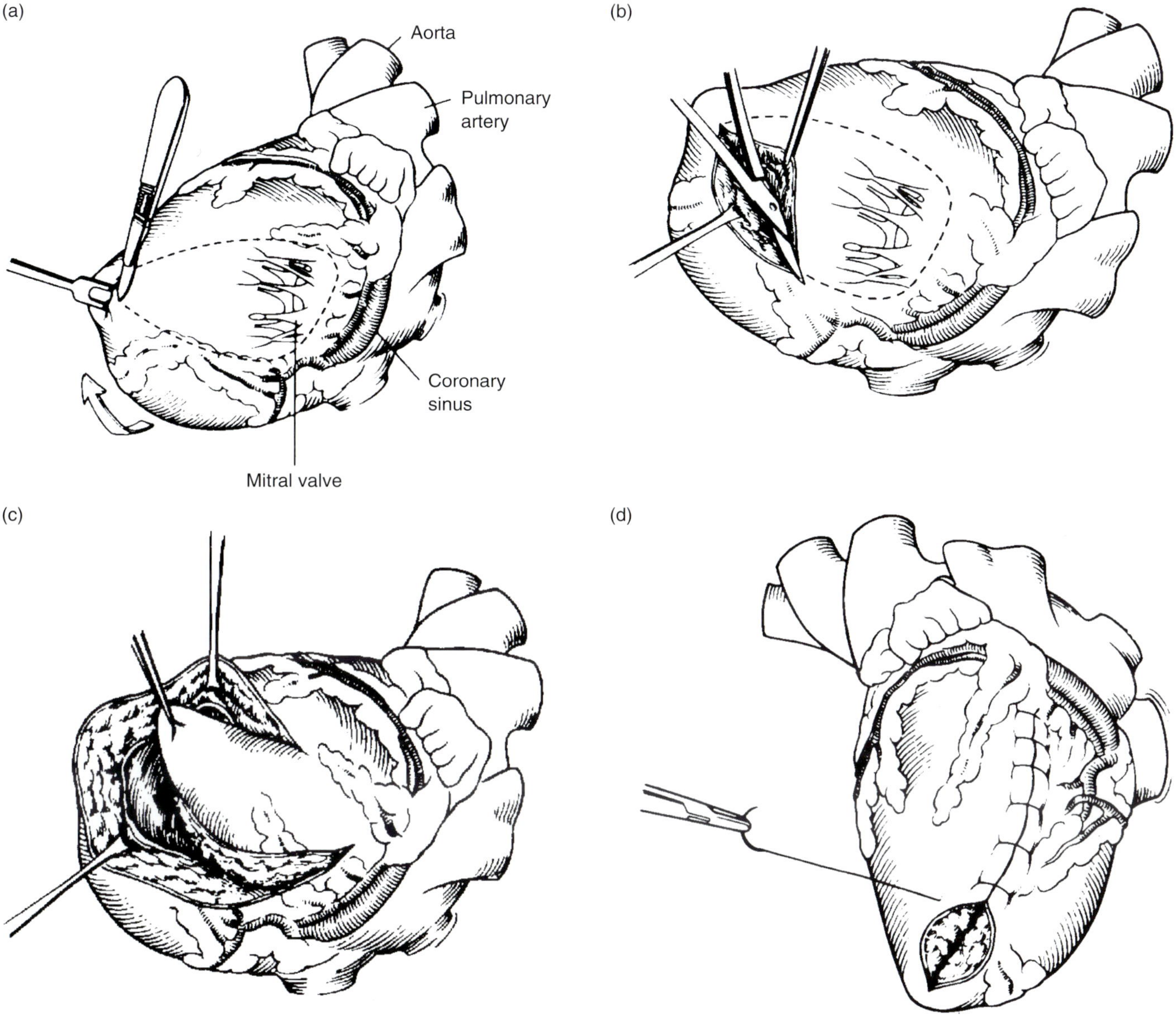


**Figure 34.16** *Partial left ventriculectomy (the Batista operation), (a) extent of myocardial resection in the territory of the circumflex marginal coronary artery, (b) and (c) excision of inferolateral myocardium between the papillary muscles, (d) reconstitution of the left ventricular cavity by continuous suture.*

**Table 34.2** Patient summary in six series of partial left ventriculectomy operations

| Author | *n* | Age mean (range) | Patient's profiles | Transplant candidacy |
|---|---|---|---|---|
| McCarthy | 53 | 53 (17–72) | DCM (idiopathic, familiar, valvular) | Yes |
| Stolf, Moreira | 37 | 46 (28–72) | DCM (non-ischaemic), LVEF ≤ 25% | Yes |
| Gradinac, Popovic | 22 | 50 (20–66) | DCM (non-ischaemic) LVEDD ≥ 7cm | Yes |
| Batista, Salerno | 120 | 53 (11–74) | DCM | Yes (Batista) |
| Angelini | 14 | 65 | DCM (idiopathic, ischaemic, valvular) | Yes |
| Suma | 30 | 47 (14–67) | DCM (idiopathic, valvular, with ARVD, sarcoidosis) | No |
| Total | 276 | 52 (11–74) | | |

ARVD = arrhythmogenic right ventricular dysplasia, DCM = dilated cardiomyopathy, LVEDD = left ventricular end-diastolic diameter, LVEF = left ventricular ejection fraction.

criteria overlap with those of cardiac transplantation, but very few centres attempted PLV for ischaemic cardiomyopathy, potentially the largest group of eligible patients [24] (Fig. 34.17a, b). Most were discouraged by the incidence of fatal postoperative ventricular dysrhythmias.

## Mechanisms of symptomatic improvement

The underlying principle of PLV for dilated cardiomyopathy is to reduce the volume but not the mass of the chamber, thereby reducing left ventricular wall stress. Chamber enlargement in heart failure results in elevated peak systolic wall stress (by Laplace's law) followed by compensatory myocardial hypertrophy in an attempt to normalize wall stress. Despite remodelling, myocardial stress persistently outweighs mass in dilated cardiomyopathy [25].

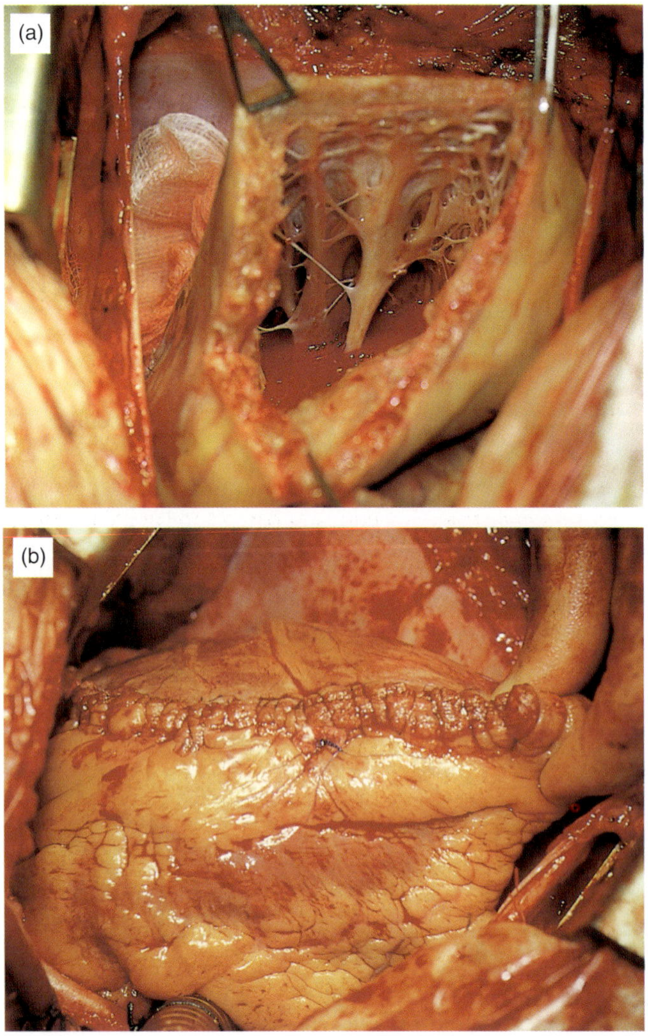


**Figure 34.17** *Partial left ventriculectomy in ischemic cardiomyopathy: (a) left ventricular resection preserving the papillary muscles, (b) direct closure to produce a much smaller elliptical ventricle.*

Little is known about the relationships between intrinsic myocardial contractile function, muscle mass and overall left ventricular performance after PLV in the non-ischaemic dilated ventricle.

The Columbia group devised a multiple compartment elastance model to simulate the effects of reduction in cardiac mass by PLV, in an attempt to predict the effects on end-systolic and end-diastolic pressure–volume relations (ESPVRs and EDPVRS), stress–strain relations, LVEF and overall pump performance (Frank–Starling relationship) [26]. They showed that a progressive increase in muscle excised was associated with a leftward shift in ESPVR and EDPVR; the magnitude of the volume-axis shifts were identical for both relations. These changes were associated with only minor alterations in filling pressure, stroke volume, peak systolic pressure, or overall loop shape (Fig. 34.18). The stroke work/left ventricular end-diastolic pressure (LVEDP) relation showed improved systolic left ventricular function.

Mass reduction caused increases in both end-systolic elastance, LVEF and diastolic chamber stiffness, but decreases in left ventricular end-diastolic volume (LVEDV). Mass reduction also caused a decrease in myocardial afterload stress for any given ventricular pressure. Consequently, to generate a fixed pressure within the left ventricle, a lower wall stress was required after mass reduction.

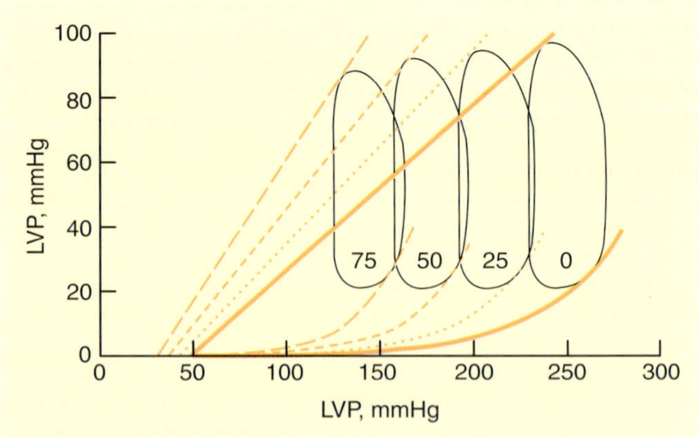


**Figure 34.18** *Left ventricular pressure–volume loops (LVP and LVV) are shown at each of the four levels of mass reduction (0, 25, 50 and 75 g of tissue removed). The pressure–volume loops shifted to the left in response to mass reduction. As masses reduced from 0 to 75 g the ESPVR (straight lines that intersect the end-systolic point of the respective pressure–volume loop) slope increases and the curvature of the EDPVR (curvilinear relations that intersect the end-diastolic point of the respective pressure–volume loop) increases. Both relations tend to move in a parallel fashion (reprinted with permission from the American Association for Thoracic Surgery).*

The relationship between filling pressure and stroke volume (Frank–Starling curves) exhibited a downward and rightward shift in response to mass reduction suggesting a slight reduction in overall pump performance (Fig. 34.19).

Decreased afterload stress following mass reduction has several important implications. Myocardial hypertrophy in heart failure is believed to occur in response to increased wall stress. In turn, myocardial hypertrophy contributes to contractile dysfunction. Reduction in wall stress might therefore lead to regression of hypertrophy and potential clinical benefit. However, after PLV, improvements in haemodynamic indices are based on the geometric rearrangement and not underlying myocardial function. The beneficial effects would not be immediate, since regression of hypertrophy occurs only after weeks or months, provided that the afterload reduction was sustainable.

PLV itself changes the unloaded end-systolic and end-diastolic ventricular shapes and creates regional stiffness in and around the surgical repair site. As a consequence, end-systolic elastance (ESPVRs) and diastolic compliance (EDPVRs) are altered and improve from preoperative status.

Ratcliffe and colleagues developed a finite element model of a dilated LV with impaired contractility, in which the effects of PLV were simulated [27]. Their findings were basically the same as those of the Columbia group, PLV shifted end-systolic elastance and diastolic compliance leftwards on the pressure–volume diagram. Their results suggest that PLV increases the slope of the stoke work/LVEDV relationship (preload recruitable stroke work) and decreases the slope of the Starling relationship.

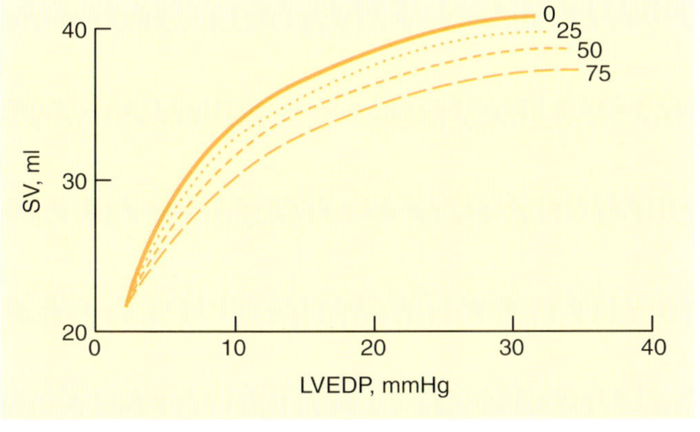


**Figure 34.19** *Frank–Starling relationship at the four mass reduction conditions (0–75 g of tissue excision). Mass reduction is associated with downward shift of the Frank–Starling curves indicating a reduction in pump function. SV=stroke volume, LVEDP=left ventricular end-diastolic pressure (reprinted with permission from the American Association for Thoracic Surgery).*

The shape and physical properties of a cylinder, such as the LV dictate that significant wall stress exists, even in the absence of intracavity pressure [28]. This residual stress has not been measured in dilated cardiomyopathy, but may have a significant impact on PLV, which increases residual prestrain and stress. Left ventricular pressure during the relaxation (filling) phase is not only determined by the visco-elastic properties of the myocardium, but also by an active muscle-borne restoring force, which provides 'diastolic suction'. Restoration of a smaller end-systolic volume (ESV), with an increase in elastic recoil, can aid in ventricular filling. A significant enhancement of contractile performance will also benefit by reinstituting the active diastolic filling phase. This suggestion by Kresh and Wechsler remains unproven and needs supportive laboratory data; however, it may explain how end-diastolic compliance is improved in some patients, despite reduction in chamber size and a relatively thickened wall [29].

## Surgical technique

Effective myocardial protection is particularly important in this operation since preoperative left ventricular function is poor. Batista's original approach employed cardiopulmonary bypass, with moderate hypothermia (33–34°C) and continued myocardial perfusion. Others including the Cleveland Clinic group preferred cardioplegic arrest [30].

In most reports PLV is performed according to Batista's original suggestion. A wedge of posterolateral LV is resected between (and often including) the papillary muscles, extending from the apex of the heart up to 2–3 cm from the mitral annulus (Fig. 34.16). The incision begins at the apex of the ventricle and extends toward the base. The interior of the LV is inspected and the distance between the anterior and posterior papillary muscles determined. The resection proceeds irrespective of the coronary anatomy and usually excises the obtuse marginal branches of the circumflex coronary. The left ventricle is then repaired along its long axis with an over-and-over suture, buttressed by felt or pericardial strips. McCarthy and colleagues modified this technique with an incision beginning approximately 2 cm lateral to the LAD artery and 3 cm from the apex. The incision circumscribes and removes the whole apex, then extends to the base of both papillary muscles and towards the mitral annulus (Fig. 34.20) [30]. The apico-anterior

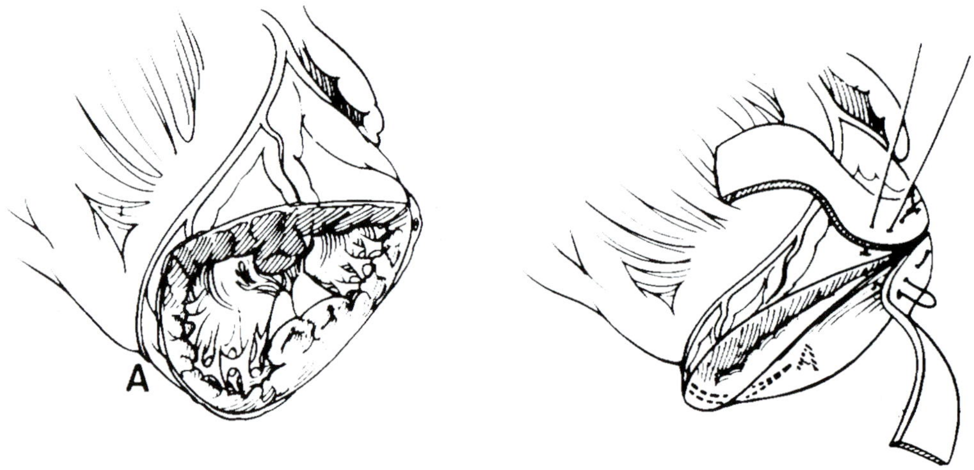


**Figure 34.20** *McCarthy's modification of the Batista operation. The incision circumscribes and removes the whole apex, then extends to the base of both papillary muscles and towards the mitral annulus. The apico-anterior and postero-lateral aspects of the left ventricle are thereby removed.*

and posterolateral aspects of the LV are thereby removed. For ischaemic cardiomyopathy patients, Westaby directed PLV towards the antero-lateral aspect where most punctate scarring was situated (Fig. 34.17a, b) [24]. Westaby also performed PLV on infants with idiopathic dilated and ischaemic cardiomyopathy from anomalous left coronary artery from the pulmonary artery who could not be weaned from cardiopulmonary bypass (Fig. 34.21a, b). (These procedures provided excellent long-term outcome.)

There is surprisingly little information on the amount of ventricle to be excised. The Cleveland group weighed the resected specimen, which ranged from 30 to 290 g (mean 96 g) [30]. The São Paulo group reports a resected posterolateral area measuring 10.9 ± 2.5% [21].

In some patients a more radical approach is necessary to achieve sufficient reduction in left ventricular cavity dimensions. This involves resection of both papillary muscles followed by mitral valve replacement. Approximately half of McCarthy's patients had the base of one or both papillary muscles resected on the basis of preoperative echocardiographic measurements or intraoperative inspection of the ventricle [30]. Rather than replace the valve with a prosthesis, the heads of the resected papillary muscles were reimplanted with multiple transfixation sutures and approximated to each other at ventriculotomy closure. Gradinac described a modification where the attachments of both papillary muscles were kept in continuity with the ventricle, but partially rotated and pulled

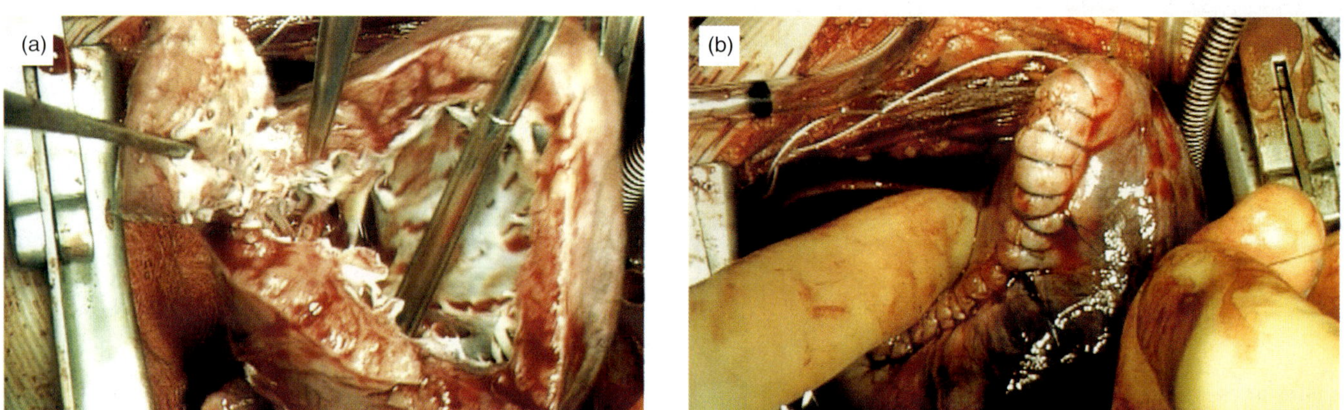


**Figure 34.21** *Partial left ventriculectomy in a 3-month-old infant with anomalous left coronary artery from the pulmonary artery. The procedure was performed after reimplantation of the left main coronary artery, following which the infant could not be weaned from cardiopulmonary bypass. (a) The left ventricular resection showing extensive endomyocardial fibrosis, (b) closure of the left ventricle producing a smaller elliptical left ventricular cavity. The infant was then weaned from cardiopulmonary bypass and 2 years later has normal left ventricular function and a patent left coronary artery.*

toward the apex by anchoring sutures during closure [22]. Their aim was to improve the orientation of the tension apparatus after radical geometric transposition.

## Management of the mitral valve

More than 80% of patients require concomitant mitral valve surgery. Direct repair after PLV closely approximates the papillary muscles, unless they are reimplanted at a different site (Fig. 34.22). This re-orientation may create a redundant length of the chordae and mitral valve prolapse. Batista addresses this problem by joining the midportion of the anterior and posterior mitral leaflets with a single suture. This produces a dual-channel mitral orifice, as described by Alfieri and colleagues [31] (Fig. 34.23). The method is simple and quick, with acceptable early results. McCarthy employed ring annuloplasty and emphasizes the importance of reducing the mitral annulus, to remodel the left ventricular inflow [30]. Gradinac and colleagues combined the Alfieri repair with eccentric commisural annuloplasty with or without plication of the posterior mitral leaflet and annulus with a purse-string suture [22]. Suma employed flexible ring annuloplasty for all mitral repair cases [23].

Most centres employ tricuspid annuloplasty for moderate to severe tricuspid regurgitation. Individual incidence of the repair ranged from 19% to 57% (average 43%). The De Vega annuloplasty was used exclusively by most authors. Batista has also performed adjunctive right ventricular reduction by de-roofing the conal part of the right ventricle. The papillary muscles were left intact.

## Early mortality

The early mortality (in-hospital or 30 day) has ranged from 1.9% to 27%, with an average of 17.4% (Table 34.3). Causes of death were poorly defined for most patients. They included persistent or progressive heart failure, surgical bleeding, stroke, and ventricular dysrhythmia. Suma reported significantly higher mortality in emergency cases (86%), as compared with elective cases (8.7%, $p < 0.0003$) [23].

Mechanical circulatory support was required in 20% of patients. The incidence of circulatory support for individual series ranged from 0 to 35% [21–23]. The Cleveland

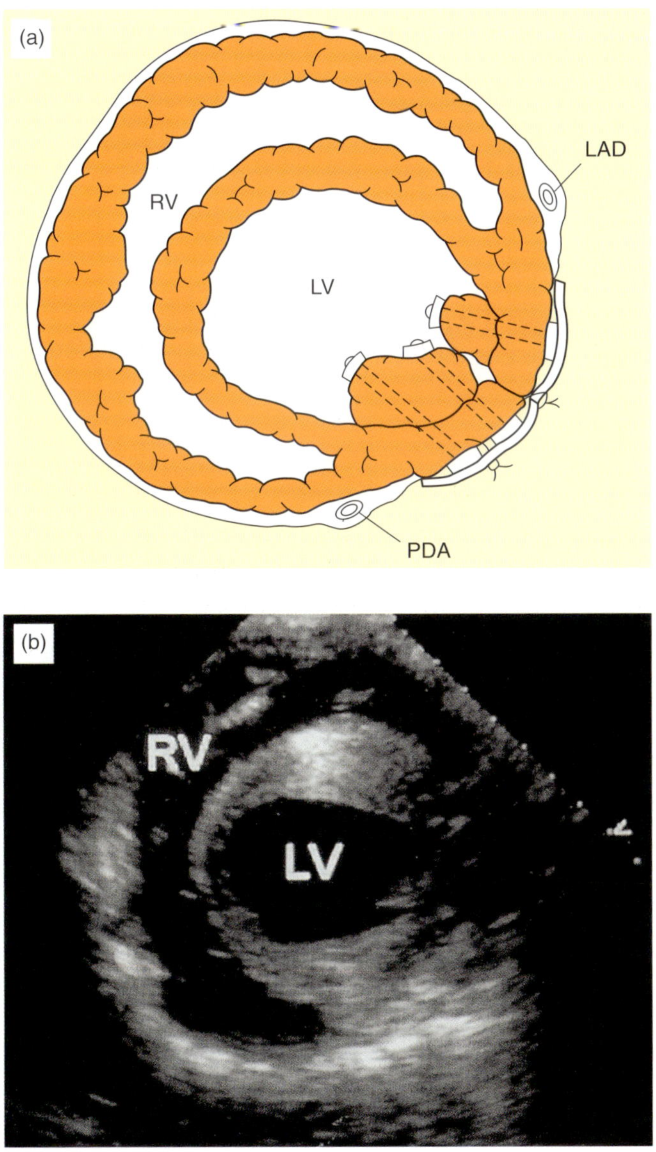


**Figure 34.22** *Diagram and two-dimensional echocardiogram following partial left ventriculectomy illustrating close approximation of the papillary muscles and virtual circumferential wrap of the left ventricle by the right ventricle.*

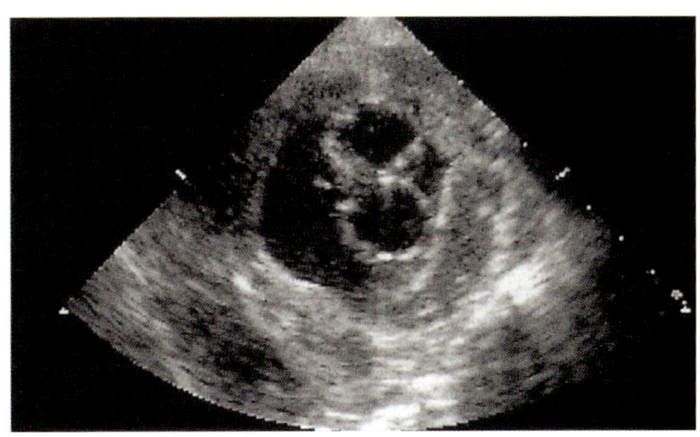

**Figure 34.23** *Two-dimensional echocardiogram illustrating the Alfieri stitch to restore competence to the mitral valve. This results in a double channel mitral orifice.*

**Table 34.3** Early and late mortality in six series or partial left ventriculectomy

| Author | *n* | Early death (%) | Late death (%) | Total (%) |
|---|---|---|---|---|
| McCarthy | 53 | 1 (1.9) | 4 (7.5) | 5 (9.4) |
| Stolf | 37 | 7 (18.9) | 9 (24) | 16 (43) |
| Gradinac | 22 | 3 (13.7) | 4 (18) | 7 (32) |
| Batista[a] | 120 | 26 (22) | – | |
| Angelini | 14 | 3 (21.4) | 1 (7.1) | 4 (29) |
| Suma | 30 | 8 (35) | 3 (10) | 11 (37) |
| Total | 276 | 48 | 17.4 | |

[a]Details not given.

Clinic patients were carefully selected dilated cardiomyopathy patients [30]. Without long-term LVADs the hospital mortality would have been 15%. Hospital-stay ranged from 6 to 31 days, averaging 13–19 days.

## Late mortality

Late deaths (>30 days) were reported in 16% of hospital survivors. Causes of death were progressive heart failure in 38%, sudden or arrhythmic death in 38%, stroke, and transplant heart failure, sepsis and hepatic failure [21–23, 30]. There is little information on risk factors for death after PLV. Gradinac and colleagues carried out a multifactorial analysis on perioperative variables, including age, preoperative NYHA class, heart rate, atrial fibrillation, pulmonary capillary wedge pressure, cardiac index, grade of mitral regurgitation, circumflex artery dominance, 6 min walking test distance, LVEF and LVESV [22]. None of these were predictive of death. The San Paulo group reported greater myocyte diameter to be related with unfavourable outcome during the first 7 months of follow-up [21]. Risk of death, or urgent heart transplantation in that period increased exponentially (achieving values >40%) when the mean myocyte diameter was >22 $\mu$m. The 2-year survival of patients with mean left ventricular myocardial cell diameter < 22 $\mu$m, was 73.6% ±10.1% versus 31.2% ± 11.5% for those >22 $\mu$m.

Late ventricular dysrhythmia is an important concern. New scarring occurs in viable muscle and may promote dysrhythmia with an incidence from 5 to 21.6%. This suggested the need for aggressive antidysrrhythmic therapy and the elective use of an implantable defibrillator.

## Volumetric data and ejection performance

Tables 34.4 and 34.5 summarize the effect of PLV on LV volume and dimensions. After PLV, there is a significant

**Table 34.4** Changes in LVEDV (ml) or index[a] (ml/m$^2$)

| | | Follow-up | | | | | |
|---|---|---|---|---|---|---|---|
| Author | Preoperative | 1 week | 2 weeks | 1 month | 6 months | 7 months | 12 months |
| McCarthy | 319 (14) | 142.9 (40)[a] | | | | | |
| Moreira | 495 (124) | | | 352 (108)[b] | 384 (95)[c] | | 380 (70)[b] |
| Gradinac | 165 (38) | | 102 (25)[c] | | | 102 (18)[c] | |
| Suma | 203 (43) | | 103 (25) | | | | |

All values are mean (standard deviation). [a]$p < 0.001$ versus preoperative, [b]$p < 0.05$ versus preoperative, [c]$p < 0.0001$ versus preoperative.

**Table 34.5** Changes in left ventricular end-diastolic diameter (cm)

| | | Follow-up | | | | | | |
|---|---|---|---|---|---|---|---|---|
| Author | Preoperative | Early | 1 week | 2 weeks | 1 month | 3 months | 6 months | 12 months |
| McCarthy | 8.1 (1.0) | | 6.4 (0.6)[a] | | | | | |
| Moreira | 8.18 (0.87) | | | | 6.85 (0.76)[b] | | 7.02 (0.7)[b] | 7.7 (0.66)[b] |
| Angelini | 7.88 (0.79) | 6.1 (0.85)[c] | | | 6.16 (0.81)[d] | 6.5 (0.9) | | |
| Suma | 7.9 (0.8) | | | 6.0 (0.8) | | | | |

All values are mean (standard deviation). [a]$p < 0.001$ versus preoperative, [b]$p < 0.05$ versus preoperative, [c]$p < 0.0003$ versus preoperative, [d]$p < 0.003$ versus preoperative but not significant versus early postoperative.

decrease in both end-diastolic and end-systolic volume (indices). Moreira showed that volume reduction was sustained at 6 months, but with a slight increase in end-diastolic chamber size (not statistically significant) [32]. At 12 months both LVEDV and EDD were still significantly less than the preoperative value (LVEDV; preoperative value 495 ± 124 ml versus 12-month value 380 ± 70 ml; $p < 0.05$, EDD; preoperative value 8.18 ± 0.87 cm versus 12-month value 7.7 ± 0.66; $p < 0.05$) Gradinac showed similar status of both LVEDVI and LVESVI after 2 weeks and 7 months of follow-up [22].

Whilst LVEF initially improved in all study groups (Table 34.6), observations at 12 months failed to show statistically-significant differences between preoperative LVEF (17.7 ± 4.6) and late LVEF (23.7 ± 6) in matched patients. Similarly, there was no difference in LVEF at between one (23.7 ± 8.8) and 12 months. Gradinac reported that reduction in heart size persisted in their patients, but the mean LVEF declined by 3.9% between 2 weeks and 7 months [22]. Though deteriorating, the 7-month LVEF was nevertheless better than preoperative values.

The suggested mechanism for improvement in LVEF is reduction of LV systolic wall stress. Popovic and colleagues observed an inverse relationship between the decrease of circumferential end-systolic stress and increase in LVEF (Fig. 34.24) [33]. This concept is supported by previous studies, all of which suggest that the improvement in LVEF is predominantly due to reduction in stress, rather than a change in LV contractility. A decrease in LV mass did not increase LVEDP, or wall stress, to maintain the stroke work; in contrast, equivalent stroke work is performed at significantly lower EDP and wall stress (Fig. 34.25).

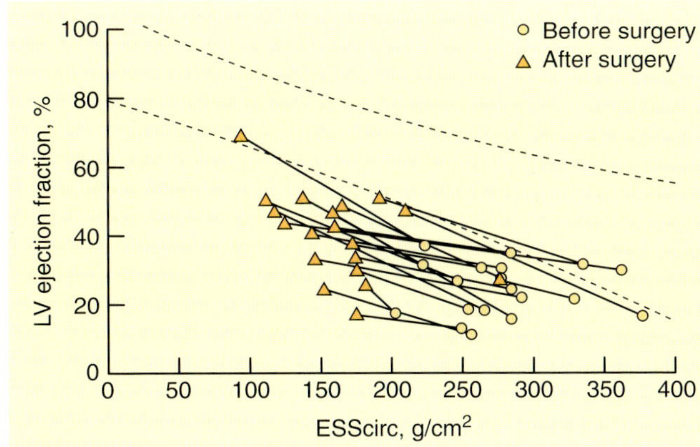


**Figure 34.24** *Relationship between left ventricular circumferential end-systolic stress (ESScirc) and left ventricular ejection fraction before and after PLV. The normal limits (± 2 SEE, dashes) for the control patients are shown for their relation. The figure shows that ventricular reduction shifts LVEF-endsystolic relations in a parallel to control data (reprinted with permission from the American College of Cardiology).*

In the majority of patients both the reduction in chamber size (both EDV and ESV) and improvement in LVEF were sustained up to 6 months. After that there is very little reliable information.

## Haemodynamic results and functional status

Important improvements have been observed in the patients' functional status. In most centres all preoperative patients (without LVADs) were NYHA class III or IV. Afterwards, 67–90% of hospital survivors improved to class I or II [22,30]. By 12 months most patients who remained in NYHA class III or IV were dead or transplanted. In the San Paulo series all surviving patients at 9 and 12 months after PLV were NYHA Class I or II [21]. Late changes

**Table 34.6** Changes in LVEF (%)

| | | Follow-up | | | | | | | |
|---|---|---|---|---|---|---|---|---|---|
| Author | Preoperative | Early | 1 week | 2 weeks | 1 month | 3 months | 6 months | 7 months | 12 months |
| McCarthy | 13.7 (6.2) | | 23.4 (7.9)[a] | | | | | | |
| Moreira | 7.17 (4.6) | | | | 23.7 (8.3)[b] | | 24.1 (8.3)[b] | | 23.7 (6) |
| Gradinac | 23.9 (6.8) | | | 40.7 (12.5)[c] | | | | 34.8 (7.7)[c] | |
| Angelini | 19.3 (7.0) | 30.6 (11.9)[a] | | | 28.3 (10.9)[d] | 30.0 (5.4)[e] | | | |
| Suma | 18 (6) | | | 31 (5) | | | | | |

All values are mean (standard deviation). [a]$p < 0.001$ versus preoperative, [b]$p < 0.05$ versus preoperative, [c]$p < 0.0001$ versus preoperative, [d]$p < 0.008$ versus preoperative but not significant versus early postoperative, [e]$p < 0.04$ versus preoperative but not significant versus early postoperative.

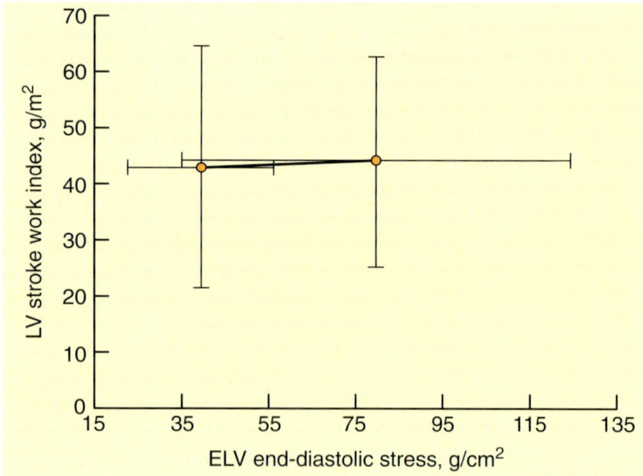


**Figure 34.25** *Relationship between left ventricular stroke work index (LVSWI) and end-diastolic stress before and after PLV. Although there was no improvement in LVSWI, it was performed at significantly lower preload (P=0.0014), compared with the values before PLV (reprinted with permission from the American College of Cardiology).*

(>12 months) of NYHA class with time have not been described.

There is limited data on haemodynamic change. Intraoperative measurements at the Cleveland Clinic showed no change in cardiac index [30]. This may reflect a decrease in stroke volume, since the heart rate increased (from 92 ± 17 to 102 ± 16: $p$ = 0.001). Others have reported a modest increase. Ventricular filling pressures (LAP, PCWP, LVEDP) fall significantly though stroke volume may not change.

Gradinac reported that pulmonary capillary wedge pressure had fallen below preoperative values by 6 weeks postoperatively (from 22 ± 8.6 to 1.51 ± 5.5 mmHg 2 weeks postoperatively; $p < 0.05$); by the 6-month follow-up examination, it had again increased toward preoperative values (18.8 ± 8.0 mmHg) [22]. Similar observations were made in follow-up studies on matched patients in the San Paulo series, where pulmonary capillary wedge pressure had returned to preoperative values by 12 months postoperatively and continued to rise [21]. These changes were associated with a steady decrease in cardiac index and stroke index.

These data suggest that the Frank–Starling relationship may improve in the short term, but begins to deteriorate within 6 months of operation. However, the assessment of LV end-diastolic properties immediately following surgery should be interpreted cautiously, as they are sensitive to loading conditions, myocardial stiffness, changes in ventricular interdependence and pericardiotomy [34].

Since LV size tends to remain constant, a steady elevation of filling pressure from 1 month after operation suggests early deterioration of global left ventricular function. The ventricle compensates for this increase in preload and the patients' functional status is not affected. Certainly the LV starts failing except perhaps after PLV in infancy.

It is still unclear as to why marked improvements in NYHA class occur despite only modest changes in haemodynamics. One concern is that the determination of NYHA class has been made solely on an observational basis and has not been reinforced by documentation of peak $VO_2$ on exercise. It is curious that, by 12 months, the São Paulo series showed the same PCWP as preoperatively, but with persistently-elevated stroke index and reduced LVEDV [21]. This does not fit with laboratory models of PLV where filling pressures and stroke volume showed downward and rightward shift in response to mass reduction implying a reduction in LV performance.

## Consensus on partial left ventriculectomy

Results of ongoing clinical trials suggest that PLV reduces LV volume without a significant change in stroke volume thereby improving LVEF. This is initially accompanied by a simultaneous increase in cardiac index and a decrease in LV filling pressure. The geometric rearrangement leads to a reduction in wall stress for a given level of pressure generation, thus implying an increase in the efficiency with which wall stress is transduced into intraventricular pressure. Although these geometric improvements (LVEDV, LVEF) may be sustained up to 12 months (but not identified afterwards), overall pump function (Frank–Starling) relationships seem to deteriorate after 6 months, perhaps with the exception of infants. The first evidence for this is a rise in LV filling pressure. This discrepancy between LV geometry and sustainability of mechanical function stems from the fact that mass reduction may cause changes in diastolic ventricular properties. Effective adjuncts, such as ACE inhibitors, or beta-blockers are employed to promote the improvement of pump function and sustainability of reduced LV volumes.

Twenty per cent of patients required mechanical circulatory support for survival. It is therefore strongly suggested that the PLV operation should be performed with extreme caution in centres without mechanical support programmes. A high incidence of late ventricular dysrhythmia warrants aggressive antidysrhythmic therapy and perhaps the elective use of an implantable defibrillator.

In reality, most centres who enthusiastically embraced the Batista operation have now cut back dramatically in the numbers being performed. As for the early days of cardiac transplantation, many units who performed only a small number of unsuccessful cases have stopped the operation altogether. Nevertheless, the experience has prompted greater interest in other heart failure procedures, such as mitral annuloplasty and the Dor operation. The eventual role of PLV itself remains to be seen.

## The influence of mitral valve repair on left ventricular remodelling

Mitral regurgitation is an important complication of end-stage cardiomyopathy and further contributes to volume overload of the dilated left ventricle For patients with dilated cardiomyopathy increased chamber sphericity and the presence of mitral regurgitation are markers of poor prognosis [4]. One-year mortality for dilated cardiomyopathy patients with LVEF <25% and moderate to severe mitral regurgitation ranges between 50% and 70% [3].

In dilated cardiomyopathy mitral regurgitation develops in the presence of a structurally normal valve through progressive dilatation of the mitral annulus and altered ventricular geometry with restricted leaflet motion (Fig. 34.1) [35]. As more mitral leaflet tissue is utilized for coverage of the enlarging mitral valve orifice, a critical reduction in leaflet coaptation causes a central regurgitant jet of functional insufficiency. Given that the most significant determinants of mitral valve coaptation are annulus size and left ventricular dimensions, both are amenable to surgical restoration.

In ischaemic cardiomyopathy the mechanisms of mitral regurgitation are similar, but include papillary muscle ischaemia [36]. This results in unsuccessful coordination of the entire subvalvar apparatus rather than an isolated problem with a single papillary muscle. Again, the result is failure of the leaflets to close the mitral orifice during systole.

The issues regarding management of patients with mitral regurgitation and impaired left ventricular function are controversial. This is partly due to the difficulty in assessing ventricular function through the favourable unloading effect of regurgitation into the low pressure left atrium. Virtually all measures of systolic function, including LVEF tend to over estimate ventricular performance. Despite this LVEF remains an important determinant of long-term survival after mitral surgery. Patients with normal preoperative LVEF have excellent postoperative survival, whereas those with moderate to severe reduction are at considerable risk [37].

Attempts to replace the mitral valve in patients with end-stage cardiomyopathy during the 1970s and early 1980s resulted in prohibitive mortality so that patients with poor ventricular function and mitral regurgitation were denied corrective surgery. Death was thought to occur because the unloading effect of regurgitation into the left atrium was removed. However, these early valve replacements were undertaken with excision of the sub-valvar apparatus (Fig. 34.26). This provided a further deterioration in compromised left ventricular function [38]. Division of all chordae tendonae results in a marked elongation of a normal left ventricle accompanied by a 47% reduction in $LVE_{max}$ (Fig. 34.27a–c). In contrast the preservation of chordal, annular, and sub-valvar continuity maintain the geometric relationships of the left ventricle and promote improvement of left ventricular function when volume overload is corrected.

Bolling has shown that patients with poor ventricular function (LVEF < 25% on angiography or radionuclide studies) can be managed by mitral valve repair alone with acceptable morbidity and mortality [39]. Bolling's patients

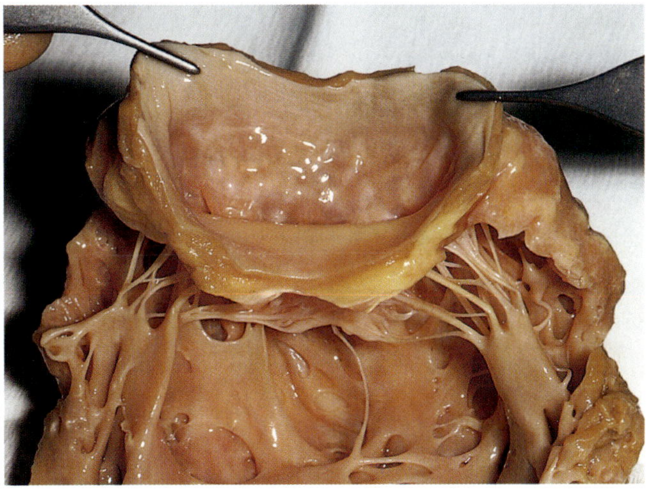

**Figure 34.26** *Dissection of the left ventricle to show the papillary muscles and chordae which constitute the mitral subvalvar apparatus.*

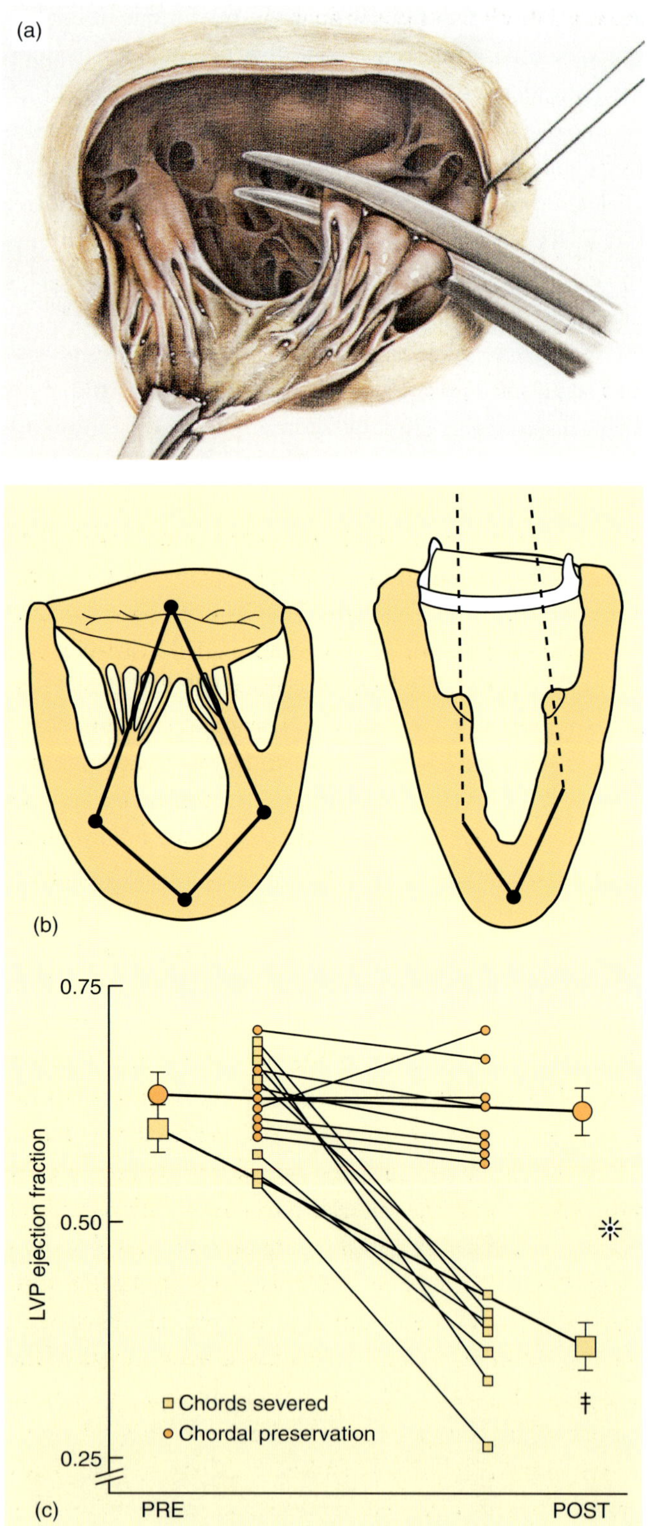


**Figure 34.27** *Excision of the mitral subvalvar apparatus used to be standard procedure during mitral valve replacement, but results in substantial deterioration in left ventricular function. (a) The surgical approach, (b) elongation of the left ventricle through interruption of continuity between the papillary muscles and annulus, (c) reduction in left ventricular ejection fraction after resection of the subvalvar apparatus in a number of mitral replacement patients.*

had NYHA class III or IV (mean 3.9 ± 0.2) congestive heart failure despite maximum medical treatment and preoperative ejection fraction ranging from 8 to 25% (mean 16% ± 3%). Mean age was 63 ± 6 years with a mean duration of cardiomyopathy of 4 ± 6 years (range 0–16). All patients underwent mitral annuloplasty using an undersized flexible remodelling ring (Fig. 34.28). One-half of the patients also required a tricuspid annuloplasty. Remarkably hospital mortality was <2%. Only trivial regurgitation persisted in a small number of patients and the mean transmitral gradient by intra-operative transoesophageal echocardiography was 3 ± 1 mmHg. Postoperatively all patients were maintained on medical therapy for congestive heart failure, and were in NYHA class I or II (mean 1.8 ± 0.4) with a mean LVEF of 26% (Table 34.7). One- and 2-year actuarial survival were 82% and 72%. Peak exercise $VO_{2\ max}$ rose significantly from a mean of 14.5 ml to 18.6 ml $O_2$/kg/minute. Echocardiography at 2 years showed a marked reduction in sphericity, regurgitant volume and regurgitant fraction with significantly improved LVEF, LVEDV and LVESV. Late deaths occurred from continued heart failure or sudden ventricular arrhythmia. Bolling suggests that mitral valve reconstruction leads to improved function in myopathic hearts by remodelling the base of the heart with an undersized valve ring. This may help restore an ellipsoid shape to the left ventricular cavity.

The great majority of patients subject to the Batista procedure also undergo mitral valve repair. This poses the question as to whether the beneficial effect is due to PLV or the mitral repair procedure. Mitral valve reconstruction in cardiomyopathy restorates a more normal ventricular mass-to-volume ratio, but with larger left ventricular volumes than have been reported after PLV. In Bolling's experience the average left ventricular volume 24 months after mitral repair remained >200 ml (still markedly abnormal) whilst partial PLV provides an acute reduction in left ventricular volume to approximately 90–100 ml at the time of operation. However, since there is no loss of ventricular mass with mitral repair, a more appropriate mass/volume ratio is still obtained and with less risk of surgical mortality.

The Cleveland Clinic Group have looked at patients subject to mitral valve repair with poor left ventricular function in comparison to their PLV patients [40]. Mitral repair provided a trend towards a small less spherical ventricle with increased stroke volume and LVEF. During 2-year follow-up they found no progression in ventricular dysfunction

**Table 34.7** Mitral repair in dilated cardiomyopathy. Left ventricular function and flow before and after annuoplasty

| Variable | Preoperative | Postoperative | Change (%)[a] | $p$ value |
|---|---|---|---|---|
| End-diatolic volume (ml) | 335 ± 107 | 307 ± 103 | −8 ± 9 | 0.06 |
| End-systolic volume (ml) | 277 ± 101 | 237 ± 98 | −15 ± 14 | 0.03 |
| Stroke volume (ml) | 58 ± 13 | 70 ± 21 | + 12 ± 10 | 0.02 |
| Ejection fraction (%) | 18 ± 5 | 24 ± 10 | +31 ± 24 | 0.03 |
| Mitral inflow (l/mm) | 12.4 ± 5.3 | 5.4 ± 0.5 | −49 ± 22 | 0.02 |
| Forward cardiac output (l/min) | 3.2 ± 1.0 | 4.7 ± 0.9 | +52 ± 38 | 0.01 |
| Regurgitant volume (l/min) | 9.2 ± 5.4 | 0.8 ± 0.6 | 88.6 ± 10.1 | 0.01 |
| Regurgitant fraction (%) | 70 ± 14 | 15 ± 11 | −79 ± 15 | <0.001 |

[a]Percentage change from preoperative study at 4–6 months postoperatively. The NYNA class fell significantly from 3.9 ± 0.4 to 1.8 ± 0.5 ($p < 0.001$). From Bolling *et al.* (1998) *J Thorac Cardiovasc Surg* **115**: 381–8.

probably through correction of volume overload and preservation of the mitral subvalvar apparatus which provides better physiological remodelling than achieved by PLV. However, whilst all the Cleveland Clinic patients were receiving maximal antifailure drug therapy, only one-third were in NYHA class III or IV. The PLV patients were much sicker with 44% receiving preoperative inotropic support and 95% transplant listed. The PLV patients had worse LVEF and larger left ventricles than the patients undergoing mitral repair. Consequently there is little to be gained by comparing outcomes in the disparate groups. The Cleveland Clinic results of mitral repair or replacement with preservation of the subvalvar apparatus, in patients with advanced left ventricular dysfunction support those of Bolling. Hospital mortality was 2.3% and 1-, 2- and 5-year survival rate was 89, 86 and 67%, respectively. Progressive

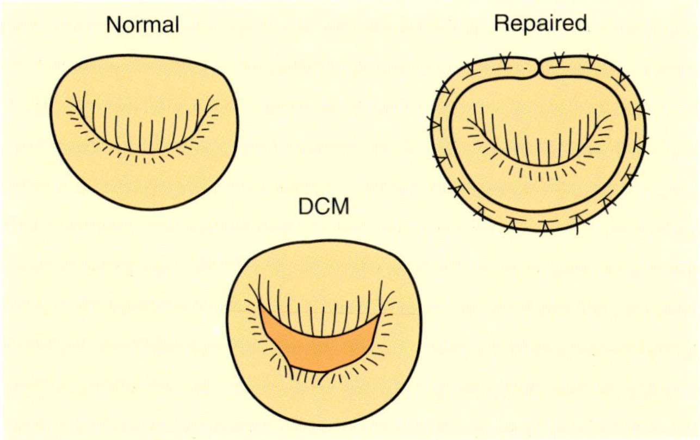


**Figure 34.28** *Dilatation of the mitral annulus in dilated cardiomyopathy (DCM) increases the area to be covered by the mitral leaflets. Ventricular enlargement in turn causes restricted leaflet motion. Mitral regurgitation can be eliminated by mitral valve repair using an undersized valve ring, which remodels the base of the left ventricle and improves left ventricular function.*

heart failure or sudden death accounted for 62% of the late deaths. NYHA class improved from 2.8 ± 0.8 preoperatively to 1.2 ± 0.5 at follow-up ($p < 0.0001$). Every patient in this group had previously been hospitalized between one and six times for heart failure management (mean 2.3 ± 1.5). Postoperative freedom from re-admission for heart failure was 88, 82 and 72% at 1, 2 and 5 years, respectively. Whilst these results appear to show better outcome over medical management alone a prospective study randomizing matched patients towards surgical correction or medical therapy is required.

In the meantime new surgical strategies are being applied in ischaemic mitral regurgitation [41]. Animal models of acute myocardial infarction (before left ventricular dilatation) show the mitral leaflets to close at annular level with only a trace of incompetence. However, 8 weeks after infarction, despite comparable LVEF, ventricular volumes are greatly increased and the mitral leaflets are apically tented away from the anterior annulus, restricting leaflet closure, and allowing mitral regurgitation to develop. In a sheep model Liel-Cohen and colleagues of the Harvard Medical School used plication of the infarct region with mattress sutures to reduce the paradoxical movement of the scar [41] (Fig. 34.29). Neither muscle excision nor cardiopulmonary bypass were required. Plication brings the posteriorly and radiolaterally shifted papillary muscles back toward the relatively fixed anterior mitral annulus. The extent of plication was guided by manual compression of the paradoxically moving infarct to determine how much reduction in bulging would eliminate mitral regurgitation, (imaged by colour Doppler from the apex). Although LVEF was unchanged, the valve leaflets were able to close at annulus level with only a trace of regurgitation.

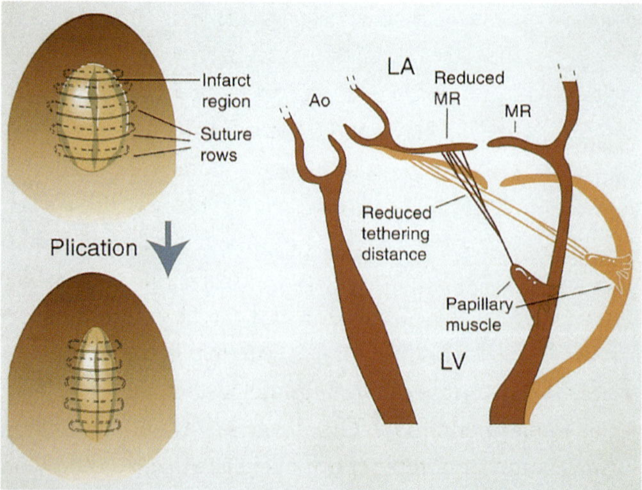


**Figure 34.29** *Experimental left ventricular remodelling by infarct plication to bring a displaced papillary muscle tip back towards the anterior annulus. In the animal model this reduced mitral regurgitation. LA indicates left atrium; AO aorta (from ref. 41).*

These results showed that acute left ventricular contractile dysfunction failed to produce mitral regurgitation in the absence of ventricular dilatation. Mitral regurgitation developed over time without change in LVEF as the ventricle remodels and the annulus dilates. The fact that simply plicating the infarct zone to reduce apical tenting can reduce or eliminate mitral regurgitation highlights the importance of the papillary muscle tip to annulus distance in determining mitral valve behaviour. This also suggests that the cause of ischaemic mitral regurgitation is not left ventricular dysfunction *per se*, but rather the geometric changes, which can be reversed surgically.

## Reverse ventricular remodelling during left ventricular assist device support 'mechanical bridge to myocardial recovery'

One of the great revelations of the past 5 years is the finding that patients with end-stage heart failure deemed irreversible still have myocardium that can restored to near normal structure and function. This has been learned from moribund patients sustained with a left ventricular assist device (LVAD) in the bridge to transplantation setting. Burch (1968) first suggested that a reduction in cardiac workload by strict prolonged bedrest could produce symptomatic improvement [42]. This approach was limited by the effects of inactivity on the skeletal muscles, vascular tone and autonomic nervous system. Modest reversal of left ventricular remodelling is sometimes seen after treatment with ACE inhibitors, nitroglycerine, and chronic beta-blockade [43]. These agents decrease systemic vascular resistance which may reduce left ventricular mass and improve left ventricular shape. However, the extent to which reverse remodelling and functional recovery can be achieved by haemodynamic unloading with an LVAD is of greater interest. When myocardial rest is combined with whole body exercise training the benefits of both become apparent. These are the conditions achieved during long-term bridge to transplantation with the ThermoCardio Systems and Novacor LVADs, which function in series with the patients own left ventricle. The improved systemic blood flow reverses multi-organ failure and enables resumed physical activity whilst the left ventricle is completely offloaded and the aortic valve remains closed [44]. Use of an LVAD in so-called status I patients awaiting transplantation increases survival both before the donor organ becomes available and after transplantation [45]. Hepatic and renal function improve whereas serum aldosterone plasma renin, atrial natriuretic and norepinephrine levels revert to normal.

Until recently in the United States, transplantation was mandatory for all patients committed to an LVAD. However, at the time of transplantation it became clear that some chronically support hearts had reverted towards normal size and weight.

One of the first Texas Heart patients had a 5-year history of chronic heart failure before LVAD insertion. He was a large blood type O patient and after 505 days support suffered a stroke after inadvisably discontinuing Warfarin. After brain herniation the device was turned off, but his cardiac function remained stable. He demonstrated a marked improvement of both cardiac function and myocardial histology compared to that at the time of LVAD insertion [46].

In patients with dilated cardiomyopathy normalization of left ventricular pressure volume relations and regression of left ventricular hypertrophy have been reported together with decreased, myocardial fibrosis, apoptosis and reduction in myocardial matrix metalloproteinase expression [47, 48]. Frazier and colleagues studied 31 patients with either idiopathic dilated cardiomyopathy or ischaemic cardiomyopathy bridged to transplantation for more than 30 days [47]. Tissue samples were taken from the apical core of left ventricular myocardium removed to accommodate the inflow cannula and compared with adjacent myocardium from the explanted heart at transplantation. Mean duration of support was 137 days (range 31–505 days). Echocardiographic measurements (serially with the LVAD switched off) showed a significant decrease in left ventricular end-diastolic dimensions and improvement in LVEF with time. Cardiac index improved progressively, whereas pulmonary capillary wedge pressure and pulmonary vascular resistance fell. The histological sample showed reduction in myocytolysis and regression of myocyte hypertrophy as well as normalization of calcium metabolism in the sarcoplasmic reticulum. Calcium channel studies show more efficient calcium flux, little leakage and normalized phospholipid and fatty acid levels. This suggested reversal of the deranged membrane and organelle function by prolonged ventricular offloading.

Levin and coworkers studied end-diastolic pressure volume loops in excised hearts from transplantation recipients with idiopathic dilated cardiomyopathy [48]. Hearts treated with maximal medical therapy were compared with those that had been offloaded with an LVAD for an average of 4 months. Reversed remodelling was found in the LVAD hearts whose end-diastolic pressure/volume relations were shifted towards much lower volume in comparison to the medically treated hearts. The left ventricular mass of LVAD hearts was reduced and regression of myocyte hypertrophy was accompanied by normalisation of fibre orientation. Others have confirmed these findings (Fig. 34.30) and even demonstrated that LVAD malfunction (valve regurgitation) can interfere with reverse remodelling [49, 50]. Together these reports demonstrate that chronic left ventricular offloading in end-stage heart failure can decrease myocyte necrosis and apoptosis, reverse myocytolysis and improve myocardial contractility.

Given the incontrovertible shortage of transplant organ donors, the prospect of permanent mechanical circulatory assistance or circulatory support as a therapeutic option is compelling. The success of early LVAD bridge to transplantation programmes was a powerful argument for the use of the electric 'HeartMate' and Novacor LVADs as an alternative to transplantation [51]. Patients moribund with heart failure can improve to NYHA class I and return to the community with these devices, though quality of life is currently restricted by the size of the blood pump, drive line infection, stroke or device failure. Although the scope for a bridge to recovery programme is obvious, there are certain requirements before this strategy has a chance for success. The first is a user-friendly LVAD for patients of all sizes. This must be simple to implant and remove without the risk of drive line infection, and easier for the patient to control. The new axial flow impeller pumps are promising in this respect [52]. Second the LVAD must be implanted early before diffuse fibrosis renders ventricular remodelling irreversible. Strategies to promote myocardial recovery with pharmacology, growth factors, gene therapy and inhibitors of apoptosis are under investigation and markers for sustainability of myocardial recovery explored. The Berlin group has used the disappearance from the serum of the autoantibody against the beta1 adrenergic receptor, suggesting that this reflects an immune process causing functional impairment [53]. The Texas Heart group suggest normalization of norepinephrine levels. Also axial flow or centrifugal blood pumps allow more consistent and realistic weaning protocols [45].

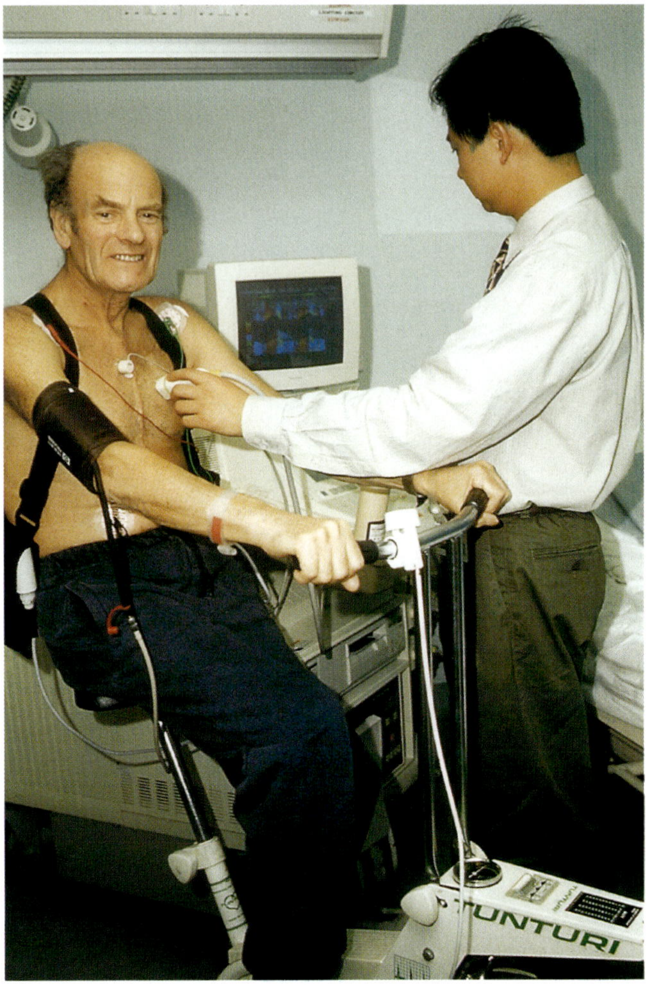


**Figure 34.30** *Exercise two-dimensional echocardiogram in a patient 8 weeks after implantation of a TCI LVAD for end-stage dilated cardiomyopathy. Marked improvement in native left ventricular function was apparent and led to the concept of bridge to myocardial recovery.*

Several major questions remain. Which types of myocardial disease will prove amenable to cardiac recovery? What degree of recovery reached during the assist period is consistent with the prospect of well-sustained cardiac function? What types of supportive therapy will promote or support the maintenance of restored cardiac function? The type of LVAD also seems to be important because complete drainage of the left ventricle appears to be mandatory to enable the heart to recover. This has been the case with the Novacor and TCI systems which both have large bore inlet cannulas at the apex of the left ventricle (Fig. 34.31). Atrial drainage appears to be unsuitable whereas the new apically positioned axial flow impeller pumps are as effective as the pusher-plate devices [54].

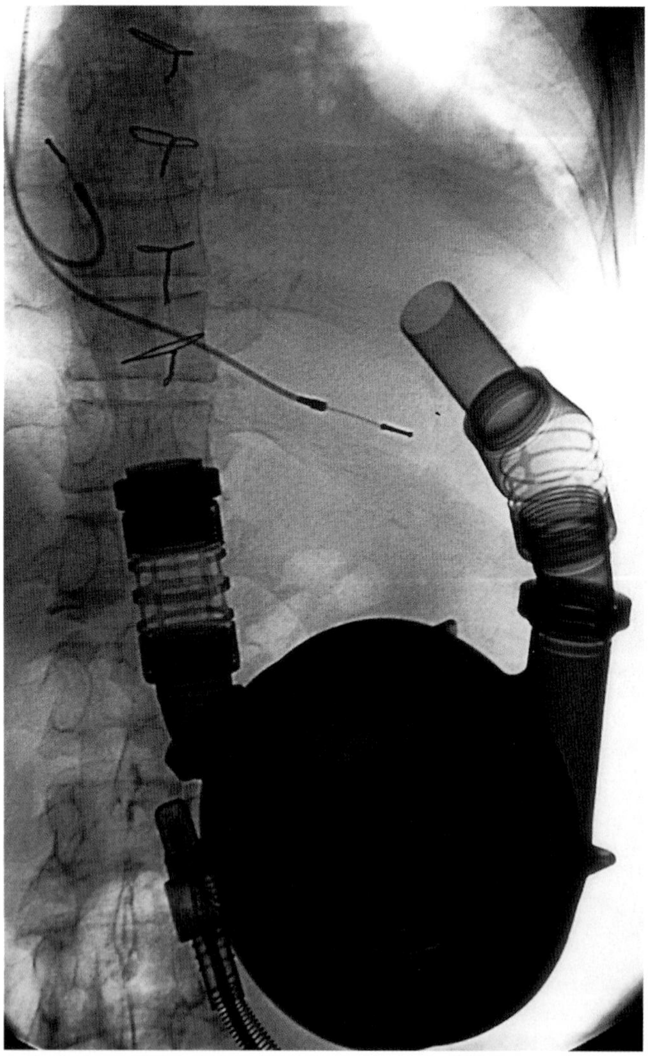

**Figure 34.31** *TCI LVAD in situ with a large inflow cannula in the apex in the left ventricle. Wide-bore apical drainage allows complete offloading of the native left ventricle.*

Hetzer and colleagues have recently published the largest series of bridge to recovery patients [54]. In the their busy transplant centre between June 1994 and January 1999, 84 patients with end-stage heart failure were supported with either a Novacor or a TCI LVAD with a view to transplantation. Of this group 65 patients had idiopathic dilated cardiomyopathy and were studied with a view to bridge to myocardial recovery. Twenty-three patients had near complete restoration of left ventricular function during a decompression period of between 30 and 794 days. This group underwent elective removal of the LVAD when on repeated echocardiography the left ventricular end-diastolic dimension had dropped below 60 mm and the LVEF had risen to >40%. Device removal was undertaken leaving the heart as undisturbed as possible. Thus for patients with the Novacor and TCI LVADs the pump housing pocket in the left upper abdominal wall was entered. The inflow and outflow dacron grafts were transected and oversewn, leaving the cannula in the left ventricular apex and the ascending aortic graft in place. Postoperatively the patients were anticoagulated with warfarin for 6 months in an attempt to avoid thromboembolism from the residual cannulas. Beta-blockers, ACE inhibitors and spironolactone were administered permanently.

Of the 23 patients 13 had stable cardiac function without signs of deterioration for between 3 months and 4 years (mean 23 ± 14 months). Three other patients have manifest some decline in cardiac function, but without clinical relevance. Seven patients had recurrent heart failure beginning between 4 months and 2 years (mean 11 ± 7 months) after pump explantation. These patients were transplanted. Four patients suffered chronic infections within the pump pocket. These resulted in the death of two from exanguination and severe infection.

At the time of LVAD implantation there were no significant differences between those patients with sustained recovery and those who relapsed into heart failure with regard to age, haemodynamics, LVEF, left ventricular internal diameter in diastole, or autoantibody against the betadrenergic receptor. However, those patients who relapsed had longer histories of heart failure and more prolonged duration of assist. Those with sustained recovery demonstrated more rapid improvement in left ventricular function (LVEF and decrease of left ventricular internal diameter) and the duration of support was shorter.

The degree of left ventricular recovery at the time of explantation was also more complete in these patients. Younger age at the time of device implantation was the only factor to correlate with duration of mechanical assist. The fact that probability of heart failure recurrence was influenced by shorter duration of preoperative left ventricular failure undoubtedly relates to the ultra-structure of the myocardium. The 42 patients with dilated cardiomyopathy who were not electively explanted improved to a mean LVEF of 25% ± 8% and LV internal dimension of 59 ± 6 mm which was deemed insufficient for safe removal of the LVAD.

In summary younger patients with shorter duration of heart failure have a better chance of recovery and lower probability for recurrence of heart failure requiring transplantation. Lasting recovery correlates with a shorter history and a more rapid restoration of normal heart function on mechanical support. This probably reflects the fact that recovery is more likely in disease processes with an on-going inflammatory component (chronic myocarditis). Certainly patients with acute viral myocarditis can recover completely even from biventricular failure with cardiac arrest [55, 56] (Fig. 34.32a–c). However, no reliable predictors have been found to pin-point which patients with dilated cardiomyopathy might be candidates for an unloading and weaning protocol before device implantation. From the Berlin experience it appears that approximately 25% of dilated cardiomyopathy patients who require LVAD support can be safely weaned and expect durable mid-term stable cardiac function.

## LVAD unloading followed by partial left ventriculectomy

Frazier has suggested the combination of left ventricular unloading followed by PLV for patients unsuitable or unlikely to receive a transplant [57]. Theoretically the improvement in left ventricular morphology induced by prolonged ventricular unloading may increase the likelihood of success after PLV. Frazier's first patient was a 6 ft 6 in, 240 lb male who was clearly unlikely to obtain a donor heart. He received an electric TCI LVAD and was discharged from hospital 4 weeks later to await transplantation. One year later he was readmitted with recurrent heart failure despite maximum medical therapy. The left ventricle had redilated after early failure of the prosthetic tissue valve within the LVAD. It was then decid-

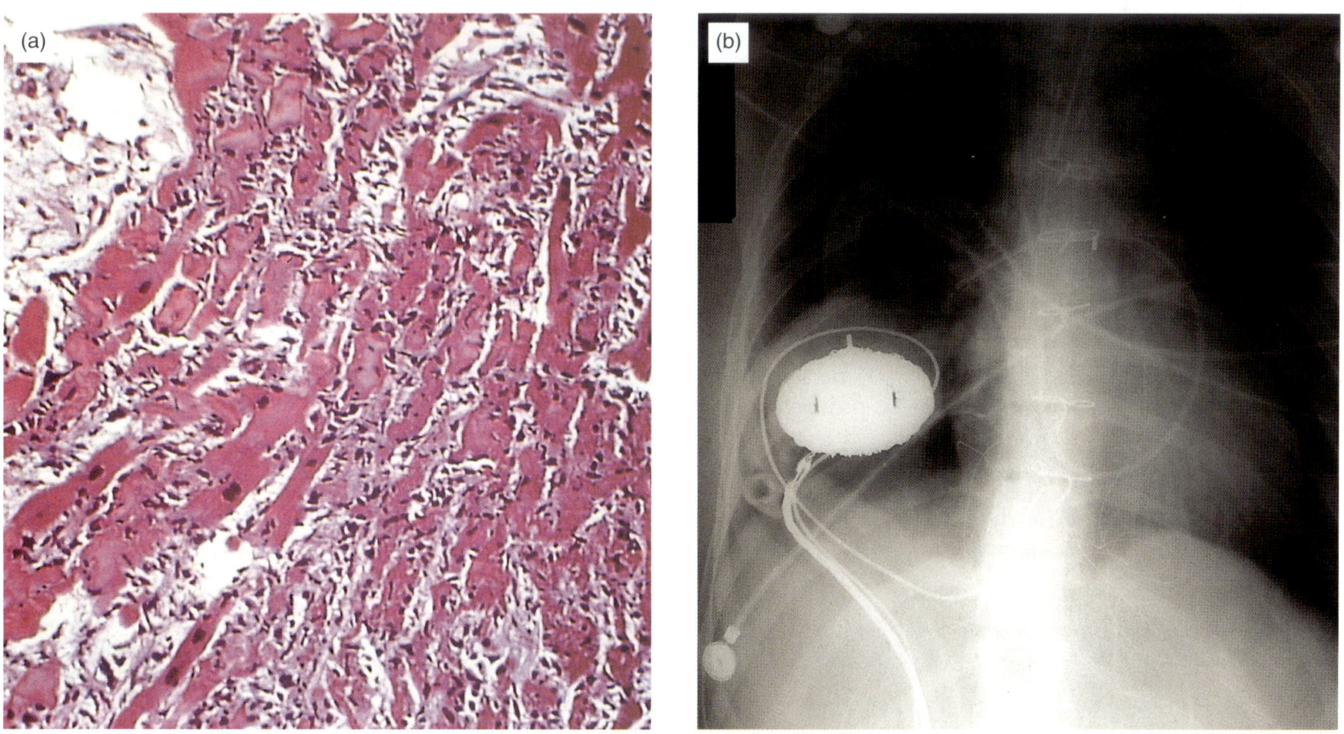


**Figure 34.32** *Bridge to myocardial recovery after cardiac arrest in fulminant viral myocarditis. (a) Histology from the left ventricle at the time of LVAD implantation, (b) Plain chest X-ray to show the AB 180 centrifugal pump implanted in the left pleural cavity. This drained the left atrium and pumped blood to the ascending aorta, (c) shown over the page.*

(c)

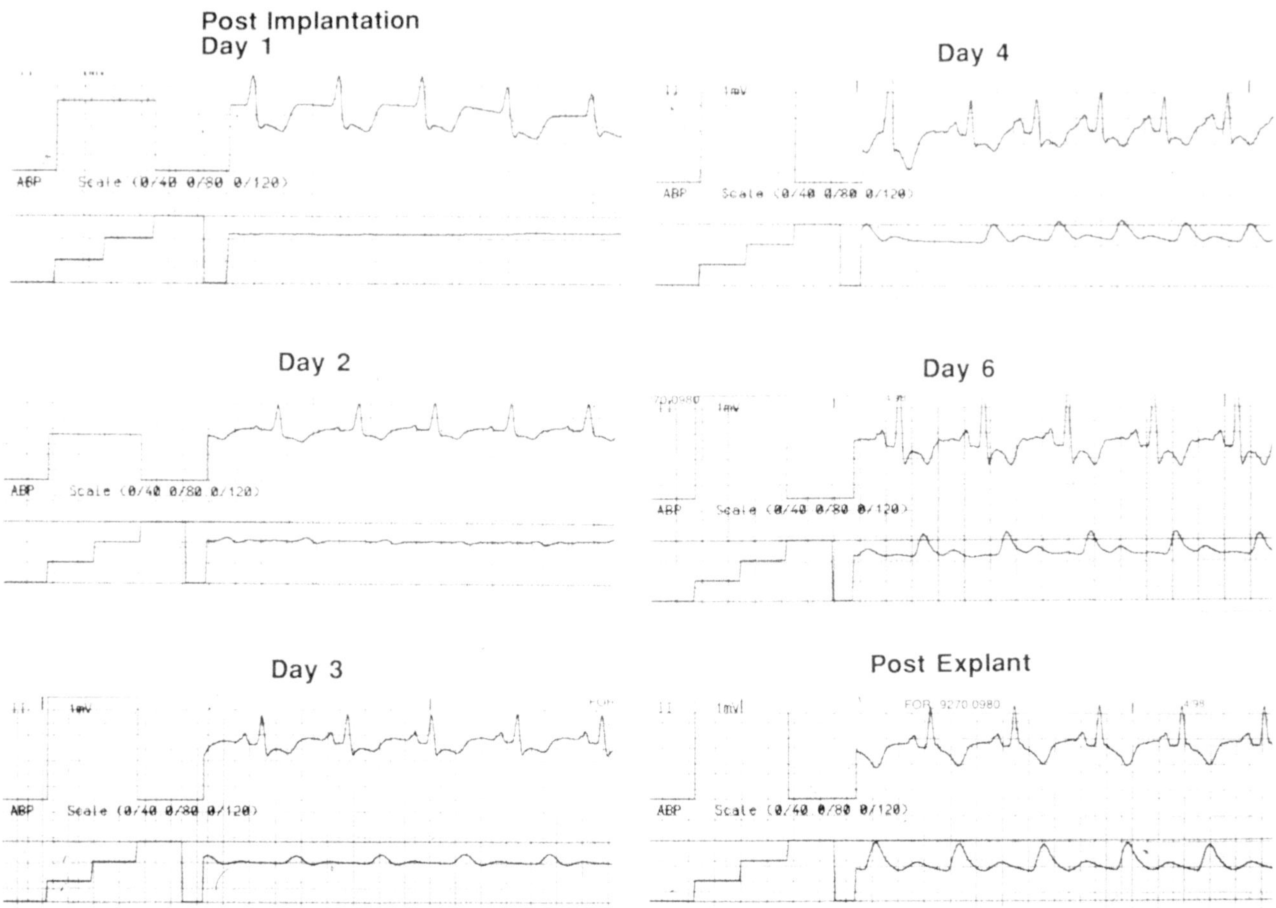


**Figure 34.32** *Bridge to myocardial recovery after cardiac arrest in fulminant viral myocarditis* (continued). *(c) The course of myocardial recovery. The patient, a 21-year-old female required cardiopulmonary bypass to sustain life during LVAD implantation. For the first 2 days of support there was virtually no left ventricular ejection and she was anuric. Subsequently the electrocardiogram began to improve during steroid therapy and ventricular ejection was noted on the arterial trace. Acute tubular necrosis then resolved. By day six, left ventricular function had improved substantially and the device was removed. Two years later she is NYHA 1 with an LVEF of 45%.*

ed to remove the LVAD and perform PLV. This resulted in dramatic improvement of left ventricular function. No inotropic support was used, indeed arterial dilators were required to keep the blood pressure down. At follow-up 1 year later the patient remained NYHA class I and had returned to work. Another 24-year-old female patient underwent 156 days of LVAD support for dilated cardiomyopathy during which her cardiac index improved from 1.2 to 2.7 $l/min/m^2$. Again, the device was removed and PLV performed. One year later she was in NYHA class I. Whether restoration of improved myocardial architecture by LVAD offloading can influence the long-term success of PLV is an intriguing question which remains to be answered.

## Novel methods to attenuate progressive left ventricular remodelling

Conceptually an exciting principle, dynamic cardiomyoplasty failed to augment cardiac output at some considerable cost to the patient (Fig. 34.33). Mortality in NYHA class III and IV was prohibitive whilst those less debilitated can derive just as much symptomatic relief from improvements in medical therapy [58]. An appropriately titled editorial, ‘Dynamic cardiomyoplasty, time to wrap it up’ heralded the demise of the procedure though many remained convinced of beneficial effects [59]. Although intact skeletal muscle could not replace myocardium, the wrap had a tendency to prevent passive left ventricular

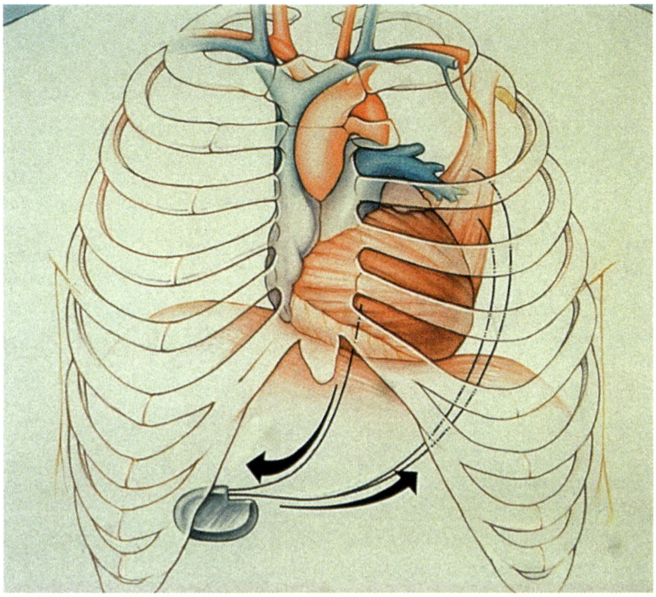

**Figure 34.33** *Diagram illustrating the cardiomyoplasty operation where the Latisimus dorsi muscle was mobilized and transferred into the chest to wrap the failing heart. Pacing was used in an attempt to augment left ventricular contraction. The procedure did not improve cardiac output, but may have delayed progressive left ventricular enlargement in some patients.*

dilatation. So could the same result be achieved with a less invasive operation?

The Laplace principle dictates that increased chamber size contributes to afterload and limits the heart's ability to translate wall tension into stroke volume. The vicious downward spiral, which triggers genetic and neurohormonal changes, could possibly be attenuated by passive ventricular restraint to prevent sphericity. This is the hypothesis underlying the development of four new surgical products, each presented to the American Heart Association in November 2000. A substantial amount of animal research was undertaken in an effort to convince the sceptical.

### *The Acorn Cardiac Support Device*

The Acorn Cardiac Support Device is a mesh-like polyester jacket surgically placed around the ventricles in order to prevent further dilatation by passive mechanical constraint (Fig. 34.34). In a dog model Sabbah and co-workers used multiple intracoronary microembolization to produce heart failure (LVEF 30–40%) [60]. Six dogs then underwent surgical implantation of the Acorn jacket via median sternotomy. Three months later parameters of left ventricular function were compared. Control animals suffered an increase in LVEDV (67 ± 5 ml to 83 ± 8 ml) and decrease in LVEF (36 ± 1% to 28 ± 2%). In contrast the dogs treated with the Acorn jacket improved in status with a decrease in LVEDV (68 ± 4 ml to 61 ± 4 ml) and increase in LVEF (34 ± 1% to 41 ± % $p<0.05$). Histology from the hearts showed cardiomyocyte cross-sectional area (reflecting hypertrophy) to be smaller in treated dogs (791 ± 51 versus 987 ± 37 mm$^2$, $p=0.011$). Functional mitral regurgitation disappeared after use of the polyester net, but worsened in untreated dogs. This group also isolated myocytes from treated and control animals and demonstrate that use of passive constraint resulted in improved intrinsic contraction and relaxation in treated animals.

Power and colleagues implanted a transonic cardiac output flow-probe around the pulmonary artery of 12 adults sheep then induced heart failure by rapid right ventricular pacing for 21 days (190 beats/min creating a 10% decrease in cardiac output) [61]. The animals were then randomized to polyester jacket or control group and

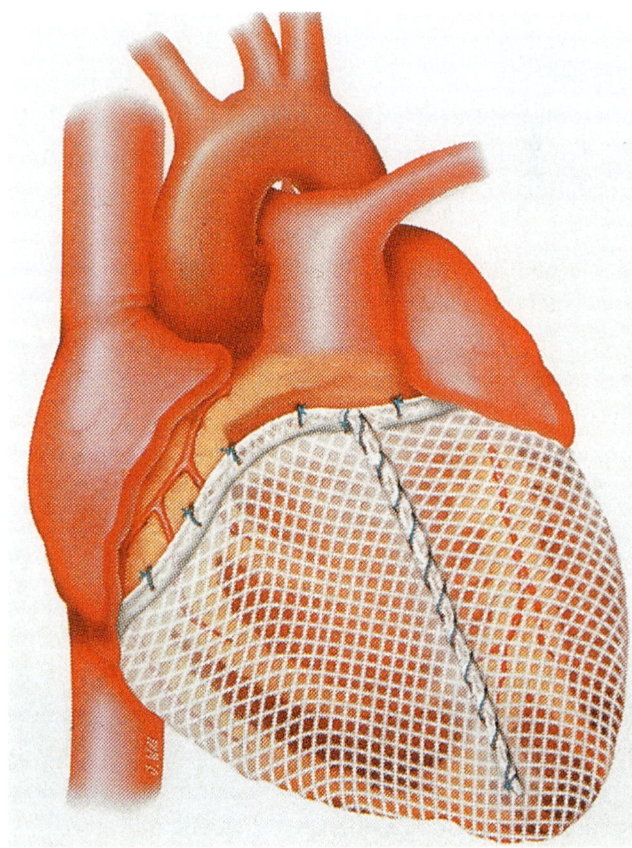

**Figure 34.34** *The Acorn device wrapped around the ventricles to prevent progressive dilatation.*

pacing recommenced at a higher rate to induce a further 10% decrease in cardiac output for 28 days. At termination of pacing the treated group showed significant improvement in left ventricular fractional shortening ($p$=0.007), lower mitral regurgitation ($p$=0.006) smaller left ventricular long axis area ($p$=0.01) and better contractility ($p$=0.008). Pathological examination of the hearts showed no significant inflammatory reaction to the jacket except for mild adhesions and no constriction the of epicardial coronary arteries. These authors concluded that passive ventricular constraint prevented the progression of heart failure in pacing induced dilated cardiomyopathy.

Rahman subsequently reported use of the Acorn device in five NYHA III patients revascularized for ischaemic cardiomyopathy with mean LVEF 27% [62]. However, four of these patients underwent left ventricular aneurysm resection, so changes in ventricular dimensions were meaningless. Even so, it was noticeable that there was no significant increase in MVO2 on exercise at 6 months despite the fact that the patients were reported to be NYHA class I. Perhaps the only finding of significance was that the device did not have negative effect on the bypass conduits. Konertz and colleagues from Berlin used the device on 27 stable NYHA class II or III patients with dilated cardiomyopathy [63]. Again, 59% of these patients had concomitant procedures, predominantly mitral valve repair. Of the 11 with isolated use of the polyester jacket changes in left ventricular dynamics were frankly modest over 6 months during which cardiac medication remained virtually unchanged. However, the device did not produce restrictive cardiomyopathy and the patients did not deteriorate over the relatively short follow-up period. Clearly more information is required before passive left ventricular constraint can be deemed successful.

## The Myosplint

McCarthy and the Cleveland Clinic group have developed a different approach to ventricular dilatation based on Laplace's law. The Myosplint (Myocor Inc., Plymouth MN, USA) consists of a set of three rods with wide buttons at either end [64]. The rods are inserted through the left ventricular cavity and the buttons approximated to change the globular left ventricular shape to a bilobular one, thereby reducing the radius of curvature and resulting stress (Fig. 34.35). The device was tested in a dog heart failure model in Cleveland and a bovine model in Lausanne, Switzerland [65]. As the myosplint was tightened progressively left-sided filling pressures and LVEDP decreased significantly at every stage, wall thickening index and peak rate of wall thickening increased significantly. None of the haemodynamic parameters or contractility worsened at any stage with the myosplint. McCarthy then studied acute changes in wall stress in end-stage heart failure patients submitted for transplantation. Five NYHA class IV patients underwent surgical implantation of the myosplint immediately prior to heart transplant to produce a symmetric bilobular left ventricle. Using the short axis echo view at the mid-papillary muscle level, the left ventricular pressure, end-systolic and end-diastolic meridional wall stresses were measured at baseline and after tightening the device. The measurements showed these indices to decrease significantly (−27% and −37%, respectively, $p<0.001$), which suggests that the concept of reshaping towards a bilobular configuration has the potential to improve patients with congestive heart failure. The procedure can be performed without cardiopulmonary bypass, but is not free from risk of bleeding or mitral subvalvar injury.

## The CardioClasp

This product employs two structural elements to geometrically remodel the left ventricle into two widely communicating lobes of smaller radius thereby reducing wall stress. Shimzu and colleagues tested this device in nine dogs with heart failure induced by 4 weeks of rapid ventricular pacing (210 bpm for 3 weeks and 230 bpm for 1 week) [66]. Left ventricular function was then assessed *in vivo* using echocardiography, pressure and aortic flow measurements. The CardioClasp decreased anteroposterior left ventricular dimension by 23 ± 2%. Left ventricular diastolic cross-sectional area decreased (12.0 ± 0.9 to 10.4 ± 1.3 $cm^2$, $p < 0.05$) while the fractional area of contraction increased (0.12 ± 0.01 to 0.26 ± 0.2, $p < 0.05$). LVEDP decreased only slightly (17.4 ± 2.8 to 16.4 ± 2.0 mmHg, $p<0.05$) whilst cardiac output and peak LV systolic pressure were unaltered. The findings show that the CardioClasp can passively reshape the left ventricle thereby reducing the load placed on the myocardium. This leads to improved indices of systolic performance at high levels of ventricular volume, without decreasing contractile mass.

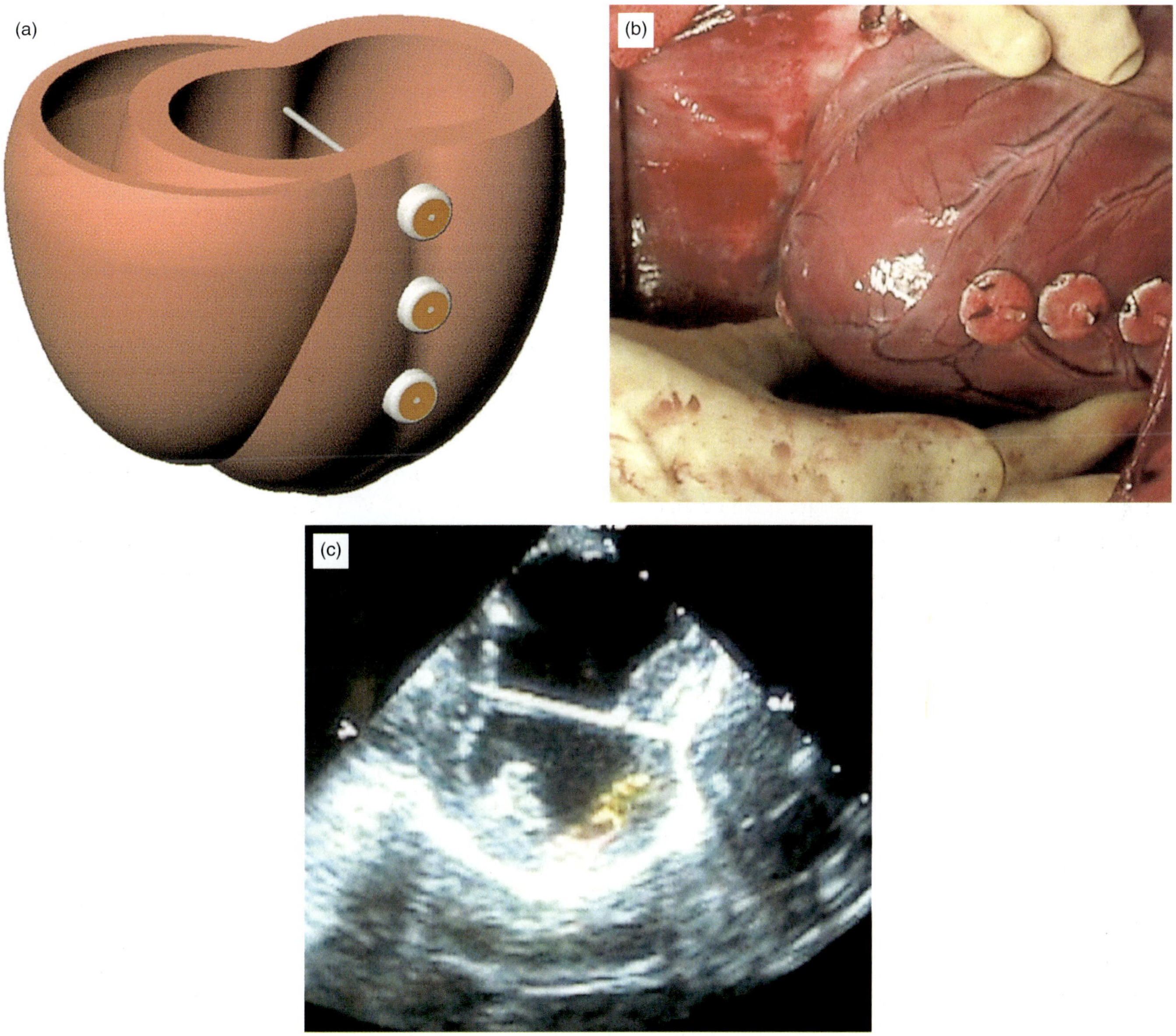


**Figure 34.35** *The Myosplint concept whereby three transventricular rods are used to produce a bilobular configuration to the left ventricle and reduce wall stress. (a) Diagram of the concept, (b) a clinical case, and (c) echocardiography showing the bilobular shape.*

## The MyoTech cardiac restoration system (Hearten Medical Inc., Tustin, CA)

This extraordinary principle of radiofrequency heating to areas of chronic myocardial infarction is based on the fact that scar expansion leads to left ventricular remodelling and ventricular dilatation predicts mortality in congestive heart failure. Previous studies in a sheep model of myocardial infarction demonstrated that bipolar radiofrequency heating of a left ventricular aneurysm with the MyoTech system causes scar shrinkage and sustained left ventricular volume reduction. Based on encouraging animal results, a pilot study of safety and efficacy was carried out by Victal and colleagues in Guadalajara, Mexico [67]. Ten coronary bypass patients with previous myocardial infarction and echocardiographic evidence of akinetic or dyskinetic scar with heart failure and LVEF $< 40\%$ were studied. Baseline and serial cardiac catherizations were performed together with radionucleide ventriculograms and exercise treadmill tests were performed.

After general anaesthesia and sternotomy the MyoTech device was applied to the area of scar on the beating heart before commencing cardiopulmonary bypass. Intraoperative digital photography of the scar demonstrated a remarkable 39% acute reduction in scar area ($p=0.01$) and trans-oesophageal echocardiography performed under the same loading conditions demonstrated a 19% acute reduction in left ventricular end-diastolic volumes ($p=0.002$). Contrast left ventriculography at baseline and 180 days after treatment demonstrated a persistent decrease in LVEDV (28%, $p=0.002$) and LVESV (36%, $p<0.001$), preserved stroke volumes and increased LVEF (26%, $p=0.01$). The investigators concluded that application of the MyoTech device results in acute reduction in scar area and ventricular volumes, which are well maintained 6 months after the intervention. Whether this less invasive intervention can rival or improve on surgical left ventricular restoration remains to be seen.

These new, relatively simple and less invasive approaches aimed at reversal of left ventricular remodelling reflect the substantial current interest in a surgical solution for heart failure patients. The non-transplant treatment of heart failure is an evolving speciality, which requires dedicated centres set apart from transplant units to evaluate these potentially high risk operations. It is important not to allow widespread commercially driven application of these procedures until properly evaluated.

## References


1. Hausmann H, Topp H, Sinaiwski H *et al.* (1997) Decision making in end stage coronary artery disease: revascularization or heart transplant. *Ann Thorac Surg* **64**: 1296–301.
2. Lee KS, Marwick TH, Cook SA *et al.* (1994) Prognosis of patients with left ventricular dysfunction, with and without viable myocardium after myocardial infarction. Relative efficacy of medical therapy and revascularization. *Circulation* **90**: 2687–94.
3. Blondheim DS, Jacobs LE, Kotler NN *et al.* (1991) Dilated cardiomyopathy with mitral regurgitation: decreased survival despite a low frequency of left ventricular thrombus. *Am Heart J* **122**: 763–71.
4. Bach DS, Bolling SF (1996) Improvement following correction of secondary mitral insufficiency in end stage cardiomyopathy with mitral annuloplasty. *Ann J Cardiol* **78**: 966–9.
5. Arais J, Alpret NR, Machennan DH *et al.* (1993) Alterations in sarcoplasmic reticulum gave expansion in human heart failure: a possible mechanism for alterations in cystolic and diastolic properties of the failing myocardium. *Circ Res* **72**: 463–9.
6. Yodshida F, Gould KL (1993) Quantitative relation of myocardial infarct size and myocardial viability log position emission tomography to left ventricular rejection fraction and 3 year mortality with and without revascularization. *J Am Coll Cardiol* **22**: 984–97.
7. Francis GS, Cohn JN, Johnson G *et al.* (1993) Plasma norepiphidrine, plasma renin activity and congestive heart failure: relations to survival and the effects of therapy with V-He FT II. *Circulation* **87** (suppl V): V140–V148.
8. Foxon DP, Myers WO, McCabe CH *et al.* (1986) The influence of surgery on the natural history of angiographically documented left ventricular aneurysm: the coronary artery surgery study. *Circulation* **74**: 100–8.
9. Dor V, Saab M, Coste P *et al.* (1989) Left ventricular aneurysm: a new surgical approach. *J Thorac Cardiovasc Surg* **37**: 11–19.
10. Cooley DA, Collins HA, Morris GG, Chapman DW (1958) Ventricular aneurysm after myocardial infarction: surgical incision with use of temporary cardiopulmonary bypass. *JAMA* **167**: 557–60.
11. Mickleborough LL, Maruyana H, Liu P, Mohamed S (1994) Results of left ventricular aneurysectomy with tailored scar excision and primary closure technique. *J Thorac Cardiovasc Surg* **107**: 690–8.
12. Dor V (1998) Repair of ventricular aneurysm. *Adv Card Surg* **10**: 25–41.
13. Di Donato M, Sabatier M, Dor V *et al.* (1997) Akinetic versus dyskinetic post infarction scar: relation to surgical outcome in patients undergoing endoventricular circular patch platy repair. *J Am Coll Cardiol* **29**: 1569–75.
14. Dor V, Sabatier M, Di Doonato M *et al.* (1998) Efficacy of endoventricular patch platy in large postinfarction akinetic scar and ventricular dysfunction: comparison with a series of large dyskinetic scar. *J Thorac Cardiovasc Surg* **116**: 50.
15. Athanasulsas CL, Stanley AWH, Buckberg GD (1998) Restoration of contractile function in the enlarged left ventricle by exclusion of remodelled akinetic anterior segment. *J Card Surg* **13**: 418–28.
16. Yamaguchi A, Ino T, Adachi H *et al.* (1998) Left ventricular volume predicts postoperative course in patients with ischemic cardiomyopathy. *Ann Thorac Surg* **65**: 434–8.
17. Spotovitz HM, Spotnitz WD, Cottrell TS *et al.* (1974) Cellular basis for volume related wall thickness charges in the rat left ventricle. *J Mol Cell Cardiol* **6**: 317–31.
18. Mickleborough LL, Maruyama H, Yasushi T *et al.* (1995) Results of revascularization in patients with severe left ventricular dysfunction. *Circulation* **92** (suppl II): II73–II79.
19. Batista RJV, Verde J, Nery P *et al.* (1997) Partial left ventriculectomy to treat end-stage heart disease. *Ann Thorac Surg* **64**: 634–8.
20. Angelini GD, Pryn S, Mehta D *et al.* (1997) Left-ventricular-volume reduction for end-stage heart failure. *Lancet* 350–489.
21. Stolf NAG, Moreira LFP, Bocchi EA *et al.* (1998) Determination of mid-term outcome of partial left ventriculectomy in dilated cardiomyopathy. *AnnThorc Surg* **66**: 1963–8.
22. Gradinac S, Miric M, Popovic Z *et al.* (1998) Partial left ventriculectomy for idiopathic dilated cardiomyopathy: Early results and six-month follow-up. *Ann Thorac Surg* **66**: 1963–8.
23. Suma H, Isomura T, Horii T *et al.* Two-year experience of the Batista operation for nonischemic cardiomyopathy. *J Cardiol* **32**: 269–76.
24. Katsumata T, Westaby S (1997) Left ventricular reduction operation in ischemic cardiomyopathy: a note of caution. *Ann Thorac Surg* **64**: 1154–6.
25. Douglas PS, Morrow R, Ioli A, Reichek N (1989) Left ventricular shape, afterload and survival in idiopathic dilated cardiomyopathy. *J Am Coll Cardiol* **13**: 311–15.
26. Dickstein MIL, Sponitz HM, Rose EA, Burkhoff D (1997) Heart reduction surgery: an analysis of the impact on cardiac function. *J Thorac Cardiovasc Surg* **13**: 1032–40.
27. Ratcliffe MB, Hong J, Salahieh A *et al.* (1998) The effect of ventricular volume reduction surgery in the dilated, poorly contractile left ventricle: A simple finite element analysis. *J Thorac Cardiovasc Surg* **116**: 566–77.

28. Fung YC (1997) *Biodynamics–circulation*. New York. Springer, 73–81.
29. Kresh JY, Wechsler AS (1998) Heart reduction surgery can reconstitute the residual stress–strain state of the left ventricle (Letter). *J Thorac Cardiovasc Surg* **116**: 1084–6.
30 McCarthy PM, Starling RC, Wong J *et al.* (1997) Early results with partial left ventriculectomy. *J Thorac Cardiovasc Surg* **114**: 755–6.
31. Fucci C, Sandrelli L, Pardini A *et al.* (1995) Improved results with mitral valve repair using new surgical techniques. *Eur J Cardiothorac Surg* **9**: 621–7.
32. Moreira LFP, Stolf NAG, Bocchi EA *et al.* (1998) Partial left ventriculectomy with mitral valve preservation in the treatment of patients with dilated cardiomyopathy. *J Thorac Cardiovasc Surg* **15**: 800–7.
33. Popovic Z, Miric M, Gradinac S *et al.* (1998) Effects of partial left ventriculectomy on left ventricular performance in patients with nonischemic dilated cardiomyopathy. *J Am Coll Cardiol* **32**: 1801–8.
34. Glantz SA, Parmley WW (1978) Factors which affects the diastolic pressure volume curve. *Circ Res*.
35. Dec GW, Fuster V (1994) Idiopathic dilated cardiomyopathy. *N Eng J Med* **331**: 1564–75.
36. Komeda M, Glasson JR, Bolger AF *et al.* (1997) Papillary muscle-left ventricular wall comples. *J Thorac Cardiovasc Surg* **113**: 292–301.
37. Carpentier A, Chaurand S, Fabiani JN *et al.* (1980) Reconstructive surgery of mitral valve incompetence: ten year appraisal. *J Thorac Cardiovasc Surg* **79**: 338–48.
38. David TE, Ho WC (1986) The effect of preservation of chordae tendinae on mitral valve replacement for postinfarction mitral regurgitation. *Circulation* (suppl I) **I**: 116–20.
39. Bolling SF, Pagani FD, Deeb GM, Bach DS (1998) Intermediate term outcome of mitral reconstruction in cardiomyopathy. *J Thorac Cardiovasc Surg* **115**: 381–8.
40. Bishay ES, McCarthy PM, Cosgrove DM *et al.* (2000) Mitral valve surgery in patients with severe left ventricular dysfunction. *Eur J Cardiothorac Surg* **17**: 213–21.
41. Liel-Cohen N, Guerrero L, Otsuji Y *et al.* (2000) Design of a new surgical approach for ventricular remodelling to achieve ischemic mitral regurgitation. *Circulation* **101**: 2756–63.
42. Burch GE, DePasquale NP (1968) On resting the human heart. *Am J Med* **44**: 165–7.
43. Pfeffer MA, Braunwald E, Moye LA *et al.* (1993) The SAVE investigators. Effect of captopril on mortality and morbidity infarction: results of the Survival and Ventricular Enlargement Trial. *N Engl J Med* **327**: 669–77.
44. Frazier OH, Rose EA, Macmannus Q *et al.* (1992) Multicenter clinical evaluation of the Heartmate 1000 IP left ventricular assist device. *Ann Thorac Surg* **53**: 1080–90.
45. Frazier OhH, Rose EA, McCarthy P *et al.* (1995) Improved mortality and rehabilitation of transplant candidates treated with a long term implantable left-ventricular assist system. *Ann Thorac Surg* **222**: 327–38.
46. Frazier OH (1994) First use of an untethered, vented electric left ventricular assist device for long-term support. *Circulation* **89**(6): 2908–16.
47. Frazier OH, Benedict CR Radovanceric B *et al.* (1996) Improved left ventricular function after chronic left ventricular unloading. *Ann Thorac Surg* **62**: 675–81.
48. Levin HROZMC, Chen JM *et al.* (1995) Reversal of chronic ventricular dilation in patients with end stage cardiomyopathy by prolonged mechanical offloading. *Circulation* **91**: 2717–20.
49. McCarthy PM, Nakatani S, Vargo R *et al.* (1995) Structural and left ventricular histologic changes after implantable LVAD insertion. *Ann Thorac Surg* **59**: 609–13.
50. Moazami N, Argenziano M, Kohmoto T *et al.* (1996) Inflow valve regurgitation interferes with reverse remodelling during LVAD support (Abstract). *Circulation* **94**(suppl I): 293..
51. Catanese K.A, Goldstein DJ, Williams DL *et al.* Outpatient left ventricular assist device support: a destination rather than a bridge.
52. Westaby S, Katsumata T, Houel R *et al.* (1998) Jarvik 2000 heart: potential for bridge to myocyte recovery. *Circulation* **98**: 1568–74.
53. Muller J, Wallukat G, Weng Y *et al.* (1997) Weaning from mechanical support in patients with dilated cardiomyopathy. *Circulation* **96**: 542–9.
54. Hetzer R, Muller JH, Weng YG *et al.* (2000) Midterm follow-up of patients who underwent removal of a left ventricular assist device after cardiac recovery from end-stage dilated cardiomyopathy. *J Thorac Cardiovasc Surg* **120**: 843–55.
55. Martin J, Sarai K, Schindler M *et al.* (1997) MEDOS HIA-VAD biventricular assist device for bridge to recovery in fulminant myocarditis. *Ann Thorac Surg* **63**: 1145–6.
56. Hertzer R, Loebe M, Potapov EV *et al.* (1998) Circulatory support with pneumatic paracorporeal ventricular assist device in infants and children. *Ann Thorac Surg* **66**: 1498–506.
57. Frazier OH (1999) Left ventricular assist device as a bridge to partial left ventriculectomy. *Eur J Cardiothorac Surg* **15**(suppl. I): S20–S5.
58. Furnary AP, Jessup M, Moreira LFF for the American Cardiomyoplasty group. (1996) Multicentre trial of dynamic cardiomyoplasty for chronic heart failure. *J Am Coll Cardiol* **28**: 1175–80.
59. Leier CV (1996) Cardiomyoplasty: is it time to wrap it up. *J Am Coll Cardiol* **28**: 1181–2.
60. Sabbah HN, Chaudhory PA, Paone G *et al.* (1999) Passive ventricular constraint with the Acorn prosthetic jacket prevents progressive left ventricular dilatation and improves ejection fraction in dogs with moderate heart failure (Abstract). *J Am Coll Cardiol* **33**(suppl A): A207.
61. Power JM, Raman J, Byrne M, Alferress C (2000) Passive ventricular constraint in advanced heart failure prevents a further decline in cardiovascular function (Abstract). *J Am Coll Cardiol* **35**(suppl A): A233.
62. Rahman J, Power JM, Buxton B *et al.* (2000) Ventricular constrainment as an adjunctive procedure in ischemic cardiomyopathy. Early results. *Ann Thorac Surg* **70**: 1124–6.
63. Konertz W, Rombeck B, Hotz H *et al.* (2000) Short term safety of the Acorn Cardiac Support Device in patients with advanced heart failure (Abstract). *J Am Coll Cardiol* **35**(suppl A): A182.
64. McCarthy PM, Fukamachi K, Takagaki M *et al.* (2000) Left ventricular shape change reduced left ventricular wall stress in patients with dilated cardiomyopathy (Abstract). *Circulation* **102**(suppl II): II683.
65. Muller XM, Tevaearai HJ, Tucker OP, vonSegesser LK (2000) An alternative to left ventricular volume reduction (Abstract). *Circulation* **102**(suppl II): II501.
66. Shimizu J, Wang J, Yi G-H *et al.* (2000) Improved systolic performance by passive remodelling in experimental heart failure (Abstract). *Circulation* **102**(suppl II): II683.
67. Victal O, Gaxiola E, Najar S *et al.* (2000) Radiofrequency heating of chronic myocardial infarction in patients with congestive heart results in sustained left ventricular volume reduction (Abstract). *Circulation* **102**(suppl II): II503.

# Towards permanent mechanical circulatory support



S. WESTABY, S. SAITO AND O. H. FRAZIER

Since the early 1970s, investigators have worked to develop a reliable, implantable, long-term substitute to replace the left ventricle. At time cardiac transplantation was performed only under an experimental protocol; and cyclosporin, which was introduced to clinical transplantation in the 1980s, was investigational. Twenty years later, cardiac transplantation as a treatment for end-stage heart disease has reached clinical and logistical limitations [1].

A new direction is now needed to address the vast numbers of increasingly elderly patients with advanced left ventricular failure. For the majority the need for total cardiac replacement is questionable. Excision of the native heart is irrecoverable, and it is difficult to decide when this should occur. Many symptomatic patients with dilated or ischaemic cardiomyopathy live for years with reasonable quality of life on modern medical therapy. Long-term mechanical circulatory support supplemented by interventions to improve native heart function is a new direction for the near future. The fact that mechanical off-loading is known to induce myocardial recovery in some patients is exciting [2]. Adjuvant therapies such as revascularization of hibernating myocardium and autogenous skeletal myoblast or stemcell transfer into scar tissue may offer an alternative to complete cardiac replacement [3].

The first use of the artificial heart and left ventricular assist devices (LVADs) in the 1960s demonstrated their feasibility, both as bridges to transplant and as bridges to recovery in the post-cardiotomy patient. Early devices were far from user friendly (Fig. 35.1). In an article published in *Scientific American* (1981) Robert Jarvik, an active researcher who developed the first permanent artificial heart, commented, 'If the artificial heart is ever to achieve its objective, it must be more than a pump, it must be more than functional, reliable and dependable, it must be forgettable'. The supposition that a pulsatile system is required to produce stroke volume and pulse pressure dictates that implantable blood pumps must be large bulky devices, unsuitable for smaller adults and children. The relevance for pulsatility is now questioned. During permanent support with continuous axial flow pumps, synergy develops between the native heart and the LVAD [4]. The circulation is not completely dependent on either, and pump flow as well as native cardiac function can be switched up or down according to metabolic requirement [5]. The continuous flow pump, by lowering the left ventricular pressure as well as left ventricular volume

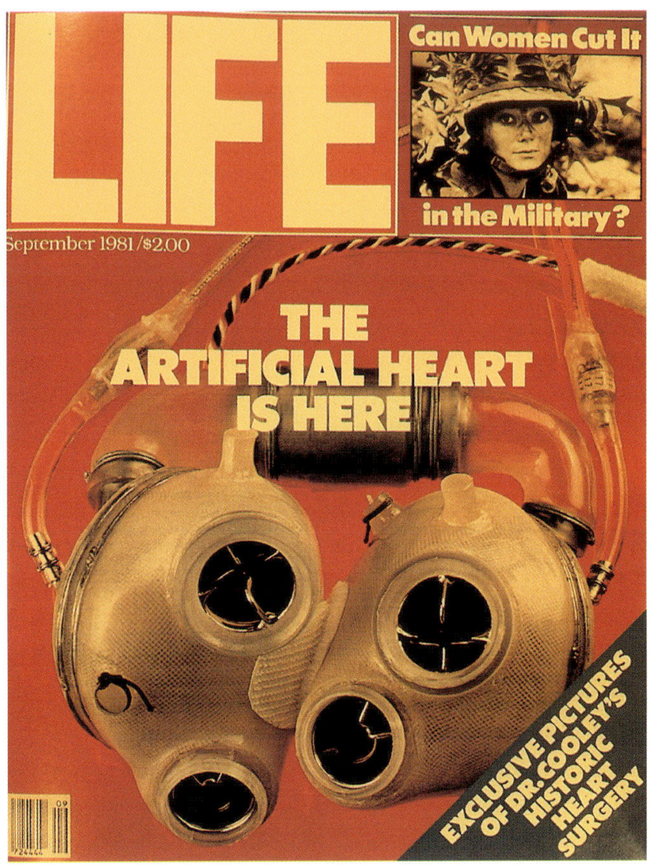


**Figure 37.1** *The front page of* Life *magazine heralding the era of the total artificial heart.*

throughout the cardiac cycle, allows for a return to Starlings's physiology, thereby resulting in improved cardiac function in response to increased blood return to the heart.

The ideal circulatory support system for chronic refractory heart failure must be miniaturized and available for patients of all ages, cost effective, easy to implant and capable of providing a physiologic level of blood flow. With improved devices, the patients should not be left to reach a moribund state with multi-organ failure before a mechanical option is considered. Existing devices such as the pacemaker and implantable defibrillator are already widely accepted and considered cost effective. Within the next 10 years new LVADs will achieve the same status.

## A brief history of blood pump development

By 1900 experiments were already beginning to elucidate the bioengineering principles of cardiac assistance. These involved the displacement of blood from a pumping chamber by means of compression. The chamber then refilled by suction and gravity. In 1930, O.S. Gibbs devised a small rubber bellows with inflow and outflow valves and two separate circuits for the systemic and pulmonary circulation. In 1937 Demikhov produced an artificial heart in Moscow. The device about the size of a normal heart consisted of two membrane pumps side by side primed with physiological saline solution. Demikhov inserted the inflow cannulas to the atrial appendages of a dog and tied them in place with ligatures. The outflow cannulas were introduced into the aorta and pulmonary artery with clamps after which ligatures were tied tightly around the base of each ventricle and the ventricles excised as the pump was switched on. The machine was driven by an electric motor outside the body with the drive shaft of the pump passing through the chest wall. The longest survival in the dogs was 5.5 hours during which cerebral perfusion and respiration were maintained. Demikhov regarded this as a useful method to maintain the organs of a dead donor pending preparation of a transplant recipient [5].

With the development of cardiopulmonary bypass by Gibbon in 1953, heart disease became increasingly amenable to surgical treatment with a need for more prolonged cardiac support when it was impossible to wean from the extracorporeal circuit. In 1958 Atsumi of Tokyo University developed a hydraulically driven plastic heart which maintained a dog's circulation for 6 hours. Two years later this group successfully provided biventricular support for 13 hours with a completely different roller pump device driven by a miniature motor. The main problem with these early machines was thrombosis. The Japanese team attempted to avoid this by building a bellows type of pump lined with silicone rubber. With this they succeeded in keeping one dog alive for 27 hours, although the majority died from pulmonary oedema or cerebral embolism. Atsumi soon identified the complex problems of achieving a physiological circulation with a mechanical blood pump. In particular, the human heart does not influence venous return or systemic arterial pressure, but accommodates changes in both. These workers identified the need for a sophisticated control system in an artificial heart so that appropriate mechanical responses could accommodate hormonal, biochemical and physiological pressure changes.

In 1959 Kolff (the pioneer of renal dialysis) and his Japanese colleague (and cardiac surgeon) Tetsuzo Akutsu implanted a pendulum type of artificial heart into a dog. The ventricles of this pump emptied alternatively maintaining a blood pressure >80 mmHg for 5 hours. Three days later they implanted a different type of biventricular roller-pump device with a valve on each side corresponding to the aortic and pulmonary valves. By 1965 this team had developed a one-piece, four-chambered heart (Fig. 35.2) which was implanted orthotopically into the pericardial sac of a calf which lived for 31 hours. At the same time the Argentinian physician Domingo Liotta developed an interest in artificial heart technology during postgraduate surgical training in France. He returned to the

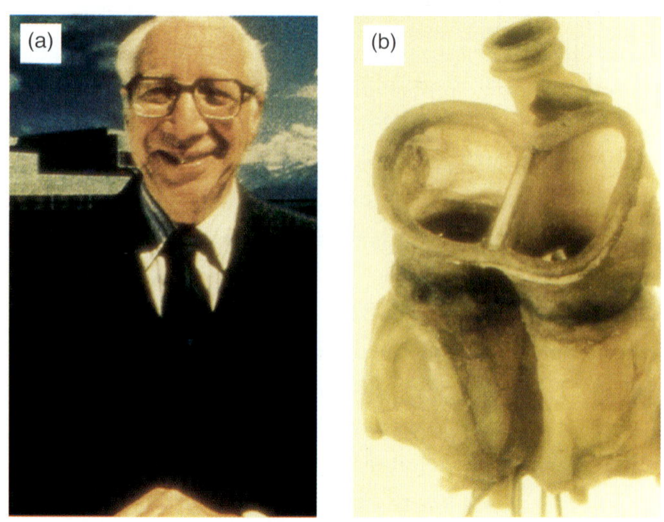


**Figure 35.2** *(a) Kolff and (b) his first total artificial heart.*

University of Cordoba and established his own artificial heart research programme using plastics obtained from an aeroplane factory run by immigrant German generals. With financial backing from the Ministry of Health Liotta constructed one of the world's first implantable artificial hearts and presented the work at the American Society for Artificial Organs (1960). Kolff invited Liotta to work at the Cleveland Clinic, but had difficulty in attracting research funds. When De Bakey learned of Liotta's device he offered him financial backing and extensive laboratory facilities at Baylor University.

DeBakey initiated work on an implantable left ventricular support device, feeling that more immediate clinical applicability would be possible with this technology. The first pump to be used clinically took blood from the left atrium to the descending aorta using a reinforced Dacron silastic tube-type pump. Ball valves at each end provided unidirectional flow produced by a second surrounding tube connected to an external source of compressed air. The pump sequence was syncronized with the 'R' wave of the electrocardiogram. This apparatus successfully supported the left ventricle of experimental animals without significant haemolysis. In 1963 De Bakey first used the LVAD to sustain a postoperative patient who had suffered a cardiac arrest and hypoxic cerebral damage. The LVAD worked successfully for 4 days, but it was determined that the patient had suffered irreversible brain damage, and support was discontinued.

Meanwhile Harken in Boston explored the concept of the diastolic counter pulsation to reduce cardiac after-load and augment blood flow during diastole. Harken's pump was a large extra-corporeal device, which was first used clinically by the De Bakey team in 1966. Counter-pulsation assisted weaning from cardiopulmonary bypass, but was insufficient to prevent death after several days of support. The principles of diastolic counterpulsation were later developed by Harken and Kolff at the Cleveland Clinic and adapted by the Kantrowitz and Mouloupolos in the form of a balloon catheter, which could be introduced into the aorta and inflated during diastole. The intra-aortic balloon pump is now widely used for postcardiotomy support and the treatment of cardiogenic shock.

De Bakey then reverted to his original pulsatile LVAD (Fig. 35.3) now lined with velour cloth to prevent clotting.

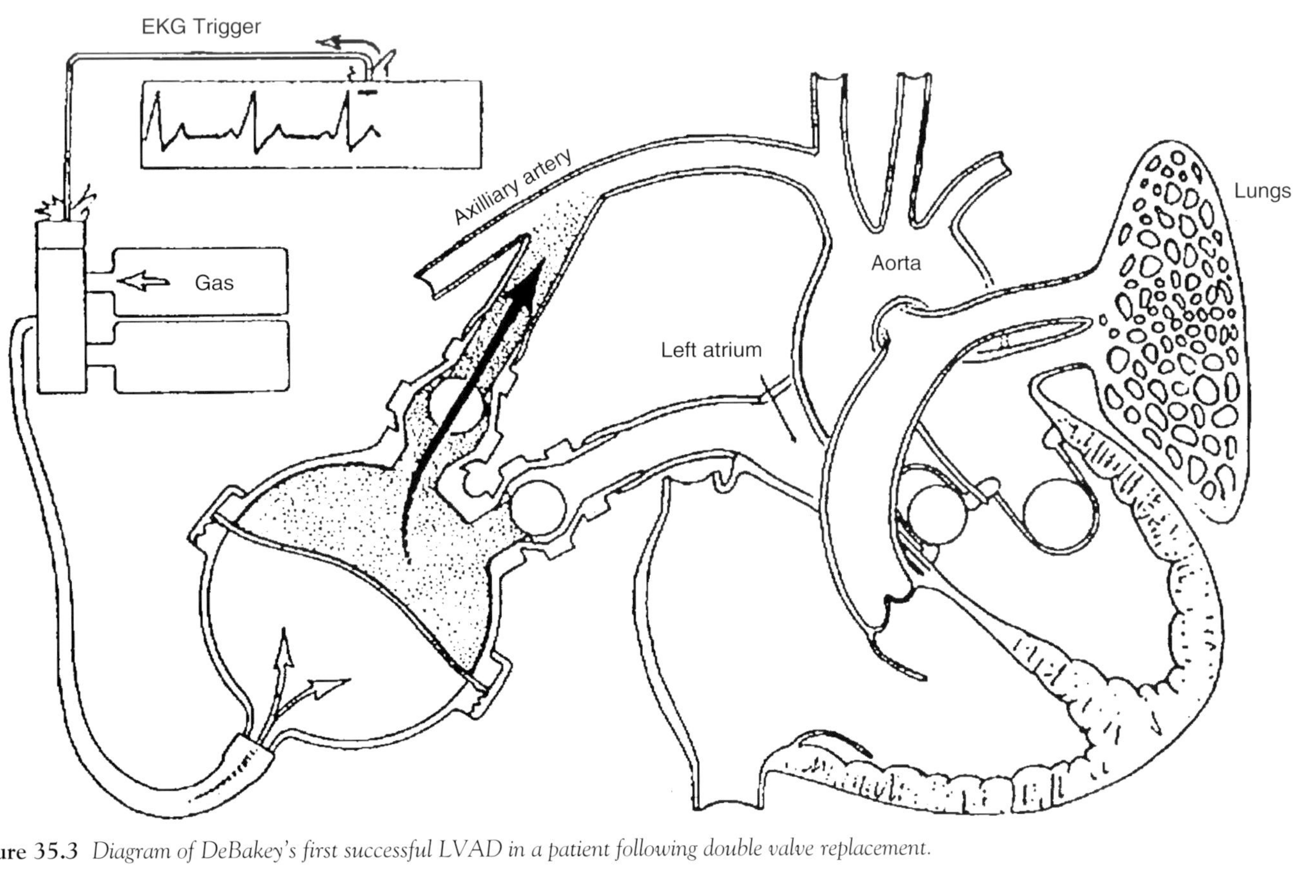


**Figure 35.3** *Diagram of DeBakey's first successful LVAD in a patient following double valve replacement.*

On 8 August 1966 the pulsatile tube device was used in a 37-year-old female who was critically ill with rheumatic aortic and mitral valve disease. After double valve replacement she could not be weaned from cardiopulmonary bypass and the LVAD was used with great success.

The pump maintained a physiological blood flow and after 10 days of support the patient was weaned from the device and discharged from hospital. This was the first successful use of an LVAD for postcardiotomy bridge to recovery [6].

The following year Barnard demonstrated that the human heart could be removed and replaced with a donor organ [7]. By August 1968 Cooley's transplant team at the Texas Heart Institute had overtaken all other units including Cape Town. When donor hearts became scarce, Cooley encouraged Liotta to resurrect his total artificial heart consisting of two airdriven diaphragm reciprocating pumps consisting of Dacron impregnated silastic (Fig. 35.4). The pumps were activated by two external power units with a pulse timer to determine ventricular rate. Uni-directional flow was regulated by the recently designed Wada/Cutter hingeless mechanical valve prosthesis. On Good Friday, 4 April 1969 the first clinical total artificial heart implant was performed by the Cooley team as bridge to transplantation, when the patient's own heart could not be weaned from cardiopulmonary bypass after left ventricular aneurysm resection. The total artificial heart maintained both the systemic and pulmonary circulation for 3 days until a donor heart was implanted. In the interim the patient developed acute renal failure and progressive anaemia due to haemolysis. The donor heart obtained in desperation failed 32 hours later and the patient died. In the *Herald Tribune* (14 July 1969), Kolff wrote 'the implantation of an artificial heart in Houston, Texas on April 4 was a step forward in medical history'. Cooley, Liotta and others kept the patient alive for 64 hours with a mechanical heart before he received a donor heart. Whilst the patient eventually died of infective complications after the second operation, the important fact is that the Houston doctors proved that an artificial heart can indeed replace a natural one in man [11].

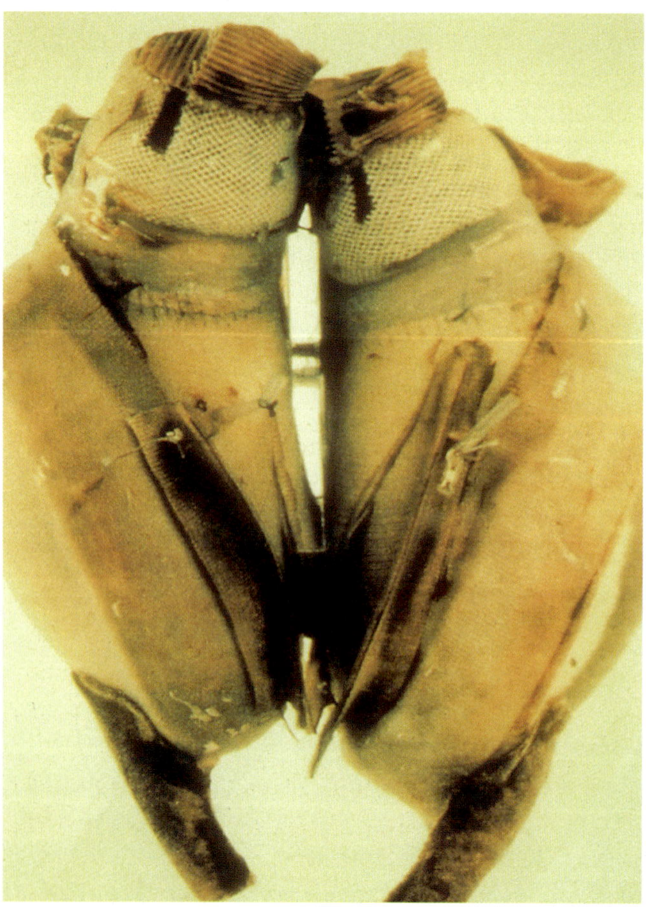

**Figure 35.4** *The Liotta double ventricle heart.*

In 1970 Jarvik joined Kolff's artificial heart programme, now at the University of Utah. The Utah team switched the emphasis from electrically driven hearts to pneumatically powered devices with an intensive programme to refine biocompatibility and durability. The Jarvik 7 Heart consisted of two ventricles made of polyurethane supported on an aluminium base (Fig. 35.5). Rings of polycarbonate supported Bjork–Shiley disc valves. For the animal implants the natural ventricles were excised and polyurethane cuffs sutured to the atrial remnants, the transected aorta and the main pulmonary artery. The procedure essentially

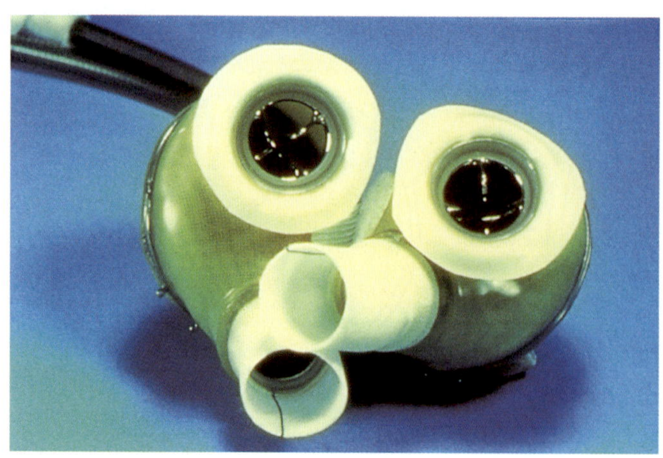

**Figure 35.5** *The Jarvik 7 total artificial heart.*

mimicked cardiac transplantation, but with a mechanical device. The separate left and right ventricles of the device were then snapped on to the polyurethane cuffs and connected to an external driving system by means of two tubes traversing the thoracic wall. Survival up to 221 days was achieved with the longest surviving calf growing from a weight of 200 lb to more than 350 lb (Fig. 35.5). The calf was able to walk on a treadmill for an hour even though it was twice the size of an intended recipient human. Biochemical parameters of renal and hepatic function remained normal for most of the calf's existence.

In December 1982 after more than $160 million of Federal funds had been invested in artificial heart development, the University of Utah team led by the surgeon DeVries, performed the first operation to deliberately replace a human heart with a permanent mechanical device [8]. There were many problems both during and after the surgery. At the end of the operation the chest could not be closed over the device, but despite this the patient regained consciousness in 3 hours and moved all extremities on command. On the 4th and 5th postoperative days haemolysis caused progressive renal failure. A programmed increase in cardiac output to 12 l/min. caused epileptic convulsions. On day 13 the rapid onset of pulmonary oedema heralded acute mechanical heart failure following strut fracture of the Bjork–Shiley mitral valve. The patient was returned to the operating table and the valve replaced. Death eventually occurred through multi-organ failure on the 112th postoperative day (Fig. 35.7) The programme was subsequently continued in Louisville with private funding by the Humana Hospital group. The longest surviving patient with any single artificial devices was Bill Schroeder, who lived longer than 2 years before dying of a stroke. More than 160 further Jarvik 7 Hearts were used for bridge to transplantation and one female patient was sustained for 620 days [9].

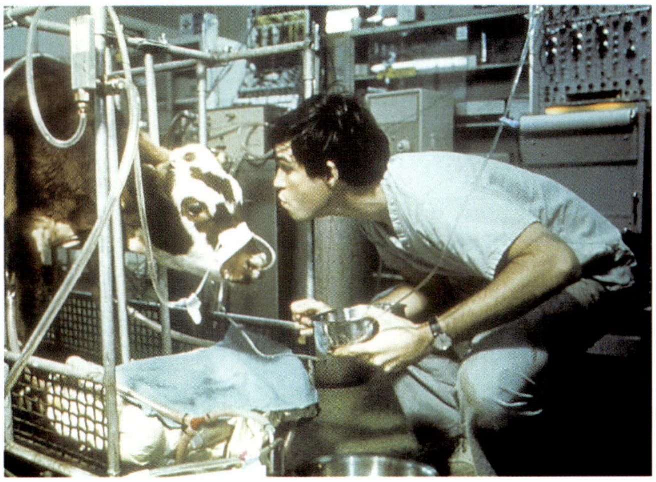

**Figure 35.6** *Young Robert Jarvik with a calf in Utah.*

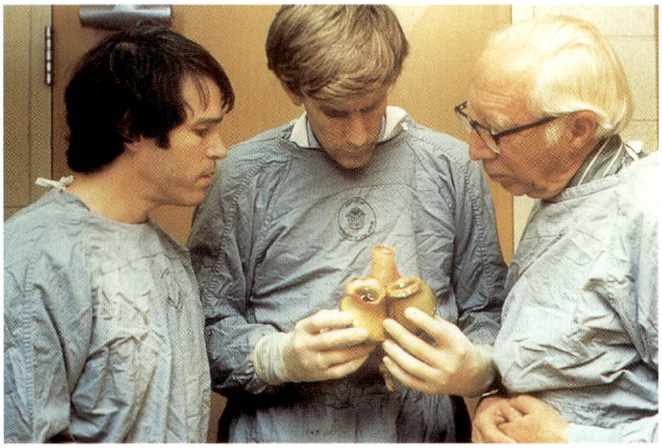

**Figure 35.7** *Jarvik, De Vries and Kolff examine the explanted Jarvik 7 heart.*

During the early 1970s Pierce and coworkers at the Pennsylvania State University designed a successful external artificial ventricle comprising of a thin-walled blood sac of segmented polyurethane housed in a spheroidal-shaped polysulphate casing (Fig. 35.8) [10]. A membrane dissected the mid-part of the spherical chamber and was inflated and deflated by a pneumatic drive control unit syncronized with the R-wave of the electrocardiogram. The forerunner of the Thoratec system, the Pennsylvania State device was used clinically by withdrawing blood either from the apex of the left ventricle or from the left atrium with return to the aorta. For right ventricular assistance the inflow cannula was placed in the right atrium and the outflow graft anastomosed to the pulmonary artery. Between 1976 and 1982 Pierce's group employed left ventricular assistance in 22 patients, right ventricular assistance in two and biventricular support in six. Fourteen patients were successfully separated from the pump with nine survivors. The Thoratec system is now commonly used for bridge to transplantation and is a less expensive, but effective alternative to the implantable LVADs.

In 1978 the Texas Heart team undertook the first implantation of an LVAD for staged cardiac transplantation. The patient was a 21-year-old man who had developed ischaemic ventricular contracture immediately after undergoing double valve replacement. His heart never

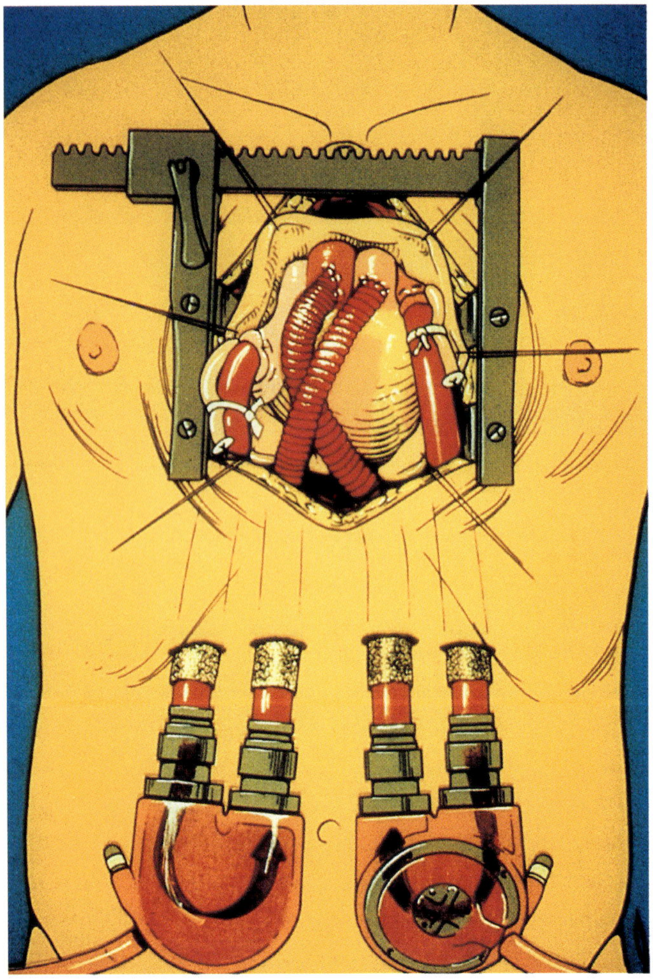

**Figure 35.8** *The Pennsylvania State University external biventricular support system, the forerunner of the Thoratec system.*

recovered so an abdominally positioned single chambered externally powered LVAD was implanted and supported the circulation for 5 days. A suitable donor heart was found and transplantation performed thereby proving the potential for LVADs in the bridge to transplant setting. Akutsu then joined Cooley in Houston and developed a biventricular polyurethane total artificial heart with Bjork–Shirley mechanical valves. This (Fig. 35.1) was air driven by an external electrical power supply and a drive console with a sophisticated monitoring system. Cooley implanted the artificial heart into a patient on 23 July 1981 after an unsuccessful coronary bypass operation. The device maintained the cardiac output between 3.5 and 4 l/min, but its bulk compressed the left-sided pulmonary veins causing pulmonary oedema and hypoxia. Sixty hours later transplantation was undertaken, but the patient died from multi-organ failure. Soon afterwards *Time* announced that 'the Artificial Heart' was here (Fig. 35.1) but it was clear to many in the field that total heart replacement with a biventricular device and pneumatically powered external console would be difficult on both quality of life and economic grounds.

The concept of long-term implantable left ventricular assistance was stimulated by the failure of the broad application of cardiac transplantation in the first era centred around broad-spectrum immune suppression with Imuran and steroids. The one use of the total artificial heart by Cooley in 1969 also demonstrated limitations of this technology in a contaminated patient with a broad-based bone marrow suppressant like Imuran. Because of this, research was directed toward the development of a fully implantable device for left chronic left ventricular support. This seemed more achievable from an anatomic, economic, and physiologic standpoint than a total artificial heart. The elements of this programme, were outlined in the LVAD conference at the NHLBI in 1974 and were further defined with the RFPs issued in 1977 (Request for Proposal RFP NHLBI-HV-77-8. Left Heart Assist Blood Pumps; and RFP NHLBI-77-9. Development of Electrical Energy Converters to Power and Control Left Heart Assist Devices) and with the assignment of John Watson and Frank Altieri to direct the NHLBI support of this effort. In 1980, a final RFP for the development of a fully implantable, chronic left ventricular assist device was issued (RFP NHLBI 80-3). The basic technologies currently being used clinically evolved from this proposal. The new LVADS were characterized by two important features, implantability and pulsatility. The major goals were mechanical durability and reliability exceeding 2 years with a tether-free system. One of the major problems in designing implantable, electrically powered, moving diaphragm type pumps for long-term use was the means to compensate for changes in air volume within the motor housing. Unless the system was satisfactorily vented a negative pressure would develop behind the pumping diaphragm and prevent its movement. Venting could be achieved by a percutaneous tube open to the atmosphere or an implantable compliance chamber where air is displaced into a bag within the thoracic cavity. Implanted compliance chambers were tested, but failed when fibrous tissue encapsulated the exterior of the chamber and decreased their flexibility, or gas within the chamber gradually escaped. The longest these devices were maintained experimentally was less than 200 days.

With the introduction of the immunosuppressive cyclosporin in the 1980s, cardiac transplantation evolved from a controversial experimental operation to an accepted therapeutic strategy for a broader patient group. Cyclosporin, unlike Imuran (or azathioprine) spared the non-specific immune system, allowing infected and contaminated patients to be successfully transplanted [11].

Since donor organs were not always available for these critically ill patients, it became apparent that the newly developed implantable LVADs could be used for these patients to allow support and survival until transplantation became possible. Frazier and coworkers at the Texas Heart Institute collaborated with the ThermoCardio Systems (TCI) group to develop and externally vented pusher plate LVAD with a portable power source (Fig. 35.9).

On 5 September 1984 Oyer at Stanford University implanted the electric Novacor LVAD (Fig. 35.10) into a moribund 51-year-old man with ischaemic cardiomyopathy. The patient was transplanted 9 days later and survived a stormy postoperative course to become the first successful bridge to transplant with an implantable LVAD designed for long-term use.

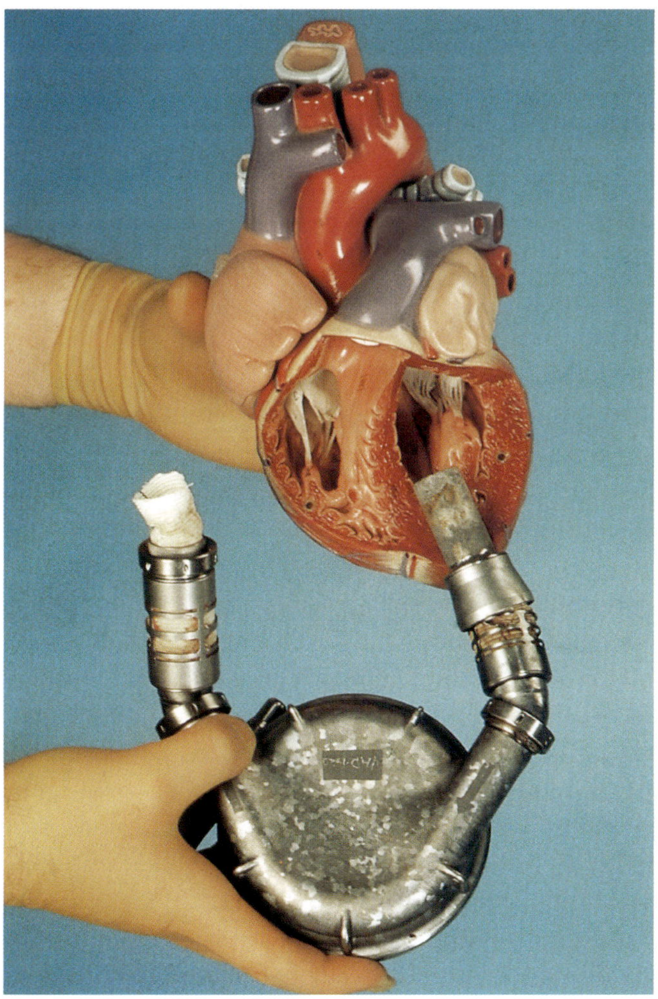

**Figure 35.9** *The ThermoCardio Systems (TCI) externally vented pusher plate LVAD.*

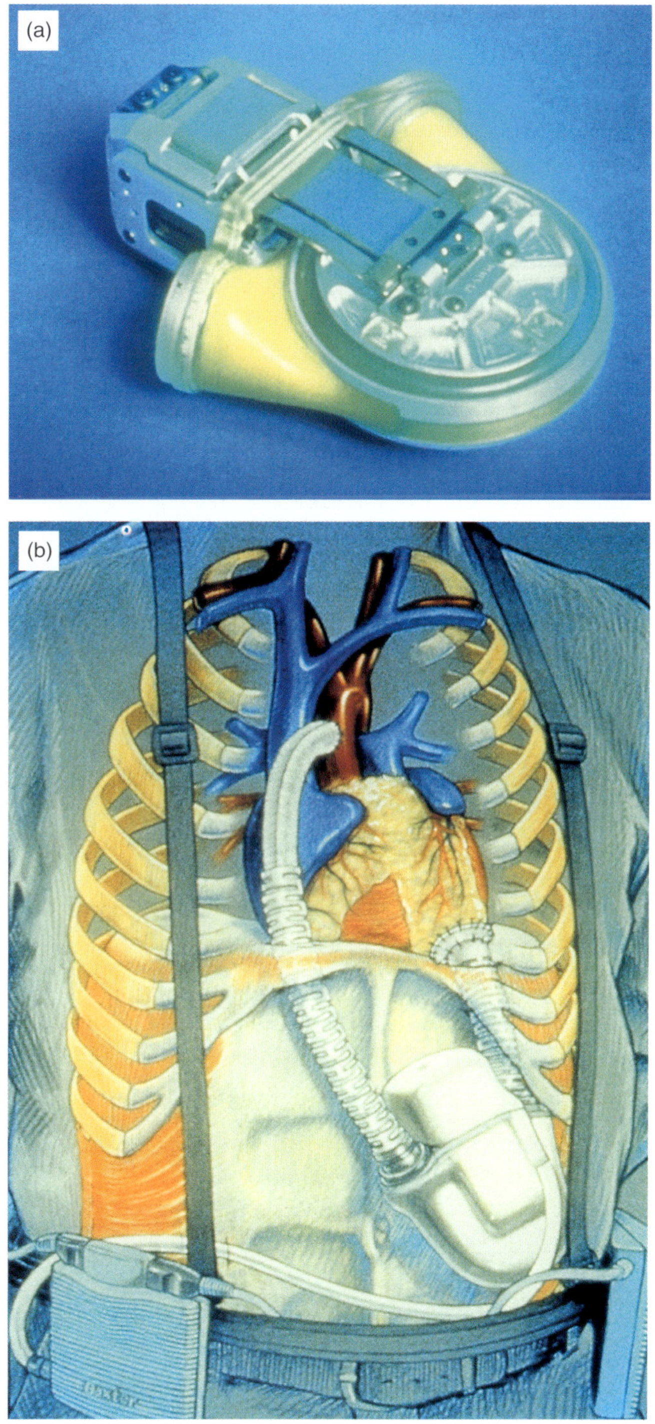


**Figure 35.10** *(a) The Novacor LAD, (b) diagram illustrating the Novacor LVAD* in situ.

On 6 September 1984 Hill at Pacific Medical Centre, San Francisco used the external pneumatic Pierce Donachy LVAD from Thoratec Laboratories to support a 47-year-old man with postinfarction cardiogenic shock. The man was transplanted and survived after a protracted and complicated course. On 6 March 1985 Vaughan and Copland excised a failed orthotopic transplant from a 33-year-old man and used the Jarvik 7 total artificial heart for 36 hours prior to a second transplant. Whilst this patient succumbed from bleeding and pulmonary oedema, the same team (on 29 August) used the Jarvik 7 in a 25-year-old man with cardiomyopathy and cardiogenic shock. The device sustained the patient for 9 days after which cardiac transplantation was successful and he became the first patient to leave hospital after use of an orthotopic total artificial heart. In 1986 the Food and Drugs Administration (USA) gave permission for the pneumatic TCI LVAD to be used in patients. The first device was air driven through a line attached to a 73 lb external console, which the patient could on a cart (Fig. 35.11).

In the meantime engineers at ThermoCardio Systems developed an electrically powered version that could be used with a battery pack small enough to be worn by the patient. The electrically powered version has an identical pumping chamber to the pneumatic device featuring a textured centred titanium surface, which proved resistant to thromboembolism (Fig. 35.12). The electric motor sits in a chamber below the flexible diaphragm and makes one revolution for each heart beat. The first electric TCI LVAD was implanted by Frazier for bridge to transplantation on 9 May 1994 [12]. Westaby then used the electric TCI LUAD as a permanent support device for non-transplant eligible patients in the UK.

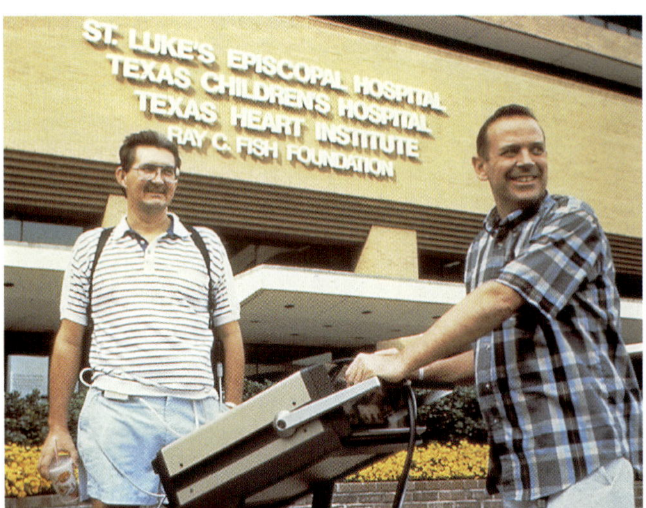


**Figure 35.11** *Patients with the TCI LVAD at the Texas Heart Institute.*

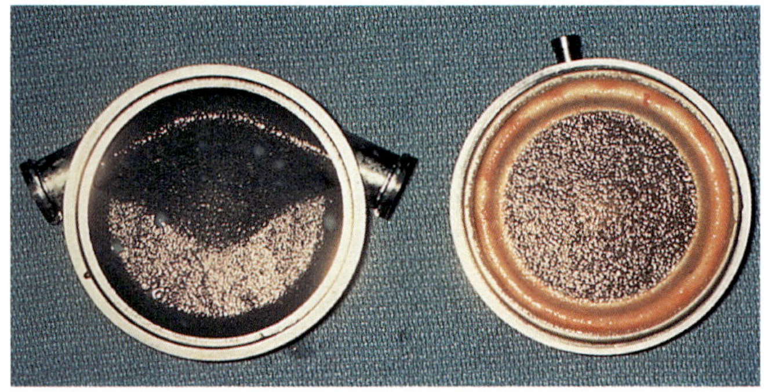

**Figure 35.12** *The textured internal surface of the pumping chamber of the TCI LVAD designed to promote an endothelial lining in order to reduce thromboembolism.*

In 1992 and 1993 the United Network for Organ Sharing (USA) gave the mean waiting times for donor hearts of all blood types as 208 and 245 days, respectively. Long waiting times were often fatal, particularly for male patients with type O blood group weighing more than 200 lb who would wait a mean of 595 days for a donor heart. At least one-third of these highly selective patients under 60 years of age died on the waiting list. Whilst the cost of an LVAD and maintenance were considerable, these proved less than a median waiting time of 75 days in an intensive care unit.

Bridge-to-transplant experience soon demonstrated dramatic physiological rehabilitation and reduced mortality for patients awaiting transplantation with an LVAD [13]. Resolution of renal and hepatic dysfunction improved the patients, physical capacity and quality of life. As experience with bridges to transplant grew it became clear that post-transplant survival of patients treated with an LVAD was better than survival for those who waited without [14]. As LVAD patients improved to NYHA I status they were transferred out of the intensive care unit to a regular floor and eventually discharged from the hospital to wait at home for their transplant. This experience was soon paralleled in European transplant units. Survival beyond 2 years with both the TCI 'HeartMate' and Novacor LVADs confirm the ability of these pumps to support the circulation artificially for extended periods. Nevertheless complications in the form of drive-line infection (Fig. 35.13), thromboembolism and mechanical failure accounted for substantial morbidity with these devices [15–17]. The full

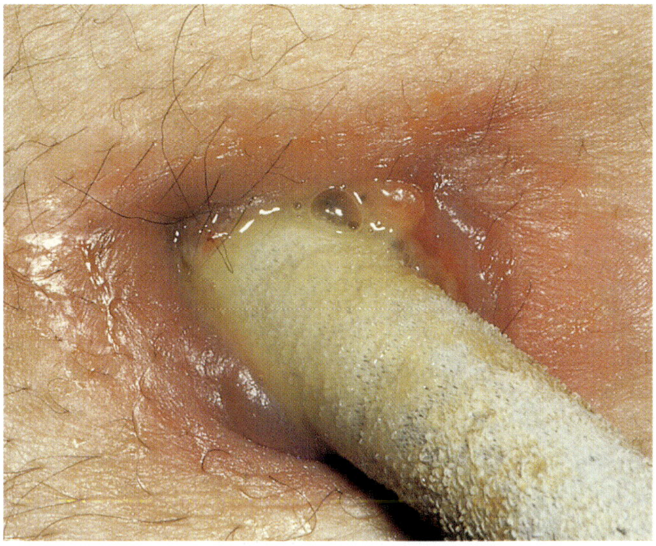

**Figure 35.13** *Drive-line infection in a TCI LVAD.*

range of mechanical cardiac assist systems available for clinical use up to the end of 1998 are shown in Table 35.1. Recently a new fully implantable pusher plate LVAD with transcutaneous energy delivery (Figs 35.14) has been introduced by Arrow. This 'Lionheart' LVAD was first implanted by Korfer in Bad Oyenhausen.

## The physiology of left ventricular support

The TCI and Novacor LVADs both employ a pusher plate mechanism (Fig. 35.15) to eject blood in a pulsatile manner providing stroke volume similar to that of a vigorous left ventricle. The Novacor has a smooth polyurethane blood sac and utilizes bovine pericardial valves to provide unidirectional blood flow. The pump has a maximum stroke volume of 70 ml and can pump in excess of 10 l/min at rates as high as 240 beats/min. The patients are anti-coagulated with both warfarin and aspirin to minimize thromboembolism from the inflow conduit or smooth blood sac. Electrical energy is converted into hydraulic work, which ejects blood from the pump. The electric power cable is brought out percutaneously from the right lower quadrant of the abdomen and connects to an extra-corporeal control console and battery power system.

The interior of the pumping chamber of the TCI 'HeartMate' promotes formation of a pseudoneointima on the blood contacting surface, which lowers the risk of thromboembolism so that anticoagulation with warfarin is unnecessary [18]. This pump has a stroke volume of 85 ml and a maximum pump output of 11 l/min. It is operated at

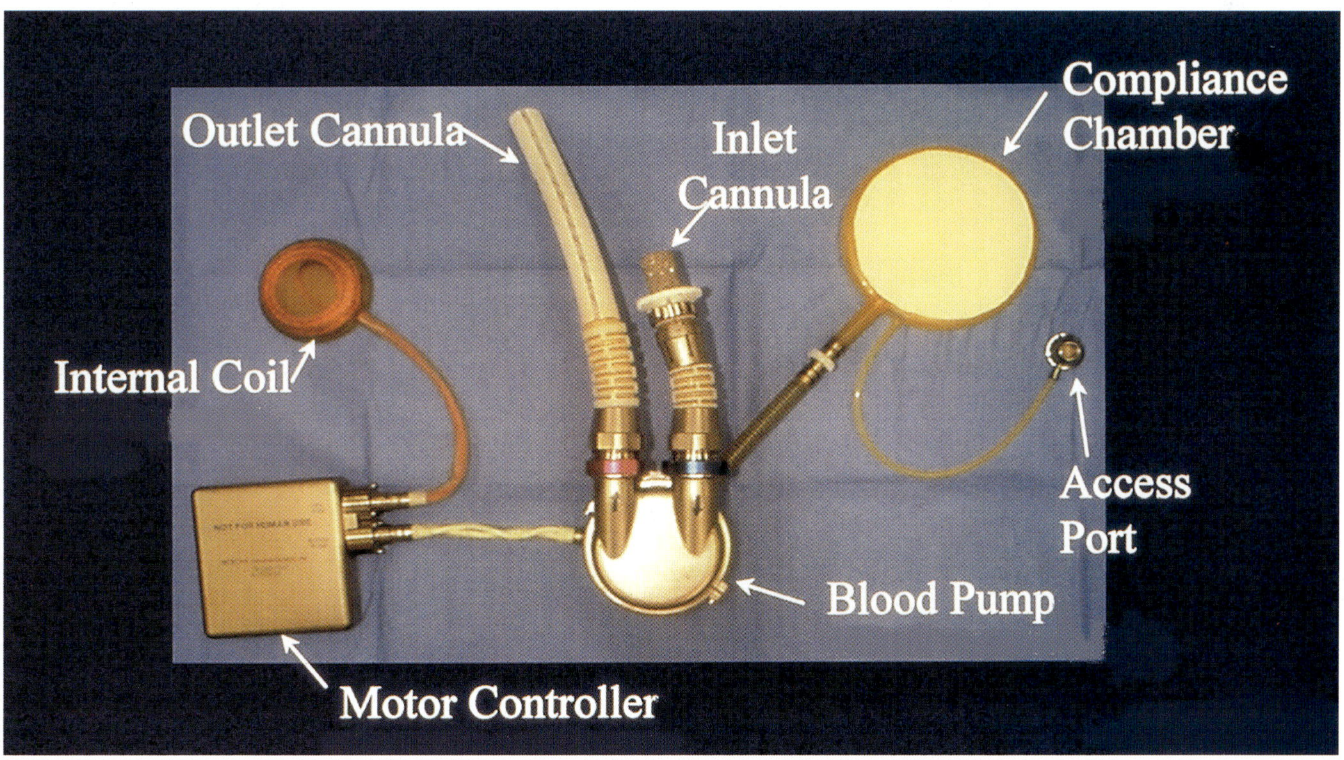


**Figure 35.14** *The 'Lionheart' implantable LVAD with compliance chamber and transcutaneous power induction.*

**Table 35.1** Range of mechanical cardiac assist systems (2000)

| System | Implantation site | Energy source | Nature of flow | Level of assist | Flow rate | Bridge to | Adult or paediatric |
|---|---|---|---|---|---|---|---|
| IABP (Intra-aortic balloon pump) | Intra-aortic | Pneumatic | Pulsatile | Partial | NA | Recovery | Adult |
| ECMO/CPS (Extracorporeal membrane oxygenation. cardiopulmonary support system) | Extracorporeal | Electrical | Continuous | Partial | 2 1/min | Recovery | Adult/paediatric |
| **Rotary pumps** | | | | | | | |
| Biomedicus (Medtronic)<br>Delphin (Sarns 3M)<br>Lifestream (St Jude)<br>HiFlow (Medos) | Para-corporeal (uni- or bi-ventricular) | Electrical | Continuous/ pulsatile | Partial | 5 l/min | Recovery (Tx*) | Adult/paediatric |
| **External heterotopic ventricles** | | | | | | | |
| Abiomed BVS-5000 | Para-corporeal (uni- or bi-ventricular) | Pneumatic | Pulsatile | Partial or total | 2–5 l/min | Recovery (Tx) | Adult |
| Nippon Zeon | | | | | 2–6 l/min | Tx (recovery) | Adult |
| Thoratec | | | | | 1.3–7 l/min | Tx (recovery) | Adult |
| Berlin Heart | | | | | 0.6–7 l/min | Tx (recovery) | Adult/paediatric |
| Medos | | | | | 0.6–7 l/min | Tx (recovery) | Adult/paediatric |
| **Orthotopic total artificial heart** | | | | | | | |
| CardioWest | Intra-corporeal | Pneumatic | Pulsatile | Total | 4–10 l/min | Tx | Adult |
| **Internal heterotopic ventricles** | | | | | | | |
| TCI Heartmate | Intra-corporeal (uni-ventricular) | Pneumatic electrical | Pulsatile | Total | 4–10 l/min | Tx/recovery | Adult |
| Novacor | Intra-corporeal (uni-ventricular) | Pneumatic electrical | Pulsatile | Total | 4–10 l/min | Tx/recovery | Adult |
| Lionheart | Fully implanted (univentricular) | Electrical | Pulsatile | Total | 4–10 l/min | Tx/recovery/ permanent | Adult |
| **Axial flow pumps** | | | | | | | |
| Jarvik 2000 Heart | Intra-corporeal | Non-pulsatile | Continuous | Partial | 2–8 l/min | Tx/recovery permanent | Adult |

Adapted from Alain Pavie M.D. Frontiers in Heart Failure Treatment, 1998.

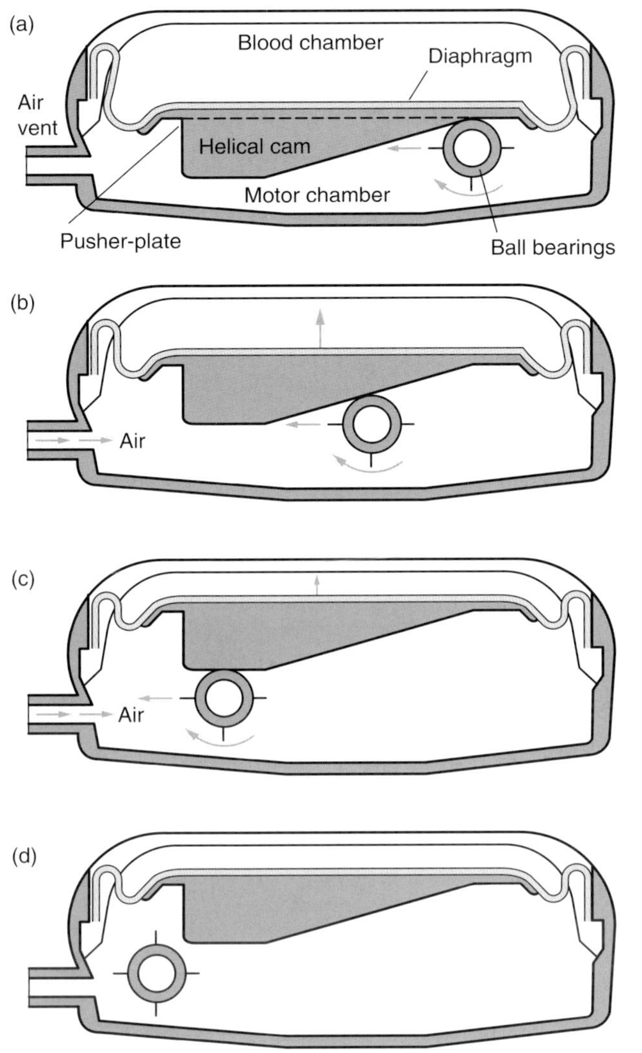


**Figure 35.15** *The pumping mechanism of the TCI pusher plate LVAD.*

either a fixed number of beats per minute or more commonly in automatic mode, which follows venous drainage similar to normal physiology. In automatic mode the device ejects when the blood sac has reached 90% filling and with activity the pump automatically increases. Blood flows in one direction determined by 25 mm porcine xenograft valves located in the inflow and outflow conduits. Typically both pumps capture all transmitral flow via the apex of the left ventricle so that aortic valve does not open. Pump output to the ascending aorta is therefore equivalent to the cardiac output. However, after a period of support the native left ventricle may improve in function and eject blood through the aortic valve in addition to pump output. These powerful mechanical blood pumps eliminate wall tension from the off-loaded ventricle and approximately double flow over preoperative values in heart failure patients. Because the native right and left ventricles function in series the increased flow to the systemic circulation causes increased venous return to the right ventricle. Consequently the right ventricle must boost its cardiac output to the amount being pumped by the LVAD. In practice, right ventricular overload and congestive heart failure are ameliorated by the positive effects of an LVAD on the pulmonary circulation [19]. Left ventricular failure causes substantial passive pulmonary hypertension secondary to elevated left atrial and pulmonary venous pressures. Right ventricular performance is after-load dependent so that pulmonary congestion impairs right ventricular function even in patients with normal pulmonary vascular resistance. LVADs produce a dramatic reduction in right ventricular after-load by reversing passive pulmonary hypertension. This is the direct result of reduced left heart filling pressures as the LVAD conveys blood from the pulmonary veins to the systemic circulation.

Decreased right ventricular after-load has an important beneficial effect on right heart function during LVAD support particularly in patients with relatively normal pulmonary vascular resistance (Fig. 35.16). In those with fixed elevated pulmonary vascular resistance from chronic obstructive airways disease or blood transfusions, this benefit may not be as apparent. Pulmonary pressures may remain elevated with increased flow through the fixed resistance.

Left ventricular unloading during LVAD support results in a reduction in left ventricular volume and pressure. This causes a marked leftward shift of the inter-ventricular septum as a result of changes in the transseptal pressure gradient. Right ventricular compliance improves and enhances right ventricular stroke work [20]. However, the contribution of the left ventricle to right ventricular contractility is reduced and the net result is a balanced effect on right ventricular performance. The anatomic systolic interaction between the unloaded left and right ventricles is determined by the compliance of the interventricular septum. Systolic interaction is decreased when the interventricular septum is hypertrophied and enhanced when the intraventricular septum is thinned in dilated cardiomyopathy. Experience shows that right ventricular ischaemia, bi-ventricular infarction, cardiomyopathy or severe pulmonary hypertension are the major factors that cause right ventricular failure. The net effect of an LVAD is to sustain the systemic circulation, eliminate left

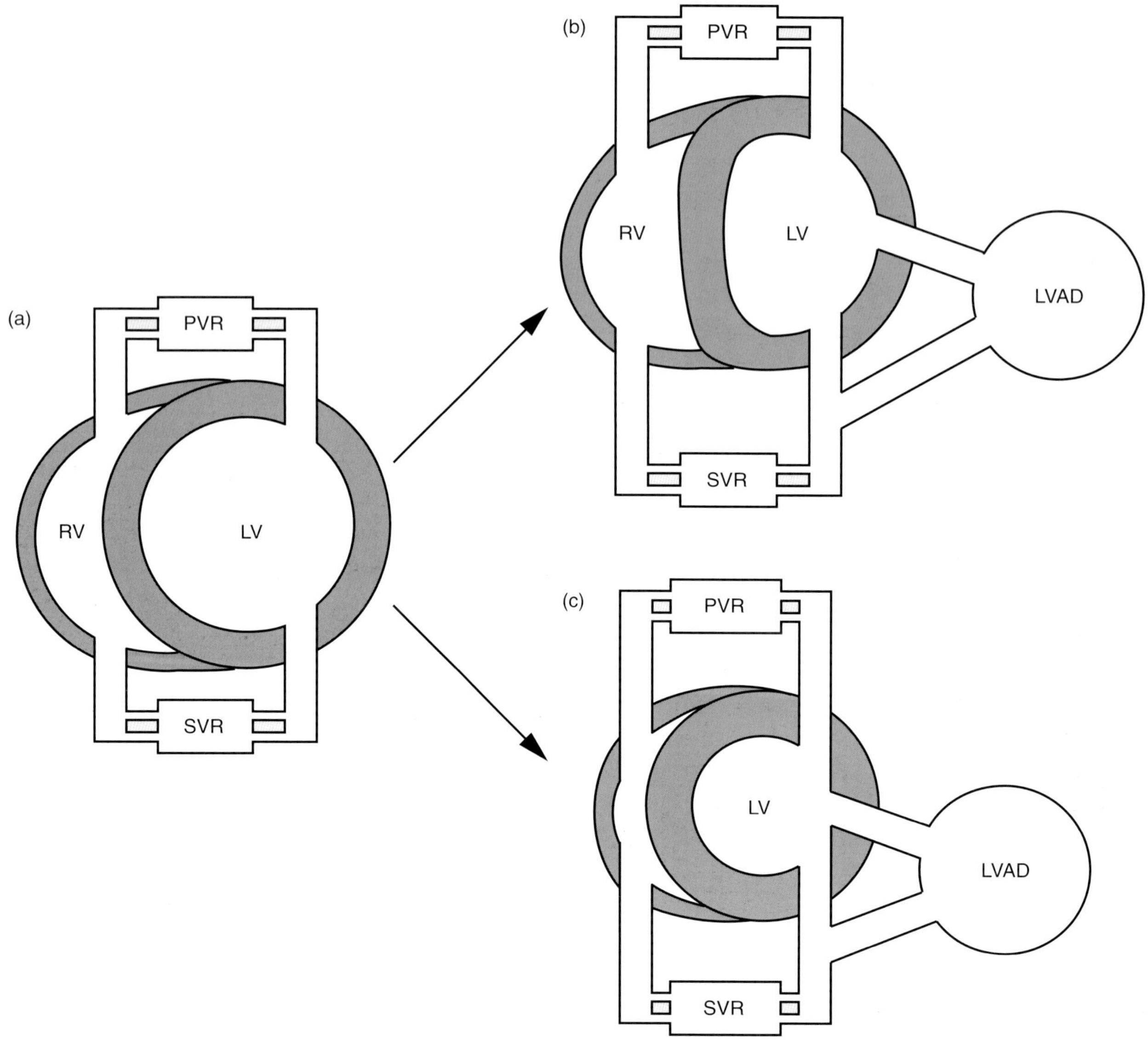


**Figure 35.16** *Influence of the LVAD on right ventricular function. Haemodynamic ventricular interactions are due to the right (RV) and left (LV) ventricles being in series connected by the systemic (SVR) and pulmonary (PVR) vascular resistance. Chronical interactions are due to a systemic coupling provided by the shared interventricular septum and common muscle fibres of the RV and LV (a). An LVAD in parallel with the LV (b and c) can increase venous return and reduce RV after-load by shifting blood volume from the pulmonary to the systemic vascular systems. An LVAD that offloads the LV (b) produces a leftward septal shift by reducing the transeptal pressure gradient, potentially improving RV filling, but decreasing the systolic LV contribution to RV contraction. If the pulmonary arterial and RV pressures are also reduced during LVAD support then both ventricles can become dimensionally unloaded (c). (From Farrar DJ, ref. 18.)*

ventricular wall tension (thereby reducing oxygen demand), increased coronary perfusion and enhance right ventricular function. This causes rapid resolution of the symptoms and signs of heart failure. Both renal and hepatic function improve through increased cardiac index and decreased pulmonary vascular resistance.

This dramatic effect on heart failure symptoms together with prolonged experience in some bridge to transplantation patients soon led to the suggestion that these LVADs could be used as permanent alternatives to cardiac transplantation [21].

## Complications in first-generation implantable LVADs

The pusher-plate LVADs are relatively large foreign bodies that directly connect with the skin via their drive-lines. Infection is frequent and is related to placing the device in the muscle layers and contamination from the skin exit site of the driveline. Although infections have decreased, they will remain a problem as long as external venting is necessary [22–24].

All current circulatory assist devices produce some degree of consumptive coagulopathy, but the overall thrombotic stimulus varies with different biomaterials and rheologic attributes. The total thrombotic stimulus cannot be measured and probably varies between patients and the different device flow rates. Bleeding is a major complication of LVAD implantation, but most patients are desperately ill with pre-existing intravascular thrombi, organ dysfunction, infections and deficiencies in coagulation or anti-infective proteins, which directly or indirectly affect haemostasis. However, markers of platelet activation and thrombin generation show fibrinolytic activity to persist for weeks after implantation, indicating an ongoing consumptive coagulopathy [25]. The intensity of coagulopathy varies inversely with the level of anticoagulation, the more anticoagulation, the less thrombin generation and fibrinolysis.

The incidence of thrombo-embolism and stroke varies markedly between current blood pumps. The 'HeartMate' LVAD appears to produce the weakest overall thrombotic stimulus with a 2–4% incidence of clinical thrombo-embolism without anticoagulation [26]. The Novacor LVAD has a higher incidence and generally requires long-term anticoagulation first with heparin, then with both Warfarin and platelet inhibitors. In warfarinized patients, Pennington observed thrombus formation in 28% and a stroke rate of 20% [27]. Others have documented up to 47% incidence of cerebral embolization in anticoagulated patients on the Novacor LVAD. However, when platelet inhibitors are added to the anticoagulation protocol, the incidence of stroke decreases to 1% without increasing bleeding. Pennington found a thrombosis rate of 15% and a stroke rate of 3% in 106 anticoagulated patients on the Thoratec system [27, 28].

Other complications occur with the pusher plate LVADs. Porcine xenografts fail earlier when subject to the substantial pressure differentials within the mechanical environment (Fig. 35.17). Constant movement of these large devices within the abdominal pocket can lead to graft erosion and profound haemorrhage.

Myocardial recovery, first demonstrated clinically in the TCI bridge-to-recovery patients, has been confirmed in patients with both Thoratec and Novacor pumps [11]. A more user-friendly technology could allow earlier implementation of support for these patients with the hope that subsequent transplant would not be required.

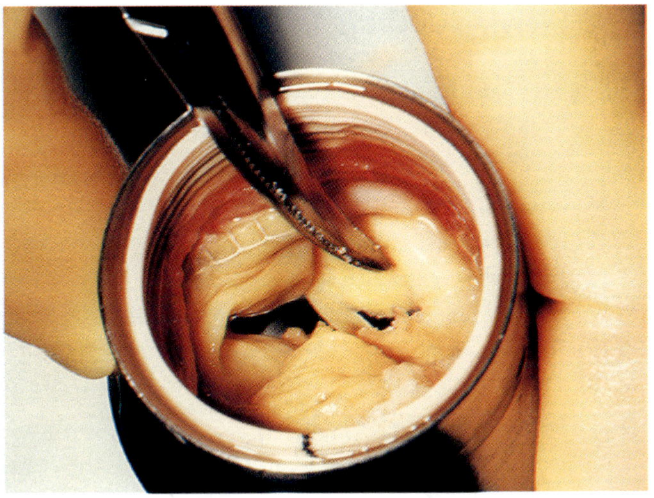

**Figure 35.17** *Failed porcine bioprosthesis in the TCI LVAD.*

## Second-generation LVADS

The design characteristics thought necessary to permit widespread application of a new cardiac assist device are as follows:

- small size and weight, which allow the pump to be implanted within the thoracic cavity in patients of all sizes
- a small biocompatible blood contact surface area to decrease activation of the Contact System of plasma
- a simple silent blood propulsion system with few movable parts, capable of providing the whole left-sided output, but should be able to be turned down safely to work synergistically with the native left ventricle
- a reliable control and power delivery system that is easily portable and manageable by the patient and relatives and with a high probability of freedom from infection.

Powerful miniaturized continuous flow pumps have been available for fluids such as oil and water for many years, but it was always thought that rapid acceleration of blood through a narrow channel would result in haemolysis or thrombosis. The axial flow impeller pumps have been developed over the past 10 years to address the physiological and biocompatibility requirements of a second-generation LVAD.

## The Jarvik 2000 Heart

The Texas Heart Institute (Houston) and the Oxford Heart Centre (UK) are collaborating to evaluate the Jarvik 2000 Heart (Jarvik Heart Inc., New York). This compact device is inserted through an apical cuff into the body of the left ventricle (Fig. 35.18). An impervious Dacron graft conveys blood to the descending thoracic aorta. The adult model measures 2.5 cm in diameter × 5.5 cm in length (Fig. 35.19). The weight is 85 g and the displacement volume 25 ml. The size approximates to that of the inflow cannula of the TCI LVAD. A smaller pediatric model under development measures 1.4 cm in diameter × 5 cm in length. One-fifth of the size of the larger model, it weighs only 18 g with a displacement volume of 5 ml. The electromagnetic pump consists of a rotor (Fig. 35.20) with impeller blades encased in a titanium shell supported at each end by blood immersed ceramic bearings <1 mm in diameter. The rotor is the sole moving part and all blood contact surfaces are titanium. Coils embedded in the titanium shell generate a magnetic field that powers the impeller across the gap through which the blood flows. Power is delivered from external batteries by a fine percutaneous wire and regulated by a pulse width/modulated, brushless, DC motor controller that determines pump speed. For the human model pump speed will eventually be responsive to heart rate, but is currently adjustable by the patient according to activity level. *In vitro* studies show the adult device to provide 10 l/min blood flow at 14 000 rpm. At normal operating speeds of 8000–12 000 rpm, flow rates of between 4 l/min and 6 l/min are obtained at a mean aortic pressure of

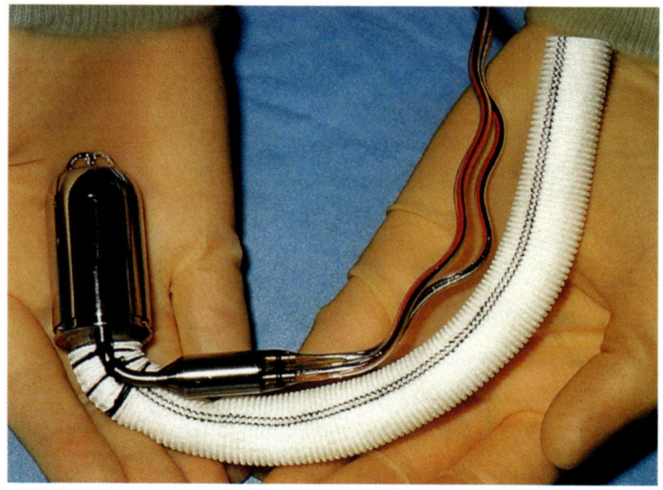

**Figure 35.19** *The thumb-sized Jarvik 2000 Heart with the outflow graft and power cable.*

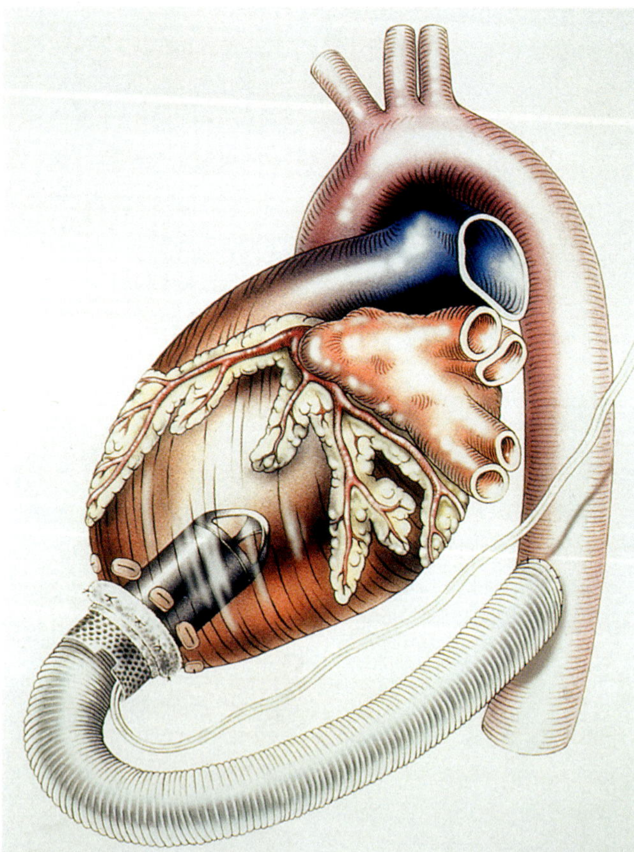

**Figure 35.18** *Diagram illustrating the Jarvik 2000 Heart implanted into the apex of the failing left ventricle and offloading to the descending thoracic aorta. The intraventricular position unique to the Jarvik 2000 Heart conveys distinct advantages over axial flow pumps with an apical inflow cannula. Alignment within the left ventricle persists during left ventricular offloading and there is no inflow cannula to suffer malalignment, a precursor to haemolysis. There is no external pocket for the device itself and encapsulation within the left ventricle and circulation provides an infection resistant environment.*

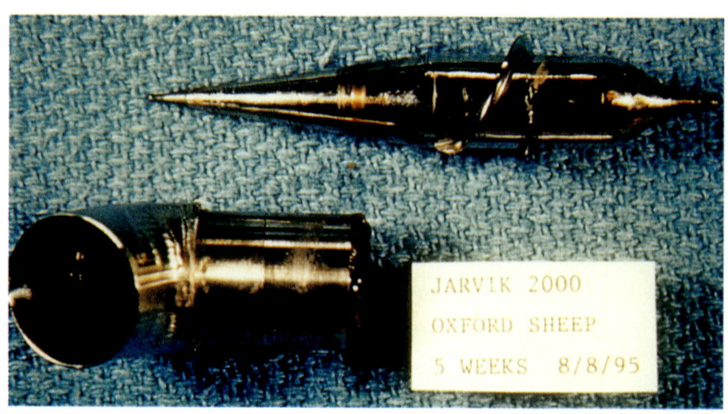


**Figure 35.20** *The impeller is suspended within the electromagnetic by blood immersed microceramic bearings and rotates at between 8000 and 12 000 rpm.*

80 mmHg and a power requirement of 7–10 watts. The device is silent to the unassisted ear, but can be heard through a stethoscope. Long-term implants have been achieved for more than 6 months in both sheep and calves.

In Oxford, 22 sheep survived between 3 and 198 days (mean 52 ± 12 days) with a functioning device [31]. With the adult pumps speed was set at between 10 000 and 12 000 rpm with 14-volt DC power. This pump speed provided a flow of 5–6 l/min. The mean energy consumption remained constant at 6.3 ± 1.1 watts during intra-operative measurements and 6.9 ± 1.0 watts at day 90. Three paediatric devices provided blood flow of between 2–3 l/min using 5–8 watts at a continuous speed of 12 000 rpm. With increasing non-pulsatile flow the aortic pulse pressure falls progressively from 40 ± 4 mmHg (pump off) to 11 ± 4 mmHg at 10 000. Above 10 000 the pump captures all blood flow through the mitral valve (Fig. 35.21) so that the aortic valve remains closed with the left ventricle fully unloaded (systemic vascular resistance averaged 1190 ± 170 dyne s cm$^5$). At 12 000 rpm the cardiac output was augmented by 33% (1.9 ± 0.5 l/min) over preimplantation values. Very low degrees of haemolysis were found in both sheep and calves. Plasma free haemoglobin levels ranged from 6.4 ± 2.9 mg/dl at 4 weeks to 7.9 ± 3.4 mg/dl at 12 weeks for sheep and 8.7 mg dl at 70 days to 7.5 mg/dl at 162 days for the calf.

The latest system consists of the Jarvik 2000 pump with a microprocessor-based automatic motor controller to respond to physiological demands. An external rate responsive controller alters pump speed and flow by modulating motor current in response to heart rate. Pump rotor speed response corresponds with heart rate in a linear function. The external batteries and controller are carried on a belt and are of similar size and weight to a portable telephone (Fig. 35.22). The Houston group is pursuing a totally implantable system that uses transcutaneous energy delivery (Fig. 35.23). For bridge to transplantation Houston apply a simple Dacron velour covered power line which

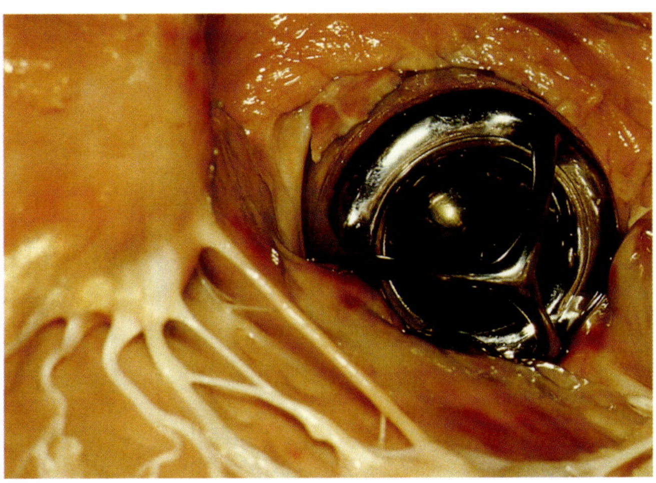

**Figure 35.21** *View of the intraventricular device through the mitral annulus. With complete unloading, all transmitral flow enters the pump and the native aortic valve remains closed.*

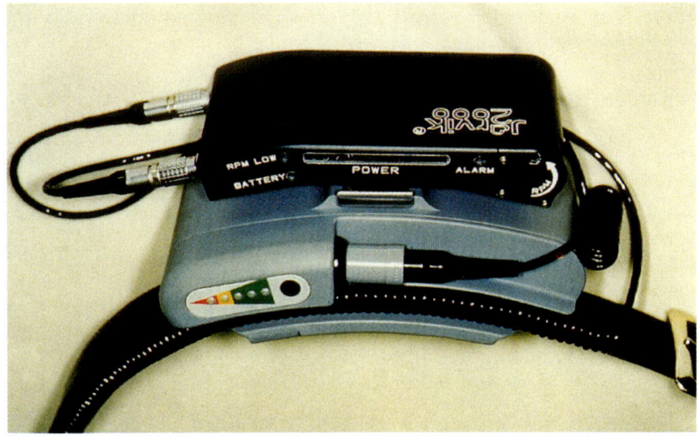


**Figure 35.22** *The external power system of the Jarvik 2000 Heart comprising the controller with single knob to control pump flow and the separate battery, both of which can fit onto a belt.*

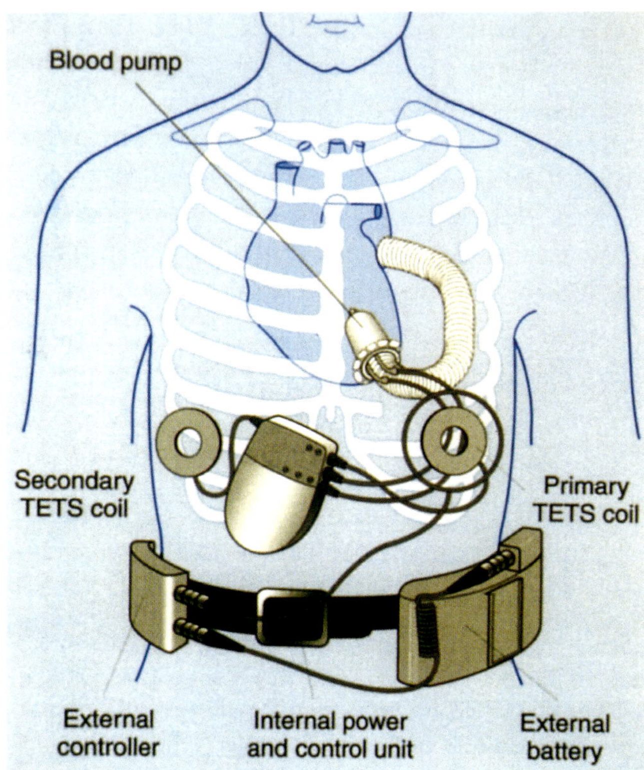


**Figure 35.23** *Diagram illustrating the totally implantable Jarvik 2000 system with transcutaneous energy delivery.*

exits the abdominal wall. In an innovative approach to power delivery for permanent implants the Oxford group bring the internal electric wires through the left pleural cavity to the apex of the chest and then subcutaneously across the neck to the skull [32]. Here a rigidly fixed percutaneous titanium pedestal transmits the fine electric wires through the skin of the scalp (Fig. 35.24). The combination of immobility and highly vascular scalp skin is known to resist infection in long-standing cochlear implant technology (artificial hearing) [33]. The Oxford group have also performed elective removal of the device with survival in sheep to test the feasibility of bridge to myocyte recovery.

Both laboratory and clinical experience suggest that the intra-ventricular position of the Jarvik 2000 Heart has distinct advantages. The device is virtually surrounded by the left ventricular cavity, so there is no external pocket with the potential for haematoma formation and infection.

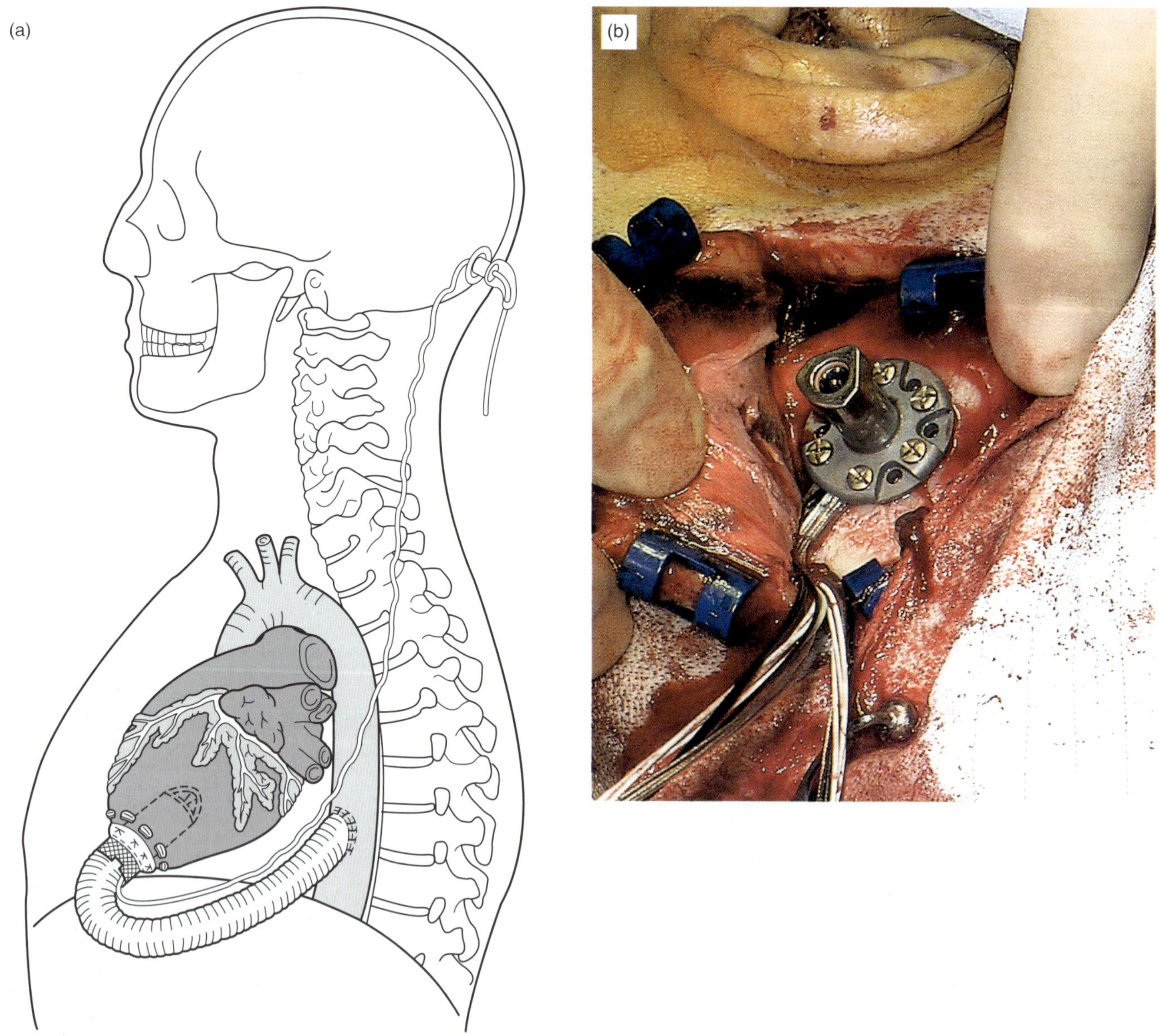


**Figure 35.24** *Power delivery based on the skull mounted pedestal for permanent Jarvik 2000 implants. (a) The power cable is brought through the pleural cavity out through the first posterior intercostal space and up the neck to the skull. The titanium pedestal screwed into the skull transmits the power cable through the skin. The combination of immobility and highly vascular scalp skin is resistant to infection as demonstrated by cochlear implant technology. (b) Skull-mounted pedestal in an Oxford permanent implant 3 months postoperatively. If the external power cable (which plugs into the skull mounted pedestal) is damaged, it can be replaced.*

Only the left pleural cavity is entered and the vascular graft delivers blood to the descending aorta. This leaves the anterior mediastinum untouched pending transplantation. Because there is no inflow cannula the device itself remains well aligned within the ventricle even when the heart is decompressed and changes position (Fig. 35.25). Other devices with an inflow cannula, a tethered apex and an external pocket have suffered malalignment and severe haemolysis when the shape and position of the ventricle changes. Though the device has been remarkably free from thrombus formation and thromboembolism, any emboli delivered to the descending thoracic aorta are less likely to enter the carotid arteries.

Retrograde flow to the upper body ending in the coronary arteries is less likely to produce the 'blind pocket' syndrome in the aortic root, than when an ascending aortic graft directs blood flow towards the head. A continuously closed aortic valve has the propensity for fusion of the cusps and thrombus formation in the aortic sinuses. For this reason the speed of the Jarvik impeller can be reduced to allow antegrade ejection through the aortic valve as well as offloading through the pump.

Data from the Oxford and Texas Heart 'Safety and Efficacy' studies led to approval for permanent implants in non-transplant eligible patients by the Medical Devices Agency (UK) and bridge to transplant by the Food and Drugs Administration (USA). The first implant took place on humanitarian grounds before investigational device exemption in December 1999. The patient, a 17-year-old male, had undergone multiple operations for aortic regurgitation and prosthetic valve endocarditis resulting in advanced heart failure and the need to close off the left ventricular outflow tract. Exit from the left ventricle was provided by a TCI LVAD with a view to bridge to myocardial recovery, then substitution of the LVAD with an apico aortic conduit. The LVAD then became infected and the plan was to replace the infected LVAD with a Jarvik 2000 Heart, thereby avoiding further sterno-laparotomy. Preceding the attempt he had suffered both focal and diffuse cerebral injury and had been recumbent in a hospital bed for more than 6 months. The ambitious clinical strategy was justified on the grounds of young age and reinforced by the fact that his only sibling had died months before in an accident.

The operation proved predictably difficult, but the device was successfully implanted following amputation of the inflow cannula of the TCI LVAD. The outflow graft of the TCI LVAD was ligated to prevent reflux of blood from the ascending aorta, but the body of the device was not removed for 24 hours when the secondary procedure was performed in a more stable patient. This staged operation allowed the remarkable X-ray (Fig. 35.26) showing first and second generation LVADs in the same patient.

The Jarvik 2000 Heart captured all transmitral flow and provided non-pulsatile systemic blood flow with a mean

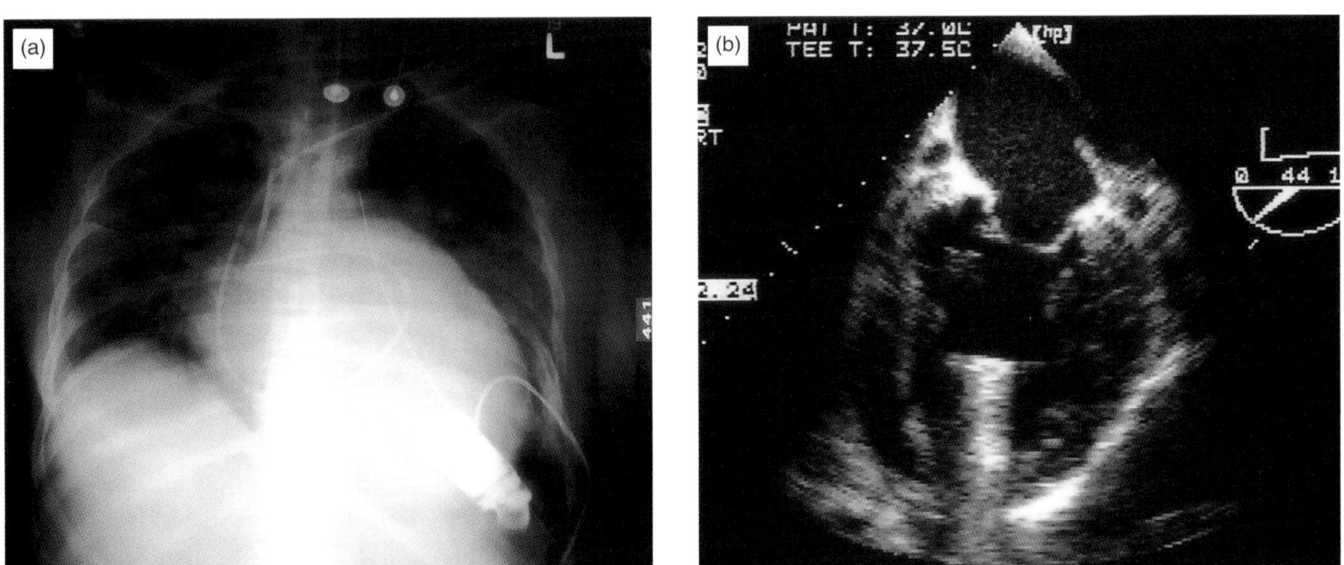


**Figure 35.25** *(a) Plain chest X-ray in a patient with dilated cardiomyopathy. The Jarvik 2000 Heart is well positioned in the apex of the left ventricle. (b) Two-dimensional echocardiography shows the pump in an in ideal position within the offloaded left ventricle.*

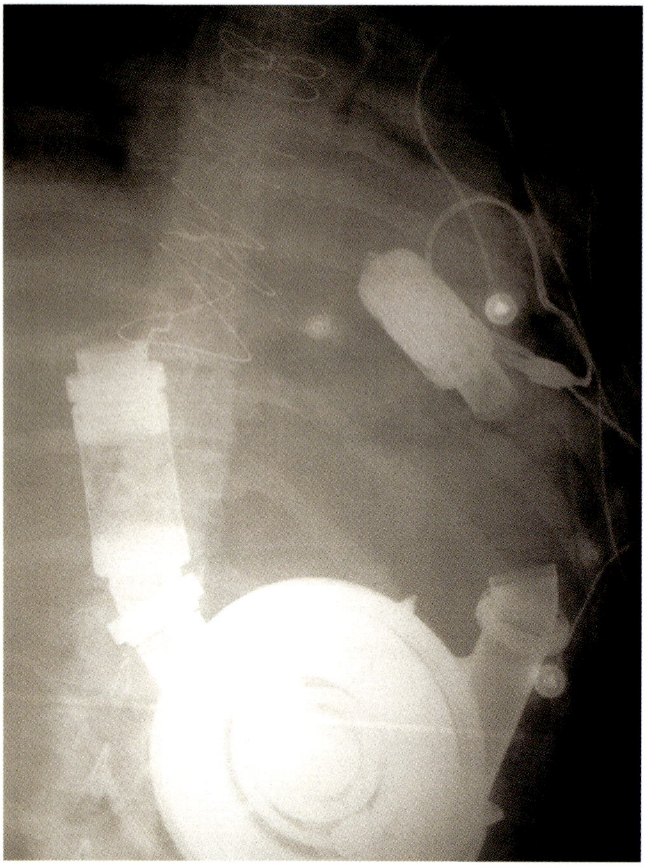

**Figure 35.26** *Unique plain X-ray film following the first Jarvik 2000 implant. This patient had an infected TCI LVAD, which was removed the following day. The Jarvik 2000 Heart is seen to be virtually the same size as the amputated TCI LVADinflow cannula.*

pressure of 60–70 mmHg (Fig. 35.27). Adequacy of tissue perfusion was determined by measuring mixed venous oxygen saturation (60–70%), acid base balance and urine output. The systemic pressure was adjusted by pharmacological vasodilatation or vasoconstriction. Over the course of both surgical procedures more than 100 units of blood were required together with platelet transfusions and clotting factors. He subsequently developed bilateral pulmonary infiltrates and renal failure after which high ventilation pressures resulted in recurrent pneumothoraces. Three weeks after the implant when survival was deemed impossible the Jarvik 2000 Heart was switched off. Throughout the whole postoperative course the systemic and pulmonary circulation were sustained by the pump which proved reliable and very simple to use.

Subsequently by 10 bridges to transplantation (according to the FDA protocol) have been very successful. For the second Houston implant total postoperative blood loss was 160 ml and pump speeds between 8000 and 10 000 rpm provided a cardiac output of 6 l/min with a pulse pressure of between 10 and 20 mmHg transmitted from the offloaded left ventricle through the device to the systemic circulation (Fig. 35.28a, b). Extubation took place 18 hours postoperatively and on the second postoperative day the patient was able to sit out in a chair. She could not hear the pump or feel any internal vibration. By 1 week all haematological and biochemical values were within normal limits. By 3 weeks she was NYHA I and remained in excellent condition until successful transplantation 13 weeks later. There have been no device related complications during the bridge to transplantation experience and at explantation of the native heart there was no thrombus formation within the left ventricular cavity, the device itself or the vascular graft.

The first permanent Jarvik 2000 Heart implant took place in Oxford in June 2000 [34]. In this case the 62-year-old male patient (115 kg, 2.1 $m^2$ BSA) had a 3-year history of idiopathic dilated cardiomyopathy and advanced heart failure (NYHA IV) on maximal medical therapy. At the time of referral his exercise tolerance was <10 yards. He had five-pillow orthopnoea, hepatomegaly, ascites and brawny leg oedema to the thighs. He was in chronic atrial fibrillation and had pulmonary hypertension (PAP 45/28, PVR 7 wood units). Cardiorespiratory exercise test showed an $MVO_2$ of 5.7 mm/min/kg at peak exercise. Transthoracic echocardiography showed a grossly dilated left ventricle with an end-systolic dimension of 7 cm and ejection fraction of <10%. Creatinine clearance was between 35 and 40 ml/min in repeated tests. Collectively these measurements suggested a prognosis <3 months. Renal impairment ruled him out as a transplant candidate irrespective of his age, blood group and the presence of a fungal skin infections.

After successful implantation of the device (Fig. 35.29) and weaning from cardiopulmonary bypass, inhaled nitric oxide was used to reduce the pulmonary vascular resistance and adrenalin infusion as an inotrope for the right ventricle. Trans-oesophageal echocardiography was used to assess left ventricular offloading, right ventricular filling and myocardial contractility. Elevation in systemic vascular resistance caused a decrease in pump output and was managed with hydralazine and beta-blockade. We maintained a pump output > 5 l/min with a mean arterial pressure of 40–60 mmHg. During the first 48 hours the systemic blood flow was provided entirely by the pump and

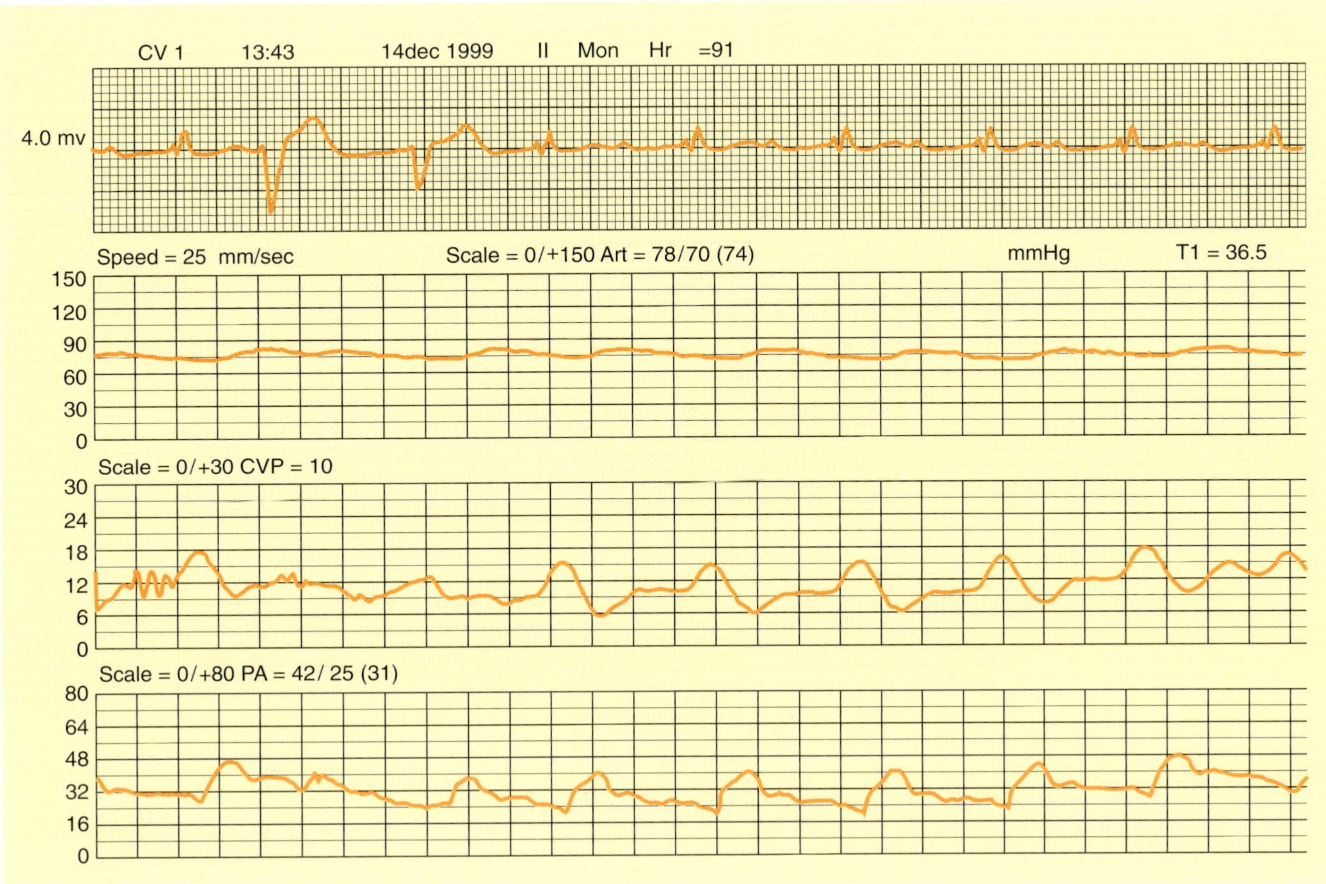


**Figure 35.27** *ECG and pressure recordings from a Jarvik 2000 patient. There is non-pulsatile flow in the systemic circulation, but a pulsatile trace from the right atrium and pulmonary artery.*

the aortic valve remained closed. A pulse pressure between 10–15 mmHg was detected when contraction of the native left ventricle increased preload to the device. Lower heart rate increased pulsatility in the circulation by increasing left ventricular filling time. During the next 2 weeks the patient's condition improved markedly. At rest the impeller speed was maintained at 9000 rpm and progressively increased to 12 000 rpm during activity and exercise. There was no significant haemolysis, the pump itself was inaudible and imperceptible to the patient. Exercise tolerance increased and was accompanied by a fall in body weight and disappearance of peripheral oedema and ascites. After 2 weeks there was no further need for diuretic therapy and he could sleep lying flat. Trans-thoracic echocardiography showed gradual improvement in both left ventricular and right ventricular function. As a result pulsatility returned to the circulation at all pump speeds (Table 35.2).

The patient soon learned to regulate pump speed according to physiological requirements and to change the batteries. With the pump switched off for 5 minutes aortic regurgitation retrogradely through the vascular graft was about 10% of total cardiac output and was well tolerated. Repeat cardiorespiratory exercise testing at 6 weeks showed a 75% improvement on baseline (Table 35.3). Twenty-four days after the implant he left the hospital for a half-way house accompanied by family members. Having ascertained that the family could manage the electrical system in the event of an emergency he was discharged home 6 weeks postoperatively and remains NYHAI 14 months later. His native heart has reverted to sinus rhythm. Clinical indices of heart failure and device function are presented in Table 35.3. There has been no sign of infection around the skull mounted pedestal (Fig. 35.30), which has proven inobtrusive for the patient. This patient has now lived at home

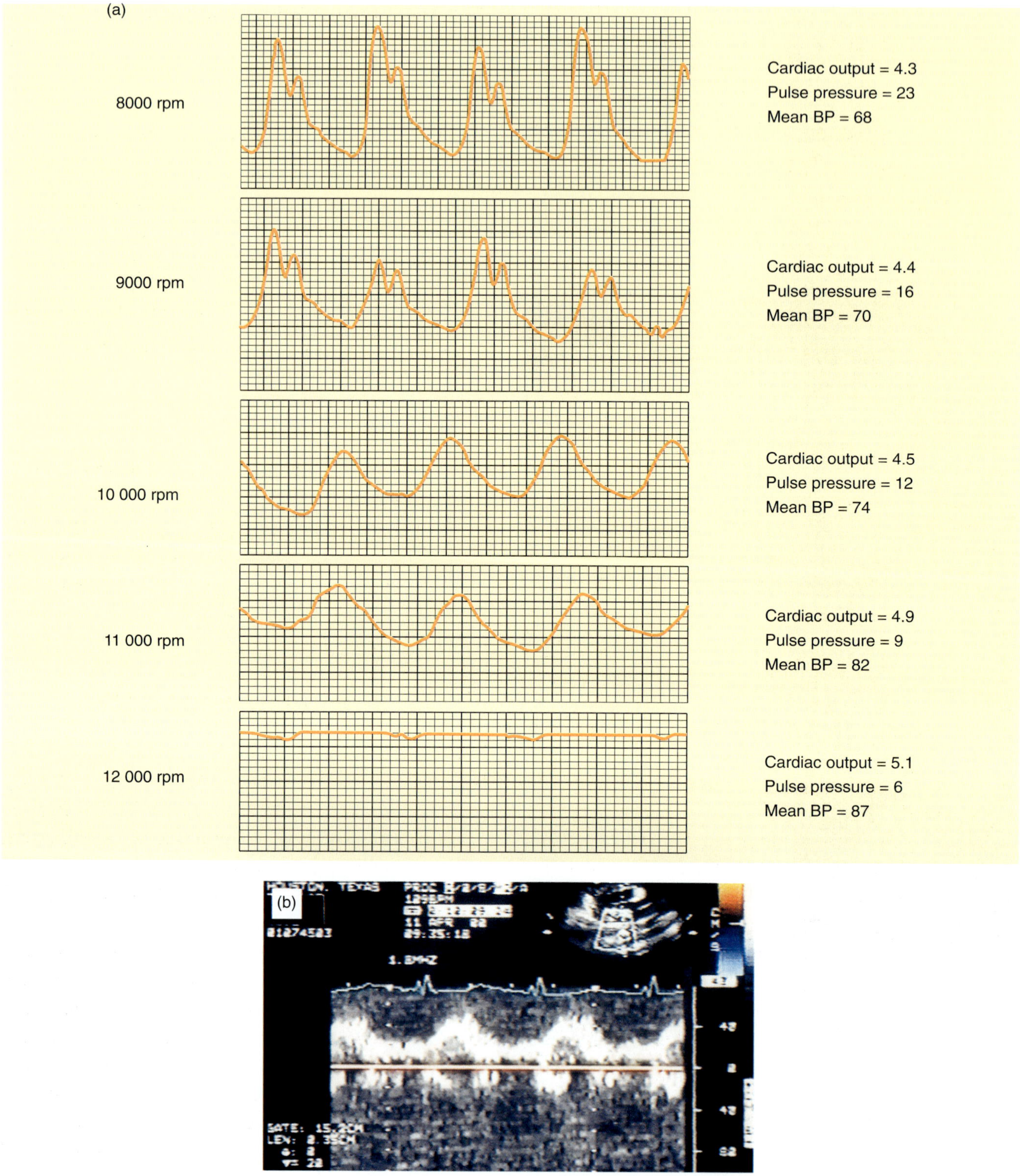


**Figure 35.28** *(a) The relationship between the Jarvik 2000 pump speed and arterial pressure trace. At 12 000 rpm the left ventricle is completely offloaded and systemic flow is non-pulsatile. At 11 000 and 10 000 rpm pulsatility appears in the circulation even though the aortic valve remains closed. This is because the contracting, but offloaded left ventricle increases preload to the device, which is transmitted as pulse into the systemic circulation. With the device switched down to 9000 rpm, native left ventricular ejection opens the aortic valve and produces a diacrotic notch in the arterial trace. Under these circumstances with lower pump flow blood is ejected by the native left ventricle as well as pumped by the device. At 8000 rpm the device acts as a valve within the system preventing functional aortic regurgitation from the descending thoracic aorta. The native left ventricle accounts for most of the cardiac output. (b) pulse in the Dacron outflow graft detected by Doppler echocardiography over the graft.*

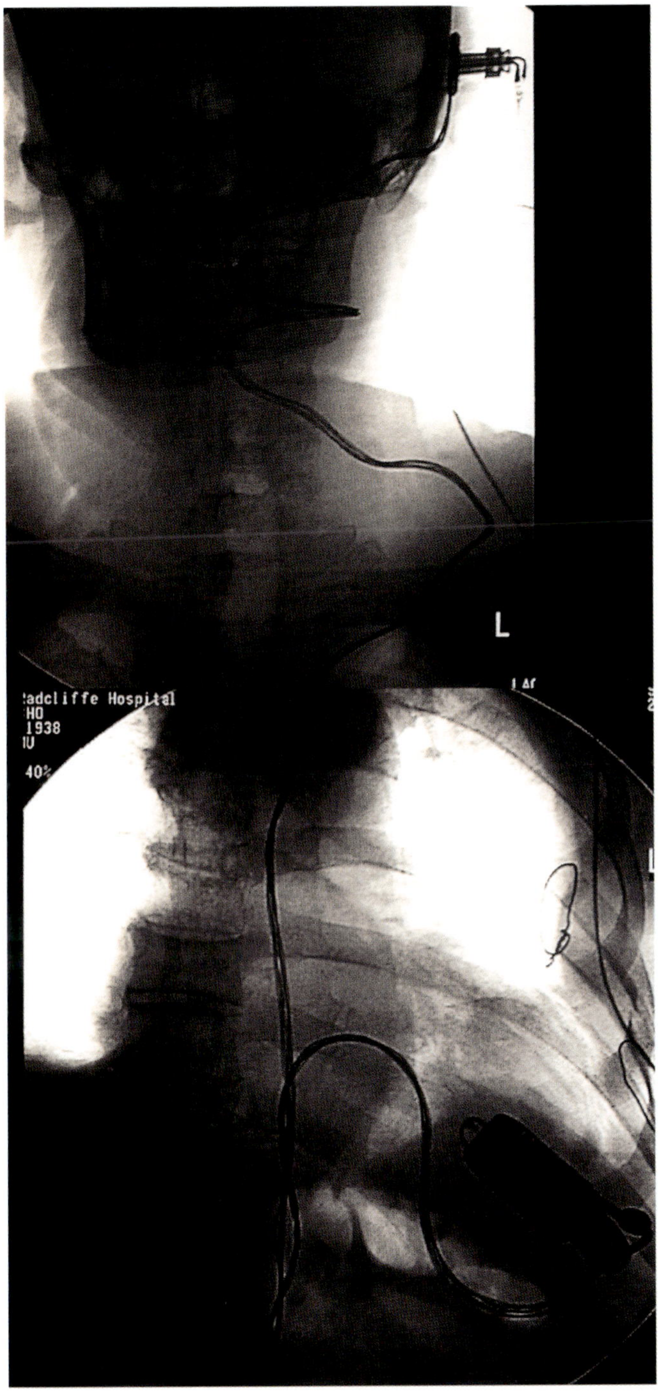

**Figure 35.29** *Subtraction plain X-ray films showing the Jarvik 2000 Heart in the apex of the left ventricle and the power cable passing through the neck to the skull-mounted pedestal.*

for 1 year and is NYHAI without diuretics. He has excellent quality of life and travelled abroad for a family vacation and regained his drivers' license. On a shopping trip a thief snatched his controller bag and detached the power cable from the skull. The alarm sounded, the thief dropped the bag and the patient plugged himself in again without adverse effects.

**Table 35.2** Relationship between pump speed and pulse pressure in the systemic circulation

| Day 4 | | Six weeks | |
|---|---|---|---|
| Pump speed (RPM) | Pulse pressure[a] (mmHg) | Pulse pressure[b] (mmHg) | Echo doppler graft flow velocity (m/sec) |
| Pump off | 32 | 36 | –0.14[c] |
| 8000 | 26 | 34 | 0.29 |
| 10 000 | 0 | 28 | 0.52 |
| 12 000 | 0 | 26 | 0.78 |

[a]Invasive arterial line measurement. [b]Non-invasive cuff pressure measurement. [c]Denotes reverse flow (functional aortic regurgitation) through the vascular graft. (Westaby S. *et al. Lancet* 2000, **356**: 900–3, with permission.)

Three similar patients have since received the Jarvik 2000 Heart as a permanent implant. Our limited but encouraging experience of this device in the outpatient setting suggests its use as an 'off the shelf' alternative for non-transplant eligible patients.

## The De Bakey MicroMed LVAD

This axial flow pump was developed jointly by the National Aeronautic and Space Administration (NASA) and Baylor College of Medicine after a NASA engineer underwent cardiac transplantation at Baylor [35]. The device is a miniaturized electromagnetically actuated titanium axial flow pump, which propels blood from the left ventricle into the ascending aorta. A titanium inflow cannula connects the pump to the apex of the left ventricle and an impervious vascular graft connects the outflow conduit to the ascending aorta (Fig. 35.31). The pump itself is small (30 × 76 mm, 93 g) and can pump in excess of 10 l/min. It consists of a flow straightener, inducer/impeller and diffuser, which are fully enclosed in a titanium flow tube (Fig. 35.32a, b). The pump is driven by a brushless direct current motor stator, which is contained in the stator housing. The inducer/impeller is the only moving part of the pump. It has six blades with magnets hermetically sealed in each blade. The inducer spins at 7500–12 500 rpm. The power supply is provided by an extracorporeal controller, which is connected with the pump via a percutaneous cable. Two external 12 watt DC batteries provide 6–8 hours of operation.

**Table 35.3** Clinical indices of heart failure and device function

| | Before surgery | After 2 weeks | After 6 weeks |
|---|---|---|---|
| Weight (kg) | 114 | 109 | 102 |
| NYHA class | IV | II | I |
| Minnesota 'Living with Heart Failure' questionnaire (max 100) | 89 | 55 | 40 |
| Mini mental state examination | 30/30 | – | 30/30 |
| Cardio-thoracic ratio (%) | 65 | 62 | 56 |
| Cardio-respiratory exercise test | | | |
| Peak load (watts) | 45 | – | 85 |
| Exercise duration (min) | 4.0 | – | 8.0 |
| $MVO_2$ (ml/min/kg) | 5.7 | – | 8.8 |
| Renal function | | | |
| Serum Cr (mmol/l) | 152 | 120 | 112 |
| Cr clearance (ml/min) | 35 | – | 61 |
| Indices of haemolysis | | | |
| LDH (IU/l) | 237 | 481 | 380 |
| Plasma Hb (mg/dl) | 5.8 | 7.1 | 6.8 |
| Medication (total daily dose) | Lisinopril 30 mg<br>Digoxin 250 mg<br>Frusemide 120 mg<br>Spironolactone 50 mg<br>Warfarin 5.0 mg | Lisinopril 20 mg<br>Amiodarone 200 mg<br>Bisoprolol 1.25 mg<br>Warfarin 3.0 mg | Lisinopril 20 mg<br>Amiodarone 200 mg<br>Bisoprolol 2.5 mg<br>Warfarin 3.0 mg |

Cr: creatinine (70–150 μmol/l), Creatinine clearance (95–140 ml/min). LDH: serum lactate dehydrogenase (110–250 IU/l). Plasma Hb: plasma free haemoglobin (1.5–8.5 mg/dl). $MVO_2$: maximum oxygen consumption rate (normal level > 20 ml/min/kg) (Westaby S. *et al. Lancet* 2000, **356**: 900–3, with permission).

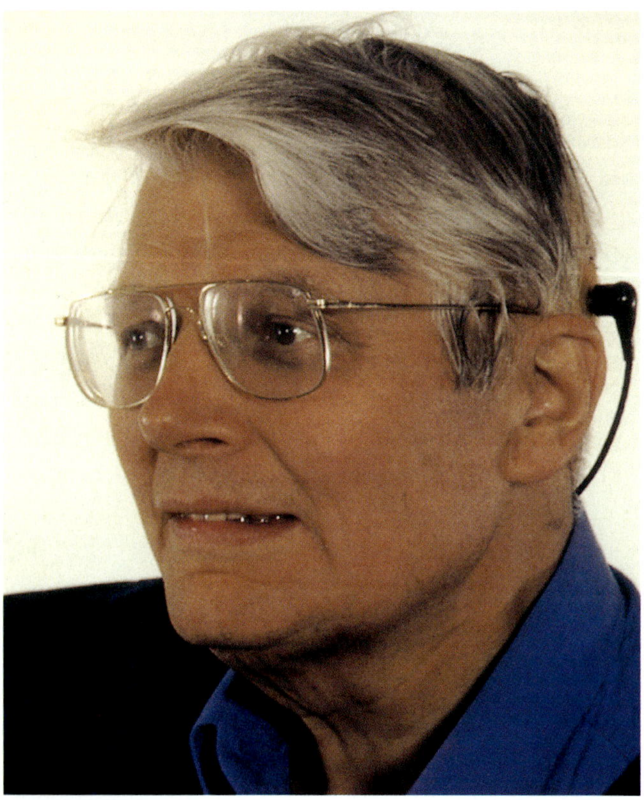

**Figure 35.30** *The Jarvik 2000 Heart patient with skull-mounted pedestal and external power cable.*

A transit time flow meter placed around the outflow conduit provides continuous read-out of pump flow. The measured pump flow is displayed either on the external LVAD controller or when connected on the clinical data acquisition system together with pump speed, power consumption and current signals from the pump. Following animal experiments at Baylor and Salt Lake City a limited phase I clinical trial of bridge to cardiac transplantation was approved by the FDA to take place in European centres at the end of 1998.

The method of implantation is different from the Jarvik 2000 Heart. The approach is via a median sternotomy using normothermic cardiopulmonary bypass via femoral arterial and venous cannulation. The left hemidiaphragm is detached in its anterior portion to provide a preperitoneal pocket for the pump. With the heart beating the sewing ring is attached to the avascular portion of the left ventricular apex with interrupted sutures. A coring tool is then used to excise the segment of myocardium within the sewing ring and then the inflow cannula is inserted into the left ventricle taking care to achieve an optimal position free of any trabecular obstructions. The inflow cannula should point straight to the aortic valve to provide an unim-

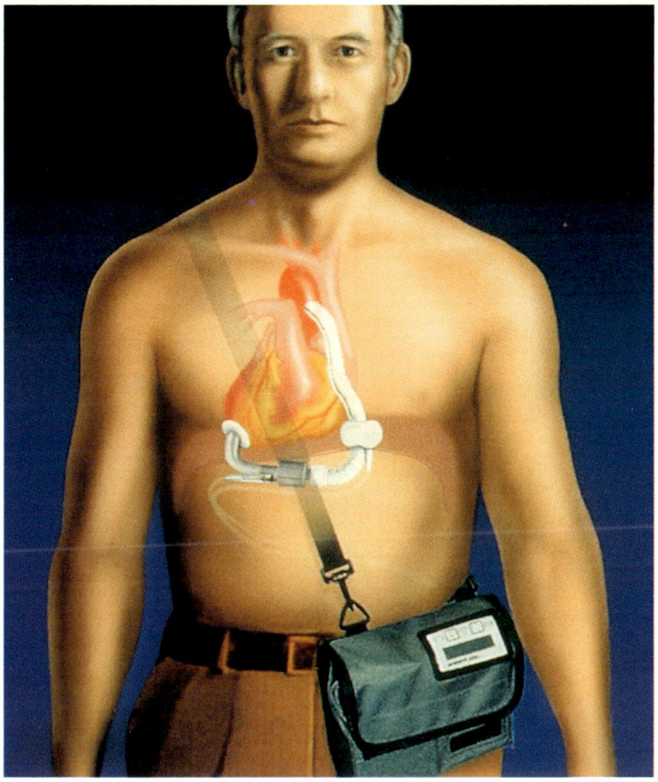

**Figure 35.31** *Diagram to show the De Bakey LVAD* in situ.

peded blood inflow during ventricular contraction. The Dacron graft is connected to the ascending aorta and the device de-aired before switching on. The patient is then weaned from cardiopulmonary bypass and the LVAD pump speed increased. Inhaled nitric oxide is used to reduce pulmonary vascular resistance though effective left ventricular off-loading causes the pulmonary arterial pressure to fall. The aortic valve remains closed.

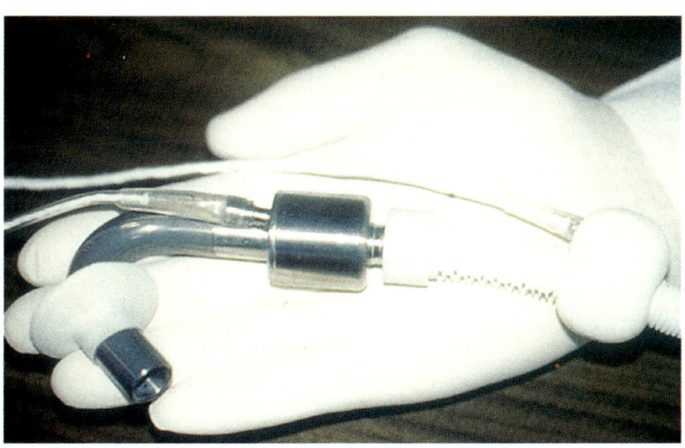

**Figure 35.32** *The De Bakey LVAD with inflow cannula and outflow graft with flow meter.*

Catecholamine support may be required for the right ventricle. Heparin is given 6–8 hours after the end of the operation when surgical bleeding is under control (15 000 units/day). Oral warfarin therapy is used to achieve an INR of 3.0–3.5. This is usually supplemented with aspirin 100 mg/day.

The De Bakey LVAD has been used for bridge to transplantation with mixed results. The outcome for the first 47 implants was presented by Turina at the European Society of Cardiothoracic Surgery in September 2000. At that time 44 pumps had been used in Europe and three at Baylor. Hospital mortality exceeded 30%. The average assist period was 63 ± 2 days. The pump speed was usually set at 9000–10 500 rpm and kept constant. The average pump flow in an awake supine patient was 4.8 ± 0.88 l/min. Indices of haemolysis in the Zürich patients showed an average plasma free haemoglobin of 13 mg/dl and an LDH of 1776 u/l. Severe haemolysis has been encountered in other patients probably related to an adverse position and partial obstruction of the inflow cannula within the left ventricle (Fig. 35.33). The problem with a rigid inflow cannula and a device fixed in an external pocket is that the off-loaded heart changes shape and the position of the apex may move, but remains tethered.

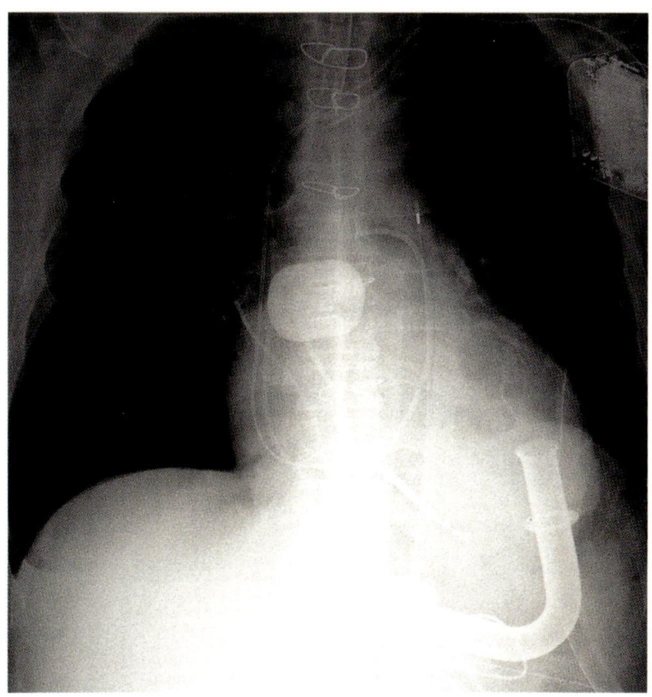

**Figure 35.33** *De Bakey LVAD in situ with poor position of the inflow cannula against the left ventricular wall. This caused severe haemolysis.*

With fully ambulatory patients stress exercise has been performed and demonstrates that the pump can practically double the flow rate without adjustment of pump speed. This occurs through increased ventricular filling and applies equally to the Jarvik 2000. Indices of heart failure including renal hepatic and neurologic function normalized rapidly in survivors with normal pump function. A positive nitrogen balance was achieved after 4–6 weeks. An inherent weakness with this pump is the development of massive aortic regurgitation into the left ventricle if the pump stops. This has caused mortality through acute left ventricular failure and is different from the Jarvik 2000 Heart where the 'pump off' situation is well tolerated for 5 minutes. As for the Jarvik 2000 pulsatility occurs in the systemic circulation through native left ventricular contraction, which is transmitted through the device [36]. Pulsatility gradually increases with improvement in ventricular function. Whilst recognized as a significant advance over pusher plate technology, the De Bakey LVAD has had a mixed reception from European surgeons.

## The HeartMate II left ventricular assist system

ThermoCardio Systems acquired the Nimbus/Pittsburgh axial flow blood pump, which has been under development at the University of Pittsburgh since 1992 [37]. This pump (Fig. 35.34a, b) consists of three major elements, an integrated pump/rotor, an inflow and outflow cannula set and an external controller and power supply. The device is manufactured from corrosion resistant titanium alloy. It has an overall length of 7 cm and an outer diameter of 4.0 cm and a displacement volume of 62 ml. However, the weight of the device is 370 g, considerably more than the Jarvik 2000 and De Bakey LVADs. The inflow cannulas are made from commercially available 40F wire reinforced polyurethane. The outflow cannula is a 14 mm reinforced extended polytetrafluoroethylene vascular graft bonded to a titanium fitting that threads to the pump outflow port with a step free interface. The system was designed for univentricular or biventricular support. For left ventricular assist the inflow and outflow cannulas are configured for connection to the left ventricular apex and the ascending aorta. The pump is then placed under the left costal margin beneath the left rectus abdominus muscle as for the De Bakey LVAD. The inflow cannula leaves the left ventricular apex to cross

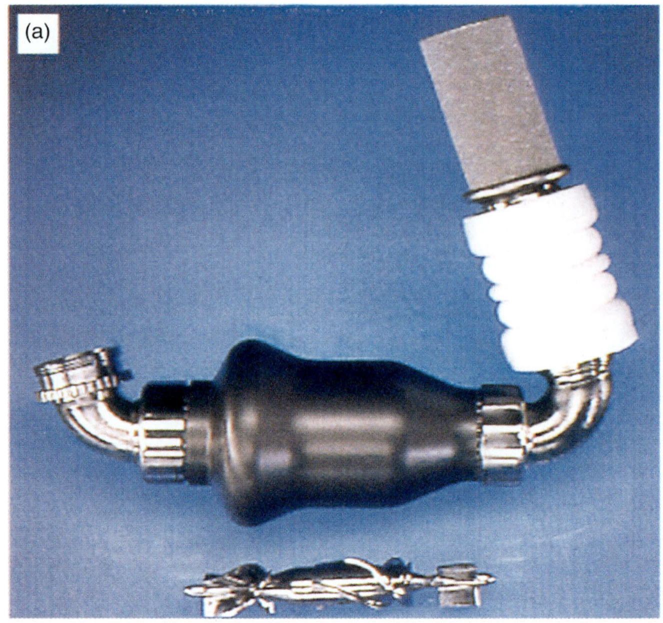


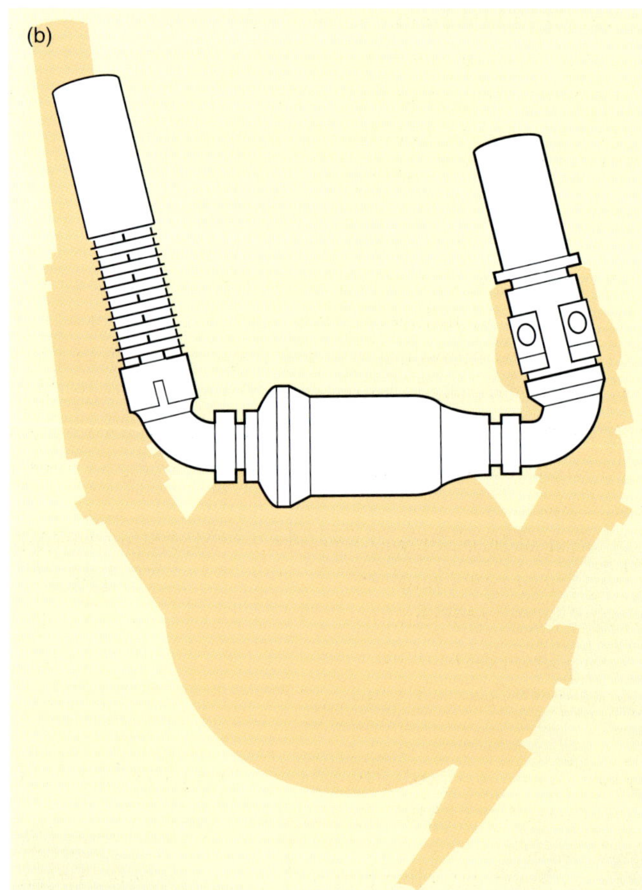


**Figure 35.34** *(a) The TCI II (Nimbus/Pittsburgh) axial flow pump. (b) Comparison in size of the TCI pusher plate (red) and axial flow pumps.*

**Table 35.4** Serial echocardiographic measurements

| | Before surgery | After 2 weeks | After 6 weeks |
|---|---|---|---|
| Heart rate (bpm) | 106 | 95 | 90 |
| LVED diameter (mm) | 67 | 63 | 64 |
| LVES diameter (mm) | 62 | 61 | 56 |
| LVEF(%)* | <10 | 10 | 30 |
| RVEF(%) | 20 | 30 | 60 |

*Ejection fraction determined by two dimentional echo cardiographic imaging using Simpsons formula (averaging 5–7 beats) with pump speed at 11 000 rpm. LVED: left ventricular end diastolic. LVES: left ventricular end systolic. LVEF: left ventricular ejection fraction. RVEF: right ventricular ejection fraction.

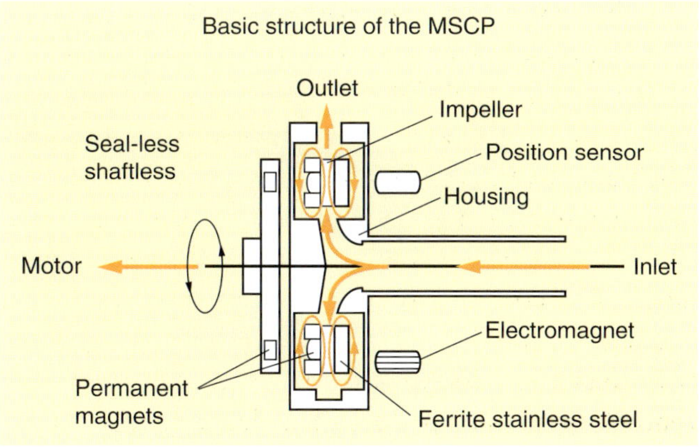


**Figure 35.35** *Diagram of the Terumo magnetically suspended centrifugal blood pump.*

the diaphragm in the costo-phrenic angle. It then enters the sub-rectus pocket to attach to the pump. The outflow cannula is tunnelled back under the sternum to the ascending aorta. For right ventricular assist the cannulas can be inserted in the right atrium and the main pulmonary artery. The blood contacting surfaces are textured (as for TCI pusher plate LVAD) in an attempt to reduce the incidence of thromboembolic complications and the need for systemic anticoagulation. Pump speed ranges between 3000 and 15 000 rpm, but is normally maintained between 10 000 and 12 000 to produce a flow >6 l/min. In short-term sheep studies the maximum plasma free haemoglobin was 27.5 mg/dl, but was less than 15 mg/dl for animals free from inflow obstruction. The controller system is expected to modulate the pump speed in response to varying physiological demands and a pulsatile mode is said to be included. A transcutaneous power system with implantable induction coils is currently under development.

A clinical implant was attempted in Israel and widely publicized during October 2000. Bleeding and haemolysis were said to be problematic and the patient died soon afterwards. A second implant by Koerfer at Bad Oyenhausen, Germany in April 2001 has been successful.

## The Terumo magnetically suspended left ventricular assist system

The axial flow impeller pumps have inflow and outflow bearings. Though these have indefinite lifespan on bench testing, they potentially restrict long-term durability and can be the site of heat generation and protein denaturation. Since 1995 the Terumo Corporation have worked to develop a magnetically suspended centrifugal blood pump (MSCP) without a drive shaft or seal [38]. The impeller of this device is suspended between the casings with magnetic forces produced by permanent magnets and electromagnets. The impeller rotates by a magentic coupling between it and the motor and is suspended by three electromagnetics (Fig. 35.35). Three position sensors keep the impeller free floating at the centre of the pump housing. The blood contacting surfaces and the inflow and outflow cannulas are modified with a heparin immobilization technique. The pump has a displacement volume of 196 ml and a weight of 400 g (Fig. 35.36). Because this is a seal-less rotor pump providing contact free rotation without any material wear, it is expected to be one of the most durable blood pumps with a theoretical life-span of decades. Early

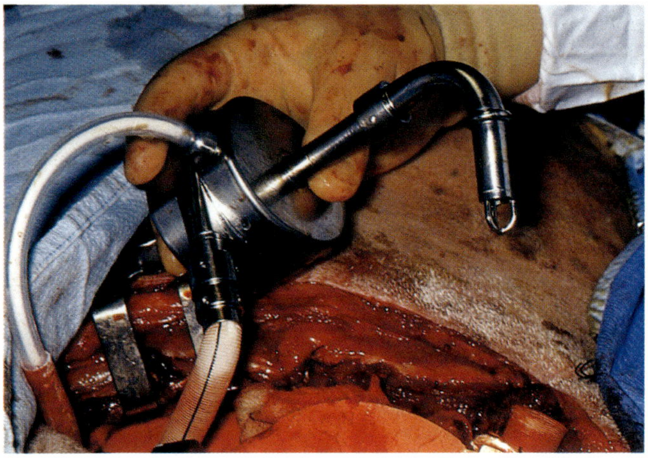

**Figure 35.36** *Terumo magnetically suspended centrifugal blood pump during implantation.*

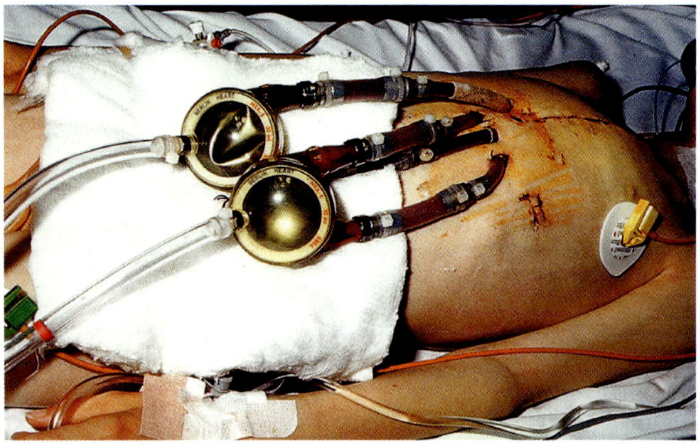

**Figure 35.37** *The Berlin Heart, an external pneumatic device for 'bridge to transplantation' or recovery. This device has been used very successfully in children with myocarditis.*

prototypes have already operated for more than 2 years in an extra-corporeal sheep model with plasma-free haemoglobin levels remaining within the normal range for all animals up to 864 days. Experience in Oxford shows the device to be effective with 5–6 litres blood flow at pump speeds of 2000 and 3000 rpm. We have maintained 20 sheep in excellent condition free from haemolysis or thromboembolism without any angicoagulation for up to 12 months. All device related parameters are recorded continuously by computer. During this time the systemic circulation has been entirely pulseless and has sustained normal endorgan function. The only detectable differences with non-pulsatile circulation are increased plasma renin activity, a 5–10 mmHg elevation of mean pressure over baseline and virtually complete abolition of baroreceptor responses. Histology from the aortic wall after prolonged non-pulsatile flow suggests thinning of the medial layer.

Although this device has yet to be used in patients, the remarkable prospect for anticoagulation free circulatory support is encouraging. This Japanese technology should be available for clinical testing by 2002.

## Management of patients with continuous flow LVADs

Animal pumping systems, epitomized by the mammalian heart, produce pulse by intermittent contraction, stroke volume, and one-way valves. Given this mechanism for blood propulsion, pulse is as obligatory as a resting phase for the myocyte. But is pulsatility necessary for normal organ function? There is no evidence that pulsatility is required for the energy exchange that occurs at the capillary level. In fact the pulse is so dampened at capillary level that it is essentially non-pulsatile. The pulsatile cardiac cycle is seemingly required only for energy delivery to the mammalian heart. The small continuous flow LVADs offer a much wider range of applicability that the current pulsatile LVADs. These devices, if properly applied, will continuously offload a functioning but failing heart and allow the native ventricle to perform with improved efficacy. This characteristic provides the potential for the axial flow pumps to become the first long-term ventricular assist devices. In effect, the pulsatile pumps capture the output of the left ventricle and, as such, are more properly termed left ventricular replacement devices than left ventricular assist devices.

Until recently there were no studies of long-term non-pulsatile flow in humans. The closest is with ECMO in children for several weeks, though the native heart provides some pulse pressure in these cases. There is already substantial evidence that the non-pulsatile blood pumps do provide pulsatility in the circulation as function improves in the off-loaded left ventricle. Experience with both the Jarvik 2000 Heart and De Bakey LVAD in patients confirms virtually normal systemic pulsatility with well-preserved hepatic and renal function [34]. More forceful contractions of the unloaded left ventricle provide pressure changes at the pump inlet, which accelerate and modulate the flow through the pump to provide pulsatile flow in the outflow graft and aorta (Fig. 35.28). Gradual elevation of pulse pressure in the circulation reduces sympathetic nervous activity in the heart failure patient. Pulsatility occurs while the native aortic valve remains closed and does not appear to be consistently dependent on pump flow, blood pressure or systemic vascular resistance. However, whilst small size is clearly beneficial in a blood pump, this limits the torque developed at impeller speeds compatible with not damaging red blood cells. Consequently axial flow pumps are much more sensitive to the differential pressure across the pump (afterload). This has significant influence on the haemodynamic management of patients with the continuous flow pump.

The continuous flow LVADs must be viewed and managed differently from conventional left ventricular assist devices. Axial flow pumps are non-phasic and yet are working with the phasic cardiac cycle. Care must be taken not to disrupt the cardiac cycle too greatly. If continuous flow results in a negative pressure throughout the whole cardiac cycle, then septal shift will occur. This results in impaired right ventricular function and decreased blood flow through the lungs to the pump and systemic circulation. We have observed this clinically in all of the patients who died with continuous flow assist devices. Therefore, synergy must be maintained between the cardiac cycle of the native heart and the continuous flow of the ventricular assist device. The optimal situation is when pulsatile flow is maintained by the native left ventricle, and the heart failure (manifest by low cardiac output) is corrected by the offloading and a contribution to flow by the assist device. This synergic approach is most challenging in the immediate postoperative period when blood loss and high pulmonary vascular resistance further compromise blood delivery to the left side. In this period, the patient must be supported by cardiotonics as well as nitric oxide and other agents to reduce pulmonary vascular resistance.

Off-loading with the Jarvik 2000 Heart brings the ventricle back towards its normal Frank–Starling curve. At low pump speed (8000–10 000 rpm), cardiac output is partly derived from the pump itself, but boosted by stroke volume ejection through the aortic valve. Under these circumstances, pulse can normally be felt in the carotid, radial or femoral arteries. Whether this strategy encourages left ventricular recovery (in comparison to complete unloading) remains to be seen. On one hand, complete offloading may lead to atrophy. On the other hand, it seems that complete off-loading is required before pressure work index is significantly reduced, and this is probably a key factor in left ventricular recovery [39]. As the patient recovers, it is becoming increasingly apparent that the left ventricle recovers as well. It seems, in our limited experience, that the ventricle recovers more with the continuous flow pump than with complete off-loading by a conventional pulsatile pumps. The native heart is able to respond to increased physiologic demands by increasing native cardiac output. Concerns for the necessity of an automated feedback system in the continuous flow pumps (to allow automatic increase in rpm and output) appear to be redundant. Even set at a constant flow the pump can increase its output as the left ventricle recovers. This is sufficient to meet the normal demands of the patient for instance when climbing stairs or taking a walk.

## Prospects for the future

The outlook is gradually improving for the heart failure patient. The new axial flow pumps are the next generation of LVADs and probably the first realistic artificial hearts for widespread use. There are three mechanical support strategies for which these blood pumps can be used. These are:

- bridge to myocardial recovery for a limited number of patients with recoverable disease
- bridge to transplantation for those with irrecoverable disease, who fit the selection criteria
- permanent circulatory support for non-transplant candidates with irreversible disease.

By far the most exciting prospect is for bridge to myocardial recovery. To-date the incidence of recovery has been relatively small in patients treated with pusher plate LVADs [40]. However, those studied have been absolutely end-stage transplant candidates with ischaemic heart disease or dilated cardiomyopathy with myocardial fibrosis. Though systemic rehabilitation is dramatic with an LVAD, cardiac morphology and genetics determine the potential for myocardial recovery. To attain recovery in a much wider population a user friendly and easily removable LVAD must be employed earlier in the disease process. For instance, we do not wait for a patient with heart block to suffer multiple syncopal attacks and irreversible cerebral injury before implanting a pacemaker. In support of this strategy the Berlin group have shown younger age (Fig. 35.39) and shorter duration of heart failure to be predictors of successful weaning from the LVAD and sustainability of myocardial recovery [39]. They have defined the optimum time for weaning to be 8–12 weeks (though Frazier disputes this). This coincides with the disappearance of the autoantibody again the beta-adrenergic receptor in dilated cardiomyopathy patients (Fig. 35.38). Histology from patients subjected to much longer duration of support in Berlin suggested that myocyte atrophy can interfere with successful weaning, though atrophy is partially reversed by ventricular loading in progressive increments. Whereas this can be achieved with an axial flow pump it is not easy to wean from a pusher plate LVAD without risk of stasis and thromboembolism.

There are a number of potential adjunctive therapies to promote sustainable recovery. These include stimulation of

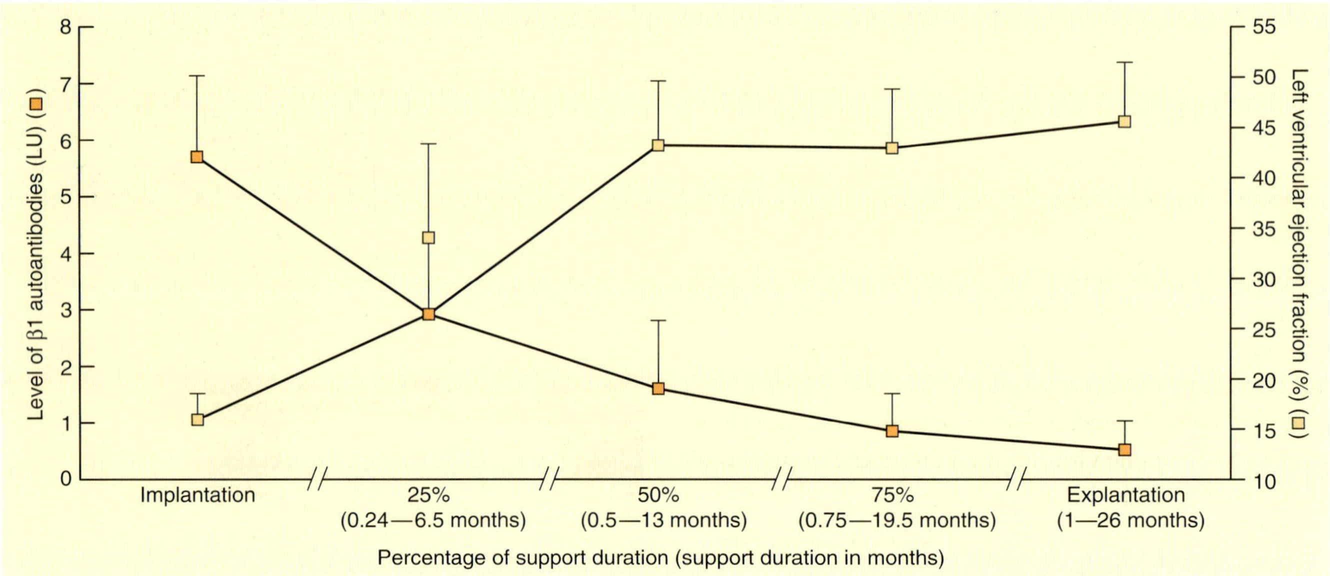


**Figure 35.38** *Course of autoantibody levels directed against the beta-adrenoreceptor versus cardiac ejection fraction. As the autoantibody level decreased over time, left ventricular ejection fraction improves. The pump was removed with sustained recovery in some patients (courtesy of Professors Hertzer and Müller, Berlin Heart Centre).*

cardiac protein synthesis by growth factors, such as insulin, Clenbutarol (which can induce myocardial hypertrophy) or growth hormone [40, 41]. Other suggestions include gene therapy to inhibit apoptosis, myocyte culture and transfer or neoangiogenesis in the ischaemic myocardium [41]. Changes in the cardiac workload and heart failure in particular, are associated with the regression to the foetal pattern of gene expression within the myocardium. The apoptotic process is a central mechanism in embryonic development and is implicated in the changes associated with modulation of cardiac workload [42].

The fact that a failing heart reverts to foetal gene expression suggests that adaptation of myocardial genetics may prove to be a future therapeutic strategy [43]. Left ventricular overload accounts for many of the alterations in cardiac and myocyte phenotype resulting from different clinical conditions. These include valve disease with increased after-load or preload, and ischaemic heart disease with quantitatively reduced myocardium after myocardial infarction. Thus over-load provides a unifying mechanism for the progression heart failure, the final common pathway for most of these disease entities. It has now been shown that LVAD therapy reverses the changes in myocardial gene expression compatible with a decreased susceptibility of apoptosis and partial improvement in calcium regulatory determinants [44]. The same German investigators have also shown that augmented endothelin receptor expression in failing human myocardium normalizes with mechanical off-loading. The potent vasoconstrictor endothelin 1 is known to be involved in the progression of heart failure and local synthesis of ET1 occurs in the endocardium, myocardium and coronary endothelium [45]. A functional significance of ET1 is suggested by the positive correlation between elevated plasma ET1 and increased mortality in human heart failure. In turn, inhibition of myocardial endothelin pathway can improve survival in heart failure.

The ability of mechanical left ventricular unloading to alter basic mechanisms of myocyte biology and arrest the underlying process of heart failure progression points to a new management strategy for patients with cardiomyopathies of differing etiology. Consequently we have taken a step beyond the use of blood pumps solely to sustain life pending cardiac transplantation. The new miniature devices are suitable for trials of long-term circulatory support as an alternative to transplantation, but are an even more valuable tool with which to initiate the 'keep your own heart' strategy. Molecular biology and blood pump technology are now advancing side by side towards a potential solution to the pandemic of congestive heart failure.

The financial consequences of widespread LVAD use could be considerable in a State-funded system. Congestive heart failure now affects 1% of the Western world and engenders increasing consternation from the governments that are obliged to provide expensive treatments for patients who are often terminal. At present LVADs are only used routinely in insurance-based health care systems, such as those in Germany and the United States. However, LVADs can prove cost effective by reversing hepatorenal dysfunction and liberating the heart failure patient from intensive care facilities. An implantable user friendly LVAD could greatly reduce the cost of drug therapy and multiple hospital admissions required during decompensation in the final few years of life. Left ventricular off-loading may even arrest the disease process in some conditions.

Accordingly, we predict that in 10 years' time new blood pumps will be applied for heart failure in the same way as is the pacemaker for heart rhythm problems (Fig. 35.39). Adjuncts to left ventricular recovery will proliferate and evolve into a new pharmacological and genetic engineering industry. Scare human donor hearts will be reserved for patients without alternative therapy.

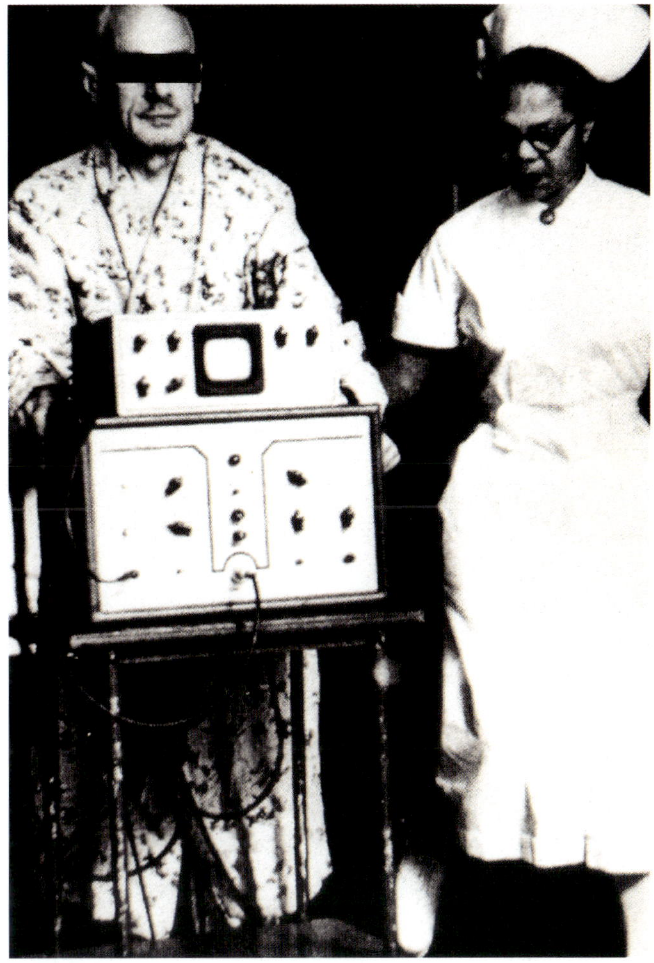

**Figure 35.39** *Pacemaker in the 1950s. Improvement in blood pump technology now parallels the development of the pacemaker from a large external system to a miniature fully implanted device.*

# APPENDIX

## Design of clinical trials to assess artificial heart technology: Modified from the Bethesda conference for the design of clinical trial to study circulatory support devices for chronic heart failure [50])

Clinical trials designed to assess new long-term circulatory support devices must be scientifically sound, clinically meaningful and achievable in a finite time frame at reasonable expense. Patients enrolled in these investigations must have severe sustained congestive heart failure despite optimum medical treatment. All patients should be under the supervision of a team experienced in the management of severe heart failure. The target population should include male and female patients with coronary artery disease and non-ischaemic cardiomyopathy and include an appropriate number of female patients.

The objective of implanting a device is to improve survival and quality of life when compared to alternative therapy. Device safety is also an important end-point. Assessment of device safety requires documentation of the incidence of adverse effects as outlined at the end of this appendix. Basic trials designs may include the following:

- a pilot study of safety and efficacy in otherwise terminal patients not amenable to other medical or surgical treatments
- randomization against maximum medical therapy for non-transplant candidates (an approach which may include other surgical therapies)
- randomization against intention to treat by transplantation in potential transplant candidates. Randomization of terminally ill patients is already controversial given the proven efficiacy of first generation LVADs.

The trial design must include sufficient numbers of patients to provide enough events to allow end-point comparison with statistically and clinically meaningful data. The primary end-points to be measured include:

- all cause mortality
- health-related quality of life
- haemodynamic status
- quantitated exercise capacity
- functional cardiac status, including cardiovascular mortality
- device reliability and adverse events.

The determination of sample size in any clinical trial is based upon the differences in the primary outcome event, which the investigator is attempting to establish. For comparisons with medical treatment sample size must be sufficient to establish clinical utility. For example the study might be designed to establish a 33% survival gain and improved quality of life by 2 years with a significance level of 0.05 with 80% power. A goal of 33% reduction in mortality is equivalent to double the effect obtained by ACE inhibitors for heart failure and thrombolytic drugs for acute myocardial infarction. Where feasible, randomization is preferable to ensure equitably constituted comparative groups. Since practical considerations dictate relatively small sample sizes in LVAD studies, the efficacy of the device must be high if it is to have a meaningful impact on survival and quality of life.

Current exclusion criteria for LVADs for include:

- anatomical contraindications to device implantation
- the presence of active systemic infection
- presence of a bleeding or coagulation disorder
- the presence of severe end-organ dysfunction deemed irreversible by improved cardiac output
- inability of the patient to communicate effectively with the investigators or follow instructions, or to be legally competent to give informed consent
- other conditions that in the opinion of the investigators would disqualify the patient from inclusion.

The duration of the study should be sufficient to establish survival of the control group and to document improvement in quality of life and survival of the recipient population. This duration may be too short to monitor device failure. With LVADs it is impossible for the investigator to be blinded to the nature of treatment prescribed. Equally sham operations performed in support of the concept of a blinded trial cannot be justified.

## Assessment of the device itself

The LVAD is implanted into patients with end-stage heart disease in order to reverse cardiogenic shock and improve end-organ function by improving systemic blood flow. As a minimum requirement the device must provide a cardiac index $\geq 2.2$ l/m$^2$/min with a pulmonary wedge pressure $\leq 18$ mmHg. The design of the device should allow increased blood flow with exercise or other physiological demands. For this reason the LVAD must either accommodate variations in preload or allow external adjustment so that output can be increased when needed. During the peri-operative period the effects of transient right heart dysfunction, reduced preload, tamponade or other surgically related problems may interfere with the ability of the LVAD to meet these demands. These are deemed as patient-related failures and not failure of the blood pump. It is also recognized that during exercise an implantable LVAD may reach maximum pump output after which the patient's own heart can eject blood through the aortic valve and further increase total cardiac output. Equally when a patient has recovered from surgery with a well functioning LVAD, exercise capacity may still be limited by the chronic systemic effects of heart failure, including skeletal muscular atrophy or pulmonary dysfunction. These problems only improve with by rehabilitation and physical training.

Aspects of cardiovascular function to be kept under review include:

- the minimally acceptable degree of circulatory support provided by the LVAD
- the effects of the device on native heart function
- changes in exercise capacity over time.

In the presence of a well-functioning LVAD, residual right ventricular dysfunction may compromise exercise capacity. The effects of LVAD support on the right ventricle and right-sided circulation are not always predictable. Elevated pulmonary vascular resistance or impaired right ventricular contractility may result in decreased left atrial pressure, an underfilled LVAD and decreased LVAD flow. The most important goal of LVAD support is to provide the patient with improved quality of life. Objective measurement of exercise capacity ($MVO_2$ ml/min/kg) can demonstrate that the patient has improved physical capacity. Other aspects of quality of life can be assessed by the Minnesota 'Living with heart failure questionnaire'.

## Transplant or non-transplant candidates?

It is widely recognized that donor hearts are a scarce commodity and that intention to treat by transplantation often includes a prolonged waiting period or intervening death. An undefined number of potential transplant candidates are never listed because of the shortage of donor hearts. In clinical trials separation of transplant candidates from non-transplant eligible patients is an important strategy to minimize the incidence of cross-over from device therapy to transplantation or vice versa. Cross-over confounds the analysis of trial results and reduces statistical power of the trial to detect effects. In contrast the competing risk of death may confound analysis of non-fatal events.

In the case of patients who are not candidates for transplantation, it is feasible to conduct prospective randomized control trials with a parallel study design. A non-randomized concurrent control group can also be considered. However, those patients who are not transplant candidates are often older and sicker with more chronic end-organ dysfunction. They are recognized to be at greater risk of complications and death during the perioperative period when compared to transplant eligible patients.

Transplant candidates improved by LVAD support have better outcomes. It should therefore be justifiable to conduct a prospect randomized trial of prospective transplant recipients to axial flow pumps or continued medical therapy. A trial to demonstrate the utility of devices in ambulatory patients might include all those with a particular disease (e.g. dilated cardiomyopathy) or be limited to patients with a low probability of being transplanted (large type O patients or those with multiple antibodies). This may necessitate a non-randomized prospective cohort study. The LVAD group might then consist of transplant candidates with a low likelihood of being transplanted while the controls would be selected from the general pool of candidates.

An independent clinical evaluation committee, preferably based in a separate hospital should review the inclusion data for each patient and audit the completeness and accuracy of data collection. The nature of adverse events must be clearly defined. Those recommended by the Bethesda Conference Report on Circulatory Support Devices and accepted by the FDA are provided in the following section.

## Definition of adverse events in LVAD patients

1. *Bleeding:* Blood loss resulting in:
   (a) death
   (b) reoperation
   (c) red blood cell transfusion (greater than or equal to 6 units within 24 hours) or
   (d) treatment or intervention for bleeding.

2. *Haemolysis:* Three plasma free haemoglobin values >40 mg/dl (measured by standard clinical pathology or laboratory medicine methods). The final two readings taken within 12 hours of each other as confirmation of the first reading.
3. *Cardiac tamponade*: Accumulation of undrained fluid resulting in haemodynamic compromise requiring reoperation or intervention.
4. *Reoperation:* Any unscheduled return to the operating room.
5. *Wound dehiscence*: Disruption of the opposed surfaces of a surgical incision, excluding infectious aetiology.
6. *Infection:*
   (a) Local infection: Positive tissue or swab culture (from the device or other sites) requiring intervention.
   (b) Systemic infection: any instance in which intravenous (IV) antimicrobial treatment is instituted (excluding routine prophylactic treatment dictated by hospital protocol). This includes treatment of culture negative symptoms.
   (c) Bacterial, viral, fungal, or protozoan infection (documented by standard clinical pathology or laboratory medicine methods), treated with antimicrobial agents (excluding routine prophylactic treatment dictated by hospital protocol).
7. *Myocardial infarction:* The presence of two of the following three criteria:
   (a) Creatine phosphokinase (CPK) (measured by standard clinical pathology or laboratory medicine methods) greater than the normal range for that hospital with a positive MB fraction;
   (b) ECG with a pattern or changes consistent with a myocardial infarction;
   (c) A history and timing consistent with either of the above events.
8. *Arrhythmias:* Any documented arrhythmia that requires intervention or results in the signs and symptoms of vital organ hypoperfusion, such as dizziness, syncope, or lightheadedness.
9. *Hypotension:* Hypotension requiring treatment or manifesting signs and symptoms of vital organ hypoperfusion, such as dizziness, syncope, or loss of peripheral pulses.
10. *Hypertension:* A blood pressure greater than or equal to 140/90 mmHg, measured on three separate days.
11. *Right heart failure*: Cardiac index less than 2.2 $l/min/m^2$, for greater than or equal to 6 hours, resulting in death, or requiring intervention, in the absence of anatomical structural reasons, left-sided dysfunction, or hypovolaemia.
12. *Left heart failure:* Cardiac index less than 2.2 $l/min/m^2$, for grater than or equal to 6 hours or resulting in death, or requiring intervention, in the absence of anatomical structural reasons, right-sided dysfunction, or hypovolaemia.
13. *Device malfunction:* Any instance when any component of the system fails to perform according to specifications. To use these data in calculating reliability for the device, an event must be evaluated using the definitions for failure that are included in the ASAIO-STS Long Term Blood Pump Reliability Recommendation.
14. *Device system failure:* The inability of the device system, including redundant, external back-up components, to provide adequate circulatory support. For example, the inability to provide pump output of X for Y period of time under ZZZ conditions (e.g. rest, exercise). The definition may be modified to address the indicated use of a specific device. However, the definitions must include measurable criteria, and must be applicable to the *in vitro*, *in vivo*, and clinical environment in order to use the data in calculating the reliability of the device.
15. *Renal failure:* Abnormal kidney function requiring haemodialysis or haemofiltration in patients who did not require these procedures prior to mechanical circulatory support/transplant/medical therapy. Renal function laboratory data (measured by standard clinical pathology or laboratory medicine methods) will be collected and recorded as part of specific protocols.
16. *Hepatic failure:* Greater than two times increase above baseline values in any two of the four liver function studies (bilirubin, SGPT, SGOT, or LDH), measured by standard clinical pathology or laboratory medicine methods, or if hepatic dysfunction is the primary cause of death.
17. *Respiratory failure:* Impairment of respiratory function requiring reintubation or tracheostomy, or inability to discontinue ventilatory support after postoperative day 6.
18. *Neurological dysfunction:* The advent of a neurological deficit, whether it be transient or prolonged, that is not present at baseline as determined by a standard neurological examination and appropriate special investigations. The investigation of new neurological deficits will be determined by the clinical presentation. However, should a new event occur and the clinical

features indicate a cerebral localization, particularly in the case of a stroke-like syndrome, a repeat computerized axial tomographic (CT) scan of the head will be indicated. A CT scan of the head and clinical examination to be carried out at entry, and this together with a further neurological examination will be repeated at appropriate intervals (interval determined by sponsor).

19. *Psychiatric problems:* Any change in mood or behavior that requires an intervention that is outside the standard management protocol.
20. *Rejection*: A clinical event, usually but not always accompanied by an abnormal myocardial biopsy, which results in augmentation of a patient's immunosuppression.
21. *Cardiac allograft vasculopathy:* An accelerated form of cardiac allograft coronary vascular disease leading to retransplantation, death or therapy for cardiac allograft dysfunction.
22. *Post-transplantation lympho-proliferative disorder*: Lymphocyte tumor in patients receiving chronic immunosuppression.
23. *Hyperlipidaemia:* A total serum cholesterol (measured by standard clinical pathology or laboratory medicine methods) or 200 mg/dl.
24. *Glucose intolerance:* An adverse event manifested by new onset of diabetes mellitus or pre-existing diabetes mellitus requiring increased intensity of medical intervention.
25. *Obesity:* A weight 20% greater than ideal body weight, For patients meeting the definition of obesity at baseline, an increase in body weight of greater than 10% from baseline will qualify as an adverse event.
26. *Osteoporosis:* Any decrease in bone density compared to baseline, determined by nuclear bone densitometry.
27. *Reproductive system dysfunction:* Any new sexual or menstrual dysfunction.
28. *Malignancy:* Occurrence of any malignancy (excluding squamous or basal cell of the skin) not present at time of entrance into the study.
29. *Pain:* Necessity for chronic pain medication or other pain management interventions.
30. *Thrombotic vascular complications (excluding central nervous system events):* Any mural thrombus or thromboembolism in the vasculature or device confirmed by standard clinical and laboratory testing that requires intervention.
31. *Loss of limb:* Loss of a limb or any portion thereof.
32. *Aneurysm:* Any aneurysm, pseudoaneurysm, or dissection requiring medical or surgical intervention, or resulting in death.
33. *Herniation:* Protrusion of an organ, part of an organ, or other structure through the wall of a cavity in which it normally resides.
34. *Cholelithiasis:* Gall bladder dysfunction causing clinical symptoms requiring medical or surgical intervention.
35. *Pancreatitis:* Pancreatic dysfunction causing clinical symptoms requiring medical or surgical intervention.
36. *Bowel obstruction/perforation*: Intestinal obstruction or perforation requiring intervention.
37. *Dysphagia:* Eating disorder causing symptoms requiring medical or surgical intervention.
38. *Loss of appetite:* Reduction of food intake severe enough to require hyperalimentation or nasogastric feeding that persists after 14 days of any surgical intervention.
39. *Haematoma:* A collection of clotted blood requiring aspiration or surgical *intervention.*
40. *Persistent malnutrition*: Inability to attain or maintain desired body weight due to inadequate intake of calories and protein following the intervention.
41. *Unscheduled hospital readmittance:* A readmission to the hospital that is unscheduled or outside the protocol.

In addition to these well-defined events, there are three quality of life issues, which are particularly relevant to LVAD patients. These are:

- the specific functional limitations on mobility, ambulation, sleep and body care related to the device
- cognitive functioning in the wake of heart failure and cardiopulmonary bypass
- the patients anxieties about device noise, mechanical failure or complications, such as stroke or driveline infection. In permanent LVAD patients anxiety about leaving the safety of the hospital environment may have negative effects on well being. As confidence and freedom increase so does quality of life. Left ventricular recovery and spontaneous restoration of sinus rhythm can also cause dramatic late improvement in well being and exercise capacity.

## References


1. Deng MC, De Meester JMJ, Smits JMA *et al.* (2000) Effect of receiving a heart transplant: analysis of a national cohort entered onto a waiting list, stratified by heart failure severity. *BMJ* **321**: 540–5.
2. Heerdt PM, Holmes JW, Cai B *et al.* (2000) Chronic unloading by left ventricular assist device reverses contractile dysfunction and alters gene expansion in end heart failure. *Circulation* **102**: 2713–19.
3. Pouzet B, Ghostine S, Vilquin J-T *et al.* (2000) Is skeletal myoblast transplantation clinically relevant in the era of angiotensin-converting enzyme inhibitors (abstr). *Circulation* **102**(suppl II) II682.
4. Westaby S, Banning AP, Jarvik RK *et al.* (2000) First permanent implant of the Jarvik 2000 Heart. *Lancet* **356**: 900–3.
5. Westaby S (1997) *Landmarks in Cardiac Surgery*. Isis Medical Media. Oxford.
6. DeBakey ME (1971) Left ventricular bypass pump for cardiac assistance. Clinical experience. *Am J Cardiol* **27**: 3–11.
7. Barnard CN (1967) The operation. A human cardiac transplant: an interim report of a successful operation performed at Groote Schuur Hospital Cape Town. *S Afr Med J* **41**: 1271–4.
8. Devries WC, Anderson JH, Joyce LD, Anderson FL, Hammond EH, Jarvik RK, Kolff WJ (1984) Clinical use of the total artificial heart. *N Engl J Med* **310**: 273–8.
9. Arabia FA, Copeland JB, Smith RG *et al.* (1997) International experience with the Cardio West Total Artificial Heart as a bridge to heart transplantation. *Eur J Cardiothorac Surg* **11**(Suppl): S5–10.
10. Pierce WS, Brighton JA, O'Bannon W, Donachy JH, Phillips WM, Landis DL, White WJ, Waldhausen JA (1974) Complete left ventricular bypass with paracorporeal pump: design and evaluation. *Ann Surg* **180**: 418–26.
11. Frazier OH, Cooley DA, Okereke OUJ *et al.* (1986) Cardiac transplantation in a patient with septicemia after prolonged intraaortic balloon pump support: implications for staged transplantation. *Tex Heart Inst J* **13**: 13–18.
12. Frazier OH (1994a) First use of an untethered, vented electric left ventricular assist device for long term support. *Circulation* **89**: 2908–14.
13. Frazier OH, Rose EA, MacMannus Q, Burton NA, Lefrak EA, Poirier VL, Dasse KA (1992) Multicenter clinical evaluation of the Heartmate 1000 IP left ventricular assist device. *Ann Thorac Surg* **53**: 1080–90.
14. Frazier OH, Rose EA, McCarthy P *et al.* (1995) Improved mortality and rehabilitation of transplant candidates treated with a long term implantable left ventricular assist system. *Ann Thorac Surg* **222**: 327–8.
15. Argenziano M, Cantanese KA, Moazami N *et al.* (1997) The influence of infection on survival and successful transplantation in patients with left ventricular assist devices. *J. Heart Lung Transplant* **16**: 822–31.
16. McCarthy PM, Schmitt SK, Vargo RL, Gordon S, Keys TF, Hobbs RE (1996) Implantable LVAD infections: implications for permanent use of the device. *Ann Thorac Surg* **61**: 359–65.
17. Schmid C, Wyaand M, Navabi DG, Hammel D, Deng M, Ringelstein EB, Scheld HH (1998) Cerebral and systemic embolization during left ventricular support with the Novacor N100 device. *Ann Thorac Surg* **65**: 1703–10.
18. Slater JP, Rose EA, Levin HR, Frazier OH, Roberts JK, Weinberg AD, Oz MC (1996) Low thromboembolic risk without anticoagulation using advanced design left ventricular assist devices. *Ann Thorac Surg* **62**: 1321–7.
19. Farrar DJ (1994) Ventricular interaction during mechanical circulatory support. *Semin Thorac Cardiovasc Surg* **6**: 163–8.
20. Farrar DJ, Compton PG, Hershan JJ, Hill JD (1985) Right ventricular function in an operating model of mechanical left ventricular assistance and its effects in patients with depressed left ventricular function. *Circulation* **72**: 1279–85.
21. Rose EA, Moskowitz AJ, Packer M *et al.* (1999) The REMATCH trial: rationale, design and endpoints. Randomized Evaluation of Mechanical Assistance for the Treatment of Congestive Heart Failure. *Ann Thorac Surg* **67**: 723–30.
22. Myers TJ, McGee MD, Zeluff BJ, Radovancevic B, Frazier OH (1991) Frequency and significance of infections in patients receiving prolonged LVAD support. *ASAIO Trans* 37: M283–5.
23. Termuhlen DF, Pennington DG, Roodman ST *et al.* (1989) T cells in ventricular assist device patients. *Circulation* **80**(Suppl III): III174–III182.
24. Ankersmith J, Tugulea S, Spanier T *et al.* (1999) Activation-induced T-cell death and immune dysfunction after implantation of left ventricular assist device. *Lancet* **354**: 550–5.
25. Livingstone ER, Fisher CA, Bibidakis EJ *et al.* (1996) Increased activation of the coagulation and fibrinolytic systems leads to haemorrhagic complications during left ventricular assist implantation. *Circulation* (Suppl II) II227–II234.
26. Rose EA, Levin HR, Oz MC, Frazier OH, Macmanus Q, Burton NA, Lefrak EA (1994) Artificial circulatory support with textured interior surfaces. A counterintuitive approach to minimising thromboembolism. *Circulation* **90**(Suppl II): II87–II91.
27. Pennington DG, McBride LR, Peigh PS, Miller LW, Swartz MT (1994) Eight years experience with bridging to cardiac transplantation. *J Thorac Cardiovasc Surg* **107**: 472–480.
28. Moazami N, Roberts K, Argenziano M, Catanese K, Mohr JP, Rose EA, Oz MC (1997) Asymptomatic microembolism in patients with long-term ventricular support. *ASAIO J* **43**: 177–80.
29. Goldstein DJ, Oz MC, Rose EA (1998) Implantable left ventricular assist devices. *N Engl J Med* **339**: 1522–33.
30. Griffiths BP, Kormos RL, Nastala CJ, Winowich S, Pristas JM (1996) Results of extended bridge to transplantation: window into the future of permanent ventricular assist devices. *Ann Thorac Surg* **61**: 396–8.
31. Westaby S, Katsumata T, Houel R, Evans R, Pigott D, Frazier OH, Jarvik R (1998) Jarvik 2000 Heart: potential for bridge to myocyte recovery. *Circulation* **98**: 1568–74.
32. Jarvik R, Westaby S, Katsumata T, Pigott D, Evans RD (1998) LVAD power delivery: a percutaneous approach to avoid infection. *Ann Thorac Surg* **65**: 470–3.
33. Parkin JL (1990) Percutaneous pedestal in cochlear implantation. *Ann Otol Rhinol Laryngol* 99: 796–800.


32. Jarvik R, Westaby S, Katsumata T, Pigott D, Evans RD (1998) LVAD power delivery: a percutaneous approach to avoid infection. *Ann Thorac Surg* **65**: 470–3.
33. Parkin JL (1990) Percutaneous pedestal in cochlear implantation. *Ann Otol Rhinol Laryngol* 99: 796–800.


34. Westaby S, Banning A, Jarvik RK *et al.* (2000) First permanent implant of the Jarvik 2000 Heart. *Lancet* **356**: 900–3.

35. Wiesenthaler GM, Schima H, Hiesmayr M *et al.* (2000) First clinical experience with the DeBakey VAD continuous axial-flow pump for bridge to transplantation. *Circulation* **101**: 356–9.
36. Potapov EV, Loebe M, Nasseri BA *et al.* (2000) Pulsatile flow in patients with a novel nonpulsatile implant LVAD. *Circulation* **102**: 183–7.
37. Butler K, Thomas D, Antaki J *et al.* (1997) Development of the Nimbus/Pittsburgh axial flow left ventricular assist system. Artifi. Organs. 602–610.
38. Nojiri C, Kijima T, Maekawa J *et al.* (2000) Terumo implantable left ventricular assist system: results of long-term animal study. *ASAIO J* **46**: 117–22.
39. Hetzer R, Müller JH, Weng Y-G *et al.* (2000) Mid term follow up of patients who underwent removal of a left ventricular assist device after cardiac recovery from end stage dilated cardiomyopathy. *J Thorac Cardiovasc Surg* **120**: 843–55.
40. Mann DL, Willerson J (1998) Left ventricular assist devices and the failing heart: a bridge to recovery, a permanent assist device or a bridge too far? *Circulation* **98**: 2367–9.
41. Tajima M, Weinberg EO, Bartunek J, Jin H, Yang R, Paoni NF, Lorell BH (1999) Treatment with growth hormone enhances contractile reserve and intracellular calcium transients in myocytes from rats with post infarction heart failure. *Circulation* **99**: 127–34.
42. Miklting H, Bartling B, Schumann H *et al.* (1999) Altered levels of RNA apoptosis mediating genes after mid term mechanical ventricular support in dilative cardiomyopathy-first results of the Halle Assis Induced Recovery Study (HAIR). *Thorac Cardiovasc Surg* **47**: 48–50.
43. Depre C, Shipley GL, Chen W *et al.* (1998) Unloaded heart in vivo replicates fetal gene expression of cardiac hypertrophy. *Nature Med* **4**: 1269–75.
44. Bartling B, Milting H, Schumann, H *et al.* (1999) Myocardial gene expression of regulators of myocyte apoptosis and myocyte calcium homeostasis during haemodynamic unloading by ventricular assist devices in patients with end-stage heart failure. *Circulation* **100**(Suppl II): S216–S223.
45. Galatius-Jensen S, Wroblewski H, Emmeluth C, Bie P, Haunso S, Kastrup J (1996) Plasma endothelin in congestive heart failure: a predictor of cardiac death? *J Card Fail* **2**: 71–6.
46. Mehta S, Anfiero TX, Pae WE Jr, Miller CA, Pierce WS (1995) Mechanical ventricular assistance: an economical and effective means of treating end-stage heart disease. *Ann Thorac Surg* **60**: 284–90.
47. Pac WE (1998) Bethesda Conference: conference for the design of clinical trials to study circulatory support devices for chronic heart failure. *AnnThrac Surg* **66**: 1452–65.

# Spatial orientation of the ventricular muscle band and approach to partial ventriculotomy in heart failure

36

F. TORRENT-GUASP, M. BALLESTER, J. M. CARALPS-RIERA,
L. E. SAMUELS AND J. NARULA

## Introduction

It has been proposed that the ventricular myocardium, both right (RV) and left ventricular (LV), exists as a continuous muscle band [1–4]. The band is orientated spatially as a helix formed by basal and apical loops. This unique anatomy and spatial configuration of the myocardial muscle determine the way in which the ventricular ejection and filling take place [5, 6]. Further, knowledge of this unique morphological and physiological characteristic should facilitate the development of more effective surgical procedures in congestive heart failure.

## Spatial orientation of the myocardial ventricular muscle band

### Unwrapping of the ventricular myocardial band

Careful anatomical cardiac studies have established that the ventricular myocardium can be unrolled in a continuous muscle band [3, 4]. Unwrapping occurs easily (Fig. 36.1), with least resistance, along a natural cleavage plane. Dissection of the ventricular myocardial band can be accomplished in three major steps. In the first step, the basal loop is unrolled (Fig. 36.2a). The superficial fibres of the anterior aspect of the LV are cut along the anterior interventricular sulcus (see arrow) in order to pull apart the RV free wall (RFW) (Fig. 36.2b). Dissection can then proceed posteriorly following the cleavage plane. In this way the complete basal loop is extended in its full length (Fig. 36.2c, red and green areas). In the second step (Fig. 36.2c, d), the aorta is dismounted, which involves separation along the cleavage plane (see arrow in Fig. 36.2c) defined by the two muscular strata, the fibres of the descending segment (DS, yellow) and the fibres of the ascending segment (AS, blue). The fibres of the AS and DS cross each other at the level of the septum. Following such a plane upwards to the aorta, right and left trigones are found (see *lt* and *rt* in Fig. 36.2d). After

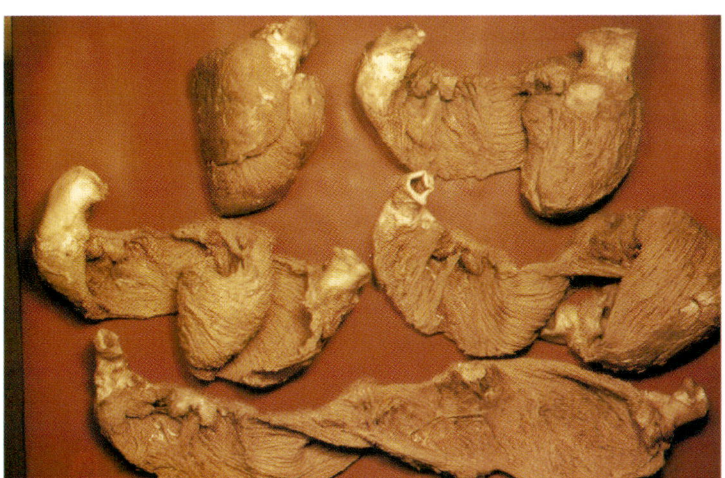

**Figure 36.1** *Consecutive stages of the unwinding of the ventricular myocardial band. See Figure 36.2 (steps a–e) for schematic representation.*

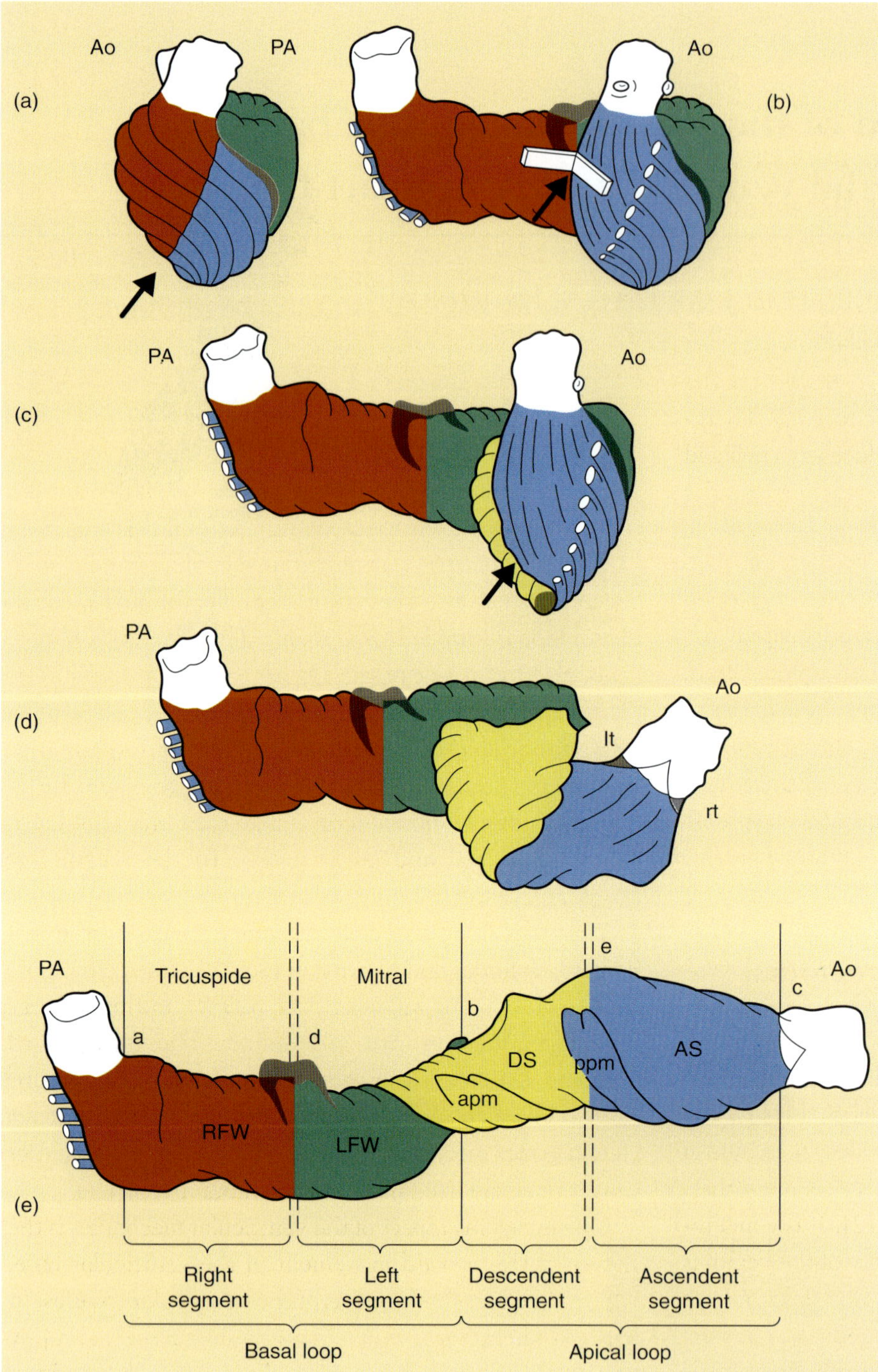


**Figure 36.2** *Schematic representation of the ventricular myocardial band (a–e) for consecutive stages of unwinding. The myocardial band can be divided into four segments (e): right ventricular free wall (RFW, red), left ventricular free wall (LFW, green), descending segment (DS, yellow) and ascending segment (AS, blue). The myocardial band extends between the pulmonary artery (PA) and the aorta (Ao). These segments spatially conform to two loops; the basal loop (from a to b), constituted by RFW (red) and LFW (green), and the apical loop (from b to c), formed by DS (yellow) and AS (blue). The spatial configuration of both loops forms a helicoid as shown in Figure 36.3. Arrows indicate the cleavage plane that provides clues for unwinding the myocardial band. apm: anterior papillary muscle; AS: ascending segment; Ao: aorta; DS: descending segment; LFW: left ventricular free wall; lt: left trigone of the aorta; PA: pulmonary artery; ppm: posterior papillary muscle; RFW: right ventricular free wall; rt: right trigone of the aorta.*

sectioning both trigones, the aorta can easily be dismounted. In the third step (Fig. 36.2d, e), the apical loop is unrolled; pulling apart the dismounted aorta, the apical loop is unrolled so that the entire ventricular myocardial band can be stretched out (Fig. 36.2e). Accordingly, the band extends from the pulmonary artery to the aorta (Figs. 36.1 and 36.2).

## Segmental anatomy of the band

At the centre of the uncoiled myocardial band, a fold can be observed that twists the band by 180°, and demarcates its basal and apical loops (Fig. 36.2e). The basal loop runs from the pulmonary artery root (a) to the central fold (b), and the apical loop runs from the central fold (b) to the aortic root (c). Both loops in turn can be divided into two segments each. The basal loop is divided into RV free wall segment (RFW, red) which extends from the pulmonary artery root (a) to the posterior interventricular septum (dotted line d), and the LV free wall segment (LFW, green) which extends from the posterior interventricular sulcus (d) to the central fold (b). Similarly, the apical loop is also divided into two segments, the descending LV segment (DS, yellow) which extends from the central fold (b) to the posterior papillary muscle (ppm, see e), which topographically coincides with the posterior interventricular sulcus when the band is wrapped, and the AS (blue) which extends from the posterior papillary muscle (e) to the aortic root (c). Therefore, the ventricular myocardial band produces two helicoid spirals. One spiral is represented by the apical loop and the other by the basal loop (Fig. 36.2). Figure 36.3 schematically represents these two spirals.

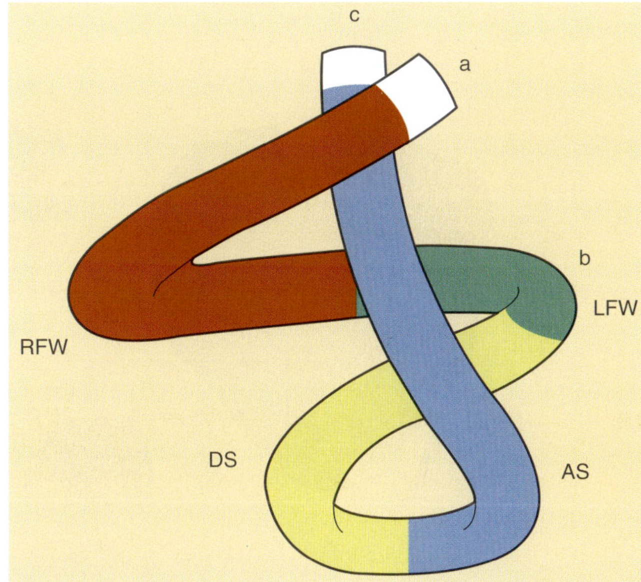


**Figure 36.3** *Schematic representation of the spatial configuration of the ventricular myocardial band as a helicoid. Abbreviations and colours as in Figure 36.2.*

## Ventricular contraction based on spatial orientation of the myocardial band

Anatomy dictates function, and it is likely that the helical anatomical configuration may contribute to ventricular performance [5–7]. In this respect, analysis of the movements of the heart in magnetic resonance imaging (MRI) studies of normal individuals demonstrates lack of movement of the apex during the cardiac cycle. Instead, the entire base of the heart (including atria and great vessels) moves downwards in systole and upwards in diastole [8–10]. Recently, using fast Fourier analysis of gated-blood pool ventriculography, it was observed that the sequence of mechanical ventricular activation follows closely the helicoid trajectory of the myocardial band; the initial segment to be activated is the basal region of the ventricle, first the RV segment then the LV, and the apical segments follow [12]. It is conceivable that the sequential contractile activity of the peculiar helicoid structure of the ventricular myocardium allows upward and downward movements. The sequence of contraction is RFW $\rightarrow$ LFW $\rightarrow$ DS $\rightarrow$ AS (Fig. 36.3). Accordingly, after contraction of the RFW segment (red) contraction of the LFW segment (green) takes place. As a result, the entire basal loop (both red and green segments) becomes a rigid external cylinder, analogous to the stiff outer shell [13]. Subsequent contraction of the descending segment pulls the ventricular base downwards, thereby shortening the long axis of the ventricular cavity, reducing its volume and allowing ventricular ejection. Contraction of the ascending segment then results in an increase in the longitudinal axis of the ventricles and an upward displacement of the base of the heart, which increases the ventricular volume. The increase in volume allows for the suction function (or diastole) of the left ventricle as previously hypothesized [14].

Therefore, the mechanics of the ventricles resembles that of a cylinder and piston of a motor engine (Fig. 36.4). The cylinder is constituted by the basal loop, the contraction of which forms an outer stiff shell which is pulled downwards by the contraction of the DS and upwards by the AS [5, 7]. Whereas the cylinder is fixed and the piston provides the mobile element in the former, the cylinder moves over the fixed piston in the human ventricle.

One intriguing aspect of the ventricular mechanics is the nature of the upward movement of the ventricular base, which elongates the long axis of the ventricular cavities. In MRI studies, the basal myocardium moves abruptly upwards in the late phase of systole [15]. The question of why the contraction of the AS should give rise to an increase in the longitudinal axis of the ventricles is intriguing. One way to explain such a movement is proposed in Figure 36.5. At the time of contraction of DS, which pulls down the entire basal loop (cylinder) of the ventricles, the AS adopts a forced ‘S’ configuration (Fig. 36.5C). However, the contraction of the AS (thicker fibres in Fig. 36.5D) implies its stiffening, which gives rise to lengthening of the long axis of the ventricular cavities. This movement is similar to the way

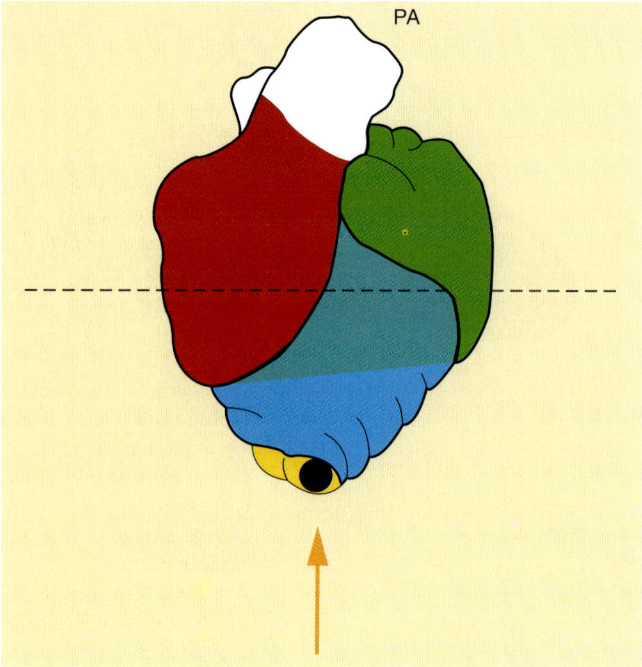


**Figure 36.4** *Orientation of the four segments of the myocardial band at the midventricular level, as seen from the base. The heart has been unwrapped, coloured by segments and wrapped to its original position to be cut at the midventricular level. Note the complexity of the segmental distribution of the segments.*

in which the contraction of the dorsal musculature of the snake is associated with lengthening and upward movement of its body structure (Fig. 36.5C–E). In the heart, an increase in the long axis of the ventricle would give rise to the suction of blood (early rapid filling phase). Owing to the spatial configuration of the AS and DS a rotational movement of the heart occurs. This confirms the echocardiographic observations of the motion of the papillary muscle (3) and motion characterization by MRI [9, 10, 11, 15]. Where a counterclockwise twist of the basal portion of the left ventricle was detected during isovolumic contraction (probably caused by contraction of the DS), whereas the base rotated clockwise during late systole (contraction of the AS). The segmental direction of the fibres of both segments shown in Figure 36.5 explains the rotational movements.

## Surgical implications of the helicoid myocardial band

Sequential contraction of ventricular muscle band, spatially distributed as a helicoid, may result in successive shortening and lengthening of the ventricles. These movements may determine the ejection and suction of blood, respectively. Such a concept proposes early diastole as an active process [14]. It should also alter the approach to surgical intervention in heart failure. Reduction ventriculectomy has been proposed as a surgical alternative in end-stage heart failure in transplant non-candidates [16]. Although theoretically logical, the technique has had a limited surgical impact [17]. It is likely that ligation of the basal and apical segment muscular planes after partial volume reduction interferes with the natural sequence of myocardial contraction, and offsets the benefit accrued from diastolic volume attenuation. It behooves us to develop surgical strategies that

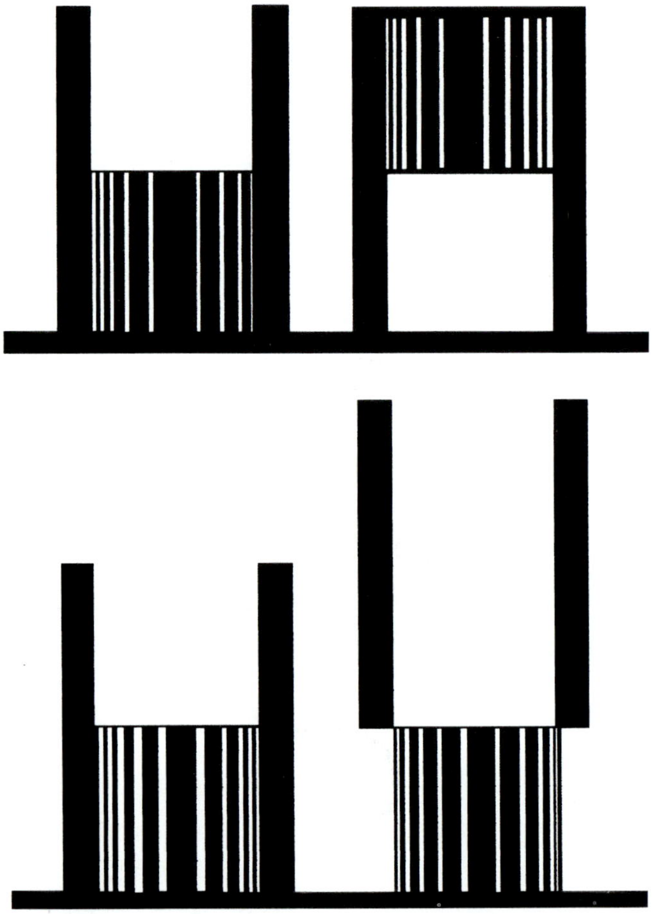

**Figure 36.5** *A mobile cylinder and fixed piston system as a representation of the proposed longitudinal movements of the myocardial band during the cardiac cycle. Top: cylinder and piston as in a motor engine;* bottom: *proposed motion in the heart: the left column represents systole, and the right column represents diastole. The cylinder is formed by the contraction and stiffening of the basal loop, i.e. RVF (red) and LVF (green) myocardial segments (Fig. 32.2). The piston is the apical loop. Contraction of the the descending segment of the apical loop pulls the cylinder down, forcing ventricular ejection. Subsequent contraction of the AS brings the base back up, creating a suction or ventricular filling.*

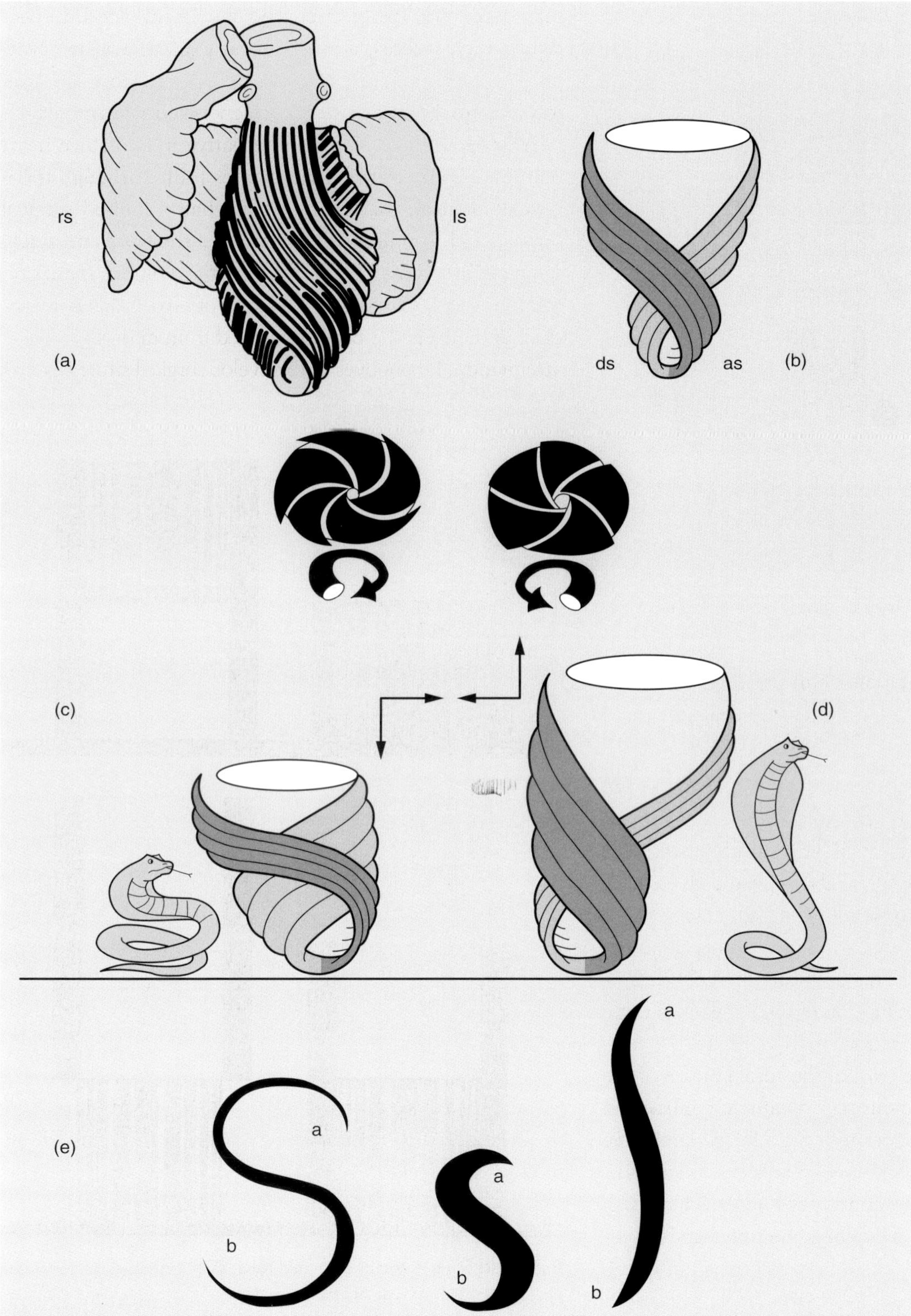


**Figure 36.6** *Proposed explanation of the late systolic upward motion of the base of the heart associated with a brisk upward movement of the base of the ventricles. (a) The basal outer shell has been removed to display the descending and ascending segments of the band, which are seen coloured in (b). (c) In early systole the base of the heart is pulled towards the apex as a result of contraction of the DS (thick bundles in yellow); such a movement forces the AS to adopt an 'S' configuration in the late systole. (d) Contraction of the AS segment (thick bundles in blue) and results in the upward movement of the base of the heart. The latter movement could be compared to the way in which contraction of the musculature of the snake elongates its body through stiffening of the muscles. (e) Scheme of the 'S' configuration of the AS* (left)*; the possibility that the DS contraction leads to a shortened 's'* (middle)*; and the likely configuration that it adopts upon its own contraction (in early diastole* (right)*. Contraction of the descending and ascending fibres also result in a rotational motion of the heart, as illustrated in the two intermediate figures which depict movement as seen from the apex.*

precisely shorten the non-overlapping regions of the ventricular muscle band [18] (Fig. 36.6–36.9).

Batista's technique is currently based on a buttonhole excision for the partial resection of the LV (Fig. 36.6b), which is usually made from basal to apical regions along the left border of the LV. With such resection, a reduction in the LV cavity volume, proportional to the amount of wall removed, is obtained. According to Laplace's law,

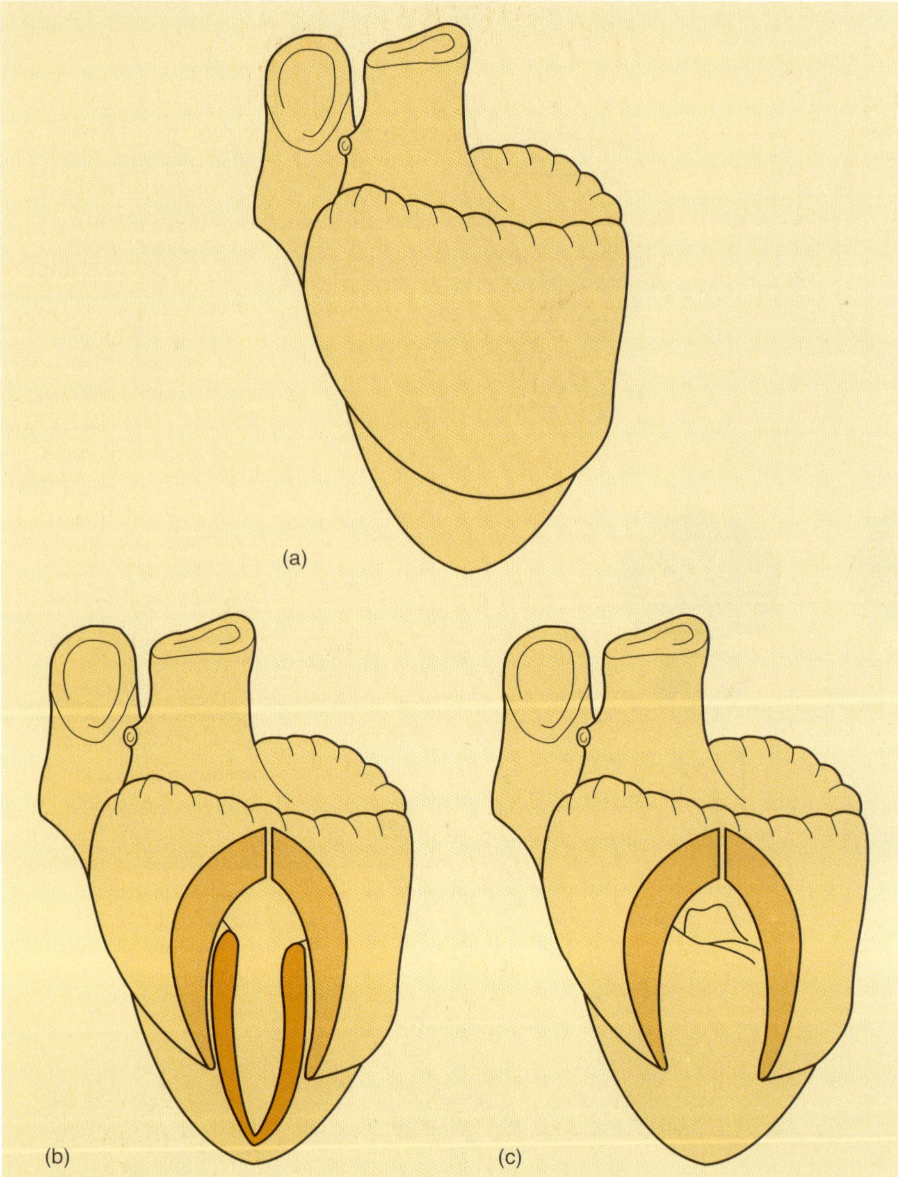


**Figure 36.7** *(a) Left border view of the left ventricle. (b) Schematic representation of Batista's procedure, which involves excision of the basal and apical loops of the ventricular myocardial band. (c) Proposed modification of the Batista procedure, in which only the basal loop is surgically excised.*

such a reduction is associated with a decreased tension in the ventricular myocardium, which improves LV ejection [18]. However, resection of the LV wall affects both the basal and apical loops of the ventricular myocardial band, disrupting the synchronized LV contraction. It may also necessitate removal of the anterior papillary muscle or even the posterior one, and concomitant mitral valve replacement.

On the basis of the knowledge of the ventricular myocardial structure, some modifications of Batista's procedure have been proposed [19]. When considering the heart as a conical structure (Fig. 36.7), it becomes evident that the decrease in volume of the cone obtained by reducing the apical half is insignificant (10%) compared with the reduction provided by excision of the basal loop (90%).

## Ventricular wall resection at the left border of the heart

An excision, as a horseshoe, may be performed in the left border of the heart on the basal loop [19] (Fig. 36.6c). In such a way, after suturing the incised edges of the ventricular band, an LV volume reduction is achieved with no damage to the apical loop. Since apical and basal loops cannot be identified in an unrolled heart, in order to avoid apical loop damage such resection should be performed at

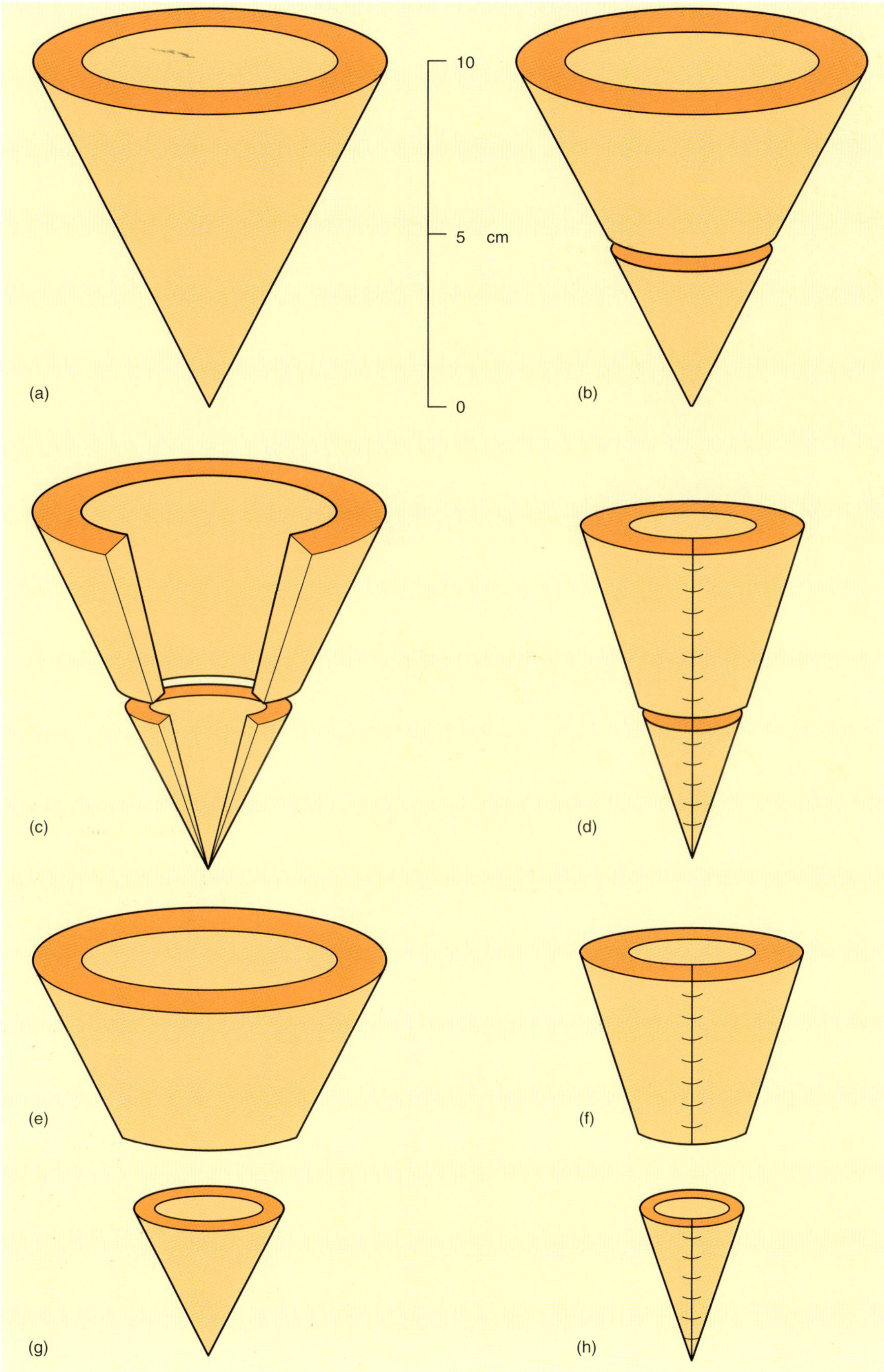


**Figure 36.8** *(a) Myocardial band anatomy represented as a cone. (b) The cone is transversely cut at its midportion to demonstrate that the proportional volume reduction provided by the excision of both basal and apical halves of the cone which correspond to the basal and apical loops of the heart (c, d). Note that the major volume reduction is related to the shortening of the diameter of the basal half (e–h).*

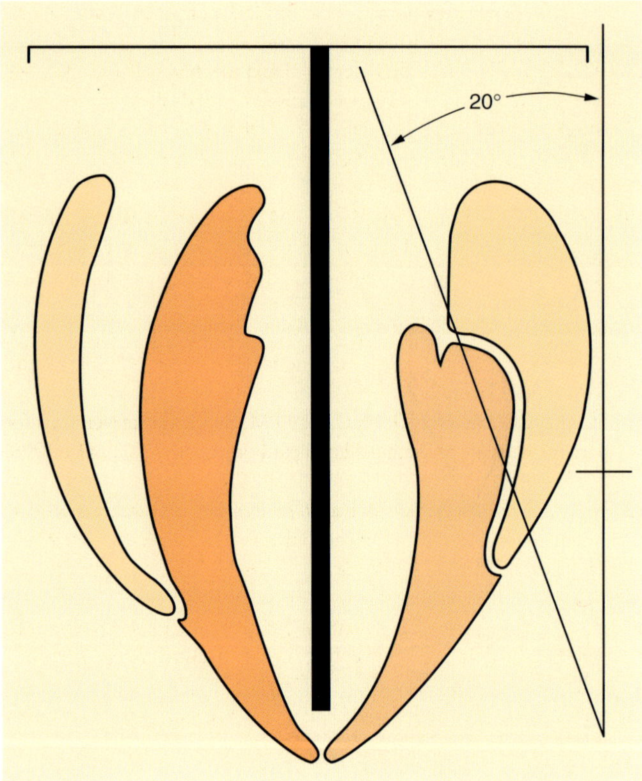


**Figure 36.9** *Longitudinal section of both ventricles wherein the overlap of both basal and apical loops is shown. Since it is not possible to differentiate basal from apical loops in the heart which is not unrolled, in the proposed modification of the Batista procedure the surgical excision must be made at an angle of 20° from the lateral border of the left ventricle predominantly to remove myocardial band of the basal loop.*

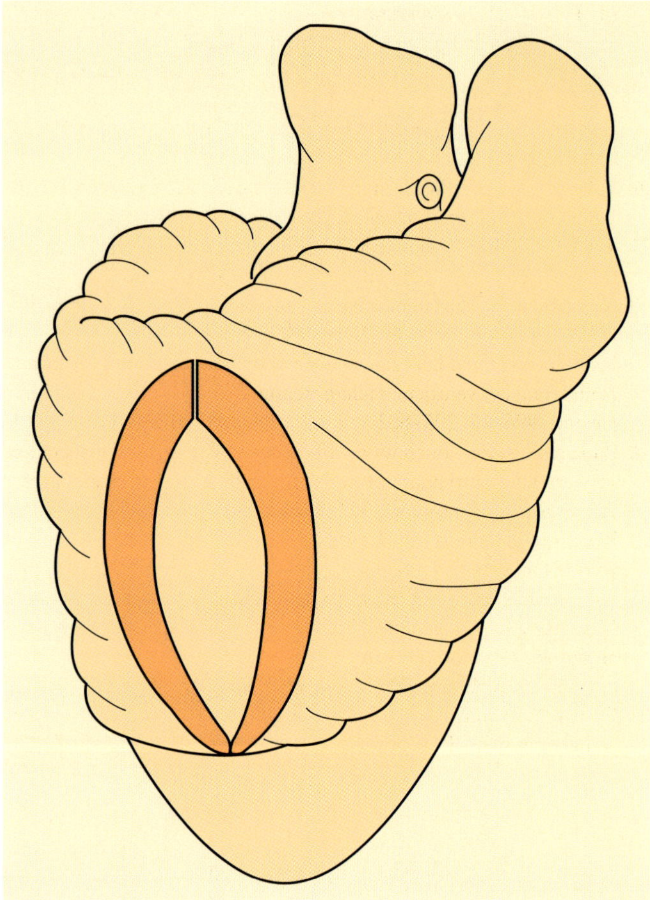

**Figure 36.10** *A buttonhole excision of the right ventricular free wall should also offer an effective reduction in left ventricular volume.*

about a 20° angle in relation to the longitudinal axis of the LV (Fig. 36.8).

### Ventricular wall resection at the right border of the heart

The basal loop circumscribes the apical loop, thus delineating both ventricular cavities and their basal halves. Since continuity exists between the RV and LV segments of the basal loop, it is hypothesized that volume reduction of the LV would be similarly achieved by means of a buttonhole excision in the RV segment (Fig. 36.9). In sparing the anatomy and function of the LV, the reduction in volume would appear to be mechanically advantageous.

## Conclusions

The two surgical modifications hypothesized, aimed at reducing the left ventricular volume of patients with end-stage dilated cardiomyopathy, appear as a means to spare the anatomy and function of the left ventricle in Batista's procedure. Such modifications spare the apical loop from the excision in a way that the papillary muscles, which generate from this loop, are not included in the surgical procedure, thus avoiding the possibility of mitral valve replacement. The fact that the apical loop remains untouched implies that the downward–upward movement of the heart should be preserved, allowing for physiological restoration of ventricular function.

## References

1. Torrent-Guasp F. *Anatomía functional del corazón*. Madrid: Paz-Montalbo, 1957.
2. Streeter DD, Torrent-Guasp F. Geodesic paths in the left ventricle of the mammalian heart. *Circulation* 1973; 48: 471–7.
3. Streeter DD, Powers WE, Ross MA, Torrent-Guasp F. Three-dimensional fiber orientation in the mammalian left ventricular wall.

In: J Barin, A Noordergraf, J Raines (eds) *Cardiovascular system dynamics*. Cambridge, MA: MIT Press, 1978, 73.

4. Torrent-Guasp F. La estructuración macroscópica del miocardio ventricular. *Rev Esp Cardiol* 1980; 133: 265–87.
5. Torrent-Guasp F. Estructura y función del corazón. *Rev Esp Cardiol* 1998; 51: 91–102.
6. Torrent-Guasp F, Whimster WF, Redmann K. A silicone rubber mould of the heart. *Technol Health Care* 1997; 5: 13–20.
7. Torreut-Guasp F, Ballester M, Ferreira A *et al.* Spatial orientation of the ventricular muscle baud vis-à-vis cardiac function! New vine in old bottle or old vine in new bottle? *J Cardiovasc Surg* 2001; (in press).
8. Karwatowski SP, Brecker JD, Yang GZ *et al.* A comparison of left ventricular myocardial velocity in diastole measured by magnetic resonance and left ventricular filling measured by echocardiography. *Eur Heart J* 1996; 17: 795–802.
9. Rademakers FE, Buchalter MB, Rogers WJ *et al.* Dissociation between left ventricular untwisting and filling. Acceutuation by catecholaunives. *Circulation* 1992; 85: 1572–81.
10. Rogers WJ, Shapiro EP, Weiss JL *et al.* Quantification of card correction for left ventricular long-axis shortening by magnetic resource tissue tagging and XXXX isolation. *Circulation* 1991; 84: 721–31.
11. Moore CC, Lugo-Olivieri CH, McVeith ER *et al.* Three-diureusionae systolic strain patterns in the normal human left ventricle characterization with tagged MR imaging. *Radiology* 2000; 214: 453–66.
12. Flotats A, Torrent-Guasp F, Ballester-Rodés M *et al.* Fourier analysis based display of the onset of myocardial contraction: correlation with the sequential contraction in the continuous ventricular myocardial band. *J Nucl Cardiol* (in press).
13. Armour JA, Randall WC. Electrical and mechanical activity of the papillary muscles. *Am J Physiol* 1970; 218: 1710–17.
14. Brutssaert DL, Sys SU, Gillebert TC. Diastolic failure: pathophysiology and therapeutic implications. *J Am Coll Cardiol* 1993; 22: 318–25.
15. Lorenz CH, Pastorek JS, Bundy JM. Delineation of normal left ventricular twist throughout systole by tagged cine magnetic resonance imaging. *J Cardiovasc Magnetic Resonance* 2000; 2: 97–108.
16. Batista RV, Santos JL, Takeshita N *et al.* Partial left ventriculectomy to improve left ventricular function in end-stage heart. *J Card Surg* 1996; 11: 96–7.
17. Starling RC, Sedira NG, McCarthy PM. Surgical interventions for patients with uouinchemic dilated cardiomyopathy. *Card Dev* 1998; 6: 334–44.
18. Belloti G, Moraes A, Bocchi E *et al.* Efeitos da Ventriculectomia Parcial nas Propiedades Mecanicas, Forma e Geometria do Ventrículo Esquerdo em Portadores de Cardiomiopatía Dilatada. *Arq Bras Cardiol* 1996; 67: 395–400.
19. Torrent-Guasp F, Caralps-Riera JM, Ballester M. Cuatro propuestas para la remodelación ventricular en el tratamiento quirúrgico de la miocardiopatía dilatada. *Rev Esp Cardiol* 1997; 50: 682–8.
20. Kass DA. Ventriculectomy. A direct application of Laplace's law. *Arq Bras Cardiol* 1996; 67: 401–2.

# Relentlessly progressive congestive heart failure: can it be prevented?

37

J. T. WILLERSON, R. DELGADO AND D. MANN

Congestive heart failure (CHF) usually occurs because of an important injury to the heart with a subsequent reduction in systolic function and/or as a result of an impaired ability of the heart to relax normally in diastole, increasing ventricular filling pressures and causing pulmonary congestion. Extracardiac factors explain some forms of heart failure as well, including very high output demands placed on the heart in conditions such as thyrotoxicosis and severe anaemia, and in large arteriovenous shunts. This chapter discusses the treatment and ultimately the prevention of the progressive systolic dysfunction that occurs in many patients with heart failure, which leads to progressively more severe symptoms following initial injury to the heart [1–4]. From an improved understanding of the biological or basic factors associated with progressive systolic dysfunction following such injury will come improved therapies, and hopefully ones that slow or stop pregression of this disease.

Systolic dysfunction and heart failure occur following injury to the heart and are then often progressive with symptoms developing slowly but relentlessly over time. On occasion, the initial injury results in a loss of functioning cardiac myocytes, such as occurs with acute myocardial infarction, and a consequent inability of the heart to maintain adequate cardiac output. In other circumstances, the development of heart failure may be more insidious and follow a long history of excessive alcohol intake, remote viral infection of the heart, longstanding systemic arterial hypertension, chronic coronary artery disease, valvular heart disease, a chronic autoimmune phenomenon, or increased heart rates for a prolonged period. In other cases, heart failure develops in families with obvious genetic risk. With acute myocardial infarction or viral myocarditis, the development of heart failure is often sudden, severe, and rapidly progressive, leading to an early demise. However, with other causes of injury, the patient remains asymptomatic for extended periods, gradually developing symptoms of heart failure in association with a progressive decline in systolic function, culminating in very severe heart failure.

It has been well demonstrated that a series of systemic compensatory mechanisms occurs with injury to the heart and subsequent depression in systolic function, and often, these are adequate to support the circulation so that the patient remains asymptomatic for some period (Fig. 32.1) [5–10]. Compensatory and adaptive mechanisms that have been identified include increases in salt- and water-retaining hormones, activation of the sympathetic nervous system, and systemic release or local effects of diuretic and vasodilator substances, including atrial naturetic hormone, selected prostaglandins, endothelin, and nitric oxide [5–12]. While these systemic biological responses help to maintain the patient in an asymptomatic state for months to years, they eventually cause worsening of cardiac dysfunction and the development of overt CHF.

It remains clear what mediates the progression of heart failure after the initial injury and how it may be influenced. Previous studies in animal models and humans have provided some answers [4, 13–33]. Specifically, alterations in excitation–contraction coupling that result from decreased sarcoplasmic reticulum calcium release and/or storage, alterations in sodium/calcium exchange across the sarcolemmal membrane, myofilament slippage, progressive loss of myofilaments, increase in β-myosin heavy chain expression, depletion of myocardial catecholamines, decreases in myocardial β-adrenergic receptor numbers, and loss of normal coupling of β-receptor stimulation to G protein intracellular signalling have been described in experimental animal models and humans. Each of these altered biological responses may play a role in the progression of heart failure. Progressive myocyte loss through

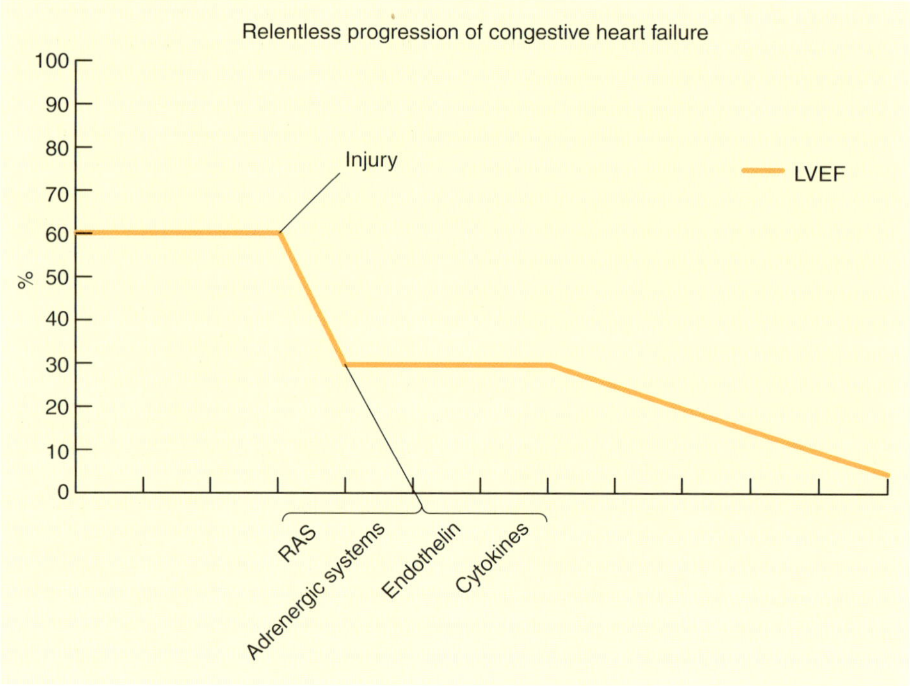


**Figure 37.1** *Relentlessly progressive reduction in contractile performance of the heart (ejection fraction, vertical axis) following an initial injury. The efforts of the renin–angiotensin system (RAS) and others initially to compensate for the reduction in systolic function are also shown on the horizontal axis.*

apoptosis has been demonstrated [4, 25–27] and adverse left ventricular remodelling [27–31] has also been shown. Scattered areas of myocardial necrosis with fibrosis are invariable findings with dilated cardiomyopathies and progressive heart failure. Concentrations of systemic catecholamines, angiotensin II, and endothelin are increased [5–7, 12, 16, 17, 32, 33], which increase the resistance or afterload against which the heart contracts, leading to further dilatation and failure of the heart. This increase may also cause direct myocardial injury and necrosis.

More recent and intriguing findings show that there is an increase in selected cytokines in the heart that may contribute to the progression of myocardial dysfunction. Specifically, the accumulation of tumour necrosis factor-α (TNF-α) [19, 34] and increased oxidative stress have been shown to cause depression of left ventricular function and to be involved in the development of apoptosis [23]. It is clear that activation of matrix metalloproteinases also occurs in animal models and probably in humans with progressive CHF [28, 29]. The metalloproteinases are a family of enzymes involved in the degradation of the extracellular matrix, which might contribute to the remodelling (i.e. progressive enlargement of the heart), myocyte slippage, and thinning that are invariably found in severely dilated hearts. In addition, there appear to be genetic mechanisms that influence the progression of heart failure which are not yet well elucidated but presumably play roles in disturbed homoeostasis of excitation–contraction coupling in the heart [30, 31]. The elucidation of these genetic abnormalities will be useful in identifying patients at risk for heart failure within families and ultimately aid in their treatment.

If important roles for TNF-α, oxidative stress, or activation of selective metalloproteinases could be confirmed in the failing human heart, certain therapeutic possibilities would become evident, including the use of inhibitors of TNF-α [34], free radical scavengers to diminish the oxidative stress burden, or inhibitors of selected metalloproteinases. Possible therapeutic agents to prevent the relentless progression of CHF include antibodies, soluble receptors, synthetic peptides, or low molecular weight inhibitors of TNF-α and metalloproteinases, and some form of gene therapy that alters and improves β-adrenergic intracellular signalling. Preliminary information from studies done by Mann and co-workers [34] in humans suggests that soluble TNF-receptor fusion protein appears to improve symptoms and functional capacity for some patients with heart failure. Lefkowitz and colleagues [35] demonstrated that transgenic mice developed to have a larger number of myocardial β-adrenergic receptors have enhanced cardiac output and heart rates. They have also shown functional β-adrenergic receptor uncoupling and upregulation of the β-adrenergic receptor kinase (β-ARK1) in cells from failing rabbit hearts. An inhibitor of β-ARK1 restored β-adrenergic receptor signalling [36], suggesting the potential to modulate detrimental alterations in the β-adrenergic system in failing heart, with consequently improved function. Transfer of adequate numbers of normally functioning myocytes or myoblasts may also be a potential therapy for heart failure in the future; such cells might provide contractile support or be vectors for relevant gene delivery.

The development and clinical application of such intervention may occur in the near future, including a clear determination of their efficacy and importance in treating and preventing the relentless progression of heart failure in humans.

## References


1. Cohn JN. Structural basis for heart failure: ventricular remodelling and its pharmacological inhibition. *Circulation* 1995; 91: 2504–7.
2. Cohn JN. Physiological variables as markers for symptoms, risk, and interventions in heart failure. *Circulation* 1995; 87: VII-110–14.
3. Lowes BD, Minobe W, Abraham WT *et al.* Changes in gene expression in the intact human heart. Down regulation of α-mysion heavy chain in hypertrophied, failing ventricular myocardium. *J Clin Invest* 1997; 100: 2315–24.
4. Narula J, Haider N, Virmani R *et al.* Apoptosis in myocytes in end-stage heart failure. *N Engl J Med* 1996; 335: 1182–9.
5. Eisenhofer G, Friberg P, Rundqvist B *et al.* Cardiac sympathetic nerve function in congestive heart failure. *Circulation* 1996; 93: 1667–76.
6. Hasking GJ, Esler MD, Jennings GL *et al.* Norepinephrine spillover to plasma in patients with congestive heart failure: evidence of increased overall and cardiorenal sympathetic nervous activity. *Circulation* 1986; 73: 615–21.
7. Dzau VJ, Colucci WS, Hollengerg NK, Williams GH. Relation of the renin–angiotensin–aldosterone system to clinical state in congestive heart failure. *Circulation* 1981; 63: 645–51.
8. Francis GS, Benedict CR, Johnstone DE *et al.* Comparison of neuronedocrine activation in patients with left ventricular dysfunction with and without congestive heart failure. *Circulation* 1990; 82: 1724–9.
9. Packer M. The Neurohormonal Hypothesis: a theory to explain the mechanism of disease progression in heart failure. *J Am Coll Cardiol* 1992; 20: 248–254.
10. Bristow MR. The adrenergic nervous system in heart failure. *N Engl J Med* 1984; 311: 850–1.
11. Dzauu VJ, Packer M, Lilly LS *et al.* Prostaglandins in severe congestive heart failure: relation to activation of the renin-angiotensin system and hyponatremia. *N Engl J Med* 1984; 310: 347–52.
12. Weber KT, Sun Y, Guarda E. Structural remodeling in hypertensive heart disease and the role of hormones. *Hypertension* 1994; 23: 869–77.
13. Tan LB, Jalil JE, Pick R *et al.* Cardiac myocyte necrosis induced by angiotensin II. *Circ Res* 1991; 69: 1185–95.
14. Mann DL, Kent RL, Parsons B, Cooper G IV. Adrenergic effects on the biology of the adult mammalian cardiocyte. *Circulation* 1992; 85: 790–804.
15. Bozkurt B, Kribbs S, Clubb Jr *et al.* pathophysiologically relevant concentrations of tumor necrosis factor-α promote progressive left ventricular dysfunction and remodeling in rats. *Circulation* 1998; 97: 1382–91.
16. SOLVD Investigators. Effect of enalapril on survival in patients with reduced left ventricular ejection fractions and congestive heart failure. *N Engl J Med* 1991; 325: 293–302.
17. SOLVD Investigators. Effects of enalapril on mortality and the development of heart failure in asymptomatic patients with reduced left ventricular ejection fraction. *N Engl J Med* 1992; 327: 685–91.
18. Bristow MR, Gilbert EM, Abraham WT *et al.* Carvedilol produces dose-related improvements in left ventricular function and survival in subjects with chronic heart failure. *Circulation* 1996; 94: 2807–16.
19. Torre-Amione G, Kapadia S, Benedict C *et al.* Proinflammatory cytokine levels in patients with depressed left ventricular ejection fraction: a report from the studies of left ventricular dysfunction (SOLVD). *J Am Coll Cardiol* 1996; 27: 1201–6.
20. Packer M, Bristow MR, Cohn JN *et al.* The effect of carvedilol on morbidity in patients with chronic heart failure. *N Engl J Med* 1996; 334: 1350–5.
21. Beuckelmann DJ, Nabauer M, Erdmann E. Intracellular calcium handling in isolated ventricular myocytes from patients with terminal heart failure. *Circulation* 1992; 85: 1046–55.
22. Bristow MR, Ginsburg R, Minobe W *et al.* Decreased catecholamine sensitivity and β-adrenergic-receptor density in failing human hearts. *N Engl J Med* 1982; 307: 205–11.
23. Olivetti G, Abbi R, Quaini F *et al.* Apoptosis in the failing human heart. *N Engl J Med* 1997; 336: 1131–41.
24. Leri A, Claudio PP, Li Q *et al.* Stretch-mediated release of angiotensin II induces myocyte apoptosis by activating p53 that enhances the local renin–angiotensin system and decreases the Bcl-2- to Bax protein ratio in the cell. *J Clin Invest* 1998; 101: 1326–42.
25. Cheng W, Li B, Kajstura J *et al.* Stretch-induced programmed myocyte cell death. *J Clin Invest* 1995; 96: 2247–59.
26. Weber KT. Extracellular matrix remodeling in heart failure. A role for *de novo* angiotensin II generation. *Circulation* 1997; 96: 4065–82.
27. Tyagi SC, Kumar S, Voelker DJ *et al.* Differential gene expression of extracellular matrix components in dilated cardiomyopathy. *J Cell Biochem* 1996; 63: 185–98.
28. Tyagi SC, Campbell SE, Reddy HK *et al.* Matrix metalloproteinase activity expression in infarcted, noninfarcted and dilated cardiomyopathic human hearts. *Mol Cell Biochem* 1996; 155: 13–21.
29. Thomas CV, Coker ML, Zellner JL *et al.* Increased matrix metalloproteinase activity and selective upregulation in LV myocardium from patients with end-stage heart failure. *Circulation* 1998; 97: 1708–15.
30. Anderson B, Christer S. The DD genotype of the angiotensin–converting enzyme gene is associate with increased mortality in idiopathic heart failure. *J Am Coll Cardiol* 1996; 28: 162–7.
31. Olson TM, Keating MT. Mapping a cardiomyopathy locus to chromosome 3p22-p25. *J Clin Invest* 1996; 97: 528–32.
32. Mulder P, Richard V, Dernmeaux G *et al.* Role of endothelin in chronic heart failure: effect of long-term treatment with an endothelin antagonist on survival, hemodynamics, and cardiac remodeling. *Circulation* 1997; 96: 1976–82.

33. Pönicke K, Vogelsary M, Heinnoth M *et al*. Endothelin receptors in the failing and nonfailing human heart. *Circulation* 1998; 97: 744–51.
34. Deswai A, Seta Y, Blosch CM, Mann DL. A phase I trail of tumor necrosis factor receptor (p75) fusion protein (TNPR:Fc) in patients with advanced heart failure. *Circulation* 1997; 96 (Suppl I): I-1802.
35. Milano CA, Allen LF, Rockman HA *et al*. Enhanced myocardial function in transgenic mice overexpressing the beta 2-adrenergic receptor. *Science* 1994; 264: 507–8.
36. Akhter SA, Milano CA, Shotwell KF *et al*. Transgenic mice with cardiac overexpression of alpha 1B-adrenergic receptors. *In vivo* alpha-1 adrenergic receptor-mediated regulation of beta-adrenergic signalling. *Proc Natl Acad Sci USA* 1997; 94: 12 100–5.

# Index